W9-CXZ-796

The Art & Science of Cytopathology

To Gail, with love

Maria Thomas MD

The Art & Science of Cytopathology

Exfoliative Cytology

Richard M. DeMay, MD
Professor of Clinical Pathology
Director of Cytopathology
University of Chicago

ASCP Press
American Society of Clinical Pathologists
Chicago

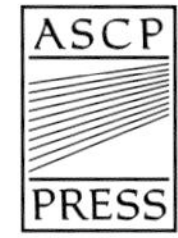

Publishing Team
Jeffrey Carlson (senior designer/production)
Andrea Meenahan (illustration/production)
Michael Methe (production)
Beena Rao (editorial)
Philip Rogers (senior editor)
Jennifer Schima (editorial)
Joshua Weikersheimer (publishing direction)

Notice
Trade names for equipment and supplies described herein are included as suggestions only. In no way does their inclusion constitute an endorsement or preference by the American Society of Clinical Pathologists. The ASCP did not test the equipment, supplies, or procedures, and, therefore, urges all readers to read and follow all manufacturers' instructions and package insert warnings concerning the proper and safe use of products.

Library of Congress Cataloging-in-Publication Data
DeMay, Richard M.
The art and science of cytopathology / Richard M. DeMay
p. cm.
Contents: v. 1. Exfoliative cytology — v. 2. Aspiration cytology
Includes bibliographical references and indexes.
ISBN 0-89189-322-9 (hardcover)
1. Cytodiagnosis. 2. Pathology, Cellular. I. Title.
[DNLM: 1. Pathology. 2. Cytological Techniques. QZ 4 D373a 1995]
RB43.D45 1995
616.07'582—dc20
DNLM/DLC 95-22364
for Library of Congress CIP

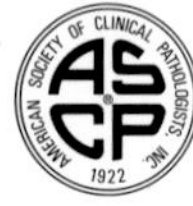

00 99 98 97 96 5 4 3 2 1

Printed in Hong Kong

Volume I
Exfoliative Cytology

Volume II
Aspiration Cytology

Table of Contents

Volume I

Exfoliative Cytology

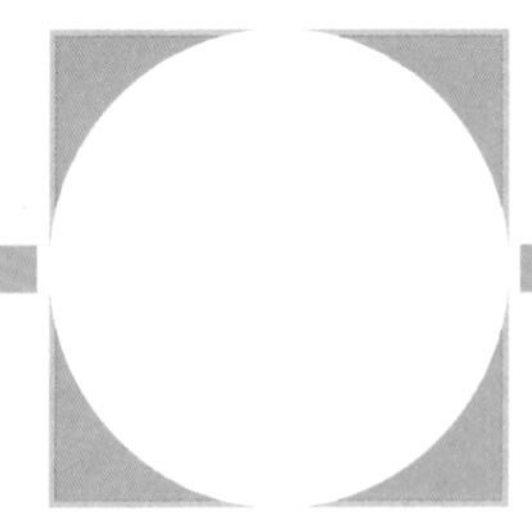

Abbreviations

ACTH: adrenocorticotropic hormone
AdCA: adenocarcinoma
αFP: alpha-fetoprotein
AGUS: atypical glandular cells of undetermined significance
AIDS: acquired immunodeficiency syndrome
AILD: angioimmunoblastic lymphadenopathy
AIM: atypical immature metaplasia
ALH: atypical lobular hyperplasia
ASCUS: atypical squamous cells of undetermined significance
BAC: bronchioloalveolar carcinoma
BCG: bacillus Calmette-Guérin
BFH: benign fibrous histiocytoma
βhCG: beta–human chorionic gonadotropin
BLL: benign lymphoepithelial lesion
BPH: benign prostatic hyperplasia
CEA: carcinoembryonic antigen
CIN: cervical intraepithelial neoplasia
CIS: carcinoma in situ
CMV: cytomegalovirus
CNS: central nervous system
CSF: cerebrospinal fluid
DCIS: ductal carcinoma in situ
DES: diethylstilbestrol
DFSP: dermatofibrosarcoma protuberans
D-MINs: double-mirror image nuclei
DNA: deoxyribonucleic acid
DPAS: diastase-resistant periodic acid–Schiff
DRE: digital rectal examination
EBV: Epstein-Barr virus
EH: epithelioid hemangioendothelioma
EIC: epidermal inclusion cyst
EM: electron microscopy
EMA: epithelial membrane antigen
EMH: extramedullary hematopoiesis
ER: estrogen receptor
ERCP: endoscopic retrograde cholangiopancreatography
FAB: French-American-British classification
FNA: fine needle aspiration
FNH: focal nodular hyperplasia
FVHT: fibrosing variant of Hashimoto's thyroiditis
GBM: glioblastoma multiforme
GCT: germ cell tumor
GFAP: glial fibrillary acidic protein
GI: gastrointestinal
H&E: hematoxylin-eosin
HCC: hepatocellular carcinoma
HCG: human chorionic gonadotropin
HCGs: hyperchromatic crowded groups
HIV: human immunodeficiency virus
HPV: human papilloma virus
HSV: herpes simplex virus
ICL: intracytoplasmic lumen
ILC: infiltrating lobular carcinoma
IM: infectious mononucleosis
INCI: intranuclear cytoplasmic invagination
K-SCC: keratinizing squamous cell carcinoma
LCA: leukocyte common antigen
LCIS: lobular carcinoma in situ
LEEP: loop electrosurgical excision procedure
LGBs: lymphoglandular bodies
LHAs: lymphohistiocytic aggregates
LL: lymphocytic lymphoma
LP: lymphocyte predominant
LT/SRH: lymphocytic thyroiditis with spontaneously resolving hypothyroidism
MALT: mucosa-associated lymphoid tissue
MEC: mucoepidermoid carcinoma
MFH: malignant fibrous histiocytoma
MG: myasthenia gravis
MG bodies: Michaelis-Gutmann bodies
MGH: microglandular hyperplasia
MI: maturation index
MNG: multinodular goiter
MTC: medullary thyroid carcinoma
N/C: nuclear/cytoplasmic
NHL: non-Hodgkin's lymphoma
NK-SCC: nonkeratinizing squamous cell carcinoma
NOS: not otherwise specified
NSE: neuron-specific enolase
NSG: neurosecretory granule
PAP: prostatic acid phosphatase
PAS: periodic–acid Schiff
PCC: proliferation center cell
PD: poorly differentiated
PDA: poorly differentiated adenocarcinoma
PIN: prostatic intraepithelial neoplasia
PLAP: placental alkaline phosphatase
PLAT: paraganglioma-like adenoma of the thyroid
PMA: progressive multifocal leukoencephalopathy
PMNs: polymorphonuclear neutrophils
PNET: primitive neuroectodermal tumor
PR: progesterone receptor
PSA: prostate-specific antigen
PTAH: phosphotungstic acid hematoxylin
PTC: papillary thyroid carcinoma
PTLD: posttransplant lymphoproliferative disorders
PVNS: pigmented villonodular synovitis
RBC: red blood cell
RCH: reserve cell hyperplasia
RNA: ribonucleic acid
RS: Reed-Sternberg
SCC: squamous cell carcinoma
SHML: sinus histiocytosis with massive lymphadenopathy
SIL: squamous intraepithelial lesion
TBMs: tingible body macrophages
TCC: transitional cell carcinoma
TDLU: terminal duct lobular unit
TGI: thyroid growth immunoglobulin
TRUS: transrectal ultrasound
TSI: thyroid-stimulating immunoglobulin
UC: undifferentiated carcinoma
VHL: von Hippel-Lindau
WHO: World Health Organization
WBC: white blood cell

Preface

Have nothing in your house which you do not know to be useful or believe to be beautiful.
—William Morris

And that should go for your library as well. *The Art & Science of Cytopathology* has been developed with both usefulness and beauty in mind. So many medical books seem to uphold a notion that science is science and art is art and ne'er the twain shall meet. But that seems blind to the broader historical perspective that urged Vesalius to study drawing in order to better convey anatomy and Leonardo to examine cadavers to perfect the art in his human figures. Though not the first, the ever-graceful Horace memorably teaches that *useful* knowledge is best assimilated when rendered *sweet* to the reader: *miscuit utile dulci*. So we've heightened the utility of the discussions and various heuristic tools (rules of thumb) by careful attention to the form of the page and the sweetening elements thereon.

The primary drive has been to make the elements of cytopathology immediate and memorable for the reader. Discussions are studded with summary lists, tables, graphs, and illustrations (with distinctive color and type treatment). All photomicrographs are in color (cytopathology is such a colorful pathologic discipline), are at a magnification appropriate to show detail, and display use of conventional and (selectively) special stains. Chapter determinations reflect some untraditional topic treatments, eg, Statistics, Pap Smear, A MICROmiscellany, the Gut Course, that attempt to better answer everyday practice needs, which is why new techniques are treated primarily within diagnostic discussions (again, where useful) and not in a separate chapter on "New Techniques and Diagnostic Modalities," or something like. The book itself is logically divided into a volume on exfoliative cytology (blue spine) and a volume on aspiration cytology (red spine)—so you always know which volume to take off the shelf. And, as in a good workshop or lecture, the discussion is sometimes punctuated with a little levity to sweeten the pot.

In other ways this book boldly goes where older books have gone before. For instance, traditional approaches to Pap smear diagnosis and nomenclature have not been abandoned, but rather are integrated with the current Bethesda System. References are exhaustive: older works of grace and utility have not been deleted just because there are newer works. After all, fine red wines have to mature before they are recognized as great; hence, a good cytopathologist should avoid sampling only this year's vintage. Likewise, this book is unabashedly dedicated to morphologic diagnosis that relies on a trained eye and a good scope: cytopathology is still an *artful* science in this book.

Were it true that a picture is worth a thousand words, this book would be much lighter and still have the value of over 1.5 million words. Unfortunately, images can't tell the whole story, so this book has nearly a million words that work with and around some 1,500 images. Making the two work together well is hard: too many images interrupt the flow of thought in the text; too few images force the reader to rely on unanchored verbal descriptions (eg, without an image, is "chromatin with a ground glass appearance" perfectly clear?). To integrate both an atlas and a traditional textbook in *The Art & Science of Cytopathology*, we have borrowed the medieval notion of the *exemplum*—a focused icon or representation that immediately illustrates a larger point—by sampling microscopic fields to point out only the important cellular or other features that are being stressed by the author, and embedding these close-cropped sections in the center column of the text itself. Full-field images are grouped as a synoptic atlas at the end of chapters so that comparisons among entities and their context can be made easily without interrupting the flow of the text. *Exempla* are indicated by a numbered square, which will often appear near the citation for the full image, eg, [96 I6.66]. The corresponding numbered square appears right next to the appropriate *exemplum*.

Our hope is that this book has become a practical storehouse of information for everyday problems that is a pleasure to use, and will, therefore, enhance the art and science of your ongoing cytologic practice. *Let us advance knowledge so that life may be enriched.*

Mac DeMay
Author

Joshua Weikersheimer
Director, ASCP Press

Acknowledgments

My sincere thanks to:

Mary King, MD, without whose encouragement this project would never have really gotten off the ground.

Denise Hidvegi, MD, Greg Spiegel, MD, Marshall Austin, MD, William Creasman, MD, Jacob Rotmensch, MD, and Arthur Herbst, MD, for advice on the Pap Smear chapter.

Greg Spiegel, MD, for innumerable bits of information and advice.

Russ Harley, MD, for advice on the Respiratory and Lung chapters.

Luna Ghosh, MD, and Tony Montag, MD, for advice on the Soft Tissue Tumor chapter.

Julius Sagal, MD, and David Sarne, MD, for advice on the Thyroid chapter.

James Vardiman, MD, for advice on the Lymphoma chapter.

Robert Schmidt, MD, for significant help with mammography.

Fred Worsham, MD, for allowing access to his prostate slide collection.

Kent Nowels, MD, Jami Walloch, MD, and Denise Hidvegi, MD, for slides.

Elizabeth E. Sengupta, MD, for supplying most of the electron micrographs.

Ronda Washington for typing most of the bibliography.

JoAnne Kuliska, Joan Schwab, and Ann Marie Maslan—it has been my great fortune to work with the best chief technologists there could ever be.

Joan Hives, library researcher extraordinaire, for countless individual acts of help.

Blair Holladay, PhD, for access to teaching material at the MUSC School of Cytotechnology.

Jim Nicholson for photographic advice and his enormous effort in hand-mounting thousands of photomicrographs taken for this book.

Steve Combs, MD, Jami Walloch, MD, Kent Nowels, MD, Dino Vallera, MD, Clay Wilson, MD, Mike Boyd, MD, Lynne Barnes, MD, and Christa Green, MD, my most excellent former Fellows in Cytopathology, as well as Carol Czapar, MD, a special Fellow, all of whom were of immense help in running the Cytology Service.

Hector Battifora, MD, Denise Hidvegi, MD, and Jack Frable, MD, three of my best teachers.

Abel Robertson, MD, Jose Manaligod, MD, Jerry Garvin, MD, Godfrey Getz, MD, Cyril Abrahams, MD, and Jo Morello, PhD, for the trust and confidence they placed in me to run their cytology laboratories.

Joshua Weikersheimer, Director of the ASCP Press, a man of taste and patience.

The staff at ASCP Press, who have pored through everything—thank you for your gargantuan effort that went into supporting this work.

Chuck Burnett, DrPH, PhD, who is like a brother to me, and has helped me in many ways.

My dad and my mother, and my sister, Laurie, for their love and encouragement.

And, of course, my darling wife, Gail, for putting up with this book for so long, and our two wonderful boys, Alex and David, all of whom I love dearly, and with whom I hope I can now spend more time.

A Word on Illustrations

A number of illustrations in this volume have been transformed from the original for use appropriate to this book. ASCP Press gratefully acknowledges the following sources:

Chapter 1 Figures
Bartels PH: The Light Optical Microscope. In Keebler CM, Somrak TM, eds: *The Manual of Cytotechnology.* 7th ed. Chicago: ASCP Press, 395–410, 1993.

Chapter 2 Staining Procedures
Holmquist MD, Keebler CM. Cytopreparatory Techniques. In Keebler CM, Somrak TM, eds: *The Manual of Cytotechnology.* 7th ed. Chicago: ASCP Press, 411–448, 1993.
Yang GCH, Alvarez II: Ultrafast Papanicolaou Stain. An Alternative Preparation for Fine Needle Aspiration Cytology. *Acta Cytol* 39: 282–290, 1995.

F4.1
Compendium on Diagnostic Cytology. Chicago: Tutorials of Cytology, 1983.

F6.4
Wied GL: Hormonal Cytology. In Keebler CM, Somrak TM, eds: *The Manual of Cytotechnology.* 7th ed. Chicago: ASCP Press, 61–72, 1993.

F6.13
Wright TC, Kurman RJ, Ferenczy A: Precancerous Lesions of the Cervix. In Kurman RJ, ed: *Blaustein's Pathology of the Female Genital Tract.* 4th ed. New York: Springer-Verlag NY Inc, 1994.

F6.21
Bahr GF: Basic Cellular Structure and Function. In Keebler CM, Somrak TM, eds: *The Manual of Cytotechnology.* 7th ed. Chicago: ASCP Press, 17–29, 1993.

F11.1, F11.2
Rosenthal DL, Mandell DB: Central Nervous System. In Keebler CM, Somrak TM, eds: *The Manual of Cytotechnology.* 7th ed. Chicago: ASCP Press, 207–217, 1993.

The Art & Science of Cytopathology

Exfoliative Cytology

Volume I

1

The Microscope
[or Through the Looking Glass]

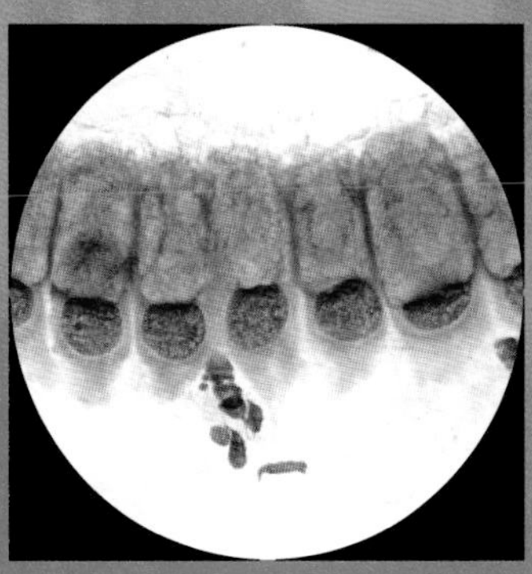

Magnification, etc
Lenses
Oculars
Objectives
Substage Condenser
Köhler Illumination

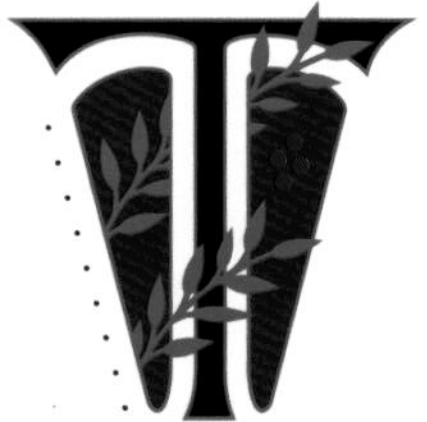

he tree of knowledge must have its roots anchored in the terra firma of basic principles; therefore, we begin with the use of the microscope. The microscope is like a crystal ball in which you can behold the existential secrets of the cell: What is it (gland, squamous, etc)? Where did it come from (cytogenesis)? What is it doing here now (normal, inflamed, metaplastic, dysplastic, neoplastic)? Where is it going (prognosis)?

The microscope can reveal the clues needed to answer these questions, *if* you know how to use it. As in any field of endeavor, the practitioner must master the "tools of the trade." *When making a microscopic diagnosis, on which important clinical decisions will be based, the diagnostician should—at the very least—know whether the instrument is working properly.*

The microscope is an optical instrument that enlarges images of objects too small to be seen with the unaided eye. The microscope makes the invisible visible. This magic is, in essence, an optical illusion, brought to you through the physics of light and lenses, a science known as Optics.

F1.1 **Near Point and Magnification**

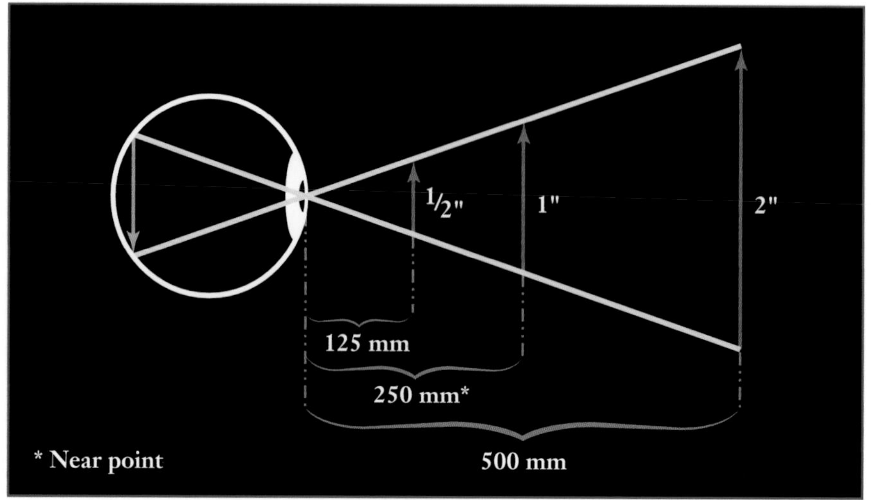

A 1-inch object viewed at 250 mm appears the same size as a 2-inch object viewed at 500 mm, because they both cut the same viewing arc at the eye. Similarly, a half-inch object viewed at 125 mm also appears the same size.

Magnification, Resolution, and Contrast

The story of the microscope begins with the eye. As objects get closer to the eye, they appear larger and finer details are made visible. But there is a limit to how close an object can be brought to the eye. Moreover, the closest *comfortable* viewing distance is around 250 mm or about 10 inches. (You are probably viewing this page at about this distance.) This viewing distance is known in microscopy as the near point. By definition, an object held at 250 mm and viewed with the unaided eye is seen unmagnified and undiminished (ie, 1× magnification). If the object is held at 500 mm and viewed with the unaided eye, the object will appear diminished by one half. If the object is viewed, instead, at 125 mm (which only the nearsighted can do), it will be magnified twofold. The reason for these perceived differences in size is fundamentally important: the eye sees size in terms of angles, hence the term *viewing angle*. At 500 mm, a 2-inch object appears the same size as a 1-inch object seen at 250 mm because they both cut the same viewing arc at the eye. The fundamental function of a microscope is to increase the viewing angle in such a way as to give the (optical) illusion of holding the object ever closer to the eye [F1.1].

There are physical limits to how small something can be and still be seen, or resolved, at the near point. For a small object to be seen clearly, its image must have sufficient resolution, magnification, and contrast.

Resolution is the ability to discern that two points close together are actually separate. The closest that parallel lines can be spaced and still be resolved as separate (by the unaided eye at 250 mm) is approximately 0.075 mm, or about 1 minute of arc. The eye cannot resolve finer detail, because the retina is made up of light receptors (rods and cones) that have finite dimensions. This limit, however, strains the eye, and 0.25-mm spacing is more comfortable for sustained viewing. Fortunately, the limit of resolution of the eye can be overcome by the use of a microscope. The microscope can improve upon 0.25 mm at 250 mm, by making the impression on the retina larger, ie, increase the viewing angle [F1.2].

There is no theoretical limit to how much an object can be magnified. However, magnification without accompanying resolution is worthless (so-called empty magnification). Unfortunately, there is a physical limit to resolution. Just as the resolution of the eye is limited by the physical dimensions of its light receptors, the physical nature of light itself limits resolution even with the microscope because light waves also have finite dimensions, known as the wavelength. The ultimate resolving power of the microscope is about one half the wavelength of the illuminating light (or 0.612 λ) (see Abbe formula). If two points are closer together than 0.612 λ, the points will be seen as one point, even with the best light microscope. The design of microscopes approached this physical limitation more than a century ago. Subsequent improvements have mostly focused on using other kinds of "light," such as electron beams.

How much *magnification* is needed to appreciate the available resolution can now be easily determined with the

F1.2 Viewing Angle

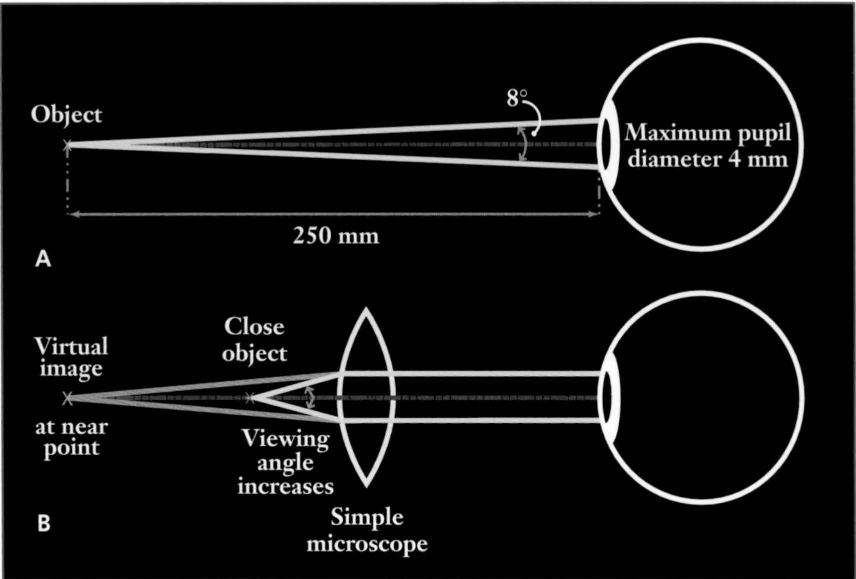

(A) The maximum viewing angle of the unaided eye, even with maximal pupil dilatation at the near point (250 mm) is relatively small, about 8°. (By comparison, an oil immersion lens has a maximum viewing angle of nearly 180°.) Bringing the object closer to the eye increases the viewing angle, but there are physical limits, not to mention eye strain. (B) A lens, or microscope, can overcome the physical limitations of the eye (up to a point). The lens increases the viewing angle (magnifies the image), at the same time producing the optical illusion that the object is at the near point.

following formula. The necessary magnification, M, is calculated as follows:

$$M = \frac{\text{Resolving power eye}}{\text{Resolving power microscope lens}}$$

This magnification makes the smallest resolvable detail large enough that the eye can comfortably see it. The maximum magnification can also be calculated:

$$\frac{0.25 \text{ mm}}{2.5 \times 10^{-4} \text{ mm}^*} = 1{,}000\times$$

*This is the limit of resolution of a "high dry" microscope lens.

Therefore, the limit of useful magnification with the light microscope and the best lens is about 1,000×.

As a rule of thumb, an image should be magnified at least 500×, but not more than 1,000×, the numerical aperture of the lens. With less magnification, the image is too small to appreciate the resolved details. With more magnification, the image is merely enlarged, without adding more detail (empty magnification). Two points to be emphasized: first, the resolving power of the eye depends on the individual—some people, especially the young, can see better than others. Second, simply because an object is not resolved does not necessarily mean that it cannot be seen at all, but rather that it cannot be seen clearly.

Finally, the object must have sufficient contrast to be seen: where there is no contrast, there is no useful image. In summary, in order to finally see an object, the microscope must not only be able to *resolve* fine details and *magnify* them sufficiently, but must also provide sufficient *contrast.*

Lenses

A lens collects light to form an image of an object. The simplest "lens" is a pinhole. When light reflects off an object, the reflected light emerges in every direction. With a pinhole, only a certain small proportion of the reflected light is collected. This light can be imaged (projected) on a piece of tissue paper, for example. With a small hole, the image will be sharp, but dim. With a bigger hole, the image will be brighter, but fuzzy [F1.3].

The problem is how to get an image that is both bright and sharp. The solution is a lens made of glass or other transparent material. A glass lens has the ability to bend light. So, it

F1.3 Pinhole and Glass Lenses

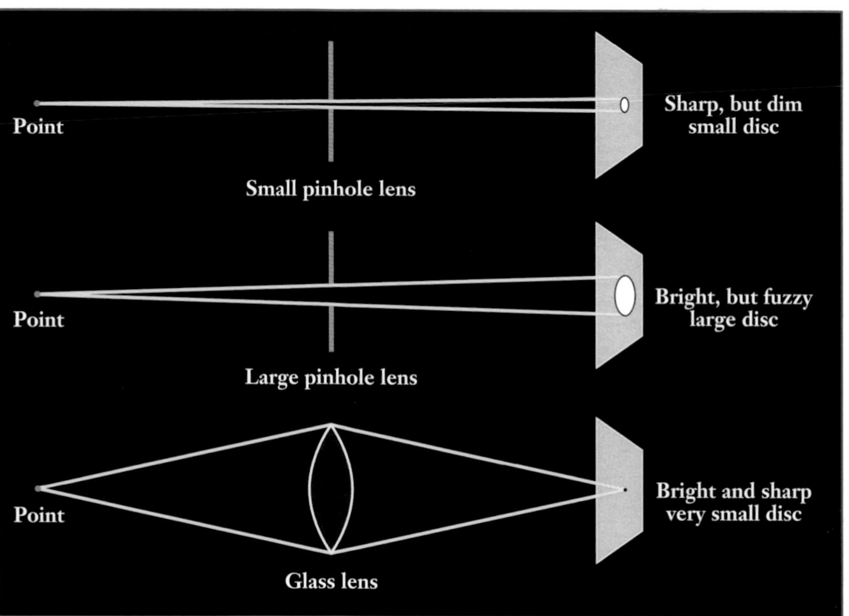

can take in a lot of light through a big hole and then bend the rays to form a sharp, clear image (within limits).

The purpose of the lens is to form an exact point-to-point correspondence between the object and the image using light (or other form of electromagnetic radiation). Unfortunately, lenses have limitations. First, the simple geometry of viewing angles points up that the largest portion of a three-dimensional object that can be viewed with an ordinary lens is one half of the emitted light rays, 180°. To view more than that would be like seeing the dark side of the moon from the earth. The same is true with objects viewed through a lens. We can only see, at most, one half of the emitted light rays, a simple but important concept. Therefore, when constructing the image of an object, we can only deal with, at most, one half of the information emitted from it.

The second limitation, the ultimate physical limitation of lenses, is the phenomenon of diffraction. Light, like Janus, has two natures: particulate and wave, the "wave-particle duality." Neither is sufficient by itself to explain the behavior of light. Unfortunately, because of diffraction phenomena related to the wave nature of light, forming an exact image of an object is impossible.

Diffraction is the breaking up of (light) waves as they pass by an obstruction, eg, a hole or aperture, or around objects. The word "diffraction" is derived from the Latin and means to break apart or shatter. Think of dropping a pebble in a pond. Wavelets move outward in concentric rings until they encounter an obstacle, then they are bent ("diffracted"). In the same way, light is diffracted by obstacles, which include lenses and apertures [F1.4].

Diffraction makes an exact point-to-point correspondence between the object and the image impossible. A point on the object becomes a bright central dot, surrounded by halos (diffraction rings) in the image: a point is imaged as a disc. This bull's-eye structure is known as the circle of minimum confusion, or the Airy disc [F1.5].

Diffraction is an inherent property of light. As such it is the ultimate limiting factor in resolution with any optical instrument. As will be shown, diffraction limits the resolving power of the microscope to the diameter of the first diffraction ring of the Airy disc's bull's eye. If two points are very close together, the Airy discs in the image will overlap and the objects (points) will appear as one—perhaps oblong—fuzzy disc (not two). That is, they are not resolved as separate because diffraction limits resolution.

F1.4 **Diffraction**

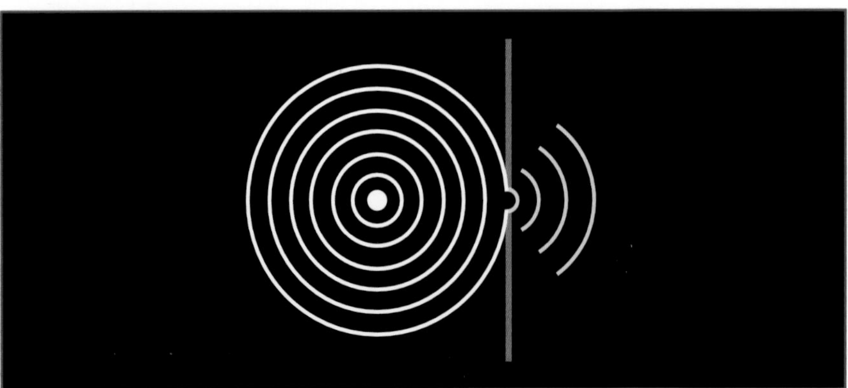

F1.5 **Airy Disc**

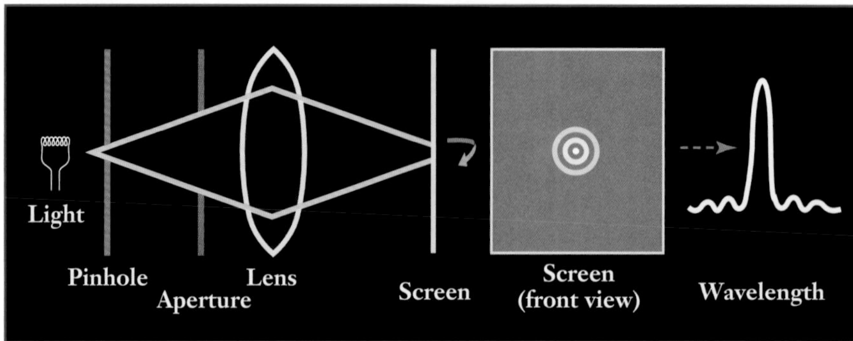

If a point source of light is focused by an apertured lens on a screen, the resulting image is not a point of light, but rather a bright central dot surrounded by diffuse rings of light, known as the Airy disc or Airy ring. The Airy disc forms by diffraction when light is impeded by an obstacle, such as the aperture of a lens, and even the lens itself.

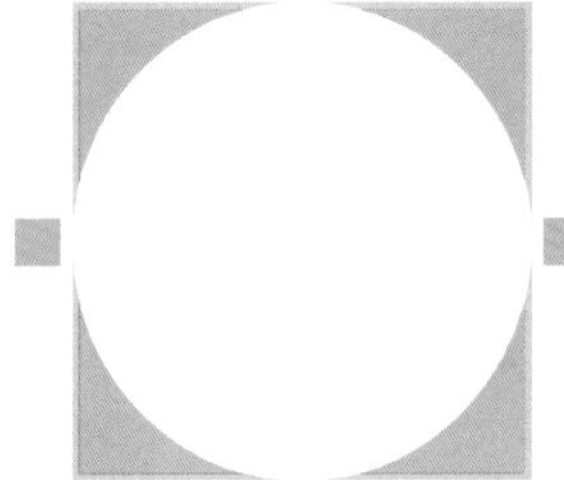

When a wave meets a medium of higher density, such as when light strikes the surface of a lens, its speed is slowed to varying degrees, causing the wavefront's direction to be changed (*refracted*). Part of the wavefront, or light, may also be reflected away from the surface of the lens. The proportion of refraction and reflection depends on the nature of the surface (dull vs polished), the nature of the material of the lens (quantified as refractive index), the wavelength of the light, and the angle of incidence of the light. A lens bends light by the property of refraction. The amount of refraction (bending) is reproducible and measurable. According to Snell's Law:

Sine of angle of incidence = Constant × Sine of angle of refraction, or $\sin \alpha = n \sin \beta$

The constant can be measured and is known as the refractive index of the medium, n.

$$n_{medium} = \frac{\text{Velocity}_{\text{light in vacuum}}}{\text{Velocity}_{\text{light in medium}}}$$

The refractive index of air (or more precisely, of a vacuum) is therefore 1.00. Glasses of various indices of refraction are available to the lens maker. The change in direction of light as it goes from one medium to another is related to changes in the speed of light in the different media as well as the angle of incidence. Bending (refraction) occurs only at interfaces, ie, surfaces (assuming uniform density of the media). Since refraction varies with the angle of incidence, lenses are ground to control the angle of incidence. If light rays are needed to converge (positive lens), the lens is ground so that the surfaces curve away from the incident light (convex lens). If light rays are needed to diverge (negative lens), the lens is ground to curve toward the light (concave) [F1.6]. The distance between the center of the lens and the focal point is the focal length. The focal length is a measure of the strength of the lens: the shorter the focal length, the stronger the lens (ie, more magnification).

Numerical Aperture

A lens accepts an inverted cone of light from each point on the object. The maximum angle of this cone, measured from the central optical ray (optical axis) to the last ray still captured, is defined as the *aperture angle*, designated α. (Alternatively, α could be thought of as one half of the total angle of the cone.) The amount of light a lens can accept, ie, its light-gathering capacity, is related to this aperture angle [F1.7].

The *aperture* of the lens is defined as the sine of the aperture angle (thus, aperture = sin α). The product of the lens aperture, sin α, and the index of refraction of the medium, n, is known as the *numerical aperture* (NA) of the lens, ie:

$$NA = n \sin \alpha$$

(Notice the similarity to Snell's law.)

F1.6 **Positive and Negative Lenses**

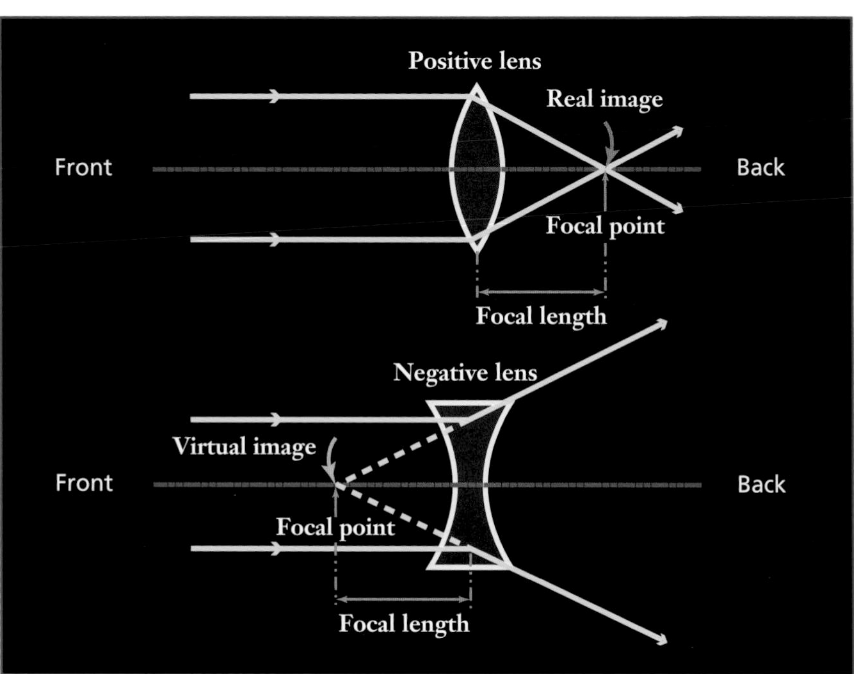

F1.7 **Aperture Angle**

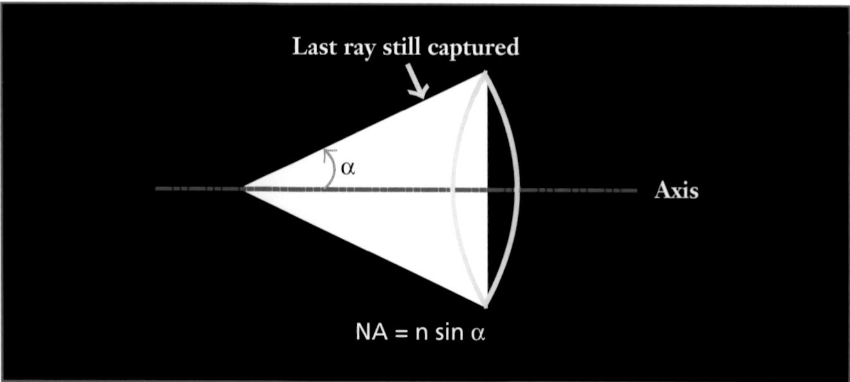

Using this formula, the magnitude of the aperture angle is indicated not in degrees, but rather in the form of a sine value, ie, a numerical value: hence, the term *numerical aperture*.

The NA is a measure of the light-gathering capacity of the lens and its ability to resolve fine detail. The larger the aperture of the lens, the more of the highly diffracted image forming rays the lens can capture (up to the maximum of 180°), and the better the resolution. Resolving power depends on NA (see Abbe's formula). Unfortunately, as you will recall, there are theoretical limits to resolution. The *maximum* viewing angle possible is 180°, which is an aperture angle (α) of 90°. Thus the complete calculation of NA for conventional microscopic viewing, or the maximum light that can be captured, is determined as follows:

$$NA = n \times \sin \alpha$$

n_{air} = 1.00; sin 90° = 1.00 NA_{air} = 1.00 × 1.00 = 1.00 (dry lens)
n_{oil} = 1.51; sin 90° = 1.00 NA_{oil} = 1.51 × 1.00 = 1.51 (oil lens)*

*Immersion oil is chosen with a refractive index similar to glass, or 1.515.

These are the theoretical limits of dry and immersion lenses. Optical lenses are so good that they approach these theoretical limits: 0.95 for dry and 1.45 for oil. The more of this theoretical maximum of light that the lens can capture, the more information about the object being viewed can be used to make an image, and the better the detail can be resolved [F1.8].

Now one of the fundamental formulas of microscopy can be considered. It is the formula defining the limits of resolution of a microscope. Ernst Abbe of Zeiss (in Germany) developed a formula relating the diameter of the first diffraction ring (d), which is the limit of resolution, to the wavelength of light (λ), the index of refraction of the medium (n), and the aperture angle of the illuminating light (α). Abbe's formula follows:

F1.8 Index of Refraction

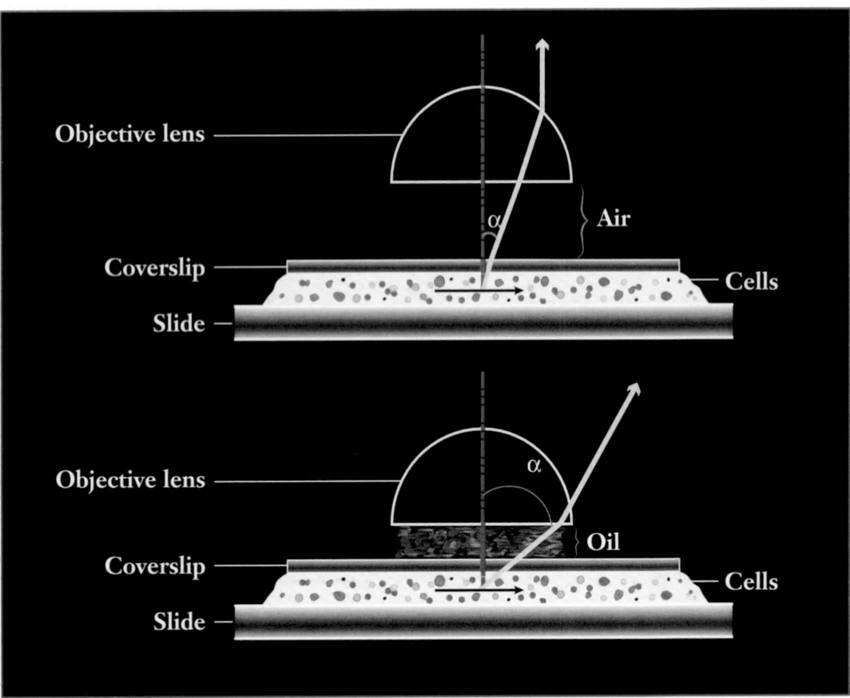

$$d = \frac{0.612\,\lambda}{n \sin \alpha} \cong \frac{0.612\,\lambda}{NA} \cong \frac{\lambda}{2NA}$$

The significance of this formula is that it relates diffraction effects, as given by the diameter of the first diffraction ring, d, to the wavelength of light and the NA. If the first order diffraction rings of two points do not overlap, then they are resolvable as two separate points [F1.9]. If they do overlap, then the two points appear as one and they are not resolved [F1.10].

Two points will be *just* resolvable, ie, distinctly seen as separate, if they are separated by a distance of at least d. Therefore, d is equal to the resolving power of the microscope. From Abbe's formula, the shorter the wavelength of light (smaller λ), the smaller the diameter of the first diffraction ring (d), and the greater the resolution (ie, the shorter the wavelength of light, the higher the resolution). The shortest visible wavelength is blue light of about 400 nm, so resolution is limited to about 0.25 μm in an optical microscope. (Immersion lenses can improve somewhat on this limit. Electron lenses can improve substantially on this limit. The wavelength of an electron accelerated to 50 kilovolts is 0.005 nm. In theory, resolution could be increased nearly 100,000 times. However, electromagnetic lenses are so poor in comparison with optical lenses, that in routine practice only a thousand-fold increase is realized.)

Notice that magnification does not enter into Abbe's formula for the definition of the limits of resolution. Magnification must account for an entirely different problem, ie, making the final image large enough to allow the resolution to be seen by the eye. Just as actual detail in an object can be too small to be seen, so resolved detail in the image of the object may not be large enough to be appreciated.

Also, as in a camera, the wider the aperture of the lens, the shallower the depth of field. This means that with a low-power, low NA objective, the entire thickness of the tissue or cell being studied may be in focus at once. But with a high-power, high NA lens, only a part of the cell might be in focus. This is depth of field, and it is one reason why it is so important to constantly be changing the focus of the microscope, up and down, when examining structures at high magnifications.

To summarize, properties inherent in the nature of light limit resolution. Also, objects reflect light in an infinite number of directions. Lenses can only intercept part of the emanating radiation and lenses can only form an image from that part. These factors are expressed in numerical terms in Abbe's formula. A lens simply cannot improve upon these limits.

Aberrations

There are also specific defects of lenses themselves that limit resolution: aberrations. Because of these aberrations, lenses are unable to produce exact point-to-point correspondence between the image and the object, ie, the image is blurred. Aberrations are broadly classified as chromatic and spherical. They are independent of one another. The smallest possible circle of confusion, d, is defined by the limit of resolution related to diffraction. Aberrations cause the circle to widen to various degrees, decreasing resolution.

Chromatic aberration causes color fringes around edges of objects. Light of different wavelengths is bent (refracted) to different degrees when passing through a lens—the classic

F1.9 Two Points Resolved

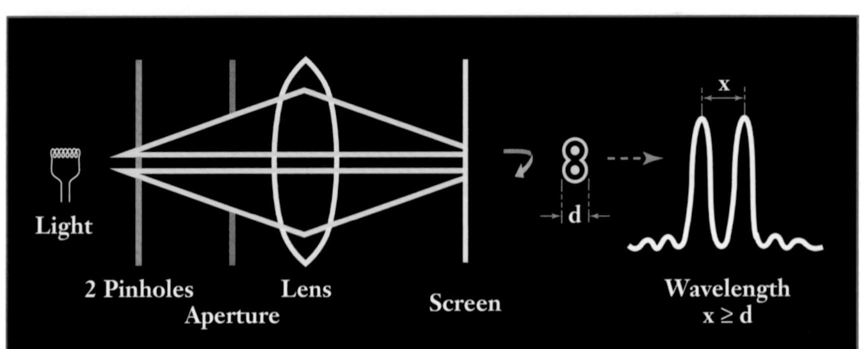

Abbe's formula gives the diameter of the first diffraction ring, d. If the distance between two points, x, is great enough that these rings do not overlap ($x \geq d$), then they are resolved as two separate points.

F1.10 Two Points Not Resolved

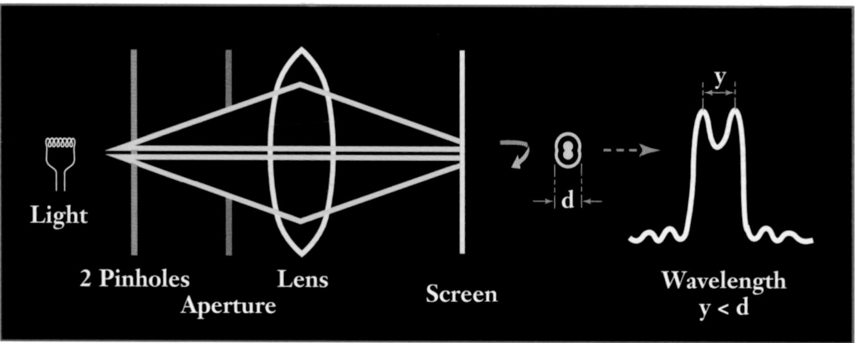

If the diffraction rings of the two points (see F1.9) do overlap (y < d), then they are not resolved, and appear as one point.

example is passing white light through a prism and producing a rainbow. Dispersion is the difference in refractive index of glass for different wavelengths. Blue light is slowed more than red light in glass. Therefore, blue light is brought to focus closer to the lens than red [F1.11].

This also means that blue light is magnified more than red, since the focal length is shorter for blue. Longer wavelengths are deviated less. In other words, light of different colors (wavelengths) passing through the same part of the lens is focused in different planes. Chromatic aberration can be decreased by using light of only one color, typically green. Chromatic aberration varies linearly with NA.

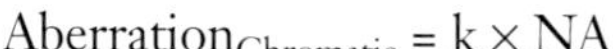

$$\text{Aberration}_{\text{Chromatic}} = k \times NA$$

Spherical aberration is due to the inability of a lens to bring all entering rays, even of one color (monochromatic rays), to a common focal point. For a lens to refract rays of light to form a perfect image, the curvature of the lens must be correct. Unfortunately, the necessary curvature is not exactly a sphere surface, rather it is more complex and cannot be created by a simple grinding process, which usually produces a portion of a spherical surface, hence "spherical aberration." An image formed by spherical surface lenses will be defective because peripheral rays are bent more than central rays [F1.12].

A point source will spread over a short distance in the axis of the image. The rays do not converge to a point, instead they converge on the axis to form a disc of minimal diameter, the "circle of minimal confusion." This disc is "focus." Spherical aberration varies with the cube of the NA.

$$\text{Aberration}_{\text{Spherical}} = k \times NA^3$$

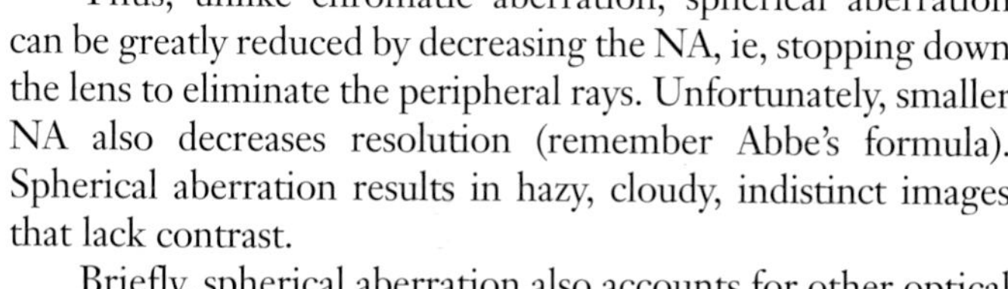

Thus, unlike chromatic aberration, spherical aberration can be greatly reduced by decreasing the NA, ie, stopping down the lens to eliminate the peripheral rays. Unfortunately, smaller NA also decreases resolution (remember Abbe's formula). Spherical aberration results in hazy, cloudy, indistinct images that lack contrast.

Briefly, spherical aberration also accounts for other optical difficulties: coma (magnification differs according to the part of the lens through which light passes), astigmatism (different appearance in different planes), curvature of field (image of flat object projected onto a curved surface, thus, eg, the center of the field may be in focus while the periphery is not), and distortion. These interfere with image shape.

Chromatic aberration also includes chromatic difference of spherical aberration and chromatic difference of magnification. These interfere with image color. Neither spherical nor chromatic aberrations can be identified individually without special techniques and are simply perceived by the eye as a degraded, blurry image. By combining positive and negative lenses, and using glasses of different indices of refraction and dispersion, lenses can be constructed to overcome, to varying degrees, the effects of chromatic and spherical aberration, until finally the theoretical limit of resolution caused by the nature of light (diffraction) is approached.

A word or two about contrast is in order. Radiation bearing no relevant information ("noise") interacts with a specimen by passing through it. After emerging from the specimen, the radiation carries information ("music") about the specimen, which can be processed by the eye (seen) and the brain (interpreted). The eye is sensitive to changes in light intensity (amplitude contrast, akin to loudness) and wavelength (color contrast, like pitch).

The four fundamental processes that take part in formation of an image are:

1. Absorption (amplitude contrast). This is the most important. Light is captured by the specimen, directly causing a change in light intensity the eye can see.
2. Interference (phase contrast). The eye is completely insensitive to this, and interference must be converted to absorption to be appreciated.

F1.11 Chromatic Aberration

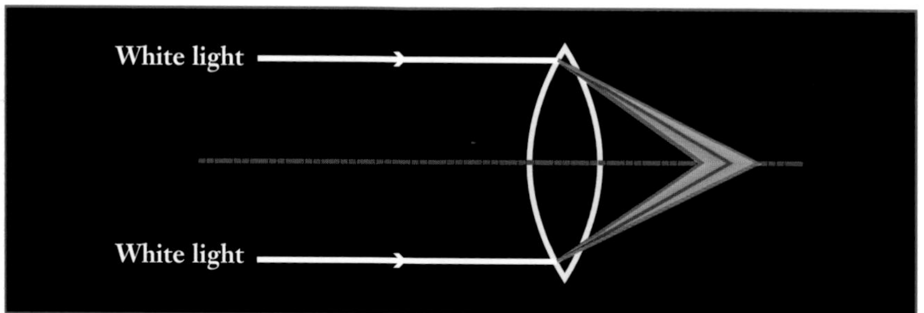

***F1.12* Spherical Aberration**

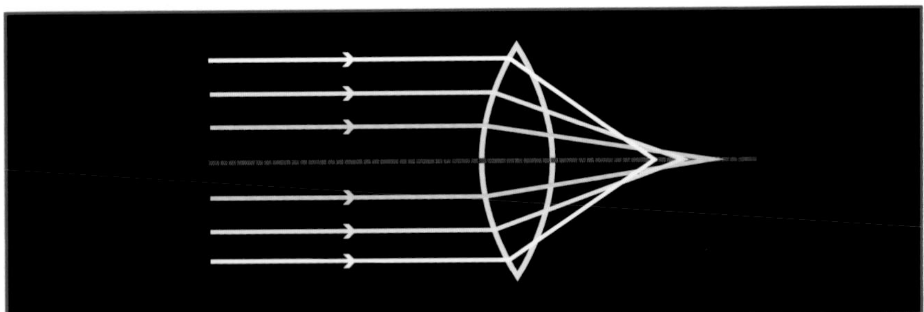

3. Diffraction. This degrades the image, but may enhance contrast. The same fringes and halos that decrease resolution may make the image edges easier to see.
4. Scattering. Scattered light degrades the image, like watching a movie in a lighted room.

Information is transferred from the specimen to the light beam that passes through it by removal of light from the beam. This removed light is absorbed or diffracted. The absorbed light is gone for good, captured by the specimen. But the diffracted light has to go somewhere. If it goes through the objective lens, this random light contributes no information, but degrades the image by decreasing the contrast. The smaller the NA, the fewer of these nonsense rays get in and the better the contrast. Unfortunately, reducing the NA also lowers the resolution (again, remember Abbe's formula). Thus, a balance must be struck between contrast and resolution.

The depth of field (Df) also depends on the wavelength of light, the index of refraction of the medium, and, most importantly, the NA. The longer the wavelength, the greater the depth of field. Unfortunately, this is the opposite of what is needed for high NA and resolution. However, the greater the refractive index, n, as with oil for example, the greater the depth of field and the higher the resolution. But the NA is more important than either wavelength or refractive index in determining the depth of field—the lower the NA, the greater the depth of field.

$$Df = \frac{\lambda \sqrt{n^2 - NA^2}}{NA^2}$$

The substage condenser diaphragm controls the NA of the system, which in turn affects resolving power, depth of field, and contrast. By adjusting this diaphragm, a compromise is made between resolving power and depth of field, as well as between resolving power and contrast. Resolving power must be sacrificed to increase both contrast and depth of field.

A final wrinkle is the working distance, the distance between the front lens of the objective and the top of the coverglass. Like depth of field, working distance decreases rapidly with increasing NA. It also is related to the thickness of the coverglass, increasing with thin coverglasses (or no coverslip at all) and decreasing with thick coverglasses, possibly to the point where the specimen cannot be brought into focus because the objective lens is physically barred from being brought close enough to the object.

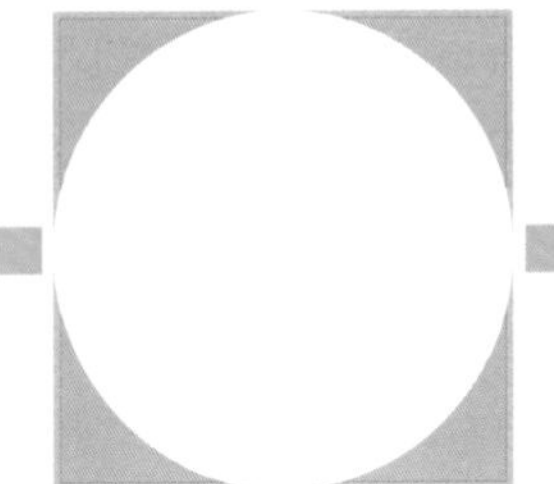

The microscope is further complicated by being two interrelated optical systems: one to illuminate an object and one to visualize it. Both systems follow the fundamental optical laws described above. The illuminating system consists of everything between the lamp and the object, including the light and substage condensers and the glass slide. The visualizing system consists of everything between the object and the eye, including the coverglass, objective, and ocular (eyepiece). Perhaps surprisingly, both the glass slide and the coverglass (which includes the thickness of the mounting medium) act like lenses. Microscopes are designed for rather exact thicknesses of these elements. Too much mounting medium will significantly degrade the microscopic image, especially with high-power dry lenses. The thickness of the coverglass with which the objective lens is intended to be used is often engraved on the casing or specified in the owner's manual. Usually, this thickness is 0.17 mm. The ideal situation is to use a No. 1.5 coverglass (0.17 ± 0.01 mm) with the object to be viewed mounted directly on the underside. Cells grown, or spread like a blood film, directly on a coverglass would be an example. Unfortunately, this is seldom possible. Therefore, thinner No. 1 coverglasses (0.10 ± 0.01 mm) are used with as little mounting medium as practical. In cytology, a very common error that compromises microscopic examination is using too much coverslipping material. [F1.13].

The viewing system is the magnifying/resolving part of the microscope. A simple microscope, like a hand lens, is a single lens unit (which may comprise more than one lens) that forms an enlarged image of an object by effectively increasing the viewing angle. An inverted ocular from a microscope makes a very good and convenient hand lens.

***F1.13* Effective Coverslip Thickness**

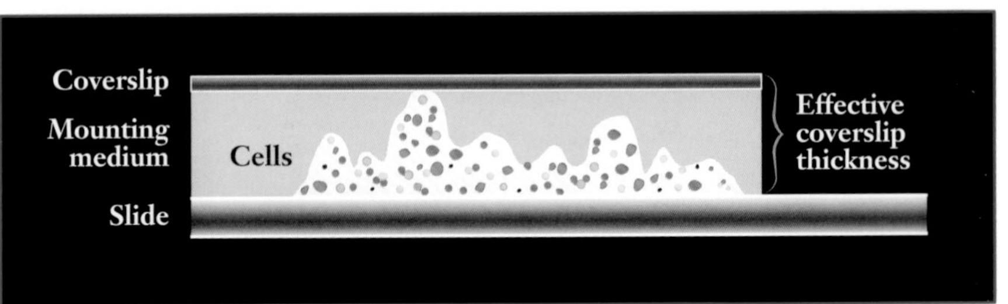

Note that the "coverslip thickness" includes not only the coverslip itself, but also the underlying mounting medium.

F1.14 Compound Microscope

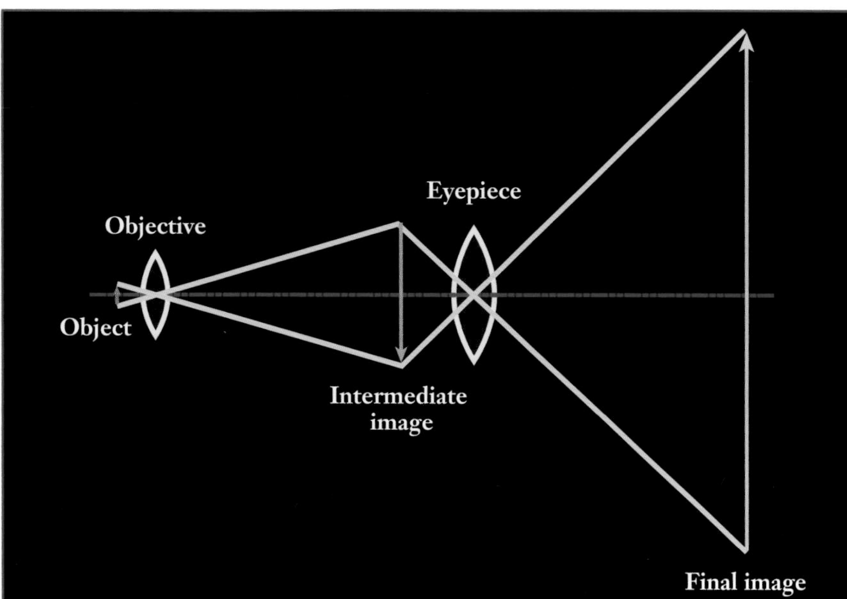

A compound magnifying system (compound microscope) magnifies in two stages. The first enlarged image, from the objective, is the object of the second lens system, the ocular, which produces a greatly enlarged image for the eye to see [F1.14].

The total magnification achieved by a compound microscope is the product of the magnification of each lens system.

Total Magnification = 1st Lens Magnification × 2nd Lens Magnification

The shorter the focal length, the greater the magnification. Therefore, high magnification is possible with relatively short path lengths, which allows for relatively compact microscopes.

The first lens of the visualizing system is the "objective" lens, since it is near the object. The second lens is the ocular, since it is near the eye. The objective lens produces the first, primary, image about 1 cm from the end of the body tube of the microscope. The distance from the shoulder of the objective to the primary image is known as the optical tube length. Most microscopes have an optical tube length of 160 mm (some are 170 mm, and some are actually adjustable).

Oculars

The ocular forms the secondary, virtual, image that the eye sees. The distance from the eyepoint (the point above the

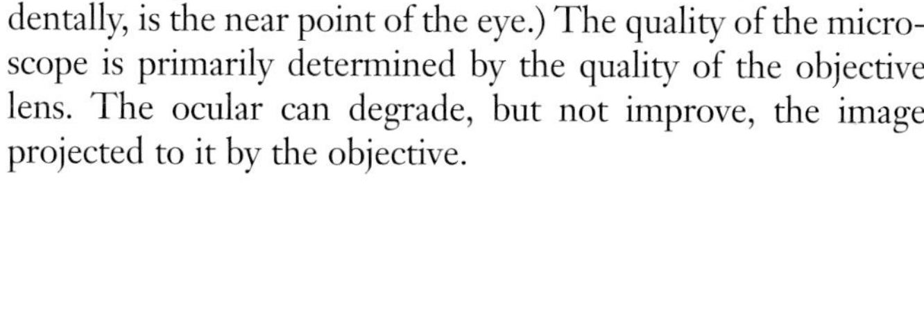

ocular where the image intersects the lens of the eye) to the virtual image is 250 mm. (Sound familiar? This, not coincidentally, is the near point of the eye.) The quality of the microscope is primarily determined by the quality of the objective lens. The ocular can degrade, but not improve, the image projected to it by the objective.

Objectives

There are three basic categories of objective lenses: achromat, fluorite, and apochromat. All of these would project a curved field, but they can be corrected to project a flat field, in which case the lens name is preceded by the prefix "plan" for flat, eg, planachromat. Flat fields are especially important in photomicroscopy so that the whole is in focus at once, not just the center or just the periphery.

Achromatic lenses are the most common and least expensive lenses currently available. The misnomer "achromatic" results from wishful thinking on the part of early microscopists. Such lenses do, however, correct for chromatic aberration in two colors, usually red and blue (opposite ends of the visible light spectrum). Spherical aberration is corrected for only one wavelength, usually green. The advantages of achromatic lenses include a good working distance (the space between the slide and the objective), a moderate NA and resolution, and easy use that is adequate for routine microscopy. The disadvantages include color fringes around the outer margin of the image, resulting in a fuzzy image, particularly in black and white photography. A sharper image for photography can be obtained by using a light source of one color (monochromatic light) to reduce chromatic aberration. Green light is usually selected because of best correction for spherical aberration. Longer or shorter wavelengths result in an inferior image.

Fluorite lenses are also known as semi-apochromatic lenses. Chromatic and spherical aberration are corrected for two wavelengths. Therefore, spherical aberration is more corrected with these lenses than with achromatic lenses. The major advantage is that this correction allows a higher NA (remember, spherical aberration in uncorrected lenses varies with the *cube* of the NA). The higher correction is made possible by use of fluorite (calcium fluoride) instead of glass to construct the lens. Disadvantages include the need to use specially matched compensating eyepieces, since the final correction of aberration actually takes place in the ocular, and high purchase price.

Apochromatic lenses are the finest available, but they are difficult to work with. Particularly at high power they require exact coverslip thickness (or a compensating adjustable mechanism in the objective itself, so that the objective and the microscope must be tediously focused against each other). Also, they have very short working distances, so that in some cases, the object will not be able to be brought into focus at all because the objective physically hits the slide. This increases the risk of damage to these expensive lenses. Finally, apochromatic lenses have a very short depth of field, so only a small portion of a cell or other object will be in focus at high power. This makes focusing, especially for photography, difficult. Apochromatic lenses are the most highly corrected lenses. They are corrected for chromatic aberration in three colors (red, green, and blue) and spherical aberration in two colors (red and blue). Consequently, they have the highest NA and resolution, resulting in the sharpest, crispest images possible in light microscopy. Like fluorite lenses, apochromatic lenses also require matched compensating eyepieces. These are the best lenses to use for color photomicroscopy, but they are not recommended for routine cytologic diagnosis [T1.1].

F1.15 Substage Condenser

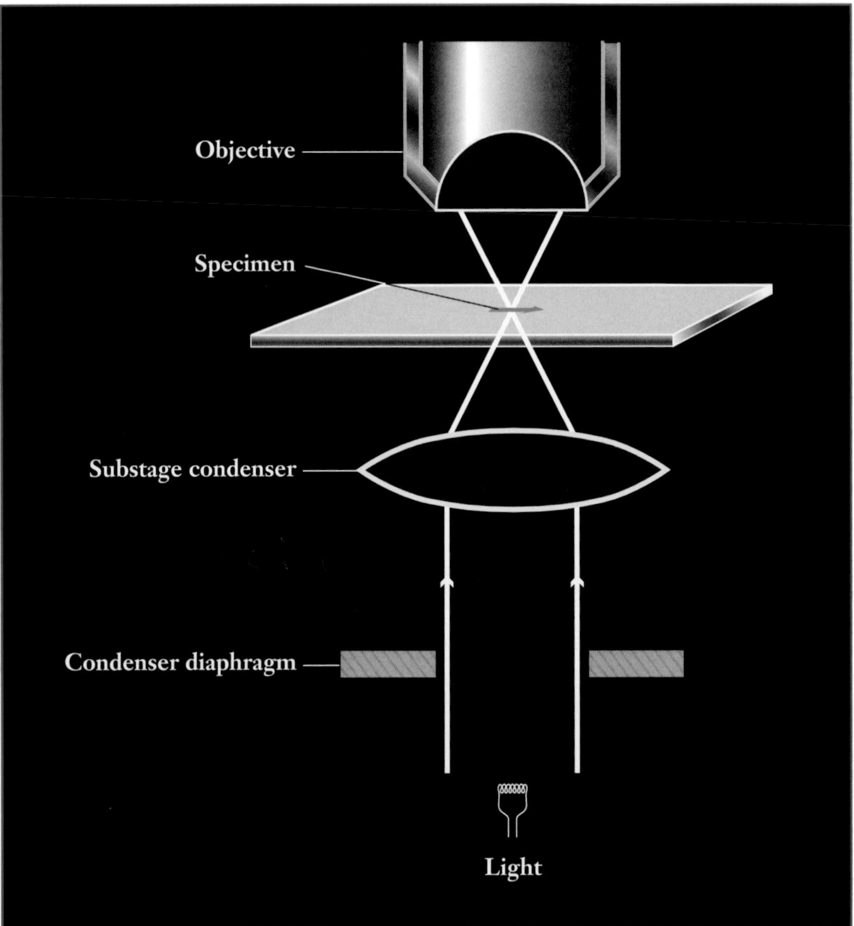

Substage Condenser

The most important part of the illumination system is the often neglected substage condenser. It is generally the least understood and most misused part of the microscope. Even the best objectives perform poorly if the object is not properly illuminated; the substage condenser controls illumination. In forming an image, the objective can only use rays of light that reach it from the object. The rays reaching the object are controlled by the condenser. The rays of light sent from the condenser are the basic material from which the objective produces an image. If these rays are insufficient to produce an image of the quality the objective is capable of forming, the image will fall short by the degree of condenser inadequacy.

So, the function of the substage condenser is to properly illuminate the object. This has little to do with light intensity and a lot to do with the angular relationship of the cone of light formed by the condenser to the aperture of the objective [F1.15].

Light from the condenser converges (focuses) on the specimen, then diverges on passing through the specimen to form an inverted cone of light to fill the front lens of the objective, picking up information about the object on its way. The angle of this illuminating cone is controlled by the substage condenser diaphragm. The substage condenser must be properly focused and properly opened. Like the weakest link in a chain, the overall NA of the microscope, and hence its resolution, is limited by the lowest NA in the system. Since the highest NA in air is about 1.00 (0.95), then objective lenses with NA greater than 1.00 will not be fully utilized unless the condenser also has an NA greater than 1.00 and the objective lens as well as the condenser lens are *both* immersed in oil. Using oil only between the slide and the objective, and not between the condenser and the slide, the highest possible NA is 1.00, that of air, even though the NA of the objective is higher, eg, 1.25. The air is responsible, in this case, for the weakest link in the chain.

Like other lenses, condensers can be chromatically and spherically corrected. Abbe condensers are the cheapest and most common. They are uncorrected for spherical and chromatic aberration. Aplanatic (aspheric) condensers focus light in one plane (ie, spherical aberration is corrected). Achromatic/

T1.1 Comparison of Lens Type, Numerical Aperture, and Corrections

Lens Type	Numerical Aperture	Chromatic	Spherical
Achromat	Good	2 λ	1 λ
Fluorite	Better	2 λ	2 λ
Apochromat	Best	3 λ	2 λ

λ = wavelength, or color.

aplanatic condensers correct for both chromatic and spherical aberration. Slide thickness is as important to the condenser as coverglass thickness is to the objective. Like the objective lens, a condenser of high NA has a short working distance. If the slide is too thick, the condenser may not be able to properly illuminate the specimen. Most condensers are designed for a glass slide thickness of 1.0 mm.

Köhler Illumination

The nature of light in general and the components of the visualizing and illuminating systems in particular have now been considered. To get the most out of these individual systems, it is necessary to coordinate their activities into one integrated whole. The most common method of doing this is called Köhler illumination. Its primary advantage is in providing uniform critical illumination for a large field from a nonuniform light source, such as a light bulb filament. Köhler illumination images the light condenser in the plane of the object, where of course the visualizing system is also focused, thereby coordinating the two [F1.16].

The substage condenser forms an image of the light directly in the plane of the object (specimen). By stopping down, or closing, the substage condenser diaphragm until the cone of light from the condenser is just equal to the cone that can be accepted by the objective, perfect illumination is theoretically provided. This is known as critical illumination. The resolution of the system is determined by the resolution of both the substage condenser and the objective. Without a condenser, the resolution of the system is perhaps half to two thirds as good as possible. On the other hand, the NA of the condenser should not exceed that of the objective, since the excess light degrades the image.

If the light source is at the focal point of the light condenser, the light rays emerge parallel. When the parallel rays reach the substage condenser, they are brought to focus to form an image of the point on the light source from which they originated. Since the substage condenser is also focused on the specimen, any inhomogeneities in the light source will be seen when the object is viewed. This is a form of critical illumination.

If the light condenser is moved away from the light source, instead of parallel rays emerging, the rays can be made to focus at the substage condenser diaphragm instead of the substage condenser. This is Köhler illumination. Since the substage condenser diaphragm is located near the focal point of the substage condenser, the rays from the light source emerge parallel from the substage condenser to form a *disc* of light in the plane of the object. Thus, each point of light on the light source forms a relatively large disc of illumination for the object (specimen), with each of these discs overlapping the other. Therefore, any inhomogeneity in the light source would make little difference in the uniformity of the illumination of the object. The light condenser has, in effect, become the source of light. Therefore, anything, including dust, in front of the light condenser would show as a dark spot in the image of the object. The total diameter of the illuminated area is determined by the diameter of the light condenser, which is the effective light source, and this can be controlled by the field diaphragm.

F1.16 Köhler Illumination

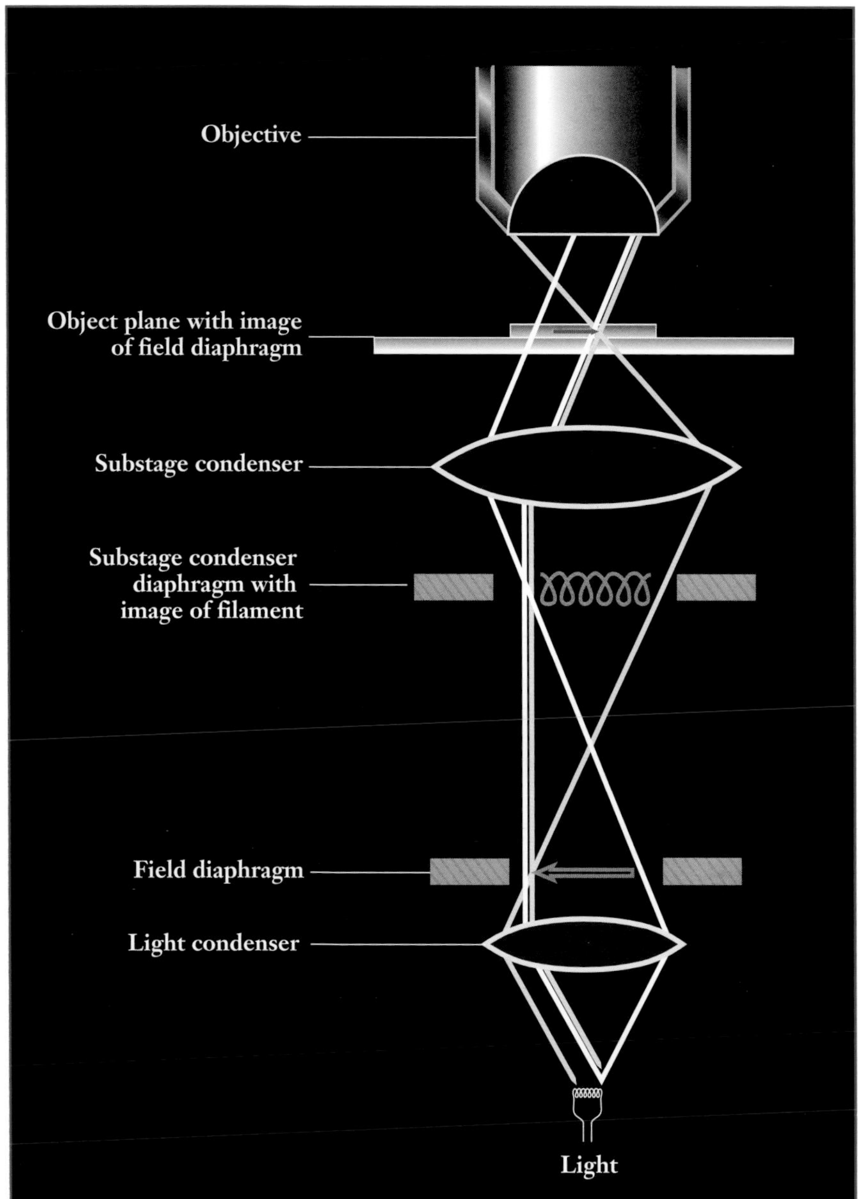

White: illuminating ray path; yellow: image forming ray path.

In summary, the field diaphragm controls the size of the field illuminated. The field diaphragm should be opened until the edges go just beyond the field of view (the back of the objective lens is filled). The substage condenser diaphragm controls the NA of the system, by controlling the angle of the cone of light transmitted to the objective. This is important because the NA of all the other lenses is fixed. The substage condenser diaphragm can be closed to increase contrast and depth of field, or opened to increase resolution. It is usually opened to about three quarters of the NA of the objective lens to achieve the optimum balance among resolution, contrast, and depth of field.

The theory of Köhler illumination may be a little confusing, but in practice it is easy to achieve in just a few seconds. To achieve Köhler illumination, simply focus the microscope on the specimen as you normally would. Then, still looking through the oculars, close the field diaphragm (not the substage condenser diaphragm) until it fills the outer one third of the field. Next, raise or lower the substage condenser until the edges of the field diaphragm are in focus. Take this opportunity to center the beam. Then, open the field diaphragm until its edges just clear the field of view. You are now in perfect Köhler illumination. Unfortunately, any dust in the light path will also be in focus; therefore, in practice, lower the substage condenser slightly to defocus any dust. (Of course, there shouldn't be any dust on your microscope, but that's only in another [dust-free] universe.)

2

Stains
[or Now You See It]

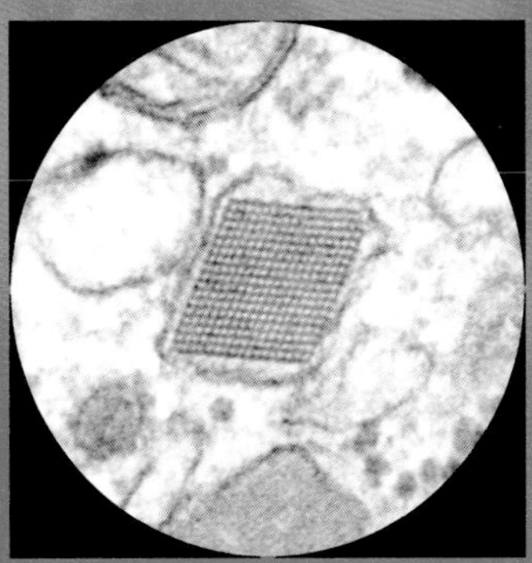

Papanicolaou Stain
Romanovsky Stain
Other Special Stains
Enzyme Reactions
Immunocytochemistry
Other Cell Markers
Electron Microscopy
Flow Cytometry
Polymerase Chain Reaction
Staining Procedures

PAPANICOLAOU STAIN has three cytoplasmic dyes, orange G, eosin Y, and light green, plus hematoxylin, for nuclear detail. Bismarck brown, a basic dye, was present in the original Papanicolaou stain but is no longer used. The Papanicolaou stain can stain cells blue or blue-green (basophilia, cyanophilia), pink (acidophilia, eosinophilia), orange (orangeophilia), or indeterminate (gray-blue) [Akura 1991, Bartels 1974, Drijver 1983, Gill 1974, Hollander 1975, Marshall 1983, Papanicolaou 1942]. Cytoplasmic cyanophilia is associated with metabolically active cells, staining ribonucleic acids, including ribosomes. Free ribosomes in the cytoplasm are associated with protein synthesis for internal consumption, and are often seen in rapidly proliferating or neoplastic cells. Ribosomes can also be bound to endoplasmic reticulum, ie, the rough endoplasmic reticulum. Rough endoplasmic reticulum produces proteins for export, including Ig-secreting plasma cells and collagen-making fibroblasts. Cytoplasmic acidophilia is associated with an abundance of nonribosomal organelles (mitochondria, lysosomes, neuroendocrine granules, filaments, and smooth endoplasmic reticulum). The structural proteins of these cytoplasmic organelles (including cell membranes) often have a chemically basic composition, and, therefore, are "acidophilic" [Chang 1992].

Orange G and eosin Y are acid dyes that stain basic proteins such as prekeratin. Cytoplasmic orangeophilia is associated with keratinization. However, cellular degeneration can result in intense eosinophilia or orangeophilia, even in nonsquamous-derived cells. Light green has an affinity for ribonucleic acids in ribosomes. Prekeratinized cells possess abundant free ribosomes in the cytoplasm for the synthesis of the prekeratin subunits (tonofilaments). As the cells differentiate, the cell organelles are broken down by hydrolytic lysosomal enzymes. True keratinization occurs when the sulfhydryl groups form insoluble disulfide bonds between adjacent cysteine molecules of prekeratin polypeptides, forming a tonofilament: amorphous matrix complex, ie, tonofibrils or keratin. Orange G has a strong affinity for this complex.

As cells keratinize, the glassy cytoplasm progresses from blue–green (abundant free ribosomes and prekeratin) to pale orange (prekeratin, few free ribosomes) to intensely orange (true keratin, or tonofibrils). Cytologically, the tonofibrils can be recognized as "rings of keratinization" in the cytoplasm.

Thus, the Papanicolaou stain is a "special stain" for keratin that is capable of detecting minimal or focal evidence of squamous differentiation in a poorly differentiated tumor. Such poorly differentiated squamous features may be impossible to detect using a H&E stain. Therefore, squamous elements in tumors may be more accurately detected cytologically than histologically, not only because individual cells can be examined to better advantage (looking for dense cytoplasm, distinct cell boundaries, rings of keratinization, etc), but also because the Papanicolaou stain is relatively specific and much more sensitive to the presence of keratin than a simple H&E stain [Hess 1981].

Fixation

Alcohol is a coagulative fixative. Alcohol-fixed cells tend to contract, and appear more rounded, almost spherical, like a boiled egg, due to coagulation [Linehan 1983]. Alcohol fixation can cause up to 70% shrinkage of the cells [Beyer-Boon 1979, Gey 1936, Schulte 1987]. (Formalin, a cross-linking fixative, causes 30% shrinkage of tissue [Jacobsen 1983].) Air drying is a form of fixation, although the cells are usually postfixed in alcohol fixative [Schulte 1986]. Interestingly, air-dried cells can be rehydrated (in tap water or normal saline) with preservation of nuclear detail, provided they have not been postfixed before rehydration [Chan 1988, Ng 1994]. Air-dried cells tend to spread out and flatten, like a fried egg, as they dry and are pulled by surface tension. In a study of small cell carcinoma, the mean nuclear area in air-dried material was 1.75 times the nuclear area in paired, alcohol-fixed (Papanicolaou-stained) slides [McCool 1992]. Air drying distorts cells to be stained by Papanicolaou stain, making interpretation difficult or impossible.

Romanovsky Stain

An advantage of Romanovsky stains (eg, Diff-Quik®) is that air drying is not a problem since air drying is usually the first step in fixation. (However, air drying is not essential for Diff-Quik staining, which can also be applied to alcohol-fixed material, resulting in excellent cytologic detail and stromal definition [Hirschowitz 1994].) Air drying significantly increases cell adherence to slides [Beyer-Boon 1978]. In contrast, alcohol causes cells to fall off slides (sometimes almost all of them), not only reducing the available cellularity for diagnosis but also resulting in "floaters" in the stains.

Air-dried slides are stained with a Romanovsky stain (Diff-Quik) like that used for peripheral blood films [Silverman 1990]. Diff-Quik staining is simple, and can be performed more rapidly than the more complex routine Papanicolaou stain (although rapid Papanicolaou stains have been developed [Yang 1995]). Rapid staining is useful for on-the-spot assessment of aspirates (adequacy, diagnosis). The primary uses of the Romanovsky stain [T2.1] are to stain cytoplasm and extracellular substances (like mucin, ground substance, colloid, young collagen, etc); enhance pleomorphism (air-dried cells expand, alcohol causes shrinkage); display glandular acini (which when air dried, open up like a flower blossom); and make lymphoreticular and hematopoietic lesions akin to bone marrow aspirates. Unlike the Papanicolaou stain, Romanovsky is a metachromatic stain, which acts something like a "general special stain" by producing a metachromatic reaction with a variety of diagnostically important entities such as various mucins and neurosecretory granules. Also, when

T2.1 **Comparative Advantages of Pap Stain vs Romanovsky Stain**

Papanicolaou	Romanovsky Stain
Nuclear detail	Cytoplasmic features
Transparent	Background substances
Keratinization	Mucin, neurosecretory granules
Squamous differentiation	Gland and lymphoreticular differentiation
Hyperchromasia	Metachromasia
Necrotic lesions	Microbiologic agents
Akin to histology	Akin to bone marrow

looking at the Romanovsky-stained slides wet and uncoverslipped (ie, before going through alcohols and xylene), fat or lipid can be visualized as glistening oily droplets. Chromatin in malignant cells may appear more metachromatic than that in benign cells [Frable 1982]. Microbiologic agents, such as bacteria or fungi, may be easier to spot in Romanovsky-stained material.

The primary uses of the Papanicolaou stain [T2.1] are for crisp nuclear detail; transparency (useful for thick smears or so that cells in three-dimensional aggregates can be seen); and squamous lesions (keratinized cells stain bright orange). Hyperchromasia is a term used for Papanicolaou stain, which differentially stains heterochromatin and euchromatin. Diff-Quik stains both more or less equally. Also, the Papanicolaou stain is more useful in examining necrotic lesions. Viral changes are usually easier to appreciate in Papanicolaou stain. The nature of the alcohol-fixed cells and hematoxylin stain make Papanicolaou-stained material more comparable to tissue morphology than air-dried Romanovsky-stained material.

As discussed in Chapter 4, the nucleus provides information about the state of health of the cell (normal, inflamed, hyperplastic, dysplastic, neoplastic); the cytoplasm provides information about the functional differentiation and origin of the cell. Perhaps surprisingly for the classical cytologist, fine nuclear detail is not always needed to render a fine needle aspiration biopsy diagnosis. In Pap smears, one is confronted with a sea of normal cells in which there are little islands of abnormal cells. In this situation, the nuclear features are critical for diagnosis and the Papanicolaou stain is preferred. However, in aspiration biopsy cytology, the situation is different. Here the slide may be almost overflowing with obviously malignant cells. The nuclear detail may not be nearly as critical. The questions now are different: what is the origin (genesis) of this tumor, "where's the primary," what is the grade of differentiation, etc. These are primarily cytoplasmic features and, therefore, Romanovsky stain may be more useful.

Other Special Stains

Periodic acid–Schiff (PAS) stains carbohydrate moieties. Predigestion with diastase (DPAS) eliminates any staining due to glycogen. Glycogen is associated with renal cell carcinoma as well as germinoma and embryonal carcinoma, among many others, including some squamous cell carcinoma, melanomas, and sarcomas. Glycoproteins, neutral mucins (such as in adenocarcinomas), some sialomucins, and immunoglobulins (such as in B-cell lymphomas) are PAS positive. Also, various kinds of hyaline globules (such as in hepatocellular carcinoma or sarcomas) may be PAS positive. PAS also stains basement membrane and reticulin as well as fungi and parasites.

PAS Stain

Carcinomas: Variably positive
Sarcomas: Usually negative, except:
- Rhabdomyosarcoma
- Smooth muscle tumors
- Ewing's sarcoma
- Chondrosarcoma
- Alveolar soft-part sarcoma
- Occasionally liposarcoma, angiosarcoma, epithelioid, and synovial sarcoma (in glands)

Melanoma: Variably positive
Lymphoma: Usually negative, but Ig can be positive
Mesothelioma: Usually positive
Germ cell tumors: Positive, especially germinomas

**Alcian blue*, at pH 2.5, stains weakly acidic sulfated mucosubstances, hyaluronic acid, and sialomucins dark blue. When used in combination with PAS, it stains acid mucins blue, PAS-positive acid mucins or mixtures of neutral and acid mucins purple, and neutral mucins magenta. Alcian blue positivity removed by predigestion with hyaluronidase is characteristic of mesothelioma and chondrosarcoma.

**(Alcian blue has been declared a carcinogen by the FDA.)*

Mucicarmine stains epithelial (neutral) mucin variably positive in carcinoma. It is negative in mesothelioma and sarcomas (except synovial sarcoma [relatively common], glands of malignant schwannoma [very rare], and chordoma [extracellular]).

Fat stains, such as oil red O or Sudan black, are generally not too helpful in differential diagnosis of tumors. Practically any cell can contain minute fat globules, often degenerative in nature and nonspecific. However, when fat globules tend to coalesce, displace the nucleus, and scallop its borders, this is indicative of a lipoblast, which is characteristic of liposarcoma. Certain epithelial malignancies (including adenocarcinomas of the kidney, breast, lung, and prostate) are associated with lipid in the cytoplasm (see Chapter 14). Oil red O can be used to demonstrate lipid-laden macrophages, as seen in, eg, lipid pneumonia.

Masson's trichrome stains myofibers, indicating skeletal or smooth muscle differentiation (vs nonmuscle fibers). Also, myofibroblasts, which may be seen in most fibroblastic tumors, have myofibers; thus, the presence of myofibrils does not necessarily imply pure smooth muscle differentiation.

Melanin is helpful in differentiating spindle cell melanoma from spindle or pleomorphic sarcomas. Also, clear cell sarcoma, probably the soft-tissue counterpart of melanoma, is frequently melanin positive.

Argentaffin and *argyrophil* are silver stains for neurosecretory granules. Argyrophil is similar to argentaffin, but adds a reducing agent.

Congo red stains for amyloid as seen in medullary carcinoma of the thyroid and amyloidosis. Amyloid stains "brick red" and shows "apple green" birefringence under polarized light.

Methyl green pyronine (*MGP*) binds to RNA; therefore, cells with abundant rough endoplasmic reticulum or prominent nucleoli will stain in the cytoplasm or nucleus, respectively. In lymphoid cells, MGP positivity indicates plasmacytoid differentiation, such as in plasmacytomas or plasmacytoid lymphomas, and indicates reactive lymphoid cells, eg, in transplant rejection.

Phosphotungstic acid–hematoxylin (*PTAH*) stains mitochondria.

Copper accumulation in liver FNA biopsy can be demonstrated using special stains (rubeanic acid, rhodanine, or orcein) that demonstrate a coarse, green-brown pigment, which is seen perinuclearly. Increased hepatocytic copper levels may be seen in such diseases as Wilson's disease, Indian childhood cirrhosis, primary biliary cirrhosis, and other chronic cholestatic liver diseases [Kobayashi 1988, Sipponen 1980].

Enzyme Reactions

Acid phosphatase is used to mark high activity in adenocarcinoma, which suggests prostatic carcinoma.

Alkaline phosphatase is a nonspecific reaction. In adenocarcinoma, it favors lung, endometrial, ovary, or kidney origin, and rejects gastrointestinal origin. Angiosarcoma and osteoblastic osteosarcoma react positively.

Aryl sulfatase reaction in adenocarcinoma suggests gastrointestinal origin [Koudstaal 1975].

Aminopeptidase reaction in adenocarcinoma suggests stomach, bile duct, bladder, or kidney origin.

Lysozyme reacts in myelomonocytic leukemia and "true" histiocytic lymphoma.

Brown Stains and "Magic Markers" (Immunocytochemistry)

Immunocytochemistry can be helpful in evaluating a variety of tumors that are difficult to classify. The method can be applied to cytologic specimens [Chess 1986, Dabbs 1995, Flens 1990, Gherardi 1992, Myers 1989, Nadji 1980,1990]. A word of warning: With the current state of the art, these stains can be as misleading as they are helpful. As of this writing, the majority of these reagents remain unapproved by the FDA and are available for research and investigational use only. However, pathologists may use these reagents for clinical purposes if such use is the consequence of their best medical judgment based on the needs of the patient. Such use should be confirmed by another medically established diagnostic product or procedure [CAP 1995]

Filaments

As a general rule, epithelial tumors are keratin positive and vimentin negative, while soft tissue tumors are vimentin positive and keratin negative, although exceptions are well known [Battifora 1988, Nguyen 1988]. For example, coexpression of keratin and vimentin may be observed in synovial sarcoma, epithelioid sarcoma, and mesothelioma, as well as renal cell carcinoma, Wilms' tumor, thyroid, endometrial, and ovarian carcinomas, and pleomorphic and monomorphic salivary gland adenomas [Domagala 1988, R Gupta 1992, Saleh 1994].

Filaments

- Thin (~6 nm)
  - Actin
- Intermediate (~10 nm)
  - Keratin
  - Vimentin
  - Desmin
  - Glial fibrillary acidic protein
  - Neurofilament protein
- Thick (microtubules, ~25 nm)
  - Myosin

Cellular expression of filaments is useful in the differential diagnosis of small blue cell tumors of childhood. Rhabdomyosarcomas are desmin positive, malignant lymphomas contain only vimentin, and neuroblastomas show positivity for neurofilaments. However, exceptions do occur.

Keratin is a complex group of intermediate filaments (~10 nm) that can, for simplicity, be divided into two groups: low- and high-molecular weight forms. Low-molecular weight keratin is expressed in all cell lines with epithelial differentiation, including endodermal, neuroectodermal, mesenchymal, or germ cell origin. High-molecular weight keratin is expressed in squamous cell carcinoma and mesothelioma.

A spectrum of keratins can be tested for, using a cocktail of low– and high–molecular weight antikeratin antibodies, such as AE1/AE3. Negative staining does not exclude epithelial differentiation and must be interpreted in context of other stains, eg, leukocyte common antigen positivity. Keratin tests positive in synovial sarcoma (particularly in glands), chordoma, and rhabdoid tumor. It is also positive in epithelioid sarcoma, which may help differentiate this tumor from granulomatous inflammation, which is negative. Unexpected keratin staining can occur in nonepithelial tumors such as smooth muscle, nerve sheath, fibrohistiocytic tumors, and even lymphoma (rare) [Swanson 1991]. Small blue cell tumors such as small cell carcinoma, Ewing's sarcoma, and Merkel cell tumor, but not lymphomas, usually test positive. Melanoma sometimes stains, although it usually tests negative for keratin.

Vimentin is an intermediate filament (~10 nm) associated with mesenchymal cells and their tumors. It is found in virtually all types of sarcomas, but can also be found in many carcinomas (including renal cell carcinoma and papillary thyroid carcinoma), melanoma, mesothelioma, and lymphomas. Vimentin is of little help in subclassification of soft tissue tumors.

Desmin is an intermediate filament (~10 nm) found in muscle of all kinds (cardiac, skeletal, smooth). Desmin is more sensitive to skeletal than to smooth muscle; therefore, most rhabdomyosarcomas are positive, while many leiomyosarcomas are negative [Truong 1990]. Also, desmin is usually negative in mesothelioma, malignant fibrous histiocytoma, malignant schwannoma, and melanoma. Some lymphomas may be unexpectedly positive.

Glial fibrillary acidic protein (*GFAP*) is intermediate filament (~10 nm) present in astrocytes, ependymal cells, and oligodendroglial cells. GFAP is positive in peripheral nerve sheath tumors as well as in pleomorphic adenomas. Sarcomas, germinomas, lymphomas, and carcinomas are usually negative.

Neurofilaments are intermediate filaments (~10 nm) of neurons that test positive in neuronal tumors, including neuroblastoma, medulloblastoma, and retinoblastoma. They also may be positive in neuroendocrine tumors, including paragangliomas, pheochromocytomas, carcinoids, islet cell tumors, and Merkel cell tumors.

Actin is a thin (~6 nm), ubiquitous contractile protein, found in virtually all cells. There are various forms of actin, some of which are found only in muscle (muscle-specific actin) and related contractile cells, myoepithelium and myofibroblasts, and their tumors.

Myoglobin

This oxygen-binding heme protein is found in skeletal and cardiac muscle. It is more specific, but less sensitive, than desmin as a marker for rhabdomyosarcoma (only about half of rhabdomyosarcomas are myoglobin positive) [De Jong 1984]. Tumors with rhabdomyoblastic differentiation, such as triton tumors and mixed müllerian tumors test positive, but malignant rhabdoid tumor tests negative.

S100

S100 is a calcium-binding protein that takes its name from being 100% soluble in ammonium sulfate [Kahn 1983]. Almost all melanomas are S100 positive, but many other tumors are also positive (ie, the test is sensitive, but not specific). In particular, neural tumors react positively (schwannoma, neurofibroma, malignant schwannoma, neuroectodermal tumors, and granular cell tumor). Sustentacular cells of paragangliomas react with S100 antibodies. In addition, certain adenocarcinomas are commonly positive, including those of ovary, endometrium, kidney, breast, colon, stomach, lung, and thyroid Hürthle cell tumors. Also, myoepithelial, chondroid, skeletal muscle, and fat cells and their tumors may test positive. S100 is used in combination with keratin to aid in differentiating melanoma (usually keratin negative) from adenocarcinoma (usually keratin positive). Although S100 is a marker for Langerhans' histiocytes, ordinary histiocytes may contain phagocytosed S100-positive material.

Epithelial Membrane Antigen

Epithelial membrane antigen (EMA) is a glycoprotein derived from human milk fat globule membrane that stains many carcinomas, but is less sensitive and specific than keratin. Hepatocellular carcinoma, adrenal cortical carcinoma, and germ cell tumors do not react, but melanoma, mesothelioma, meningioma, certain soft-tissue tumors (synovial sarcoma, epithelioid sarcoma, chordoma, some leiomyosarcomas, rarely others), and even plasma cells and lymphomas (especially T-cell and Ki-1 types) may stain for EMA.

Factor VIII

Factor VIII is an endothelial cell marker [Sehested 1981] comprising two components: "C" = antihemophiliac factor, and "R" = von Willebrand's factor (localized to Weibel-Palade body). It marks not only endothelial cells, such as vessels and vascular tumors (mostly benign), but also platelets, megakaryocytes, and mast cells. Factor VIII is nonreactive in Kaposi's sarcoma (except for supporting vessels).

Neuron-Specific Enolase

Neuron-specific enolase (NSE) is a marker for neuronal and neuroendocrine cells. Enolases are enzymes in the glycolytic pathway. They are dimers with α, β, and γ subunits. NSE is the γ portion of γ-γ or γ-α dimer that is particularly found in neuronal cells and cells of the dispersed neuroendocrine system [Tapia 1981]. NSE marks neuroblastomas, paragangliomas, carcinoids, and other neuroendocrine neoplasms, as well as melanoma. Because so many cells test positive for NSE (including breast carcinoma, renal cell carcinoma, and non–small cell lung carcinoma, as well as lymphocytes, smooth or skeletal muscle, and others), it known colloquially as "nonspecific enolase" [Schmechel 1985].

Synaptophysin

Synaptophysin tests positive for nerves, axons, neuroendocrine cells, and their tumors, including small cell (neuroendocrine) carcinoma. Synaptophysin is a protein found in the presynaptic vesicles. Synaptophysin staining is more sensitive than chromogranin, and is apparently highly specific with no known cross-reactions with other cell types.

Oncofetal Antigens

α-*Fetoprotein* (α*FP*) is a glycoprotein of the fetus synthesized by liver and yolk sac [Kuhlmann 1981]. The oncofetal protein is found in hepatocellular carcinoma, yolk sac tumor, and often, other germ cell tumors. Negative staining does not exclude hepatocellular carcinoma.

Carcinoembryonic antigen (*CEA*) is an oncofetal antigen, a heterogeneous group of glycoproteins associated with glycocalyx of fetal mucous glandular cells. CEA is associated with adenocarcinoma, particularly of gastrointestinal origin, and pancreas, but also lung and breast, and can help differentiate them from tumors usually not associated with CEA production, such as prostate, kidney, thyroid, and endometrium [D'Cunha 1994]. Hepatocellular carcinoma shows characteristic canalicular staining. CEA is also found in squamous cell carcinoma and some neuroendocrine tumors. Mesothelioma and sarcomas are usually nonreactive (except biphasic synovial sarcoma, chordoma, and focally, some leiomyosarcomas and malignant nerve sheath tumors). CEA shares antigens with nonspecific cross-reacting antigen (NCA), which is often found in neutrophils (including granulocytic sarcoma).

Serum Proteins

α_1-*Antitrypsin* (α*AT*) is synthesized by liver, histiocytes, and monocytes. αAT is an acute-phase reactant that neutralizes various proteolytic enzymes including trypsin. Levels increase in infections, as found in body fluids. αAT may be demonstrable in hepatocellular carcinoma and fibrous histiocytic lesions, particularly malignant fibrous histiocytoma, but can also be found in many other sarcomas, as well as carcinomas and melanoma, and therefore is nonspecific.

Immunoglobulins test positive in B-cell lymphomas, myeloma, and plasmacytoma, and negative in carcinomas, etc. Monoclonality favors neoplastic proliferation of lymphocytes.

Hormones

β *Human chorionic gonadotropin* is a marker for choriocarcinoma, seminoma/dysgerminoma, embryonal carcinoma, and some anaplastic carcinomas [Heyderman 1985].

Calcitonin is associated with medullary carcinoma of the thyroid, but can also be positive in nonthyroidal neoplasms, including lung, pancreas, and colonic adenocarcinomas.

Thyroglobulin tests positively in follicular thyroid cells, including follicular. and Hürthle cell neoplasms, and papillary thyroid carcinomas; colloid also stains. Giant and spindle cell carcinoma is variably stained but often negative. Medullary carcinoma is usually negative [Burt 1979, Franklin 1982, Panza 1987].

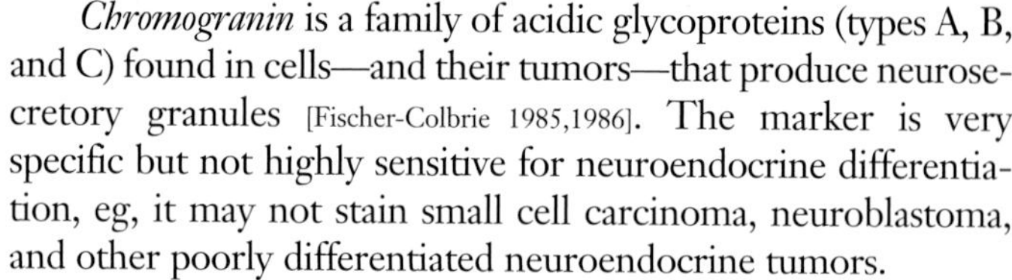

Chromogranin is a family of acidic glycoproteins (types A, B, and C) found in cells—and their tumors—that produce neurosecretory granules [Fischer-Colbrie 1985,1986]. The marker is very specific but not highly sensitive for neuroendocrine differentiation, eg, it may not stain small cell carcinoma, neuroblastoma, and other poorly differentiated neuroendocrine tumors.

Other endocrine hormones include insulin and gastrin and can be used to subclassify neuroendocrine tumors, eg, islet cell tumors. However, neuroendocrine differentiation often may only be a component of a tumor, rather than the primary cell type.

Other Cell Markers

Leukocyte common antigen (*LCA*) is a marker for B and T lymphocytes, histiocytes, and neutrophils. Interestingly, plasma cells usually do not stain. LCA is a very useful marker for lymphoid cells and lymphomas in general, but of limited use in subclassification of lymphoreticular proliferations. However, not all lymphomas mark, including lymphoblastic, Ki-1, "histiocytic," and occasionally immunoblastic types. Also, myeloma/plasmacytoma usually tests negative. False-positive staining in nonlymphoid malignancy also occurs occasionally.

Placental alkaline phosphatase (*PLAP*) is associated with trophoblasts. Most germ cell tumors, including seminoma/dysgerminoma, embryonal carcinoma, and yolk sac tumors, test positive for PLAP. Carcinomas of lung, endometrial, ovary, kidney, and gastrointestinal origin may also stain.

Prostatic acid phosphatase is associated with lysosomes in the prostatic glandular cells. Positivity in adenocarcinoma suggests prostatic carcinoma in men, but can also be positive in other tumors, including renal cell carcinoma, neuroendocrine tumors, breast carcinoma, and adenocarcinoma of the bladder, and may not be positive in poorly differentiated prostatic carcinoma.

Prostate-specific antigen (*PSA*) is more specific than prostatic acid phosphatase; it is the current method of choice for identifying prostatic origin of cells.

Leu–7 marks a subset of natural killer cells and a subset of T lymphocytes, myelin-associated glycoprotein in neuroectodermal tissue, and small cell lung carcinomas, as well as normal, hyperplastic, and neoplastic prostate tissue.

Leu-M1 (*CD 15*) marks epithelial tumors, Reed-Sternberg cells, and dermatofibroma. Immunoblasts and mesothelioma are negative.

B72.3 is derived from the membrane fraction of metastatic breast carcinoma and serves as a marker of adenocarcinomas and is usually negative in benign cells. Unfortunately, it has turned out to be neither sensitive nor specific in the diagnosis of cancer.

T2.2 **Summary of Reactions of Soft-Tissue Tumors**

Tumor	Reaction
Malignant fibrous histiocytoma	Vimentin stains positive, specific markers stain negative
Embryonal rhabdomyosarcoma	Desmin > muscle-specific actin > myoglobin
Pleomorphic rhabdomyosarcoma	Myogenic markers
Epithelioid leiomyosarcoma	Muscle-specific actin
Pleomorphic liposarcoma	Vimentin and S100 stain positive
Monophasic synovial sarcoma	Keratin and EMA
Angiosarcoma	UEA stains positive, MEMA and keratin stain negative
Epithelioid sarcoma	Keratin stains positive
Clear cell sarcoma	HMB-45, S100, and vimentin stain positive
Malignant lymphoma	LCA

[Wick 1988]

HMB-45 is a very specific but in cytology, less sensitive cytoplasmic antigen associated with melanoma. Positive staining may be focal [Ordonez 1988, Pelosi 1990]. Renal angiomyolipoma, pulmonary lymphangiomyomatosis, and clear cell "sugar tumor" of the lung are also usually positive for HMB-45 [Bonetti 1994]. Rarely, breast carcinoma and plasmacytoma, and possibly others, may be (misleadingly) positive [Bonetti 1989, Kornstein 1990].

Monoclonal antibodies are being developed all the time, and certain newer antibodies may be found useful in differential diagnosis [T2.2].

Given a poorly differentiated tumor, we recommend that you "round up the usual suspects," and test the panel of markers, with a few differentiating follow-up protocols [T2.3].

Uranyl Acetate and Lead Citrate Stain (Electron Microscopy)

Electron microscopy (EM) is a technique that can be applied to cytologic specimens, including FNA biopsy specimens [Akhtar 1981, Collins 1981, Dabbs 1988, Dardick 1991, Kindblom 1983, Nordgren 1982, Ravinsky 1993, Sehested 1987, Strausbauch 1989, Wills 1987, Young 1993]. For many years, EM was the mainstay of differential diagnosis of diagnostically difficult tumors. With the advent of immunocytochemical techniques, its use has been declining. However, EM offers at least one significant advantage over immunocytochemistry: When there is limited material available for study, EM can potentially provide a much wider range of information in a "one shot" attempt at diagnosis. In addition, immunocytochemistry, at least currently, is less than perfect, and unexpected, misleading, or uninterpretable results are too often obtained, as many can attest. EM is less prone to provoke this kind of frustration ("seeing is believing," if you will). However, an important caveat for any biopsy technique, which particularly applies to the minute samples examined by EM is: *Absence of proof is not proof of absence.* It cannot be unequivocally stated that a feature is absent merely because it was not detected. Rather, it is more appropriate to state that it could not be found in the sections examined. (It may be a good idea to specifically state how many sections were examined, and perhaps even for how long.)

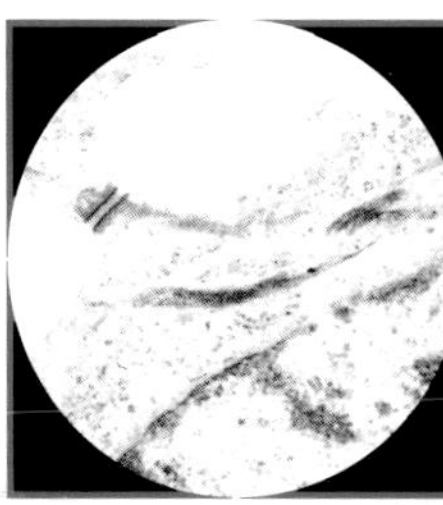
1

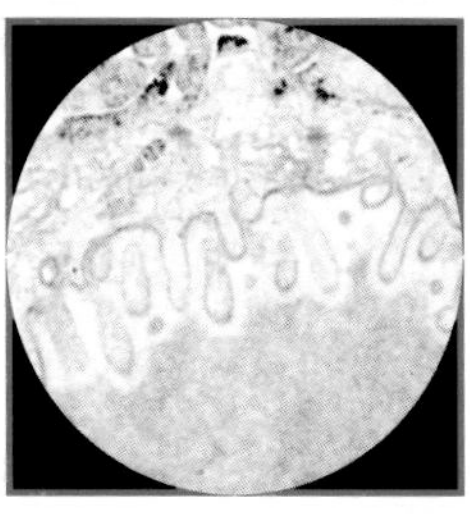
2

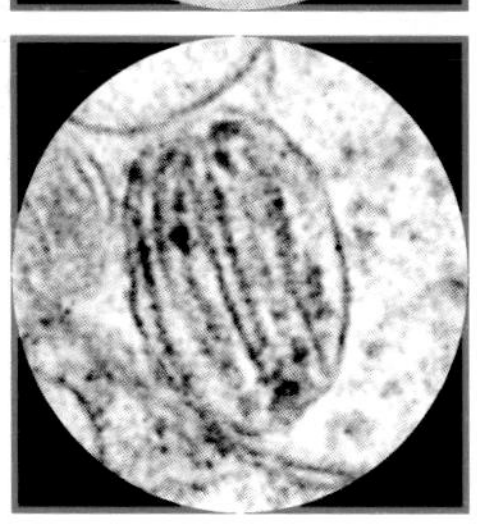
3

Carcinoma

General EM features of carcinoma include *external lamina* that tends to surround groups of cells as opposed to individual cells [I2.1] and *desmosomes* that may be well formed.

Squamous cell carcinoma [1 I2.2] features include tonofilaments, especially in bundles (tonofibrils or keratin); desmosomes (especially well developed); and microvilli attached at their tips by desmosomes (intercellular bridges).

In *adenocarcinoma*, inter- and intracellular lumens are most characteristic. Intercellular lumens show junctional complexes at the luminal aspect, forming an acinus with a central hollow space lined by microvilli [I2.3]. Intracellular lumens show an intracytoplasmic space lined by microvilli, probably formed by invagination of the cell surface membrane, which is often filled with flocculent secretory product (ie, mucin) [2 I2.4].

"Specific" Features That Indicate Origin of Adenocarcinoma

Colon: Microvilli, glycocalyceal bodies, terminal web, apical mucin [I2.6] [Herrera 1985]
Lung: Lamellar (surfactant) bodies [I2.7], multivesicular bodies
Breast: Intracellular lumens [I2.4]
Ovary: Staghorn microvilli
Renal: Tubulofilamentous cytoplasmic structures

The following evidence of secretion, or the machinery necessary to make it, supports a diagnosis of adenocarcinoma: well-developed endoplasmic reticulum, large Golgi, secretory granules (eg, mucin [I2.3, I2.4] or zymogen [I2.5]).

In *oncocytoma*, the cytoplasm is stuffed with mitochondria to virtual exclusion of other organelles [I2.8].

In *neuroendocrine carcinoma*, neurosecretory granules are seen (see neuroblastoma).

In *mesothelioma*, long microvilli and desmosomes are seen (see Chapter 8).

Melanoma

Premelanosomes and melanosomes [3 I2.9] are typical EM features of melanoma. They are also seen in clear cell sarcoma, pigmented neuroectodermal tumor, malignant schwannoma, and, rarely, other neural crest derived tumors.

T2.3 Immunocytochemical Panels for Poorly Differentiated Tumors

Recommended Panel of Magic Markers (Typical Reactions)

	Carcinoma*	Lymphoma	Sarcoma	Melanoma	Germ Cell†
Keratin	+	–	±	–	±
Vimentin	±	+	+	+	–
CEA	±	–	–	–	–
S100	±	–	±	+	–
HMB-45	–	–	–	+	–
LCA	–	+	–	–	–

* Breast, ovary, endometrial carcinoma: Positive estrogen/progesterone receptor.
Prostate carcinoma: Positive prostate-specific antigen.
Hepatocellular carcinoma: Positive αFP, α_1-antitrypsin.
Small cell carcinoma: Positive neuron-specific enolase.
† Positive αFP, βHCG. Keratin is negative in germinoma, positive in embryonal carcinoma among others.

Panel for Small Blue Cell Tumors

	Keratin	Vimentin	NSE	LCA	Actin/Desmin	Synaptophysin*
Lymphoma	–	+	–	+	–	–
Small cell carcinoma	+	–	±	–	–	+
Neuroblastoma	–	–	+	–	–	+
Rhabdomyosarcoma	±	+	±	–	+	–
Ewing's sarcoma/PNET	–	+	±	–	–	±
Wilms' tumor	+	±	–	–	±	–

* Also chromogranin.

Mesothelioma vs Adenocarcinoma

	Mucin*	HAB†	CEA	Leu M1	AE1	AE3‡
Mesothelioma	–	+	–	–	+	+
Adenocarcinoma	+	–	+	+	+	±

* DPAS/Mucicarmine.
† Hyaluronidase-sensitive alcian blue positivity.
Positive implies hyaluronic acid is present.
‡ High molecular weight keratin is more characteristic of mesothelioma.

Hepatocellular Carcinoma vs Adenocarcinoma

	αFP	CEA	AE1	AE3	HBsAg
Hepatocellular carcinoma	+	+*	–	+	+
Adenocarcinoma	–	+	+	–	–

* Canalicular.

Lymphoma

An EM feature that is consistent with lymphoma is complete lack of intercellular junctions. There are no specific ultrastructural features.

Sarcoma

Sarcomas lack well-formed desmosomes on EM [T2.4]. However, poorly formed junctions may be seen, particularly in synovial sarcoma, smooth muscle tumors, nerve sheath tumors, and hemangiopericytoma. External lamina tends to surround *individual* cells. No intracellular lumens, tonofibrils (bundles of tonofilaments), or neurosecretory granules are seen. (Note: The mere presence of mesenchymal cells in a tumor by no means proves it to be a sarcoma. Myofibroblasts are particularly likely to be encountered in a wide variety of epithelial and mesenchymal lesions, nonneoplastic and neoplastic, benign and malignant.)

T2.4 **Electron Microscopic Features of Sarcoma**

Leiomyoma/Sarcoma
- External lamina
- Pinocytotic vesicles
- Attachment plaques
- Thin filaments
- Dense bodies

If any are missing, suggests malignancy.

Rhabdomyosarcoma [I2.10]
- Minimum for diagnosis: Both thick and thin (myo)filaments; possible Z band material

Neuroblastoma [I2.11]
- Neurites
- Synaptic vesicles
- Neurosecretory granules
- Neuro(micro)tubules

Malignant Schwannoma
- Neuro(micro)tubules and neurofilaments
- Elongated nontapered cell processes
- External lamina
- Luse bodies (long spacing collagen)

Liposarcoma
- Lipoblasts with lipid in fat-producing organelles

Ewing's Sarcoma [I2.12]
- Glycogen
- Rudimentary cell junctions
- No other specific features

Malignant Fibrous Histiocytoma
- Fibroblast-like cells
  - Extensive rough endoplasmic reticulum (RER)
  - Fat may be present in RER
- Histiocyte-like cells
  - Lysosomes, filopodia

Fibrosarcoma and Other Fibroblastic Tumors
- Dilated RER filled with flocculent material—precollagen
- Smooth muscle features may also be seen (myofibroblastic tumors)

Hemangiopericytoma
- Perivascular tumor cells
- Intermediate cell junctions
- Microfilaments, pinocytotic vesicles, glycogen, external lamina

Synovial Sarcoma
- Fibroblast-like cells w/poorly formed junctions, no external lamina
- Epithelioid cells forming microvillous lined spaces w/cell junctions and external lamina

Angiosarcoma
- Weibel-Palade bodies

Granular Cell Tumors
- Numerous tertiary or phagolysosomes [I2.13]

Alveolar Soft-Part Sarcoma
- Rhomboid crystals [I2.14]

Flow Cytometry

Flow cytometry is a technique for measuring multiple characteristics of single cells in a moving fluid stream. Cell size, internal structure, antigens, DNA ploidy, and cell cycle analysis can be studied. Clinical applications are increasingly numerous and summarized below.

Pap Smear

Aneuploidy is associated with high-grade squamous intraepithelial lesions (SILs) and does not specifically identify invasive squamous cell carcinoma. Traditionally diagnosed low-grade SIL may also show aneuploidy.

Respiratory Cytology

Flow cytometry can complement conventional cytology in the diagnosis of lung carcinoma by detecting aneuploidy or high S-phase fraction. The false-positive rate is similar to the false suspicious rate of routine cytology.

Body Cavity Fluids

The utility of flow cytometry is currently limited because false-negative rates range up to 38% and false-positive rates up to 14% in various studies. However, flow cytometry may be helpful in diagnosis of lymphoreticular malignancies in body cavity fluids.

Gastrointestinal Cytology

DNA ploidy analysis can be helpful in diagnosis of high-grade dysplasia in ulcerative colitis.

Urine Cytology

Flow cytometry can usually detect carcinoma in situ and invasive transitional cell carcinoma by the presence of aneuploidy in exfoliated cells. Grade I lesions, however, are characteristically diploid.

Cerebrospinal Fluid

Although hindered by low volume of fluid, flow cytometry can enhance tumor detection, with a low false-positive rate.

Fine Needle Aspiration Biopsy

Unfortunately, aneuploidy has been reported in a wide variety of benign conditions and even normal tissue. Therefore, caution is warranted in interpreting results. However, there are certain uses for flow cytometry. For example, DNA ploidy may be a predictor of prognosis in breast cancer. Flow cytometry is useful in diagnosis and predicting prognosis in certain hematologic malignancies. Also, it is useful in prognostication of neuroblastoma, medulloblastoma, and acute lymphoblastic leukemia of childhood.

Polymerase Chain Reaction

Structural changes in DNA occur in neoplasia and infection. Characteristic mutations have diagnostic importance. The advantage of the polymerase chain reaction (PCR) is that it can amplify single copies of gene sequences to easily detectable levels, but the disadvantage is that the morphology is lost. PCR can be applied to cytologic specimens [Kühler-Obbarius 1994, Pestaner 1994].

Staining Procedures

Papanicolaou Staining Procedure, Progressive Method

95% ethanol (fixative)	15 min
80% ethanol	6-8 dips
70% ethanol	6-8 dips
50% ethanol	6-8 dips
Water, distilled	6-8 dips until glossy look disappears
Harris hematoxylin,* undiluted	45 sec
Water, distilled	Rinse
Water, distilled	Rinse
Water, distilled	Rinse
50% ethanol	6-8 dips
Ammonium hydroxide NH_4OH (1.5% in 70% ethanol)	1 min
70% ethanol	6-8 dips
70% ethanol	6-8 dips
80% ethanol	6-8 dips
95% ethanol	6-8 dips
OG-6	1-1/4 min
95% ethanol	Rinse
95% ethanol	Rinse (do not allow slides to remain in alcohol)
EA-50 or -65	3 min
95% ethanol	Rinse gently
95% ethanol	Rinse gently
95% ethanol	Rinse gently
100% ethanol	6-8 dips
100% ethanol (if large volume)	6-8 dips
100% ethanol:xylene (1:1)	6-8 dips
Xylene	6-8 dips
Xylene	6-8 dips
Xylene	Until ready to mount

[Keebler 1993]

* Undiluted stock to which 4 mL glacial acetic acid per 100 mL of stain has been added.

Papanicolaou Staining Procedure, Regressive Method

95% ethanol (fixative)	15-30 min
80% ethanol	6-8 dips
70% ethanol	6-8 dips
50% ethanol	6-8 dips
Water, distilled	15 sec-2 min until glossy look disappears
Harris hematoxylin: distilled (1:1) stock solution diluted with an equal volume of distilled water	6 min
Distilled water	Rinse to remove excess stain
Distilled water	Rinse
Aqueous hydrochloric acid solution HCl (0.25% aqueous)	6 dips
Gentle running tap water (lukewarm)	6 min
50% ethanol	6-8 dips
70% ethanol	6-8 dips
80% ethanol	6-8 dips
95% ethanol	6-8 dips
OG-6	1-1/2 min
95% ethanol	Rinse off excess stain
95% ethanol	Rinse (do not allow slides to stand in the alcohol as it will decolorize them)

EA-36, -50, or -65	1-1/2 min
95% ethanol	Rinse gently (do not leave slide in alcohol)
95% ethanol	Rinse gently (do not leave slide in alcohol)
95% ethanol	Rinse gently (do not leave slide in alcohol)
100% ethanol	6-8 dips
100% ethanol (if large volume)	6-8 dips
100% ethanol:xylene (1:1)	6-8 dips
Xylene	6-8 dips
Xylene	6-8 dips
Xylene	Until mounted

[Keebler 1993]

Diff-Quik Staining for Air-Dried Smears—Modified Wright-Giemsa

Fixative (aqua)	25-30 dips
Solution I (orange)	5-10 dips
Rinse (water)	5-10 dips
Solution II (purple)	30-90 dips (depending on thickness of smear)
Rinse (water)	5-10 dips
Solution I (orange)	5-10 dips
Rinse (water)	5-10 dips
Solution II (purple)	5-10 dips
Rinse (water)	5-10 dips

Examine wet and uncoverslipped to assess staining reaction. Allow to thoroughly dry, dip in xylene, coverslip.

Note: The Diff-Quik stain was originally developed to stain peripheral blood films to provide a quick differential cell count. Blood films are very thin and stain rapidly. When adopting the stain to FNA biopsy sections, which may be considerably thicker, the staining times need to be modified. In particular, solution II (purple) does not penetrate rapidly and, therefore, the slide must be left longer in this stain (the amount of time depends on the thickness of the smear, up to 1-1/2 min). Unfortunately, this results in everything appearing too purple. The secret to obtaining a good stain, with good differentiation, is to go back through the stains (not the fixative) a second time, and this time follow the manufacturer's directions (ie, a few dips in solution I and a few dips in solution II). Look at the slides wet and uncoverslipped (the water works like a coverslip). If the slides are understained, one can go right back into the staining solutions. Although it is relatively difficult to overstain, should this happen, alcohol, including the fixative supplied, will destain.

Ultrafast Papanicolaou Stain

Normal saline	30 sec
95% ethanol (optional, for storage/transport)	
Alcoholic formalin	10 sec
Water	6 slow dips
Richard-Allan Hematoxylin 2*	2 slow dips
Water	6 slow dips
95% ethanol	6 slow dips
Richard-Allan Cytostain†	4 slow dips
95% ethanol	6 slow dips
100% ethanol	6 slow dips
Xylene	10 slow dips
Mount and coverslip	
Total time	90 sec

Reprinted with permission [Yang 1995].

* Richard-Allan Inc (Richland, Mich).

† Alcoholic mixture of orange G, eosin Y, light green, and aniline blue.

I2.1
Carcinoma. Note the external lamina. In carcinoma, the external lamina characteristically surrounds groups of cells. In sarcoma, the external lamina tends to surround individual cells.

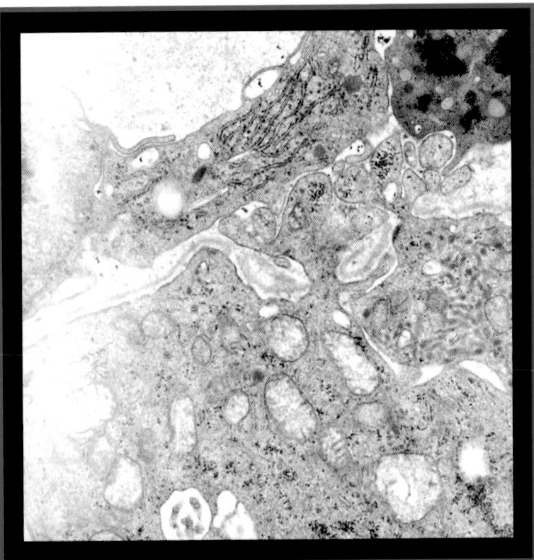

I2.2
Squamous cell carcinoma. Note tonofibrils and well-formed desmosomes. Causes dense, waxy cytoplasm characteristically seen in light microscope.

I2.3
Adenocarcinoma. Intercellular lumen and mucin vacuoles.

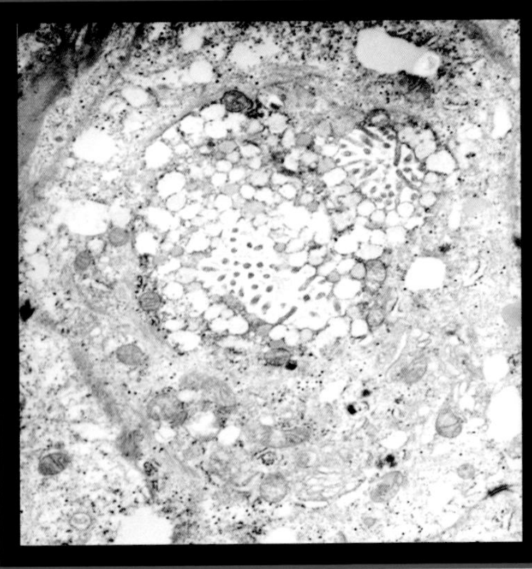

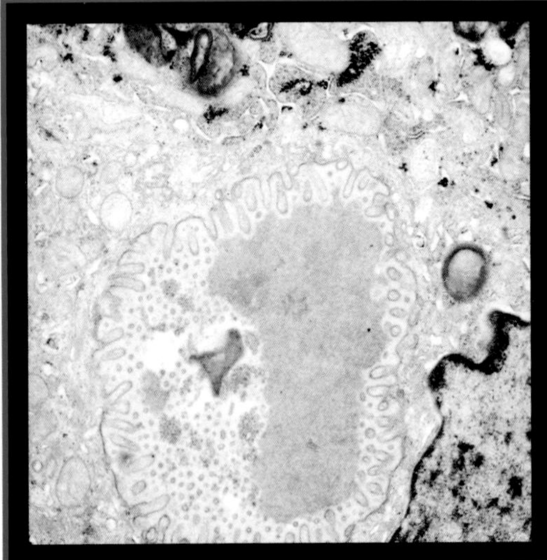

I2.4
Adenocarcinoma. Intracytoplasmic lumen as commonly seen in breast carcinoma, but not specific. Microvilli are too small to be resolved in light microscope, but cause lumen to appear sharply outlined.

I2.5
Adenocarcinoma. Zymogen granules (acinar cell tumor of pancreas). Cytoplasm would appear granular in light microscope.

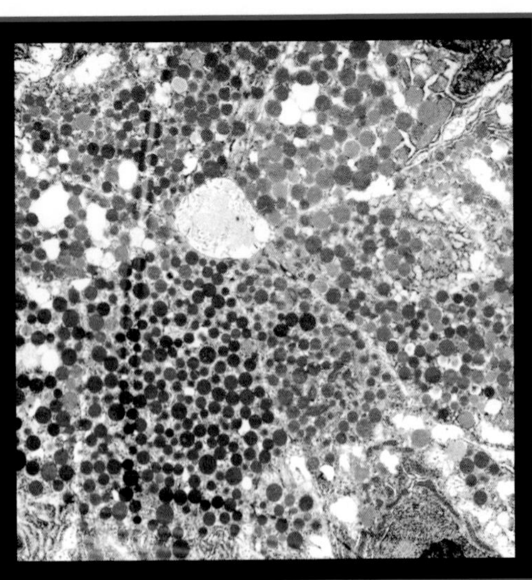

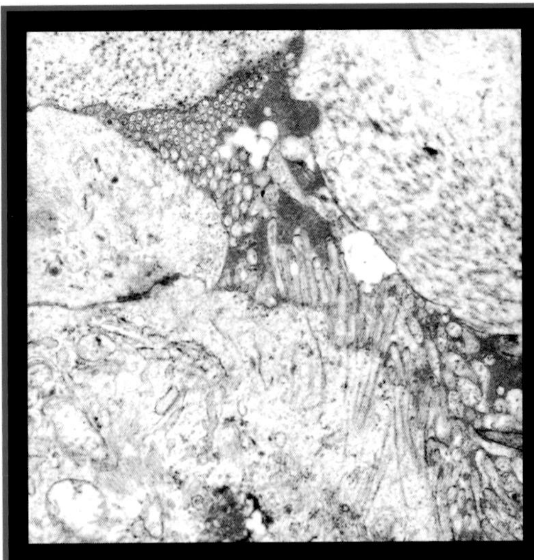

I2.6
Adenocarcinoma. Microvilli and long rootlets characteristic of colonic adenocarcinoma. Causes "terminal bar–like" appearance in light microscope.

I2.7
Adenocarcinoma. Lamellar (surfactant) body characteristic of bronchioloalveolar carcinoma of lung.

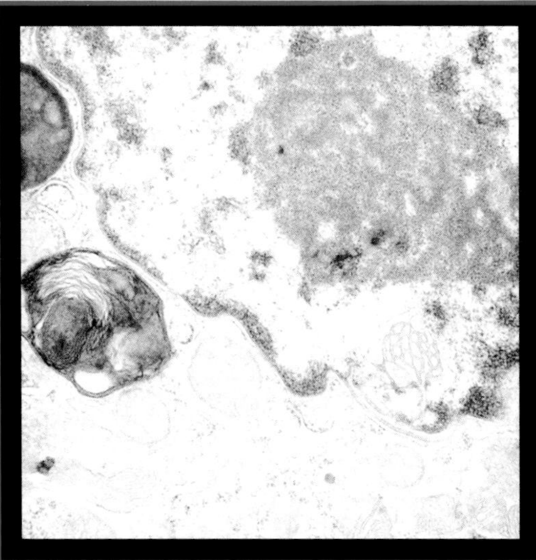

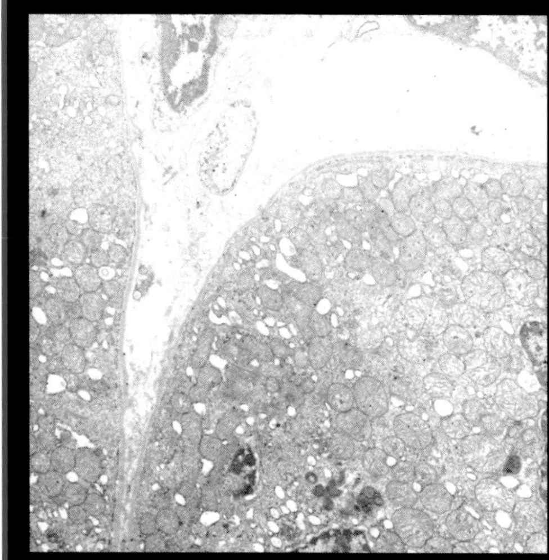

I2.8
Oncocytoma. Cytoplasm stuffed with mitochondria. Causes fine cytoplasmic granularity in light microscope. Note external lamina.

I2.9
Melanoma. Note characteristic premelanosomes. Another cause of cytoplasmic granularity in light microscope.

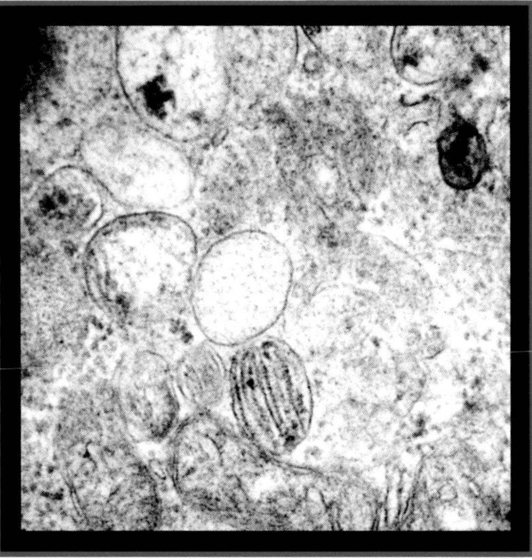

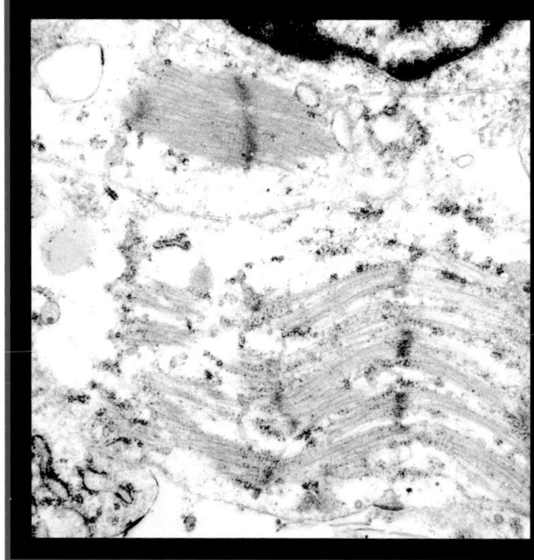

I2.10
Rhabdomyoblast. Note presence of both thick and thin filaments, also Z band material. Usually, the contractile apparatus is randomly oriented in malignancy; therefore, cross striation is rarely observed in light microscope.

I2.11
Neuroblastoma. Note neurosecretory granules and neurites (thin cytoplasmic processes). Neurites causes fibrillar appearance in light microscope.

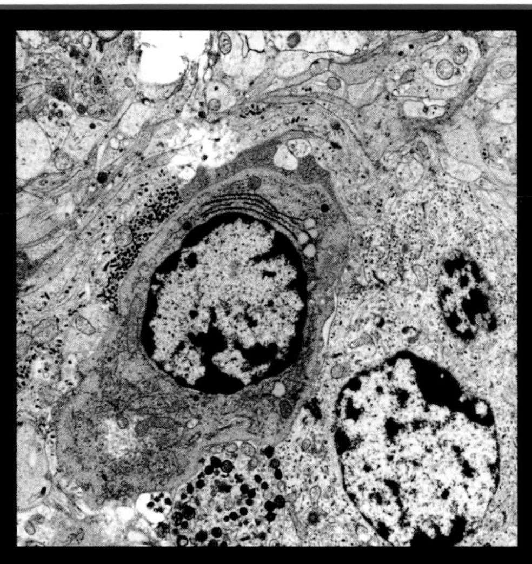

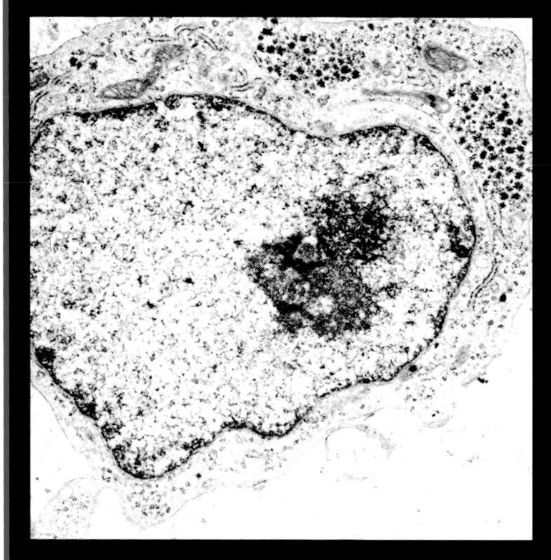

I2.12
Ewing's sarcoma. Note presence of glycogen ("rosettes" of dark cytoplasmic granules), but absence of other specific features. The tumor cells may have a clear appearance in the light microscope.

I2.13
Granular cell tumor. Cells stuffed with phagolysosomes. Yet another cause of cytoplasmic granularity.

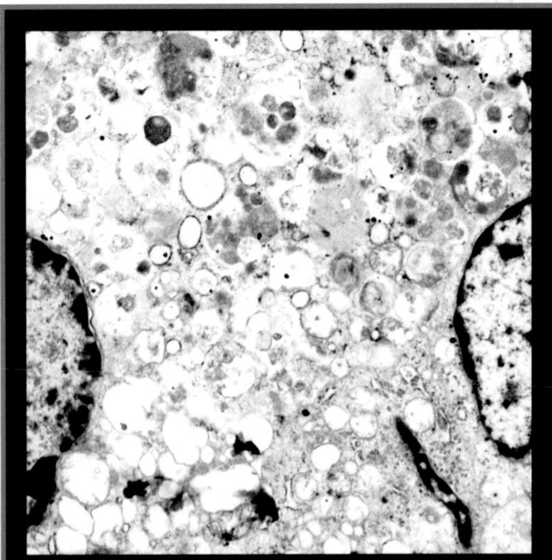

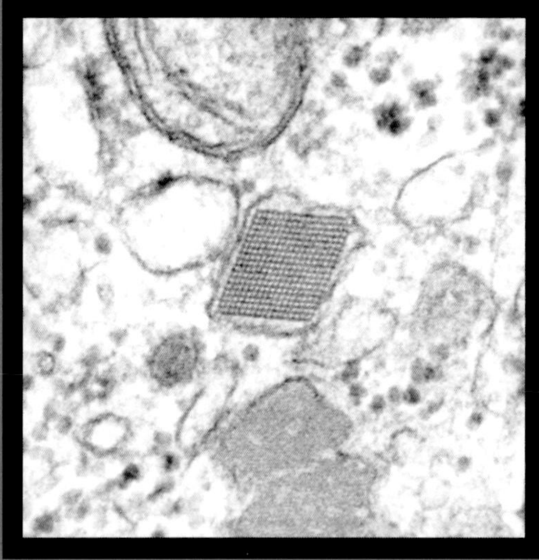

I2.14
Alveolar soft part sarcoma. Characteristic rhomboid crystal.

References

Akhtar M, Ali MA, Owen EW: Application of Electron Microscopy in the Interpretation of Fine-Needle Aspiration Biopsies. *Cancer* 48: 2458–2463, 1981.

Akura K, Takenaka M: Modified EA Staining Solution Using Fast Green in the Papanicolaou Method. *Diagn Cytopathol* 7: 317, 1991.

Bartels PH, Bahr GF, Bibbo M, et al: Analysis of Variance of the Papanicolaou Staining Reaction. *Acta Cytol* 18: 522–531, 1974.

Battifora H: Clinical Applications of the Immunohistochemistry of Filamentous Proteins. *Am J Surg Pathol* 12(S): 24–42, 1988.

Beyer-Boon ME, Voorn-den Hollander: Cell Yield Obtained With Various Cytopreparatory Techniques for Urinary Cytology. *Acta Cytol* 22: 589–594, 1978.

Beyer-Boon ME, Van Voorn-den Hollander MJA, Arentz PW, et al: Effect of Various Routine Cytopreparatory Techniques on Normal Urothelial Cells and Their Nuclei. *Acta Pathol Microbiol Scand [A]* 87: 63–69, 1979.

Bonetti F, Colombari R, Manfrin E, et al: Breast Carcinoma With Positive Results for Melanoma Marker (HMB-45). *Am J Clin Pathol* 92: 491–495, 1989.

Bonetti F, Pea M, Martignoni G, et al: Sarcomatoid Tumors of the Kidney. *Diagn Cytopathol* 10: 305–306, 1994.

Boon ME, Kok LP: An Explanation for the Reported Variability of Nuclear Areas in Air-Dried Romanowsky-Giemsa-Stained Smears of Follicular Tumors of the Thyroid. *Acta Cytol* 31: 527–530, 1987.

Burt A, Goudie RB: Diagnosis of Primary Thyroid Carcinoma by Immunohistological Demonstration of Thyroglobulin. *Histopathol* 3: 279–286, 1979.

CAP: Questions and Answers on Immunohistochemical (IHC) Reagents [Letter to Members], 1995.

Chan JKC, Kung ITM: Rehydration of Air-Dried Smears With Normal Saline: Application in Fine-Needle Aspiration Cytologic Specimens. *Am J Clin Pathol* 89: 30–34, 1988.

Chang A: Oncocytes, Oncocytosis, and Oncocytic Tumors. *Pathol Annu* 27 (1): 263-304, 1992.

Chess Q, Hajdu SI: The Role of Immunoperoxidase Staining in Diagnostic Cytology. *Acta Cytol* 30: 1–7, 1986.

Collins VP, Ivarsson B: Tumor Classification by Electron Microscopy of Fine Needle Aspiration Biopsy Material. *Acta Pathol Microbiol Scand* [A] 89: 103–105, 1981.

Dabbs DJ, Silverman JF: Selective Use of Electron Microscopy in Fine Needle Aspiration Cytology. *Acta Cytol* 32: 880–884, 1988.

Dabbs DJ, Hafer L, Abendroth CS: Intraoperative Immunocytochemistry of Cytologic Scrape Specimens. A Rapid Immunoperoxidase Method for Triage and Diagnosis. *Acta Cytol* 39: 157–163, 1995.

Dardick I, Yazdi HM, Brosko C, et al: A Quantitative Comparison of Light and Electron Microscopic Diagnoses in Specimens Obtained by Fine-Needle Aspiration Biopsy. *Ultrastruct Pathol* 15: 105–129, 1991.

D'Cunha S, Pinto MM: Cytologic Examination and Carcinoembryonic Antigen Assay of Fine Needle Aspirates of Bone Tumors. *Acta Cytol* 38: 543–546, 1994.

De Jong ASH, Van Vark M, Albus-Lutter Ch E, et al: Myosin and Myoglobin as Tumor Markers in the Diagnosis of Rhabdomyosarcoma: A Comparative Study. *Am J Surg Pathol* 8: 521–528, 1984.

Domagala W, Weber K, Osborn M: Diagnostic Significance of Coexpression of Intermediate Filaments in Fine Needle Aspirates of Human Tumors. *Acta Cytol* 32: 49–59, 1988.

Drijver JS, Boon ME: Manipulating the Papanicolaou Staining Method: Role of Acidity in the EA Counterstain. *Acta Cytol* 27: 693–698, 1983.

Fischer-Colbrie R, Frischenschlager I: Immunological Characterization of Secretory Proteins of Chromaffin Granules: Chromogranins A, Chromogranins B, and Enkephalin-Containing Peptides. *J Neurochem* 44: 1854–1861, 1985.

Fischer-Colbrie R, Kilpatrick L, Winkler H: Chromogranin C: A Third Component of the Acidic Proteins in Chromaffin Granules. *J Neurochem* 47: 318–321, 1986.

Flens MJ, van der Valk P, Tadema TM, et al: The Contribution of Immunocytochemistry in Diagnostic Cytology: Comparison and Evaluation With Immunohistology. *Cancer* 65: 2704–2711, 1990.

Frable WJ: Needle Aspiration Biopsy of Pulmonary Tumors. *Semin Resp Med* 4: 161–169, 1982.

Franklin WA, Mariotti S, Kaplan D, et al: Immunofluorescence Localization of Thyroglobulin in Metastatic Thyroid Cancer. *Cancer* 50:939–945, 1982.

Gey GO. The Maintenance of Human Normal Cells and Tumor Cells in Continuous Culture. *Am J Cancer* 27: 45–76, 1936.

Gherardi G, Marveggio C: Immunocytochemistry in Head and Neck Aspirates: Diagnostic Application on Direct Smears in 16 Problematic Cases. *Acta Cytol* 36: 687–696, 1992.

Gill GW, Frost JK, Miller KA: A New Formula for a Half-Oxidized Solution That Neither Overstains nor Requires Differentiation. *Acta Cytol* 18: 300–311, 1974.

Gupta RK, Naran S, Dowle C, et al: Coexpression of Vimentin, Cytokeratin and S-100 in Monomorphic Adenoma of the Salivary Gland; Value of Marker Studies in the Differential Diagnosis of Salivary Gland Tumors. *Cytopathology* 3: 303–309, 1992.

Herrera GA, Wilkerson JA: Ultrastructural Studies of Malignant Cells in Fluids. *Diagn Cytopathol* 1: 272–285, 1985.

Hess FG Jr, McDowell EM, Trump BF: The Respiratory Epithelium: VIII. Interpretation of Cytologic Criteria for Human and Hamster Respiratory Tract Tumors. *Acta Cytol* 25: 111–134, 1981.

Heyderman E, Chapman DV, Richardson TC, et al: Human Chorionic Gonadotropin and Human Placental Lactogen in Extragonadal Tumors: An Immunoperoxidase Study of Ten Non-Germ Cell Neoplasms. *Cancer* 56: 2674–2682, 1985.

Hirschowitz SL, Mandell D, Nieberg RK, et al: The Alcohol-Fixed Diff-Quik Stain. A Novel Rapid Stain for the Immediate Interpretation of Fine Needle Aspiration Specimens. *Acta Cytol* 38: 499–501, 1994.

Hollander DH: De Gustibus Non Disputandum: An Examination of Papanicolaou Staining. *Acta Cytol* 19: 404–406, 1975.

Jacobsen GK, Gammelgaard J, Fuglo M: Coarse Needle Biopsy Versus Fine Needle Aspiration Biopsy in the Diagnosis of Focal Lesions of the Liver: Ultrasonically Guided Needle Biopsy in Suspected Hepatic Malignancy. *Acta Cytol* 27: 152–156, 1983.

Kahn HJ, Marks A, Thom H, et al: Role of Antibody to S100 Protein in Diagnostic Pathology. *Am J Clin Pathol* 79: 341–347, 1983.

Keebler CM, Somrak TM: *The Manual of Cytotechnology.* 7th ed. Chicago: ASCP Press: 434-435, 1993.

Kindblom L-G: Light and Electron Microscopic Examination of Embedded Fine-Needle Aspiration Biopsy Specimens in the Preoperative Diagnosis of Soft Tissue and Bone Tumors. *Cancer* 51: 2264–2277, 1983.

Kobayashi TK, Nukina S, Nishida K, et al: Diagnosis of a Case of Wilson's Disease by Cytochemical Staining of Fine Needle Aspirates of the Liver. *Acta Cytol* 32: 123–125, 1988.

Kornstein MJ, Franco AP: Specificity of HMB-45. *Arch Pathol Lab Med* 114: 450, 1990.

Koudstaal J: The Histochemical Demonstration of Arylsulphatase in Human Tumors. *Eur J Cancer* 11: 809–813, 1975.

Kühler-Obbarius C, Milde-Langosch K, Löning T, et al: Polymerase Chain Reaction—Assisted Evaluation of Low and High Grade Squamous Intraepithelial Lesion Cytology and Reappraisal of the Bethesda System. *Acta Cytol* 38: 681–686, 1994.

Kuhlmann WD: Alpha-Fetoprotein: Cellular Origin of a Biological Marker in Rat Liver Under Various Experimental Conditions. *Virchows Arch Pathol Anat* 393: 9–26, 1981.

Linehan JJ, Melcer DH, Strachan CJL: Rapid Outpatient Detection of Rectal Cancer by Gloved Digital Scrape Cytology. *Acta Cytol* 27: 146–424, 1983.

Marshall PN: Papanicolaou Staining—A Review. *Microsc Acta* 87: 233–243, 1983.

Martin AW, Carstens PHB, Yam LT: Crystalline Deposits in Ascites in a Case of Cryoglobulinemia. *Acta Cytol* 31: 631–636, 1987.

McCool JW, Lee T-K, Silverman JF: Nuclear Morphometry of Small Cell Carcinoma in Fine Needle Aspiration Biopsies of the Lung: A Comparison of Diff-Quik and Papanicolaou Stain. *Acta Cytol* 36: 591–592, 1992.

Myers JD: Development and Application of Immunocytochemical Staining Techniques: A Review. *Diagn Cytopathol* 5: 318–330, 1989.

Nadji M: The Potential Value of Immunoperoxidase Techniques in Diagnostic Cytology. *Acta Cytol* 24: 442–447, 1980.

Nadji M, Ganjei P: Immunocytochemistry in Diagnostic Cytology: A 12-Year Perspective. *Am J Clin Pathol* 94: 470–475, 1990.

Ng WF, Choi FB, Cheung LLH, et al: Rehydration of Air-Dried Smears With Normal Saline. Application in Fluid Cytology. *Acta Cytol* 38: 56–64, 1994.

Nguyen G-K: What is the Value of Fine-Needle Aspiration Biopsy in the Cytodiagnosis of Soft-Tissue Tumors? *Diagn Cytopathol* 4: 352–355, 1988.

Nordgren H, Akerman M: Electron Microscopy of Fine Needle Aspiration Biopsy From Soft Tissue Tumors. *Acta Cytol* 26: 179–188, 1982.

Ordonez NG, Sneige N, Hickey RC, et al: Use of Monoclonal Antibody HMB-45 in the Cytologic Diagnosis of Melanoma. *Acta Cytol* 32: 684–688, 1988.

Papanicolaou GN: A New Procedure for Staining Vaginal Smears. *Science* 95: 438–439, 1942.

Panza N, Lombardi G, De Rosa M, et al: High Serum Thyroglobulin Levels: Diagnostic Indicators in Patients With Metastases From Unknown Primary Sites. *Cancer* 60: 2233–2236, 1987.

Pearse AGE: The Cytochemistry and Ultrastructure of Polypeptide Hormone-Producing Cells of the Apud Series and the Embryologic, Physiologic and Pathologic Implications of the Concept. *J Histochem Cytochem* 17: 303–313, 1969.

Pelosi G, Bonetti F, Colombari R, et al: Use of Monoclonal Antibody HMB-45 for Detecting Malignant Melanoma Cells in Fine Needle Aspiration Biopsy Samples. *Acta Cytol* 34: 460–462, 1990.

Pestaner JP, Bibbo M, Bobroski L, et al: Potential of the *In Situ* Polymerase Chain Reaction in Diagnostic Cytology. *Acta Cytol* 38: 676–680, 1994.

Ravinsky E, Quinonez GE, Paraskevas M, et al: Processing Fine Needle Aspiration Biopsies for Electron Microscopic Examination. Experience Implementing a Procedure. *Acta Cytol* 37: 661–666, 1993.

Saleh H, Masood S, Wynn G, et al: Unsuspected Metastatic Renal Cell Carcinoma Diagnosed by Fine Needle Aspiration Biopsy. A Report of Four Cases With Immunocytochemical Contributions. *Acta Cytol* 38: 554–561, 1994.

Schmechel DE: γ-Subunit of the Glycolytic Enzyme Enolase: Nonspecific or Neuron Specific? *Lab Invest* 52: 239–242, 1985.

Schulte E: Air Drying as a Preparatory Factor in Cytology: Investigation of Its Influence on Dye Uptake and Dye Binding. *Diagn Cytopathol* 2: 160–167, 1986.

Schulte E, Wittekind C: The Influence of the Wet-Fixed Papanicolaou and the Air-Dried Giemsa Techniques on Nuclear Parameters in Breast Cancer Cytology: A Cytomorphometric Study. *Diagn Cytopathol* 3: 256–261, 1987.

Schulte EKW: Standardization of Biological Dyes and Stains: Pitfalls and Possibilities. *Histochemistry* 95: 319–328, 1991.

Sehested M, Hou-Jensen K: Factor VIII Related Antigen as an Endothelial Cell Marker in Benign and Malignant Diseases. *Virchows Arch* [Pathol Anat] 391: 217–225, 1981.

Sehested M, Juul N, Hainau B, et al: Electron Microscopy of Ultrasound-Guided Fine-Needle Biopsy Specimens. *Br J Radiol* 60: 351–353, 1987.

Silverman JF, Frable WJ: The Use of the Diff-Quik Stain in the Immediate Interpretation of Fine-Needle Biopsies. *Diagn Cytopathol* 6: 366–369, 1990.

Sipponen P, Pikkarainen P, Vuori E, et al: Copper Deposits in Fine Needle Aspiration Biopsies in Primary Biliary Cirrhosis. *Acta Cytol* 24: 203–207, 1980.

Strausbach P, Neill J, Dabbs DJ, et al: The Impact of Fine-Needle Aspiration Biopsy on a Diagnostic Electron Microscopy Laboratory. *Arch Pathol Lab Med* 113: 1354–1356, 1989.

Swanson PE: Heffalumps, Jagulars, and Cheshire Cats: A Commentary on Cytokeratins and Soft Tissue Sarcomas. *Am J Clin Pathol* 95(S1): S2–S7, 1991.

Tapia FJ, Barbosa AJA, Marangos PJ, et al: Neuron-Specific Enolase is Produced by Neuroendocrine Tumours. *Lancet* (i): 808–811, 1981.

Truong LD, Rangdaeng S, Cagle P, et al: The Diagnostic Utility of Desmin: A Study of 584 Cases and Review of the Literature. *Am J Clin Pathol* 93: 305–314, 1990.

Weintraub J, Redard M, Wenger D, et al: The Application of Immunocytochemical Techniques to Routinely-Fixed and Stained Cytologic Specimens: An Aid in the Differential Diagnosis of Undifferentiated Malignant Neoplasms. *Pathol Res Pract* 186: 658–665, 1990.

Wick MR, Swanson PE, Manivel JC: Immunohistochemical Analysis of Soft Tissue Sarcomas: Comparisons With Electron Microscopy. *Appl Pathol* 6: 169–196, 1988.

Wills EJ, Carr S, Philips J: Electron Microscopy in the Diagnosis of Percutaneous Fine Needle Aspiration Specimens. *Ultrastruct Pathol* 11: 361–387, 1987.

Wright RG, Castles H: Variability of Thyroid Cell Nuclear Size With Romanowsky Stains. *Acta Cytol* 31: 526–527, 1987.

Yang GCH, Alvarez II: Ultrafast Papanicolaou Stain. An Alternative Preparation for Fine Needle Aspiration Cytology. *Acta Cytol* 39: 55–60, 1995.

Yazdi HM, Dardick I: What Is the Value of Electron Microscopy in Fine-Needle Aspiration Biopsy? *Diagn Cytopathol* 4: 177–182, 1988.

Young NA, Naryshkin S, Katz SM: Diagnostic Value of Electron Microscopy on Paraffin-Embedded Cytologic Material. *Diagn Cytopathol* 9: 282–290, 1993.

Zaharopoulos P, Wong JY: Hemoglobin Crystals in Fluid Specimens From Confined Body Spaces. *Acta Cytol* 31: 777–782, 1987.

3

Statistics
[or Lies, More Lies, and...]

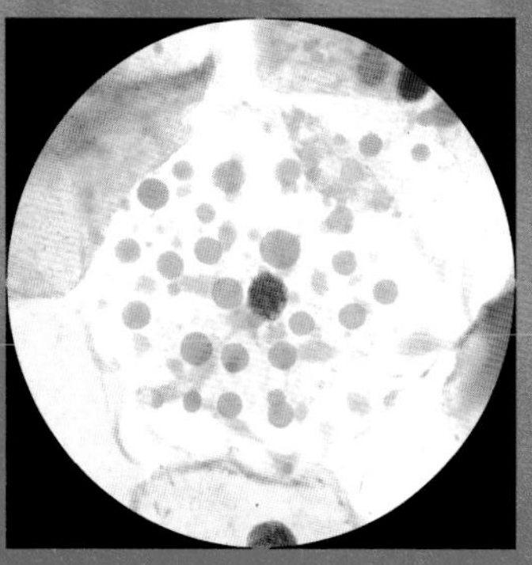

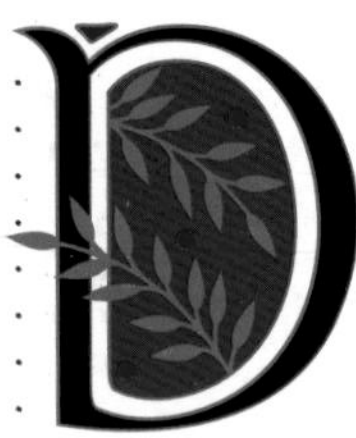

iagnosis is just another name for opinion. "The clinician cannot subdivide the general problem of the individual patient into different sectors, based on statistical probabilities; the individual's problem cannot be grasped by statistics as long as a method is not 100 per cent valid, which in biology is a daydream." [Grunze 1973]

What Is Normal?

Normal has many definitions, but a statistical definition is values that lie within the mean, ± two standard deviations, which encompasses 95% of the population. Other statistical terms for normal are *confidence limits* or *reference interval*. An interesting consequence of statistical definitions of normal is that given enough tests, abnormal results will be found in normal people. For example, if twenty (independent) tests are administered to a genuinely normal person, there is a 64% chance of finding at least one abnormal result.

Chance of abnormal result = $1.00 - (0.95)^{20} = 0.64$, or 64%

Thus, normal people are more likely to be found abnormal than normal, by a factor of nearly two to one.

What Does a Diagnosis Really Mean?

Diagnosis is the act of identifying a disease. But how does one *know* when the disease has been identified? Unfortunately, many clinicians believe that pathologic diagnosis is a matter of black and white—yes or no—when, in fact, it is mostly shades of gray. Although some diagnoses are almost black and some almost white, an absolutely pathognomonic diagnosis is rare. Given that there is almost never a 100.00% certainty in medicine, how sure of a diagnosis does one have to be to proceed clinically? The answer depends at least in part on the consequences of action vs inaction. For example, one loathes doing radical surgery for benign disease, but on the other hand, one loathes doing nothing for malignant disease. Thus, there is a constant balancing act, juggling many parameters (including the virulence of the disease, possible outcomes, degree of diagnostic certainty), always concentrating on what is best for the patient.

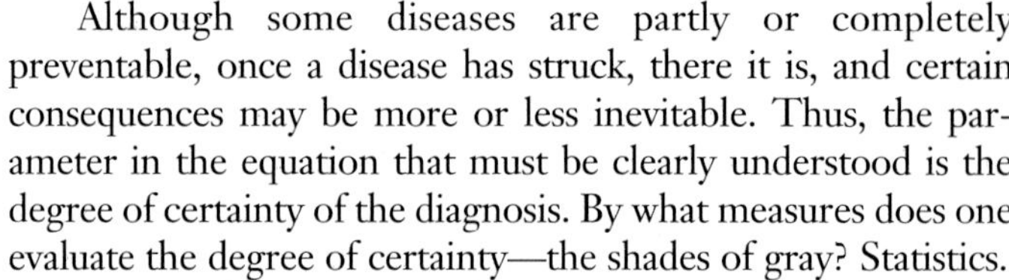

Although some diseases are partly or completely preventable, once a disease has struck, there it is, and certain consequences may be more or less inevitable. Thus, the parameter in the equation that must be clearly understood is the degree of certainty of the diagnosis. By what measures does one evaluate the degree of certainty—the shades of gray? Statistics.

Among the parameters that can be measured are true and false positive and negative diagnoses. From these, diagnostic sensitivity, specificity, predictive values, and accuracy can be calculated. (These will be discussed in more detail.) But the only way to determine which test results are *true* and which are *false* is to have a second test for verification, which is generally accepted as proof, ie, the true test, or "gold standard" [Raab 1994]. Thus, *the test to be tested (the test test) must be tested against a time-tested test (the true test).* In cytology, histologic diagnosis ("tissue confirmation") is often taken to be the gold standard against which the cytologic diagnosis is tested. However, "proof" could also include the clinical course, clinical impression, x-rays, scans, blood tests, etc (sometimes even a simple repeat of the cytology), alone or in combination. But a valid question arises: What proof do we have of the validity of the gold standard?

The Gold Standard

By what standard does one ultimately judge a diagnosis to be true or false? Generally, as we have said, histopathology is considered the gold standard of morphologic diagnosis. What *proof* is there of the accuracy of histopathology? Precious little may be the answer [Frable 1989]. Cytology has been shown to be more accurate, in some cases, than histology, ie, a truer indication of what is actually going on with the patient [Weisbrod 1987]. For example, what is *apparently* a false positive on cytodiagnosis may in *reality* be a false negative on tissue examination (ie, a false false positive cytologic diagnosis) [Cagle 1993, Kreuzer 1978, Tao 1984,1986]. (It has even been known to occur that a false-positive cytologic result was "confirmed" by a false-positive histologic result, which might be considered the false false false positive [Lopes Cardozo 1964]!)

Cytology can be more *sensitive* than histology. For example, it is quite possible to have a breast cancer patient with a "positive" pleural effusion (cytology), but "negative" pleural biopsy (histology). Is this necessarily a cytologic false-positive result? No. Patients have been described with positive cytologic findings but negative tissue biopsy findings, and who later return with incurable cancer [Loux 1969, Maimon 1974]. Also, a positive cytologic diagnosis could be followed by therapy (eg, radiation), and, consequently, the subsequent tissue biopsy may be negative—hardly an example of a true false positive. Moreover, clinical findings are not absolutely reliable, either. For example, in the gastrointestinal tract most "false-positive" cytologic diagnoses occur in patients with known premalignant diseases such as ulcerative colitis or familial polyposis, and have a clinically undetected neoplasm [Winawer 1976]. Several tissue biopsies, or even autopsy, may be needed to confirm a positive cytologic result [Sandler 1961]. *A positive cytologic result cannot be ignored, but rather should be actively followed up.*

In addition, cytology can be more *specific* than histology [Weisbrod 1987]. For example, careful electron microscopic studies of lung cancer have shown that the majority of primary pulmonary malignancies have combined glandular and squamous differentiation. Cytology, using the Pap stain, can readily detect many of these mixed tumors. However, routine histology is *incapable* of accurately diagnosing most of these tumors, misclassifying them as pure adenocarcinoma, pure squamous cell carcinoma, or large cell undifferentiated carcinoma. Thus, cytology is superior to histology (ie, more specific) in typing at least some common cancers [Hess 1981a,b,c]. Yet, histology is without qualification given the status of the gold standard!

In the few studies that do relate directly to the accuracy of histopathology, a high false-negative diagnostic rate has been found in some cases [Nichols 1968, Pickren 1963, Wilkinson 1978]. A false-positive diagnosis may never be discovered—the "lucky" patient having apparently been "cured" by therapy. Nevertheless, although false-positive histologic diagnoses are rare, they are well known to occur, and have occasionally been reported in, eg, analyses of frozen sections [De Rosa 1993].

The Statistical Importance of Clinical History

Clinicians commonly seem to think that clinical information should be withheld from pathologists so as not to "bias" the microscopic diagnosis. Is there any proof, one way or the other, regarding this possible "bias" and the outcome on patient care? Yes—in a certain way—and there is an explanation for it as well. First, the explanation. Clinical information, including history and physical examination—the foundations of the practice of medicine—together with other laboratory and radiologic results, will have vastly reduced the universe of all *possible* diagnoses (to a small subset of *probable* diagnostic entries). Stated in statistical language, providing clinical information has the effect of substantially increasing the *prevalence* of (a particular) disease in the patient population being examined. The diagnostic benefit gained by increasing the prevalence of disease is *independent* of the quality of the test itself (ie, its sensitivity and specificity). In essence, the more refined the question, the more refined the answer.

And now the proof. Looking at it mathematically, the higher the index of clinical suspicion, the more "accurate" the test (or the higher the predictive value, PV[+]). For example, the prevalence of carcinoma of the breast in the general female population is, let us say, about 1 in 1,000. However, if patients with clinically suspicious palpable breast masses and abnormal mammograms are selected for biopsy, the prevalence in this selected population may be as high as 1 in 2. Using *constant* sensitivity and specificity, eg, each 95%, observe the difference in the diagnostic "accuracy" (ie, PV[+]) when the prevalence of disease changes from 1/1000 to 1/2:

$$\text{PV}(+) = \frac{(\text{prev})(\text{sens})}{[(\text{prev})(\text{sens})] + [(1 - \text{prev})(1 - \text{sens})]}$$

$$\text{PV}(+)_{(1/1000)} = <2\%$$
$$\text{PV}(+)_{(1/2)} = 95\% \text{ (an almost } \textit{50-fold} \text{ increase)}$$

Thus, the prevalence of disease, and by extension, the clinical information *can be the single most important factor in the reliability of a test* [Ongphiphadhanakul 1992].

It is clear that the best results in fine needle aspiration (FNA) biopsy examination occur when one physician sees the patient, performs the biopsy, and interprets the smears (see Chapter 12). There are many reasons for this, ranging from ensuring that the correct area is sampled to ensuring high-quality smear preparation, but it can be asserted that one key factor is the gathering of clinical information at the time of the biopsy. In summary, if any "bias" is introduced by having access to clinical history, it is to the significant benefit of the patient!

And then my doctor said, "We're going to admit you to the hospital for a 'few tests.'"

There is another aspect to the statistical problem regarding the prevalence of disease, one which is being seen with increasing frequency in medicine today. As more and more investigations are performed, an inevitable consequence is that more and more *incidental* abnormalities will be detected (remember the 64% chance of abnormality in "normal" people), which often require further investigation, sometimes including major surgery. Not only is there an inherent risk of morbidity and even mortality, there is also substantial financial cost for these "unnecessary" procedures. Moreover, because the prevalence of serious disease, such as cancer, in these incidental lesions is low, the finding of incidental abnormalities can wreak havoc on diagnostic "accuracy," costing still more to sort out the conflicting results.

For example, patients undergoing surgery are routinely subjected to numerous tests as part of their preoperative evaluation. In a study of men undergoing prostatic surgery, asymptomatic space-occupying lesions of the kidney (suspicious for renal malignancy) were detected in 15% of patients. There was a much lower rate (4.6%) of such lesions identified in all patients in whom excretory pyelograms were obtained. And only 0.4% of all patients admitted to the hospital during the same period had space-occupying renal lesions detected [Lang 1973]. There seems to be an almost linear relationship between the use of screening tests (in this case, excretory urography) and the discovery of lesions that need further investigation. (It makes sense, though: "the harder one looks, the more one finds.") However, the prevalence of malignancy in the renal lesions detected was only about 5%! Plug 5% prevalence of disease into the predictive value (PV) equation and see what happens. With sensitivity and specificity of 95%, the PV(+) is 50%—the equivalent of a coin toss. Another well-known example of this problem is the so-called "incidentaloma" which has become increasingly frequent in modern medicine (see Chapter 26).

Subjective Objectivity, or the Art and Science of Cytopathology

A larger question is what percent of what we do in cytologic diagnosis is subjective: 1%? 10%? 90%? It can be argued that microscopic diagnosis is 100% subjective. Our *interpretations* of what we see are *certainly* subjective; the *criteria* by which we judge what we see are *probably* subjective; and the *metacriteria* (eg, quality assurance) by which we assess our criteria are *possibly* subjective. To argue that one ought not be subjective in diagnosis is like arguing that a fish ought not get wet in the water.

Thus, we sink or swim in a sea of subjectivity. This is the *art* of cytopathology. The criteria by which we make a microscopic diagnosis are not altogether different from those by which we judge fine art (eg, elements of contour, proportion, and light). *The art of cytology consists in refining our visual diagnostic criteria much as the connoisseur refines his or her taste.*

In science, nothing is proven until the results can be reproduced: reproducibility is the essence of scientific proof. When we can develop our subjective cytodiagnostic criteria to the point that other observers can arrive at the same conclusion in a high proportion of cases, we have a *science* of cytopathology. Further, the most satisfying solution to a problem is what is called an "elegant proof." An elegant proof consists in cutting the Gordian knot, providing the simplest solution to a vexing problem. Thus, *the science of cytopathology consists in building simple, reproducible diagnostic criteria.* Which raises a further question: What are the minimal criteria by which a diagnosis can be made? Well, this is where I must invite you to read the rest of the book.

Of True and False Negative and Positive Tests [T3.1]

A *true positive* test result is a genuine indication of the presence of disease: the sick diagnosed as sick.

T3.1 **True and False Negative and Positive Tests**

Test Result	Patient (With Disease)	Patient (Without Disease)	Totals
+	TP	FP	All (+)
–	FN	TN	All (–)
	All with disease	All without disease	All results

$$\text{TP} = (\text{Prevalence}) \times (\text{Sensitivity})$$
$$\text{Probability} = (1 - \text{Sensitivity}) = \text{FN}/(\text{TP} + \text{FN})$$

A *true negative* test result is a genuine indication of the absence of disease: the healthy diagnosed as healthy.

$$\text{TN} = (1 - \text{Prevalence}) \times (\text{Specificity})$$
$$\text{Probability} = (1 - \text{Specificity}) = \text{FP}/(\text{TN} + \text{FP})$$

A *false positive* test result occurs in a person without the disease: the healthy diagnosed as sick (a type II or β error, which is an error of commission).

$$\text{FP} = (1 - \text{Prevalence}) \times (1 - \text{Sensitivity})$$
$$\text{Probability} = \text{Specificity}$$

A *false negative* test result occurs in a patient with the disease: the sick diagnosed as healthy (a type I or α error, which is an error of omission).

$$\text{FN} = (\text{Prevalence}) \times (1 - \text{Specificity})$$
$$\text{Probability} = \text{Sensitivity}$$

Of Sensitivity and Specificity

Sensitivity (α) *speaks to the presence of disease*, or TP/(TP + FN). The term refers to the ability to detect the presence of disease, ie, detection rate or diagnostic yield. Sensitivity answers the question: If a person has a disease, how likely is it that the test is positive or what is the proportion of positive results among all patients with disease (all patients with disease = disease prevalence)? Sensitivity relates to the ability to detect true positives, at the expense of including false positives.

The following is a highly illustrative story of a 100% sensitive test—one that "never misses a single case of disease." The unscrupulous Dr X says he has developed a remarkable "cancer stain" that he then advertises in the *Journal of Pathological Results* as 100% sensitive to the presence of cancer. In fact, Dr. X even guarantees it will be positive in every single case of cancer or double your cancer back. Many skeptical, but curious, pathologists order this expensive special stain for their laboratories, only to find out that it has a peculiar resemblance to hematoxylin. (When you go back and read the fine print, you discover that not only does it stain all cancer cells, but it also stains all other cells with a nucleus. Therefore, although the test is *extremely sensitive*, it is *completely nonspecific*.)

Specificity (β) *speaks to the absence of disease*, or TN/(TN + FP). The term refers to the ability to exclude the presence of disease. Specificity answers the question: If a person does not have a disease, how likely is the test to be negative, or what is the proportion of negative results among all people without disease (all people without disease = 1 – disease prevalence)? (Note: Specificity can also refer to the ability to diagnose the particular type of disease present, cytotyping accuracy.)

The following is another highly illustrative story, this time of a 100% specific test—one that "never mistakes a healthy person for a diseased patient." Suppose our unethical (but apparently enterprising) Dr X decides to open a "Pap mill" and that Dr X is smart enough to screen mostly healthy, low-risk women (perhaps by charging a high price?) in whom the prevalence of cervical cancer or high-grade dysplasia is very low, let's say, 0.1%. Now imagine that Dr X does not screen or even process the cases, but simply generates a "within normal limits" report, never once issuing a positive diagnosis in some 100,000 women. The local newspaper decides to investigate. Dr X says the statistics will *prove* that the lab is doing a fantastic job, that the results are 100% specific as well as 99.9% "accurate." And, this is (more or less) correct.

Among these 100,000 low-risk women, only 100 (100,000 × 0.1%) would be expected to have significant cervical pathology (as defined above). Therefore, there will be, on average, 100 false-negative diagnoses among 99,900 true-negative diagnoses, and no false-positive diagnoses (no "positives" at all, in fact). Thus, the Pap smear diagnoses are 100% specific [99,900/(99,900 + 0) = 100%]: not a single women was mistakenly diagnosed as having significant cervical pathology. Furthermore, the lab's Pap smear results have an "accuracy" of 99.9% [99,900/(99,900 + 100) = 99.9%]. And even if an order of magnitude (ie, 10 times) more women actually had significant cervical pathology, the results would remain 100% specific and still be 99% "accurate." But keep in mind that in this case, "accuracy" is the predictive value of a negative test [TN/(TN + FP)] (keep reading). Note, however, that the sensitivity is zero and predictive value of a positive test cannot be calculated.

Here's a similar real life problem: the case of malignant cysts. It is known that, for example, 99 of 100 aspirated thyroid cysts are benign, but for those unlucky patients who actually have a cystic thyroid cancer, FNA biopsy will only be able to diagnose about half of them (cells too diluted or distorted to make a diagnosis). One might say that this is one of those "good news, bad news" deals for the patient. Let's say you aspirate a patient's thyroid, it turns out to be a cyst, and you give it a benign cytologic diagnosis. The good news is that there is a very good (99%) chance that the benign diagnosis is correct (without even examining the fluid, by the way). Unfortunately, for the unlucky one in 100 *with* cystic thyroid cancer, there is no better chance than flipping a coin that cytology would be able to diagnose it. Therefore, the bad news is that there is also a good chance (~50%) that a cystic malignancy will go undetected until clinically apparent—perhaps metastatic. A similar story could be told about other cysts, eg, cystic breast cancer, where as many as three quarters of cystic cancers may not be diagnosable by cytology [Tabár 1981].

Predictive Value and Accuracy

Positive Predictive Value

Positive predictive value [TP/(TP + FP)] refers to the chance of a positive test result being a true positive, ie, how reliable a positive test is in predicting the presence of disease. Positive predictive value answers the question: What is the chance that a positive test result is real, not false, and that the patient with a positive test is in fact afflicted with the disease, ie, what is the proportion of real positives among all positive results issued by the lab?

An examination of the implications of predictive value formulations can be unsettling. For example, assume that a pregnancy test is 98% "accurate," ie, if a woman is pregnant, the test will be positive 98% of the time and if she is not, the test will be negative 98% of the time. Assume that 5 women in 1,000 are pregnant. Now let's say that someone you know has a positive pregnancy test, how sure can she be that she is pregnant?

Suppose the pregnancy test is taken by 10,000 randomly selected women. On average, 50 women would be expected to be pregnant (5/1,000 × 10,000 = 50). 98% of these 50 pregnant women will test positive, or 49 positive results. Of the 9,950 women who are not pregnant, 2% will also test positive, resulting in 199 positive results (2% × 9,950 = 199). Altogether there are 248 positive results (49 + 199). Therefore, the great majority (199/248) of positive tests are *false*-positive results and the probability that your friend is pregnant, even though she tested positive, is only about 20% (49/248 = 19.8%)! That is, the predictive value of a positive test in this example is ~20%. In summary, paradoxically, if your friend has a positive pregnancy test, she is four times more likely *not* to be pregnant than she is to be pregnant (at least in this hypothetical example)! (Now assume that your insurance company wants you to take an AIDS test or your employer wants to do a drug test. What would you say to them?)

Here is something else for a cytologist to keep in mind about testing for a disease. When a disease is highly prevalent, as it may be in a preselected patient population, no matter *what* tests are administered, the results are likely to correlate with the presence of disease (even if not directly related). For example, in (highly preselected) patients with jaundice, abdominal pain, and a dilated gall bladder, but without gallstones, even a positive patellar tendon (knee jerk) reflex is quite likely to be "predictive" of pancreatic carcinoma.

Negative Predictive Value

Negative predictive value [TN/(TN + FN)] refers to the chance of a negative test result being a true negative, ie, how reliable a negative result is in predicting the absence of (excluding) the disease. Negative predictive value answers the question: What is the chance that a negative result is real, not false, and the person with a negative test is in fact free of disease, ie, what is the proportion of real negatives among all negative results issued by the lab? A short story will quickly expose the principle: the prevalence of malignant disease in patients undergoing transthoracic needle biopsy has been reported to be as high as 93%. In such a highly diseased population of patients, *most* negative results are likely to be *false* negative; thus the predictive value of a negative test is likely to be low (only 28% in this case) [Simpson 1988].

Efficiency

Efficiency (aka accuracy) [(TP + TN)/(TP + TN + FP + FN)] refers to the overall ability of a positive or negative test result to genuinely indicate the state of the patient. Efficiency seeks to answer the question: What is the chance that a result is real, not false, and the test is an accurate reflection of the actual state of the patient, ie, what is the proportion of real results among all results issued by the lab?

Summary

- *Sensitivity:* If the patient has a disease, how likely is he/she to have a positive test?
- *Specificity:* If the patient does *not* have the disease, how likely is he/she to have a negative test?
- *Positive predictive value:* If the patient has a positive test, how likely is he/she to have the disease?
- *Negative predictive value:* If the patient has a negative test, how likely is he/she to *not* have the disease?

As the prevalence of a disease in the population increases, there is a tendency for the predictive value of a positive test to also increase but for the predictive value of a negative test to *decrease*, and these statistical factors are *independent* of the quality of the test itself (ie, independent of the test's sensitivity and specificity).

Screening vs Diagnostic Tests

Because there is almost inevitably some degree of diagnostic uncertainty and overlap between categories of normal and disease, there is a trade-off between diagnostic sensitivity and specificity: we can increase one, but at the expense of the other. In essence, there are two kinds of tests, screening and diagnostic. Screening tests are used to find cases of possible disease, diagnostic tests are used to definitively label a patient as sick. Thus, screening tests should be sensitive and diagnostic tests should be specific. For example, the Pap smear is a screening test, and as such, should find all patients with neoplasia, at the risk of including some patients with only inflammatory atypia. On the other hand, breast needle biopsy is often used as a diagnostic test followed by mastectomy and, therefore, no cases of benign disease should be included in the positive category (ie, highly specific). However, sometimes the use of the test changes, and then we can change the parameters of sensitivity and specificity. For example, if the next step after breast FNA biopsy is to be tissue biopsy or perhaps lumpectomy, we would not want to miss any cases of cancer and would adjust our diagnostic criteria (ie, make them more sensitive), at the risk of a (small, we hope) increase in the number of benign biopsies.

Significance of "Suspicious" Findings and Unsatisfactory and Nondiagnostic Specimens

Contrary to popular belief, the categories of "suspicious," "unsatisfactory," and "nondiagnostic" do provide some diagnostic information. According to one study, the overall positive predictive value of an inconclusive (atypical/suspicious) diagnosis averages about 80%, and ranges from 57% to 93%, depending on the anatomic site [Coogan 1994]. For example, in respiratory cytology it has been found that the majority of patients, about 60% to 75%, with suspicious or inconclusive cytologic diagnoses did indeed have respiratory tract malignancy [Caya 1985, Coogan 1994, Johnston 1982]. However, the diagnostic efficiency of a suspicious diagnosis is low, on the order of 50% in this example [Caya 1985]. Similarly, in prostate aspirations with cytologic atypia suggestive of cancer, about half of patients may be found to have carcinoma on follow-up aspiration biopsy. Patients with mild atypia are subsequently positive in about one third of cases, while patients with highly atypical cells yield a subsequent diagnosis of carcinoma in about three fourths of cases [Eble 1992]. Suspicious diagnoses are most useful for detecting disease (ie, in screening tests, like the Pap smear), but least useful in firmly establishing a diagnosis (ie, in diagnostic tests, like effusion cytology).

Perhaps surprisingly, unsatisfactory and nondiagnostic biopsies can also sometimes provide meaningful diagnostic data—but within limits. For example, in many series, about 80% of unsatisfactory breast FNA biopsies derive from *benign* disease [Bell 1983, Dundas 1988, Fessia 1987, Norton 1984, Russ 1978, Young 1986]. Remarkably, 98% to 99% of patients with unsatisfactory thyroid FNA biopsy have benign disease [Ashcraft 1981a,b]. Similarly, nondiagnostic biopsies may correlate with a strong likelihood of benign disease. For example, in a series of FNA biopsies of the liver, three quarters of nondiagnostic specimens were from patients with benign disease [Leiman 1989]. Therefore, these apparently nebulous categories of "unsatisfactory" or "nondiagnostic" do contain at least some diagnostic information, although the predictive value may not be great enough to preclude the need for further investigation [Giard 1990,1992]. For example, the thyroid statistic just given reflects a high incidence of benign thyroid disease (and low incidence of thyroid carcinoma), particularly a high incidence of benign cysts (which usually yield "unsatisfactory" specimens). However, given a predominantly cystic papillary thyroid carcinoma, as many as 50% may be missed by FNA biopsy; thus, the predictive value is low.

Unlikely Events and Their Concurrence

How many times have you noticed that, from time to time, there seems to be a run on, say, synovial sarcomas, or some other rare diagnosis? You've diagnosed two already this week, and there's a rumor of another one on its way. There must be an epidemic. Or is there?

What is the likelihood of the concurrence of two unlikely events? To simplify the discussion, consider the "birthday problem": What is the likelihood of at least two people in a group of 30 having been born on the same day of the year (ie, the concurrence of two unlikely events)? Is the chance of such a shared birthday high, medium, or low? If there are 365 days in a year, and 30 people, then the chance must only be:

$$\frac{30}{365} \times \frac{30}{365} = 0.00675, \text{ or less than } 1\%$$

In other words, fat, slim, or no chance...right?

Wrong! The chance is actually quite high. Look at the problem from another point of view: what is the chance of *nonconcurrence* of the two unlikely events (ie, the chance of two people in the group *not* having at least one shared birthday). The chance of only one person not having a shared birthday is 365 out of 365 or 100% (since there would be no one with whom to share the birthday). Next, the chance of two people *not* having a shared birthday is:

$$\frac{365}{365} \times \frac{364}{365} = 99.7\%$$

The chance of three people *not* sharing a birthday is:

$$\frac{365}{365} \times \frac{364}{365} \times \frac{363}{365} = 99.2\%$$

and so on up to, in this example, 30 people. If you do the calculation, the chance of 30 people *not* having a shared birthday is 29.4%. Thus, the chance of *having* a shared birthday is 100% – 29.4% = 71.6%. So, there is better than a two out of three chance that at least two people in a group of 30 will have a birthday on the same day of the year. With forty people, the chance is nearly 9 out of 10 that at least two people will share a birthday!

What is the nonmathematical explanation for this? The reason is that the *specific* rare event, in this case a specific day, eg, October 30, was not specified in advance. Had it been, the chance of two or more people having a birthday on that *particular* day would, indeed, be very small. But since it could be *any* rare event (ie, any day of the year), not specified in advance, the chance of concurrence of two rare events is not low, but rather *expected* to occur with some regularity!

The birthday problem is a scientific explanation for having runs of rare cases in pathology. Had one asked in advance what the chances were that next week we would have two or more cases of synovial sarcoma, the chance would practically approach zero. But the chance of having two or more cases of *something* rare is quite high, and in fact, happens "all the time."

Another problem: A deck of cards is honestly shuffled, and you are dealt a fair 13-card hand of bridge. You calculate that the chances of having been randomly dealt that *particular* hand are less than one in 600 billion. It would be absurd to conclude that since your chances of having been dealt that hand are so slim, the cards must be someone else's—although you may wish they were. This is another example of not specifying in advance what the rare event might be.

Epidemiologic Studies

According to Dr. Denis Burkitt, cases of colonic carcinoma have increased dramatically in Africa as the people have become more "Westernized." He observed, in a private (and tongue in cheek) epidemiologic survey, that the number of women who carried various items in pots on their heads had decreased, while the number of men who carried briefcases had increased. Since either of these changes could affect posture, and therefore the internal environment of the colon, perhaps diminished pot carrying or increased briefcase use was related to the observed increase in colonic cancer.

Of course, we regard this as nonsense, and prefer a dietary explanation for the observed increase in colonic carcinoma, but the point is well taken: *Epidemiologic studies prove nothing* (although we do not "like" theories that don't fit the epidemiologic data). Even in more traditional epidemiologic studies, which seem to make more sense, the results can still be difficult to interpret. For example, in some studies it was found that birth control pill use seemed to afford some degree of protection from cervical cancer. However, since women who use the pill must go to a physician for a prescription, they are much more likely to receive annual Pap smears than women who use other forms of birth control. Since annual Pap smears provide a high degree of protection from cervical cancer, the question became: does the pill protect from cancer, or is it the effect of the Pap smear? Subsequent studies, controlling for various factors, including Pap smear use, have shown that there may actually be an *increased* risk of developing invasive cervical cancer among pill users. Even so, since it is a fact that pill users are likely to get regular Pap smears, the question, at least at the population level, remains: Does use of the pill increase or decrease risk?

Of Order and Chaos

Many read horoscopes to "see" the future. When we peer into the future scientifically, we often use statistics (though some say, sadistics). Statistics is the science of predicting the future based on the past, by gathering data to determine probability. That definition itself raises an interesting question: Are the laws of nature universal and enduring or are they merely statistical aberrations?

Consider the classic case of flipping an "honest" coin, ie, one that is unbiased. We would predict that, *on average*, the coin will come up heads 50% of the time and tails 50% of the time, based on our past experience with coin flipping. But we also have learned that there will be some variation in the sequence of heads and tails, ie, we do not expect that we will get a perfect order of heads, tails, heads, tails, heads…ad infinitum. Rather, we expect some randomness and, furthermore, given enough flips, there will be sequences where only heads (or only tails) will come up in long series, eg, heads, heads, heads, heads….

Now, what if the universal laws of nature only amount to so many zillions of eons of coin flipping, and what seems from our limited perspective to be *order* is, in reality, *randomness?* What happens when, and if, tails comes up again? Linearity would fail utterly, and nothing would be for certain. Even within our perspective, the Heisenberg Uncertainty Principle predicts that *randomness is the order of the day*. But then, that was the point of statistics in the first place.

References

Ashcraft MW, Van Herle AJ: Management of Thyroid Nodules. I: History and Physical Examination, Blood Tests, X-Ray Tests, and Ultrasonography. *Head Neck Surg* 3: 216–230, 1981a.

Ashcraft MW, Van Herle AJ: Management of Thyroid Nodules. II: Scanning Techniques, Thyroid Suppressive Therapy, and Fine Needle Aspiration. *Head Neck Surg* 3: 297–322, 1981b.

Bell DA, Hajdu SI, Urban JA, et al: Role of Aspiration Cytology in the Diagnosis and Management of Mammary Lesions in Office Practice. *Cancer* 51: 1182–1189, 1983.

Cagle PT, Kovach M, Ramzy I: Causes of False Results in Transthoracic Fine Needle Lung Aspirates. *Acta Cytol* 37: 16–20, 1993.

Caya JG: Respiratory Cytology: Significance of "Suspect" Results in a Series of 435 Patients. *South Med J* 78: 701–703, 1985.

Coogan AC, Wax TD, Johnston WW: Clinical Significance of an Inconclusive Cytopathologist Diagnosis. I. Positive Predictive Value. *Acta Cytol* 38: 193–200, 1994.

De Rosa G, Boschi R, Boscaino A, et al: Intraoperative Cytology in Breast Cancer Diagnosis: Comparison Between Cytologic and Frozen Section Techniques. *Diagn Cytopathol* 9: 623–631, 1993.

Dundas SA, Sanderson PR, Matta H, et al: Fine Needle Aspiration of Palpable Breast Lesions: Results Obtained With Cytocentrifuge Preparation of Aspirates. *Acta Cytol* 32: 202–206, 1988.

Eble JN, Angermeier PA: The Roles of Fine Needle Aspiration and Needle Core Biopsies in the Diagnosis of Primary Prostatic Cancer. *Hum Pathol* 23: 249–257, 1992.

Fessia L, Botta G, Arisio R, et al: Fine-Needle Aspiration of Breast Lesions: Role and Accuracy in a Review of 7,495 Cases. *Diagn Cytopathol* 3: 121–125, 1987.

Frable WJ, Paxson L, Barksdale JA, Koontz WW Jr: Current Practice of Urinary Bladder Cytology. *Cancer Res* 37: 2800–2805, 1977.

Frable WJ: Needle Aspiration Biopsy: Past, Present, and Future. *Hum Pathol* 20: 504–517, 1989.

Giard RWM, Hermans J: Interpretation of Diagnostic Cytology With Likelihood Ratios. *Arch Pathol Lab Med* 114: 852–854, 1990.

Giard RWM, Hermans J: The Value of Aspiration Cytologic Examination of the Breast: A Statistical Review of the Medical Literature. *Cancer* 69: 2104–2110, 1992.

Grunze H: Cytologic Diagnosis of Tumors of the Chest. *Acta Cytol* 17: 148–159, 1973.

Hess FG Jr, McDowell EM, Trump BF: The Respiratory Epithelium: VIII. Interpretation of Cytologic Criteria for Human and Hamster Respiratory Tract Tumors. *Acta Cytol* 25: 111–134, 1981a.

Hess FG Jr, McDowell EM, Resau JH, et al: The Respiratory Epithelium: IX. Validity and Reproducibility of Revised Cytologic Criteria for Human and Hamster Respiratory Tract Tumors. *Acta Cytol* 25: 485–498, 1981b.

Hess FG Jr, McDowell EM, Trump BF: Pulmonary Cytology: Current Status of Cytologic Typing of Respiratory Tract Tumors. *Am J Pathol* 103: 321–333, 1981c.

Johnston WW: Ten Years of Respiratory Cytopathology at Duke University Medical Center: III. The Significance of Inconclusive Cytopathologic Diagnoses During the Years 1970 to 1974. *Acta Cytol* 26: 759–766, 1982.

Kreuzer G: Aspiration Biopsy Cytology in Proliferating Benign Mammary Dysplasia. *Acta Cytol* 22: 128–132, 1978.

Lang EK: Roentgenographic Assessment of Asymptomatic Renal Lesions: An Analysis of the Confidence Level of Diagnoses Established by Sequential Roentgenographic Investigation. *Radiology* 109: 257–269, 1973.

Leiman G, Leibowitz CB, Dunbar F: Fine-Needle Aspiration of the Liver: Out of the Ivory Tower and Into the Community. *Diagn Cytopathol* 5: 35–39, 1989.

Lopes Cardozo P: Cytologic Diagnosis of Lymphnode Punctures. *Acta Cytol* 8: 194–205, 1964.

Loux HA, Zamcheck N: Cytological Evidence for the Long "Quiescent" Stage of Gastric Cancer in 2 Patients with Pernicious Anemia. *Gastroenterology* 57: 173–184, 1969.

Maimon HN, Dreskin RB, Cocco AE: Positive Esophageal Cytology Without Detectable Neoplasm. *Gastrointest Endosco* 20: 156–159, 1974.

Mavec P: Cytologic Diagnosis from Tumor Tissue Using the "Quick Method" During Operation. *Acta Cytol* 11: 229–230, 1967.

Nichols TM, Boyes DA, Fidler HK: Advantages of Routine Step Serial Sectioning of Cervical Cone Biopsies. *Am J Clin Pathol* 49: 342–346, 1968.

Norton LW, Davis JR, Wiens JL, et al: Accuracy of Aspiration Cytology in Detecting Breast Cancer. *Surgery* 96: 806–814, 1984.

Ongphiphadhanakul B, Rajatanavin R, Chiemchanya S, et al: Systematic Inclusion of Clinical and Laboratory Data Improves Diagnostic Accuracy of Fine-Needle Aspiration Biopsy in Solitary Thyroid Nodules. *Acta Endocrinol* 126: 233–237, 1992.

Page DL, Hough AJ Jr, Gray GF Jr: Diagnosis and Prognosis of Adrenocortical Neoplasms. *Arch Pathol Lab Med* 110: 993–992, 1986.

Pickren JW, Burke EM: Adjuvant Cytology to Frozen Sections. *Acta Cytol* 7: 164–167, 1963.

Raab SS: Diagnostic Accuracy in Cytopathology. *Diagn Cytopathol* 10: 68–75, 1994.

Russ J, Winchester DP, Scanlon EF, et al: Cytologic Findings of Aspiration of Tumors of the Breast. *Surg Gynecol Obstet* 146: 407–411, 1978.

Sandler HC: The Detection of Early Cancer of the Mouth by Exfoliative Cytology. *Acta Cytol* 5: 191–194, 1961.

Simpson RW, Johnson DA, Wold LE, et al: Transthoracic Needle Aspiration Biopsy: Review of 233 Cases. *Acta Cytol* 32: 101–104, 1988.

Tabár L, Péntek Z, Dean PB: The Diagnostic and Therapeutic Value of Breast Cyst Puncture and Pneumocystography. *Radiology* 141: 659–663, 1981.

Tao L-C, Weisbrod G, Ritcey EL, et al: False "False-Positive" Results in Diagnostic Cytology. *Acta Cytol* 28: 450–456, 1984.

Tao LC, Sanders DE, Weisbrod GL, et al: Value and Limitations of Transthoracic and Transabdominal Fine-Needle Aspiration Cytology in Clinical Practice. *Diagn Cytopathol* 2: 271–276, 1986.

Weisbrod GL, Cunningham I, Tao LC, et al: Small Cell Anaplastic Carcinoma: Cytological-Histological Correlations From Percutaneous Fine-Needle Aspiration Cytology. *J Can Assoc Radiol* 38: 204–208, 1987.

Wilkinson EJ, Gnadt JT, Milbrath J, et al: Breast Biopsy Evaluation by Paraffin Block Radiography. *Arch Pathol Lab Med* 102: 470–473, 1978.

Winawer SJ, Melamed M, Sherlock P: Potential of Endoscopy, Biopsy and Cytology in the Diagnosis and Management of Patients With Cancer. *Clin Gastroenterol* 5: 575–594, 1976.

Young GP, Somers RG, Young I, et al: Experience With a Modified Fine-Needle Aspiration Biopsy Technique in 533 Breast Cases. *Diagn Cytopathol* 2: 91–98, 1986.

4

The Cell
[and the Four Elements of Cytology]

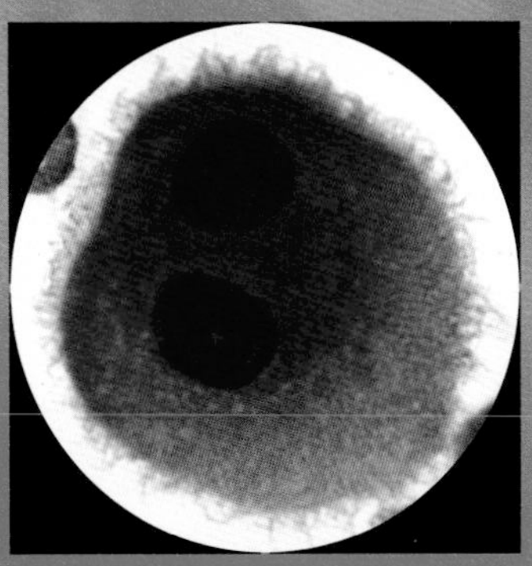

The Cell in Health and Disease
The Nucleus
The Cytoplasm
The Cell Membrane
The Extracellular Matrix
Diagnostic Features of Malignancy

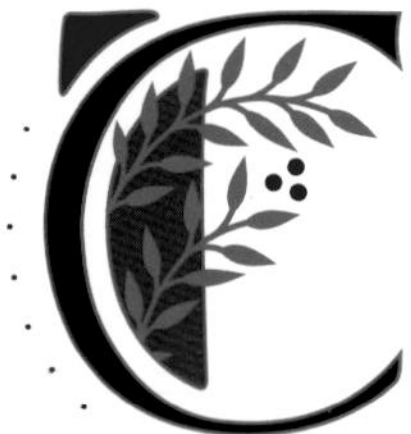

ytology, derived from the Greek word *kytos* ("hollow vessel"), is defined as the study of cells, their structure and function. The word "cell" was first used in a biologic sense in 1665 by Robert Hooke in his classic *Micrographia.* It derives from the Latin *cella* ("little room"). In ancient temples, the cella was the most holy inner sanctuary, the sanctum sanctorum, containing the sacred shrine—which in the biologic cell is synergistically the essence of life. Although the cell is more than the sum of its parts, for cytologic purposes, it can be broadly divided into the nucleus and cytoplasm, with its outer limits defined by the cell membrane, and also including the extracellular matrix, the milieu in which the cell lives. These four elements (*nucleus*, *cytoplasm*, *membrane*, and *extracellular matrix*) comprise the basis of the study of diagnostic cytology.

Since Schleiden and Schwann proposed the cell theory in 1838, it has become recognized as a fundamental truth that all plants and animals are composed of cells. *The cell is the unit of life.* Later, Rudolf Virchow, the first cellular pathologist, focused the study of *disease* at the cellular level. The cell can become, then, the unit of disease. Today, we can recognize diseases of subcellular organelles and even the cell's molecules. Still, it is the cell or its components, that are the basis of health and disease.

Disease is a disruption of the cell's normal homeostasis or steady-state, rather than a de novo cellular feature. When studying cells, whether sick or healthy, it is important to remember that their living reality has been distorted by being fixed in space and time and unnaturally stained to allow us to see them better. But living cells are dynamic structures, and do not normally exist pickled and dyed. Of course in histopathology, the cells have undergone the further ignominy of having been boiled in oil (paraffin embedded) and sliced like a salami.

When appropriate throughout this book, an attempt will be made to correlate the cell with its tissue of origin to help illustrate the relationship between cytology and histology. In this chapter, however, descriptions of cytologic features that can be observed by the light microscope will be correlated with the corresponding ultrastructural features. Also, the way in which ultrastructural features correlate with, or indeed may be the cause of, disease will be pointed out. Pathologists have directly correlated a particular disease with virtually every lack or malfunction of an ultrastructural component of the cell that has been described.

The Cell in Health and Disease

Cells are living machines and have often been described as self-contained manufacturing plants. Some cells, like amoebas, are capable of entirely self–sufficient, independent function. However, cells often do not function as individuals, but rather form ordered groups (ie, tissues), each specialized in a relatively limited number of functions, for mutual benefit. The price paid by the cell when it becomes more specialized is a loss of self-sufficiency. Thus, cells in tissue are more dependent on the proper function of other cells. For example, the viability of a given cell may be dependent on such factors as nutrient supply, neural function, or waste disposal. Specialization may make cells vulnerable to agents that affect their particular function. Also, highly specialized cells are usually less capable of self-protection, self-repair, or self-replication, so when stressed, they may either have to change into something else (metaplasia) or be replaced by scarring. Unfortunately, the replacement cells are never capable of providing all of the former specialized service. Loss of function in one cell may result in loss of function in others, each affecting still more cells, until the entire organism may suffer (disease) as a result of this cascade. The cell's internal milieu must be maintained within narrow limits, ie, normal, for proper function and homeostasis to continue.

A general principle of cytodiagnosis is that the *nucleus* reflects the state of health of a cell (normal, inflamed, or degenerated, as well as hyperplastic, metaplastic, dysplastic, or neoplastic) while the *cytoplasm* reflects the origin and functional differentiation of the cell (eg, mucus-producing glandular cell, protective squamous cell, etc). When properly evaluated, the nucleus and cytoplasm reveal a wealth of information about the cell.

The Nucleus

The nucleus is the repository for the knowledge the cell has accumulated over the course of its evolution. The information contained in the nucleus not only directs the cell's current activities but also passess the word to future generations through cellular reproduction. DNA is the scroll on which this genetic information is written (or coded). Except for a small amount of mitochondrial DNA, the nucleus contains all of the cell's DNA. DNA has the unique ability to build cells from spare parts, like amino acids. The nucleus, therefore, must see to (1) the *storage* and *replication* of DNA; (2) the *synthesis* (transcription) of a working copy (RNA) of the master DNA; and (3) the *transport* of this RNA to the cytoplasm, where ribosomes translate the words of the genetic code into protein, thereby directing the function of the cell. The nucleus is encyclopedic in its contents, with all the information for every type of cell in the organism (not unlike a set of "How to" manuals). Normal cells read only one volume, eg, how to make muscle, or how to make pancreas.

Diseased cells, however, may perform functions abnormal for their lineage, as if reading from more than one volume and conflating related information.

The nucleus is enveloped in two unit membranes, separated by a space, the *nuclear cisterna*, which is continuous with the internal space of the endoplasmic reticulum. The outer nuclear unit membrane is apparently derived from the endoplasmic reticulum and may be studded with ribosomes, like rough endoplasmic reticulum. The nuclear cisterna is normally too small to be seen with the light microscope, but in disease, eg, after radiation, it may dilate and appear as a vacuole.

The inner and outer unit membranes of the nuclear envelope fuse at many points around a central opening, the *nuclear pore*. Pores occur over areas of DNA activity and probably provide exit routes for ribosomes, the messengers from the nucleus. The pores are apparently closed by a thin diaphragm.

Just inside the nuclear envelope is a feltwork of fine fibers, the *nuclear fibrous lamina*. It may provide structural support, and may also act as a filter in nuclear-cytoplasmic exchange. The nuclear envelope and the nuclear fibrous lamina are too thin to be seen, individually, in the light microscope. However, these structures, together with attached chromatin, give rise to what is referred to in light microscopy as the "nuclear membrane." A common feature of cancer cells is so-called "thickening of the nuclear membrane." Ultrastructurally, it can be seen that what is really happening is margination and condensation of chromatin beneath the inner aspect of the nuclear envelope. Thus, "thickening of the nuclear membrane" is a manifestation of hyperchromasia and increased chromatin, features often associated with malignancy.

The nuclear sap (also known as nucleoplasm, karyoplasm, or karyolymph) contains proteins, inorganic and organic molecules, water, and ions. It also contains the *chromatin*, which is a complex formed by a type of acid-base physiochemical reaction between DNA (nucleic *acids*) plus histones (the nucleoproteins, which are *basic*) and other acidic nonhistone proteins. Chromatin accounts for about one quarter of the nuclear volume, and DNA, in turn, accounts for about 15% of the chromatin. The chromatin is present in the nucleoplasm as extremely slender threads (*euchromatin*), which here and there are tangled to form dense knots (*heterochromatin*). Heterochromatin is functionally inactive, but plays an important structural role in supporting the dispersed, or active, euchromatin during transcription of DNA to RNA. If fully extended, the chromatin of a *single* nucleus is over one meter long.

There are two major categories of nuclear proteins: histones and nonhistone proteins. *Histones* are cylindrical proteins around which the DNA coils, like thread around a spool. Histones provide protection of the DNA and assist in the condensation of chromatin to form heterochromatin. *Nonhistone proteins* are a diverse group, including initiator, regulator, and controller proteins. Heterochromatin and nonhistone proteins are acidic, and, therefore, stain basophilic (acid loves base) with the Papanicolaou stain. Together, they are responsible for the characteristic nuclear staining pattern seen with the light microscope using the Papanicolaou stain. Some bits of heterochromatin are relatively large and can be seen as distinct particles, the *chromocenters*. The highly condensed heterochromatin is functionally inactive, but plays an architectural role in supporting the dispersed, or active, euchromatin, thereby aiding in the process of transcription of DNA to RNA. In some cases, entire chromosomes may be present as inactive heterochromatin, eg, the Barr body. The Barr body is an inactive X chromosome that may be seen with the light microscope as a small, triangular or rectangular density along the inner aspect of the nuclear membrane. Diseases with too few or too many Barr bodies are well known (eg, XO [Turner's syndrome lacks Barr bodies], or XXX with extra Barr bodies). Extra Barr bodies can also occasionally be seen in malignant cells, where they are an indication of abnormal chromatin.

Euchromatin, active in the synthesis of RNA, is poorly stained in light (and electron) microscopy and therefore is seen only as a slightly basophilic space between the chromatin particles. This space is known as *parachromatin* or the parachromatin space. Normal, nonmitotic cells have a fixed amount of DNA. Hyperchromatic nuclei have more (inactive) heterochromatin, while hypochromatic nuclei have more (active) euchromatin. Therefore, perhaps surprisingly, darker nuclei are associated with fewer cell activities than paler ones. In cancer cells, however, nuclei are often hyperchromatic due to an actual increase in the amount of DNA, being polyploid or aneuploid (regular or irregular multiples, respectively, of the normal number of chromosomes). This increase in chromatin is also associated with an increase of basophilic nonhistone proteins in the nucleus.

The intensity of basophilic staining of the nucleus is roughly proportional to the amount of DNA present, but nuclear hyper- or hypochromasia depends on three factors: the amount of stainable material, the size of the nucleus, and Beer's law of absorption. The stainable material includes the chromatin and proteins that we've already discussed. Regarding nuclear size, it is important to keep in mind that the nucleus is a three-dimensional object. Thus, a small change in the linear dimension, *radius*, results in a exponential increase in *volume*. For example, if the diameter of the nucleus doubles, the volume has actually increased eightfold (volume = $4/3\ \pi r^3$)! Finally, Beer's law of absorption states that the absorption of light increases exponentially with the linear path length traversed. Thus, Beer's law and nuclear volume effects work in opposite directions and have some tendency to cancel each other out.

The size of the nucleus correlates with the functional activity of the cell: in general, the larger the nucleus, the more active the cell. Clumping of the chromatin is an important observation in cytology. Chromatin clumps may be either fine or coarse, and regularly or irregularly distributed in the nucleus [T4.1]. At one extreme, the chromatin may be gone, dissolved (karyolysis, as in an anucleate squame). At the other, it may form a compact mass (pyknosis, as in a superficial cell). Another

T4.1 **Matrix of Diagnostic Chromatin Patterns**		
	Fine	Coarse
Uniform	Normal for many cells	Carcinoma in situ, plasma cells
Irregular	Adenocarcinoma	Squamous cell carcinoma

possibility is homogenization of the chromatin (ground glass appearance) as seen in viral infections.

In early cellular degeneration, the chromatin forms *regular*, multiple, rounded particles, which may, however, vary in size. Sometimes the chromatin particles migrate either to the center or periphery of the nucleus. Cancer is also associated with chromatin clumping. However, in cancer the clumps are often *irregular* in size, shape, and distribution. In degeneration, the chromatin often appears *smudgy*, while in cancer the chromatin usually appears *crisp and distinct.* A simple way to judge chromatin distribution of a nucleus is to mentally divide the nucleus into four equal quadrants. If the amount of chromatin in the quadrants is unequal, this indicates irregular chromatin distribution and, therefore, suggests cancer. Furthermore, in cancer there is variation not only within one nucleus, but also from nucleus to nucleus. In fact, *marked variation of any cellular feature among cells is a hallmark of malignancy.* This is particularly true if the cells are attached to each other, forming groups, suggesting they are all of the same type and origin.

Another peculiar, but useful, property is the staining of the parachromatin space between the chromatin particles. In cancer, the parachromatin space is irregularly widened and clear. Thus, nuclear enlargement and hyperchromasia are likely to be *truly* indicative of malignancy when the nucleus is *blue*. On the other hand, in inflammation, the parachromatin often stains *red*, giving the nucleus a red, inflamed look and *warning* that the changes are benign, not malignant. Another nuclear change is nuclear vacuolization. Small, round, single, or multiple vacuoles may be seen compressing the chromatin. Vacuolization is particularly common after radiation.

In degenerative processes, many changes in nuclear configuration may occur. Frequently, as an early, nonspecific response to irritation (inflammation, thermal, radiation), the nucleus enlarges. However, in contrast with neoplasia, nuclear enlargement due to inflammation shows generally little or no hyperchromasia, unless induced by radiation. In addition, the cytoplasm of an inflamed cell usually exhibits changes too, eg, vacuolization. In cloudy swelling or hydropic degeneration, the nucleus enlarges and the chromatin becomes pale and homogenized, ie, the chromatin is diffuse, without distinct particles. The whole cell balloons. The nuclear enlargement may mimic dysplasia, but the nuclear features are indistinct and nondiagnostic. Similar diagnostic problems occur as a result of delayed fixation. Unfortunately, delayed fixation with consequent air drying of cells is a very common and frustrating problem in routine cytology.

Nuclear changes diagnostic of cell death are pyknosis (complete clumping of the chromatin into a single ink dot–like mass), karyorrhexis (pyknotic material breaks up into particles with dissolution of the nuclear membrane), and karyolysis or chromatolysis (in which the nuclear material dissolves). In karyolysis, a pale, empty space may be seen where the nucleus used to be: the nuclear ghost.

The idea that cancer is due to some derangement of the DNA is deeply entrenched in the dogma of oncology. Cytogenetic abnormalities have been associated with many malignancies. One example is the Philadelphia chromosome, which is associated with chronic granulocytic leukemia. Abnormalities of the number of chromosomes (polyploidy, aneuploidy, as previously mentioned) are also associated with cancer, although cancers can also be diploid. Genetic abnormalities generally cannot be seen with either the light or the electron microscope. However, highly abnormal mitotic figures correlate with aneuploidy. Unfortunately, no single microscopic feature diagnostic of cancer has ever been found. (Even atypical mitotic figures can be seen in nonmalignant lesions, such as benign mesothelial cells in serous effusions and cervical dysplasia.) Failure to find a universal marker of malignancy has been the great disappointment of cytology (as well as ultrastructural pathology and immunocytochemistry). In practice this means that no one criterion is pathognomonic of cancer, but rather a combination of criteria must be used to make a malignant diagnosis. Selections from nuclear, cytoplasmic, and cellular features must be made and added together to build a complete diagnosis. As a corollary, lack of any given feature does not guarantee the cell is benign, either. This is what makes cytology so intriguing.

Nucleoli may be the most prominent nuclear structures in some cells. They vary in size, number, and shape, but are usually small (micronucleoli), few, and round to oval. Nucleoli are composed of about 10% RNA and even less DNA, the major component being protein. Specific parts of the chromatin, the nucleolar organizing regions, are responsible for making nucleoli. A portion of the chromatin, the perinucleolar chromatin, is physically wrapped around the nucleolus. A feature useful in distinguishing a chromocenter from a nucleolus is the differential staining of nucleic acids, which are basophilic, and nucleolar protein, which is acidophilic. Since nucleoli are mostly protein, in a well-performed stain, nucleoli, unlike chromocenters, may "shine red." However, there is a certain amount of basophilic nucleus-associated nucleic acid. Thus, a small nucleolus may be surrounded by blue-staining material, obscuring the red appearance. Chromocenters are usually irregular and angular, and nucleoli are usually smooth and round.

The function of the nucleolus is the synthesis of ribosomal RNA and assembly of ribosomal subunits. Ribosomes (see below), in turn, are directly involved in protein synthesis. Therefore, there is a direct relationship between the size of the nucleolus and the rate of protein production by the cell. Nucleoli are often enlarged, multiple, and irregular in cancer cells; however, similar nucleoli can also be seen in some benign cells, such as those derived from a reparative process. So, while nucleoli are often prominent in malignancy, they are not diagnostic of it. When a nucleolus becomes as large as, or larger than, a red blood cell (ie, a macronucleolus), however, this is usually indicative of malignancy.

Diagnostic rule of thumb: "Conspicuous" nucleoli can be easily seen at high power (40× objective); "prominent" nucleoli can be seen at scanning power (10× objective); "macronucleoli" should be about the size of red blood cells (but this term is often used loosely to refer to large, prominent nucleoli).

More than six nucleoli per nucleus is abnormal. Also, marked variation in the number of nucleoli, particularly if the cells are attached to each other in groups, is suggestive of malignancy. Finally, very irregular shapes, with spicules, or points (eg, stars, bananas) suggests a diagnosis of cancer. Although irregular nucleoli are usually associated with poorly differentiated cancers, they can also be seen occasionally in atypical, but benign, reparative processes.

Nucleoli are free to roam about in the nucleus. When protein synthesis is particularly active, the nucleolus may abut the inner aspect of the nuclear membrane, in which position it is said to be "marginated." Margination of the nucleolus may facilitate nucle*olo*-cytoplasmic exchange. Nuclear membranes are often folded or convoluted in malignant cells. This has the dual effect of increasing the surface area for nucle*ar*-cytoplasmic exchange while at the same time allowing a centrally placed nucleolus to be in contact with the nuclear membrane, facilitating nucleolo-cytoplasmic exchange. The presence of irregular nuclear membranes is an important diagnostic feature of malignancy. Therefore, it is important to distinguish between malignantly folded or convoluted nuclear membranes and crenation, which is merely a degenerative change. The former have relatively smooth, convex hills and valleys, either like the brain or like cookie cutter bites; the latter have irregular, conçave spikes, like a star.

When a growing cell reaches a certain, predetermined size, usually about twice normal, this signals the cell to divide, ie, undergo mitosis. The cell's outwardly directed activities, like secretion, come to a halt. Most protein synthesis stops, too, including proteins needed for cell growth. The cell turns its attentions inward. The cell rounds up, the nucleolus disappears, and chromosomes become visible. Next, the nuclear membrane dissolves: this is *prophase*. The chromosomes first line up in the middle of the nucleus, *metaphase*, and then separate, *anaphase*. Finally, the cell itself divides, *telophase*. When the predetermined *organ* size is reached, mitosis stops.

Increased mitotic activity and particularly atypical mitotic figures are associated with malignancy. In cancer, cell division is out of control and there is a loss of coordination between the nucleus and the cytoplasm. The nucleus may divide before the cytoplasm is ready. This leads to an inadequate amount of cytoplasm for the daughter cells, and another important feature of cancer, increased nuclear/cytoplasmic ratio. Normally, the nucleolus involutes in mature or differentiated cells, but in cancer, the nucleolus remains active; therefore, a prominent or macronucleolus may be present in a small cell.

DNA is normally protected by the nuclear envelope and histones. During mitosis, however, the nuclear membrane dissolves and the DNA completely unwinds, exposing itself and making it vulnerable to carcinogens, radiation, and certain drugs (eg, chemotherapy). The normal cell has two sets of chromosomes (diploidy), but acquires four sets during division (tetraploidy). Some normal cells have other, even multiples of the diploid state, eg, octaploid transitional cells. Any deviation from these even multiples is aneuploidy, a feature often associated with malignancy. Moreover, ploidy status often varies among cancer cells, leading to diagnostically important variation in nuclear size (anisonucleosis or anisokaryosis) and staining.

An assortment of intranuclear inclusions may also be present. The most common type is the *intranuclear cytoplasmic invagination* (INCI) in which a portion of the cytoplasm pushes into the nucleus. INCIs (the so-called magenta bodies seen in Diff-Quik stain) are also known as pseudoinclusions because they remain outside the nuclear membrane and do not lie free in the nucleoplasm. Cytoplasmic organelles can often be demonstrated in these inclusions, ultrastructurally. Because INCIs are enclosed by a membrane, they appear very distinct and sharply outlined in the light microscope, which distinguishes them from artifacts like bubbles. INCIs have been seen in a large number of normal as well as hyperplastic and neoplastic cells. Sometimes they are diagnostically important, as in papillary thyroid cancer and malignant melanoma. More often, however, they are merely an interesting observation.

True intranuclear inclusions are not common. Among several types of true nuclear inclusions, the most important are crystalline arrays of viral particles, seen as Cowdry type A and B bodies (eosinophilic or red bodies in the nucleus, with or without, respectively, other associated virally induced changes in the cell).

The nucleus can undergo a variety of changes that can be seen and interpreted. Many of these have already been mentioned, like margination of chromatin and irregularities of the nuclear membrane as seen in malignancy. In response to inflammation and particularly radiation, multinucleation and multinucleated giant cells may be seen.

Examples of Multinucleated Giant Cells

Foreign body
Langhans'
Osteoclasts
Megakaryocytes
Cancer
Herpes, measles
Syncytiotrophoblast
Macrocytes, eg, radiation, condyloma
"Syncytia," eg, atrophy, carcinoma in situ

Multinucleation can result from either *endomitosis* (nuclear division without cytoplasmic division), in which case the nuclei tend to be very similar to one another (sibling image); or cell fusion, in which case the nuclei may be less similar in size and shape.

A final word about nuclei. When they lose the support of their cytoplasm, very unusual changes may occur in their appearance. Therefore, *never* unequivocally diagnose cancer based *only* on features seen in naked nuclei.

The Cytoplasm

The cytoplasm of the cell consists of everything outside the nucleus and inside the cell membrane [F4.1], including the organelles and cytoplasmic matrix. The cytoplasmic matrix, or cytosol, is a colloidal gel in which organelles and inclusions are suspended, like fruit in gelatin. The gel is mostly water. Many cellular reactions, for example anaerobic glycolysis, are catalyzed by enzymes suspended in the cell matrix. The cytosol is probably highly organized, but the structure cannot be appreciated in the light microscope. The cytoskeleton is a major factor in the architectural organization of the cell matrix and its organelles. More will be said about the cytoskeleton later, when intracellular filaments are discussed. When a living cell is examined in a phase microscope, the particles in the cell can be seen to be dancing about, in brownian motion. Certain chemicals (eg, ethanol) or heat coagulate the cell matrix, fixing the cell like a boiled egg.

Mitochondria are the proverbial powerhouses of the cell and the primary source of cellular adenosine triphosphatase (ATP), one of the cell's major energy units. Mitochondria are the site of many metabolic reactions, particularly those involving aerobic respiration and energy production, including the Krebs cycle, fatty acid cycle, and the respiratory chain enzymes, including cytochromes. Mitochondria vary in size (roughly 0.5–1.0 μm wide × 3–5 μm long), shape (cigar, club, or racquet), and number (few to hundreds, even thousands, in disease). Normally, there is a direct correlation between the number and size of the mitochondria vs the cell's metabolic activity. Cells with high metabolic activity, eg, proximal renal tubular cells, are often full of mitochondria. Cancer cells may be an exception to this rule. Tumor cells often have fewer than the expected number of mitochondria. Their mitochondria may also be more fragile than normal. Tumor mitochondria are often swollen compared with those of the parent tissue. This may be a reaction to ischemia or to a change in membrane permeability. The mitochondria may be pleomorphic, either large or small, with sparse or numerous cristae (see below). Enzyme changes are also often present in tumor mitochondria. Warburg showed that anaerobic glycolysis (which occurs in the cytosol) predominates over aerobic respiration (which occurs in mitochondria) in cancer cells. The favoring of glycolysis, then, correlates with a paucity of mitochondria in malignant cells. Glycolysis results in increased production of lactate dehydrogenase (LDH) and lactic acid, a byproduct of anaerobic glycolysis. Lactic acid, by the way, is what makes your muscles hurt (like a burning sensation) when you use them anaerobically, as when you lift weights or run fast.

F4.1 **The Cell**

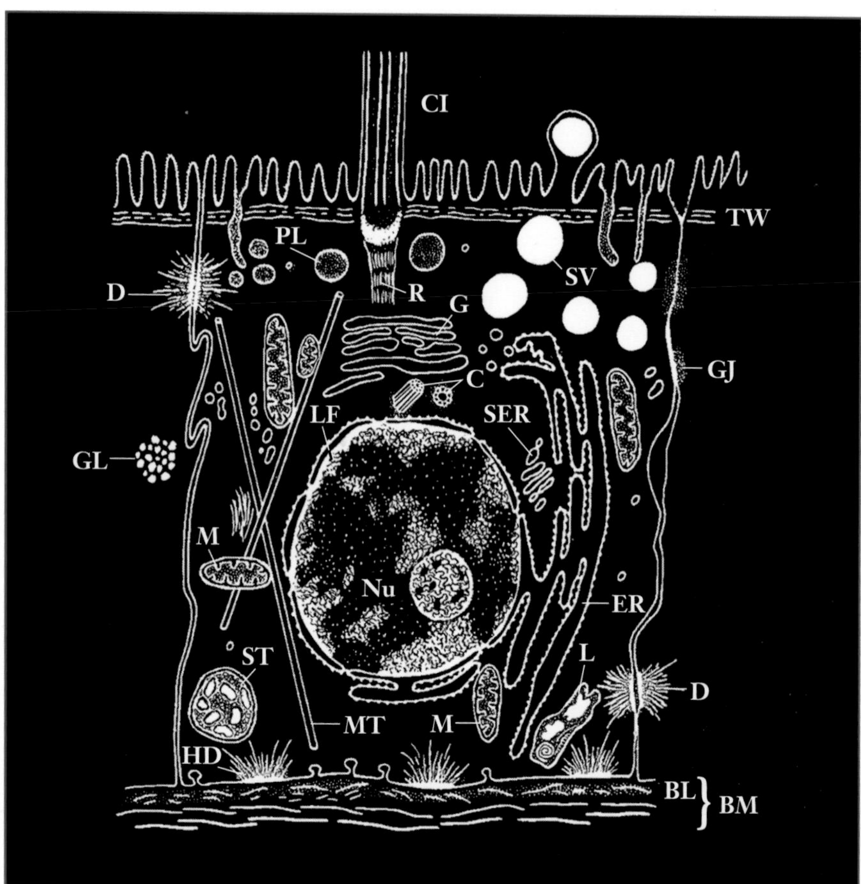

CI = cilium, R = anchoring rootlets, SV = secretory vacuole, TW = terminal web, G = Golgi apparatus, PL = primary lysosome, D = desmosomes, M = mitochondria, MT = microtubules, LF = nuclear fibrous lamina, Nu = nucleolus, C = centrioles, ER = endoplasmic reticulum, SER = smooth endoplasmic reticulum, GL = glycogen lake, ST = storage or tertiary lysosome, L = lipofuscin, GJ = gap junction, HD = hemidesmosomes, BM = basement membrane, BL = basal lamina. (Modified from *Compendium on Diagnostic Cytology*. Chicago: Tutorials of Cytology, 1983.)

Ultrastructurally, mitochondria are largely composed of two membranes. They have a smooth outer membrane (envelope). The inner membrane is complexly folded to form the mitochondrial cristae (*crista* is Latin for a crest or a ridge). The two membranes divide the mitochondria into compartments: the outer compartment, between the two membranes, and the inner compartment, which is the matrix space of the mitochondrion. The outer *membrane* contains monoamine oxidase and other enzymes. The outer *compartment* contains adenylate cyclase and nucleoside diphosphokinase. The inner *membrane* contains the enzymes for oxidative phosphorylation. The matrix, or inner *compartment*, has the enzymes for the citric acid (Krebs) cycle, as well as DNA, RNA, and divalent calcium ions. Mitochondria also have glycogen, ribosomes, and calcium containing crystals.

All mitochondrial DNA is inherited from the mother via the cytoplasm of the ovum. Mitochondrial DNA codes for membrane-bound proteins and some, but not all, mitochondrial RNA. Various types of muscular dystrophies have been associated with deficiencies of mitochondrial genes. However, most mitochondrial proteins are imported from the cell as soluble precursor subunits, which are then assembled to make complete proteins and enzymes. There are many inherited diseases related to specific lack of imported mitochondrial enzymes.

The outer mitochondrial membrane, like the cell membrane, is composed of lipids and proteins. Much of the membrane protein consists of enzymes involved in energy production. The inner membrane, however, is not like that of other eukaryotic cells, in that it has more acidic phospholipid, but no cholesterol, making it more like that of a bacterium. Moreover, mitochondrial DNA is circular, lacks histone proteins, and is not contained in a nucleus (features of a prokaryotic or bacterial cell). Thus, the hypothesis has been made that mitochondria may be parasites living in symbiosis with the host cell. It is suggested that the outer membrane represents a phagosome supplied by the host cell, while the inner membrane represents the original bacterial cell membrane.

Pathologic swelling of mitochondria is often caused by ischemia, which floods the mitochondria with water. Surgical anoxia, cell injury, and cloudy swelling due to vascular or metabolic disturbances (or delayed fixation) may all lead to mitochondrial swelling. The outer membrane may rupture. The inner membrane also degenerates and the matrix becomes dense. Pathological swelling is one of the earliest observable ultrastructural features of irreversible cell injury and imminent cell death.

Some metaplastic and neoplastic cells become stuffed with innumerable mitochondria and are then known as *oncocytes*; their tumors are called oncocytomas. The mitochondria are biochemically defective, so their increase may represent compensatory hyperplasia. These mitochondria often have abnormal cristae. By light microscopy, oncocytes have abundant, very finely granular cytoplasm, the granules being the mitochondria. Mitochondria can be stained with iron hematoxylin, phosphotungstic acid hematoxylin (PTAH), or acid fuchsin.

Sometimes giant mitochondria are seen in cells, particularly in hepatocytes of patients with alcoholic hepatitis or cirrhosis. These mitochondria, which can approach the size of a red blood cell, may be very abnormally shaped. Giant mitochondria can also be seen in some nutritional deficiencies, skeletal muscle myopathies, and tumors such as hepatocellular carcinoma.

Ribosomes are found in most cells because they are intimately involved in protein synthesis, a major function of any cell, including proteins for growth and division or extracellular secretion. Ribosomes are made up of two subunits, one larger than the other. Each subunit is composed of roughly equal parts of ribosomal RNA and protein. One subunit sits on the other, like a snowman, and they are joined together by messenger RNA (mRNA). Directed by mRNA from the nucleus, ribosomes receive amino acids from the cytosol that are specifically labeled by transfer RNA (complementary to mRNA). The ribosomes bind the amino acids together in the sequence specified by mRNA to form proteins.

Most (80%) of the total RNA of a cell is in the form of ribosomes. Ribosomes are basophilic, being largely composed of nucleic acid, and are responsible for blue staining cytoplasm in cells actively making proteins, known in classical microscopy as ergastoplasm (*ergaster* is the Greek word for workman). A special stain for RNA, methyl green pyronin, is useful in demonstrating ribosomes (and nucleoli). Cells rich in ribosomes, such as plasma cells and plasmacytoid lymphocytes (red is the positive reaction), can be made to stand out in a field of morphologically similar cells by applying this stain. This stain is useful in determining the phase of inflammation, eg, in evaluation of possible transplant rejection.

Ribosomes can either be free in the cytoplasm, forming rosettes or chains, known as polyribosomes, or bound to the outer membrane of the endoplasmic reticulum, in which case it is referred to as "rough" endoplasmic reticulum.

Polyribosomes synthesize proteins for growth and maintenance of the cell. Polyribosomes are prominent in immature or undifferentiated cells and cancer cells, cells which are specialized for growth and division. Thus, abundant polyribosomes correlate with rapid cell growth and go hand-in-hand with marginated and hypertrophied nucleoli, as well as increased mitotic rate. The individual ribosomes of polyribosomes are attached to one another by messenger RNA, just as the subunits are linked together, in the cleft between the two subunits. Polyribosomes are found randomly dispersed in the cytoplasm.

The *endoplasmic reticulum*, along with the nucleus, mitochondria, Golgi apparatus, and the outer cell membrane, are largely composed of unit membrane. The endoplasmic reticulum consists of anastomosing or branching tubules, flattened parallel sacs (cisternae), or vesicles, forming a *reticulum* (network) in the *endoplasm* of the cell. A large part of the cytoplasm of most metabolically active cells consists of endoplasmic reticulum. The endoplasmic reticulum may be either smooth (without attached ribosomes, characteristic of steroid producing or drug detoxifying cells) or rough (studded with ribosomes, as previously mentioned, characteristic of protein exporting cells).

The endoplasmic reticulum is in continuity with the nuclear envelope and Golgi apparatus, but probably not the outer cell membrane. It forms a continuous membrane-bound space that is isolated from the rest of the cytoplasmic matrix. Any surface ribosomes are, however, in contact with the endoplasm so they can capture amino acids and messenger RNA from the cytosol.

Rough endoplasmic reticulum (RER) is the site of synthesis of many proteins, which will eventually be exported from the cell or enclosed in membranes to form, for example, lysosomes. Therefore, RER is particularly well developed in cells that synthesize these proteins, such as plasma cells (immunoglobulins), acinar/acinic cells of pancreas and salivary glands (digestive enzymes), fibroblasts (collagen), osteoblasts (osteoid or uncalcified bone matrix), melanocytes (melanin), and hepatocytes (numerous different products, including clotting factors and albumin). RER more or less persists in tumors of these cells, and so may be an important feature in their diagnosis. On the other hand, RER is seldom well developed in immature or undifferentiated cells, such as stem cells, blasts, and poorly differentiated tumors. Also, in mechanically specialized cells, like squamous cells, and their tumors, RER is poorly developed.

Protein newly manufactured by the ribosomes embedded in the surface of the RER is extruded into the lumen of this organelle. Here the proteins are stored, condensed, and eventually passed (as if on a conveyer belt) to the Golgi apparatus for packaging and eventual export (secretion) from the cell.

The *smooth*, or *agranular*, *endoplasmic reticulum* (SER) lacks ribosomes. It usually appears more bubbly or vesicular than the cisternae of the RER ultrastructurally. Although lacking ribosomal granules, the SER is nevertheless rich in enzymes involved in the manufacture of steroid hormones and the metabolism of some drugs and chemicals. SER is also involved in the production of lipids and glycogen. Hepatocytes, especially with long-term exposure to certain drugs such as phenobarbital or alcohol, often have a proliferation (compensatory hyperplasia) of the SER. Abundant SER can be seen in the light microscope as a ground-glass appearance of the cytoplasm of affected hepatocytes. Viral hepatitis can cause similar ground glass cytoplasm.

In chronic cell injury, material may accumulate in the endoplasmic reticulum due to defective transport. For example, immunoglobulin glycoproteins may accumulate in plasma cells (which are rich in RER) as Russell bodies, giving rise to the light microscopic appearance of "constipated plasma cells with Russell bodies." Russell bodies are small, homogeneous, rounded, eosinophilic hyalin (from the Greek *hyalos*, glassy) bodies frequently found in plasma cells in chronic inflammation, giving the appearance of a mulberry.

The *Golgi apparatus*, together with the endoplasmic reticulum, contains a major portion of the unit membrane of a cell. Like the RER, it is best developed in secretory cells. In some cells, such as plasma cells, the Golgi is so well developed that it can be seen in the light microscope as a pale area next to the nucleus known as the *perinuclear hof* (hof is German for court or courtyard). Conversely, the Golgi apparatus is poorly developed in cells specialized for mechanical function, like muscle and squamous cells. The function of the Golgi apparatus is modifying, condensing, and especially packaging of material to form secretory granules. The Golgi also manufactures carbohydrates, which are then added to proteins to form glycoproteins. The Golgi apparatus is usually located near the nucleus. It is a series of membrane-bound spaces, stacked like soup bowls, that in section are thin at the center and progressively dilate to become bulbous at the ends. The convexity points toward the nucleus. The concave, or product-forming side, is continuous with the RER, from which it receives the material to be packaged. The product-forming portion is rich in enzymes and is the site where most of the synthetic activity of the Golgi takes place. The product is packaged and leaves the Golgi apparatus through the product-maturing, enzyme-poor side closest to the nucleus. The packaged cell products for export (secretion) are pinched off as membrane bound vesicles from the lateral, bulbous ends of the cisternae of the Golgi.

Immature or undifferentiated cells, like stem cells and blasts, have poorly developed Golgi complexes. A fast growing tumor will also usually have a poorly developed Golgi. There is some correlation between cellular differentiation and the size of the Golgi in any given tumor type. Benign and well-differentiated malignant tumors generally have a well-developed Golgi, *if* the parent cell also did. Occasionally, marked hypertrophy, dilatation, and distortion of the Golgi is seen in tumors.

In summary, the pathway of secretory protein synthesis is the following. DNA sends a coded message to the cytoplasm, via mRNA. The mRNA finds a ribosome and transfer RNA transports amino acids from the cytoplasm to the ribosome. Here, the amino acids are sequentially linked to form proteins. If the protein is for use in the cell, the ribosomes float free in the cytosol as polyribosomes. However, if the protein is for export, it is synthesized by the ribosomes of the RER. These newly formed proteins are transferred into the cisternae of the ER, where they are isolated from the remainder of the cytoplasm. The secretory proteins are then conveyed to the Golgi apparatus. The Golgi may add carbohydrate to some proteins to form glycoproteins. It then concentrates and packages the product into membrane-bound secretory vacuoles, which migrate to the surface of the cell. Here the vacuolar membranes fuse with the outer cell membrane and the product is released from the cell, ie, secreted.

Secretory granules can be extremely useful in the identification of the cell of origin (cyto- or histogenesis) of a tumor. For example, dense core granules (an ultrastructural observation, known to contain polypeptide hormones) imply neuroendocrine differentiation. Malignant melanoma is characterized by the presence of melanosomes, and especially, premelanosomes. Zymogen, or proenzyme, granules are helpful in diagnosis of metastatic pancreatic (acinar) carcinoma. Many of these cellular products can be demonstrated by special stains and seen with the light microscope. Specific identification of cell products (and other antigens) via immunocytochemistry is of growing importance. In fact, immunologic techniques have replaced electron microscopy in many applications. They have several advantages, including use of the ordinary light microscope, comparative ease of preparation, ability to use archival cases, relative ease of interpretation of results, and much greater specificity.

Lysosomes are rounded, membrane-bound structures containing a wide variety of hydrolytic enzymes. These enzymes catalyze chemical breakdown of substances into simpler compounds, eg, starch to maltose, fat to glycerol, and protein to amino acids, by the addition of the elements of water (H+ and OH–). Acid phosphatase is particularly common. These enzymes are synthesized in the RER and packaged in the Golgi. Ultrastructurally, lysosomes are quite heterogeneous in appearance, reflecting the presence of different kinds of materials undergoing digestion.

There are three basic types of lysosomes: primary, secondary, and tertiary (aka residual bodies). Primary lysosomes are storage vacuoles containing enzymes that have not previously been used for digestion. Primary lysosomes become secondary lysosomes by fusing with phagosomes (membrane-bound ingested extracellular particulate matter) or with worn out cytoplasmic organelles (aka autophagic vacuoles). Active digestion takes place inside secondary lysosomes. Because not all material is degradable, undigested debris may remain inside a vacuole. These vacuoles are known as tertiary lysosomes, or residual bodies. Residual bodies often contain undigested lipids, especially phospholipids and unsaturated fats of cell membranes. These become oxidized to form pigmented materials like lipofuscin, that are periodic acid–Schiff (PAS) and fat positive. Lipofuscin accumulates with age and therefore is also known as the "wear and tear" pigment. A common example of residual bodies is the brown lipofuscin pigment seen in hepatocytes, which may remain in the cell for a long time or be ejected (emiocytosis, cell vomiting). Presence of lipofuscin in a cell implies that the cell is slow growing and benign, because it takes a relatively long time for this pigment to accumulate.

Lysosomes are associated with a variety of diseases, which can be divided into three groups. The first group of lysosomal diseases is associated with normal lysosomal function. The lysosome tries to digest something that it cannot, eg, silica. This causes release of the lysosomal enzymes from the cell. Leaking lysosomal enzymes may damage neighboring cells, leading to tissue destruction and eventual repair with fibrous scar tissue. Sandblasters, for example, may inhale excessive silica dust and ultimately develop pulmonary fibrosis. A second group of lysosomal disease is associated with abnormal release of normal lysosomal enzymes, eg, some types of allergic reactions, arthritis, and muscle diseases. Finally, there are lysosomal storage diseases that are the result of abnormal lysosomes. Lysosomal storage diseases usually result from a deficiency or defect of a single lysosomal enzyme, which causes its substrate to accumulate in the lysosome. Affected lysosomes vary greatly in size as they become stuffed with indigestible substrate. The abnormal lysosomes may eventually occupy so much of the cell that they interfere with the normal cellular functions. Lipids and glycoproteins (mucopolysaccharides) are often involved because of their complicated metabolic pathways, involving many enzymes. In lipidoses, eg, Tay-Sachs disease, lipid accumulates in the brain and other organs, causing blindness and mental retardation. In the glycogen storage diseases, glycogen accumulates, especially in liver and muscle cells. Mucopolysaccharidoses, eg, Hurler's disease (gargoylism, referring to those grotesque human or animal figures on buildings), take several forms, including dwarfism, enlarged liver and spleen, skeletal deformities, and mental retardation.

Changes in lysosomes may also occur in neoplasia. The lysosomes are often smaller and different in appearance from their normal counterparts. In adenocarcinoma, they may be more numerous than normal. In neoplasia, and sometimes in cysts, lysosomes (phagolysosomes) may contain large amounts of phagocytosed debris, giving rise to large eosinophilic cytoplasmic inclusions that are visible with light microscopy. In some tumors, lysosomes may be virtually absent, eg, hepatocellular carcinoma. At the other extreme, granular cell tumor is packed with lysosomes.

Peroxisomes, also known as *microbodies*, are similar to lysosomes in both structure and function. They are found predominantly in the liver and renal tubular cells. Peroxisomes contain several enzymes related to the production and destruction of hydrogen peroxide: oxidase and catalase, respectively. They are important in the metabolism of lipids. Microbodies assist in elimination of drugs from the cell and in defense against bacterial and viral infections.

Cells have the ability to store substances. Some are produced in the cell. Some are stockpiles for use in building things or for energy production, eg, glycogen and lipid. Some, as mentioned, are waste products and abnormal accumulations. Many are nonfunctional inclusions, or *intracellular pigments*, some of which have already been mentioned. Pigments can be helpful in the diagnosis of tumors. Many, however, are nonspecific. *Hemosiderin* is a golden brown, refractile crystalline pigment. Hemosiderin is a storage form of iron, often obtained from degradation of red blood cells. Thus, the presence of hemosiderin may indicate old bleeding and possibly the presence of cancer. Hemosiderin is largely composed of ferritin. Ferritin contains carbohydrates and so can be seen with special stains for carbohydrate groups, like PAS. Ferritin is formed in the intestinal mucosa. It is the principal storage form of iron in the body, and is primarily found in the reticuloendothelial cells of the liver, spleen, and bone marrow. *Hematoidin*, like hemosiderin, derives from hemoglobin, but does not contain iron. Hematoidin is closely related to *bilirubin*. These two pigments are bright orange yellow to golden brown. When eliminated from cells (via exocytosis), bilirubin forms amorphous masses, while hematoidin forms crystals, most characteristically, small "cockleburrs." *Hematin* is identical to heme, except that it contains ferric rather than ferrous iron. It is usually a formalin fixation artifact that occurs in bloody tissue and is seen as a precipitate of brown-black pigment. Its formation can be prevented by using neutral-buffered formalin. Lipofuscin, the golden brown "wear and tear" pigment, has been previously mentioned.

Anthracotic pigment, derived primarily from carbon compounds, is usually seen as granular, black particles. This pigment is frequently present in macrophages residing in the alveoli of the lung (so-called "dust cells"). It is practically ubiquitous in the urban environment, and its accumulation is a consequence of living in an industrialized society. However, smokers may have a marked increase in this pigment.

Melanin is a normal pigment in skin and hair. It really is a group of pigments that are yellow, brown, and black to violet. Melanin occurs in the cytoplasm as melanosome, a special kind of lysosome. The presence of melanin in malignant cells is characteristic of malignant melanoma. Melanin must be distinguished from hemosiderin. The best way to do this is with special stains. Although Fontana Masson stains melanin nonspecifically, the presence of melanin can be confirmed using melanin bleach to see if the staining goes away. Prussian blue stains the iron in hemosiderin and is easier on the cells than the Fontana Masson stain. However, a "quick and dirty" test that can be done before the special stains are available is to partially close the substage condenser diaphragm of the microscope. Hemosiderin is a refractile crystal and will sparkle. Melanin will only get darker. Melanin also tends to be finer (the size of lysosomes) than hemosiderin crystals. This is not completely reliable and should be confirmed with the special stains.

Crystalloids of various sorts are rare inclusions. Proteins and polysaccharides may crystallize, eg, Reinke crystals, seen in some gonadal tumors. Viral particles can also form arrays, or crystals.

The *cytoskeleton* consists of a variety of filaments, including microfilaments, intermediate filaments, microtubules, myofilaments, and the microtrabecular system. The cytoskeleton permeates the cell, determining its shape and providing support for its organelles. All microtubules are similar; however, filaments vary considerably in type. Filaments are often involved in motility of both intracellular organelles and the cell as a whole. Normal cells show contact inhibition of cell motility and proliferation, but cancer cells do not. They will move, pile up, and divide indefinitely. This lack of contact inhibition may be related in some way to cell filaments.

Microfilaments are a heterogeneous group, both functionally and chemically. They are about 5 to 7 nm in diameter. Most of these filaments are actin; however, some are myosin. The diameter compares with true muscle myosin, which is about 15 nm. An important contractile protein, actin is concentrated in the ectoplasm, just under the cell membrane, where it forms a terminal web. The inner leaflet of the cell membrane, as well as microvilli if present, inserts into this web. Actin adds elasticity to the cell. Although present in all human cells, actin is particularly abundant in muscle and myoepithelial cells. Myoepithelial cells occur around gland acini and ducts: the contraction of myoepithelial cells may aid in the process of secretion. Myoepithelial cells are also important in aspiration biopsy because their presence suggests that the glandular cells were completely contained in their space and are, therefore, probably benign.

Intermediate filaments are also a heterogeneous group. They average about 8 to 10 nm in diameter. Many of the filaments in this group are diagnostically important, including neurofilaments, glial filaments, and tonofilaments. However, intermediate filaments are prominent in many cell types, particularly epithelial cells. Keratin, vimentin, and desmin filaments are "sticky" at both ends, and attach to various cell structures, forming part of the cytoskeleton in various types of cells. Intermediate filaments also guide movement of intracellular organelles. Some of these filaments are composed of the protein related to prekeratin and keratin.

Intermediate Filaments (8–10 nm)

Cytokeratin: Positive in all epithelial cells
Vimentin: Positive mainly in mesenchymal cells
Desmin: Positive in smooth and skeletal muscle
Glial fibrillary acidic protein: Positive in localized glial cells
Neural filaments: Positive in most neurons

Note: Coexpression of multiple filaments is rare normally, but can be seen in some neoplasms, eg, pleomorphic adenoma, renal cell carcinoma, and mesothelioma.

Microtubules are about 25 nm in diameter. They are found in all lines of cells because they are important in mitosis, forming the mitotic spindle. Microtubules are dynamic structures made of filamentous subunits, which are composed of the globular protein tubulin. Microtubules can form bridges between cellular structures. They also help form cilia and flagella. As part of the cytoskeleton, they help maintain cell shape. Microtubules also direct movement of cell organelles and inclusions within the cell.

Myosin is about 15 nm in diameter and is located in the A band of striated muscle. Although myosin is most prominent in skeletal muscle, it is present in almost all cells, usually in the form of microfilaments. Myosin is a contractile protein that helps in cell motility. Compared with normal cells, cancer cells often have increased amounts of contractile proteins.

The *microtrabecular system* consists of a network of filaments less than 2 nm in diameter. It is ubiquitous, and all cell components are caught in its web. It is responsible for the gel state of the cytoplasm, which allows the cell to change shape but at the same time gives it enough support so that the contents of injured cells do not flow out of their membrane, like water out of a broken balloon. Due to its minute size, even using the electron microscope, special techniques are required to visualize the microtrabecular system. It is not currently diagnostically important.

Some intracytoplasmic filaments occur in highly ordered arrangements, like the actin and myosin filaments of skeletal muscle cells. Other filaments occur in loosely ordered groups, like the bundles of tonofilaments (tonofibrils) of keratin in squamous cells or in attachment plaques of desmosomes. Increased intracytoplasmic filaments are often noted in disease, especially in cells that normally contain many filaments. However, even cells that normally do not contain filaments, such as lymphocytes, may develop them in disease or after therapy, eg, radiation. Intracytoplasmic filaments are diagnostically important in some tumors, particularly in squamous cell carcinoma. (The quantity of filament bundles—keratin—directly correlates with the degree of differentiation of squamous cells.) Cytoplasmic filaments may be an indication of increased metabolic activity in neoplastic cells. On the other hand, they may also represent a sign of degeneration and impending necrosis. Unfortunately, they are often nonspecific and rarely can be relied on as the sole diagnostic criterion.

The *cell shape*, then, depends on the balance of internal and external forces, eg, surface tension, viscosity of the cytoplasm, rigidity of the cell membrane, and pressure of surrounding structures. Most cells tend to round up when surrounding tissue support is lost, particularly when released into fluids, like effusions. Therefore, roundness of a cell, particularly in a fluid, is a nonspecific feature. The cell membrane is elastic and contracts, resulting in increased intracellular pressure. Molecules inside the cell try to get out and those outside the cell try to get in (osmotic pressure). When there is an imbalance of these forces, the cell may expand or contract. The internal cytoskeleton acts to help maintain the cell shape. Forces outside the cell are also active in maintaining cell shape. Cells are supported by one another in tissue, and these forces are reinforced by cell junctions and basal lamina.

The Cell Membrane

The cell membrane serves two basic functions: the barrier or boundary function, which distinguishes the cell from its environment, and organizing structural support for certain portions and enzymes. Intracellular membranes also define various compartments within the cell. Membranes are only semipermeable, and can facilitate or impede transmembrane movement of various substances. Deep folds in the cell membrane may occur, eg, in transitional epithelium, to allow the cell to expand.

Ultrastructurally, and this can only be appreciated at very high resolution, cellular membranes are trilaminar. The membrane is seen as two dense lines, each about 2 to 3 nm thick, separated by a lucent zone about 3 to 4 nm thick, giving a total membrane thickness of 7.5 to 10 nm. This is far below the resolution of a light microscope, and even in routine electron microscopic diagnosis, the cell membrane appears only as a single thin line.

Cell membranes are made of lipids, protein, and carbohydrates. The major component is phospholipid, which has the special property of having both a water soluble end, the hydrophilic phosphate, and a lipid soluble, hydrophobic tail. These form a double layer, with the lipid tails of each layer facing each other. Cholesterol lends some rigidity to the membrane. Proteins are embedded in the inner or outer surfaces, and some go through the entire membrane. The proteins float in the lipid and are able to move around in the membrane. The function of the membrane largely depends on its proteins. The proteins are responsible for enzymatic activity, selective ion and molecule transport, and also structure and contractility. Another component of cell membranes is carbohydrate, linked to proteins (glycoproteins) or lipids (glycolipids).

Membranes have receptor molecules that are composed of protein, carbohydrates, or lipid. Receptors are able to trap specific molecules from the microenvironment that may be needed for cellular metabolism to direct cellular function (eg, hormone receptors). Receptors combine with their particular complementary molecule, like a lock and key, inducing a physiochemical change that results in a functional response of the cell. Receptors participate in enzyme reactions, active transport, intercellular recognition and communication, and immunologic properties. There are also other types of immunologic "markers" that are similar to receptors, but may have no other known receptor function. A, B, and O blood groups and other antigenic proteins and glycoproteins are examples. They are present in the outer cell membrane.

The barrier function of the membrane is associated with the membrane lipids. Gas gangrene is a disease of loss of barrier function due to disruption of cell membranes. It is caused by the bacterium *Clostridium perfringens*, which produces a variety of toxins. One of these, phospholipase C, breaks down phospholipids of cell membranes. This results in leakage of intracellular ions and enzymes, uptake of water with cell swelling, and interference with mitochondria energy production (oxidative phosphorylation). Cell death and necrosis rapidly become widespread.

Cell membranes help maintain the homeostasis of the cell. This requires energy, making the cell vulnerable to interruptions in the supply line of energy sources. Since the cell membrane is also involved in intercellular recognition, disorders of the membrane may be important in cancer, eg, loss of contact inhibition. Most cells grow to fill their place; further growth is inhibited by contact with their neighbors. Contact inhibition is characteristic of benign cells but not cancer. Cancer continues to grow (loss of contact inhibition) and even abandons its place; it invades and metastasizes.

The cell membrane is a dynamic structure. It sends out ruffles, blebs (outpouches of cytoplasm), and vacuoles from the surface of the cell. These surface projections are the result of changes in electrical charges, in the cytoskeleton, in membrane composition, and in pressure. They can be useful in diagnosis, eg, pinocytotic vesicles are a common ultrastructure feature in smooth muscle; microvilli are associated with glandular lumens; and cilia are almost always associated with benign cells. Ruffles are cytoplasmic flaps. Histocytes and cells in effusions have them. They precede the cell in locomotion, and assist in cell attachment and in phagocytosis. Cell membranes may also fuse, forming multinucleated (giant) cells.

Endocytosis is a general term that refers to a cell's taking up extracellular material by invagination of the cell membrane and pinching it off to form a vesicle or vacuole. If the material is dissolved or suspended in fluid, this is known as pinocytosis

(Greek *pinein*, to drink). (Water, however, moves primarily by simple osmosis.) If the material is relatively solid, it is known as phagocytosis (Greek *phagein*, to eat). If a part of the cell itself is taken up, in this case by a membrane of the endoplasmic reticulum, rather than the cell membrane, this is autophagy.

Microvilli are uniform, finger-like projections forming a fringe at the cell surface, usually at its apex. This markedly increases the surface area for absorption or secretion. Individual microvilli are usually too fine to be seen separately with the light microscope. However, masses of them can be seen as a dense line. Renal tubular cells have relatively long microvilli (~2 μm) forming a "brush border," which is visible in the light microscope. Cells lining the small intestine also have prominent microvilli, about 1 μm long, which are seen as parallel lines or striations known as the "striated border."

Ultrastructurally, the microvilli have a core of fine filaments that are attached to the cell membrane at the tip of the microvillus, and extend from its base to anchor into the terminal web in the ectoplasm of the cell. The filaments contain actin, which not only adds support, but since it is a contractile protein, is probably involved in movement of the microvilli. Microvilli are long and prominent on mesothelial cells (and mesothelioma), squamous cells (and squamous cell cancers—the better the differentiation, the longer the microvilli), melanomas, large cell lymphomas, and hairy cell leukemia.

Cilia and *flagella* are specialized structures concerned with motion. Cilia usually help move substances like secretions along cells lining a surface. Flagella help provide locomotion for single cells such as *Trichomonas* or sperm. Both are projections from the cell surface. Cilia are about 0.2 μm in diameter, and can just barely be seen individually in the light microscope, in contrast with microvilli, which cannot. Both cilia and flagella have a core composed of nine microtubule pairs (doublets) arranged in a circle around two single microtubules in the center, all enclosed in the cell membrane. This "9 + 2" arrangement is characteristic of *all* cilia and flagella. The peripheral doublets terminate in basal bodies. The central tubules anchor into a dense granule. Attached to the doublets is a pair of dynein arms, involved in generating energy for movement of the organelle. A disease in which the dynein arms are missing, known as immotile cilia syndrome, is characterized by lack of movement of the organelle, and its effects produce immotile sperm, chronic bronchitis, and sinusitis. The patients have frequent acute respiratory infections due to failure of ciliary assisted movement of mucus in the respiratory tract.

By electron microscopy, it has been observed that a wide variety of tumors can develop cilia. These are usually single and only present on a few tumor cells. Thus, a *solitary* cilium is a nonspecific ultrastructural finding that is usually invisible in the light microscope. On the other hand, the presence of numerous cilia, which would be visible in the light microscope, virtually guarantees that a cell is benign. Only very rare exceptions occur, eg, certain well-differentiated carcinomas of the ovary, endometrium, pancreas, and stomach. Aside from these few cases, in practice, *when cilia are visible, the cell is benign until proven otherwise.*

Centrioles and *basal bodies* are morphologically similar. They are composed of nine triplets of microtubules arranged in a circle forming a cylinder. Centrioles, which occur near the nucleus at the "cell center," are paired structures. One part of the pair is larger. The other, nearly identical, satellite body is oriented at a right angle to its mate. Centrioles play a key role in cell division, being associated with the development of the mitotic spindle. Division of the centriole is the earliest observable step in mitosis, heralding the onset of cell division. Abnormal division of centrioles may be responsible for abnormal multipolar mitoses. Basal bodies serve the purpose of anchoring cilia and flagella.

Changes in the cell membrane occur in neoplasia. For example, surface microvilli in adenomatous polyps or adenocarcinoma of the colon become diminished in both size and number. Membranes interdigitate extensively in Schwann cells (nerve sheath cells) and their tumors (schwannomas). Intercellular and intracellular glandular lumina, formed by a group of cells or within one cell, respectively, are characteristic of tumors of glandular origin, adenomas and adenocarcinomas. The lumina are lined by microvilli and may contain secretory products like mucin.

The *cell coat*, or *glycocalyx*, is present on virtually every cell, but varies from one cell type to another. It is, for example, highly developed on intestinal cells. The glycocalyx is a fuzzy lining on the exterior of the cell membrane that can only be appreciated by electron microscopy. It helps protect the cell, helps material attach to the cell, thereby facilitating absorption, and helps in cell-to-cell interaction. Changes in the cell coat in cancer may have something to do with the ability of cancer cells to invade and metastasize.

Epithelial and endothelial cells have specialized structures of neighboring cell membranes known as junctional complexes. Junctional complexes play a role in cell adhesion (so cells can form tissues that do not fall apart, like a handful of sand); sealing off extracellular spaces, such as gland or vascular lumens; and intercellular communication. Junctional complexes are named according to their size and nature. *Macula* refers to a spot or disc; *zonula*, to a line, which extends like a belt or band around the entire cell; and *fascia*, to a sheet, which covers part of the cell, like a patch. The function of the junction is closely related to the width of the space that separates the adjacent attached cells.

There are also three functional categories of junctions: occludens, adherens, and gap. Closely apposed cells are normally separated by a 15 to 20 nm space. In the occludens-type junction, the outer leaflets of the cell membranes fuse or touch, occluding the extracellular space between cells. It is seen as a single line ultrastructurally and is also known as a tight junction. These junctions seal the space between cells, preventing passage of material between the cells. They are usually associated with gland lumina and are of the zonula configuration, to completely close off the extracellular lumen from the rest of the tissue. Therefore all substances in the lumen must either come from, or must pass through, the cells without bypassing them.

In gap junctions, the membranes very closely approach one another, but are separated by a narrow space, or gap, of about 2 nm. Gap junctions are always small plates. They are thought to be important in intercellular communication, by providing a pathway for the flow of small molecules or electrically charged ions (electrical coupling) between cells. Gap junctions help coordinate cellular activity, eg, they help ciliated respiratory cells "do the wave" (coordinate the beating of the cilia in waves to move mucus in the respiratory tree).

In adherens junctions the cell membranes are actually slightly farther apart than usual, about 20 to 25 nm separation. Adherens junctions are located just beneath the occludens junctions in gland cells, and since the membranes do not fuse, material can pass between the cells at this point. Adherens junctions are generally of two sizes, zonula or macula. Ultrastructurally, there is an electron-dense plaque just beneath the cell membrane. Intracytoplasmic intermediate filaments approach the plaques but then make a hairpin turn away, without actually inserting into them. The filaments form an anchor for the junction. The filaments do not extend into the extracellular space; however, the space does contain a laminated glycoprotein that probably acts as a glue that binds the cells together.

The desmosome, or macula adherens, is essentially a spot weld holding cells together. They are focally distributed along cell membranes. Desmosomes are especially numerous and well formed in epithelial, but not in mesenchymal, cells. Squamous cells are attached to one another by desmosomes at the end of long, finger-like microvillous projections. This configuration allows the squamous plates to give when movement is needed. The long projections can be seen with the light microscope as *intercellular bridges* and the desmosome can sometimes be seen as a minute (0.5 μm) density in the center of the bridge, known as the Granule of Ranvier or the Node of Bizzozero. Hemidesmosomes attach cells to extracellular materials, like basement membrane, and are essentially half desmosomes.

Morphologic changes occur in junctions in cancer. Desmosomes may lose some of their characteristic structure. With dedifferentiation of a tumor, desmosome anchoring fibrils decrease in number. Finally, only focal thickening of adjacent membranes is seen. These junctions are then properly referred to as primitive cell junctions, rather than desmosomes.

Well-formed junctional complexes are characteristic of epithelial, endothelial, and mesothelial cells. Intercellular junctions are completely absent in cells of hematopoietic and lymphoreticular origin, and are usually poorly formed, at best, in cells of mesenchymal origin and their neoplasms. Intercellular junctions, although usually too small to be seen with the light microscope, play a very important role in cytologic diagnosis. Epithelial cells and their tumors usually form at least some groups (although decreased intercellular cohesion is a feature characteristic of malignancy). In contrast, lymphomas and leukemias form no groups at all. Sarcomas and melanomas usually form few or no groups of cells; any groups present are usually only loosely cohesive.

The Extracellular Matrix

Cells, in tissue, are usually supported, like bricks in a building, on a framework made of connective tissue, composed mainly of different types of collagens. *Fibronectin* is a kind of molecular cement that binds cells to collagen fibers and to each other. The location of a cell in tissue affects both its structure and function.

The *basal lamina* is a neutral polysaccharide-rich layer at the base of various epithelia, serving as a support, and made by the epithelial cells. It is about 50 to 100 nm thick, and consists of a central dark lamina and a lucent zone on either side. The basement membrane of light microscopy consists of the basal lamina plus the underlying collagen fibers. The basement membrane provides mechanical support, primarily from the collagen, and may have a filtering function, primarily from the basal lamina. Basal lamina is manufactured by the epithelial cells, while the collagen is produced by the underlying fibroblasts in the stroma. Groups of epithelial cells are characteristically surrounded by basal lamina as they form structures such as glands. In contrast, mesenchymal cells tend to lie free in the extracellular matrix. Some may have a polysaccharide-rich coat or layer around them, similar to basal lamina (known as external lamina, since basal vs apical orientation is not relevant), but others do not. This can be important in distinguishing a carcinoma, in which groups of cells are invested with reticulin fibers, from sarcomas, in which individual cells may be invested with reticulin. A special silver stain can be used to demonstrate reticulin.

The extracellular material may be represented on the cytology slide as the background. The background may reflect a normal, inflammatory, dysplastic, or neoplastic process. A great deal of information can be gained by carefully observing the background of a slide, the milieu in which the cell exists. Intact red and white blood cells are nonspecific, though numerous inflammatory cells usually indicate inflammation. An inflammatory background, or inflammatory diathesis, as seen in *Trichomonas* infection, for example, is usually finely granular and basophilic. A tumor diathesis represents the host response to the invasive tumor. It is an adverse host reaction that indicates a destructive process is occurring. A tumor diathesis consists of fresh and old blood, fibrin, and necrotic cellular debris. Conditions other than cancer may produce a similar exudate, eg, cervical stenosis or pyometra. A watery background, or transudate, can be seen in Pap smears of women with carcinoma of the endometrium or fallopian tube. Metastatic carcinomas typically lack a diathesis.

Summary of Diagnostic Features of Malignancy

Cells
- Usually numerous
- Disorganized, crowded groups (chaotic architecture)
- Single intact atypical cells
- Cannibalism (cell-in-cell pattern)
- Pleomorphism, anisocytosis
- Abnormal shapes
- Increased nuclear/cytoplasmic ratio

Nucleus
- Disorderly: loss of polarity, piled up, crowded
- Enlargement
- Pleomorphic size and shape, including abnormal shapes
- Multinucleation
- Naked
- Molding
- Irregular nuclear membrane
- "Thick" nuclear membrane
- Hyperchromatic
- Irregular, abnormal chromatin
- Prominent, multiple, irregular, or macro-nucleoli
- Mitotic figures, particularly abnormal

Cytoplasm
- Pleomorphism
- Loss of cell boundaries
- Abnormal staining, eg, polychromasia, orangeophilia
- Abnormal cellular products, eg, keratin, mucin

Background
- Necrosis
- Blood, hemosiderin
- Tumor diathesis

Marked variation of features from cell to cell is characteristic of malignancy.

In general:

- Malignant: More cells, poor cohesion, disorderly.
- Benign: Fewer cells, cohesive, orderly.
- Cells with cilia are almost always benign.
- Cells with atypical mitoses are almost always malignant (or dysplastic).

The above represents a smorgasbord of diagnostic criteria. It is up to the cytologist to choose wisely among the selections to arrive at a well-balanced diagnosis. *No single feature is diagnostic of malignancy*, and virtually any feature listed can be found from time to time in benign cells. The cytologist must evaluate the whole pattern of the smear and assess the content of the slides in light of the clinical context. A corollary of this is that *failure of the clinician to provide pertinent clinical data may compromise the cytologic diagnosis.*

5

A MICROmiscellany

[of Microbiology]

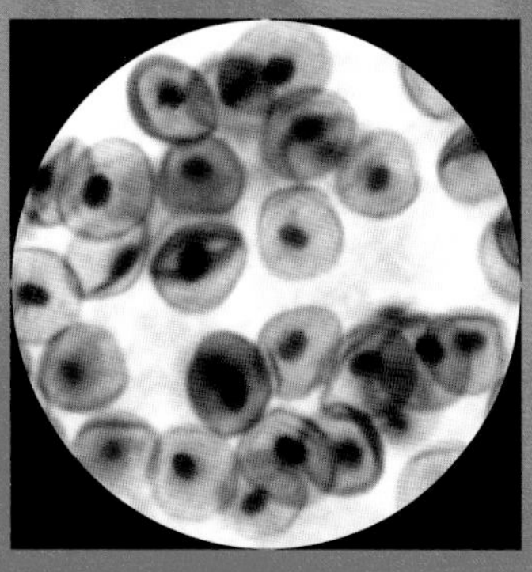

Viruses	Parasites
Bacteria	Arthropods
Fungi	Contaminants

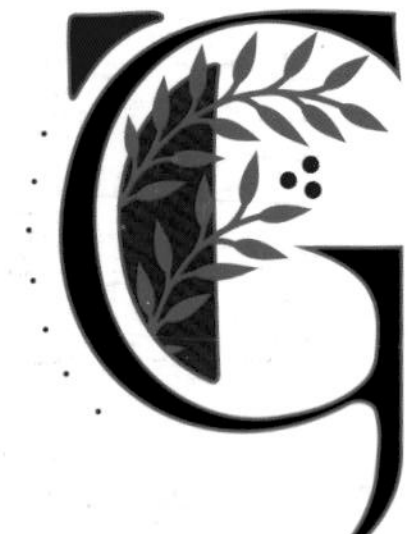

enerally, infectious agents are discussed in requisite depth within chapters devoted to the cytology of particular organs. This chapter was devised with those needing a very quick reference example (or those in the unenviable position of cramming for examinations, whether Boards or some sort of proficiency testing) in mind. Readers wanting a quick reference image and brief discussion of selected features of various common and a few notable but exotic microbiologic entities will find them herein. The chapter is something of a "rogues' gallery" of microbiologic agents; for those needing more information, please consult a microbiology textbook. For still more images of diagnostic morphology, subtle variations and differential diagnostic representations, see appropriate illustrated books.

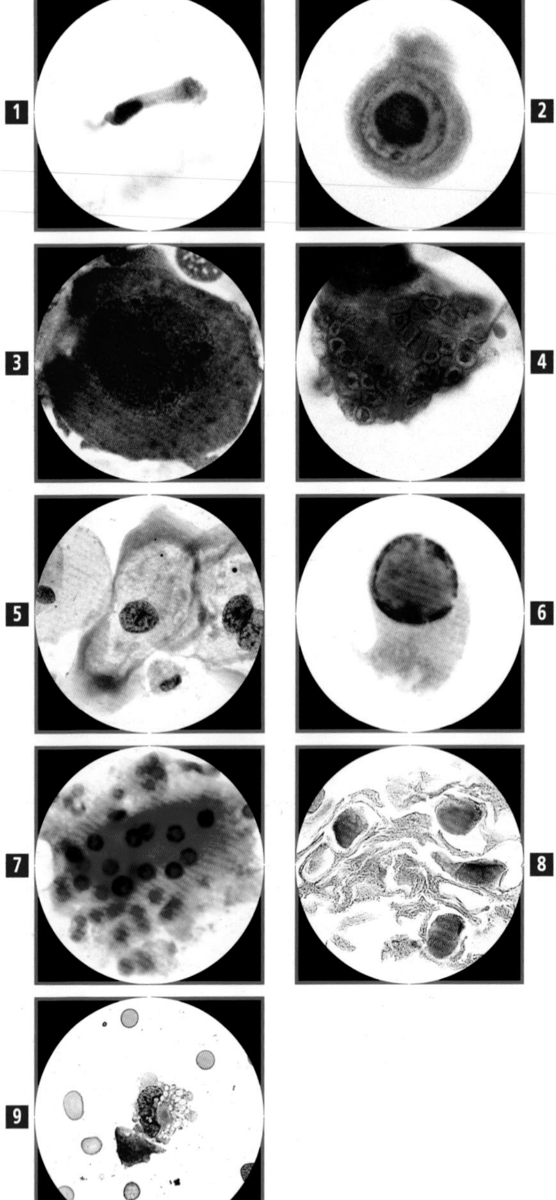

Viruses

Adenovirus is marked by intranuclear inclusions in bronchial cells. The initially small red body with a halo becomes a homogeneous blue body that fills the nucleus, giving rise to a "smudged" appearance **1**. Infected cells are enlarged, but retain basic configuration. While cilia may be retained, adenovirus (like parainfluenza virus, respiratory syncytial virus, and cytomegalovirus) may cause cells to undergo ciliocytophthoria (when cells "flip their wigs" in this fashion, only the cilia may be found).

Cytomegalovirus is marked by the finding of large cells, usually with a single nucleus (occasionally multinucleated, but not molded as in herpes), and large, smooth, amphophilic intranuclear inclusions **2**. The inclusion sports a very prominent halo, and thin strands of chromatin connect the inclusion with the inner nuclear membrane. Small, satellite cytoplasmic inclusions sometimes occur and are better visualized with a Romanovsky stain **3**.

Herpesvirus (simplex or zoster) produces infected cells that may have either a single, enlarged nucleus, or more commonly, multiple nuclei that exhibit prominent molding (adjacent nuclei compress one another). The chromatin tends to marginate beneath the nuclear envelope ("thickened nuclear membrane"), resulting in a ground glass appearance in the remainder of the nucleus. Eosinophilic intranuclear viral inclusions (Cowdry type A) surrounded by a pale halo are commonly seen. These are said to be characteristic of secondary (ie, recurrent) infection. Intracytoplasmic inclusions are not seen. A mnemonic device is the 3M's: Multinucleation, molding, margination with ground glass chromatin, and eosinophilic intranuclear inclusions **4** (see also Chapter 6). Herpesvirus infections are associated with ulceration and evidence of epithelial repair. The atypical, pleomorphic, virally infected cells with giant "macronucleoli" (actually, viral inclusions), together with atypical reparative cells, in a necrotic background could possibly result in a false-positive diagnosis of carcinoma.

Human papilloma virus is marked by the finding of koilocytes. Koilocytes are mature squamous cells with nuclear "dysplasia" and cytoplasmic "halos," and are pathognomonic of condyloma and HPV infection. To be a diagnostic koilocyte, the cytoplasmic vacuole must be clear and well defined, with condensation of the peripheral cytoplasm **5**. The nucleus must also appear abnormal (ie, enlarged and dark). Binucleation is common (see Chapter 6).

Human polyoma virus is marked by decoy cells, which have large, dark, smudgy nuclear inclusions **6**. They are usually found in transitional cells and, rarely, other cell types (see Chapter 10).

Measles virus produces Warthin-Finkeldey multinucleated giant cells, which feature tiny eosinophilic nuclear and cytoplasmic inclusions and scant cytoplasm. The appearance is sometimes like a bunch of grapes **7**.

Molluscum contagiosum is a pox virus that causes a skin disease (that in the case of sexual transmission can involve both vulva and vagina) characterized by large cells filled with dense, red, or polychromatic intracytoplasmic inclusions (ie, molluscum bodies) that compress the degenerated or pyknotic nucleus to the periphery of the cell **8**.

Respiratory syncytial virus produces giant cells (>100 μm) that are formed by syncytial aggregation of respiratory cells. The large, basophilic cytoplasmic inclusions have wide halos **9**. This infection may be quite difficult to distinguish from cytomegalovirus infection.

Bacteria

Mycobacteria are not visible with Papanicolaou or Romanovsky stain, although one may see a negative image with Romanovsky stain **10** when organisms are abundant (as they may be in AIDS patients) [Ang 1993, Urban 1994]. Negative images are not specific [Silverman 1993], but use of acid-fast stain yields long, red *beaded* rods **11**. Unfortunately, *M tuberculosis* appears to be showing up with greater frequency. The sensitivity of cytology alone in suspected cases is low; mycobacterial culture is recommended for conclusive diagnosis.

Gram-positive and negative bacteria can be seen in Papanicolaou and Romanovsky-stained smears. You can identify shape (eg, coccoid, bacillary, etc) and groupings (eg, clusters, strings, etc), but you cannot determine whether a bacterium is gram-positive or negative without Gram stain.

Haemophilus influenzae is a gram-negative encapsulated small coccobacillus **12**.

Neisseria meningitidis is a gram-negative intracellular diplococcus **13**.

Escherichia coli is a gram-negative rod **14**.

Streptococcus pneumoniae is a gram-positive diplococcus **15**.

Streptococci are gram-positive cocci that occur in chains; staphylococci are gram-positive cocci that occur in grape-like clusters.

Lactobacilli, aka Döderlein bacilli and *Bacillus vaginalis*, are a heterogeneous group of rod-like bacteria that are a component of the normal vaginal flora. Enzymes of these bacteria may cause cytolysis, leaving naked nuclei strewn in the background of the smear **16** (see Chapter 6).

Gardnerella vaginalis produces a velvety coating of small coccobacilli on random squamous cells, the so-called clue cells, which are clues to the presence of *Gardnerella*. Clue cells often appear with background clumps of small rods. This bacterium may be a normal finding, but also may be associated with vaginosis **17** (see Chapter 6).

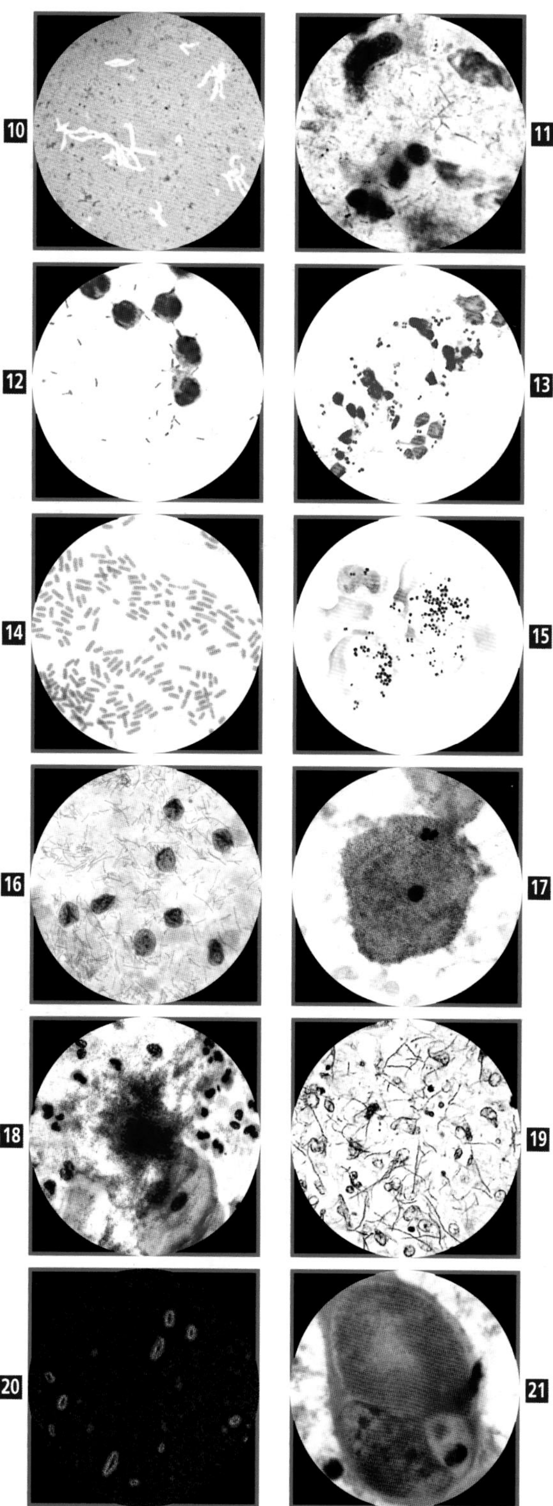

Actinomyces may be no more than a saprophyte from tonsils, but it may just as well represent invasive disease (becomes abscess with "sulfur granules" followed by scar). The clusters of branching filamentous bacteria tend to stain red, with club-shaped ends that are due to the Splendore-Hoeppli phenomenon (antigen–antibody reaction), forming radiate arrays. and associated with other bacteria (blue staining) **18**.

Nocardia are delicately branched, gram-positive filaments. They are generally acid-fast, though an irregular acid-fastness may give the filaments a somewhat beaded appearance **19**. Though most infections are acquired by inhalation of soil saprophytes, disseminated nocardiosis is becoming a more frequent finding in central nervous system and other subcutaneous tissues.

Legionella (micdadei) are extremely small, gram-negative rods. Because the organisms are not distinctive in Papanicolaou stain, use of Dieterle silver stain, or better yet, immunofluorescent stain using anti-*Legionella* antisera **20**, is necessary to demonstrate them. Neutrophilia is often characteristic of *Legionella* pneumonia in the otherwise healthy individual; however, the patients at particular risk for it often have profound neutropenia, which eliminates an otherwise useful clue.

Chlamydia trachomatis is a very small intracellular microorganism that is notoriously difficult to diagnose by Pap smear alone. Culture produces verification of the "real McCoy" (as would monoclonal antibodies or enzyme-linked immunoassays). Cellular changes include the formation of vacuoles with distinct outlines, which occur with cyanophilic granular inclusions **21**.

Fungi

Alternaria is usually a stain contaminant, and only occasionally a pathogen [Lobritz 1979, Radio 1987]. Its most characteristic feature is a "snowshoe"-like appearance **22**. *Alternaria*, like other organisms producing phaeohyphomycosis, also features characteristic natural brown pigmentation.

Aspergillus (fumigatus, niger) is characterized by 45° angle branching of true, septate hyphae of 3 to 6 µm uniform width **23**. Rarely observed fruiting heads (conidiophores) clinch the diagnosis **24**. The form of the conidiophore gives the fungus its name (Latin *aspergillum*: hand-held device used for sprinkling holy water). *Aspergillus* (especially *A niger*) may be associated with calcium oxalate crystals [Farley 1985]. These needle-like crystals are birefringent and may form rosettes or wheat sheaf–like clusters. Aspergillosis can also produce cellular atypia or be associated with cancer. Uniform thickness and septa differentiate this organism from *Mucor*; true hyphae and septa differentiate it from *Candida*.

Blastomyces (dermatitidis) organisms are 8 to 15 µm in diameter. Its thick, refractile cell wall tends to a double contour **25**. The granular cytoplasm and single, *broad-based budding* are characteristic. No hyphae are found. The infection is marked by a suppurative granulomatous inflammation.

Candida (albicans, and other species*)* is a common inhabitant of the oropharynx and female genital tract. Probably the most commonly encountered fungus, it is often of little or no clinical importance, but may be a nuisance and occasionally is life-threatening. Both pseudohyphae and inflammatory background should be observed to be certain of infection (infestation). Some remember the pattern of pseudohyphae and yeasts as "sticks and stones" (respectively). The yeast form is typically 2 to 4 µm in diameter, and forms buds. Pseudohyphae (ie, elongated yeasts) occur with additional buds to form what look like "balloon dogs" **26**. It is important to remember that no true hyphae or septa are found. *Candida* (formerly, *Torulopsis*) *glabrata* is a small yeast-like fungus, *without* pseudohyphae.

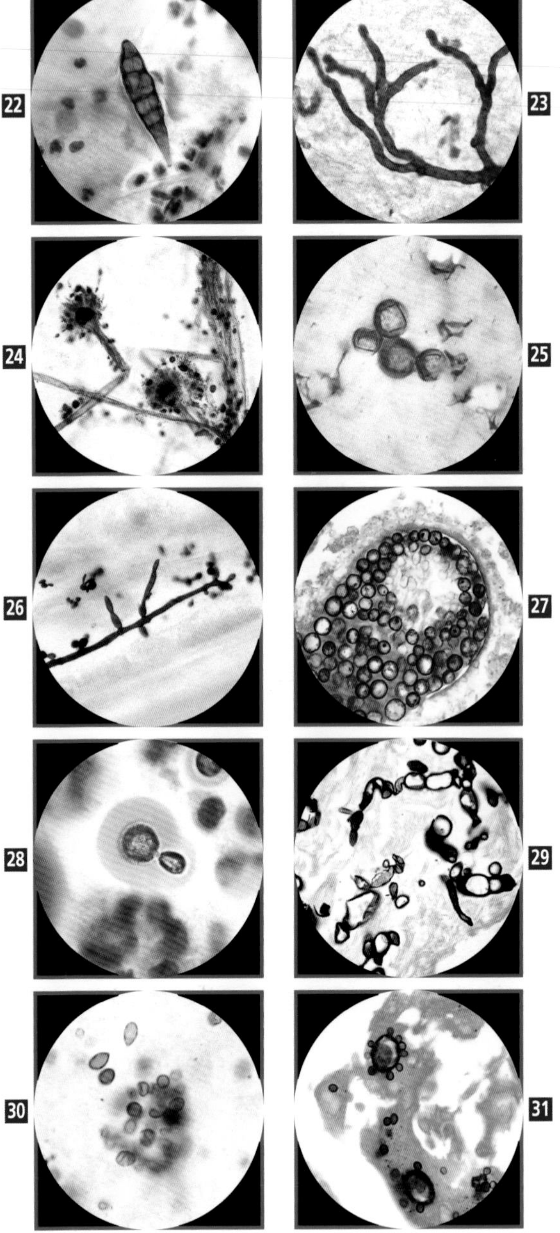

Coccidioides (immitis) is marked by spherules and endospores. Spherules are nonbudding, thick-walled, and measure 20 to 60 µm, occasionally larger than 100 µm. They may be empty or contain round, nonbudding endospores measuring 1 to 5 µm. A full spherule resembles a bag of marbles, which when it endosporulates, ruptures **27**. Take care not to confuse empty spherules of *Coccidioides* with *Blastomyces*. Arthrospores, similar in appearance to those of *Geotrichum*, or hyphae may also occur.

Cryptococcus (neoformans) organisms measure 5 to 20 µm, but are most commonly on the small end of that range. A very thick, gelatinous capsule (clear zone) may render it almost invisible (ergo, the name "crypto") without special stains, such as mucicarmine, alcian blue, or PAS. The mucoid capsule stains red (with variable intensity) with mucicarmine **28**. Single, teardrop-shaped budding is characteristic. Infestation may elicit little or no inflammatory response, or a granulomatous one.

Geotrichum (candidum) produces septate hyphae, spheric cells, and rectangular arthrospores, and may branch (at a 90° angle) from the midportion of the hypha without an intervening septum **29**. Because *G candidum* is endogenous and not particularly virulent, its isolation in sputum or feces is not a cause for concern in an asymptomatic person.

Histoplasma (capsulatum) is a small organism, measuring 1 to 5 µm. It is a round to oval, budding yeast, which must be identified within cytoplasm of a histiocyte or neutrophil to be diagnostic, and to differentiate it from similar appearing, but extracellular, contaminants. GMS stain is helpful because the organism is not well visualized with routine stains **30**.

Paracoccidioides (brasiliensis) is a round to oval yeast, 4 to 60 µm in diameter (though most are in the 5–30 µm range), with distinctive blastoconidial "ship's wheel" multiple budding **31**. In addition to the unique budding formation, which is often inconspicuous because single and nonbudding cells are more frequent, the marked size variation is strongly characteristic.

Zygomycetes (*Mucor*, *Rhizopus*, etc) exhibit broad (from 5–20 µm), irregular, thin-walled, ribbon-like, and pauciseptate hyphae that branch at irregular intervals, often at 90° angles 32. The thin walls often allow for extensive folding, twisting, and wrinkling of the hyphae.

Pneumocystis (carinii), though commonly classified as a parasite, is now thought to be a fungus [Edman 1988]. Formerly rare, the organism is now a common problem with the AIDS epidemic. Organisms are often seen in foamy/flocculent alveolar casts (rounded masses of organisms) [Tregnago 1993]. Casts stain eosinophilic to basophilic in Papanicolaou stain (the organisms also show green-yellow autofluorescence [Wehle 1991,1993]) 33. Organisms themselves stain poorly or not at all in Papanicolaou stain, although you may see overlapping ringlets. The alveolar casts are virtually diagnostic, but their appearance can be closely mimicked, eg, by red blood cell ghosts [Wasdahl 1993]; therefore, a special stain should be used to confirm. In GMS, the cell wall of a cyst stains black, often with a central dark dot 34. Cysts are 4 to 8 µm in diameter (slightly smaller than RBCs) and spherical or cup shaped. The cell wall does not stain in Romanovsky stain (you see a negative image against purple background). Trophozoites, up to 8 per cyst, are about 0.5 to 1.0 µm in diameter. Trophozoites stain in Romanovsky (tiny purple dots) 35 but not in GMS. Infestation is seldom associated with an inflammatory response.

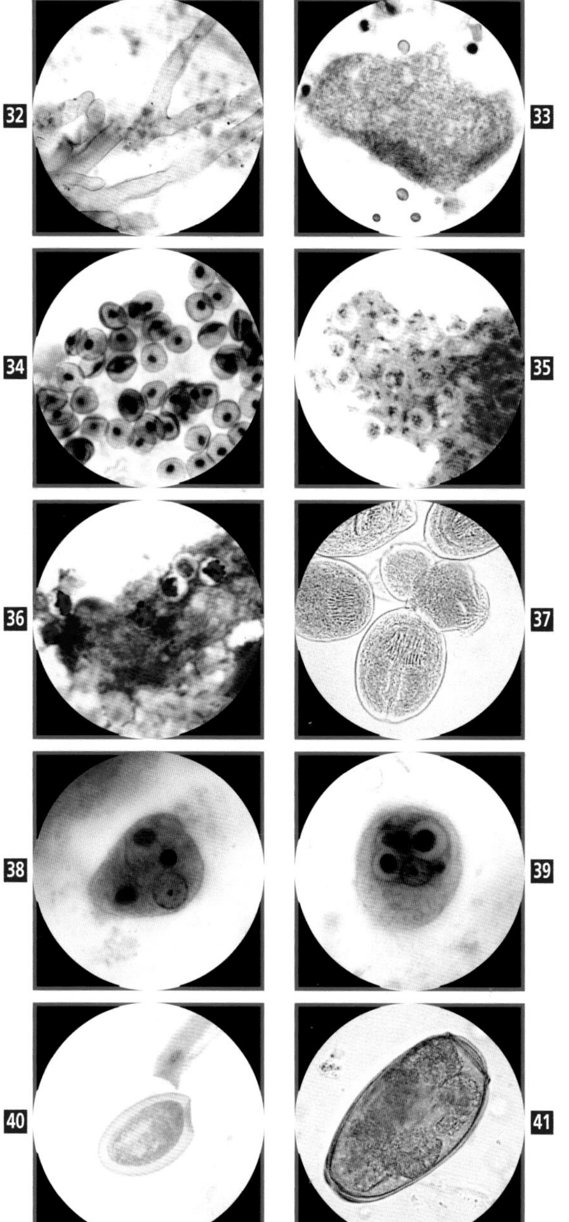

Parasites

Cryptosporidium is a round, basophilic protozoal organism, normally encountered as oocysts, measuring 2 to 4 µm, that may resemble platelets (which tend to clump) or yeasts (which may bud). The organisms can be visualized with Papanicolaou stain, but are better appreciated with an acid-fast or Romanovsky stain. Oocysts stain vividly red with acid-fast stain. Note the presence of black granules within the oocysts 36. The organism is associated with the brush border of gastrointestinal tract cells.

Echinococcus granulosus (hydatid disease) is often considered a contraindication due to possible anaphylaxis, but it has been aspirated inadvertently with fine needle with no untoward effects (see Chapter 14). Carmine-stained hydatid "sand" aspirated from a hydatid cyst shows both scoleces of *Echinococcus* and their hooks 37. Hydatid cysts may form in any tissue, but are most common in liver, lung, and the central nervous system.

Entamoeba histolytica is an ameba whose trophozoites characteristically display a prominent vesicular nucleus with a dot-like central karyosome. Cytoplasm is finely granular. A finding of ingested red blood cells is considered diagnostic 38. Trophozoites are most often encountered in the colon and cecum, though invasive forms may be found in a number of organs, including liver, lung, and brain.

Entamoeba gingivalis, like *E histolytica*, produces trophozoites, usually recovered from the oral cavity (it has rarely been reported to occur also in vaginal and cervical smears), that have a small nucleus with a dot-like central karyosome. Unlike *E histolytica*, however, only ingested white blood cells will be found, which may sometimes push the nucleus into an eccentric position 39.

Enterobius vermicularis (the common human pinworm) is often found as eggs (~20 × 60 µm), which are ovoid, with a double-walled shell that is distinctly flattened on one side 40. Adult worms may also occasionally be encountered.

Paragonimus (kellicotti, westermani) eggs are found in fecal matter and also in sputum (and occasionally as a vaginal contaminant). They measure approximately 100 µm long, are golden yellow, oval, and have a flattened, thick operculum at one end and a rounded thickened shell at the opposite end 41.

Strongyloides (stercoralis) is usually identified in the form of rhabditoid larvae (180-380 μm long) in human feces. However, filariform (infective-stage) larvae have been recovered from sputum in some cases of hemorrhagic pulmonary infection. Filariform larvae measure 400–500 μm, and have a closed gullet and an often hard to detect notched tail **42** [Marsan 1993].

Trichomonas (vaginalis) is a pear-shaped organism with an elliptical nucleus, red cytoplasmic granules, and flagella. The diagnostic rule of thumb is: you *must* see the nucleus for diagnosis, you *may* see the red granules in the cytoplasm, but you will never see the flagellum in Pap smears **43**. *Trichomonads* are customarily observed with *Leptothrix*, but the two do not necessarily occur concurrently.

Trichuris trichiura eggs (~25 × 50 μm) are barrel-shaped, thick-shelled, and yellow-brown, with unmistakable mucoid polar prominences that are simply called "polar plugs" **44**. They are rarely found outside the large intestine, cecum, and appendix.

Toxoplasma gondii trophozoites are oval to crescent-shaped and measure from 4-8 μm long and 2-3 μm wide. They have rather large nuclei. Tissue cysts measure between 5-50 μm and take different shapes: they are spherical in the brain **45** and more elongated in cardiac and skeletal muscle. Organisms are best visualized by Romanovsky, PAS, or immunohistochemical stain.

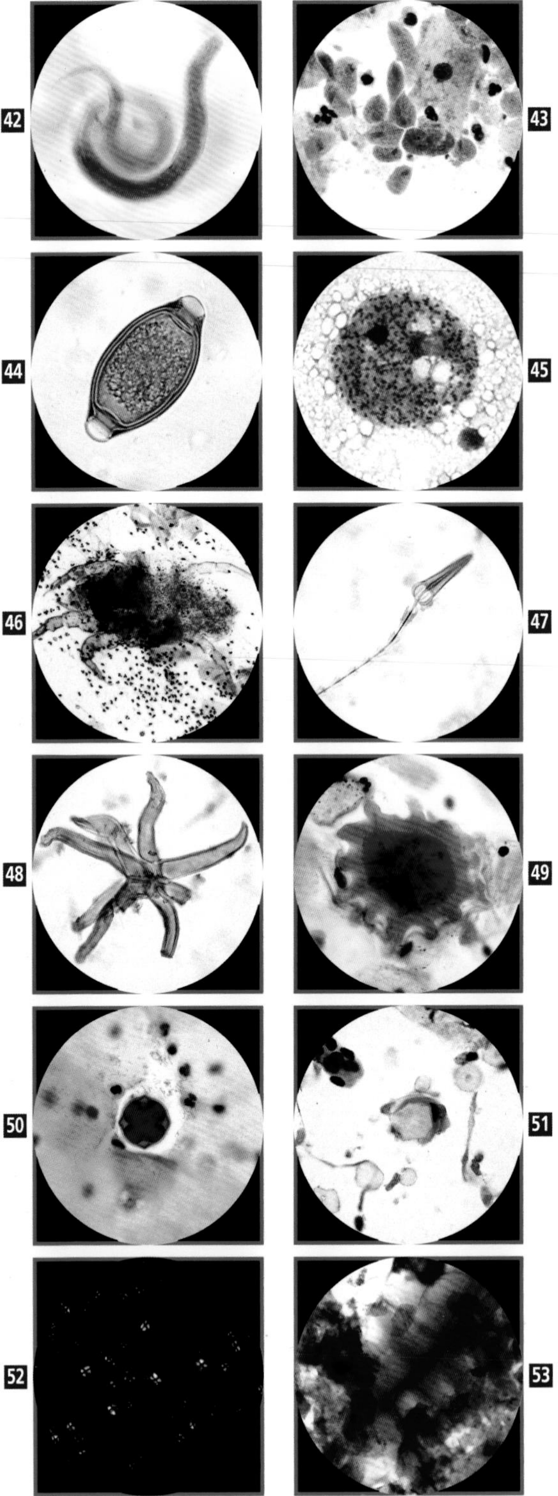

Arthropods and Contaminants

Arthropods, such as this mite, which looks every bit like a tiny crab **46**, sometimes find their way into cytologic samples.

Carpet beetle parts, can be found in a Pap smear, may be introduced as a contaminant, eg, from a cotton applicator or tampon **47** [Ahmed 1981, Bechthold 1985, Bryant 1994, Cormia 1948, Johnson 1989, Ludolph 1988].

Trichomes are derived from leaves and stems of *Viburnum dentatum* (arrowwood). The large starfish-like, stellate structures stain pale yellow-pink, with thick cell walls and hollow centers. Many plants may contain trichomes of different size, shape, and color **48**.

Asterosclereid is another contaminant derived from a tree **49**.

Pollen can be a most attractive contaminant. Note the cell wall with spikes **50**.

Glove powder is now made up of starch crystals (talc is no longer used). This contaminant may obscure cells, when abundant, or may be phagocytosed by cells, producing a signet ring–like appearance **51**. Maltese cross birefringence is also characteristic of starch granules **52**.

Lubricant is a sticky, purple-staining material that can interfere with screening. Clinicians should note that the speculum should be lubricated only with warm water before taking the Pap smear **53**.

References

Ahmed A, Razzaque MR, Barr RA, et al: Carpet Beetle Dermatitis. *J Am Acad Dermatol* 5: 428–432, 1981.

Ang GAT, Janda WM, Novak RM, et al: Negative Images of Mycobacteria in Aspiration Biopsy Smears From the Lymph Node of a Patient With Acquired Immunodeficiency Syndrome (AIDS): Report of a Case and a Review of the Literature. *Diagn Cytopathol* 9: 325–328, 1993.

Ash L, Orihel T: *Atlas of Human Parasitology, 3rd ed.* Chicago: ASCP Press, 1990.

Bechthold E, Staunton CE, Katz SS: Carpet Beetle Larval Parts in Cervical Cytology Specimens. *Acta Cytol* 29: 345–352, 1985.

Bryant J, Maslan AM: Carpet Beetle Larval Parts in Pap Smears: Report of Two Cases. *South Med J* 87: 763–764, 1994.

Chandler FW, Watts JC: *Pathologic Diagnosis of Fungal Infections.* Chicago: ASCP Press, 1987.

Cormia FE, Lewis GM: Contact Dermatitis From Beetles, With a Report of a Case Due to the Carpet Beetle (*Anthrenus scrophulariae*). *N Y State J Med* 48: 2037–2039, 1948.

Edman JC, Kovacs JA, Masur H, et al: Ribosomal RNA Sequence Shows *Pneumocystis carinii* to be a member of the Fungi. *Nature* 334: 519–522, 1988.

Farley ML, Mabry L, Munoz LA, et al: Crystals Occurring in Pulmonary Cytology Specimens: Association With Aspergillus Infection. *Acta Cytol* 29: 737–744, 1985.

Geisinger K, Silverman J, Wakely P: *Pediatric Cytopathology.* Chicago: ASCP Press, 1994.

Johnson FP, Batchelor J: Carpet Beetle Larval Hairs in a Sputum Cytology Specimen. *Acta Cytol* 33: 286, 1989.

Keebler C, Somrak T: *The Manual of Cytotechnology*, 7th ed. Chicago: ASCP Press, 1993.

Kjeldsberg C, Knight J: *Body Fluids, 3rd ed.* Chicago: ASCP Press, 1993.

Lobritz RW, Roberts TH, Marraro RV, et al: Granulomatous Pulmonary Disease Secondary to Alternaria. *JAMA* 241: 596–597, 1979.

Ludolph ED, Naylor B: Carpet Beetle Larva in Cervical Smear. *Acta Cytol* 32: 131–132, 1988.

Mann JL: Autofluorescence of Fungi: An Aid to Detection in Tissue Sections. *Am J Clin Pathol* 79: 587–590, 1983.

Marsan C, Marais MH, Sollet JP, et al: Disseminated Strongyloidiasis: A Case Report. *Cytopathology* 4: 1234–126, 1993.

Medak H, Burlakow P: Stellate Structures in Oral and Vaginal Smears. *Acta Cytol* 24: 269–270, 1980.

Osborne PT, Giltman LI, Uthman EO: Trichomonads in the Respiratory Tract: A Case Report and Literature Review. *Acta Cytol* 28: 136–138, 1984.

Raab SS, Silverman JF, Zimmerman KG: Fine-Needle Aspiration Biopsy of Pulmonary Coccidioidomycosis: Spectrum of Cytologic Findings in 73 Patients. *Am J Clin Pathol* 99: 582–587, 1993.

Radio SJ, Rennard SI, Ghafouri MA, et al: Cytomorphology of Alternaria in Bronchoalveolar Lavage Specimens. *Acta Cytol* 31: 243–248, 1987.

Silverman JF, Holter JF, Berns LA, et al: Negative Images Due to Clofazimine Crystals in a Bronchoalveolar Lavage Specimen. *Diagn Cytopathol* 9: 534–540, 1993.

Stanley MW, Davies S, Deike M: Pulmonary Aspergillosis: An Unusual Cytologic Presentation. *Diagn Cytopathol* 8: 585–587, 1992.

Tregnago R, Xavier RG, Pereira RP, et al: The Diagnosis of *Pneumocystis carinii* by Cytologic Evaluation of Papanicolaou and Leishman-stained Bronchoalveolar Specimens in Patients With the Acquired Immunodeficiency Syndrome. *Cytopathology* 4: 77–84, 1993.

Urban A, Llatjos M, Romeu J, et al: Our Experience With Negative Images of Bacilli in Fine-Needle Aspiration Biopsies (FNAB) From Lymph Nodes of Patients With Acquired Immunodeficiency Syndrome (AIDS). *Diagn Cytopathol* 10: 196–197, 1994.

Wasdahl DA, Goellner JR, Scheithauer BW: Red Blood Cell "Ghosts" as Look-Alikes for Infectious Organisms. A Report of Two Cases. *Acta Cytol* 37: 100–102, 1993.

Wehle K, Blanke M, Koenig G, et al: The Cytological Diagnosis of *Pneumocystis carinii* by Fluorescence Microscopy of Papanicolaou Stained Bronchoalveolar Lavage Specimens. *Cytopathology* 2: 113–120, 1991.

Wehle K, Kupper T, Marzahn S, et al: Identification of Phagocytosed *Pneumocystis carinii* in Human Pulmonary Macrophages. *Cytopathology* 4: 225–229, 1993.

Zaharopoulos P, Wong JY: Cytologic Diagnosis of Rhinoscleroma. *Acta Cytol* 28: 139–142, 1984.

The ASCP Press could accomplish nothing without a little help from our authors and friends.
We thank the following for generously contributing images for this chapter:

Images 1, 12, & 25 are courtesy of Kim Geisinger, MD and Jan Silverman, MD

Images 7 & 37 are courtesy of Bernard Naylor, MD

Image 8 is courtesy of Fadi Abdul-Karim, MD

Images 13 & 15 are courtesy of Carl Kjeldsberg, MD

Images 19, 27, & 31 are courtesy of Francis Chandler, DVM and John Watts, MD

Image 20 is courtesy of Karen Honeycutt, MT(ASCP) via James Linder, MD

Images 36, 38, 39, 41, & 44 are courtesy of Lawrence Ash, PhD

Image 42 is courtesy of William W. Johnston, MD

Image 45 is courtesy of Denise Hidvegi, MD

6

The Pap Smear

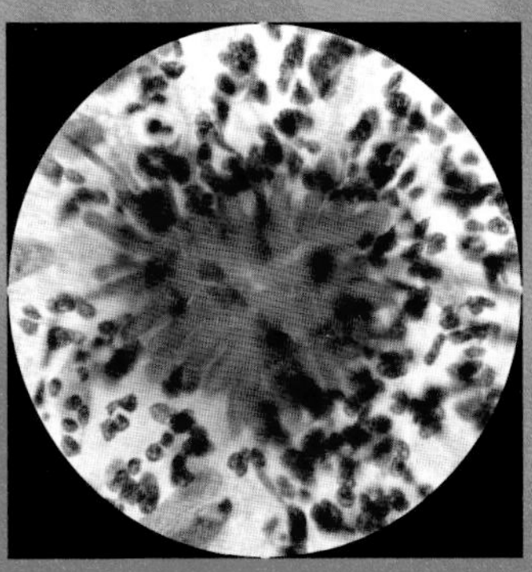

Brief History of the Pap Smear
Squamous Differentiation
Carcinogenesis
CIN or Dysplasia and CIS
Squamous Cell Carcinoma
Condyloma and HPV Infection
Nomenclature
Cytoplasm and Nucleus
ASCUS
Epithelial Changes
Endocervical Cells
Microglandular Endocervical Hyperplasia
Endometrial Cells
Endometrial Adenocarcinoma
Endocervical Carcinoma
The Cells of Pregnancy
Small Cell Cervical Cancers
Sarcomas
Melanoma
Clinical Management
Failure of the Pap Smear
Toward a Practice Standard
Specimen Adequacy
General Categorization
Descriptive Diagnosis
Diagnostic Criteria for the Bethesda System

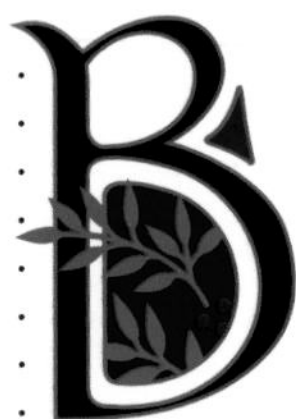

Before the Pap smear was introduced into clinical practice, carcinoma of the cervix was the leading cause of cancer-related deaths among American women (and it still is a leading cause of cancer deaths in countries where Pap smear screening is not widely available [Parkin 1988, Pisani 1993]). Because the Pap smear can detect treatable precursor lesions, its use has correlated with a remarkable reduction in the morbidity and mortality of squamous cell carcinoma of the uterine cervix [Adami 1994, Benedet 1992, Devesa 1989, Koss 1989a, van der Graaf 1990]. Lack of Pap smear screening is a major risk factor for development of cervical cancer [Brinton 1987, Christopherson 1976, E Clarke 1979, Herrero 1992]. In fact, *no other test has been as successful as the Pap smear in eradicating cancer!*

Unfortunately, the Pap smear is not perfect. Sources of failure of the Pap smear in cervical cancer prevention include problems with sampling, interpretation, and effective clinical follow-up. Certain types of cancers are difficult to diagnose by the Pap smear, such as adenocarcinoma, which is an increasingly common cervical cancer, and the most common invasive uterine cancer [Kim 1991, Mitchell 1993a]). There may well be a subset of rapidly developing cervical cancers that can arise in the interval between Pap smear screenings. Consequently, some women will develop cervical cancer in spite of appropriate screening [Kurman 1994, Wied 1981]. Yet, the most important reason for failure of the Pap smear is inadequate screening [Janerich 1995].

Three Key Points Pertaining to the Pap Smear

1. Excellent, but not perfect, test to prevent cervical carcinoma; no other test has been so successful in eradicating cancer!
2. Works by detecting treatable precursor lesions (ie, dysplasia/CIS, CIN, SIL)
3. Not a good screening test for glandular lesions, which are the most common uterine cancers

A Simplifying Synopsis

The Pap smear is the "bread and butter" of cytology, but it is also one of the most difficult and complex types of specimens to diagnose—often far more challenging than a fine needle aspiration biopsy. Although this chapter attempts to dissect, analyze, and simplify the diagnostic concepts, the reader must keep in mind that when dismantling a clock to see how it works, you sometimes end up with a lot of parts, and it may not always be obvious how they go back together. This synopsis is presented so that you, the reader, will know where we're going, ie, how the major parts fit together.

During normal maturation, the squamous epithelium of the uterine cervix can be conceptualized as differentiating from basal/reserve cells to parabasal cells to intermediate cells to superficial cells. These four cells (the "Icons") are the keys to the most common daily diagnostic problem in cytology, ie, "Is it, or isn't it, dysplasia?" (or cervical intraepithelial neoplasia [CIN], or squamous intraepithelial lesion [SIL], etc—these terms will be used interchangeably, as appropriate to their definitions, throughout the chapter) [T6.1]. Dysplasia mimics these four cell types. The intermediate cell, or more precisely, its nucleus, is particularly important because it serves as a benchmark for nuclear size and chromatin quality (texture and staining) [1 I6.4]. Compare the nucleus in question with an intermediate cell nucleus; in essence, if it's big and it's dark—it's dysplasia.

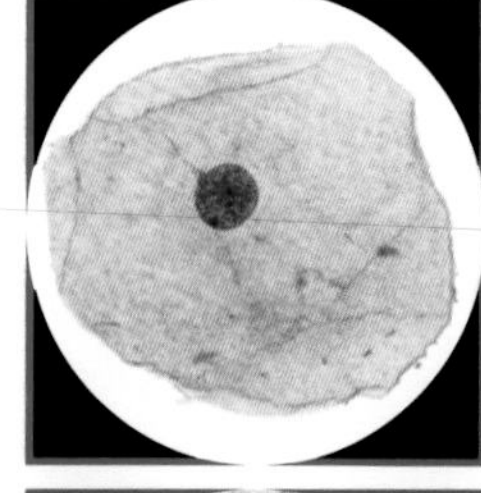
1

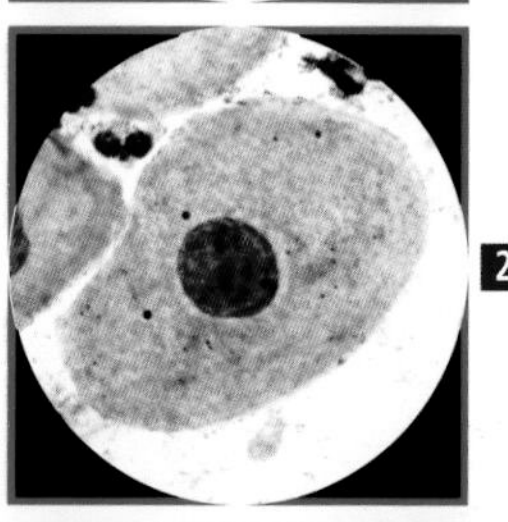
2

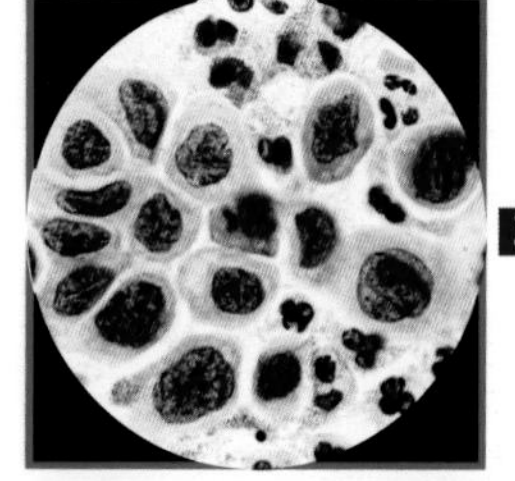
3

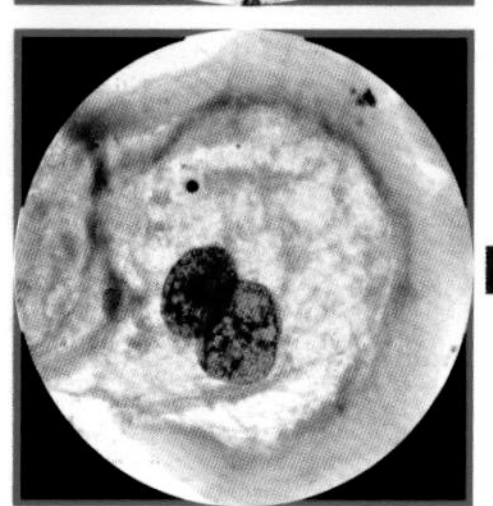
4

To make an oversimplification [T6.2]: most mild dysplasia (CIN I, low-grade squamous intraepithelial lesion) resembles mature cells (ie, intermediate to superficial cells with "big, dark" nuclei [2 I6.85]); most moderate dysplasia (CIN II, low end of spectrum of high-grade squamous intraepithelial lesion) resembles metaplastic cells (parabasal-sized cells with "big, dark" nuclei [I6.86]); and most severe dysplasia/carcinoma in situ (CIN III, high end of spectrum of high-grade squamous intraepithelial lesion) resembles basal/reserve cells (with "big, dark" nuclei [3 I6.87, I6.89]). High-grade dysplastic lesions can also be characterized by pleomorphic, abnormally keratinized cells [I6.88]. Koilocytes (ie, mature cells with very well-defined cytoplasmic vacuoles/halos and atypical—big, dark—nuclei) are diagnostic of condyloma/human papilloma virus (HPV) infection, a form of low-grade squamous intraepithelial lesion [4 I6.73].

Perhaps surprisingly, the largest nuclei are found in mild dysplasia (CIN I, low-grade SIL). Both squamous atypia (a form of atypical squamous cells of undetermined significance [ASCUS]) and more advanced dysplasia (and even cancer) have smaller nuclei. Therefore, low-grade SILs have the biggest, "ugliest" nuclei and occur in the largest (most mature) cells; therefore, they tend to "stand out" conspicuously in the Pap smear. On the other hand, high-grade dysplasias may be represented by minute cells with subtle cytologic abnormalities that can be difficult to detect in the first place ("no-see-ums"), and difficult to interpret once detected (resemble immature metaplasia or even histiocytes) [I6.141]. A clue to the diagnosis: high-grade dysplasias usually have irregular nuclear membranes, resulting in characteristic "raisinoid" nuclei.

It is important to search for, and carefully evaluate, crowded groups of hyperchromatic cells ("hyperchromatic crowded

T6.1 **Rosetta Stone for Deciphering Various Diagnostic Terminologies**

Traditional Nomenclature	CIN Nomenclature	Bethesda System Nomenclature (SIL)
Squamous atypia	Squamous atypia	ASCUS
Condyloma	Condyloma	Low-grade SIL
Mild dysplasia	CIN I	Low-grade SIL
Moderate dysplasia	CIN II	High-grade SIL
Severe dysplasia	CIN III	High-grade SIL
CIS	CIN III	High-grade SIL

T6.2 **Synoptic Oversimplification for Understanding the Pap Smear**

Low-Grade SIL		High-Grade SIL		
HPV/ Condyloma	Mild Dysplasia	Moderate Dysplasia	Severe Dysplasia	CIS
Koilocytes (cytoplasmic halos, nuclear atypia)	Mature (intermediate to superficial) cells	Metaplastic (parabasal-sized) cells	Basal/reserve cells; also pleomorphic, abnormally keratinized cells	HCGs, associated dysplasia

REMEMBER: IF THE NUCLEUS IS BIG AND DARK, IT'S DYSPLASIA.

groups" or HCGs). Although hyperchromatic crowded groups are usually benign and include such entities as endometrial cells [5 I6.134] and severe atrophy [6 I6.133], they can also be the general cytologic appearance of a variety of serious lesions. For example, carcinoma in situ (CIS) often presents in the Pap smear as hyperchromatic, crowded groups [7 I6.89, 8 I6.137]. Look for disorderly arrangements of the cells ("loss of nuclear polarity"), coarse, dark chromatin, and mitotic figures—features that suggest neoplasia. Another diagnostic clue: squamous carcinoma in situ is usually accompanied by squamous dysplasia. Other serious lesions that can present as hyperchromatic crowded groups include invasive squamous cell carcinoma, and endocervical adenocarcinoma—in situ or invasive [Boon 1991]. Endocervical neoplasia is an increasingly important diagnostic category.

Unfortunately, there is not always a perfect, one-to-one correspondence between the cytologic diagnosis and the histologic diagnosis [Konikov 1969, Swinker 1994, Tabbara 1992, E Walker 1986]. In many cases, the cytology significantly undercalls or overcalls the lesion seen in the corresponding biopsy. For a screening test, false-negative diagnosis (substantially undercalling or entirely missing a lesion) is, of course, the most serious problem. Therefore, some diagnostic specificity may have to be sacrificed in order to enhance sensitivity (receiver-operator curves: like a teeter-totter—if sensitivity goes up, specificity goes down). Weighing the risk of missing significant lesions, against the expense of investigating all lesions, has led to considerable controversy regarding the management of patients with slightly "abnormal" Pap smears [Cuzick 1994, Herbst 1990,1992, Hunt 1994, Koss 1993b, Kühler-Obbarius 1994a, Kurman 1994, Richart 1993].

5
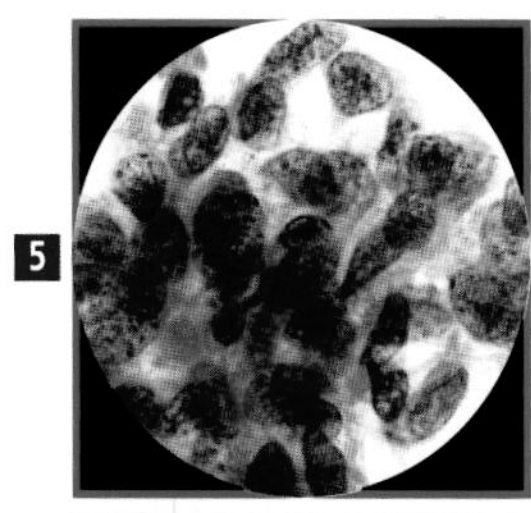

6
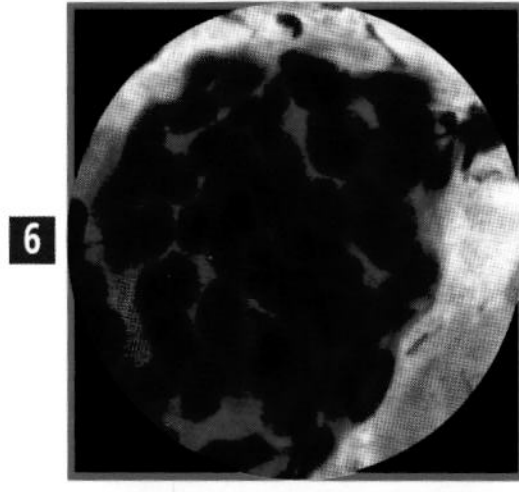

7
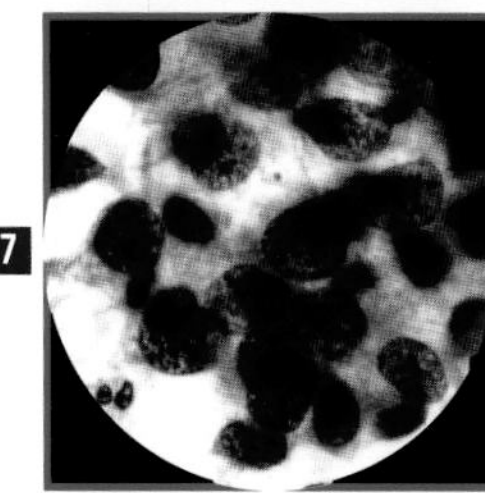

8
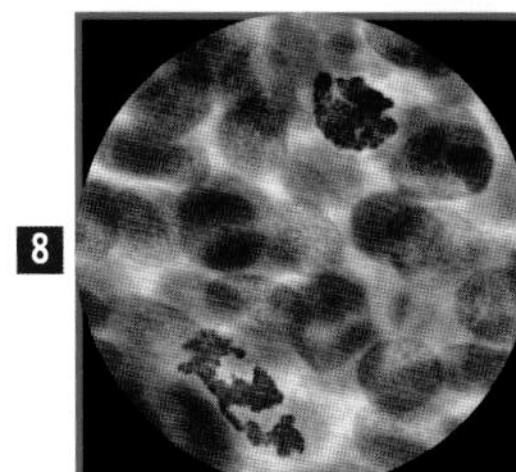

Brief History of the Pap Smear

While studying the hormonal maturation of the human vaginal mucosa, George Papanicolaou, MD, PhD, discovered that tumor cells could be found in vaginal fluid of women with cervical cancer [Barter 1992, Kyle 1977]. Papanicolaou, for whom the Pap smear is named, presented his paper entitled "New Cancer Diagnosis" at the Third Race Betterment Conference in Battle Creek, Michigan, in 1928 [Papanicolaou 1928]. Unfortunately, it reached a limited audience and came at a time when histologic techniques were being perfected and cytologic methods were on the wane. The concept of carcinoma in situ had been known since at least 1910 [Rubin 1910], the colposcope had just been invented (by Hinselmann in 1925), and the Schiller iodine test was about to be devised (1933) [Petersen 1955, Schiller 1938]. Furthermore, Aurel Babès, a Romanian pathologist, published a paper entitled "The possibility of diagnosing uterine cancer by the smear technic" in the Proceedings of the Conference of the Gynecologic Society of Bucharest of January 23, 1927 [Koprowska 1985, Wied 1964]. Babès elaborated on this paper in April 1928 in *La Presse Medicale* [Babès 1928, Douglass 1967, Grosskopf 1978] and clearly stated that his method was applicable to early cancers that had not yet penetrated the stroma. Later, in a 1931 paper, Babès made the statement that Kermauner and Schiller had used a modified vaginal smear method for the diagnosis of cervical cancer on a large scale with very good results [Babès 1931, Koprowska 1981]. Yet ironically the feeling at the time (as expressed by prominent oncologist James Ewing) was that since the uterine cervix was accessible to biopsy, the use of a cytologic examination was superfluous [Breathnach 1983, E Carmichael 1984]. Coincidentally, Martin and Ellis' first paper on needle aspiration biopsy, which also met with something less than enthusiastic response, was published about the same time, in 1930 [H Martin 1930].

Papanicolaou's discovery lay dormant for more than a decade. Then, encouraged by Joseph Hinsey, chairman of Anatomy at Cornell [Hinsey 1962], Papanicolaou again pursued the subject and published a new paper in 1941 [Papanicolaou 1941]. This was followed in 1943 by the classic monograph written with Herbert Traut, a gynecologist trained in pathology [Long 1991], and beautifully illustrated by Hashime Murayama. Entitled *Diagnosis of Uterine Cancer by the Vaginal Smear*, this slim volume (48 pages of text plus 11 color plates with descriptions) introduced the technique of diagnosing uterine carcinoma by cytology, as well as the possibility of diagnosing early cervical cancer, to a wide audience [Papanicolaou 1943]. By 1943 the concepts of early cancer and carcinoma in situ were widely understood, and the potential of the "Pap smear" for cancer prevention was finally appreciated [Ayre 1946, Foote 1948, Fremont-Smith 1947, CA Jones 1945, Pund 1947]. Physicians were enthusiastic about the possibility of conquering cervical cancer. It was actually a Canadian physician, J. Ernest Ayre, who, in the mid-1940s, described the method we know today as the Pap smear [Ayre 1947,1948]. Papanicolaou had studied vaginal pool secretions: easy to obtain, but tedious to screen. Ayre used a spatula instead—the Ayre spatula—to directly scrape cells from the cervix.

The rest, as they say, is history. By the late 1940s, cytology laboratories were opening, and by the 1950s, Pap smear screening was widespread, even before clinical trials could be performed [Koss 1993a]. When Papanicolaou published his *Atlas of Exfoliative Cytology* in 1954 [Papanicolaou 1954], it became clear that the cytologic technique could be extended to virtually any organ [Breathnach 1983]. The work of Papanicolaou and his followers has remained a dominant influence in modern cytology.

I. Cytology of the Squamous Epithelium

Simplification is the secret to understanding the sometimes bewildering array of benign and malignant proliferative conditions affecting the uterine cervix. We will consider a simple diagnostic matrix, constructed from just two basic concepts: (1) squamous differentiation and (2) carcinogenesis.

These basic concepts constitute the fundamental principles of Pap smear diagnosis. Their manifestations are seen in the cytoplasm and nucleus of the cell, respectively.

The cytoplasm provides information about the origin and functional differentiation of a cell. For this reason, cytoplasmic features are used to determine the degree of squamous differentiation. The cytologic hallmarks of squamous differentiation are distinct cell boundaries and the accumulation of dense cytoplasm.

The nucleus provides information about the health of the cell (eg, whether it is normal, inflamed, hyperplastic, or neoplastic). Nuclear features determine where in the continuum of neoplastic transformation, or carcinogenesis, the cell may be. Changes in nuclear size, configuration, and chromatin (hyperchromasia, coarsening, and, eventually, irregular distribution) and the appearance of visible nucleoli are the main nuclear features of ensuing carcinogenesis.

However, the warp and woof of possible nuclear and cytoplasmic alterations is infinite and weaves a fine fabric of possible cytologic diagnoses. To be practical, the two basic diagnostic concepts of squamous differentiation and carcinogenesis must be further simplified. Squamous differentiation (ie, cytoplasmic changes) can be arbitrarily, but usefully, divided into four cell layers, which are epitomized by the four primary cell types: *basal*, *parabasal*, *intermediate*, and *superficial*. Carcinogenesis (ie, nuclear changes) can also be divided into four stages, starting with *normal* and proceeding to *benign proliferative reactions*, then *intraepithelial neoplasia* (dysplasia/carcinoma in situ), and finally, *carcinoma* (microinvasive and fully invasive). (Note: Although the cytologic changes involved in carcinogenesis that are discussed here do have some biologic validity, they are presented in this section primarily as a morphologic "construct" to help teach the microscopic appearance of the lesions [F6.1]. Carcinogenesis per se is complex and incompletely understood, and will be discussed later.)

The Fundamental Concepts of the Pap Smear

1. Squamous differentiation (Cytoplasm)
   Accumulation of dense cytoplasm and distinct cell borders
   Cells: Basal, parabasal, intermediate, superficial
2. Carcinogenesis (Nucleus)
   Nucleus: Variation in size, shape, outline, number
   Chromatin: Hyperchromatic with varying coarseness
   Nucleoli: Abnormal number, size, shape
   Nuclear/cytoplasmic ratio alterations

Now, a simple matrix can be constructed, creating diagnostic categories [F6.2]. The nature of the cell is diagnosed by its location in the map, which is determined by the nuclear and cytoplasmic features of the cell. Remember, there are no sharp, clear-cut divisions between categories: each change is part of a continuum. Even between in situ and invasive cancer there is a gray area of microinvasive carcinoma.

Each sequence will be discussed in detail as we reconstruct this matrix step by step. First, we will consider the normal, orderly maturation of the squamous epithelium (the four primary cell types), including hormonal and Barr body cytology. Then, we will discuss carcinogenesis beginning with the benign proliferative reactions. Benign proliferative reactions mimic normal maturation and recapitulate, with slight perturbation, the maturation process shown in the four primary cell types (Icons). Next we discuss dysplasia and carcinoma in situ (also known as cervical intraepithelial neoplasia [CIN], and more recently as squamous intraepithelial lesion [SIL]), which arise in and reflect, in a distorted, disorderly way, the benign proliferative reactions. Finally, carcinoma, arising from intraepithelial neoplasia/lesion, imitates in a chaotic way the primary cell types.

Squamous Differentiation

Squamous differentiation represents a continuum of cytoplasmic change from undifferentiated, basal cells to mature fish-scale-like squamous cells at the epithelial surface. The primary

F6.1 **Sequence of Events in Carcinogenesis**

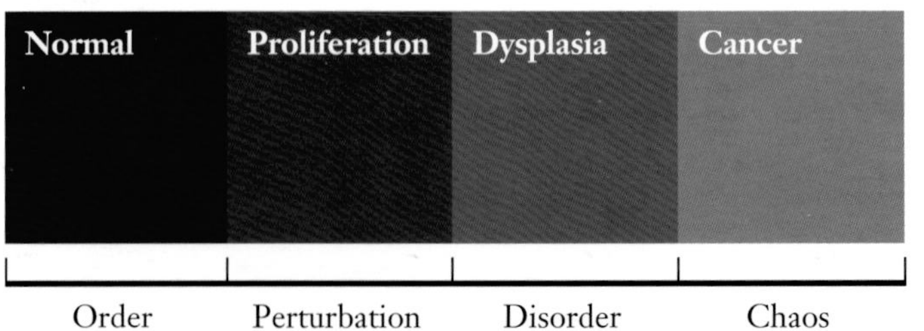

F6.2 Matrix of Diagnostic Categories

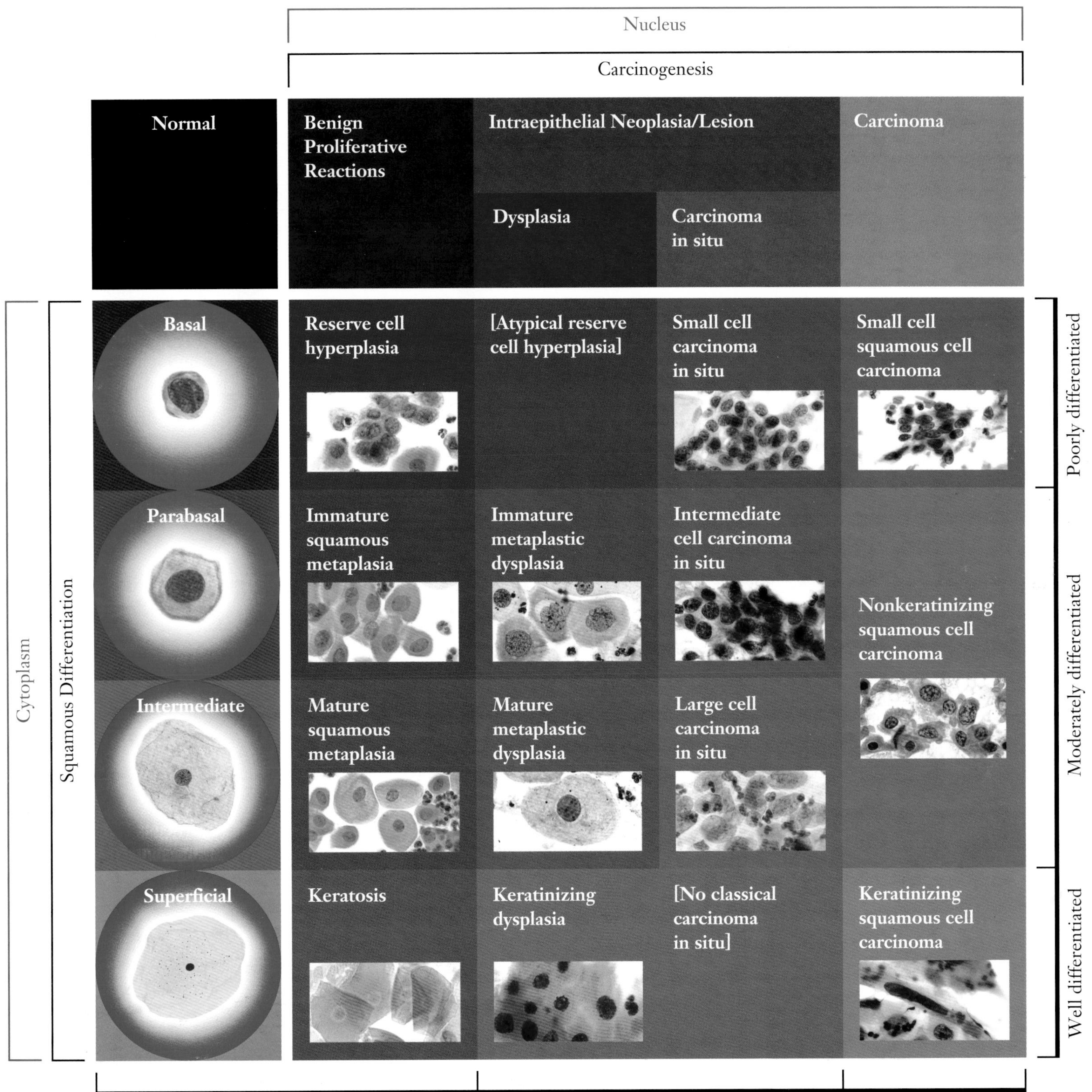

purpose of the squamous epithelium is to protect the cervix and vagina from various physical, chemical, and microbiologic assaults. The squamous mucosa may also be important in providing glycogen, and perhaps other nutrients, for sperm. The cell's journey from base to surface normally takes about 4 to 5 days.

The mucous membrane that covers the vagina and vaginal portion of the uterine cervix (portio vaginalis) is normally a nonkeratinizing, stratified squamous epithelium [9 I6.1]. The nonkeratinizing epithelium can be conceptually—and somewhat arbitrarily—divided into four cell layers that share similar morphologic features [F6.3].

Squamous cells in a Pap smear usually exfoliate from the epithelial surface. In that sense, they could all be considered superficial cells. However, the names of the four types of squamous cells are derived from their histologic counterparts in a mature epithelium. Any of these four types of cells can be seen in a Pap smear.

The Cells

Basal Cells

Basal cells are small, undifferentiated cells that measure about 10 to 12 μm in diameter. They resemble small histiocytes, particularly when occurring singly. Basal cells have a central, vesicular nucleus and a small amount of delicate cytoplasm. The nucleus is round or oval. Isolated basal cells are seldom recognized in Pap smears. Occasionally, however, basal cells can be seen in severe atrophy, as apparently syncytial aggregates (hyperchromatic crowded groups) of small cells with bland nuclei and scant cytoplasm. Basal cells can also be seen in a sample taken from the edge of an ulcer or if an entire area of epithelium is denuded by an excessively vigorous scrape. When basal cells are present in a smear, they are usually associated with the next larger cell type, the parabasal cell.

***F6.3* Normal Squamous Differentiation in Histology and Cytology**

Histology

Germinal | Deep spinous | Superficial spinous | Superficial

Basal | Parabasal | Intermediate | Superficial

Cytology

9

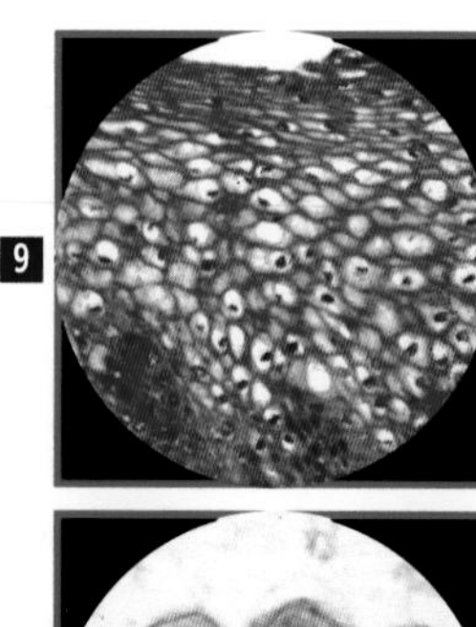

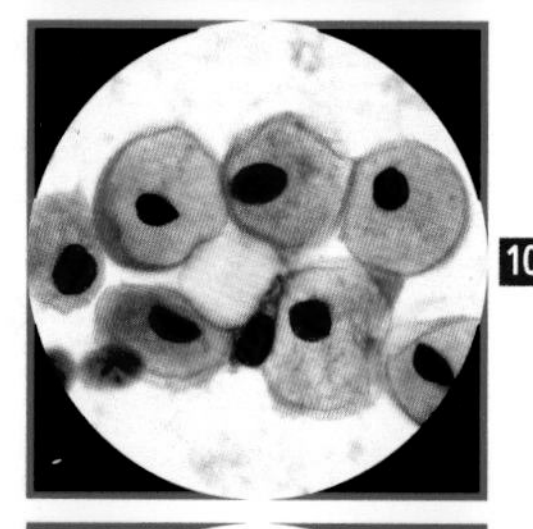

10

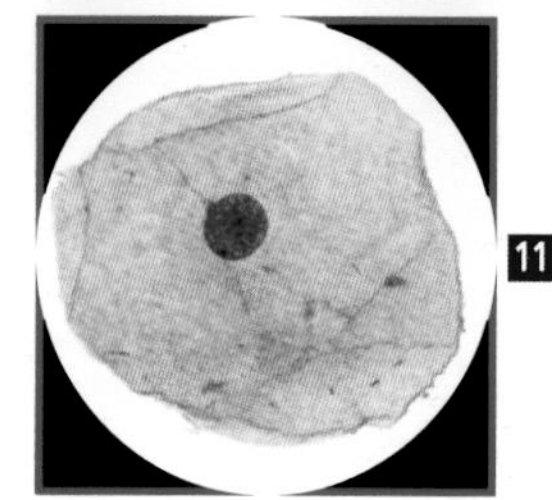

11

Basal cells serve several important functions. They are the cells that anchor the epithelium to the basement membrane by hemidesmosomes. They are also the germinative cells responsible for continually renewing the epithelium, because they are the only cells in the squamous mucosa that normally undergo cell division. When the basal cell divides, one of the daughter cells commits itself to squamous differentiation, which is manifested by dense, protective cytoplasm that gives it distinct cell boundaries. This selfless daughter cell eventually dies and is exfoliated: it serves to protect. The other daughter cell, which remains attached to the basement membrane, is an "immortal" cell (lasting for the life of the woman herself). The basal cell may also participate (by sending a signal to the stroma?) in producing a basement membrane, which separates the epithelium from the mesenchyme.

Basal Cells

Resemble histiocytes (single)
HCGs
Function:
Attachment, mitosis, differentiation, basement membrane

Parabasal Cells

Parabasal cells, the next larger cell type, are commonly observed in Pap smears [10 I6.7]. However, parabasal cells are unlikely to be found in a Pap smear of a fully mature epithelium. The presence of parabasal cells at the mucosal surface, where the Pap smear is taken, indicates that the epithelium is incompletely or "poorly" differentiated, ie, atrophic. Atrophy is a common finding during childhood, postmenopause, and postpartum.

In tissue, parabasal cells have definite squamous features, including dense cytoplasm, distinct cell boundaries, and intercellular bridges. Intercellular bridges, which are the spinous processes of the histologic stratum spinosum, correspond ultrastructurally to long microvilli attached by desmosomes. Intercellular bridges may be difficult to appreciate in cytology.

Parabasal cells are moderately large, 15 to 30 μm in diameter, and have rounded cell boundaries. The nuclei are round to oval with finely granular, evenly distributed chromatin and occasional chromocenters. Nucleoli are inconspicuous or absent, unless the cells are reactive or inflamed. The nuclear area averages about 50 μm^2, or 8 to 9 μm in diameter, which is slightly larger than a red blood cell. Parabasal cells have moderately dense cytoplasm and typically stain blue-green or gray, sometimes pink, and, rarely, orange.

Intermediate Cells

The ovoid parabasal cells begin to flatten and mature into intermediate cells [11 I6.4]. Intermediate cells range from about 35 to 50 μm in diameter, ie, from about the size of parabasal cells (low intermediate cells) to the size of superficial cells (high intermediate cells). The cytoplasm also changes from somewhat thick with rounded outlines, like that of parabasal cells, to thin with polygonal outlines, like that of superficial cells.

Intermediate cells may contain glycogen, which stains golden yellow with the Papanicolaou stain but does not stain with hematoxylin and eosin. Marked accumulations of glycogen sometimes result in elongated cells shaped like boats, the so-called navicular cells (Latin *navis* = ship) [12 I6.5]. Navicular cells can be seen late in the menstrual cycle and, especially, during pregnancy. The normal bacterial flora of the vagina use glycogen as food, producing lactic acid as a byproduct of catabolism. The lactic acid maintains the normal (acid) pH of the vagina. The action of the bacteria may cause the cells to lyse (a process known as cytolysis), leaving naked nuclei (cells stripped of their cytoplasm), strewn in the background of the smear [13 I6.46]. Cytolysis is essentially limited to intermediate cells: Superficial cells rarely cytolyse, parabasal cells almost never do. Also, dysplastic cells typically lack significant glycogen (the basis of the Schiller iodine test [Richart 1964b, Schiller 1938]) and therefore seldom undergo cytolysis.

The nucleus of an intermediate cell is centrally placed, as is characteristic of squamous cells in general. The nuclear area is about 35 µm^2, or 7 to 8 µm in diameter, which is about the size of a red blood cell, and somewhat smaller than the parabasal nucleus. The nucleus of an intermediate cell is round to oval and open and vesicular, with finely divided, evenly distributed chromatin and occasional chromocenters. Nucleoli are normally inconspicuous.

The nucleus of an intermediate cell is a touchstone in the art of cytopathology. Its size and the characteristics of its chromatin are key elements that serve as a standard reference as well as an internal control for staining and fixation artifacts. For example, the intermediate cell nucleus is an important size reference in diagnosing dysplasia. Also of major importance, when a nucleus is said to be hyperchromatic, it is generally in comparison with an intermediate cell nucleus. Similarly, when chromatin is said to be coarse, it is usually in comparison with intermediate cell chromatin.

12
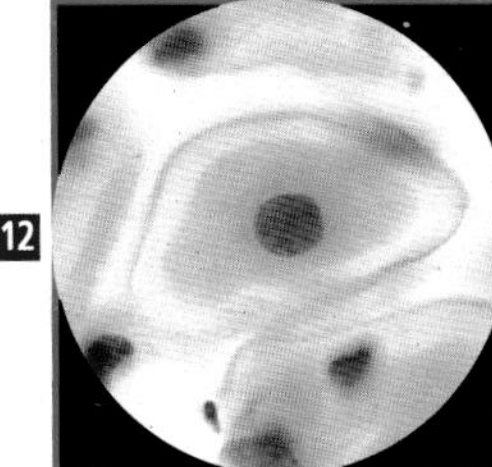

13
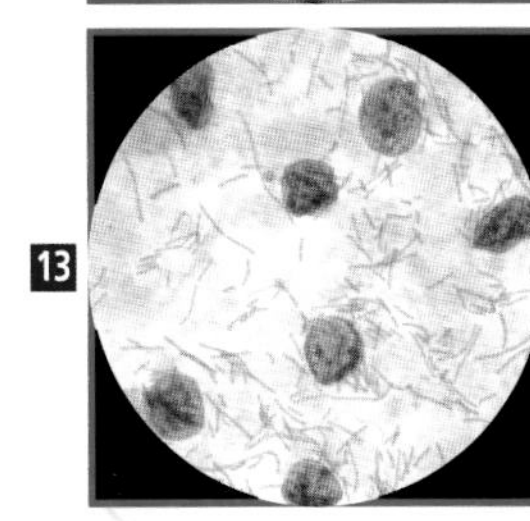

14
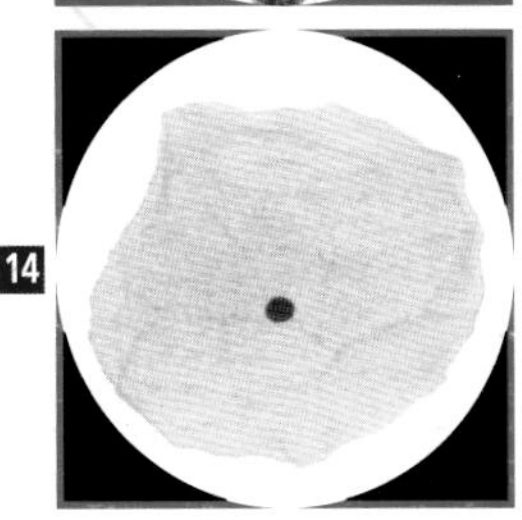

Superficial Cells

The superficial cells are the most differentiated squamous cells in a normal, nonkeratinizing squamous mucosa [14 I6.3]. They measure about 45 to 50 µm in diameter and look almost identical to the most mature intermediate cells, *except* that superficial cell nuclei are small and pyknotic, or dense, like India ink-dots. These compact nuclei are nonfunctional (ie, dead). The nucleus of a superficial cell is normally smaller than a red blood cell (<5–6 µm); if it is larger than a red blood cell, suspect dysplasia. The cytoplasm is abundant, thin, delicate, and transparent. The cell borders are well defined and have polygonal outlines. There is a tendency for superficial cells to stain pink and intermediate cells blue, but color is an unreliable basis for distinguishing the two cell types. The nuclear change from vesicular (intermediate) to pyknotic (superficial) is the key to differential diagnosis.

The Concept of the Icons

Learn the four basic squamous cell types (basal, parabasal, intermediate, superficial) by heart. These four cells are the icons on which much of what follows depends. The concept of the icons is the basis for understanding the morphology of normal squamous maturation, benign proliferative reactions, dysplasia, and cancer, each of which goes through stages that mimic these four basic cell types.

Hormonal Cytology

The cervicovaginal epithelium responds to a wide variety of stimuli, particularly hormones [F6.4] [Rakoff 1961a,b, Wied 1968]. The mucosa, particularly the vaginal mucosa, is very sensitive to estrogen and progesterone and varyingly sensitive to androgens, corticoids, thyroxin, vitamins, antibiotics, digitalis, mechanical stimulation, and inflammation. During the first half of the menstrual cycle, the follicular phase, the squamous mucosa is primarily influenced by estrogen, which promotes full maturation of the epithelium to the level of the superficial cell. During the second half, or luteal phase, of the cycle, and also during pregnancy, the epithelium is primarily influenced by progesterone. Progesterone is produced by the corpus luteum of the ovary, which is formed after ovulation. During pregnancy, progesterone is first formed by the corpus luteum, and later by the placenta. Progesterone inhibits full squamous differentiation, allowing maturation only to the intermediate, rather than the superficial, cell layer. Normal mucosal thickness is maintained by functional hyperplasia of the intermediate zone.

F6.4 Urinary Excretion of Ovarian Hormones

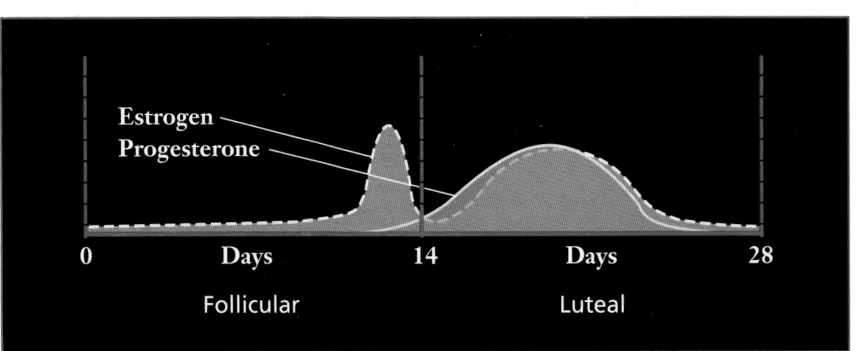

Three to five days elapse between the time the hormonal signal is received by the basal cell and the time the mature cell is formed at the surface. A Pap smear that is dominated by intermediate cells (ie, intermediate predominant maturation), therefore, is characteristic of the late luteal and early follicular phases of the cycle. Superficial cell predominance reaches its peak at the time of ovulation. Between ovulation and the late luteal phase, there is a gradual change from the superficial to the intermediate cell pattern. Obtaining parabasal cells from the scraped surface indicates that the epithelium is thin and atrophic, and has not even matured to the intermediate cell layer. Although better tests are available, the Pap smear can help assess ovarian function, including estimating the time of ovulation, as well as monitoring placental function or hormonal therapy.

There are many ways to express the degree of maturation of the vaginal epithelium, but the most reproducible and commonly used method is the Maturation Index (MI). Three hundred single (not clustered) cells are counted, and the relative percentages of parabasal, intermediate, and superficial cells are written as a ratio: parabasal %: intermediate %: superficial %, eg, 0: 80: 20. (Note: For MI assessment, basal cells are counted with parabasal cells as one cell type.)

For an MI, the smear should be taken as a *gentle* scrape (to obtain naturally exfoliated surface cells) about two thirds of the way up the lateral wall of the vagina. (Note: An ordinary Pap smear should be taken with a *vigorous* scrape.) This site is chosen because the vaginal epithelium is most sensitive to hormonal changes; smears from this area are usually clean (ie, free of inflammation, bacteria, debris, or other contaminants), and other types of cells are usually absent. Cyclic changes, including ovulation, can be appreciated only when smears are taken daily for at least one full cycle. Smears should be batched and stained together, and screened by one technologist to reduce technical artifacts.

A satisfactory specimen for hormonal evaluation should show no evidence of inflammation in the smear, because inflammation can cause nonhormonal maturation of the epithelium. Cervical (as opposed to vaginal) smears are unsatisfactory because of the frequent presence of inflammation and other confusing cell types, eg, squamous metaplasia, which can mimic ordinary parabasal cells.

Normally, only one or two cell types are represented. If all three types of cells are seen, inflammation is usually present or the smear was taken from the cervix. Such smears are unsatisfactory for hormonal evaluation. Exceptions to the "two cell rule" may occur when the epithelial maturation is changing, eg, prior to puberty, when cells from all three layers can be present normally.

The general pattern of maturation is more important than the actual values calculated. For example, there may be no significant difference between an MI of 0: 60: 40 and one of 0: 70: 30, both of which represent intermediate cell predominance. On the other hand, two women with identical MIs may have completely different causative factors for them. What may be normal for one, might be abnormal for another (eg, a maturation index of 80: 20: 0 would be normal in late postmenopause, but would suggest intrauterine fetal demise in a pregnant woman).

In summary, an MI smear should be free of inflammation, glandular cells, metaplastic cells, hyperkeratosis, and parakeratosis, as well as evidence of dysplasia; usually no more than two cell types should be present [T6.3]. The smears can only be properly interpreted in the light of adequate clinical history. This includes age, menstrual history, last menstrual period, past menstrual period, pregnancy, hormone therapy, surgery, all drugs, and radiation or chemotherapy. Finally, the report should indicate whether the MI is, or is not, compatible with the patient's history. The actual numbers are only of secondary importance.

Maturation Index

Parabasal %: Intermediate %: Superficial %

1. Complete history: Clinical; menstrual including last menstrual period, past menstrual period, regularity; pregnancies; hormonal therapy; drugs; surgery; radiation; previous neoplasia
2. Gentle scrape, two thirds up lateral vaginal wall
3. No evidence of inflammation
4. No more than two cell types present

Meaningful readings require all four conditions be met.

The Two Most Characteristic Maturation Patterns

1. Atrophy: Predominance of parabasal cells without superficial cells
2. High estrogen-like effect: Predominance of superficial cells without parabasal cells

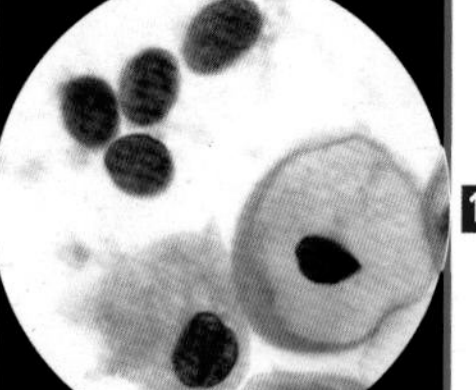

15

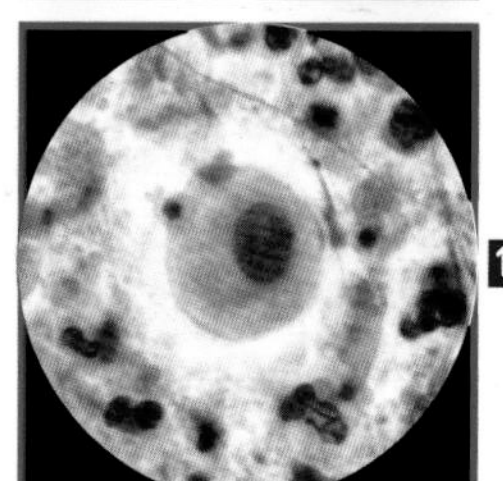

16

Parabasal Predominant Maturation Index (Atrophy)

The parabasal predominant maturation pattern indicates a poorly differentiated, or atrophic, epithelium. The squamous features of these atrophic cells, including keratin formation and intercellular bridges, are also poorly developed and the cytoplasm appears delicate rather than dense. The parabasal cells may be single or, in long-standing atrophy, in sheets. Sheets of atrophic parabasal cells often appear syncytial, because the intercellular space is too small to be resolved in the light microscope. Occasionally, the cells actually do fuse. Because atrophic cells are fragile, naked nuclei, often in clumps resembling endometrial cells, may be seen in the background of the smear [15 I6.7]. (For differential diagnosis, see "Endometrial Cells," p 123.)

Parabasal Predominant Maturation Index

Postmenopausal (classic)
Childhood (>1 month)
Postradiation
Ovarian insufficiency
Postpartum*
Lactation*
Androgens (exogenous, tumors)*
Androgenic atrophy*
Intrauterine fetal demise
Estrogen deficiency
Ulcer (cervicovaginal)
Turner's syndrome (XO)
Hypopituitarism, including starvation
Hypothyroidism (severe)
Gonadal dysgenesis
Prolactin

* Parabasal cells characteristically glycogenated.

Atrophy is frequently associated with inflammation [16 I6.9]. The atrophic epithelium is thin and the cells often lack glycogen, which is important in maintaining normal flora and pH. The lack of glycogen makes the mucosa more susceptible to various assaults.

T6.3 **Representative Maturation Patterns**

	Parabasal %	Intermediate %	Superficial %
Newborn	0	90	10
Child	80	20	0
Preovulatory	0	40	60
Postovulatory	0	60	40
Pregnancy	0	100	0
Postmenopause	80	20	0

The postmenopausal state, with its attendant decrease in sex hormones, is typically associated with a parabasal predominant, or atrophic, pattern. However, the postmenopausal MI varies significantly from woman to woman. A mature pattern may persist for many years, an occurrence that is possibly related to variable sensitivity to adrenal hormones [Efstratiades 1982, Meisels 1966a]. The atrophic pattern is also normal during childhood. A wide variety of other conditions, including starvation and anorexia nervosa, with decreased pituitary gonadotropins resulting in ovarian failure, can also be associated with an atrophic pattern.

Postpartum, upon withdrawal of placental hormones, the epithelium may become atrophic until the ovaries again begin to cycle hormonally. Postpartum atrophy is more common with lactation and usually lasts about 3 to 6 weeks, but may last up to several months, or until the infant is weaned. An atrophic pattern occurring *during* pregnancy is abnormal and suggests intrauterine fetal demise (see "Hormonal Cytology of Pregnancy," p 133).

In postpartum and lactational Pap smears, the parabasal cells are typically heavily glycogenated. Similarly, in response to androgens, the mucosa may become atrophic, and glycogenated parabasal cells will be found in the smear. This pattern (atrophy with glycogenated parabasal cells) is known as androgenic atrophy [I6.5]. The source of the androgen can be either exogenous (eg, testosterone given for treatment of lichen sclerosis) or endogenous. In a postmenopausal woman, the most common endogenous source of androgen is the adrenal gland. Rarely, androgenic atrophy may be caused by virilizing functional ovarian tumors (eg, Sertoli-Leydig, Leydig, lipid cell tumors, and rarely, ovarian stroma reactive to metastatic carcinoma).

Intermediate Predominant Maturation Index

- Newborn (~1 month)
- Postovulatory
- Pregnancy
- Early menopause
- Progesterone therapy
- Cortisone therapy
- Adrenocortical hormones
- Tetracycline (perhaps others)
- Late childhood (premenarche)
- Acromegaly
- Digitalis (premenopausal)
- Ovarian dysfunction
- Low dose estrogen therapy
- Androgens, including tumors
- Luteinized follicle
- Corpus luteum cyst

Intermediate Predominant Maturation Index

The intermediate predominant pattern is characteristic of progesterone effect, which inhibits complete maturation to the superficial cell layer [17 I6.4]. Progesterone production is associated with the postovulatory, luteal phase of the menstrual cycle as well as pregnancy. The normal, pure intermediate pattern (0/100/0) characteristic of pregnancy may take a trimester or more to develop. Progesterone also encourages glycogen accumulation and, particularly during pregnancy, navicular cells may be seen [18 I6.5].

17

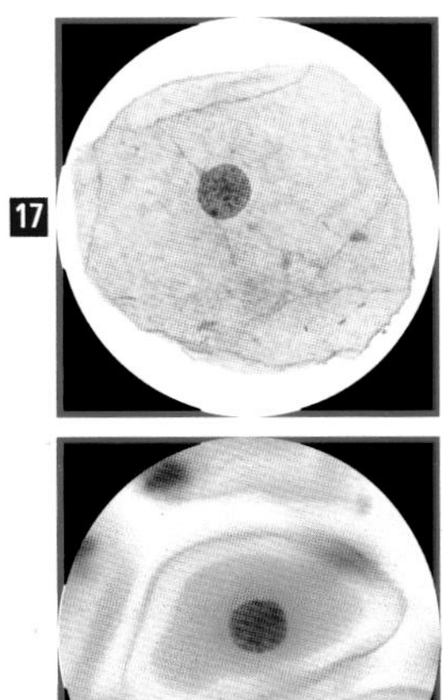

18

For about a month following birth, a newborn girl's vaginal mucosa will be under the (transplacental) influence of her mother's hormones, and will show intermediate predominance. As the maternal hormones are metabolized, the newborn's mucosa atrophies. It remains atrophic until a few years before menarche, when the atrophic pattern is gradually replaced by a noncycling intermediate predominant MI (about a year or so before actual menarche, the mucosa begins to show cyclic change).

Loss of ovarian function (postmenopause, surgery, radiation, etc) is usually associated with atrophy. However, some postmenopausal women never develop an atrophic pattern and maintain an intermediate predominant maturation, perhaps sustained by adrenal hormones. Some postmenopausal women on long-term, low-dose estrogen replacement also maintain an intermediate, rather than superficial, predominant pattern. In addition, a variety of drugs, including digitalis [Britsch 1963, Navab 1965] and broad-spectrum antibiotics, can influence the maturation of the cervicovaginal epithelium.

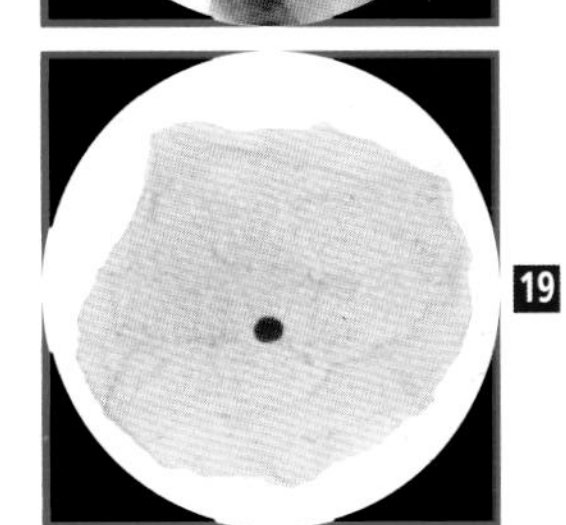

19

Superficial Predominant Maturation Index

Estrogen stimulation, either endogenous or exogenous [19 I6.3], usually produces superficial predominance, which is characteristic of the first half, or follicular phase, of the menstrual cycle. Superficial predominance reaches its peak at ovulation. Sensitivity to estrogen varies greatly; some women can develop a mature mucosa from the small amount of estrogen in some facial creams. Superficial predominance in postmenopause indicates estrogen stimulation, which is a possible risk factor for endometrial disease. Furthermore, a mature maturation pattern in a postmenopausal woman, without an exogenous source of estrogen, could be due to an ovarian tumor. The tumor itself could secrete estrogen (eg, granulosa cell tumor) or it could induce hyperplasia of the estrogen-producing ovarian stroma (eg, metastasis or endometriosis). Because androstenedione, from the adrenal gland, is metabolized in the peripheral fat into estrone, a weak estrogen, obesity can also result in increased maturation. Cirrhosis of the liver can interfere with degradation of estrogen, resulting in estrogen excess. Postmenopausal women taking digitalis for more than 2 years can develop high maturation [Navab 1965]. Paradoxically,

Superficial Predominant Maturation Index

- Preovulatory (peaks at ovulation)
- Estrogen therapy (very variable)
- Obesity
- Cirrhosis
- Excess androgens
- Testicular feminization
- Ovarian tumors
- Granulosa cell
- Thecoma
- Metastasis
- Primary endometriosis
- Digitalis (postmenopause)

tamoxifen citrate, an antiestrogen used in the treatment of breast cancer, can also cause an estrogen-like effect in postmenopausal women [Athanassiadou 1992, Eells 1990, Rayter 1994], possibly because it binds to estrogen receptors.

Barr Bodies

The Barr body is another cell feature that can be useful in diagnosis. In every female somatic cell there is normally one Barr body, which represents the second, inactivated X chromosome [Barr 1949]. Barr bodies are dense, triangular or rectangular bits of heterochromatin, about 1 µm in diameter, attached at random to the inner aspect of the nuclear membrane [**20** I6.6]. Because Barr bodies can be reliably identified only when seen on the lateral nuclear margin of a cell, even in normal females, they are identified in only 20% to 60% of cells. Multiple Barr bodies may be present not only in genetic diseases but also in intraepithelial and invasive neoplasia due to chromosomal abnormalities. (Note: A buccal smear is usually preferred for evaluation of the Barr bodies since there are fewer artifacts.) Hormonal status and Barr bodies can be evaluated together [T6.4].

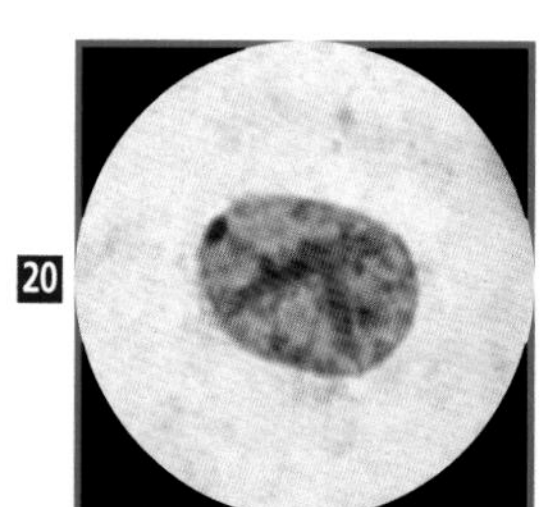
20

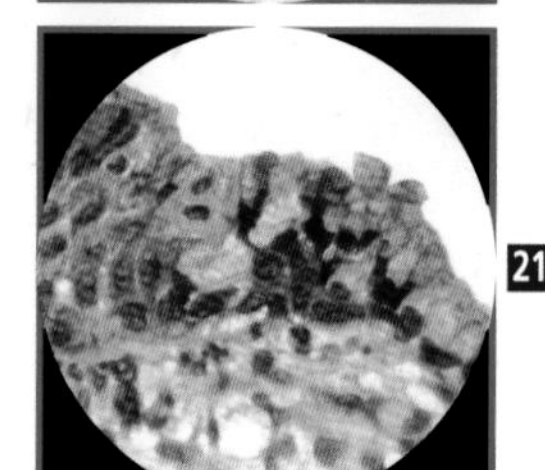
21

Carcinogenesis

Benign Proliferative Reactions

In response to various stimuli, such as pH or endocrine changes, trauma, or inflammation, the delicate glandular epithelium of the cervix changes into a squamous epithelium, by a process known as ***metaplasia.*** The primary function of squamous cells is protective. When the stress is particularly severe, the normally nonkeratinizing squamous epithelium of the cervix and vagina can also undergo *keratosis*, becoming hyperplastic, and providing a tough, skin-like epithelium. Metaplasia and keratosis are the two basic kinds of benign proliferative reactions. These epithelial proliferations, particularly metaplasia, are the milieu in which cervical carcinogenesis may begin. *Proliferation is the force that drives carcinogenesis.*

T6.4 Hormonal Status and Barr Bodies

Normal hormonal status, (+) Barr bodies
- Normal female
- Congenital atresias of genital tract (except ovaries)
- Disease/endocrinopathy (insufficient for abnormal hormonal pattern)

Note: Very few, or small, Barr bodies may indicate mosaicism or translocation.

Abnormal hormonal pattern, (+) Barr bodies
- Dysfunction of endocrine organs
  - Ovary
  - Other (eg, pituitary, adrenal, thyroid [marked hypofunction])
- Dysfunction of chromosomes
  - Down's, somatic trisomy
  - XXX (double Barr body)

Note: Rule out hormone therapy, inflammation, cervical or vulvar contamination.

Normal hormonal pattern, (–) Barr bodies
- Testicular feminization (androgen insensitivity syndrome) (= XY with feminizing male pseudohermaphroditism)

Abnormal hormonal pattern, (–) Barr bodies
- Turner's (XO)
- Other gonadal dysgenesis (XY)

Metaplastic Reactions

During fetal development most of the vagina is lined by columnar (endocervical-like) glandular epithelium of müllerian origin. Squamous epithelium normally grows in from the urogenital sinus lining the vagina and the ectocervix, and replaces the columnar epithelium through the process of metaplasia. (Diethylstilbestrol [DES] interferes with this normal process and may leave islands of this glandular epithelium in the vagina, a condition known as vaginal adenosis.) At birth, the glandular and squamous epithelium interface at the external os (Latin: mouth) of the cervix. The site of this interface is known as the "original" squamocolumnar junction, and the squamous mucosa is known as the "native" squamous epithelium.

At puberty and during pregnancy, the cervix increases in size and changes in shape, resulting in eversion of the endocervical glandular epithelium onto the portio vaginalis of the cervix. This eversion is termed an ectropion (Greek: out-turning); however, because the underlying red, vascular stroma can be seen through the delicate columnar epithelium, it may look like an erosion clinically [Briggs 1979]. Ectropion is more common and more extensive on the anterior than on the posterior lip of the cervix (the same is true of the distribution of dysplasia).

In response to the normal acid pH of the vagina, as well as a host of other possible irritants, including inflammation, polyps, and birth control pills, the everted columnar epithelium is replaced by metaplastic squamous epithelium, forming a new squamocolumnar junction. Squamous metaplasia is at its peak during fetal development, puberty, pregnancy (particularly the first), and postpartum. (Note: There is a significant drop in the vaginal pH at puberty, resulting in extensive metaplasia at this time [Briggs 1979], and possibly, increased susceptibility to carcinogenic agents, such as HPV.) Due to this metaplasia, instead of a squamocolumnar junction, there may now be a squamo-metaplastic-columnar junction. The metaplastic zone between the native squamous and glandular epithelium is known as the transition zone (also known as the transformation zone in colposcopy, or for simplicity, the "T zone") [**21** I6.2]. *The transformation zone is the site at which cervical neoplasia is most likely to arise.*

For proper cancer surveillance, the T zone is the critical area to sample. Due to squamous metaplasia, the location of the T zone changes during a woman's lifetime: the squamocolumnar junction gradually recedes proximally (ie, upward, into the endocervix). During the reproductive years, the squamocolumnar junction is usually distal to the external cervical os, and is easy to sample. However, later in life, especially postmenopause, the T zone may be found within the endocervical canal, where it can be difficult to sample. Endocervical cells, and to some degree metaplastic cells, are the best evidence that the T zone is represented in a Pap smear.

There is a gradient of maturity of the metaplastic process. Squamous metaplasia is less mature proximally and more mature distally, toward the site of the original squamocolumnar junction on the ectocervix. Indeed, squamous metaplasia on the ectocervix may be so mature as to be indistinguishable from the native squamous epithelium.

Squamous metaplasia is so common that it is considered a normal physiologic process. It is thought to begin with the endocervical reserve cell [Howard 1951, Reagan 1962], the origin of which is still controversial, but ultimately agreed to be müllerian. Endocervical reserve cells are morphologically similar to squamous basal cells. However, the reserve cell has the capacity to differentiate into either a glandular or a squamous cell, unlike the basal cell (squamous only). When the reserve cell receives the signal to undergo squamous metaplasia, the first step is proliferation, or reserve cell hyperplasia. Then, squamous differentiation begins (immature, followed by mature, squamous metaplasia). The undifferentiated reserve cell is also thought to be the ultimate source of cervical squamous cell carcinoma, adenocarcinoma, and mixed adenosquamous carcinoma [F6.5].

F6.5 **Reserve Cell Differentiation**

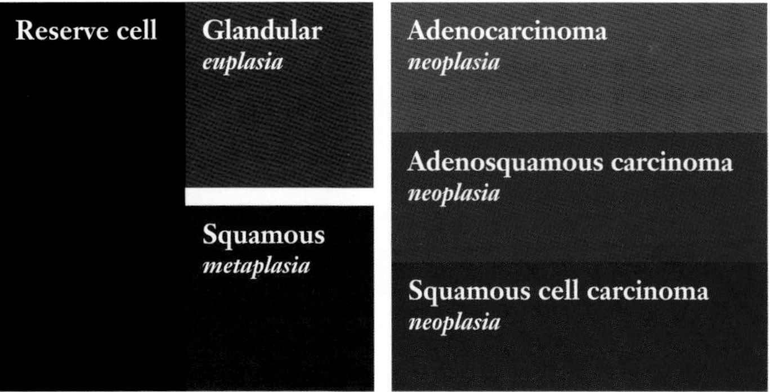

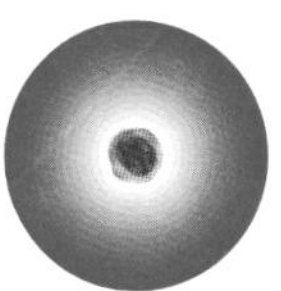

Reserve Cell Hyperplasia

Histology: In the earliest phase of nascent metaplasia, the reserve cells begin to proliferate along the basement membrane, underneath the endocervical-type glandular epithelium. Histologically, this single row of reserve cells is the first recognizable stage of reserve cell hyperplasia (RCH). Next, the reserve cells begin to pile up, forming two to five layers of undifferentiated small cells, before they start to acquire definite squamous features, such as dense cytoplasm, distinct cell boundaries, intercellular bridges, stratification, that is, before true squamous metaplasia begins. Reserve cell hyperplasia usually remains covered by glandular epithelium.

Reserve Cell Hyperplasia

- Histology (commonly observed)
  - 1 to 5 layers
  - Undifferentiated small cells
  - Indistinct cell boundaries
- Cytology (rarely recognized)
  - Syncytial-like aggregates
  - Cells: Resemble histiocytes
    - Cytoplasm: Delicate
    - Nucleus: Bland, high nuclear/cytoplasmic ratio
    - Associated with small endocervical cells
      - Immature squamous metaplasia

Cytology: Although commonly seen in tissue, reserve cell hyperplasia is rarely recognized in the Pap smear. The reserve cell closely resembles the basal cell (note the choice of icon). Individual reserve cells are indistinguishable from small histiocytes or superficial endometrial stromal cells. Reserve cell hyperplasia can most reliably be diagnosed, cytologically, when the reserve cells occur in aggregates, particularly when covered on one side by small, columnar endocervical cells.

Reserve cells are small and have high nuclear/cytoplasmic (N/C) ratios [22 I6.31]. Their cytoplasm is scanty, delicate, finely vacuolated, and cyanophilic, with poorly defined cell borders. The single, central nucleus may be round to oval, or sometimes bean-shaped, with a fold or groove in the nuclear membrane. The chromatin is fine, with occasional chromocenters, similar to the nucleus of a normal endocervical cell. Neither hyperchromasia nor nucleoli are present. Extensive immature squamous metaplasia, which usually accompanies reserve cell hyperplasia, provides supporting evidence of the diagnosis.

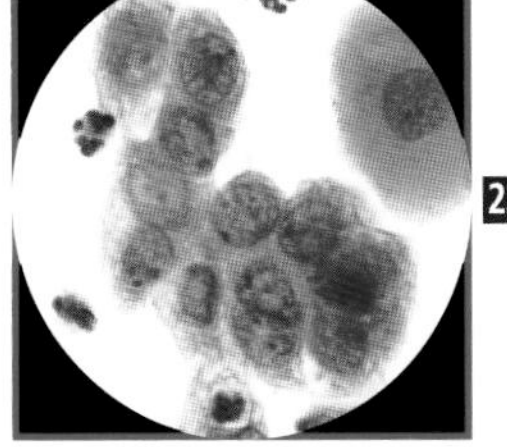

22

Differential Diagnosis: Since hyperplastic reserve cells may form layers of primitive cells, reserve cell hyperplasia could be mistaken for carcinoma in situ, particularly in tissue. In cytology, reserve cell hyperplasia is seen as apparently syncytial aggregates of undifferentiated cells with immature nuclei, features also shared with carcinoma in situ. However, the cells of reserve cell hyperplasia remain uniform and orderly, and the nuclei appear bland and benign. Carcinoma in situ, on the other hand, is disorderly, and the nuclei are clearly abnormal.

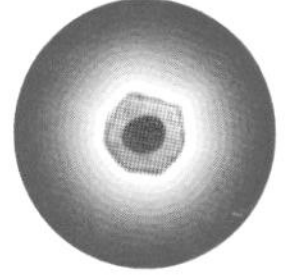

Immature Squamous Metaplasia

Histology: When the reserve cells start to acquire squamous features (ie, differentiate), bona fide squamous metaplasia begins. Squamous differentiation is recognized, cytologically, by the accumulation of dense cytoplasm and the appearance of distinct cell borders. These features develop when the cells lay down numerous intermediate-sized tonofilaments in their cytoplasm. The immature metaplastic cells become packed with tonofibrils (bundles of tonofilaments, the keratin apparatus) and round up (to achieve maximal volume in minimal space), resulting in moderately high N/C ratios.

Histologically, the cells begin to stratify and develop a well-defined basal layer, features not seen in reserve cell hyperplasia.

Intercellular bridges are not conspicuous at this point, but become prominent as the metaplasia matures. The immature metaplastic epithelium is composed of two zones, basal and parabasal. Thus, the cells at the surface are the size and shape of parabasal cells (the icon), which the immature metaplastic cells closely resemble. The border between the immature metaplastic epithelium and the native squamous epithelium is sharply defined histologically.

Immature Squamous Metaplasia

Very common
Histology
 Squamous maturation
 Stratification
 Well-defined basal layer
Cytology
 Cobblestone arrangement
 Cells: Rounded, parabasal-sized
 Cytoplasm: Dense, ectoplasmic rim; vacuolization common
 Nucleus: Vesicular
 Spider cells

Cytology: Immature squamous metaplasia is usually easily recognized in the Pap smear as parabasal-sized cells with dense cytoplasm and rounded cell borders. They are characteristically arranged in a cobblestone pattern, and tend to be single or only loosely aggregated [23 I6.32]. The cytoplasm usually stains blue-green and usually does not contain visible glycogen. The cytoplasm is particularly thick and dense and the cell borders are sharply defined ("cookie cutter" look). There is often a dense zone just underneath the cell membrane, known as the ectoplasmic rim, which is distinct from the endoplasm of the cell.

The nucleus is round to oval and has a smooth membrane, fine chromatin, and rare chromocenters. Nucleoli are not normally seen, but they may be present in reactive change, which commonly affects metaplastic cells. The nucleus measures about 50 µm², about 8 µm in diameter, which is slightly larger than either a red blood cell or an intermediate cell nucleus.

Squamous metaplastic cells are fairly variable in size and shape, depending upon the degree of maturation. If the cells have been forcibly scraped, rather than spontaneously exfoliated, from the mucosal surface, they may also show thin, spidery legs extending from the main body of the cell [Buckley 1994]. These are called spider cells [24 I6.33].

Differential Diagnosis: Layers of pleomorphic, immature squamous cells with high N/C ratios and nuclei showing reactive atypia may resemble dysplasia, histologically. Similarly, the differential diagnosis of immature metaplastic cells vs dysplasia is a common diagnostic problem in evaluating the Pap smear. Critical examination of the nucleus, particularly its size and the quality of the chromatin, is the ultimate key to the proper classification of the cells.

Immature metaplastic cells are frequently vacuolated. Vacuolated metaplastic cells with active nuclei may resemble adenocarcinoma [25 I6.143]. Vacuolated cells in a Pap smear are far more likely to be benign metaplasia than glandular cancer. The vacuoles of metaplastic cells can be of three types: (1) degenerative (degeneration is hydropic, containing only water and electrolytes and appearing crystal clear), (2) secretory (containing lightly staining mucin), or (3) phagocytic (containing stainable material or cells).

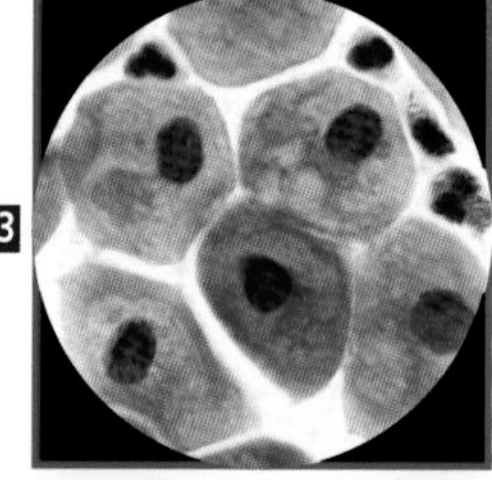
23

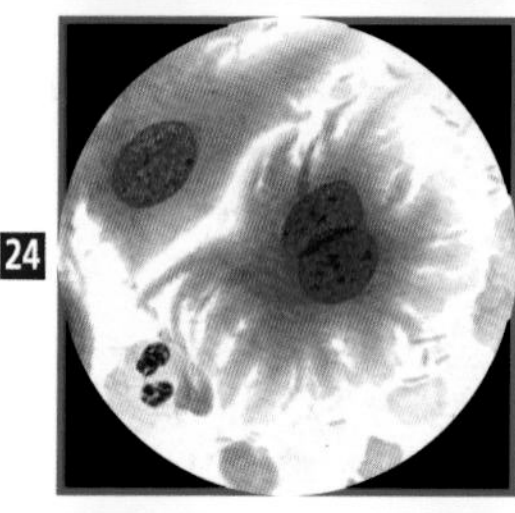
24

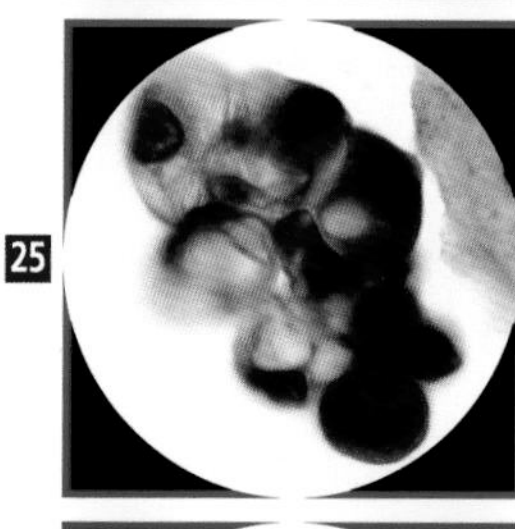
25

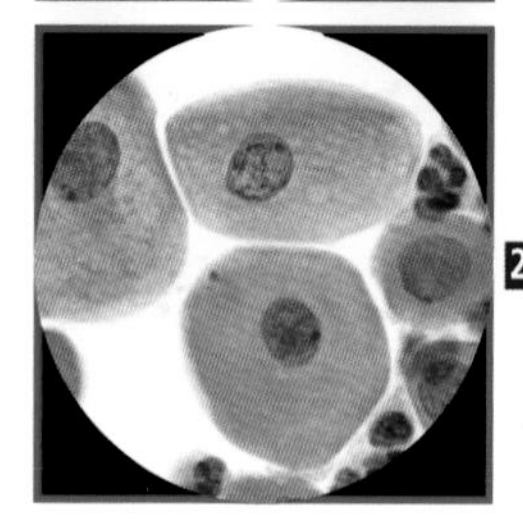
26

Differentiating parabasal-sized cells of metaplasia from those of atrophy is a common dilemma. Robust, actively proliferating metaplastic cells can be distinguished from delicate atrophic cells by the thickness and density of metaplastic cytoplasm, the presence of an ectoplasmic rim, and the cobblestone arrangement of the cells. Spidery forms are more frequent in metaplasia, while syncytial-like aggregates are common in atrophy. Immature metaplastic cells are usually intermingled with more mature metaplastic cells.

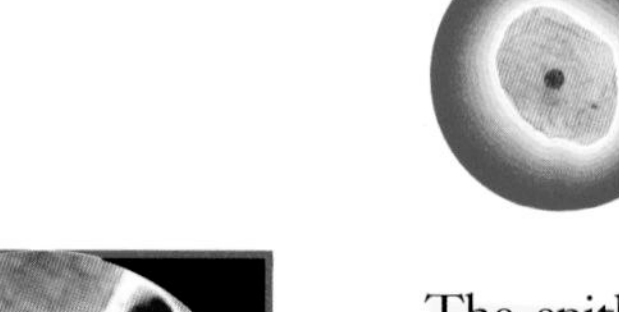

Mature Squamous Metaplasia

Histology: As the cytoskeleton (keratin) and cell membrane continue to develop, the metaplastic cell becomes a shield-like scale. The epithelium now forms three zones: basal, parabasal, and intermediate. This stage is known as mature squamous metaplasia. Histologically, the only clue to the metaplastic origin of the mature squamous epithelium may be the presence of underlying endocervical glands, indicating its endocervical source. Endocervical glands are not found directly beneath the native squamous epithelium.

Mature Squamous Metaplasia

Histology
 Similar to native epithelium
 Underlying endocervical glands
Cytology
 Intermediate-like cells
 Rounded outlines
 Slightly dense cytoplasm
 Remnants of cobblestone pattern

Cytology: The cells at the surface of the epithelium closely resemble normal intermediate cells (the icon), except that their cell outlines may be a little more rounded than polygonal and the cytoplasm may be slightly denser than mature intermediate cells [26 I6.154]. Remnants of a cobblestone arrangement of the cells may be seen cytologically. Eventually, the squamous metaplasia matures completely and becomes cytologically indistinguishable from the native squamous epithelium, including the presence of cyclic hormonal changes.

Keratotic Reactions

Estrogen stimulates complete maturation to the superficial cell, the final icon. Under certain circumstances, the normally nonkeratinizing squamous epithelium, whether native or metaplastic, can undergo further differentiation into a keratinized, skin-like squamous epithelium. This hyperdifferentiation is called keratosis, of which there are two basic kinds, hyperkeratosis and parakeratosis. Keratosis may be caused by marked irritation of the mucosa, eg, due to uterine prolapse, inflammation/infections, pessaries, radiation, or DES exposure in utero, or it may be idiopathic. In addition, some cases of keratosis are related to condyloma or dysplasia. In the Pap smear, hyperkeratosis is recognized by anucleate and granular superficial cells, and parakeratosis by miniature superficial cells.

Keratosis is usually associated with a fully mature epithelium, but it can also be found on the surface of an atrophic epithelium or, more ominously, a neoplastic epithelium. The keratotic surface looks white, which is termed leukoplakia (Greek: white plaques) clinically, or white epithelium, colposcopically. However, a white appearance can be due to a variety of conditions, including not only hyperkeratosis or parakeratosis, but also warts (condyloma), dysplasia, and even cancer.

Keratosis itself is benign. Its primary diagnostic significance lies in the fact that as a surface reaction, keratosis may cover a lesion, thereby masking it. Thus, the underlying abnormality may not be sampled when taking the Pap smear, which only scrapes the mucosal surface. However, patients with only hyperkeratosis or parakeratosis are probably not at increased risk of developing cervical intraepithelial neoplasia or condyloma (squamous intraepithelial lesions) [Andrews 1989b, Cecchini 1990c, Sorosky 1990]. However, if keratosis is combined with inflammatory changes and, particularly, squamous atypia, there may be increased risk of condyloma (low grade squamous intraepithelial lesion) [Hudock 1995]. Also, finding keratosis in a patient with a history of condyloma or dysplasia may correlate with persistence of the lesion [Kern 1991b].

Hyperkeratosis

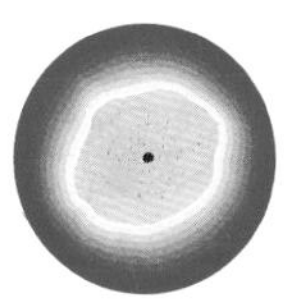

Histology: Hyperkeratosis is a proliferative process that is usually characterized by overall thickening of the epithelium with elongation of the rete pegs (acanthosis) and formation of an additional two layers of cells at the surface: the stratum granulosum and the stratum corneum [27 I6.36].

In the stratum granulosum, or the granular cell layer, the prekeratin of the superficial cell forms small, darkly staining granules of dense keratin (known as keratohyalin granules). A granular layer in a tissue biopsy (usually designated hypergranulosis, or spiegelosis [28 I6.34]) can be helpful to the clinician because it is an explanation for white epithelium that may have been seen colposcopically. In the stratum corneum, the degenerated, pyknotic nucleus of the superficial cell dissolves completely (a process known as karyolysis), forming a layer of anucleate squames.

Hyperkeratosis

Skin-like squamous mucosa
Surface reaction, may cover underlying lesion
Associated conditions

Prolapse	Inflammation/Infection
Pessaries	DES exposure in utero
Radiation	Condyloma, dysplasia, SCC

Cytology
- Anucleate squames, especially in clumps, diagnostic
- ± Nucleated cells with keratohyaline granules

Differential diagnosis of hyperkeratosis
- Contaminants: Take stain poorly

DES = diethylstilbestrol, SCC = squamous cell carcinoma.

Cytology: Cytologically, the most diagnostic feature of hyperkeratosis in a Pap smear is the presence of anucleate squames, particularly in clumps [29 I6.35]. Anucleate squames resemble superficial cells (note the icon), but lack a nucleus. However, there may be a pale area in the space that was occupied by the nucleus before it lysed. This is the nuclear ghost. Anucleate squames of hyperkeratosis usually stain yellow, orange, or pink. Nucleated cells from the granular cell layer may also be present. These cells resemble normal superficial cells, but have small, dark blue cytoplasmic keratohyalin granules.

A few uniform, polygonal anucleate squames in a Pap smear have little clinical importance. However, patients with extensive clusters should be followed more closely to rule out a hidden underlying dysplasia or cancer, particularly if there is no obvious explanation for the hyperkeratosis (eg, uterine prolapse). If the squames have irregular, abnormal outlines (tadpole, spindle, etc), colposcopy is usually indicated, because significant keratinizing dysplasia or carcinoma is associated with pleomorphic cellular shapes [Nauth 1983].

27 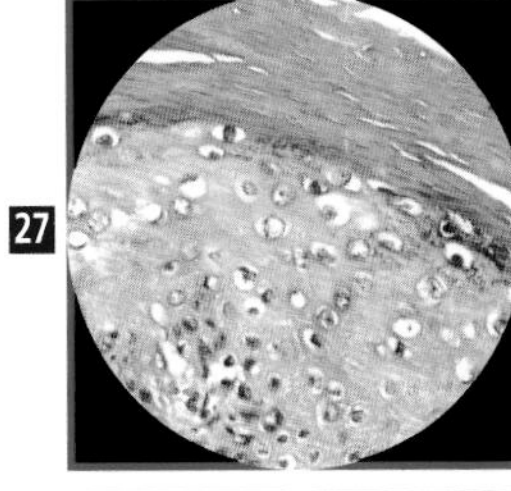

28 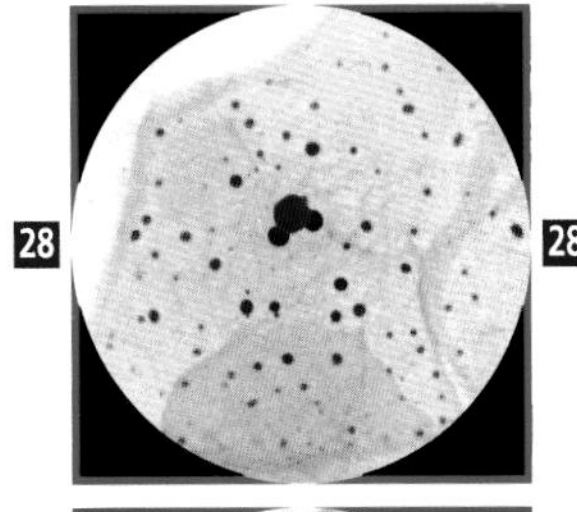 28

29 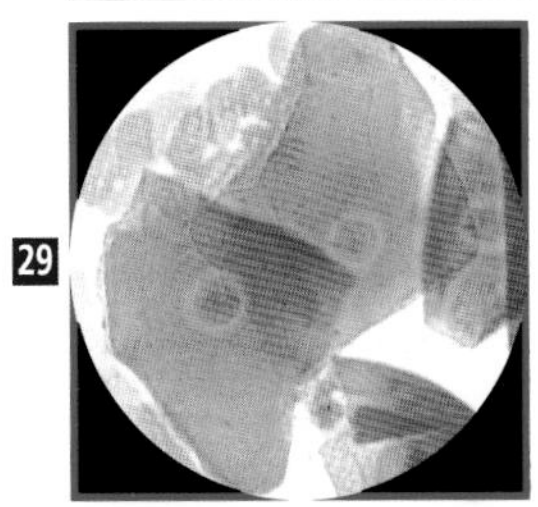

30 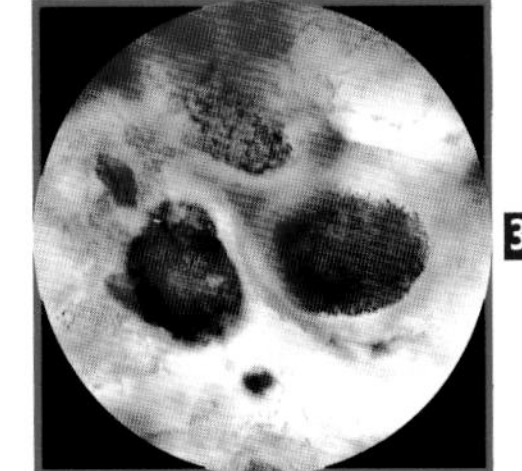

Differential Diagnosis: The Pap smear may be contaminated with anucleate squames from the skin (vulva of the patient or fingers of anyone touching the glass slide). In contrast to the squames of hyperkeratosis, which take the Pap stain beautifully, staining glorious colors of red, yellow, and orange, these contaminant squames are coated with oils from the skin and take the stain poorly, staining dirty brownish yellow or rust.

Keratohyalin granules must be differentiated cytologically from the brown artifact known as cornflakes [T6.5; 30 I6.151]. Cornflakes are caused by air bubbles trapped on top of the cell, which mark where the xylene evaporated before coverslipping. The air bubbles appear as refractile, dark golden-brown, relatively uniform, tiny dots that cover the squamous cell, giving it the appearance of a brown cornflake. The bubbles focus above the plane of the cell. Keratohyalin granules are blue-black, somewhat larger, variable in size, and focus inside the cell [28 I6.34]. Cornflakes may obscure cellular detail, in which case recoverslipping the slide may help reduce the artifact.

Parakeratosis

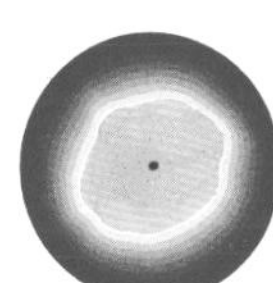

Histology: Parakeratosis is another surface keratotic reaction. Parakeratosis is benign, but like hyperkeratosis, it can conceal a significant underlying lesion, including dysplasia or cancer. Parakeratosis is brought on by the same factors that stimulate hyperkeratosis, but the former is perhaps more frequently associated with condyloma. Parakeratosis is composed of small

T6.5 **Differentiation of Keratohyalin Granules From "Cornflakes"**

Keratohyalin	Cornflakes
In cell	Above cell
Fewer (granules)	More (bubbles)
Blue-black	Golden brown
Slightly larger, variable	Minute, uniform
Indicates keratosis	May obscure cell detail

Parakeratosis

Related to hyperkeratosis
Cytology
Miniature superficial cells
Isolated, single
Layered strips
"Pearls"
Cytoplasm: Usually orange
Nuclei: Usually pyknotic

polygonal or rounded cells resembling miniature superficial cells (note the icon). It is not obvious why parakeratotic cells should be small.

Cytology: Cytologically, parakeratosis may be seen as single flat cells, layered strips of cells, or concentrically arranged "pearls" [31 I6.37, 32 I6.38, 33 I6.39]. The cells usually stain orange (but may also be yellow, red, or even blue) and typically have centrally placed, pyknotic nuclei, although some nuclei may be more open. Parakeratosis frequently coexists with hyperkeratosis.

Differential Diagnosis: Coagulative necrosis can cause any cell to condense and develop deep orange cytoplasm (a staining artifact) and pyknotic nuclei. Therefore, not every small orange cell with an ink-dot nucleus represents parakeratosis. For example, degenerative changes can be seen in endocervical cells of some women taking birth control pills [34 I6.40]. These pseudoparakeratotic endocervical cells are found in linear arrangements in the smear (see "Microglandular Endocervical Hyperplasia," p 122). Parabasal cells of atrophy also commonly undergo this degenerative change ("pseudo-pseudoparakeratosis"?). Coagulated atrophic cells are found randomly in the smear.

The clues to the correct identification [T6.6] of degenerated, pseudokeratotic cells are (1) the accompanying milieu (eg, other signs of atrophy or degeneration), (2) the rounded or columnar (not polygonal) cell contours, (3) the distribution of the cells, and (4) the foamy/granular (not waxy) cytoplasm, which is more commonly eosinophilic than orangeophilic. The degenerative changes may be more pronounced in the cytoplasm than the nucleus. Degenerated glandular cells have an eccentric nucleus.

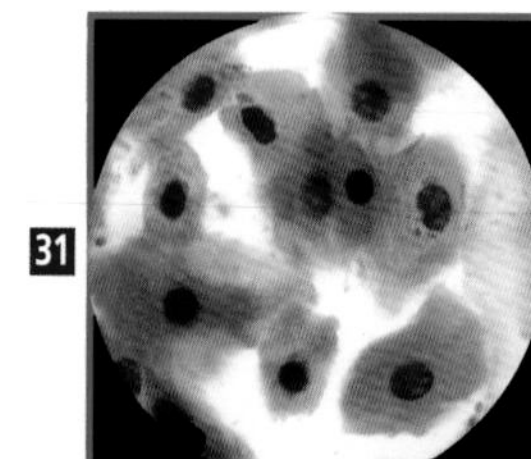
31

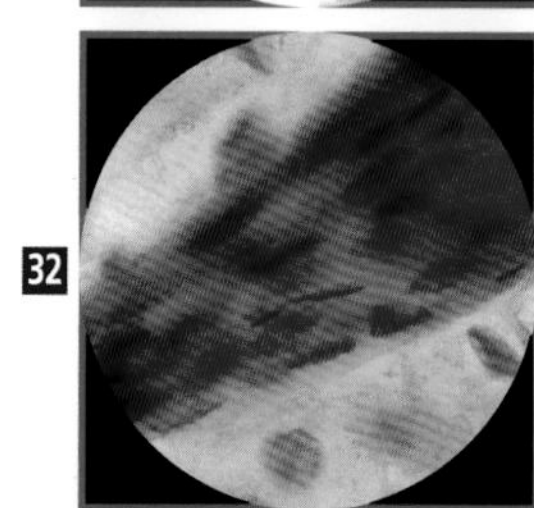
32

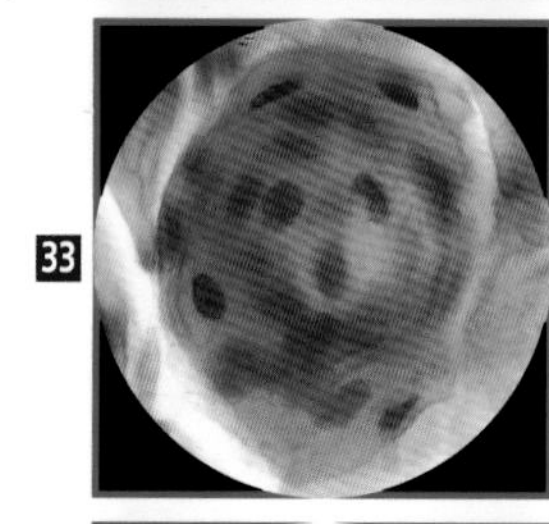
33

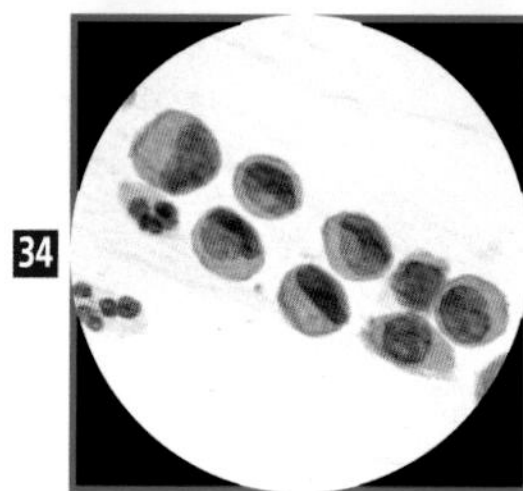
34

Atypical Parakeratosis

Atypical parakeratosis, also known as pleomorphic parakeratosis, is probably best regarded as a form of atypical squamous cells of undetermined significance (ASCUS). Atypical parakeratosis is composed of pleomorphic, miniature superficial cells; the nuclei and cytoplasm vary in size and shape. Atypical parakeratosis resembles keratinizing dysplasia, but occurs in small cells. Atypical parakeratosis is particularly important because it not only can mask an underlying lesion, but is usually associated with a more significant lesion (condyloma, dysplasia, or even squamous cell carcinoma). Similar or identical cells, called dyskeratocytes, are closely associated with condyloma. Atypical parakeratosis is a clue to the presence of a significant underlying abnormality and should be reported to the clinician if a more advanced lesion cannot be identified in the Pap smear.

Atypical Parakeratosis

Associated with neoplasia, condyloma
Cytology
Pleomorphic parakeratosis
Mimics miniature keratinizing dysplasia

T6.6 **Differentiation of Pseudokeratosis and Parakeratosis**

	Pseudokeratosis	Parakeratosis
Milieu	Atrophy (or birth control pills) Signs of degeneration	Mature Clean, keratosis
Cell	Rounded (or columnar)	Polygonal
Cytoplasm	Granular	Waxy
Distribution	Spotty (or linear)	Groups

Summary of Benign Proliferative Reactions

In summary, there are two basic benign proliferative reactions: metaplasia and keratosis, classically associated with the endocervix and ectocervix, respectively. Squamous metaplasia begins with reserve cell hyperplasia, which is composed of undifferentiated, basal-like cells that resemble histiocytes (generally covered by small endocervical cells). This begins to differentiate into immature squamous metaplasia with dense, rounded parabasal-like cells occurring in smears in a cobblestone arrangement. These cells then differentiate to mature squamous metaplasia, with cells resembling normal intermediate cells at the surface. Under the influence of estrogen, superficial cells differentiate, indicative of a fully mature nonkeratinizing squamous epithelium, identical to the native squamous epithelium of the ectocervix. The mucosa may also "hyperdifferentiate," resulting in hyperkeratosis or parakeratosis, represented in the Pap smear by anucleate or miniature superficial cells, respectively. F6.6 recaps the benign proliferative reactions.

Cervical Intraepithelial Neoplasia or Dysplasia and Carcinoma In Situ

Benign proliferative reactions are just that—benign. They are not precancerous but are the soil in which the seed of cancer may be sown. The nature of the seed is the subject of much research and speculation, and will be considered later. For the moment, it is unimportant what causes the changes about to be discussed. What is important is that cancers generally follow a recognizable pattern of development, which has been extremely well studied in the uterine cervix.

This section will take a fairly traditional approach to diagnosis of preinvasive lesions, emphasizing the familiar terminology relating to dysplasia/carcinoma in situ. Dysplasia and

F6.6 **Benign Proliferative Reactions**

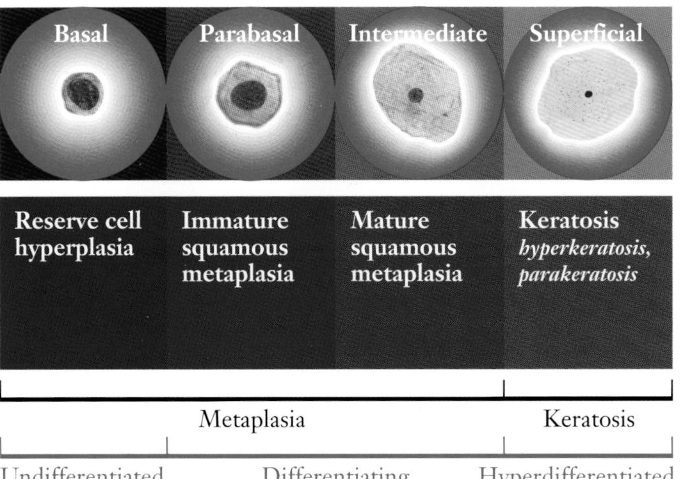

carcinoma in situ form a morphologic spectrum that is also known as cervical intraepithelial neoplasia (CIN). However, whether these lesions are truly neoplastic is controversial (see "DNA Ploidy and Prognosis," p 107). In part because of this controversy in the late 1980s, another terminology, squamous intraepithelial lesion (SIL), was introduced as part of the Bethesda System. *The various terminologies all describe essentially the same abnormalities.* Therefore, for the purposes of discussion, they will be used more or less interchangeably—as appropriate to their definitions—in the following presentation. (See "Nomenclature," p 89.)

Many of the concepts, as well as the morphometry, to be discussed are based on Patten's classic monograph, *Diagnostic Cytopathology of the Uterine Cervix* [Patten 1978]. Subsequent sections will take up newer concepts of condyloma, human papilloma virus, and carcinogenesis.

Morphogenesis

Benign proliferation indicates that the cell's machinery for division has been "revved up." Although the biologic system is perturbed, it is still under control, and will revert to normal if the inciting stimulus is removed or neutralized. Cell division is normally confined to a single layer of basal cells attached to the basement membrane. The daughter cells blossom and mature in an orderly fashion.

However, if something (eg, a virus) causing genetic injury deranges the cells while they are proliferating, they may gradually lose control of basic cellular functions, like division and differentiation, and become neoplastic. The abnormal cells remain mitotic and do not fully differentiate as they rise in the epithelium, ie, the proliferation is disorderly. *Disordered proliferation is the essence of dysplasia* (Greek: bad molding) [35 I6.82, 36 I6.83]. If the abnormality continues to progress, the cells differentiate less and less, gradually losing their squamous features until eventually the full thickness of the epithelium is made up of *undifferentiated*, atypical, basaloid cells. This stage is known as carcinoma in situ [37 I6.84]. *The essential difference between dysplasia and carcinoma in situ is the presence or absence, respectively, of any visible sign of squamous differentiation in the abnormal cells.*

It is believed that the morphology of the squamous lesion depends on the maturity of the epithelium in which the abnormal process occurs [Patten 1978]. Simply stated: *dysplasias basically resemble the benign proliferative reactions*, just as the benign proliferative reactions recapitulate normal maturation and the icons. For example, a dysplasia may arise in, or mimic, immature squamous metaplasia. The dysplastic cells resemble ordinary immature metaplasia but have abnormal nuclei (ie, parabasal-like cells with dysplastic nuclei).

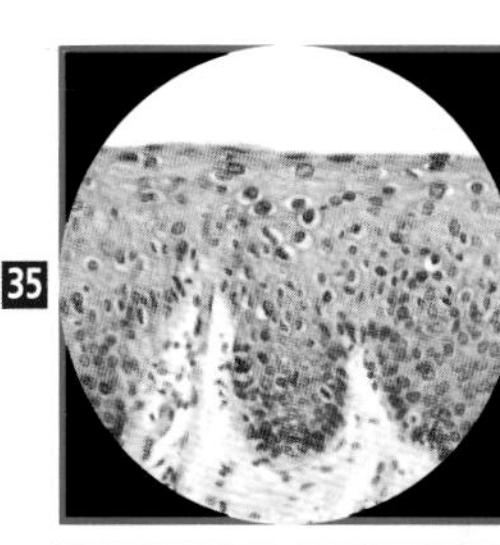

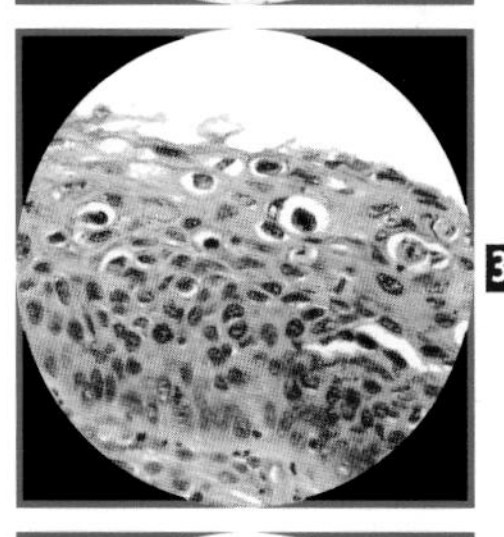

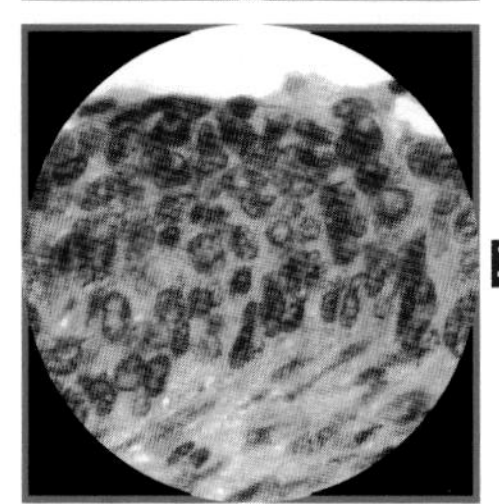

Morphology of Dysplasia and Carcinoma In Situ

The entire thickness of the epithelium is involved by the abnormal process, be it dysplasia or CIS, as it must be in order for the abnormal cells to be sampled at the mucosal surface when the Pap smear is taken. The essential difference between dysplasia and carcinoma in situ is squamous differentiation. Both dysplasia and carcinoma in situ (CIS) are characterized by abnormalities of the nucleus, including its size, shape, and outline, as well as chromatin texture and staining. (Note: Irregular chromatin distribution is a feature associated with invasive carcinoma.) Nucleoli can also be seen, in histologic section, in both dysplasia and CIS. However, they are usually not present in surface cells of either lesion; therefore, nucleoli are not usually seen in the cytology of either dysplasia or CIS, although they may be seen with inflammation as well as infiltrating cancer. Similarly mitotic figures, including atypical forms, are commonly seen in both dysplasia and CIS, in tissue. However, mitotic figures at the mucosal surface are associated with CIS, rather than with dysplasia. Therefore, mitotic figures are usually not seen in dysplastic cells in the Pap smear, but can be seen in CIS. The milieu in which the cells of intraepithelial lesions are found is either clean or inflammatory, but there is no tumor diathesis (which is associated with infiltrating cancer).

Dysplasia

Dysplasia is characterized by the presence of at least some squamous features in the cytoplasm of the abnormal cells [I6.85–I6.88]. The hallmarks of squamous differentiation are dense cytoplasm and distinct cell boundaries. Dysplastic cells in a smear are frequently single or in flat sheets, and the cells have sharply demarcated edges. Nuclear features are paramount in determining whether a cell is dysplastic. Nuclear enlargement and hyperchromasia are key in this determination (remember, compared with the intermediate nucleus, if it's big and it's dark, it's dysplasia) [38 I6.85]. Dysplasias can be graded in severity depending, in essence, on how closely the cells resemble the corresponding type of benign proliferative reaction (and its corresponding icon). The N/C ratio is a measure of the degree of maturity of a cell. The higher the N/C ratio (compared with its appropriate icon cell type) the more advanced the dysplasia. Thus, cells that closely resemble their icon, but have abnormal ("big, dark") nuclei and mildly increased N/C ratios, are mild dysplasia. (Note: Although the largest nuclei are found in mild dysplasia, mildly dysplastic cells have relatively abundant cytoplasm, which tends to preserve the N/C ratio.) Cells that barely resemble their icon, with very abnormal nuclei and very high N/C ratios, but still retain some squamous cytoplasmic features, are severe dysplasia [39 I6.87]. The chromatin in dysplasia is hyperchromatic, evenly distributed, and usually relatively fine, although chromatin clumping may occur. Nuclear membrane irregularities become more pronounced with advancing degrees of dysplasia; thus, severe dysplasia tends to have irregular, "raisinoid" nuclei. The background is clean or inflammatory, with no tumor diathesis.

Cytology of Dysplasia

Cells
- Tend to be single or in loose, flat sheets

Nuclei (big and dark)
- Enlarged and hyperchromatic
- Irregular outline
- Fine to coarse chromatin; regular distribution
- Mitotic figures not seen in cytology

Cytoplasm
- Immature, but squamous
- Increased nuclear/cytoplasmic ratio

Background
- Clean/inflammatory, no diathesis

In general, the more pronounced these features, the more advanced the dysplasia.

Carcinoma In Situ

Carcinoma in situ is the final stage of intraepithelial neoplasia [I6.89, I6.90, 40 I6.91, I6.92]. At this stage, the abnormal cells shed all visible signs of squamous differentiation. The cells of CIS devote most of their energy to cell division, rather than differentiation. In contrast with dysplasia, the undifferentiated cytoplasm characteristic of CIS is delicate, and the cells have ill-defined borders [T6.7]. Three-dimensional syncytial-like aggregates or hyperchromatic crowded groups, which are crowded clusters of disorderly, abnormal cells with hyperchromatic nuclei, are particularly characteristic of CIS. The hyperchromatic crowded groups typically show loss of nuclear polarity or "chaotic architecture," coarse, dark chromatin, and mitotic figures. Ultrastructurally, the aggregates are not true syncytia. The cells remain separate, but closely spaced, and have abundant, densely packed surface microvilli [Rubio 1976, Shingleton 1968, Williams 1973, Younes 1969].

Cytology of Carcinoma In Situ

Cells
- In hyperchromatic crowded groups
- Three-dimensional, syncytial-like aggregates
- Abnormal cells, chaotic architecture

Nuclei
- Similar to high-grade dysplasia
- Mitotic figures, prophase nuclei
- No nucleoli

Cytoplasm
- Undifferentiated, delicate
- High nuclear/cytoplasmic ratios

Background
- Clean/inflammatory, no diathesis

T6.7 **Differentiation of Dysplasia From Carcinoma In Situ**

Dysplasia	Carcinoma In Situ
Histology	
Well-defined basal cell layer	Loss of basal palisade
Some squamous differentiation toward surface	No differentiation
Some horizontal layering (stratification)	± Vertical orientation
Increasing number mitotic figures	More abnormal mitotic figures
Mitotic figures above basal layer	Mitotic figures at surface
Cytology	
Distinct cell boundaries	Syncytial appearance
Dense cytoplasm	Delicate cytoplasm, naked nuclei
Flat sheets, single	Hyperchromatic crowded groups, ± spindle, microacini
Increasing nuclear/cytoplasmic ratio	Maximum nuclear/cytoplasmic ratio
Less irregular nuclear membrane	More irregular nuclear membrane
Finer chromatin*	Coarser chromatin*
Small nucleoli possible (irritation)	Nucleoli suggest microinvasive carcinoma

* Even distribution.

38
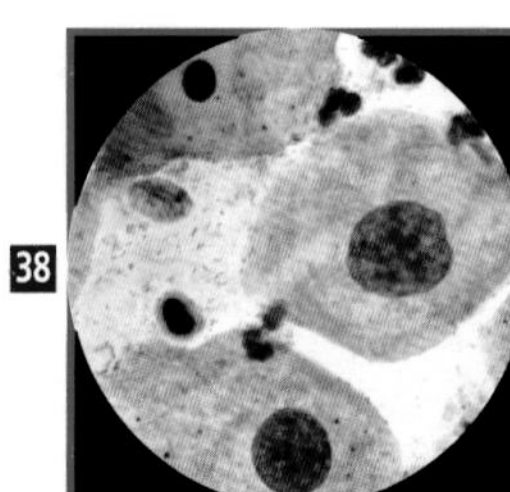

39
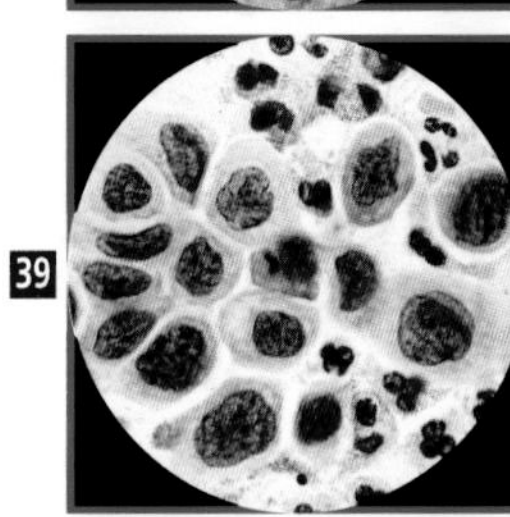

40
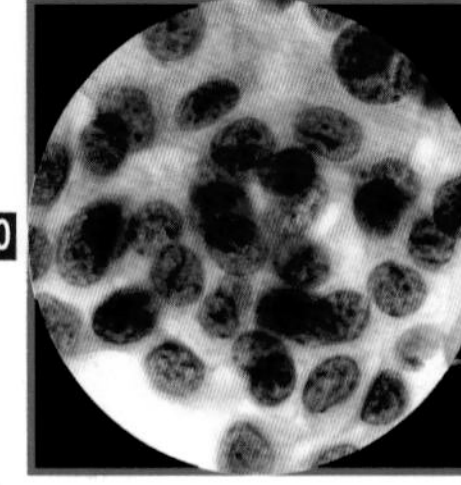

The cells of CIS are relatively small, with scant cytoplasm. The highest N/C ratios are seen in CIS: the cells are composed almost entirely of their nuclei. Nuclear abnormalities, including membrane irregularity and chromatin coarseness, tend to become more pronounced than in dysplasia. Unlike the case in dysplasia, mitotic figures, including prophase nuclei (in which the nuclear envelopes have dissolved for impending cell division), are commonly seen. Naked nuclei, which are probably related to the delicate nature of the undifferentiated cytoplasm, are often seen and provide a clue to the diagnosis of CIS [I6.90]. Oval or spindle-shaped cells may occur in CIS and are apparently caused by rapid proliferation. Rudimentary glandular differentiation (ie, microacini) are commonly seen in the syncytial-like aggregates, a feature that has been associated with endocervical glandular extension [Selvaggi 1994], but may well reflect the dual potential of the reserve cell. Nucleoli are usually sparse or absent in CIS, unless the lesion is inflamed. (Nucleoli may be an ominous finding, suggesting invasion.) The background is clean or inflammatory, with no tumor diathesis.

There is a morphologic similarity between CIS and reserve cell hyperplasia as well as between dysplasia and squamous metaplasia. In reserve cell hyperplasia, the cells are undifferentiated and often appear as syncytia. Undifferentiated cells and syncytia-like aggregates are also characteristic of CIS. In dysplasia and squamous metaplasia, the squamous features are more obvious, resulting in numerous isolated cells with dense cytoplasm and distinct cell boundaries.

Metaplastic and Keratinizing Lesions

There are two important morphologic types of dysplasia: metaplastic and keratinizing. Metaplastic and keratinizing dysplasias arise in, or mimic, the benign proliferative reactions (ie, metaplasia and keratosis), which in turn imitate their corresponding icons (basal, parabasal, intermediate, and superficial cells). Metaplastic dysplasia, by far the more common type, can be further subdivided into immature and mature types. The basic division of carcinoma in situ is simple and based on cell size: small cell, intermediate cell, and large cell. Microinvasive and fully invasive squamous cell carcinomas are considered in succeeding sections.

Metaplastic Lesions

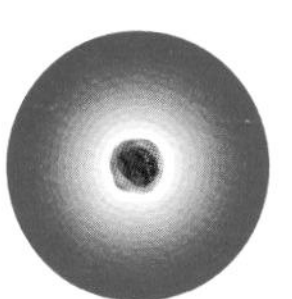

CIN Mimicking Reserve Cell Hyperplasia

Atypical Reserve Cell Hyperplasia: A carcinogenic agent (perhaps a virus) could manifest its presence in cells at the stage of reserve cell hyperplasia [F6.7]. However, reserve cell hyperplasia occurs before the onset of squamous differentiation. Therefore, an abnormality at this early stage of development would not be true squamous dysplasia, since no squamous differentiation ever occurred—ergo, the term atypical reserve cell hyperplasia. However, a lesion composed of atypical reserve cells would be indistinguishable from carcinoma in situ, because reserve cells are undifferentiated (see next section). Thus, reserve cell dysplasia or atypical reserve cell hyperplasia are, essentially, philosophic concepts, rather than actual diagnoses. Note also that atypical reserve cell hyperplasia is sometimes used as a term for cells that suggest small cell carcinoma, but lack complete diagnostic features.

Small Cell Carcinoma In Situ: Small cell carcinoma in situ is composed of atypical, undifferentiated, relatively small cells [**41** I6.91]. These atypical, reserve cell–like cells average 11 µm in diameter. They may be present singly or in characteristic "syncytia" (hyperchromatic crowded groups). The nuclei are usually oval to spindle shaped, with a high mitotic rate. Prophase nuclei are common. The mean nuclear area is about 68 μm^2 (range, 60–80 μm^2), which is about twice the area of an intermediate cell nucleus [Patten 1978]. The chromatin is hyperchromatic and evenly distributed. It is usually coarse, but may be fine, with variable chromocenter formation. Nucleoli are absent, or rare and small.

When small cell carcinoma in situ becomes invasive, it is associated with small cell, or poorly differentiated, nonkeratinizing squamous cell carcinoma, a very aggressive type. (Do not confuse small cell *squamous* cancer with small cell *neuroendocrine* carcinoma, discussed under "Rare Tumors.") Only a minority of cases of CIS are small cell type, and the incidence may be decreasing [Patten 1978].

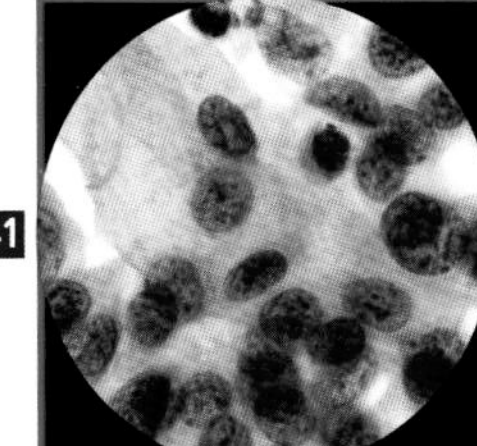

41

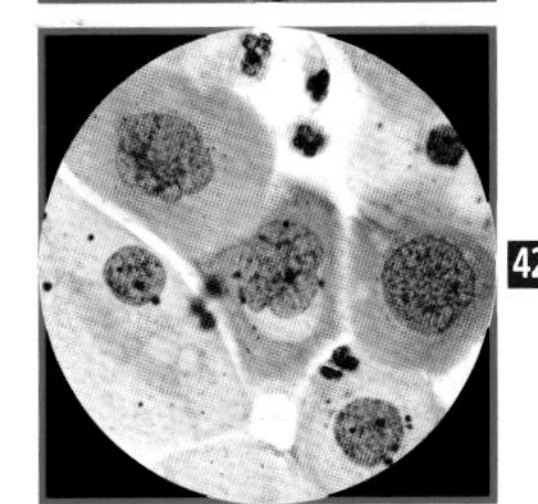

42

F6.7 Morphologic Range of the Basal/Reserve Cell

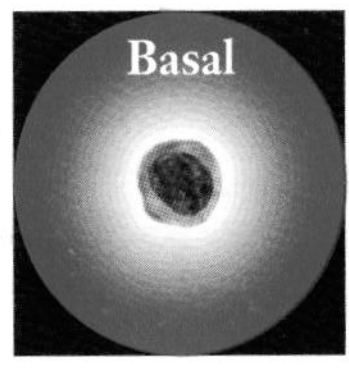

Reserve cell hyperplasia	[Atypical reserve cell hyperplasia]	Small cell carcinoma in situ	Small cell squamous cell carcinoma

CIN Mimicking Immature Squamous Metaplasia

Immature Metaplastic Dysplasia: If the squamous abnormality appears a bit later than reserve cell hyperplasia in the spectrum of proliferative reactions, ie, after squamous differentiation has begun, then this is the beginning of bona fide squamous dysplasia, and is known as immature metaplastic dysplasia, or simply metaplastic dysplasia [F6.8]. Although immature metaplastic dysplasia represents only 10% to 15% of all cases of dysplasia, it is particularly significant because it is the most likely type to progress to classical carcinoma in situ [Patten 1978]. Immature metaplastic dysplasia characteristically arises proximal to the external cervical os, in the endocervical canal.

In essence, immature metaplastic dysplasia resembles immature squamous metaplasia, but has abnormal, dysplastic nuclei [**42** I6.86]. The dysplastic cells usually occur singly, but they can also be seen in loose sheets or in cobblestone arrangements, reminiscent of ordinary immature metaplasia. Also, as in ordinary immature metaplasia, the dysplastic cells are predominantly round to oval, but may also be polygonal. They are parabasal-sized and usually stain blue-green (cyanophilic). The cytoplasm is also typical of immature squamous metaplasia (ie, very dense, with very distinct cell boundaries, the "cookie cutter" look). In contrast with benign metaplasia, however, the nuclei are enlarged and hyperchromatic ("big and dark"). The dysplastic nuclei average 156 ± 35 μm^2, which is about 2.5 to 4 times the size of a normal immature metaplastic cell's nucleus or

F6.8 Morphologic Range of the Parabasal Cell

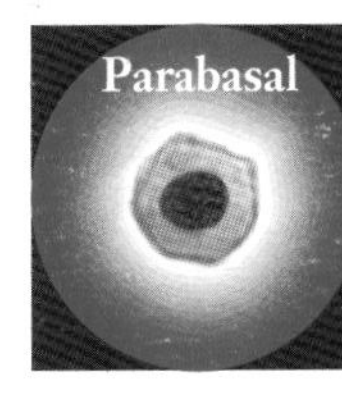

Immature squamous metaplasia	Immature metaplastic dysplasia	Intermediate carcinoma in situ	Non-keratinizing squamous cell carcinoma
	Mild, Moderate, Severe		

3.5 to 5.5 times an intermediate nucleus [Patten 1978]. The chromatin is generally moderately granular—finer than in small cell lesions, but coarser than mature metaplastic (large cell, nonkeratinizing) dysplasia. However, as the degree of dysplasia advances, chromocenter formation occurs, the chromatin progressively coarsens, and the nuclear membranes become more irregular. Nucleoli are usually absent or inconspicuous.

Differential Diagnosis: Diagnosis of metaplastic dysplasias can be challenging. The first diagnostic dilemma is distinguishing ordinary metaplasia from metaplastic dysplasia. Both can be composed of somewhat similar metaplastic cells, including immature nuclear and cytoplasmic features, as well as pleomorphism, increased N/C ratios, and atypical (reactive versus dysplastic) nuclei. Nuclear enlargement can occur in either reactive or dysplastic metaplastic cells but is usually more marked in dysplasia. Although chromatin abnormalities of immature metaplastic dysplasia can be subtle, hyperchromasia, coarse chromatin, or chromocenter formation suggest dysplasia, while fine, pale chromatin and nucleoli suggest a benign, reactive process. The presence of irregular nuclear membranes points to a diagnosis of dysplasia.

Another diagnostic problem is that the cells of high-grade immature metaplastic dysplasia are very small and immature ("very immature metaplastic dysplasia"), and may closely resemble small histiocytes [I6.87, I6.141]. The dysplastic cells sometimes hide in strands of mucus with inflammatory cells, which they may resemble, and can be so well camouflaged that they might be easily missed in screening ("no-see-ums"). Look carefully at strings of cells in mucus, as one does for small "oat" cell carcinoma in sputum. Another diagnostic clue is "like accompanies like." Severe dysplasia will usually be accompanied by lesser degrees of dysplasia (mild, moderate). Paradoxically, these less abnormal cells not only tend to be larger, and therefore easier to find, but their nuclei may be somewhat easier to evaluate (ie, bigger, darker). In contrast, benign immature metaplasia will usually be accompanied by mature metaplasia rather than by dysplasia.

Grading of immature metaplastic dysplasia can also be difficult [43 I6.85, 44 I6.86, 45 I6.87]. The N/C ratio, a measure of cell maturity, is generally one of the most useful parameters in assessing the grade of dysplasia. However, since metaplastic cells are, by definition, immature, ***the N/C ratio is elevated in both ordinary and dysplastic metaplastic cells***. Therefore, critical evaluation of nuclear features is particularly important in grading immature metaplastic dysplasia. Unfortunately, as the degree of dysplasia progresses, the nucleus becomes smaller and therefore may be more difficult to evaluate. Still, the key is that the N/C ratio increases in concert with the nuclear features of advancing dysplasia. For example, severe dysplasia usually has very high N/C ratios and very irregular nuclear membranes ("raisinoid nuclei" [I6.87, I6.141]). Smooth nuclear membranes are generally incongruous in a diagnosis of severe dysplasia.

Intermediate Carcinoma In Situ: Immature metaplastic dysplasia may develop into carcinoma in situ composed of cells

43 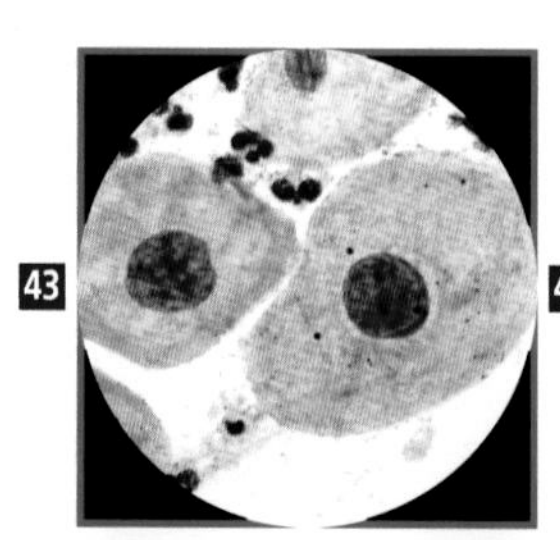 43

44 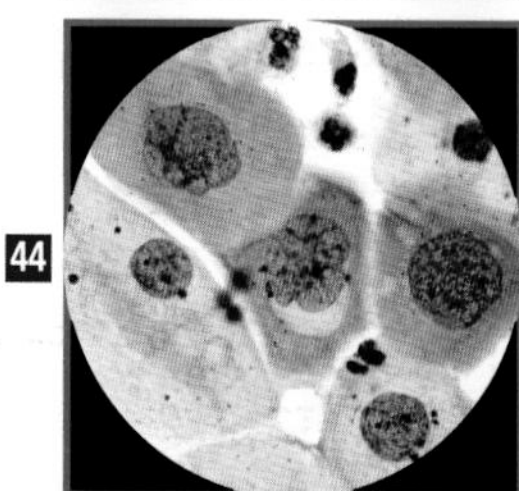

45 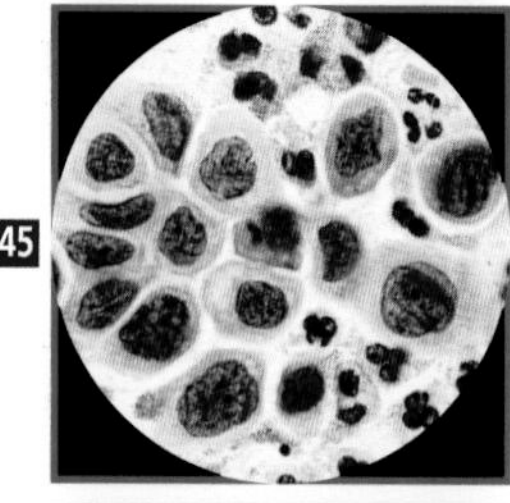

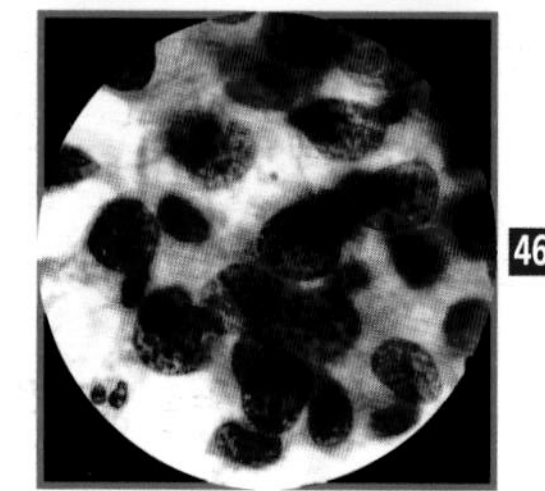 46

intermediate in size between small and large cell carcinoma in situ [46 I6.89]. Intermediate carcinoma in situ is the most common type, accounting for more than half of all cases [Patten 1978]. As usual, syncytia-like aggregates (hyperchromatic crowded groups) are characteristic. The nuclei are round to oval and average about 95 µm² (range, 80–120 µm²), about 2 to 3.5 times the size of an intermediate cell nucleus, or about twice the size of an ordinary metaplastic cell nucleus [Patten 1978]. The chromatin is hyperchromatic with variable texture (usually relatively fine, but occasionally coarse). Chromocenters are variable, too, from few to many. Nucleoli are usually absent, or rare and small. Intermediate carcinoma in situ is associated with nonkeratinizing squamous cell carcinoma when it invades.

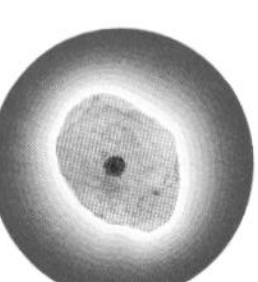

CIN Mimicking Mature Squamous Metaplasia

Mature Metaplastic Dysplasia: Mature metaplastic dysplasia, also known as large cell or nonkeratinizing dysplasia, arises in or mimics a mature squamous metaplastic process or the native nonkeratinizing squamous epithelium [F6.9] [Patten 1978]. The icon for this type of dysplasia is the intermediate cell, which the dysplastic cells resemble [43 I6.85]. Mature metaplastic dysplasia is usually found near the cervical os, in or near the transition zone of the cervix. It is by far the most common pattern of dysplasia, but as might be expected from its high degree of differentiation, the dysplasia is usually mild and is unlikely to progress to carcinoma in situ or cancer, although it can.

Mature metaplastic dysplasia is composed of cells that resemble normal intermediate cells, except that their nuclei are dysplastic (in essence, enlarged and hyperchromatic—big and dark—when compared with the normal intermediate cell nucleus). Nearly all of the cells are single and they usually have polygonal outlines, with well-defined cell borders. Most of the cells stain blue, and a few stain pink, like normal intermediate cells. However, the cytoplasm is somewhat immature and, when compared with that of normal intermediate cells, appears slightly thicker and less abundant. The nuclei are usually only slightly hyperchromatic, but can be darker. The chromatin is usually fine, reminiscent of the normal intermediate cells, with occasional chromocenter formation. Nucleoli are absent or

***F6.9* Morphologic Range of the Intermediate Cell**

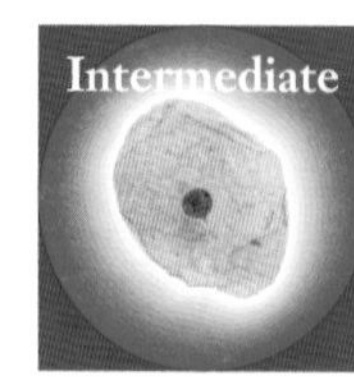

inconspicuous. The nuclei average 178 ± 32 μm², which is 4 to 6 times the size of a normal intermediate cell nucleus [Patten 1978].

When dysplasias progress, the cells become more immature. Thus, as mature metaplastic dysplasia becomes more advanced, it begins to resemble immature metaplastic dysplasia, although the cells may remain relatively large. This merging of features is to be expected, for the lesions represent a morphologic spectrum. This spectrum of morphology is emphasized by the terminology, ie, immature and mature metaplastic dysplasia, as opposed to metaplastic dysplasia and large cell, nonkeratinizing dysplasia, respectively.

Large Cell Carcinoma In Situ: Large cell carcinoma in situ (CIS) [47 I6.155] is the least common type of CIS [Patten 1978]. Like other kinds of classical carcinoma in situ, and in contrast with dysplasia, large cell carcinoma in situ lacks features of squamous differentiation. Although the N/C ratio is elevated, these cells may have somewhat more abundant cytoplasm and may not appear as crowded as other forms of CIS. The cytoplasm is usually cyanophilic, relatively delicate, and appears syncytial. Single cells are rare in large cell carcinoma in situ. The nuclei are abnormal (irregular membranes, loss of polarity, etc), and the chromatin is hyperchromatic, but rather fine, with variable chromocenter formation. The nuclei average about 164 μm² (range, 150–200 μm²) or about four to six times the size of an intermediate cell nucleus [Patten 1978]. Nucleoli are usually absent, or rare and small. With invasion, both intermediate and large cell CIS are associated with nonkeratinizing squamous cell carcinoma.

Keratinizing Lesions

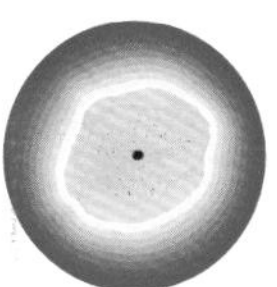

CIN Mimicking Keratosis

Keratinizing Dysplasia: Keratinizing dysplasia, and keratinizing squamous cell carcinoma which is associated with it, arises in or mimics the hyperdifferentiated benign proliferative reaction, keratosis [F6.10]. Keratinizing dysplasia tends to arise distal to the cervical os, in the ectocervical epithelium. It is less common than the metaplastic types of dysplasia, previously discussed [Patten 1978].

F6.10 **Morphologic Range of the Superficial Cell**

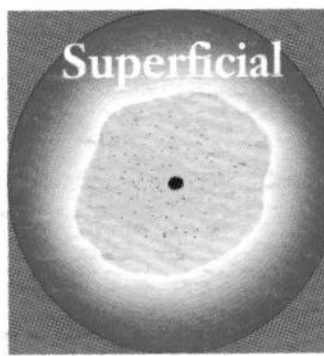

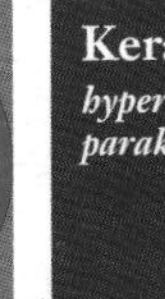

Keratosis *hyperkeratosis, parakeratosis*	Keratinizing dysplasia	No classical carcinoma in situ — *severe keratinizing dysplasia is equivalent*	Keratinizing squamous cell carcinoma
	Mild, Moderate, Severe		

47 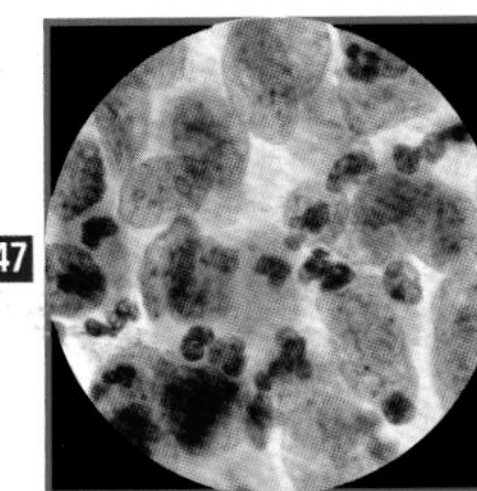

48 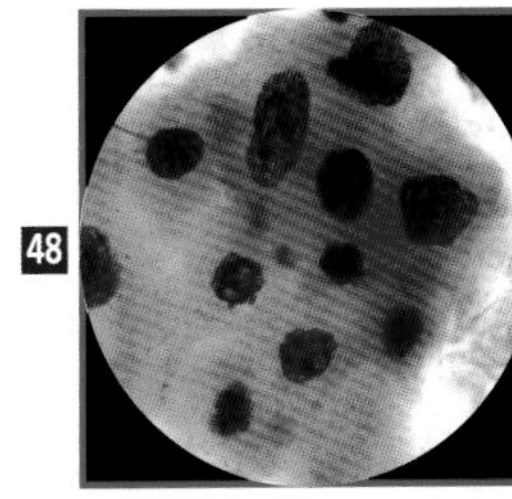

49 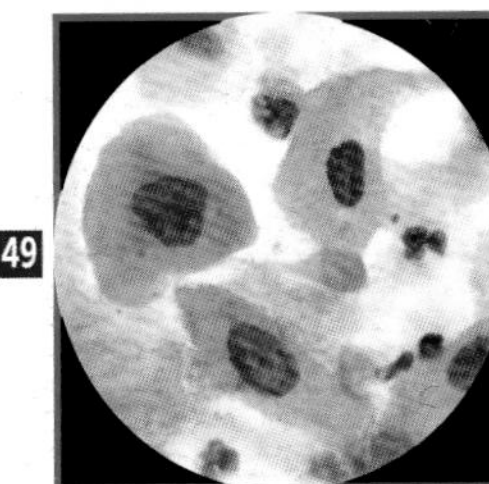

The morphology of keratinizing dysplasia echoes the morphology of the normal superficial cell, consisting of cells with dense, sometimes orangeophilic cytoplasm, and very hyperchromatic, sometimes pyknotic, nuclei [48 I6.75, 49 I6.88]. Despite the image conjured up by the word "keratinizing," orangeophilic cells may be a minor, although characteristic, component of keratinizing dysplasia. Blue, pink, or polychromatic cells are also seen. The cells are mostly single, with occasional sheets. Many of the cells, particularly in low-grade lesions, have well-defined, polygonal outlines, like normal superficial cells. As the degree of dysplasia becomes more advanced, the cells become pleomorphic (a characteristic feature), with tadpole, spindle, and irregularly shaped cells, eventually resembling keratinizing squamous cell carcinoma. Thus, a synonym for keratinizing dysplasia is pleomorphic dysplasia.

The majority of nuclei have relatively fine, but very hyperchromatic, uniform chromatin. Perhaps surprisingly, very coarse chromatin is not a common feature of keratinizing dysplasia. Pyknotic nuclei are characteristic, but are seen in only about 15% of the cells [Patten 1978]. Other signs of nuclear degeneration (eg, karyorrhexis or lysis) may also occur. The nuclei average about 169 ± 42 μm² or 3.5 to 6 times the area of an intermediate cell nucleus [Patten 1978].

Keratinizing dysplasia, which arises in the milieu of keratosis, is usually accompanied by hyperkeratosis, parakeratosis, or atypical parakeratosis [I6.76]. It may be difficult to distinguish severe keratinizing dysplasia from invasive keratinizing squamous cell carcinoma, because degenerated, pyknotic nuclei mask the typical nuclear features of cancer and a tumor diathesis may be lacking in a keratinizing squamous cell carcinoma (since the tumor tends to grow exophytically).

Keratinizing Carcinoma In Situ: By definition, the atypical cells of these dysplastic keratinized lesions always have a keratinized cytoplasm. Therefore, since keratinization is the sine qua non of squamous differentiation, there cannot be a classical keratinizing CIS, because classical CIS requires undifferentiated cells. Thus, severe keratinizing dysplasia is the direct precursor lesion of invasive keratinizing squamous cell carcinoma and can invade directly without going through a classical CIS stage. In fact, however, invasive cancer can arise from *any* degree, or type, of dysplasia, including mild, but it is much more *likely* to arise from advanced dysplasia and particularly, CIS. Severe keratinizing dysplasia can be considered the equivalent of classical CIS and both are grouped as cervical intraepithelial neoplasia, grade III.

The various types of dysplasia often coexist in one patient. The more serious lesions tend to occur farther up in the endocervical canal, especially in postmenopausal women, where the dysplasia seen in the Pap smear may be only the "tip of the iceberg" of a more advanced lesion, including invasive cancer.

Microinvasive Squamous Cell Carcinoma

As intraepithelial neoplasia progresses, the nucleus and cytoplasm are reverting to a more and more primitive state, the cells giving up the commitment to mature and giving in to the urge to reproduce. As the cells invade through the basement membrane into the cervical stroma, both nuclear and cytoplasmic changes occur. As one of the earliest visible changes, a nucleolus develops in carcinoma in situ–like cells—a nonspecific marker of increased protein synthesis. The appearance of nucleoli heralds the beginning of invasion (microinvasion) as the cells gear up to make these proteins, possibly including a "basement membranase." Then the chromatin, which has been becoming progressively coarser during the intraepithelial phase, begins to break up into shards, changing from regular to irregular in distribution. Irregularly distributed chromatin, with parachromatin clearing, is the first truly malignant morphologic change that can be recognized in the cell.

The cytoplasm is also undergoing changes with incipient invasion. In carcinoma in situ, the cytoplasm is undifferentiated. Paradoxically, with progression of carcinoma in situ to invasive cancer, the abnormal cells redifferentiate. The cytoplasm "plumps up" a little, reacquiring squamoid features. The cellular changes can be viewed as an unfolding from carcinoma in situ to microinvasion to frank carcinoma: invasive cancer germinates from seeds of carcinoma in situ. As invasion progresses, the cells become differentiated to varying degrees: poorly differentiated or small cell squamous cell carcinoma, moderately differentiated or nonkeratinizing squamous cell carcinoma, and well-differentiated or keratinizing squamous cell carcinoma. With deep invasion, the stroma is broken down, the surface ulcerates, and bleeding occurs, which results in protein, fibrin, fresh and old blood, dead cells, and debris in the background of the smear. This composes the tumor diathesis that is so characteristic of invasive cancer.

Microinvasive carcinoma is a gray area between carcinoma in situ and fully invasive squamous cell carcinoma [T6.8]. Unlike carcinoma in situ, microinvasive carcinoma is invasive. However, unlike frank cancer, microinvasive carcinoma is associated with a very low mortality rate (0%–5%). Therefore, microinvasive carcinoma can be treated more conservatively than frankly invasive carcinoma. Unfortunately, the exact definition of microinvasive carcinoma remains controversial, with both its beginning and end points in dispute. The Society of Gynecologic Oncologists suggests that questionable stromal invasion should be regarded as carcinoma in situ [Seski 1977]. Other authors arbitrarily set the deepest limits of microinvasion of the stroma between 1 and 5 mm, or even deeper [Larsson 1983]. Lymph node metastases are rare or nonexistent with less than 1 mm of invasion but occur in proportion to greater depth of invasion, increasing to 11.1% at 5 mm [Ng 1969, van Nagell 1983].

The two most widely used definitions of microinvasive carcinoma are those of the Society of Gynecologic Oncologists (SGO) and the International Federation of Gynecology and Obstetrics (FIGO) [T6.9]. The SGO limits depth of penetration to 3 mm or less, with no vascular space involvement by tumor [Seski 1977]. FIGO divides microinvasive carcinoma into two groups [FIGO 1986]. FIGO Stage Ia1 exhibits "minimal" stromal invasion (usually taken to mean microinvasive "buds," which are not specifically defined, but generally regarded as less than 1 mm deep). FIGO Stage Ia2 limits invasion to 5 mm or less with less than 7 mm in horizontal spread.

Invasion is measured from the base of the epithelium, at the basement membrane, where invasion begins, which could be from a gland [Ostor 1993b]. (Note: This is in contrast to melanomas, which are measured from the granular cell layer of the overlying epithelium.) Histologic features that help to determine prognosis are: depth of invasion, lateral extent, extension into vascular spaces, growth pattern, and host immune response (inflammation). Confluence of tumor growth is important insofar as it affects the overall extent of the tumor. Confluence generally correlates with the depth of invasion [Robert 1990].

Clinical Features: As part of the general trend in earlier cervical cancer detection, microinvasive carcinoma is being recognized with increasing frequency. Currently, as many as a quarter of all squamous cell carcinomas are microinvasive when first diagnosed, depending upon the patient population and whether the 3 or 5 mm criterion is used. Cytology is critical in the detection of this disease because up to two thirds of the patients are asymptomatic, many symptoms are nonspecific, and more than half of the patients have a grossly normal appearing cervix. However, about one third of the patients present with more specific symptoms, eg, abnormal bleeding or vaginal discharge [Kolstad 1989, Larsson 1983, Ng 1969].

***T6.8* Differential Diagnostic Features of Carcinoma In Situ, Microinvasive Carcinoma, and Squamous Cell Carcinoma**

	Nucleus		Cytoplasm	Background
	Prominent Nucleoli	Irregular Chromatin Distribution	Squamous Differentiation	Tumor Diathesis
Carcinoma in situ	(–)	(–)	(–)	(–)
Microinvasive carcinoma	(+)	(+)	(±)	(±)
Squamous cell carcinoma	(++)	(++)	(++)	(++)

***T6.9* Criteria for Microinvasive Carcinoma**

Definition	Maximum Depth	Vascular Space	Horizontal Space
SGO	3 mm	(–)	NA
FIGO	5 mm	NA	<7 mm

SGO = Society of Gynecologic Oncologists, FIGO = International Federation of Gynecology and Obstetrics.

The mean age at diagnosis of microinvasive carcinoma is midway between that of CIN III/CIS and fully invasive cancer, with each step taking nearly a decade to evolve (eg, CIN III–30, MicroCA–39, SCC–47) [Ng 1969, Paraskevaidis 1992]. More than half the cases occur in the anterior portion of the cervix, another third involve both the anterior and posterior cervix, while the posterior cervix alone is involved in only about 10% of cases, a distribution similar to cervical intraepithelial neoplasia [Ng 1969].

Histology: When the neoplastic cells penetrate the basement membrane invasion has occurred [50 I6.95]. As the tumor begins to invade the stroma the contour of the lesion becomes irregular. A host response to the infiltrating tumor is usually seen histologically and includes (1) local desmoplasia with edematous, young collagen (which is metachromatic) and (2) a chronic inflammatory reaction, which may include granuloma formation. These features are clues to the presence of a focus of invasion, histologically, but are weak or absent in some cases [Ostor 1993b]. In contrast to intraepithelial neoplasia, squamous pearls may be seen at the base of the epithelium (so-called paradoxical maturation). Paradoxical maturation is both a common and an early feature of microinvasion. The infiltrating cells begin to differentiate and accumulate eosinophilic cytoplasm. Keratinized cells abutting stroma also indicate invasion. Giant bizarre cells, large keratinized cells, keratin pearls, and necrosis all suggest invasion [Leung 1994]. Microinvasion usually (90% of cases) arises from the surface epithelium, with or without involvement of the glands. Only a minority of cases of microinvasion (<10%) are limited to the glands [Ng 1969]. There are usually (>90% of cases) two or more foci of invasion [Ng 1969]. The epithelial surface is often ulcerated in microinvasive carcinoma.

In nearly 95% of cases in which a determination can be made, the origin of the invasion is carcinoma in situ with or without dysplasia. *Invasive carcinoma almost always arises from the most advanced intraepithelial abnormalities, usually classical carcinoma in situ.* However, a few cases arise from dysplasia, and a very rare case has a histologically normal surface [Ng 1969].

Cytology: Microinvasive carcinoma is the bridge between in situ and fully invasive squamous cell carcinoma [51 I6.93, 52 I6.94]. The cells are changing from being merely neoplastic to frankly malignant. As an evolving process, microinvasive carcinoma presents a spectrum of morphologic findings. At the beginning, the cells closely resemble carcinoma in situ, but the deeper the invasion, the more microinvasive carcinoma resembles frank cancer.

"Syncytial" carcinoma in situ–like aggregates of crowded cells (hyperchromatic, crowded groups) are common in microinvasive carcinoma. There are also many single cells. The earliest cytologic change is the development of prominent nucleoli in the otherwise characteristic "syncytia": nucleoli are the harbingers of microinvasion [51 I6.93] [Patten 1978]. Therefore, it is important to examine all carcinoma in situ–like "syncytial" aggregates for prominent nucleoli, which are found in up to 25% of the abnormal cells in microinvasive carcinoma, depending on the depth of invasion. There are also many inconspicuous nucleoli or micronucleoli.

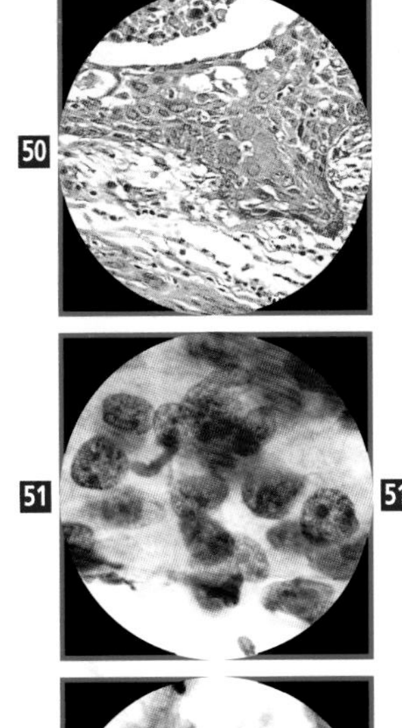

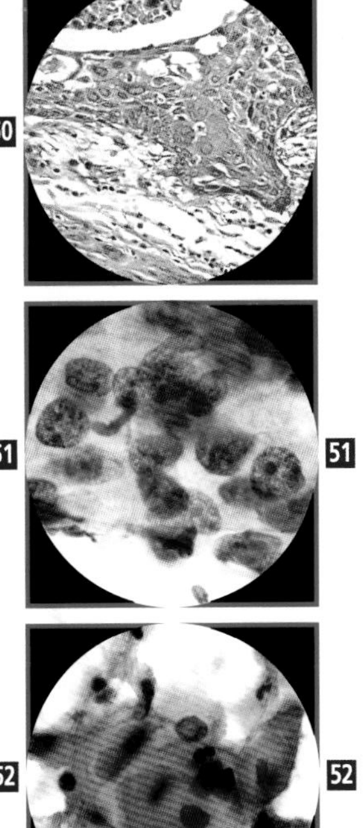

The nuclei average about $88 \pm 39.2\ \mu m^2$ in area, or about 1.5 to 3.5 times the size of an intermediate cell nucleus [Patten 1978]. The chromatin varies from fine to coarse; chromocenter formation is variable. A cytologic hallmark of the essential change to a fully malignant lesion is irregular chromatin distribution, a truly malignant feature of cells. It may be very subtle in the beginning [51 I6.93]. (Try the "four quadrant test" of chromatin distribution: mentally divide the nucleus into quarters—does each quarter have the same amount of chromatin?)

The first cells that invade the stroma are characterized by accumulating dense, acidophilic cytoplasm (apparent keratinization), ie, they "redifferentiate" from the undifferentiated state of carcinoma in situ [52 I6.94]. Differentiation is minimal at first, but becomes progressively more prominent with deeper invasion [F6.11]. The differentiated cells are larger than carcinoma in situ cells, with increased amounts of acidophilic cytoplasm, and lower N/C ratios. They are also more pleomorphic and may show abnormally heavy keratinization.

The deeper the invasion, the more the cytologic picture looks like frank cancer, including the presence of a host response, the tumor diathesis, which is characteristic of fully invasive carcinoma. Also, the greater the horizontal spread, the more the lesion resembles frank cancer [Sugimori 1987]. The cytologic features of microinvasive carcinoma are the most distinctive at 3 mm of invasion. Shallower invasion resembles carcinoma in situ, but by 5 mm of penetration, many cases of microinvasive carcinoma are cytologically indistinguishable from clear-cut cancer.

The preponderance (~80%) of cases of microinvasive carcinoma are nonkeratinizing squamous cell carcinoma, some are

F6.11 **Nucleoli in Microinvasive Carcinoma**

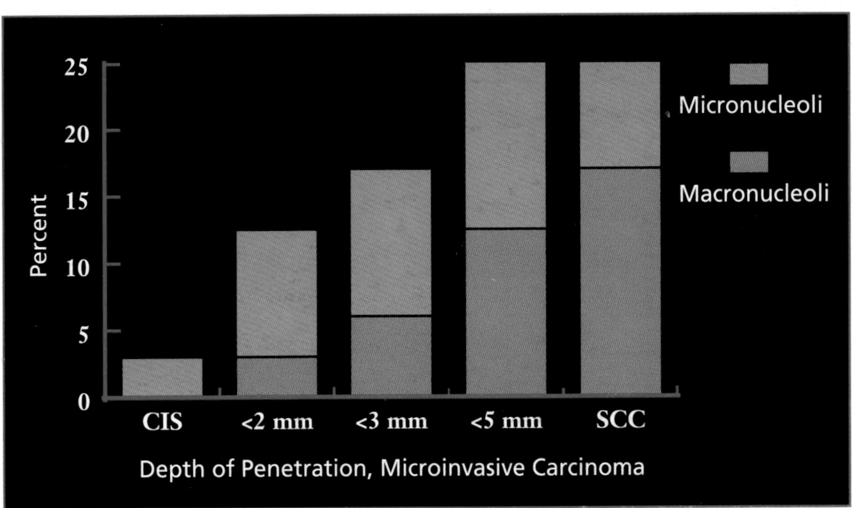

[Ng 1969]

Cytology of Microinvasive Carcinoma

Cells
- Syncytia (hyperchromatic crowded groups)
- Pleomorphism with (abnormal) differentiation

Nucleus
- Nucleoli (up to 25%, micro- and macro-)
- Irregular chromatin distribution

Cytoplasm
- More abundant than carcinoma in situ
- Acidophilic, ± evidence of keratinization

Background
- Diathesis (up to 35% of cases at 5 mm)

keratinizing (~15%), and a few are small cell (~5%) [F6.12] [Larsson 1983, Ng 1972, Tweeddale 1969]. Keratinizing microinvasive carcinoma may have the best prognosis [Larsson 1983].

The cytologic diagnosis of microinvasive carcinoma cannot be considered definitive. Although retrospective series have reported remarkable diagnostic accuracy (nearly 90%) [W Johnston 1982, Ng 1972, Nguyen 1984a], microinvasive carcinoma is ultimately a histologic, not a cytologic, diagnosis. In practice, in up to one third of cases there is neither cytologic nor colposcopic suspicion of invasion [Paraskevaidis 1992]. Conversely, virtually any of the features of microinvasive carcinoma, including prominent nucleoli, irregular chromatin, and a necrotic background, can be seen from time to time in noninvasive lesions, particularly when obtained by the endocervical brush [Covell 1992]. For therapeutic purposes the diagnosis must be based, at a minimum, on thorough examination of an adequate cone biopsy (the margins must be free of disease). The most important contribution of the cytology of microinvasive carcinoma is to detect the presence of a possibly invasive lesion. When microinvasion is suspected, a useful cytologic diagnosis is "carcinoma in situ, invasion not excluded." When microinvasive carcinoma is suspected cytologically, colposcopy and biopsy are the next appropriate steps.

Differential Diagnosis: Again, the lesion of microinvasive carcinoma must be differentiated from carcinoma in situ and fully invasive cancer. Nucleoli in carcinoma in situ–like syncytial-like aggregates are the most sensitive feature to the presence of invasion. However, *nucleoli are not specific for invasion.* For example, inflamed carcinoma in situ may show nucleoli. The presence of both nucleoli and irregular chromatin distribution is more specific for invasive malignancy. Frank squamous cell carcinoma shows more abnormal cells, with more pleomorphism, more irregular chromatin, and more prominent nucleoli, as well as a tumor diathesis in most cases.

Nonkeratinizing microinvasive carcinoma may have three-dimensional groups of cells with relatively delicate (ie, nonkeratinized) cytoplasm and many prominent nucleoli. These features may resemble those of adenocarcinoma. Furthermore, squamous carcinoma in situ may show rudimentary glandular structures (microacini), which further heighten the resemblance to adenocarcinoma [Selvaggi 1994]. Well-formed glands, columnar cells, and evidence of mucin production indicate true glandular differentiation. Some tumors are mixed adenosquamous carcinoma.

Since squamoid features of the cytoplasm are relatively common in microinvasive carcinoma, ordinary squamous dysplasia also enters into the differential diagnosis. However, in dysplasia, the chromatin is regularly distributed and nucleoli are usually absent. Furthermore, evidence of *heavy* cytoplasmic keratinization, which may be seen in either microinvasive carcinoma or fully invasive cancer, is usually not a feature of dysplasia. Finally, an inflammatory background (inflammatory diathesis) can closely mimic a tumor diathesis, in which case the key to the correct diagnosis is the presence (or absence) of definitive tumor cells. (For diathesis, see "Squamous Cell Carcinoma," p 83.)

According to an older study, the average age of patients with stromal penetration of less than 1 mm is 42.8 years; for <3 mm, 46.7 years; and for <5 mm, 50.3 years [Ng 1969]. This suggests that the tumor infiltrates at the rate of roughly about 0.5 mm per year, at least in the beginning. Early invasion may be reversible in some cases [Wentz 1962, Reagan 1967] because the immune system may work to eradicate foci of invasive carcinoma. This might even be a frequent event [Patten 1978].

A characteristic feature of invasion is cytoplasmic differentiation of the invasive cells. The differentiation of the invasive vanguard of cells resembles keratinization, but is actually due to increased production of contractile protein filaments consistent with actin and myosin [Genadry 1978], which like keratin filaments, are acidophilic. These contractile proteins are important in cell motility, hence, they could also be significant in invasion of the stroma. However, after invasion has been established, the cells undergo true squamous differentiation to varying degrees, although the invasive vanguard continues to make contractile proteins.

Therapy: Therapy for microinvasive carcinoma is as controversial as its definition. T6.10 gives a general idea of the extent of surgery. Depth of stromal penetration is but one

F6.12 **Percent of Neoplastic Cells Relating to the Depth of Stromal Penetration**

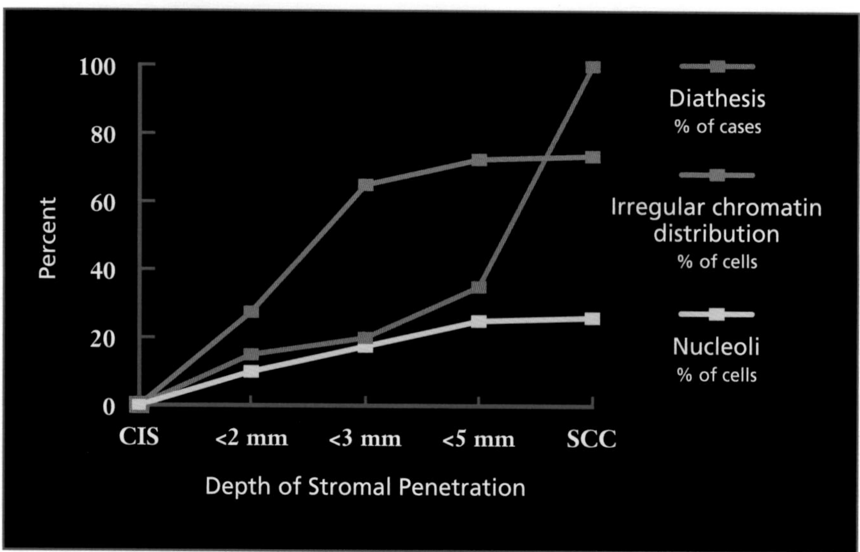

Note: Features of squamous differentiation also develop [Ng 1969, 1972]. At <1 mm, microcarcinoma resembles CIS [Nguyen 1984a], and at >5 mm, frank SCC. A diathesis is not always present in invasive SCC.

T6.10 **Therapy for Microinvasive Carcinoma**

	Extent	(+) LN	Therapy	Mortality
FIGO Ia1	<1 mm*	<1%	Cone biopsy	0
SGO	≤3 mm	~1%–2%	Hysterectomy†	≤1%
FIGO Ia2	≤5 mm	~6%–7%	Individualized	≤5%

[W Benson 1977, Burghardt 1991, Creasman 1985, Robert 1990]
* Not defined—see text.
† Simple hysterectomy; also cone biopsy with margins.

aspect of complete evaluation of the lesion. Other important factors to be considered in recommending appropriate therapy include horizontal extent or volume, confluence, vascular invasion, histologic type, and margins of cone biopsy.

There are relative indications for more extensive surgery in microinvasive carcinoma: (1) extensive or multifocal disease, (2) extensive tumor confluence, (3) true vascular involvement, especially away from the tumor, (4) positive margins in (cone) biopsy, (5) cell type (small cell, adenosquamous, etc), and (6) tumor differentiation (especially poorly differentiated adenocarcinoma or mixed).

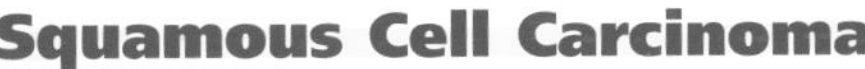

Squamous Cell Carcinoma

Squamous cell carcinoma is being diagnosed at earlier stages today than in the past, thanks to the Pap smear [J Carmichael 1984, Pretorius 1991]. As many as one quarter of cases of squamous cell carcinoma are only microinvasive at the time of diagnosis. The great preponderance (perhaps 90%) of cases are stage I or II at the time of discovery, at least in other than tertiary care hospitals. More than half of the patients are either asymptomatic or have only nonspecific symptoms, an ominous one being abnormal bleeding. Cytology plays an important role in recognizing patients with cervical cancer, but, unfortunately, by the time the patient has developed invasive cancer, the important early battle (ie, detecting preinvasive disease) has already been lost.

The cellular features are similar to microinvasive carcinoma, but more developed. The cells are fully malignant and show typical malignant features [53 I6.96, 54 I6.99; T6.11].

Tumor Diathesis

Granular background
Blood: Fresh and, particularly, old (hemosiderin)
Fibrin and protein deposits
Tissue necrosis and debris
Nuclear and cytoplasmic fragments
Fewer WBCs than in inflammatory background
Note: Variable in amount and composition

A tumor diathesis represents the host response to the invading tumor, as the stroma breaks down and bleeds [55 I6.100]. The presence of a tumor diathesis is one of the key features in the diagnosis of fully invasive carcinoma. The diathesis can be spread diffusely in the background of the smear or may only be focally present around tumor cells. In the absence of a diathesis (clean background), fully invasive carcinoma is less likely, but can occur, particularly with exophytic tumors or metastases.

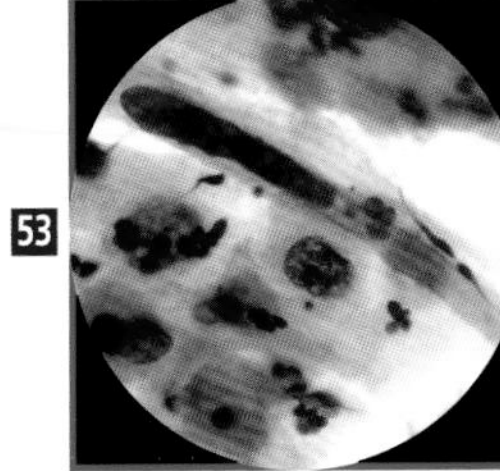
53

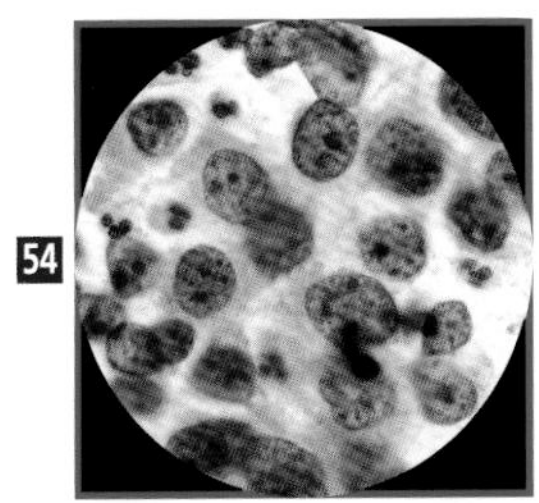
54

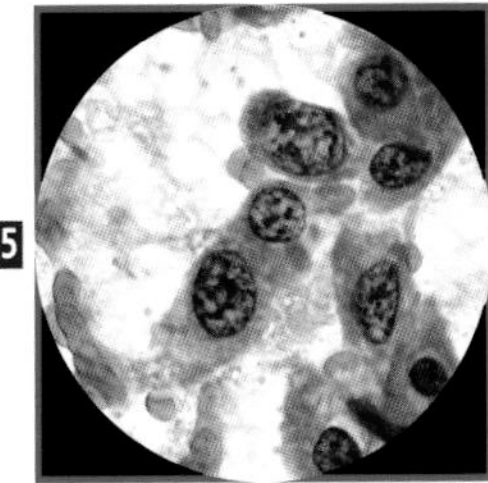
55

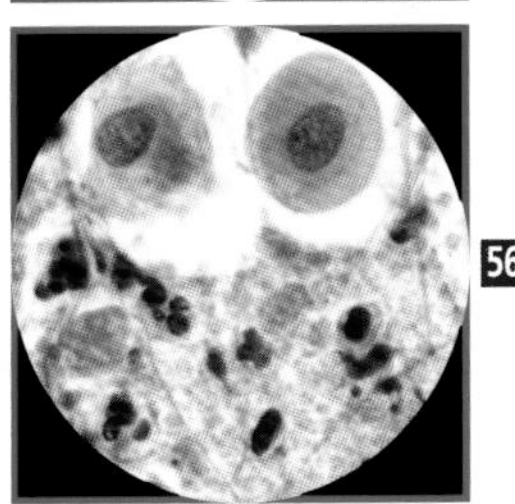
56

Although the presence of a diathesis is suspicious for infiltrating cancer, a diathesis alone is insufficient evidence to make a firm diagnosis of cancer: malignant cells must also be present. Several different benign processes can be associated with a background similar in appearance to a tumor diathesis ("benign diathesis"). For example, an inflammatory, dirty background may be seen in severe infections, particularly *Trichomonas* or herpes. A granular background resembling a diathesis is also common in severely atrophic smears from postmenopausal women [56 I6.9]. Abundant bacteria, especially cocci, can also produce a blue, granular background, mimicking a tumor diathesis. The key to differentiating a benign diathesis from a malignant diathesis is the absence of cancer cells despite careful search.

Benign Diathesis

Severe infection, eg, Trichomonas, herpes
Pyometra
Cervical stenosis
Abscess
Necrotic, ulcerated polyp
Severe atrophy
Coccoid bacteria
Key to differential diagnosis: presence or absence of cancer cells.

The prognosis of squamous cell carcinoma is primarily related to the extent of the tumor (stage) and also its type (small cell, keratinizing, or nonkeratinizing). Mixtures of nonkeratinizing and keratinizing squamous cell carcinoma are also common. The Broders' grade of squamous cancer of the cervix is of less importance in the prognosis than it is in adenocarcinoma of the cervix.

Although reported rates vary, up to one third of cases of cervical carcinoma either have a glandular component (adenosquamous carcinoma) or are pure adenocarcinomas (see "Endocervical Carcinoma," p 127). Small cell (squamous) carcinoma is a poorly differentiated, nonkeratinizing carcinoma. However, other types of small cell carcinomas, including poorly differentiated neuroendocrine carcinomas, also occur in the cervix. While it is agreed that small cell squamous carcinoma usually has the worst prognosis of the squamous cancers, there is disagreement over the prognosis of keratinizing as opposed to nonkeratinizing squamous cell carcinoma. In most body sites, keratinizing squamous cell carcinoma is associated with better differentiation and therefore, a better prognosis. However, because the cervical epithelium is normally nonkeratinizing, an argument could be put forward that nonkeratinizing squamous cell carcinomas are the better differentiated at this site [Wentz 1965]. Although the issue remains unresolved, most observers today believe there is no

Prognostic Factors for Cervical Carcinoma

Stage
- Local extent
- Vascular invasion
- Metastases

Cell type and subtype
- Squamous (large or small)
- Adenocarcinoma (origin)
- Sarcoma (type)

Broders' grade
- (Adenocarcinoma > SCC)

T6.11 General Cellular Features of Squamous Cell Carcinoma

- Single cells, loose aggregates
- Variation of features from cell to cell
- Tadpole, spindle, or heavily keratinized cells
- Nuclei
  - Average smaller than in dysplasia
    - (50–120 μm² for SCC vs 120–210 μm² for dysplasia)
  - Pleomorphic (size/shape)
  - Irregular membranes
  - Chromatin abnormalities
    - Irregular distribution
    - Increased coarseness
    - Parachromatin clearing
  - Nucleoli
    - Increased size and number
    - Irregular shapes
- Tumor diathesis
- Often associated with dysplasia/carcinoma in situ

significant prognostic difference between nonkeratinizing and keratinizing squamous cell carcinoma.

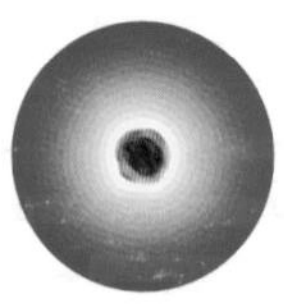

Small Cell Squamous Carcinoma

Small cell squamous carcinoma is a form of poorly differentiated nonkeratinizing squamous cell carcinoma [57 I6.102; T6.12]. (Note that not all poorly differentiated squamous cell carcinomas are small cell type.) At first glance, the cells may actually appear relatively uniform due to their small size. However, close inspection reveals that within this small size range, the cells are actually fairly pleomorphic. Characteristically, many cells are oval or spindle shaped. Syncytial-like aggregates are common. The cytoplasm is scant and evidence of keratinization is absent or minimal. The N/C ratio is very high; the cell is composed almost entirely of its nucleus. The average nuclear area is 65 ± 13 μm², which is about 1.5 to 2 times the size of an intermediate cell nucleus [Patten 1978]. The chromatin is usually coarse and very hyperchromatic. Occasional cases display fine chromatin, and pyknotic nuclei can also be seen. Nucleoli are present, but not prominent, and may be difficult to appreciate due to the small size and dense chromatin structure of the nucleus. Paradoxically, nucleoli may be more easily appreciated in microinvasive, than in fully invasive, small cell carcinoma. Naked nuclei may be present, and mitotic figures may be numerous. A tumor diathesis is seen in the background of the smear (see "Small Cell Cervical Cancers" in "Cytology of Rare Tumors").

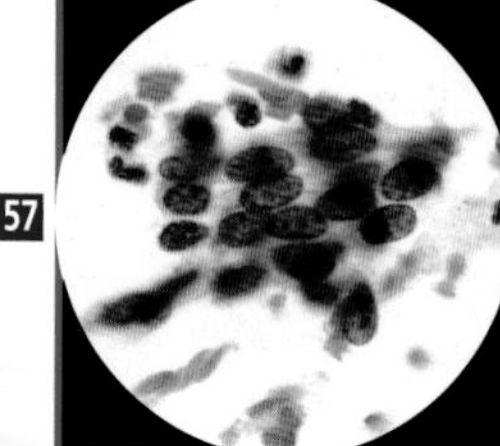

57

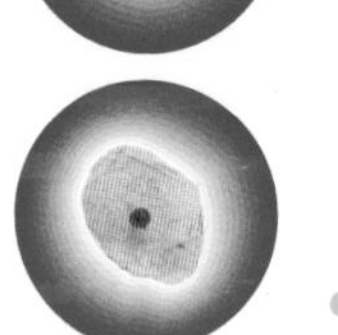

Nonkeratinizing Squamous Cell Carcinoma

Nonkeratinizing squamous cell carcinoma, sometimes also known as large cell nonkeratinizing or moderately differentiated squamous cell carcinoma, is associated with the pathways of either immature or mature metaplastic dysplasia (ie, intermediate and large cell carcinoma in situ, respectively). Nonkeratinizing squamous cell carcinoma is the most common type of cancer of the cervix. Histologically, nonkeratinizing squamous cancer usually invades with a pushing margin [I6.101].

Cytologically, apparent syncytia, as well as naked nuclei, are most common in this variant of squamous cell carcinoma [T6.12]. Nonkeratinizing squamous cell carcinoma is composed of medium to large cells: the size of the cells varies from case to case, but in any given case they are relatively uniform [I6.99, I6.100]. Marked cellular pleomorphism, including bizarre cells, is more characteristic of keratinizing squamous cell carcinoma.

The nuclei are rounded and relatively large. The nuclear area is 88 ± 30 μm², which is about two to three times the size of an intermediate cell nucleus [Patten 1978]. The hallmark of malignancy in these cells is the coarse, irregularly distributed chromatin. The chromatin particles vary considerably in size. Nucleoli are frequent and large, and some are irregular. Most cells are cyanophilic. Occasionally, individual cells may keratinize. The presence of a few of these "dyskeratotic" cells does not change the diagnosis to keratinizing squamous cell carcinoma. However, no pearls are seen in pure nonkeratinizing squamous cell carcinoma. A tumor diathesis is usually present.

Differential Diagnosis: Nonkeratinizing squamous cell carcinoma must be differentiated from a benign reparative process. Both have large cells, with altered N/C ratios, and macronucleoli, which can be multiple and irregular. However, in contrast with cancer, reparative cells (repair) occur in flat, cohesive, well-ordered sheets, with few single cells. The chro-

T6.12 Characteristic Features of Squamous Cell Carcinomas

	Small Cell SCC	Nonkeratinizing SCC	Keratinizing SCC
Background			
Diathesis	(+)	(+)	(±)
Arrangements			
Single	(+)	(+)	(++)
"Syncytia"	(+)	(++)	(+)
Cells			
Size	Small	Medium	Large
Variance	Apparently uniform	Relatively uniform	Pleomorphic
Shape	Oval	Round	Spindle/bizarre
Cytoplasm			
Density	Delicate	Moderate	Dense
Stain	Basophilic	Cyanophilic	Orange
Nucleus			
Chromatin	Very coarse	Moderately coarse	Pyknotic
Macronucleus	(+)	(++)	(±)

matin of repair is neither hyperchromatic nor coarse, and a tumor diathesis is not present.

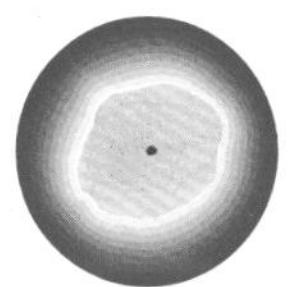

Keratinizing Squamous Cell Carcinoma

Keratinizing squamous cell carcinoma, sometimes also known as well-differentiated squamous cell carcinoma, is characterized by bizarre, heavily keratinized cells [T6.12]. Pearls are pathognomonic of keratinization [58 I6.98]. In contrast to the pushing invasion characteristic of nonkeratinizing squamous cell carcinoma, keratinizing squamous cell carcinoma usually, but not always, invades with finger-like projections and incites a desmoplastic stromal reaction.

Pleomorphism is the hallmark of this type of cancer [59 I6.96, 60 I6.97]. Cells with bizarre configurations (spindle snakes, caudate tadpoles, etc) are a characteristic feature, but form a minor, albeit important, component of the tumor. Similarly, although orangeophilia (associated with dense keratinization) is characteristic, eosinophilia may be more prominent, and many cells are cyanophilic. Most of the cells are single, although occasional syncytial-like aggregates can be seen. The nuclei are 77 ± 28 μm², which is 1.5 to 3 times the size of an intermediate cell nucleus [Patten 1978]. The chromatin is typically coarse, with many pyknotic nuclei. Macronucleoli may be present, but are rarely observed due to karyopyknosis. Keratinizing squamous cell carcinoma is usually accompanied by evidence of hyperkeratosis, parakeratosis, atypical parakeratosis, and keratinizing dysplasia.

Differential Diagnosis: The differential diagnosis between severe keratinizing dysplasia and keratinizing squamous cell carcinoma may be difficult [60 I6.97]. Theoretically, there is no intervening stage of classical carcinoma in situ (see "Keratinizing Carcinoma In Situ"). The background of all dysplasias, as well as some exophytic keratinizing squamous cell carcinomas, is clean. Therefore, the absence of a tumor diathesis does not exclude invasive keratinizing squamous cell carcinoma. Nuclear features of malignancy, eg, nucleoli and irregular chromatin clumping, can also be difficult to detect in keratinizing squamous cell carcinoma due to nuclear pyknosis. In practice, a smear in which more than 15% of the total cellularity shows high-grade "keratinizing dysplasia" should be considered suspicious for keratinizing squamous cell carcinoma. In summary, factors favoring a diagnosis of keratinizing squamous cell carcinoma over dysplasia include the following: more cells, more pleomorphism, coarse, irregular chromatin, macronucleoli, syncytial-like aggregates, and diathesis.

Another pitfall in diagnosis of keratinizing squamous cell carcinoma is atypical parakeratosis, in which individual cells may look malignant but are too small to be diagnosed as cancer. *Never unequivocally diagnose cancer based only on the presence of parakeratotic-sized cells.* While keratinizing squamous cell carcinoma is generally accompanied by atypical parakeratosis, the presence of atypical parakeratosis alone does not always imply cancer. Atypical parakeratosis can be seen in condyloma, dysplasia, and even inflammation.

58
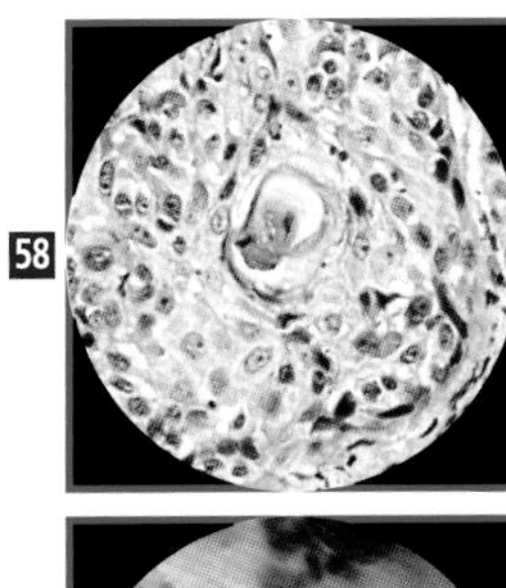

59
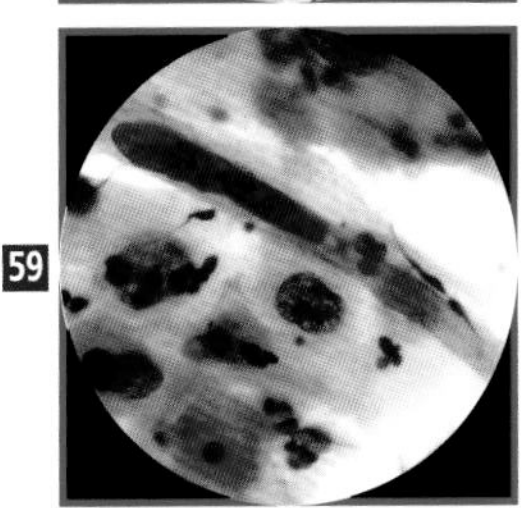

60
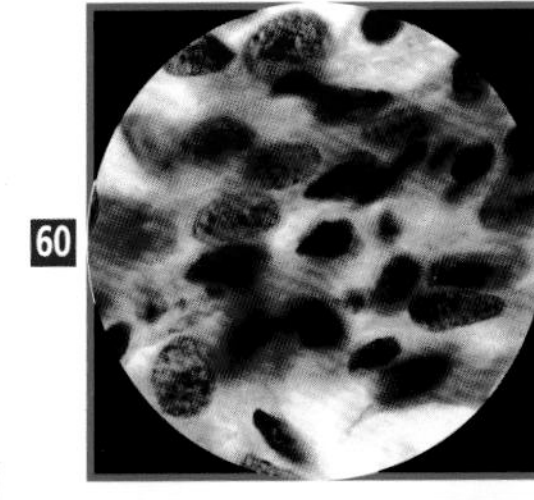

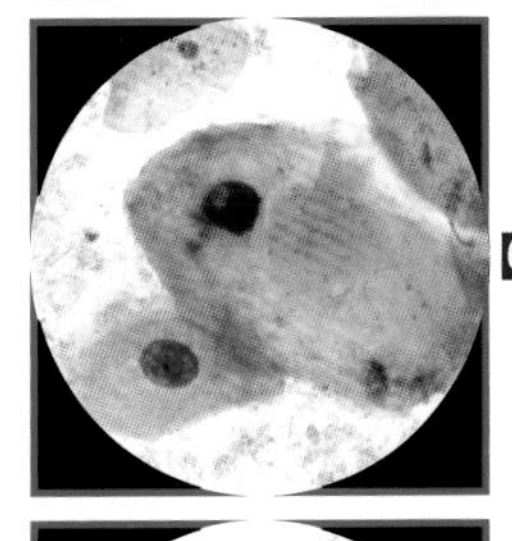
61

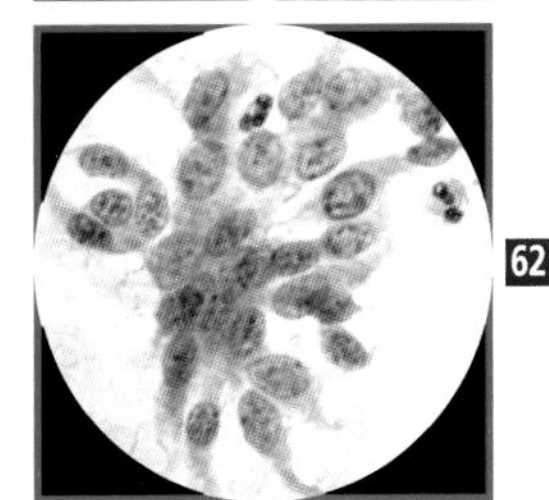
62

Nonkeratinizing squamous cell carcinoma is more common than keratinizing squamous cell carcinoma, in the uterine cervix. The incidence of nonkeratinizing squamous cell carcinoma increases with the age of the patient. Keratinizing and small cell squamous cell carcinomas are decreasing in overall frequency. Small cell carcinomas, fortunately, are rare.

Other Variants of Squamous Cell Carcinoma

Verrucous Squamous Cell Carcinoma: Characteristics of this type of squamous cell carcinoma include "papillary" growth pattern and infiltration with pushing, bulky rete peg expansion. Very well-differentiated, the cytology may only be suggestive of a low-grade cervical intraepithelial neoplasia, in a pattern of keratinizing dysplasia [61 I6.103] [Barua 1983, deTorres 1981, Inaba 1992]. Few or no koilocytes are present. In histologic section, fibrovascular cores are poorly developed compared with condyloma. This cancer does not metastasize, but frequently recurs. Radiotherapy may be contraindicated [Richart 1987].

Papillary Squamous Cell Carcinoma: Growth pattern similar to verrucous squamous cell carcinoma, but exhibits significant nuclear atypia. Has propensity for late recurrence and metastases.

Lymphoepithelioma-like Squamous Cell Carcinoma: Similar to tumor more commonly occurring in head and neck area; extremely rare in cervix. Abundant, delicate, syncytial cytoplasm, round nuclei, macronucleoli, and lymphoid infiltrate.

Spindle Squamous Cell Carcinoma: Spindly, nonkeratinized cells that may resemble sarcoma (therefore also known as pseudosarcoma) or melanoma [62 I6.104]. Stroma may be heavily fibrotic or hyalinized.

Condyloma and Human Papilloma Virus Infection

Condyloma is a sexually transmitted infection caused by human papilloma virus (HPV). Condylomas are contagious (~60% of sexual partners contract disease), have an incubation period of about 3 months (range, 3 weeks to 8 months), and tend to be multifocal [Oriel 1971]. However, they have a high regression rate, with half to two thirds of them spontaneously disappearing [A Evans 1985, Meisels 1981a]. Condyloma is more commonly diagnosed in younger women (especially <30 years) and during the second half of pregnancy [Meisels 1992].

There are two basic histologic growth patterns of condyloma: acuminatum (cauliflower-like, warty) and planum (commonly called flat, and first described in 1977 [Meisels 1977b, Purola 1977]) [I6.81]. An endophytic variety of condyloma is also recognized, but this may simply represent endocervical glandular extension of the lesion. Spike condyloma is a variant of acuminatum with multitudes of spike-like projections (known as "asperites") that give a velvety appearance to the lesion on colposcopy.

Whether a condyloma is warty or flat depends on the maturation of the involved epithelium [Crum 1984]. If a *keratinized* epithelium is infected, typical cauliflower-like venereal warts, which are called condylomata acuminata, are more likely to occur. If the virus infects a *mature metaplastic* epithelium, flat condylomas usually result [63 I6.81]. Condylomas of the cervix are most commonly flat. Flat condylomas are usually inconspicuous or invisible to the naked eye, but they can be seen on colposcopy with the application of acetic acid to enhance their visibility. The histologic types of condyloma (warty, flat) cannot be predicted cytologically: they yield identical cells.

The word condyloma is frequently used unmodified to refer to a lesion without specifying whether it is flat or warty. Condyloma, or more precisely, HPV infection, is also thought to be important in the development of cervical neoplasia. Condyloma is considered, together with ordinary CIN I (mild dysplasia), a low-grade squamous intraepithelial lesion in the Bethesda System.

In addition, the HPV may infect *immature metaplastic* epithelium, causing a noncondylomatous lesion known as atypical immature metaplasia. Finally, HPV infection can be present without any lesion being detectable clinically or morphologically (this is known as latent or subclinical infection). Such patients have apparently normal cervices, Pap smears, and biopsy specimens. Latent infections are very common. (Note: Some authors use "subclinical infection" to include *lesions* invisible to the naked eye, ie, flat condyloma or atypical immature metaplasia.)

Methods of Detection of HPV Infection

The life cycle of human papilloma virus (HPV) is tightly linked to squamous differentiation. Complete HPV replication only occurs in mature, terminally differentiated squamous cells. Permissive infection refers to those lesions that permit full viral DNA replication and capsule formation, eg, well-differentiated flat or warty condyloma (low-grade squamous intraepithelial lesions). Glandular cells, atypical immature metaplasia, latent infections, high-grade dysplasia/carcinoma in situ, and cancer do not allow full viral expression with formation of viral capsule, hence, they are considered nonpermissive infections.

Koilocytes are a specific feature of condyloma and HPV infection. Koilocytes are present in at least 80% of permissive HPV infections, histologically [63 I6.81] [Sato 1987]. However, koilocytes form predominantly in the intermediate to superficial cell layers—the surface is often covered with dyskeratotic cells; therefore, koilocytes are not very sensitive in the detection of HPV infection by the Pap smear. They occur in only about 20% to 33% of cases [Mayelo 1994, Okagaki 1992, V Schneider 1989].

63

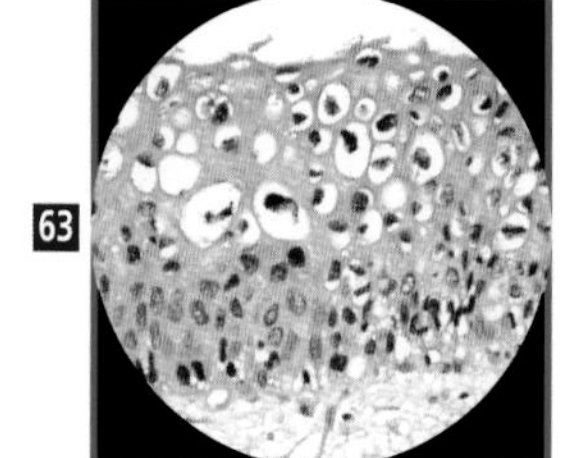

Also, the formation of koilocytes progressively decreases with increasing severity of cervical intraepithelial neoplasia, which is currently thought to be related to HPV infection. Koilocytes are usually, but not always, absent in invasive cancer (a nonpermissive lesion) [A Schneider 1989].

Electron microscopy can only detect viral particles (requires permissive infection), although they need not be completely mature [Sato 1987]. Since the tissue concentration of virions is low, electron microscopy is not very sensitive for diagnosis, unless preselected areas are examined (which amounts to confirmation of a light microscopic diagnosis by EM).

Immunocytochemical staining can detect viral capsular antigens (in permissive infections). However, viral capsule formation is a late and focal event. Therefore, immunocytochemical staining is positive in only about one half of cases of classic condyloma and mild dysplasia (ie, low-grade squamous intraepithelial lesions), and the detection rate declines as the dysplasia becomes more severe [Kurman 1983]. In practice, koilocytosis (ie, ordinary histologic diagnosis) is more sensitive than immunostaining in detection of HPV infection.

DNA hybridization techniques, by detecting HPV-DNA or RNA, are more sensitive and specific methods of diagnosing HPV infection than light microscopy, electron microscopy, or immunocytochemical staining, and, unlike those techniques, can detect nonpermissive viral infections in which the viral DNA is integrated into the host genome. Hybridization techniques can also determine the specific type of HPV. T6.13 details the sensitivity of the various DNA techniques.

HPV–DNA is detected by the extent of homology ("hybridization") with a labeled probe (purified HPV DNA or RNA labeled with a radionucleotide or biotin, etc). Filter hybridization uses denatured, single stranded DNA on a filter support, which binds the DNA. Hybridization depends on the extent of nucleic acid homology as well as the conditions under which the test is performed: the higher the degree of base pair similarity, the stronger the hybridization.

Southern blot, which is considered the "gold standard" technique for HPV diagnosis [Koutsky 1988], is a modification of the filter hybridization technique. DNA is extracted from cells and digested with restriction enzymes to cut the DNA at specific sites. The procedure separates the DNA fragments (using electrophoresis), which are then transferred to a filter support and hybridized with labeled probes [T Wright 1990]. This

***T6.13* Relative Technique Sensitivities for HPV Detection**

Method	Sensitivity	Adequate for
In situ	5–50 gene copies per cell	L SIL
Southern blot	1 copy per 100 cells	H SIL, SCC
PCR	1 copy per million cells	Latent infection

[Anonymous 1989, T Wright 1990]
L SIL = low-grade squamous intraepithelial lesion, H SIL = high-grade squamous intraepithelial lesion.

dual characterization, by migration pattern and hybridization, is highly specific [Southern 1975]. In addition, it can assess the physical state (episomal vs integrated) of the virus. Unfortunately, Southern blot technique cannot localize the individual infected cells, requires fresh or frozen tissue and relatively large amounts of DNA, and is laborious to perform.

Another method of HPV detection is in situ hybridization, in which a labeled probe is applied directly to an ordinary tissue section. In contrast with filter techniques, in situ hybridization can be applied to formalin fixed tissue and allows localization of infected cells. This allows their morphology to be studied, and gives the investigator the ability to retrospectively examine archival specimens. However, it is not as sensitive as filter hybridization.

The *polymerase chain reaction* (PCR), which uses enzymatic DNA amplification, is currently the most sensitive method of HPV detection. PCR can detect less than 1 µg of HPV–DNA [A Schneider 1989]. Such sensitivity is theoretically capable of detecting one viral particle in 10^6 cells [Anonymous 1989]. However, the extreme sensitivity of the method makes it prone to false-positive diagnoses due to contamination, thus diminishing specificity.

Diagnosis of Condyloma in the Pap Smear

Koilocytes: Human papilloma virus causes a cytopathic effect in some cells, resulting in the formation of a halo cell known as the koilocyte [64 I6.73]. Koilocytes are pathognomonic of condyloma and HPV infection, if strict diagnostic criteria are used to identify them [Boras 1989, Koss 1987b, Meisels 1981a]. However, as discussed above, koilocytes are not very sensitive in the cytologic diagnosis of condyloma and HPV infection.

In the Pap smear, koilocytes are found singly or in small clusters. The koilocyte is an intermediate or superficial cell that has a characteristic halo surrounding the nucleus [Koss 1956, Mayelo 1994, Meisels 1976a, Saigo 1986]. The halo is a relatively large space caused by the cytopathic effect of the virus. The edge of the halo is very distinct and sharply defined, and surrounded by a wall of dense, sometimes hyalin, cytoplasm. The cytoplasmic density corresponds ultrastructurally to condensation of cytoplasmic fibrils. The cytoplasm can stain pink, or blue, or both (polychromasia). Sometimes a few tiny dot-like fragments of degenerated cytoplasm can be seen floating in the space, but the halo is usually otherwise clear.

To be diagnostic for condyloma and HPV infection, the nucleus of the koilocyte must look abnormal: enlarged and hyperchromatic (big and dark). The nuclear membrane is often wrinkled and the chromatin usually appears dark, distinct, and granular. In a word, the nucleus looks dysplastic—usually to a mild or moderate degree. Sometimes, the nuclei are degenerated, with "smudgy," pyknotic, fragmented, or marginated chromatin. Nucleoli are inconspicuous or absent. Binucleation is frequent, multinucleation is less frequent, and giant nuclei can sometimes be seen [Koss 1956, Mayelo 1994, Meisels 1977b]. Although virus may be present in the nucleus [Casas-Cordero 1981], neither intranuclear nor intracytoplasmic viral inclusions are seen with the light microscope.

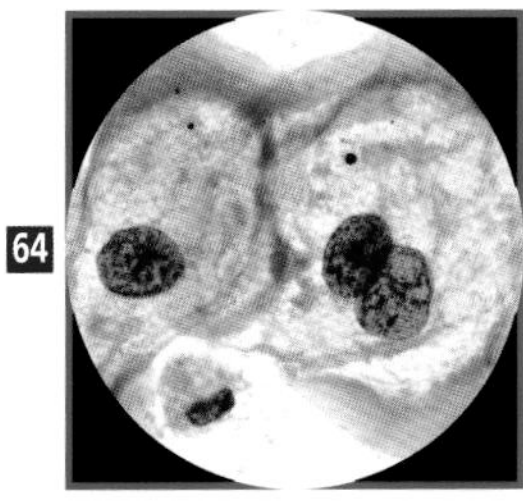
64

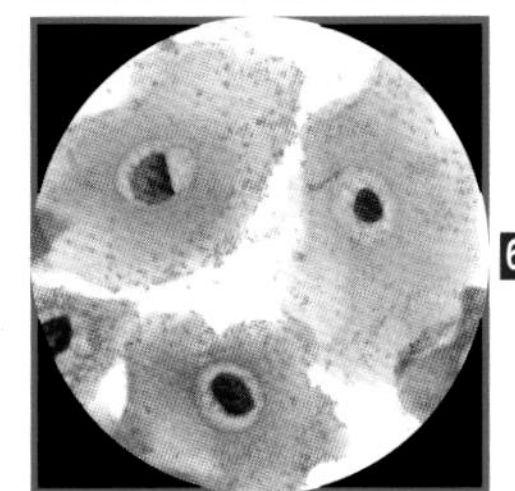
65

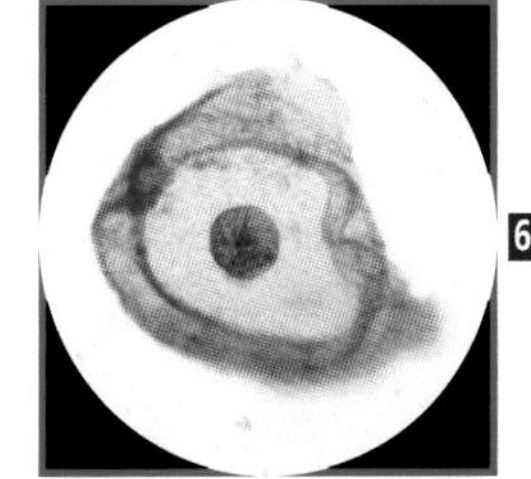
66

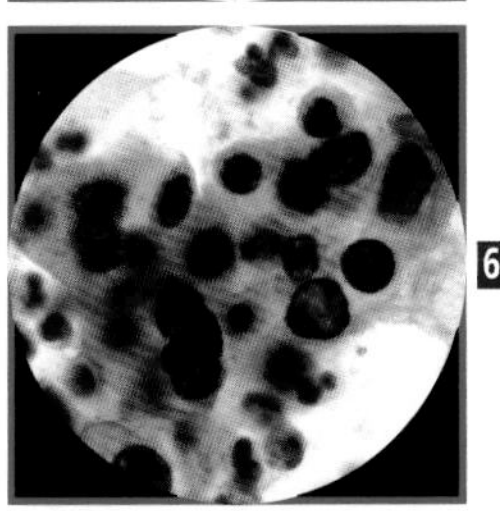
67

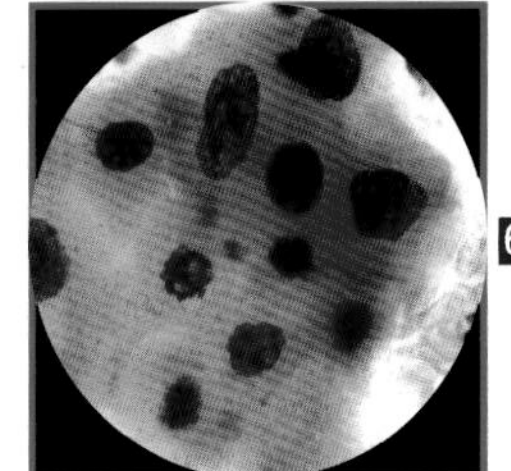
68

Differential Diagnosis of Koilocytes: Koilocytes are not the only cells in the Pap smear that can have "halos." The koilocyte halo must be distinguished from perinuclear halos seen in inflammation, especially due to *Trichomonas* infection ("trich halos") [65 I6.50]. Knowing the different mechanisms of halo formation helps in differentiating the two types of halos. The koilocyte halo, caused by *destruction* of the cytoplasm, is usually at least the width of an intermediate cell nucleus (7–8 µm). Inflammatory perinuclear halos are generally smaller. They are caused by alcohol fixation, which produces shrinkage of an enlarged, edematous, inflamed nucleus. This leaves a small clear space, usually with little or no damage or condensation of the cytoplasm. Inflammatory halos are usually less than the width of an intermediate cell nucleus.

Certain cells contain abundant glycogen in their cytoplasm (eg, navicular cells or androgenic atrophy cells), which forms a perinuclear vacuole ("halo"). This glycogen vacuole may resemble a koilocyte halo [66 I6.74]. Koilocytes usually have no visible glycogen (which stains golden yellow with the Pap stain) in the halo; what is more important, the edge of the halo in koilocytes is dense and sharply defined and the nuclei are abnormal, while glycogenated cells usually have a somewhat hazy or less distinct edge to the vacuole and the nuclei are normal.

Immature squamous metaplastic cells may have an attenuated, pale staining endoplasm with a relatively dense ectoplasmic rim, but lack the sharp demarcation and marked peripheral cytoplasmic density associated with koilocytes. Also, immature metaplastic cells are parabasal-sized cells, while koilocytes resemble intermediate or superficial cells. Immature metaplastic cells, like koilocytes, usually lack visible glycogen. And, importantly, the metaplastic nuclei are normal or reactive appearing.

In summary, if the nucleus does not appear abnormal, the halo cell is not a diagnostic koilocyte [Koss 1987b, P Ward 1990]. The presence of abnormal nuclei is also of diagnostic importance in histopathology, where it can sometimes be difficult to differentiate the normal glycogenated cells ("basket-weave pattern") from koilocytes [I6.81]. One final note: the mere presence of koilocytes does not exclude high-grade dysplasia—or even invasive carcinoma.

Dyskeratocytes: These are abnormally keratinized squamous cells, hence the term "dys-kerato-cytes." Dyskeratocytes occur on the surface of the condyloma. In the Pap smear, dyskeratocytes are characteristically found in thick groups of haphazardly arranged cells, with loss of nuclear polarity, but they can also occur singly.

Dyskeratocytes range in size from small to large [67 I6.76, 68 I6.75]. Small dyskeratocytes have orange cytoplasm, and atypical, dense or pyknotic nuclei. These cells resemble (or are identical with) atypical parakeratosis [67 I6.76]. Larger dyskeratocytes have dense orange cytoplasm, and may contain one or more enlarged, atypical nuclei, with dark and coarse, smudgy, or pyknotic chromatin. These cells are similar, or identical, to keratinizing dysplasia [I6.75].

The presence of thick, disorganized clusters of bright orange dyskeratocytes strongly suggests a diagnosis of condyloma, even in the absence of typical koilocytes [Boras 1989, Mayelo 1994, Meisels 1976a]. Note that ordinary parakeratosis, with uniform cells and maintenance of nuclear polarity (eg, well-formed pearls, linear strips), has much less significance in the diagnosis of HPV infection.

Macrocytes: Macrocytes may be more sensitive, but less specific, than koilocytes in the diagnosis of HPV infection. The macrocytes of condyloma are morphologically similar to those found in radiation or chemotherapy effect and vitamin deficiency (folate or B_{12}). Macrocytes are very large, often several times the size of intermediate or superficial cells [69 I6.77]. Their abundant cytoplasm stains pink or blue or, frequently, polychromatic. Cytoplasmic vacuolization is relatively common and the vacuoles may contain ingested particles or neutrophils, or even other squamous cells. The nuclei are usually enlarged, often multiple, and may be atypical. The N/C ratio, however, is relatively low or almost normal.

Minor Criteria for Diagnosis of Condyloma: There are a variety of other cytologic features that are suggestive, but less than diagnostic, of condyloma. These nonclassic signs (or minor criteria) include not only cytomegaly but also polka dot cells (cells with numerous small globules of condensed cytoplasm [70 I6.80]), kite cells (stretched out cells with long tails [71 I6.78]), two-tone (polychromatic) cells, cracked cells (condensed cytoplasmic filaments give the impression of cracks), balloon cells (clear cytoplasm, peripheral nucleus, resemble adipocytes [72 I6.79]), and hyalin cytoplasmic inclusions (condensed intermediate filaments), as well as binucleation or multinucleation, spindle nuclei, chromatin smudging, and karyorrhexis [Cecchini 1990b, de Borges 1989, Mayelo 1994, Schlaen 1988, A Schneider 1987b, V Schneider 1989, Shroyer 1990, Tanaka 1993]. A diagnosis of condyloma not only carries the stigma of a venereal disease, but condyloma may also be part of the spectrum of premalignant conditions. Therefore, the presence of any of these minor criteria should initiate a search for cells that are more diagnostic, but their presence alone should not lead to a report of "suspicious" for condyloma.

Atypical Immature Metaplasia: Atypical immature metaplasia is a lesion, distinct from condyloma, caused by HPV infection of immature metaplastic cells [Crum 1983b]. Atypical immature metaplasia resembles low-grade immature metaplastic dysplasia. The cells are parabasal-sized, with minimally atypical nuclei. Koilocytes are not seen in atypical immature metaplasia, unless it coexists with typical (flat or warty) condyloma. Like condyloma, atypical immature metaplasia is thought to be part of the spectrum of cervical intraepithelial neoplasia (or squamous intraepithelial lesions) and, therefore, the lesion should be removed or destroyed [Crum 1984].

In summary, condylomas exfoliate cells that appear (or are) dysplastic. Koilocytes are diagnostic of condyloma and HPV infection (low-grade squamous intraepithelial lesion). Other atypical cells that are shed often resemble keratinizing dysplasia, usually of mild or moderate degree, and can be thought of as koilocytes without halos (dyskeratocytes). Macrocytes are often present, although they are a nonspecific finding. However, the presence of macrocytes in a background of dysplasia, particularly of keratinizing type, suggests, but is not diagnostic of, condyloma. Minor criteria in condyloma are nondiagnostic, but should alert the screener to search carefully for diagnostic evidence of condyloma or dysplasia.

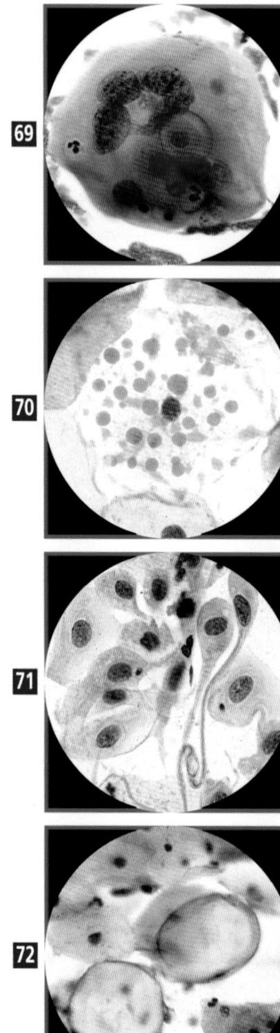
69
70
71
72

Criteria of Condyloma and HPV Infection

- Koilocytes (pathognomonic)
  - Cytoplasmic halos
  - Nuclear dysplasia
- Dyskeratocytes
  - Atypical parakeratosis
  - Keratinizing dysplasia
- Macrocytes and dysplasia (suggestive)
- Atypical immature metaplasia
- Minor (nondiagnostic) criteria
  - Cells: Macrocytes, kites, balloons
  - Cytoplasm: Polka dots, cracks, two-tone staining
  - Nuclei: Binucleation, spindling, smudging

Differential Diagnosis of Condyloma: Occasionally, the nuclei of condyloma cells in the Pap smear are markedly atypical (greatly enlarged, with very coarse, dark chromatin). Yet, despite the strikingly abnormal appearance of the cells, there can still be a high degree of differentiation in the corresponding tissue. Thus, in some cases, the degree of abnormality (or "dysplasia") of a condyloma may be overestimated in the Pap smear when it is compared with the results of tissue biopsy. Such cases have been referred to as "atypical condyloma" [Meisels 1981b]. Rarely, condyloma has almost malignant appearing nuclei, which may even be mistaken for squamous cell carcinoma [Koss 1956, Meisels 1981b].

The best clue to the grading of abnormality of a squamous lesion is the N/C ratio. The atypical nuclei of condyloma are usually found in relatively abundant cytoplasm, resulting in an N/C ratio that may only be slightly increased (akin to low-grade dysplasia). In condyloma, the chromatin of the atypical cells is regularly distributed, although it may be coarse or smudgy. Features favoring a diagnosis of squamous cell carcinoma include abnormal nuclei with frankly malignant appearing, irregularly distributed chromatin, prominent nucleoli, bizarre shaped cells, and a tumor diathesis.

Note, also, that condyloma can coexist with high-grade dysplasia or even invasive cancer. In fact, condyloma is frequently associated with "ordinary" dysplasia. Currently, condyloma and dysplasia are thought to be closely related biologically, and according to the Bethesda System, it is not critically important to make a distinction in every case.

Condyloma Redux

Condyloma has been a controversial topic. There are two basic schools of thought about it. One school makes a distinction between condyloma and dysplasia, maintaining that condyloma is only a viral infection that can cause cellular changes that mimic dysplasia, but are not genuine dysplasia. The so-called "atypical condyloma" may bridge the gap between simple infection and "true" dysplasia [Meisels 1981b]. Others believe that condyloma *is* dysplasia, or at least, that it is *indistinguishable from* dysplasia. There is also a middle ground, those who believe that condyloma is a *precursor to* dysplasia.

The Bethesda System has included mild dysplasia (CIN I) and HPV effect (condyloma) in the same category of low-grade squamous intraepithelial lesion. Reasons for the grouping of these "two" lesions are summarized below:

1. There is a high interobserver variability in the diagnosis, ie, the two lesions cannot be differentiated by light microscopy with much more accuracy than flipping a coin [D Evans 1986, Ismail 1989,1990, Kurman 1991, A Robertson 1989a,b, Sherman 1992c].
2. The molecular virology of the two lesions is similar or identical, ie, they have the same viral types: these are predominantly, but not exclusively, low-risk types, eg, HPV 6, 11 [Crum 1984, 1985, Dürst 1983, Gissmann 1982, Kadish 1986, Kurman 1991, Lörincz 1987a, Mitao 1986, Reid 1987, Richart 1987, Schiffman 1991, Willett 1989]. Moreover, both lesions may demonstrate aneuploidy [Watts 1987].
3. The lesions have similar or identical clinical behavior, ie, they have a low progression rate [Campion 1986, Kataja 1989, Kurman 1991, Nasiell 1986, Syrjänen 1988].

Whether condyloma is dysplasia, merely coexists with dysplasia, or is a transitional stage on the path to dysplasia may be controversial, but koilocytosis is not a trivial lesion [Koss 1987b, Meisels 1977b]. There is a concern that condyloma might be undertreated [Kaufman 1983b]. The presence of koilocytes does not rule out the possibility of ordinary cervical intraepithelial neoplasia (CIN). For example, a focal CIN lesion could be missed in a biopsy or smear [Selvaggi 1986]. Moreover, the mere presence of koilocytes identifies a patient who is at high risk of having or developing significant cervical neoplasia [Mitchell 1986] and who should be further investigated with colposcopy and possibly biopsy [Koss 1987a,b]. Although up to two thirds of condylomas may eventually regress [Meisels 1981a], one third of patients diagnosed with condyloma develop ordinary CIN in less than 1 year [Nash 1987]. Evidence of condyloma decreases the mean age of grades of CIN [Meisels 1981a] and shortens the time for cancer to develop [Sadeghi 1989]; in fact, patients with koilocytosis (ie, condyloma) may develop cancer rapidly.

Currently, the safest approach is to make the simplifying assumption that *if it looks like dysplasia, it is dysplasia* [Fletcher 1983]. Dysplasia, with or without koilocytes, should be diagnosed by the usual morphologic criteria. The lesions should be graded according to the degree of abnormality of the nucleus and the N/C ratio, regardless of whether HPV is thought to be present or not. A statement regarding evidence of HPV infection can be added to the report, but women with condyloma should receive the same clinical management as those with conventional forms of cervical intraepithelial neoplasia, which usually means that the lesion should be eradicated regardless of grade or virus effect [Bajardi 1986, Kaufman 1983a,b, Raymond 1987b, Richart 1987].

A Final (?) Word on Nomenclature and a Summary

Schottländer-Kermauner phenomenon; unruhige (restless) epithelium; unquiet epithelium; leucohyperkeratosis; atypical epithelium; basal cell: hyperactivity, hyperplasia, or anaplasia; precancerous metaplasia; metaplasia with atypicality; metaplasia with anaplasia; prickle cell hyperplasia; spinal cell atypia; dyskaryosis; atypical epithelial hyperplasia; dysplasia; carcinoma in situ; cervical intraepithelial neoplasia; squamous intraepithelial lesion; what next?

The controversy surrounding the best terminology to use in diagnosis of the "Schottländer-Kermauner phenomenon" (c 1912) has been raging for virtually the entire 20th century [Bottles 1991, Briggs 1979, Crum 1989a, Drake 1984, Giacomini 1983,1991, Herbst 1990, NCI 1989a,b,c, Kurman 1994, Richart 1973]. In the 1930s, Broders found that a lesion composed of undifferentiated, atypical cells—which he called carcinoma in situ—was a precursor lesion of squamous cell carcinoma [Broders 1932]. It later became apparent that similar, but less abnormal (or more differentiated) lesions also occurred, which were termed dysplasia [Reagan 1953]. Among the various systems of nomenclature, perhaps the best known and most widely understood is dysplasia/carcinoma in situ, which can also be applied without modification to many organs other than the uterine cervix.

The Papanicolaou Classification System for cytologic diagnosis was introduced in the 1950s. Although the Papanicolaou class was probably never intended to be used as a substitute for a narrative diagnosis, this unfortunately became common practice [Maguire 1988]. In its original form, the Papanicolaou class was intended to indicate the degree of certainty that cancer was present or absent. However, as the concept of precursor lesions became more widely understood, the emphasis shifted from degrees of *certainty* to degrees of *abnormality*. Consequently, the Papanicolaou system suffered modifications too numerous to count, in essence trying to fit square pegs into round holes. Moreover, the Papanicolaou class has no correlation with histopathology, and had been considered outmoded for decades [Reagan 1965]. However, a proposal has been made to combine the old Papanicolaou classification with the new Bethesda System to facilitate triage of patients [Frankel 1994].

In the late 1960s and early 1970s, prospective clinical studies and DNA ploidy analysis proved that dysplasia and carcinoma in situ were closely related; therefore, a new terminology, cervical intraepithelial neoplasia, was introduced to encompass both lesions [Richart 1973, T Wright 1990]. Prior to that time, dysplasia was too often undertreated clinically, while a diagnosis of carcinoma in situ sometimes resulted in unnecessary hysterectomy, occasionally even removing an extensive vaginal margin; in short, overtreatment [Richart 1973]. The primary purpose behind the introduction of the cervical intraepithelial neoplasia terminology was to emphasize that these lesions represent a continuum of change [Richart 1968] and that all grades are important and should be treated, but by the most conservative method indicated [Richart 1973].

Although cervical intraepithelial neoplasia was subdivided into three grades, the concept of a continuum diminishes the importance of grading. What is most important is to distinguish cervical intraepithelial neoplasia from benign, reactive atypias [Crum 1984]. Nevertheless, cervical intraepithelial neoplasia with good evidence of squamous differentiation statistically behaves better; however, even well-differentiated lesions can progress, and, rarely, may invade directly.

More recent information pointing to an apparent biologic dichotomy between mere "infection" and genuine "neoplasia" has resulted in the latest entry, the Bethesda System [Kurman 1994, NCI 1989a,b,c]. The Bethesda System terminology suggests that the disease is not a continuum, but rather a discontinuous, two-disease system, emphasized by the terminology of low- and high-grade squamous intraepithelial lesion. Low-grade squamous intraepithelial lesion is caused by a heterogeneous group of viruses, including both low-risk (eg, 6 and 11) and high-risk (eg, 16 and 18) viral types, which can produce morphologically indistinguishable, well-differentiated lesions. Low-grade squamous intraepithelial lesion is expected to have an unpredictable clinical behavior, but is less likely to progress than the other category, high-grade squamous intraepithelial lesion. High-grade squamous intraepithelial lesion is predominantly caused by high-risk virus and is expected to behave as a precursor lesion [Richart 1990].

It is almost as though we return now to the days of yesteryear, when precursor lesions were a two disease system (ie, dysplasia and carcinoma in situ)! Richart states "the current data are consistent with a two-disease system....The classical histologic distinctions between mild, moderate, and severe dysplasia and carcinoma *in situ*...reflect the proportion of 16/18 group lesions, the anticipated clinical course, and the degree of ultimate risk" [Richart 1987]. Though the concepts have now been refined to include our understanding of DNA ploidy and low- and high-risk virus, the morphology still roughly corresponds to dysplasia and carcinoma in situ (or borderline lesion and carcinoma in situ), and the degree of risk correlates with the morphologic grade of the lesion.

With each new nomenclature, there has been a "frame shift" in the line of division. At first, the split was between carcinoma in situ and severe dysplasia, then cervical intraepithelial neoplasia incorporated these two lesions into one category, cervical intraepithelial neoplasia III. Next, the Bethesda System included moderate dysplasia and cervical intraepithelial neoplasia III into one category, high-grade squamous intraepithelial lesion. These changes may be, at least in part, a reflection of a patient population willing to accept less and less risk.

Nevertheless, most invasive cancers arise from high-grade dysplasia and particularly, classical carcinoma in situ [Ng 1969]. We can pull out a portion of our original matrix to show the relationships between systems [T6.14].

Which system(s) of nomenclature to use is left to the reader. At the University of Chicago, all three systems are used together, providing the clinician with a veritable smorgasbord of diagnoses. Although probably obvious by now, it may be worth noting that the author's personal preference is the dysplasia/carcinoma in situ terminology. It can always be translated into the other systems, but the reverse is not true. When other systems of nomenclature are described, they are almost invariably compared with the dysplasia/carcinoma in situ scheme. This simple fact speaks volumes. Dysplasia/carcinoma in situ remains the most widely used diagnostic terminology (squamous intraepithelial lesion is increasing, cervical intraepithelial neoplasia diminishing) [Davey 1992b]. Dysplasia/carcinoma in situ can be utilized for tissues throughout the body, and the concept of dysplasia/carcinoma in situ is covered in most textbooks of pathology. Only with adherence to standard nomenclature will it be possible to study the natural history of disease and communicate in one language [Christopherson 1977a], but if history holds any lesson, it is that there will be still other terminologies introduced in the future. The lesions do not change, only the names.

Cytoplasm and Nucleus: Yin and Yang of Diagnosing Dysplasia

The cells exfoliated from the mucosal surface faithfully reflect the morphology of the hidden underlying epithelium. This axiom is the cornerstone of Pap smear diagnosis. The basic concepts of squamous differentiation and carcinogenesis have been presented. Their manifestations are seen primarily in the cytoplasm and the nucleus, respectively. The degree of nuclear and cytoplasmic abnormality of the cells found in the Pap smear

T6.14 **Terminology of Three Nomenclature Systems**

Dysplasia/CIS	CIN	Bethesda System	Next?
Mild dysplasia	CIN I	SIL, low grade }	Aneuploid?
Moderate dysplasia	CIN II }	SIL, high grade }	
Severe dysplasia }	CIN III }		
CIS }			

"When I use a word," Humpty Dumpty said, in a rather scornful tone, "it means just what I choose it to mean—neither more nor less."
"The question is," said Alice, "whether you can make words mean so many different things."
"The question is," said Humpty Dumpty, "which is to be master—that's all."

—Lewis Carroll, *Through the Looking-Glass*

indicates the degree of abnormality of the tissue, from dysplasia to carcinoma in situ and finally cancer.

After an arduous journey through the preceding diagnostic challenges, return now, like Odysseus to Penelope, to view in a new light the "fine fabric of possible cytologic diagnoses" that has been woven.

The Cytoplasm

Carcinoma In Situ

Carcinoma in situ can be defined as "an abnormal [neoplastic] reaction of the squamous mucosa which, in the absence of invasion, through the full thickness of the epithelium, no squamous differentiation takes place" [Wied 1962].

Dysplasia

Dysplasia can be defined as "all other similar abnormal reactions, but which show some squamous differentiation toward the surface." (Modified from an International Agreement made in Vienna in 1961 [Wied 1962].)

Squamous differentiation is manifested principally by more abundant, dense cytoplasm and the presence of distinct cell boundaries. Dysplasia can be further categorized as mild, moderate, or severe, depending on how differentiated the abnormal process is. With these intraepithelial abnormalities there is a continuum of morphologic change beginning with normal at one extreme and ending with carcinoma in situ at the other, with grades of dysplasia in between. This creates three diagnostic zones, between normal and carcinoma in situ [F6.13].

In practice, there are no sharp demarcations between the various grades of dysplasia, eg, a "high-grade" mild dysplasia is almost identical to a "low-grade" moderate dysplasia. (This, by the way, is a potential problem for the Bethesda System's squamous intraepithelial lesion terminology: there is no gray zone between low-grade squamous intraepithelial lesion [mild dysplasia] and high-grade squamous intraepithelial lesion [moderate dysplasia or worse].)

Histology: In mild dysplasia, the undifferentiated abnormal cells are confined to the lower third of epithelium; considerable squamous differentiation can occur before the cells are exfoliated at the surface [I6.82]. In moderate dysplasia, the undifferentiated cells occupy at least the lower one third, but no more than two thirds, of the thickness of the epithelium [73 I6.83]. In severe dysplasia, little squamous differentiation occurs, and only in the upper third of the epithelium, with at least the bottom two thirds of the epithelium being composed of abnormal, undifferentiated cells.

The final stage of intraepithelial neoplasia is carcinoma in situ, in which the full thickness of the epithelium is made up of undifferentiated abnormal cells [74 I6.84]. The cells at the surface may flatten a little, due to surface tension effects, but they do not truly differentiate or acquire dense squamous cytoplasm.

The severity of the lesion depends on how high the level of undifferentiated cells rises in the epithelium before the squamous differentiation, if any, begins. The transition between the undifferentiated and the differentiated cells is usually fairly well demarcated. Undifferentiated cells have delicate cytoplasm and indistinct cell boundaries; differentiated cells have dense cytoplasm and distinct cell boundaries.

Mitotic figures correlate with undifferentiated cells. Normally, mitotic figures are confined to a single layer of undifferentiated basal cells. In dysplasia, mitotic figures are seen above the basal layer, while in carcinoma in situ, they may be found at all levels of the epithelium, including the surface. Although abnormal mitotic figures can be found in mild dysplasia, they are usually associated with more advanced dysplasia and carcinoma in situ [Jenkins 1986]. Abnormal mitoses are abortive and correlate with aneuploidy.

The severity of the lesion may vary from area to area. Surface keratotic reactions (hyperkeratosis, parakeratosis) are not included in the histologic assessment of the degree of differentiation of the lesion, including carcinoma in situ. In dysplasia, a certain amount of order remains in the epithelium. In carci-

F6.13 **Precursor Lesions of Cervical Carcinoma**

In histology, as the undifferentiated cells ascend from the basal layer, the dysplasia becomes progressively more severe, until finally, at the stage of CIS, the entire thickness of the epithelium is replaced with undifferentiated cells. In cytology, as the dysplasia becomes more advanced, the cell exfoliated at the surface become progressively less differentiated, until finally, at the stage of CIS, the surface cells are undifferentiated. Of important note is that even in mild dysplasia, the entire thickness of the epithelium is abnormal, but differentiates toward the surface; in CIS, the entire thickness is both abnormal and undifferentiated. Invasive cancer usually arises from most advanced lesions, particularly classical CIS. [Modified from Wright 1994.]

73 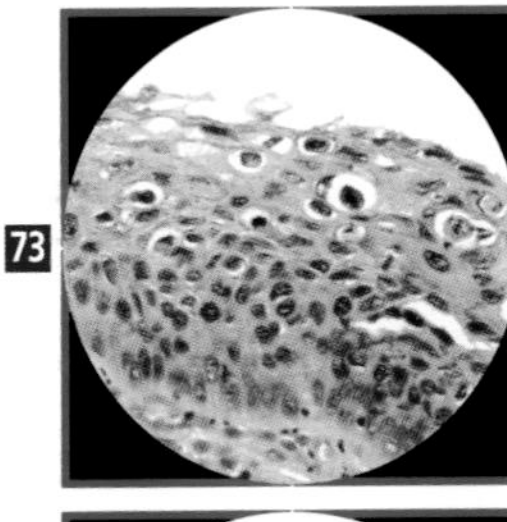

74 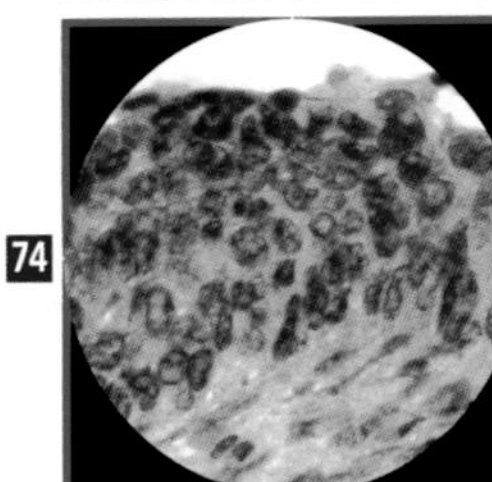

noma in situ, there is no order at all. So, in contrast with even severe dysplasia, there is no palisade of the basal layer of cells in carcinoma in situ. However, in carcinoma in situ, the cells may proliferate so rapidly they crowd each other into vertical spindle shapes. Since there is no maturation in carcinoma in situ, the epithelium looks about the same right side up as upside down, when viewed histologically. One more note: In some high-grade lesions, in which the epithelium matures poorly, the lesion may only be a few cells thick (known as "thin CIN"). The danger of thin cervical intraepithelial neoplasia is that it may be underdiagnosed or overlooked altogether in the tissue.

Cytology: Because carcinoma in situ is defined in terms of a "full thickness" abnormality of the epithelium, a common misconception is that dysplasia is not a full-thickness abnormality. But, dysplasia, even of mild degree, represents a profound biologic upheaval and derangement of the entire thickness of the epithelium, at least focally, otherwise abnormal cells would not appear at the surface. This is crucial: If it were not the case, the Pap smear would not work because only the surface of the epithelium is sampled. *The important concept is that in dysplasia, there are abnormal cells through the full thickness of the epithelium, but they differentiate toward the surface.*

Histologically, the fraction of the whole epithelium that is composed of *undifferentiated* abnormal cells determines the degree of dysplasia. Cytology has a different perspective: it looks at differentiated cells exfoliated from the surface. The two perspectives are complementary: as the undifferentiated level ascends from the basal layer (viewed histologically), there is a corresponding decrease in the degree of squamous differentiation at the surface (viewed cytologically). One could say that a glass that is "more full" (histology) is correspondingly "less empty" (cytology).

In low-grade dysplasia, considerable maturation can occur before the cells exfoliate, and therefore the abnormal surface cells appear fairly mature. In high-grade dysplasia, the undifferentiated cells ascend high in the epithelium, and little squamous maturation can occur before the cells exfoliate. Therefore, the surface squamous cells of high-grade dysplasia appear immature. In carcinoma in situ, the full thickness of the epithelium is undifferentiated; therefore, undifferentiated cells are found at the mucosal surface.

F6.14 Nuclear Areas Compared With Intermediate Cell Nucleus

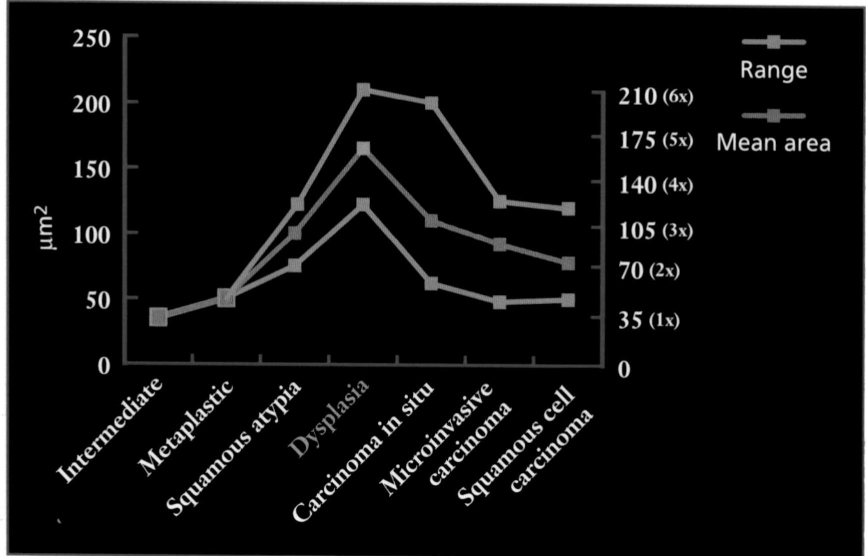

Nuclear area peaks at dysplasia (mild); x = intermediate cell nuclear area [Patten 1978].

The Nucleus

Nuclear features also undergo changes that correlate with the degree of epithelial abnormality [F6.14]. The nuclear size, shape, outline, chromatin texture, and distribution as well as the presence of nucleoli all follow a predictable pattern of development. The nucleus of an intermediate cell serves as the reference. The mean nuclear area is 35 µm², about the size of a red blood cell. The chromatin is finely granular and evenly distributed. The nuclear membrane is generally smooth, or it may have a neat fold.

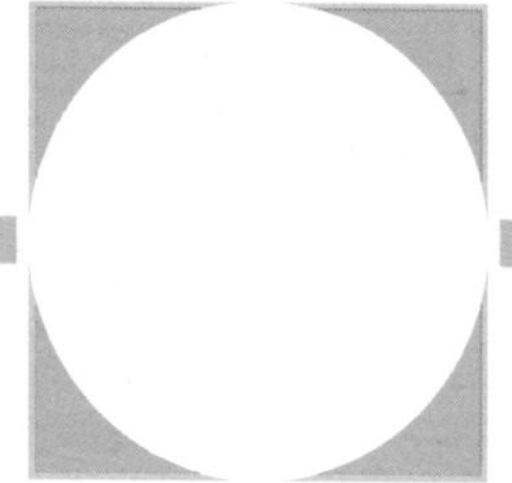

Important changes occur as cells progress from metaplastic to dysplastic to neoplastic and malignant. The nucleus of a metaplastic cell enlarges to about 50 µm², but is otherwise similar to an intermediate cell nucleus in terms of its nuclear membrane and chromatin quality.

At the next stage, dysplasia, profound changes are occurring in the nucleus. Perhaps most surprising is that the nuclei of dysplasia are, on average, the largest nuclei in the whole chain of events from benign to malignant lesions, and the largest of all are found in mild dysplasia.

Dysplastic nuclei average about 165 µm² (range, ~120–210 µm²), which is 3.5 to 6 times the size of an intermediate cell nucleus [Patten 1978]. From this point, the average nuclear size diminishes. The mean nuclear area of squamous cell carcinoma is only about 85 µm² (range, ~50–120 µm²), or up to about 2 to 3 times the size of an intermediate cell nucleus. The average nuclei of dysplasia are larger than those of invasive cancer; in fact, the smallest dysplastic nuclei are larger than the largest malignant nuclei [Patten 1978]! Compared with the life of a star, dysplasia is a red giant (in which viruses may be multiplying), and cancer a white dwarf (in which the viruses are integrated).

On the other hand, there is almost complete overlap in the range of nuclear areas of carcinoma in situ (from ~60–200 µm²) with both dysplasia and squamous cell carcinoma. This suggests that carcinoma in situ is a dynamic process in which the cells are changing from merely dysplastic to frankly malignant. The nuclei of microinvasive and fully invasive carcinoma and squamous cell carcinoma are virtually identical in size.

At the stage of mild dysplasia, with its large, ballooned nuclei, the nuclear membranes may be more or less smooth and the chromatin is often relatively fine. Recall that the volume of a sphere increases with the cube of the radius, $4/3\ \pi\ r^3$. Therefore, a small increase in the width of a nucleus may mean a marked increase in the volume of nuclear material, even when the overall staining remains relatively normochromatic. Therefore, the nuclei may need not be especially hyperchromatic in dysplasia, particularly in low-grade dysplasia and squamous atypia. Usually, however, the nuclei are at least somewhat hyperchromatic, compared with an intermediate cell nucleus. As the dysplasia progresses, the chromatin "precipitates," and tends to become coarser and darker, with chromocenter formation. At the same time, the nuclear envelope becomes wrinkled or crinkled as the nucleus crumples (like wadding up a ball of paper). By the stage of cervical intraepithelial neoplasia III, there is a small, irregular, "raisinoid" nucleus [75 I6.87, I6.141].

Judging nuclear areas and relative sizes may be difficult. To give a concrete example using ordinary objects of daily life, let's suppose that a dime represents an intermediate cell nucleus [T6.15].

N/C Ratio

In histology, the degree of dysplasia is diagnosed by the ratio of the thickness of the undifferentiated layer to the thickness of the whole epithelium (an undifferentiated/mucosal thickness ratio). In cytology, an analogous ratio is the N/C ratio: the higher the N/C ratio, the less mature the cell [F6.15]. Because the intermediate cell is a mature form, the N/C ratio is quite low. Metaplastic cells are relatively immature; therefore, the N/C ratio is higher than that of an intermediate cell. Cellular immaturity, measured by N/C ratio, reaches its peak at the stage of carcinoma in situ (completely undifferentiated cells), after which the cells "redifferentiate" as they become invasive cancer, and the N/C ratio falls. Poorly differentiated cancers have a higher N/C ratio than well-differentiated cancers. In summary, while nuclear size peaks at dysplasia, the N/C ratio peaks at the stage of carcinoma in situ.

When invasion begins, the chromatin falls apart, separating into irregular, pointed shards, with areas of clearing. A nucleolus develops. The cell acquires more cytoplasm, and redifferentiates, though abnormally. A simple matrix condenses all these features for easy comparisons [T6.16].

T6.15 An Aid to Judging Nuclear Areas and Relative Sizes

Coin	Area, μm^2	
Dime	35	Intermediate cell nucleus
Nickel	50	Squamous metaplastic nucleus
Quarter	70	Beginning squamous atypia
Half-dollar	100	Average of squamous atypia
Silver dollar	150	Range of dysplasia

T6.16 Nuclear Features Compared in Various Abnormalities

	Dysplasia	Carcinoma In Situ	Microinvasive Carcinoma	Squamous Cell Carcinoma
Nuclear size	Maximum	Variable	Minimum	Minimum
Nuclear/cytoplasmic ratio	Increases	Maximum	Decreases	Decreases
Chromatin	Finer → Coarser		Irregular distribution	Irregular distribution
Prominent nucleoli	Absent	Absent	Herald invasion	Invasion
Cytoplasm	Dedifferentiates	Undifferentiated	Abnormal differentiation	Abnormal differentiation

75
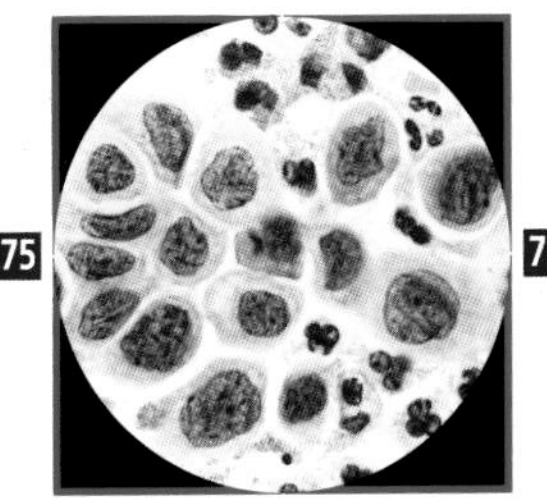
75

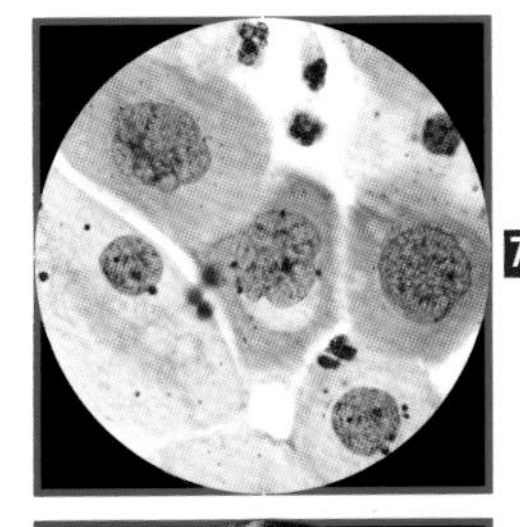
76

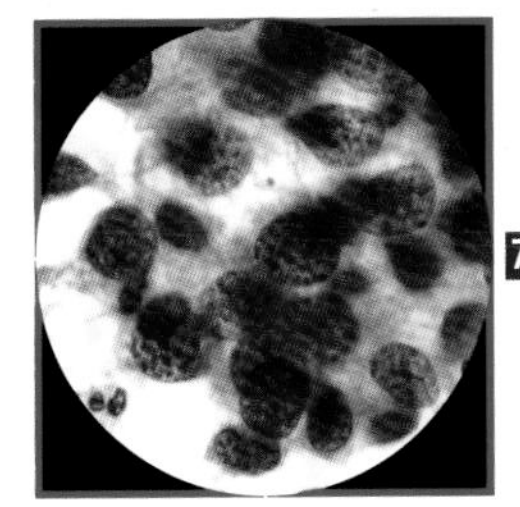
77

The Secrets of Diagnosing Dysplasia and Carcinoma In Situ

There are really only two steps to diagnosing dysplasia. First, the cell is determined to be dysplastic by virtue of its nuclear features, as previously discussed. Nuclear enlargement greater than 120 μm^2 (≥3.5 times intermediate cell nucleus) is the beginning of dysplasia [I6.85, 76 I6.86]. Nuclear enlargement in squamous atypia results in a nucleus that is two to three times the size of an intermediate cell nucleus. In essence, compare the nucleus in question with that of an intermediate cell: *If it's big and it's dark, it's dysplasia.*

Second, if the cell is determined to be dysplastic, then the N/C ratio is assessed to grade the dysplasia. The N/C ratio is a measure of cellular maturity. The higher the N/C ratio (relative to its icon), the higher the grade of dysplasia.

Nuclear changes characteristic of advancing dysplasia occur in concert with N/C ratio alterations. For example, if a cell has a high N/C ratio but the nucleus has a smooth, regular membrane, it is probably not cervical intraepithelial neoplasia III, which generally has irregular, "raisinoid" nuclei [75 I6.87, I6.141] but may be, for example, an immature metaplastic cell. Single cells, or small groups of cells, are easier to evaluate than cells found in thick groups, especially with respect to the N/C ratio. Although binucleated or multinucleated cells can be dysplastic, they are not evaluated in assessing the N/C ratio or degree of dysplasia.

Carcinoma in situ is characterized by the presence of three-dimensional syncytial-like aggregates of abnormal cells, with indistinct cell borders, and chaotic architecture (so-called loss of nuclear polarity). These cellular aggregates can be seen at low scanning power in the microscope as "hyperchromatic crowded groups" (HCGs) [77 I6.89]. It is very important to look for hyperchromatic crowded groups and carefully examine them, because these may represent a serious lesion, such as

F6.15 **Nuclear/Cytoplasmic Ratios (Relative Nuclear Area in %)**

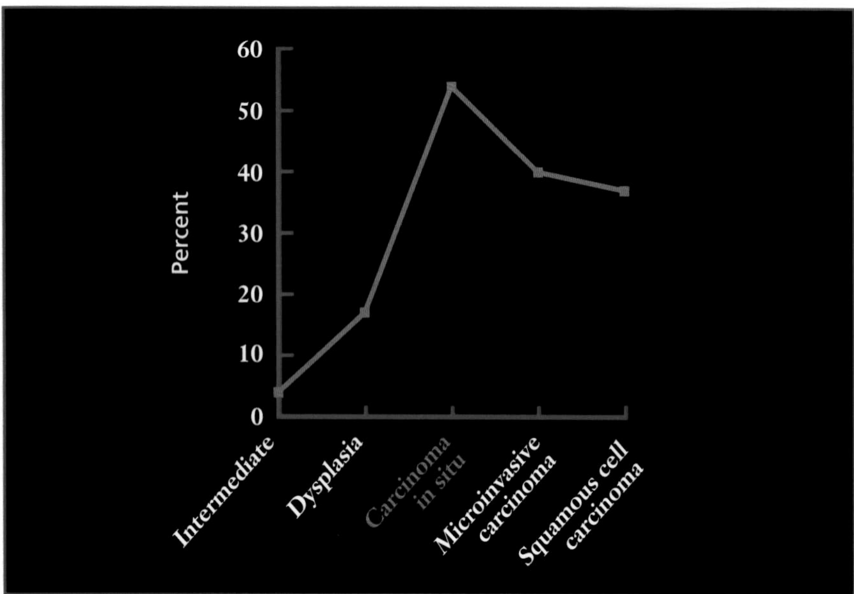

Note: The nuclear/cytoplasmic ratio of well-differentiated squamous cell carcinoma tends to be lower than the nuclear/cytoplasmic ratio of poorly differentiated squamous cell carcinoma [Patten 1978].

squamous carcinoma—in situ or invasive [Koike 1994]. However, many other benign and malignant lesions can be associated with hyperchromatic crowded groups, including endometrial cells and severe atrophy, as well as endocervical glandular neoplasia [Boon 1991]. As a rule (80% to >90% of cases), squamous carcinoma in situ is accompanied by squamous dysplasia, ranging from mild to severe ("like accompanies like"). The presence of an accompanying dysplasia is usually a good clue that the lesion in question really is carcinoma in situ and not a benign mimicker [T6.17]. Exceptionally, when the cervix is extensively involved with pure carcinoma in situ, an accompanying dysplasia will not be found. This situation is more likely to occur in postmenopausal patients.

In general, the more advanced the lesion, the more cells that are exfoliated, but cellularity alone is not a reliable diagnostic feature (eg, sampling could be a problem). Lesions are graded in the Pap smear—not by the number of abnormal cells, nor by the predominant cell type—but rather by the most abnormal cells present, even if there are only a few of them. However, it should be noted that when many abnormal cells are present, the diagnosis is more likely to be confirmed on biopsy than when there are only rare abnormal cells [S Hall 1994]. Dysplasia can be easier to diagnose by cytology than histology. For example, cytology provides exquisite nuclear detail, which facilitates the diagnosis of subtle nuclear abnormalities indicative of dysplasia. In addition, cytology, because intact nuclei are laid out in full view for direct one-to-one comparison, considerably simplifies the detection of small aberrations. And, importantly, a wider area—theoretically the entire cervix and endocervix—is sampled by cytologic methods.

Atypical Squamous Cells of Undetermined Significance

Atypical squamous cells of undetermined significance (ASCUS) is defined, according to the Bethesda System, as squamous abnormalities that are more marked than those attributable to reactive changes, but that quantitatively or qualitatively fall short of a definitive diagnosis of a squamous intraepithelial lesion. For example, when there are cells suggestive of a squamous intraepithelial lesion, but their sparsity or degeneration preclude a definitive diagnosis, the designation ASCUS can be applied. Atypical repair, atypia of atrophy, and atypical parakeratosis can also be included in the category of ASCUS. Cellular changes thought to be purely reactive in nature should not be included in the category of ASCUS. Therefore, excluded from the ASCUS category are "reactive cellular changes" including Pap class II, reactive "atypia," inflammatory "atypia," and benign "atypia." A diagnosis of ASCUS is expected for up to 4%–6% of patients in the average patient population. However, in high-risk populations, with a high prevalence of squamous intraepithelial lesions, there may be a correspondingly higher prevalence of ASCUS (up to 3 times the rate of SIL) [Hudock 1995]. Unfortunately, ASCUS can also be a wastebasket category for a variety of diagnostic problems. Although there are certainly cells that are difficult to classify, ASCUS should not be used as a diagnostic crutch every time a funny-looking cell is encountered.

Also included in the category of ASCUS are lesions that could be considered minimal dysplasia (squamous atypia, atypical squamous metaplasia). The Bethesda System defines these cells as having nuclei about two to three times normal size with normochromatic or slightly hyperchromatic nuclei, even chro-

T6.17 **Benign Conditions Mimicking Low-Grade and High-Grade CIN and Cancer**

Mimics Low-Grade CIN	Mimics High-Grade CIN	Mimics Cancer
Trichomonas, *Candida*, and most other inflammation	Herpes*	Repair
Atypia of maturity	IUD Atypia*	Reactive endocervical cells
Squamous metaplasia	Atypia of atrophy*	Arias-Stella reaction
Vitamin deficiency	Squamous metaplasia	(Also mimics of high-grade CIN)
Radiation	Endometrial cells*	
Histiocytes	Follicular cervicitis*	
Decidual cells	Histiocytes*	
	Decidual cells	
	Reserve cell hyperplasia*	

* May see hyperchromatic crowded groups.

matin distribution, and smooth or only slightly irregular nuclear membranes.

These minimally dysplastic lesions, however, rather than being of "undetermined" significance, when properly diagnosed, are of reasonably well determined significance.

Minimal Dysplasia

In practice, two basic forms of minimal, or very mild, dysplasia may be observed. The first type of minimal dysplasia occurs in mature cells and is also known as noninflammatory squamous atypia or, simply, squamous atypia. Squamous atypia resembles intermediate or superficial cells with normochromatic or slightly hyperchromatic nuclei, which are about two to three times normal size. The second type of minimal dysplasia occurs in metaplastic cells and is also known as atypical squamous metaplasia. It resembles immature (parabasal-like) squamous metaplasia with minimally enlarged, hyperchromatic nuclei. (Atypical parakeratosis can be regarded as a third form of minimal dysplasia and has been discussed previously.) The number of abnormal cells in either type is highly variable.

Squamous Atypia or Mature Minimal Dysplasia: The mature form of minimal dysplasia, squamous atypia [78 I6.71], is the easier form to diagnose. This lesion is diagnosed by finding intermediate or superficial cells with a "sick" nucleus, but usually essentially normal-appearing cytoplasm. The nuclear abnormality ("dyskaryosis") may be similar to that of mild dysplasia, but is usually somewhat less marked. The nuclei are enlarged, averaging about 100 μm² (range, 75–120 μm²), which is about two to three times the area of an intermediate cell nucleus. This compares with mild dysplasia in which the nuclei range from 120–210 μm (average, 165 μm²), ie, greater than three times normal [Patten 1978]. The nuclear membranes are smooth or only slightly irregular. The chromatin is fine, and usually at least slightly hyperchromatic, although sometimes it can be quite dark. Chromocenter formation is usually inconspicuous in either squamous atypia or mild dysplasia.

Although the degree of nuclear abnormality is the primary consideration in the differential diagnosis of squamous atypia vs mild dysplasia, subtle cytoplasmic differences may be noticed. In squamous atypia the cytoplasm tends to remain essentially normal in appearance, ie, thin, delicate, and transparent, practically identical to that of the normal mature intermediate or superficial cell. The cytoplasm may stain blue or pink or orange. In contrast, in mild dysplasia, not only is there more obvious nuclear abnormality, but in addition, the cytoplasm usually appears slightly thick and dense (ie, slightly immature) compared with normal mature intermediate or superficial cells. (In more advanced dysplasia, the cytoplasm appears still more immature, reminiscent of metaplasia, or is abnormally keratinized.)

Atypical Squamous Metaplasia or Metaplastic Minimal Dysplasia: Minimal dysplasia of immature metaplastic cells is also known as atypical squamous metaplasia [79 I6.72] and is characterized by nuclear abnormalities (size, outline, and chromatin) that are less severe than those associated with mild dysplasia. Compared with the normal metaplastic nucleus (50 μm²), the nuclei of atypical squamous metaplasia are enlarged ~1.5 to 2 times normal (range, 70–120 μm²). Chromocenters or small nucleoli may be present. The cells of atypical squamous metaplasia are intermediate in appearance between ordinary squamous metaplasia and mild (immature) metaplastic dysplasia. Atypical squamous metaplasia is much more difficult to diagnose than squamous atypia [D Jones 1987]. Since the cytoplasm of metaplastic cells is, by definition, immature, a valuable distinguishing diagnostic clue is lost (compare with squamous atypia). The nuclear abnormalities are subtle, and can be very difficult to distinguish from benign reactive changes, on the one hand, and more advanced dysplasia, on the other [T6.18].

HPV Infection and Minimal Dysplasia: The rate of HPV infection in women with benign atypia, including both squamous and inflammatory atypia, is high, about two to eight times the rate of normal controls [Bauer 1991, Borst 1991, Rader 1991, Wagner 1984]. Thus, the presence of atypia often indicates infec-

78
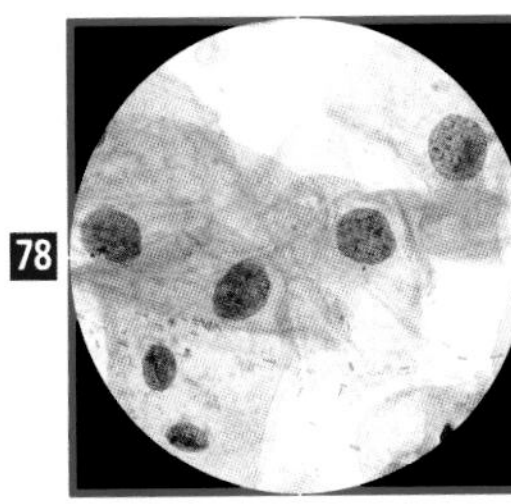

79
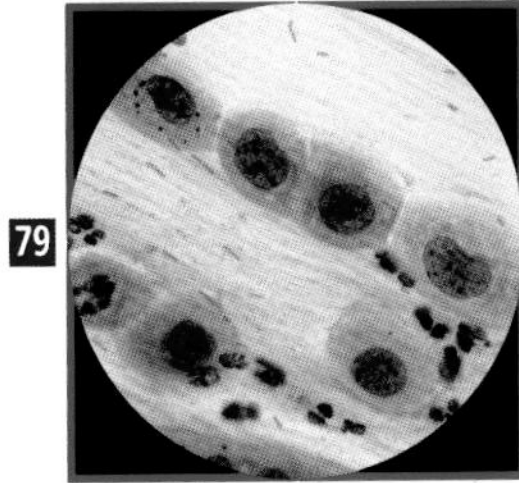

T6.18 **Criteria for Diagnosis of Minimal Dysplasia (ASCUS)**

Mature Lesions	Squamous Atypia	Mild Dysplasia
Cells	~Size and appearance of superficial or intermediate	~Same
N/C Ratio	Very slightly increased	Slightly increased
Nucleus	Moderately enlarged	Markedly enlarged (largest)
	2 to 3x normal intermediate nucleus	>3x normal intermediate nucleus
	75 to 120 μm²	120 to 200+ μm²
Membrane	Regular or slightly irregular	~Same
Chromatin	~Normal to slightly dark	Often darker
	Even distribution	Same
	Fine	Variably coarse
Chromocenters	Usually (–)	(±)
Nucleoli	Absent, inconspicuous	Same
Cytoplasm	Blue to pink to orange	Same, but slightly dense
	± Indistinct halos	Usually no halos (except koilocytes)
Metaplastic Lesions	**Atypical Squamous Metaplasia**	**Mild Metaplastic Dysplasia**
Cells	Atypical metaplastic cells	Slightly more abnormal
Nucleus	Slightly enlarged	
	1.5 to 2.5x metaplastic nucleus	
	2 to 3.5x intermediate nucleus	3.5 to 6x intermediate nucleus
Membrane	Regular or slightly irregular	~Same
Chromatin	Slight hyperchromasia	~Same
	± Chromocenters	~Same
Nucleoli	±	~Same

[G Davis 1987, Maier 1986, Noumoff 1987, Paavonen 1989, Ridgley 1988]

tion with HPV [Stewart 1993]. Macrocytes may also be present. Binucleation is common. If koilocytes are present, the diagnosis should mention condyloma, because koilocytes are pathognomonic for it.

Biologic Significance of Minimal Dysplasia: Finding these minimally dysplastic cells on the mucosal surface implies a full thickness abnormality of the epithelium at least focally. And by the time abnormalities are visible in the light microscope, a tremendous upheaval of the biologic machinery of the nucleus at the ultrastructural, and even molecular, level has already occurred. In fact, ultrastructural and biochemical abnormalities that precede visible light microscopic changes are demonstrable in cervical epithelium of animals treated with carcinogenic agents [Rubio 1981a]. DNA analysis raises the possibility that many of these lesions are aneuploid [Watts 1987]. The morphologic changes, then, may not be so minimal.

Before becoming invasive cancer, dysplasias usually progress through the recognized grades of intraepithelial neoplasia. However, as previously discussed, some cases apparently invade without going through all stages, and in (very) rare cases apparently invade from so-called minimal dysplasia. ASCUS may be the only cytologically detectable lesion preceding the development of high-grade squamous intraepithelial lesions [Sherman 1992a]. These findings support the concept of the potentially malignant nature of even extremely low-grade intraepithelial lesions. Furthermore, minimal dysplasia often coexists with more advanced dysplasia, which not only argues for its being considered true dysplasia, but also serves as a warning that a more advanced lesion may be lurking in the patient.

Clinical Significance of Squamous Atypia and Minimal Dysplasia: Evaluation of the clinical significance of squamous atypia is hampered because many studies are based on: (1) atypical (Papanicolaou class II) smears [Figge 1970, Hulka 1968, Morrison 1988, Nyirjesy 1972, Reiter 1986, Sandmire 1976, Spitzer 1987]; (2) mild "dyskaryosis" [J Robertson 1988], a British term for mild dysplasia [D Evans 1986]; or (3) koilocytotic atypia [Campion 1986], which is diagnostic of condyloma, a low-grade squamous intraepithelial lesion. By some definitions, Papanicolaou class II (atypical) Pap smears include cases of condyloma [Morrison 1988] and well-defined cervical intraepithelial neoplasia [W Jones 1986, Koss 1978], as advanced as moderate dysplasia (CIN II, high-grade squamous intraepithelial lesion) [Hulka 1968].

Even after studies that include these more advanced squamous lesions have been eliminated, "squamous atypia" or minimal dysplasia still remains a significant finding in the Pap smear. It has been shown that even one, and particularly two, Pap smears showing minimal dysplasia identifies a patient who has a manyfold (more than 5–10 times) increased risk of subsequently developing a well-defined dysplasia [Melamed 1976]. Atypical squamous metaplasia is more likely to progress to a more advanced lesion than squamous atypia (12% vs 4%), while mixed lesions are the most likely to progress (49%) [Paavonen 1989].

Bona fide minimal lesions are difficult to appreciate in a tissue biopsy, thus histologic confirmation of the cytologic diagnosis is doubtful. Therefore, in theory, *when a diagnosis of squamous atypia is made on a Pap smear, it is predicted that were a biopsy performed, the results would be "negative."* The primary importance of a diagnosis of squamous atypia lies in identifying patients who are at high risk for a significant squamous intraepithelial lesion. Unfortunately, in practice, many patients already have a significant lesion. A review of 2,765 reported cases of "squamous atypia" reveals that of patients with a Pap smear showing only this lesion, more than one quarter (28%) will have a simultaneous, biopsy-proven, well-defined squamous intraepithelial lesion (cervical intraepithelial neoplasia, condyloma) [T6.19]. And more than 10% of patients have CIN II or worse, ie, high-grade squamous intraepithelial lesion, even including rare cases of invasive cancer [August 1991, Dressel 1992, Soutter 1986]! (If Papanicolaou class II atypical smears were included, up to 4.5% of cases would show invasive carcinoma on biopsy [Hulka 1968].) Furthermore, studies focusing on human papilloma virus infection have found that patients with an initial diagnosis of squamous atypia may have extraordinarily high rates of condyloma, ranging up to 58% [August 1991, Borst 1991, Kaminski 1989a, Lawley 1990]. One study found that 85% of cases of squamous atypia were associated with high-risk viral types [Goff 1993].

Toon reported 106 cases of squamous atypia, 13 with CIN—any degree—on follow-up [Toon 1986]. Kaminski reported squamous intraepithelial lesions in 21% of pregnant patients who had an initial Pap smear diagnosis of squamous atypia [Kaminski 1992]. Walker reported 41 cases, 12 with high-grade squamous intraepithelial lesion on follow-up [E Walker 1986]. Stafl reported 713 cases in which 34 carcinomas in situ were found on biopsy samples [Stafl 1973]. In long-term follow-up of "borderline" lesions, Hirschowitz found progression to high-grade

***T6.19* Summary of Follow-up Biopsies of Patients Whose Pap Smears Indicated Only Squamous Atypia (ASCUS)**

Study	No. of Cases	Total SIL (%)	High-Grade SIL(%)
Andrews 1989a	353	55 (15.6)	19 (5.4)
M Brown 1985	104	14 (13.5)	10 (9.6)
Cunnane 1992	82	26 (31.7)	4 (4.9)
G Davis 1987	406	76 (18.7)	31 (7.6)
Goff 1993	171	28 (16.4)	5 (2.9)
D Jones 1987	256	58 (22.7)	10 (3.9)
Kaye 1993	63	31 (49.2)	9 (14.3)
Kohan 1985	86	60 (75.0)	42 (48.8)
Lindheim 1990	101	30 (29.7)	17 (16.8)
Maier 1986	429	86 (20.0)	60 (14.0)
Noumoff 1987	375	108 (28.8)	38 (10.1)
Paavonen 1989	124	51 (41.1)	17 (13.7)
Sidawy 1993	31	19 (61.3)	1 (3.2)
Slawson 1993	96	81 (84.4)	15 (15.6)
Soutter 1986	44	18 (40.9)	17 (38.6)
Tay 1987d	44	33 (75.0)	18 (40.9)
Total	2765	774 (28.0)	313 (11.3)

dyskaryosis in 22.4% of patients [Hirschowitz 1992]. Other studies, using biopsy or cytology follow-up, report generally similar findings [Davey 1994, Dressel 1992, Howell 1993, Sheils 1992].

The high-grade lesions may be focal [Stafl 1973]. The rate of abnormal biopsy findings decreases with age, with about 75% of cases occurring by age 40 years [Kaminski 1989a]. Thus, older patients with ASCUS have a significantly lower, but still real, risk of developing intraepithelial neoplasia than younger patients [Cunnane 1993, Kaminski 1989b, Symmans 1992].

The differential diagnosis of squamous atypia includes benign cellular changes, such as reactive or inflammatory "atypia." However, it is of importance that even apparently benign cellular changes are associated with squamous intraepithelial lesions in many cases [C Collins 1992]. Inflammatory "atypia" is frequently associated with dysplasia or condyloma. Up to 25% of patients with a cytologic diagnosis of inflammatory "atypia," particularly when persistent, may have high-grade squamous intraepithelial lesions on biopsy, with low-grade squamous intraepithelial lesions ranging up to 43% [Busseniers 1991, Cecchini 1990a, Frisch 1990, McLachlan 1994, Pearlstone 1992, J Wilson 1990]. Moreover, patients with endocervical glandular "atypia" also have a high rate of squamous intraepithelial lesions (up to 58% of patients [Kohan 1985]) [L Brown 1986, Goff 1992, Kohan 1985, Nasu 1993].

In summary, *patients with a diagnosis of "squamous atypia" are at high risk of either having or developing well-defined squamous intraepithelial lesions, including high-grade lesions.* Therefore, squamous atypia, or minimal dysplasia, is a significant diagnosis that should be taken seriously. However, because the numbers of cases of "squamous atypia" are abundant (as many as 15%–20% of all smears [August 1991]), the volume of patients tends to overwhelm the capacity of the colposcopy units, and follow-up of patients becomes a problem. Cervicography has been suggested for triage of these patients [August 1991].

Recommendations for Management of Patients With ASCUS: Patients at high risk for cervical neoplasia should be considered for immediate colposcopy at the first diagnosis of ASCUS (squamous atypia, atypical squamous metaplasia). For others, a reasonable clinical compromise is to treat any inflammation/infection as specifically as possible and then repeat the smear in 4 to 6 months (ie, "Treat and Repeat"). This time interval gives the less serious, or less well-established, lesions a chance to regress [Hulka 1968, Ridgley 1988]. However, such therapy may not significantly affect the rate of reversion to normal cytology [Reiter 1986]. A high proportion of repeat smears, up to 80%, in patients with squamous atypia will still be abnormal [August 1991]. And false negative diagnoses are a problem. Repeat Pap smears in patients with "squamous atypia" misses a significant number of patients who actually have a well-defined dysplasia, more advanced than indicated by the Pap smear [Andrews 1989a, G Davis 1987, Noumoff 1987]. A significant number of patients, at least 10% [Andrews 1989a, Maier 1986], who eventually have biopsy-proven dysplasia, will show two or more consecutive negative Pap smears (which may be taken as evidence that the lesion has disappeared). Two related problems are that cases of dysplasia are frequently underdiagnosed as atypia [Frisch 1987a,b] and as has been discussed, dysplasias may come and go.

Therefore, it could be argued that—since a second positive diagnosis adds no new information, but does delay proper diagnosis and treatment, and because patients with dysplasia may have a false-negative Pap smear, further complicating management—perhaps colposcopy should be performed at the first sign of any abnormality [D Jones 1987]. Patients with persistent "atypical" cells run up to a 30% chance of having CIN III on biopsy [M Brown 1985]. At least three consecutive, satisfactory negative smears should be obtained before reassuring the patient and returning to routine screening [Ridgley 1988].

In conclusion, although opinion is about evenly split regarding the need for immediate colposcopy on the first smear showing "squamous atypia," it is virtually unanimous that patients with persistent ASCUS should be referred for colposcopy.

Epidemiology of Cervical Neoplasia

In one of the first epidemiologic studies ever published, the Italian physician Rigoni-Stern analyzed the mortality records of the city of Verona. He reported, in 1842, that uterine cancer (later interpreted as mostly cervical cancer [Griffiths 1991]) was more common among married than unmarried women, and that it was rare in nuns [Kessler 1987, Stavola 1987]. By the mid-20th century, epidemiologic evidence suggested that cervical cancer was related to early marriage and low socioeconomic status of the woman [Aitken-Swan 1966, E Jones 1958, Stocks 1955, Terris 1980], with an additional component (thought possibly to be smegma or sperm) related to the man.

It is now believed that factors related to sexual behavior are at the root of those epidemiologic findings. Cervical cancer is thought to be rare in virgins and common in prostitutes (although these findings may not be as well proven as sometimes assumed [Gardner 1974, Skrabanek 1988, Towne 1955]). The strongest epidemiologic correlations have been with early age at first coitus (particularly before 18 years of age) [Aitken-Swan 1966, Boyd 1964, Brinton 1987, Kessler 1974, Koutsky 1992, C Martin 1967, Munoz 1994, Pridan 1971, Rotkin 1962,1967a, Wynder 1954], and history of multiple sexual partners (particularly more than two) [Barron 1971; Brinton 1987, Edebiri 1990, Kessler 1974, C Martin 1967, Pridan 1971, Rotkin 1973, Terris 1980]. Some increase in risk may occur in patients initiating coitus before 21 years of age [Rotkin 1967a]. Also, women who have had more than one sexual partner may increase their risk twofold to threefold compared with women who have had only one partner [Kessler 1974, Rotkin 1967a]. Which factor is more important—early sexual experience or multiple partners—is controversial [Brinton 1987, Harris 1980, Kiviat 1989, LaVecchia 1986b, Reeves 1985, Rotkin 1967a, Singer 1975].

Another strong factor is coitus with a "high-risk male," which includes men who are promiscuous [Brinton 1989b], have penile condylomas [Boon 1988], or have had previous partners with cervical neoplasia. Penile condylomas (which like the cervical counterpart, may be flat and invisible to the naked eye) are found in 70% to 90% of male partners of women with genital HPV infections [Boon 1988, Campion 1985, Sand 1986, A Schneider 1988a, Sedlacek 1986, Wosnitzer 1988], and the virus detected may be the same viral type [Barrasso 1987, A Schneider 1987c]. There is also a high prevalence of penile HPV infection in men who are the regular sexual partners of women with histologically proven cervical intraepithelial neoplasia III [Campion 1988]. A high incidence of HPV has been found in men with penile carcinomas [Boon 1989b, Varma 1991, Villa 1986]. Wives of men with penile cancer have a substantially increased risk of developing cancer of the cervix [S Graham 1979a]; a clustering of cases of cervical carcinoma in areas with high rates of penile cancer has also been noted [Li 1982]. On the other hand, circumcision status is apparently not related to development of cervical neoplasia [Rotkin 1973, Terris 1973], and whether semen or any of its various components are important in the development of cervical cancer is unknown.

Although other factors, such as early age at first pregnancy, short time between pregnancies, abortions, early age of first marriage, poor genital hygiene, and most venereal diseases [Brinton 1987, Levin 1942] may be risk factors, they seem more likely to be "confounding" variables of sexual activity [Richart 1973]. The effect of certain hormones, eg, diethylstilbestrol (DES) and birth control pills, has been controversial [Robboy 1981,1984, Vessey 1983]; however, there does appear to be an increased risk of cervical cancer among users of birth control pills, particularly among long-term users (≥5 years) [Harris 1980, Meisels 1977a, Swan 1982], who may have a twofold higher risk [Brinton 1986a]. Douching, which alters the vaginal milieu, could also be related to development of cervical cancer [Gardner 1991, S Graham 1979b, Rotkin 1968]. On the other hand, barrier methods of contraception (condom, diaphragm) decrease the risk of developing cervical cancer [Rotkin 1973, N Wright 1978] (although unconfirmed, condom use has been reported to cure intraepithelial cancer, perhaps by preventing reinfection! [Richardson 1981]).

Many other factors have also been considered, eg, menstrual patterns, use of tampons or vaginal deodorants [Brinton 1987], masturbation, even coital positions [Rotkin 1967b], but again, most are not currently thought to be causal. Other factors that are probably unrelated to development of cervical cancer include lifetime frequency of intercourse [Brinton 1987, E Jones 1958, C Martin 1967, Rotkin 1967a, Terris 1980] and age at menarche [Brinton 1987, E Jones 1958, Rotkin 1967a]. Parity, previously dismissed as a risk factor for cervical cancer [Boyd 1964, Rotkin 1967a, Wynder 1954], may in fact be related [Brinton 1989a].

The interpretation of these epidemiologic data is that a carcinogenic agent is transmitted by sexual intercourse to a female at risk, ie, *cervical cancer may be a venereal disease* [Affandi 1993, Beral 1974, Kessler 1976,1987] (everything causes cancer). The data further suggest that the patient is more susceptible to this agent at a young age and that the exposure must be maintained over a long period [Herrero 1990]. The nature of the agent has been the subject of intense investigation. Naturally, infectious agents have been suspected. Virtually every organism ever found in the female genital tract, including *Trichomonas*, *Treponema*, gonococcus, *Chlamydia*, cytomegalovirus, herpes, and most recently human papilloma virus (HPV), has had its 15 minutes of fame as the possible cause of cervical cancer. Except for HPV, and possibly herpes [Kessler 1987, zur Hausen 1982], these agents are now generally thought to be dependent variables of sexual behavior.

It has been found that smoking increases the risk of developing cervical neoplasia, independent of sexual factors [Brinton 1986b, LaVecchia 1986a, Luesley 1994, Slattery 1989, Trevathan 1983, P Ward 1990, Winkelstein 1977,1984,1990], perhaps by acting as a cancer "promoter." Smokers have about a 50% higher risk of developing cervical squamous cell carcinoma than do nonsmokers [Brinton 1986b]. The risk is dose dependent (ie, directly related to long term habit, packs per day, unfiltered cigarettes). Smoking by the male partner may also be a risk factor [Zunzunegui 1986]. Finally, failure to obtain Pap smears is also a significant risk factor (discussed in more detail later).

Incidence and Prevalence: The incidence of squamous cell carcinoma of the cervix in 1947, when the Pap smear was just being introduced, was about 2.5 times that in 1970 [Cramer 1974]. Since the 1970s, the yearly incidence has generally tended to fall, but with an upward blip in the 1990s [F6.16].

Mortality has shown a remarkable decrease, with a reduction of 70% to 80% in the same time frame [F6.16] [Boring 1991, D Fink 1988]. Before the introduction of the Pap smear, cervical cancer was the leading cause of cancer death in women. By the early 1990s, in the United States, it had declined, with a mortality of 4,800 expected in 1995 [Wingo 1995]. Today in the United States, less than 2% of cancer deaths in women, and

F6.16 Annual Incidence and Mortality of Cervical Cancer

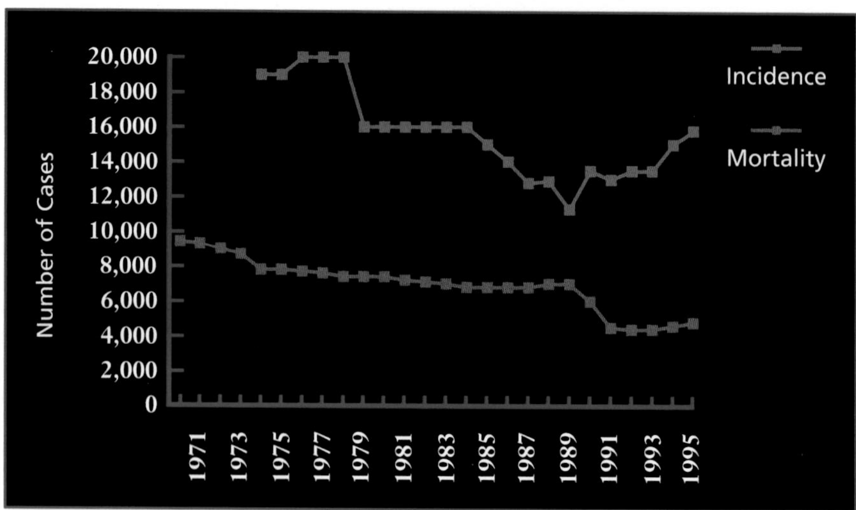

Note: Annual incidence of "carcinoma in situ" increased from ~40,000 to 65,000 over the same period, but in later years cases of CIN III and recently high-grade SIL, were included. [Source: *CA—A Cancer Journal for Clinicians*; Annual Cancer Statistics: 1970-1995.]

less than 0.5% of all (female) deaths are now attributable to cervical cancer [Boring 1994]. Unfortunately, worldwide, particularly in developing countries, cervical cancer is still a leading cause of cancer death in women, even in areas with otherwise low cancer rates [Parkin 1988, Pisani 1993].

Despite advances in medicine, the survival rate to patients with cervical cancer has remained relatively unchanged over the past 50 years [Kessler 1987]. Therefore, it is believed that the lower incidence and mortality rates for cervical carcinoma represent a triumph of the Pap smear in achieving early cancer detection [Koss 1989a]. Lesions are now being detected earlier, while they are still in a more curable, often preinvasive, state. In the early 1950s, two of three cervical cancers were invasive at the time of diagnosis. By the late 1960s, at least three of four patients were diagnosed while their lesions were still intraepithelial [Kessler 1987]. Invasive cervical cancers detected by the Pap smear are predominantly stage I (80% to 90%), compared with those presenting for reasons other than abnormal Pap smears, of which one third are stage II and one quarter stage III or IV [Carmichael 1984, Pretorius 1991].

While the incidence of invasive cancers has declined, *there has been a marked increase in histologically confirmed abnormal Pap smears* (threefold to fourfold rise from the mid-1960s to the late 1970s [Wolfendale 1983]). The incidence of carcinoma in situ has soared (at least a 300% to 500% increase from 1950 to 1970 [Kessler 1987] and is still increasing [F6.16]). By the early 1990s, carcinoma in situ was diagnosed more than three times as often as squamous cell carcinoma of the cervix (>50,000 cases); however, at least some of this increase is artificial, and reflects the replacement of the diagnosis of carcinoma in situ by CIN III, which includes cases of severe dysplasia. In the future, as high-grade squamous intraepithelial lesion replaces CIN III, another round of artificial inflation will likely occur, since cases of moderate dysplasia would be added. In fact, this is happening (>65,000 cases) [Wingo 1995].

In the 1960s, the overall prevalence of dysplasia was on the order of 5.4 to 13.3 per 1,000 [Bibbo 1971a, Stern 1969], while the overall prevalence of carcinoma in situ was about 3.8 to 6.4 per 1,000 [Bibbo 1971a, Stern 1964]. By the 1980s, the prevalence of cervical intraepithelial neoplasia (all grades) was about 23.3/1,000 [Sadeghi 1988]. Of course, the rates could be higher or lower, depending on the particular patient population screened.

In addition, there has practically been an explosion of cases of condyloma, with more than a sixfold increase in visible lesions during the 1960s and 1970s [CDC 1983]. Although condyloma was probably underdiagnosed in the past [S Bernstein 1985] and the rates may have leveled off [Mazur 1984], there has apparently been a worldwide epidemic of HPV infections and cervical intraepithelial neoplasia [T6.20] [Wolfendale 1983]. Condyloma has become the most frequent of the squamous intraepithelial lesion [Meisels 1977, Richart 1987].

Age at Diagnosis: As the incidence and prevalence of preinvasive disease has been rising, the average age has been falling. Mild dysplasia has been reported in 10-year-olds, severe dysplasia in 15-year-olds [Sadeghi 1988], and carcinoma in situ in teenagers [Ferguson 1961, Kaufman 1970, Wallace 1973]. Even invasive carcinoma has been reported as early as the teenage years [Bibbo 1971a, Chung 1982, Kling 1973]. Dysplastic lesions are common in teenagers [Feldman 1976, Hein 1977, Sadeghi 1984, Snyder 1976]. By the early 1980s, the cervical intraepithelial neoplasia prevalence rate (all grades) was 18.8 per 1,000 for ages 15 to 19 years [Sadeghi 1984].

***T6.20* Worldwide Survey of the Condyloma and Dysplasia Epidemic**

Australia [Mitchell 1990a]
- Substantial increase in CIN—all age groups
- ~Seven times increase in CIN from 1970–1988
  - Most increase in lower grades, ie, < CIN III
  - Corresponding decrease in age at diagnosis

Canada [Raymond 1987a]
- CIS in 20- to 29-year-olds doubled during 1970s

England [Beral 1986]
- Substantial increase in mild atypia
- Possible quadrupling of SCC in young patients

Finland [Syrjänen 1990]
- Estimate up to ~80% will contract HPV infections between ages 20 and 79 years

New Zealand [A Chang 1985]
- Incidence of abnormal smears ~tripled from 1973–1977 to 1978–1982

United States
- Marked increase in CIS with a precipitous drop in median age in just 3 years of the early 1970s [Creasman 1975]
- CIS increased from ~40,000 to ~65,000 cases annually from mid-1970s to 1990s (see F6.16)
- Squamous atypia and mild dysplasia increased from 2% in 1964 to 21.8% in 1989 in young, indigent patients [Costa 1991a]

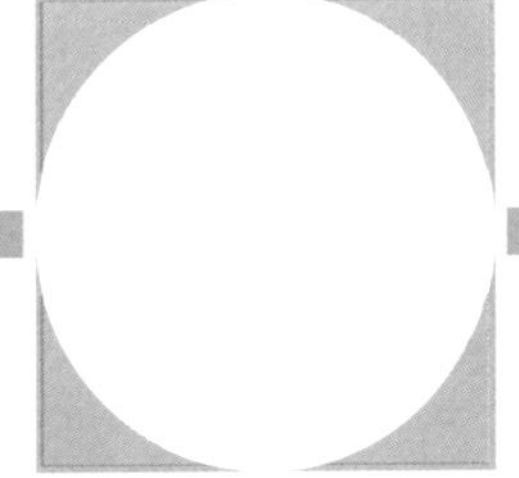

These alarming statistics are ascribed to changes in sexual behavior ("the sexual revolution"). Moreover, preinvasive disease may be progressing more rapidly than in the past, particularly in young patients [Adcock 1982, Bain 1983, Benoit 1984, Berkeley 1980, Berkowitz 1979, T Johnson 1994, Laskey 1979, LiVolsi 1984, MacGregor 1982, Paterson 1984, Pedersen 1971, Prendiville 1980, Schwartz 1988, Yule 1978]. Increased incidence and more rapid progression of precursor lesions are the basis of some concern that there may be a recrudescence of cases of squamous cell carcinoma, especially in younger patients [Beral 1974, Devesa 1987, Levine 1993]. The marked decline in the mortality rate for all age groups could conceal an increased mortality among younger patients. There is some evidence of increasing incidence and mortality of squamous cell carcinoma in young women [Anello 1979, Armstrong 1981,1983, Beral 1986, Bourne 1983, Devesa 1989, Draper 1983, Green 1978,1979, Larson 1994, L Weiss 1994, Yule 1978]. The cancers of these young patients may also be more anaplastic [Prempree 1983] and aggressive [Elliott 1989, Prempree 1983, BG Ward 1985], with earlier recurrences [Prempree 1983] and poorer prognosis [Chapman 1988, Prempree 1983, Stanhope 1980]. It must be noted, however, that several studies refute these findings and the subject remains controversial [Berkowitz 1979, J Carmichael 1986, Chu 1987, Kyriakos 1971, LaVecchia 1984a, Lowry 1989, Meanwell 1988, Mitchell 1990b, Spanos 1989].

The occurrence of condyloma, dysplasia, and carcinoma in situ rises, then falls, with age, while the occurrence of squamous

T6.21 **Mean and Peak Ages for Occurrence of Intraepithelial Lesions**

Disease	Mean Age, y	Peak Age, y
Condyloma	28.2	19
Mild dysplasia	29.0	22
Moderate dysplasia	28.3	22
Severe dysplasia	30.3	23
Carcinoma in situ	36.0	30
Squamous cell carcinoma	52.8	39

[Carson 1993, Meisels 1977b]

cell carcinoma more or less steadily increases. The mean and peak ages for condyloma, degrees of dysplasia, and carcinoma in situ are estimated in T6.21. Average age increases in more or less direct proportion to the degree of abnormality exhibited by the lesion. Today's patients may be younger [M Johnston 1988]. The presence of condyloma and cervical intraepithelial neoplasia together may lower the mean age of occurrence of cervical intraepithelial neoplasia [Zuna 1984]. Since the curves are skewed, the peak (mode) age gives a better idea than mean age of the "average" patient actually seen in daily practice [Carson 1993].

After reaching a peak in ages 20 to 39 years, the incidence and prevalence of condyloma and dysplasia progressively decrease. Visible condylomas are relatively unusual after 25 years of age [Oriel 1971], and two thirds of patients with flat condylomas are younger than 30 [Meisels 1981a]. Currently, *as many as 90% of all cases of squamous intraepithelial lesion (condyloma and cervical intraepithelial neoplasia) occur before the age of 35* [Binder 1985, Carson 1993, Meisels 1992]. Patients 50 years or older have a low prevalence of dysplasia [Bibbo 1971a, Carson 1993], but the occurrence of cervical cancer tends to increase with age [F6.17].

Natural History of Squamous Intraepithelial Lesions

Squamous intraepithelial lesions may be slowly progressive, and may also regress, but studies have found widely divergent rates. Accurate data are difficult to obtain. First, to observe the entire natural history prospectively would require allowing a patient to develop invasive cancer [Paul 1988]. Also, the disease may actually be eradicated by the very method used to investigate it (ie, biopsy). In fact, it has been found that even an incomplete biopsy can sometimes result in cure of the lesion. Apparently, the healthy mucosa is better able to replace the area that underwent biopsy, and the associated inflammatory reaction may help destroy residual disease [Koss 1963, Richart 1966b].

"Study of the natural history of a lesion such as carcinoma *in-situ* by conventional means is further bedevilled by what amounts almost to a biological uncertainty principle analogous to that in nuclear physics. The act of observation, of making the diagnosis, may interfere significantly with the thing to be observed, in this case the natural history" [Ashley 1966a].

On the other hand, it has also been shown that the dysplasia often comes back after biopsy, frequently in a different location [Koss 1963].

Though the natural history of these lesions is controversial, and still incompletely understood, the following are traditionally accepted teachings:

1. New lesions arise as mild dysplasia (CIN I, low-grade squamous intraepithelial lesion).
2. Any grade of dysplasia can progress to carcinoma in situ.
3. Most dysplastic lesions do not progress (corollary: more cases of CIN I than CIN III).
4. Many cases of carcinoma in situ will progress to cancer if left untreated.
5. Invasive carcinoma can arise without first developing classic carcinoma in situ, but this is the exception.

In essence, the more advanced the disease, the more likely it is to progress, the more rapidly it progresses, and the less likely it is to regress. Though only a small minority of all lesions advance, those that do seem to "pick up steam" as they progress to carcinoma in situ, where they may be held in check for some

F6.17 **Age Distribution of Dysplasia, Carcinoma In Situ, and Squamous Cell Carcinoma**

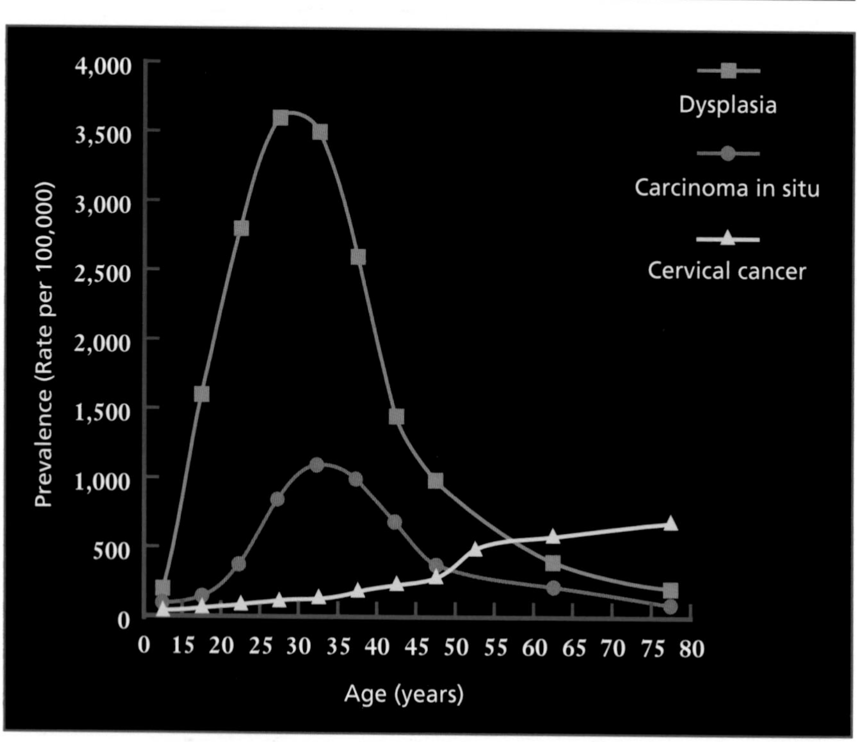

[Reid 1986]

time before invading. Invasion usually occurs from the most advanced lesions (apparently >90% from classic carcinoma in situ [Ng 1969]), and then only after many years (5–10, or more) [Barron 1978, J Dunn 1967, Fidler 1968, S Jordan 1981, Richart 1969, van Oortmarssen 1991]. However, invasive cancer apparently can arise from any degree of dysplasia, even mild dysplasia [Nelson 1989], as well as from apparently normal epithelium (though this is very rare) [Ng 1969] without first developing classic carcinoma in situ [Koss 1978].

The total duration of the disease, from incipient dysplasia to invasive cancer, may be 10 to 20 years [T6.22]. Probably less than 15% (and more like 5%–10%) of all dysplasias, left untreated, would progress to carcinoma in situ [Patten 1978]. However, a significant number of cases of carcinoma in situ (at least 10%, possibly 50%–90%) would progress to invasive cancer if left untreated [Albert 1981, Fidler 1968, McIndoe 1984, Ostor 1993a, Richart 1973].

These rates are averages and, unfortunately, the data are dirty. They have probably been affected by old definitions of low-grade dysplasia, which include lesions that would now be recognized as carcinoma in situ (ie, lesions that have already progressed) [McKay 1959, Okagaki 1962, Richart 1969]. On the other hand, the data may also be skewed in the opposite direction by low-grade squamous intraepithelial lesions caused by low-risk viral types, which may never progress. Thus, shorter transit times for those squamous intraepithelial lesions that are capable of progressing may be expected. In cases with evidence of HPV infection (condyloma), it is possible that the lesions may progress faster [Meisels 1981a, Syrjänen 1981]. The bottom line is that an accurate prediction for an individual patient cannot be made: the transit time may be slower or faster.

In some cases, cancer can apparently develop rapidly, possibly in as little as 6 months [Adcock 1982, Albert 1981, Ashley 1966a,b, Bain 1983, Bamford 1983, Benoit 1984, Berkeley 1980, J Dunn 1967,1981, Fetherston 1983, Fidler 1968, Figge 1970, Fox 1968, Hadjimichael 1989, Hammond 1968, M Jordan 1964, Laskey 1979, Liu 1967, LiVolsi 1984, Macgregor 1982, P Martin 1972, Mitchell 1990b, Paterson 1984, Pedersen 1971, R Peters 1988, Prendiville 1980, Sandmire 1976, Schwartz 1988]. However, many so-called rapidly progressive cancers, particularly those with very brief transit times (weeks or a few months) are probably not genuine, but rather represent misinterpretation of previous Pap smears, ie, previous false-negative diagnosis. A substantial increase in rapidly progressive cancers might be expected based on changes in the population structure, a general increase in cervical cancer rates, and increases in the proportion of women screened [Silcocks 1988].

T6.22 **Progression Rate Guesstimates**

From	Time, y	Progressing Fraction
Mild to carcinoma in situ	3–5	1/6 to 1/5
Moderate to carcinoma in situ	2–3	1/4 to 1/3
Severe to carcinoma in situ	1–2	1/3 to 1/2
Carcinoma in situ to carcinoma	5–10	1/2 or more?

[J Dunn 1967, McIndoe 1984, Meisels 1981a, Nasiell 1983,1986, Ostor 1993a, Richart 1969]

T6.23 **Site of Dysplasia in Relation to Cervical Os***

Type of Dysplasia	Relation to Cervical Os
(Immature) Metaplastic	Proximal
Mature Metaplastic	Near
Keratinizing	Distal

* These locations represent averages. The actual location depends on where the transition zone is located in an individual patient.

Regression and Recurrence: Regression of dysplasia is yet another matter of controversy. Most agree that lesions can regress. The overall rate of spontaneous regression for cytologically diagnosed dysplasia is in the range of 6% to more than 80% [Campion 1986, Eddy 1990, Fox 1967, Macgregor 1978, Richart 1969, J Robertson 1988, van Oortmarssen 1991]. The less advanced the lesion, the more likely it is to regress (conversely, the more advanced, the less likely) [Fox 1967, J Hall 1968]. Younger patients may have a higher rate of regression than older patients [van Oortmarssen 1991]. Why lesions should spontaneously regress is not always apparent. However, a feature of dysplastic and malignant cells is decreased cellular cohesion. Therefore, minimal trauma, possibly including taking the smear itself, as well as coitus and tampon use, could cause dislodgment of the dysplastic epithelium from the basement membrane [Berner 1980, Hellberg 1994]. There is a very high regression rate of dysplasia after childbirth, possibly as high as 50% to 75% [Kiguchi 1981], which could be related to trauma as well as to a change in immune status [Benedet 1987, Hellberg 1987]. In fact, the host immune status may be an important factor not only in cases of spontaneous regression, but also in the development of the disease in the first place. Biopsy, even with incomplete removal of the lesion, has been mentioned as a possible cure of certain dysplastic lesions. Drugs, such as antibiotics and vitamins, might also influence the course of the disease [Koss 1978].

One should keep in mind the possibility of recurrence of these lesions, which may be due to incomplete therapy, reinfection, or a reservoir of latent virus. Whatever the mechanism, once a patient has been diagnosed as having dysplasia, even if it subsequently regresses, she is still at high risk for redeveloping intraepithelial (or invasive) neoplasia. Close surveillance of this high-risk patient population with more frequent Pap smears is important.

Site: Dysplasia/carcinoma in situ or cervical intraepithelial neoplasia is usually found in the transition zone of the squamocolumnar junction, in contact with the endocervical glandular epithelium [T6.23]. This area is only a few millimeters wide. The anterior lip of the cervix is affected twice as often as the posterior lip, while the lateral margins are usually spared [Richart 1965a]. This corresponds to the location of the metaplastic epithelium on the cervix [Richart 1973].

Cervical intraepithelial neoplasia can grow by expansion to encompass the entire transition zone [Richart 1973]. The anterior lip is in a position more exposed to trauma, eg, during intercourse (which could be important in the inoculation of a carcinogenic agent) or childbirth. Condyloma, in contrast with ordinary cervical intraepithelial neoplasia, is not necessarily confined to the transformation zone [Meisels 1977b].

Beginning at the squamocolumnar junction, cervical intraepithelial neoplasia spreads out distally on the cervix, like a ripple in a pond of squamous metaplasia, stopping abruptly at the shore of the native epithelium. However, the disease can occasionally grow proximally up the endocervical canal as far as the endometrium [Ferenczy 1971] or even the fallopian tube [Kanbour 1978]. There is a gradient of differentiation of the CIN lesion, with the proximal or endocervical portion being less differentiated (higher grade), and the distal portion being more differentiated (lower grade) [Richart 1973]. The maturity of the lesions has a distribution reminiscent of the metaplastic reactions: the more immature, the higher up in the endocervical canal the change is likely to be found.

Morphologic Distribution and Degree of Dysplasia: Mature metaplastic dysplasia is the most common type of dysplasia but, as might be expected from its high degree of differentiation, it is seldom advanced (ie, seldom high grade). Keratinizing and especially mixed (keratinizing and metaplastic) dysplasias are more likely to be advanced, but are relatively uncommon. Thus, in absolute numbers, (immature) metaplastic dysplasia is the most common type of dysplasia to be advanced [F6.18].

Of cases having progressed to carcinoma in situ, the great majority (up to 90%) are preceded by (immature) metaplastic dysplasia. Mature metaplastic (or large cell, nonkeratinizing) dysplasia precedes most of the remaining cases of carcinoma in situ [Patten 1978]. Keratinizing dysplasia does not progress to classical carcinoma in situ, but can "invade directly" as keratinizing squamous cell carcinoma. Unfortunately, it is impossible to predict morphologically which dysplasias will progress in an individual patient.

Pathogenesis: The cellular origin of the disease is a matter of controversy [Richart 1973]. Does the disease arise in a field of abnormal cells and progress by transformation of other cells [Burghardt 1983]? Or does it have a unicellular origin in which a clone of cells takes over? Based on colposcopic [Richart 1965a,1966a], microscopic [Richart 1973], chromosomal [Spriggs 1971], and biochemical (X-linked enzyme [J Smith 1971]) studies, the "single bullet theory" is favored, ie, the disease represents a clone of cells deriving from a single cell or a very small group of cells. The abnormal clone of cells is thought to proliferate relatively rapidly and literally plow the normal epithelium out of the way [Richart 1963a]. Human papilloma virus (HPV) may be important in the malignant transformation of the cells, and transcriptional activity of HPV genomes in cervical tumors also suggests monoclonality [Lehn 1985]. Low-grade squamous intraepithelial lesions may be multicellular in origin. High-grade squamous intraepithelial lesions, thought to be the true precursor lesions, may begin as a small focus (unicellular) within a low-grade lesion, which gradually expands. High-grade squamous intraepithelial lesions are usually associated with a single type of HPV.

F6.18 **Dysplasia Distribution**

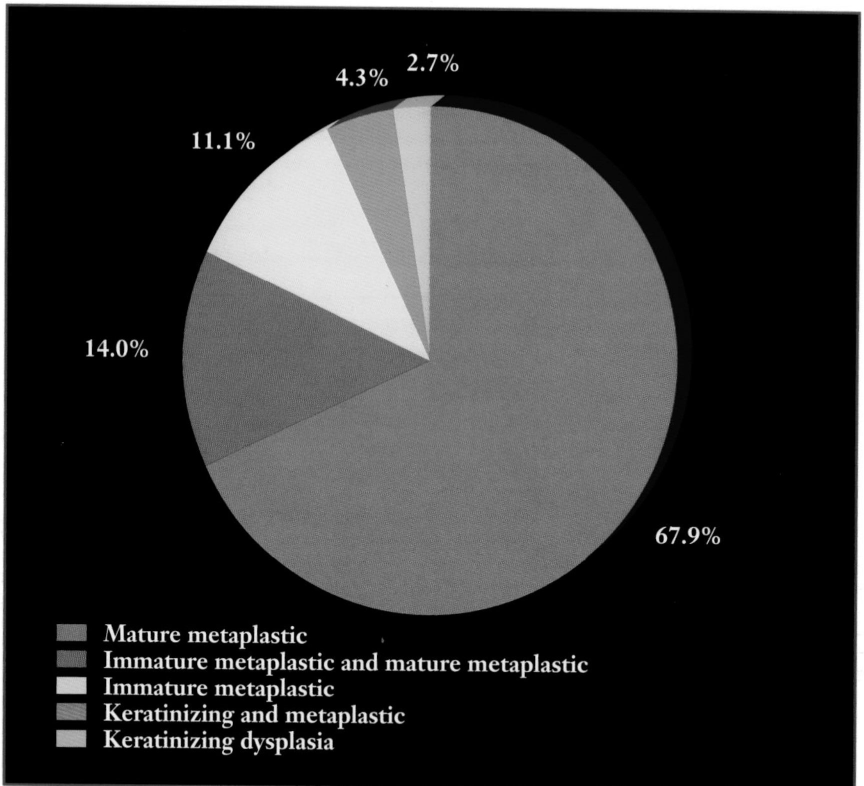

[Patten 1978]

Although the traditional view has been that lesions usually progress through stages of dysplasia to carcinoma in situ and then to invasive carcinoma, more recently an alternative explanation has been suggested. As already mentioned, high-grade lesions may develop de novo as a small focus within a low-grade lesion, and then expand in size, accompanied by apparent progression in cytologic grade [Tidbury 1992]. Cervical cancer arises from this aggressive cervical intraepithelial neoplasia III lesion—widely present on the cervix and established years before invasion—rather than as a progression of a low-grade lesion [J Robertson 1994].

Carcinogenesis is probably a multistep process [Barron 1968] that takes a considerable period to develop (years, even decades), involves a limited number of genes, is affected by host and environmental factors, and ultimately results in a malignant clone of cells. Superinfection may be important in pathogenesis. In the background of increased cellular proliferation (eg, metaplasia), at which time the cells may be more susceptible to genetic injury or mutation, it is believed that some factor(s) results in activation of oncogenes or inactivation of tumor suppressor genes (or both). These tumor-associated genes are normally involved in cellular pathways that regulate cell growth and proliferation.

Squamous metaplasia is at its peak in young patients, especially on the anterior lip of the cervix. HPV preferentially involves the immature (ie, metaplastic or reserve) epithelium of the cervix. HPV appears to infect the basal or reserve cells [Reid 1989], which are still capable of dividing, and may stimulate their proliferation. These facts possibly explain the importance of young age in cervical carcinogenesis and suggest a reason for its most common location, the transformation zone. Other, non-HPV, venereal diseases might help provide the soil for carcinogenesis to begin by inducing inflammatory reparative proliferation or metaplasia.

Viruses have the ability to usurp the host's DNA machinery in order to replicate. If a virus infects a cell and somehow manages to derange the DNA machinery while the process of proliferation is already revved up, proliferation might get out of control, become neoplastic, and eventually malignant. The host cells could begin proliferating in a disordered way, mimicking the benign proliferative reactions, and so on, down the path previously described to cancer.

It is not known what causes cervical cancer. However, the lowly wart virus is currently thought to be at least one of the culprits [Koutsky 1992, Munoz 1994, Schiffman 1993, Syrjänen 1986a, zur Hausen 1974,1981]. Evidence for this is seductive, but not conclusive.

A Brief History of HPV in Relationship to Condyloma and Cervical Carcinogenesis

Genital warts, or condylomas (Greek: knuckle), are an affliction that have been known through the ages and were described by ancient Greek and Roman writers [Lutzner 1983, Oriel 1971]. The diagnostic halo cell was first described by Ayre [Ayre 1949]. Its Greek name, koilocyte (for "hollow cell"), was derived from Koss and Durfee's description of koilocytotic atypia [Koss 1956, Meisels 1983]. They concluded "it is unlikely that the koilocytotic lesion is a part of the natural history of more than a fraction of cervix cancers" [Koss 1956]. In 1960, Ayre speculated that the koilocyte, which he called the "halo" cell, was a viral change in premalignancy. He wrote:

> "a viral nucleic acid might enter a host cell and be incorporated into the genetic structure of the cell....The viral nucleic acid...would be subject to...carcinogenic agents—which could cause it to...greatly increase its rate of replication, and thus to act as an independent functional unit. The result would be production of a mutant, perhaps cancerous, cell....The significant feature of the [koilocyte] would seem to be that it represents a steppingstone between normal cells and malignant or premalignant cells....The thought is, then, that [koilocytes] represent the earliest manifestation of malignancy in human cells, that they are caused by some nucleic acid–viral infectious activity in an estrogenic environment which produces derangement of cell metabolism and orderly replication of cells, and that they are probably a mutant deviation towards malignant cell growth" [Ayre 1960].

This essentially summarizes what we think decades later. In 1968, Dunn reported finding intranuclear viral particles in genital warts with the electron microscope [A Dunn 1968]. In 1977, Purola and Meisels independently described the flat condyloma and suggested that most "dysplasia" was really viral infection [Meisels 1977b, Purola 1977]. Prior to that time it was thought that condyloma (ie, visible condyloma acuminatum) was a relatively rare lesion on the cervix [Woodruff 1958]. In 1980 Gissman first reported partial characterization of an HPV from genital warts, which was designated HPV 6 [Gissmann 1980].

Microbiology and Molecular Biology of HPV

The human papilloma viruses are epitheliotropic: they infect specific epithelial or mucosal membranes, and often produce warts or other epithelial proliferations. HPV is thought to infect the basal cell, where it remains as a single copy episome, replicated only once per cell cycle. These infected cells may provide a reservoir of virus in morphologically normal appearing cells (latent infection) [T Wright 1990]. As the cell matures, complete, infectious virions are produced, and a specific cytopathic effect, the koilocyte, is formed in the upper cell layers (productive infection).

HPV is a nonencapsulated, icosahedral, non–lipid-containing (ie, nonenveloped) DNA virus that replicates in the nucleus of infected cells. The DNA is double-stranded, circular, and composed of about 7,900 base pairs. The viral genome is divided into two regions: a coding region (open reading frames or ORFs) and a noncoding region also known as the long control region (LCR) or upstream regulatory region [F Chang 1990].

The coding region (open reading frames) contains both early and late genes. Viral gene expression is tightly linked to host cell differentiation. Early and late refer to the time in the viral life cycle when the genes are expressed. Early genes code for regulatory proteins that control viral growth and have transforming, or oncogenic, properties [T Wright 1990]. Late genes code for structural proteins involved in viral assembly. HPVs contain seven early and two late genes. The long control region contains transcription promotors and enhancers. Promotors recognize RNA polymerase, thereby initiating RNA synthesis; enhancers modulate gene transcription.

It appears that integration of viral genetic material into the host genome is a critical event in malignant transformation of the cell. Integration appears to consistently disrupt the viral genome at the E1-E2 region [Tidy 1989b], resulting in failure to transcribe late genes. The life cycle of the virus is interrupted and complete virions are not formed (nonproductive infection). E2 codes for a protein that binds an enhancer of the long control region [Hirochika 1987], thus providing feedback regulation [Lambert 1987]. Therefore, disruption of the E2 gene could result in uncontrolled transcription of E6 and E7 genes [Tidy 1989b] and possibly malignant transformation because E6 and E7 code for proteins that regulate viral growth [Knebel Doeberitz 1988].

It has been shown that E6 and E7 are capable of immortalizing [Kaur 1989] and transforming cells in vitro [Phelps 1988] and that these genes are consistently transcribed in cervical carcinoma [Shirasawa 1987, Tidy 1989b]. E6 and E7 proteins can bind, respectively, the gene products of p53 [Werness 1990] and retinoblastoma genes [Dyson 1989, Münger 1989], effectively inactivating these tumor suppressor genes. E6 and E7 expression is associated with increased cell proliferation [Knebel Doeberitz 1988], selective growth advantage, and possibly cancer [Ambros 1990]. It is also suggested that the HPV 18 genome plays a role in *myc* expression in the later stages of carcinogenesis [Dürst 1987] and that *myc* expression has prognostic value [Riou 1987].

Viral DNA is usually not integrated in low-grade squamous intraepithelial lesions [Lehn 1988]. In contrast, in high-grade lesions and squamous cell carcinoma, the viral DNA is usually [Lehn 1988] (but not always [Dürst 1985]) integrated. Therefore, although integration is thought to be important in carcinogenesis, there may be alternative pathways involved in production of the malignant appearance of intraepithelial lesions as well as for production of malignant behavior of invasive cancer.

Evidence for HPV as the Cause of Cervical Cancer

As a transmissible agent, HPV would fit the epidemiologic data that seem to implicate sexual promiscuity and early onset of coitus in the development of the disease [Schiffman 1993, Syrjänen 1984]. HPV infections occur at a younger average age than cervical intraepithelial neoplasia (ie, condyloma precedes dysplasia) [Binder 1985, Crum 1983a, Fu 1983, Meisels 1981a, Syrjänen 1980,1981] and patients with both condyloma and cervical intraepithelial neoplasia are, on average, younger than patients with only cervical intraepithelial neoplasia [Zuna 1984]. There seems to be a progression from condyloma to dysplasia to carcinoma in situ [Meisels 1981a, Syrjänen 1985]. It is accepted that HPV is the cause of condylomas and koilocytosis [Meisels 1977b, Oriel 1971]. Koilocytes are found in up to one half of all cases of cervical intraepithelial neoplasia [Syrjänen 1979], and in almost all cervical intraepithelial neoplasia patients younger than 20 years of age [Syrjänen 1983]. Condyloma and dysplasia frequently coexist in a given patient and are found in close association on the cervix [Meisels 1981a]: dysplasia, the more advanced lesion, is generally more proximal [Saito 1987]. At least one third of patients with biopsy-proven condyloma develop ordinary cervical intraepithelial neoplasia within 1 year [Nash 1987]. Patients with evidence of both condyloma and cervical intraepithelial neoplasia progress faster than patients without evidence of condyloma [Meisels 1981a, Syrjänen 1981]. HPV can be demonstrated in both condyloma [Ferenczy 1981] and cervical intraepithelial neoplasia (by immunoperoxidase techniques [Kurman 1981, Syrjänen 1981]). There is also a strong epidemiologic association between HPV and cervical intraepithelial neoplasia [Schiffman 1993]. There is a strong association between infection with HPV 16 or 18, or both, and cervical intraepithelial neoplasia and cervical cancer, even after adjusting for other risk factors [Koutsky 1992, Munoz 1994, Reeves 1989].

As further evidence, other wart viruses are known to cause neoplasia; in fact, the Shope papilloma virus was one of the first viruses shown to be capable of causing cancer [Rous 1935]. Malignant transformation of condyloma acuminatum has been observed [Kovi 1974]. Perhaps most compelling of all is the presence of HPV–DNA in most cases of dysplasia and nearly all (>90%) cases of intraepithelial and invasive squamous cancer [de Roda Husman 1994, Kadish 1986, Kühler-Obbarius 1994b, Nagai 1987, Nelson 1989, Okagaki 1992, Richart 1987, Schiffman 1991], as well as metastases [Lancaster 1986] and recurrences [Holloway 1991]. HPV has now been found in all major types of cervical cancer, including adenocarcinoma (in situ and invasive) [Smotkin 1986, Tase 1989a, Wilczynski 1988a,b], adenosquamous carcinoma [Smotkin 1986], small cell carcinoma [Stoler 1991], and even glassy cell carcinoma [Smotkin 1986]. HPV is also associated with other, nongenital tumors, eg, laryngeal papillomatosis and squamous cell carcinoma.

Evidence Against HPV as the Cause of Cervical Cancer

On the other hand, it happens that HPV infection is extremely common, probably the single most common genital infection. HPV–DNA can be detected (by relatively sensitive hybridization techniques) in 25% to 30% of women [R Burk 1986, deVilliers 1987, Lorincz 1986, A Schneider 1987a] who have apparently normal cervices and normal Pap smears (latent infection). Many of these otherwise normal women have high-risk viral types [Pasetto 1992]. (In most reports, however, cytologic normality was based on a single Pap smear [Syrjänen 1994]. And, on reexamination, cytologic or colposcopic features of HPV infection or cervical intraepithelial neoplasia can be found in a significant number of cases [Moscicki 1991, A Schneider 1988b, Wagner 1985].) Still higher prevalences of HPV–DNA occur in some high-risk patient populations [Ritter 1988, A Schneider 1987c], including teenagers with multiple sexual partners (54%) [Rosenfeld 1989]. Recently, using the extremely sensitive polymerase chain reaction, HPV 16 (a high-risk type) has been detected in cervical scrapes in up to 90% of clinically normal women with negative Pap smear results [M Johnson 1990, A Schneider 1992, Tidy 1989a, L Young 1989]. Repeated sampling is found to increase the cumulative prevalence with an overall lifetime risk of contracting HPV infection at least once of 80% for women between 20 and 80 years of age [Syrjänen 1994]. Interestingly, positivity is more likely during the luteal phase of the menstrual cycle [A Schneider 1992].

In a given specimen, the distribution of viral DNA and its transcriptional activity are patchy and may be extremely focal [Nagai 1987, Stoler 1986]. Also, there is an inverse relation between the amount of viral DNA and the degree of abnormality of the lesion, with the lowest levels being found in invasive cancer (and the highest levels in condyloma) [A Schneider 1991]. Although the virus can immortalize cell lines, HPV 16/18 does not appear to be carcinogenic by itself [Woodworth 1988]. And, although HPV positivity diminishes with age [de Villiers 1992, Ley 1991, Melkert 1993], cervical cancers increase.

Because condyloma often follows exposure to a partner with genital warts [T Barrett 1954], and because condylomas are more common in patients with multiple partners [Daling 1986] and detection of HPV–DNA is associated with the presence of condylomas, it has been assumed that all HPV–related genital lesions are due to a recently acquired venereal infection. However, although condylomas are contagious and apparently related to sexual activity [Oriel 1971], HPV positivity may not be [Kiviat 1989]. There is evidence that high sexual activity does not increase the risk of HPV infection and that barrier contraception is not protective [Kjaer 1990]. There is no clear-cut association between sexual activity and the detection of HPV–DNA in genital tract epithelium [Kiviat 1989, Kjaer 1988, Reeves 1989]. Although cervical neoplasia is more common in prostitutes than controls, the HPV detection rate is similar in both groups [Gitsch 1991]. Polymerase chain reaction results indicate that 20% of virgins are carriers of the virus [Ley 1991], but do not show cytologic abnormalities [A Peters 1994]. The specific infectious agents implicated in dysplastic lesions may differ to some extent from those causing invasive cancer [LaVecchia 1986b]. High detection rates of HPV–DNA occur in areas with the low cancer rates, while the low rates of HPV–DNA occur in areas with the high cancer rates [Acs 1989]. Treatment of the male partner seems to have no effect on recurrence of cervical intraepithelial neoplasia [Krebs 1991]. Moreover, according to some studies, the concordance of HPV types in couples having sexual relations is surprisingly low (only 5% to 10% have the same viral type) [Syrjänen 1994]. HPV infection and cervical carcinoma may have different risk factors [Villa 1989]. Promiscuity may be too broad a risk factor; some other factor, perhaps related to promiscuity, may be important [Rogo 1990]. While the experimental evidence may suggest a role for HPV, the epidemiologic evidence is inconclusive [Munoz 1988].

Possible Cofactors in Cervical Carcinogenesis

Why a cell progresses from latent infection to clinically apparent lesions to invasive cancer is unknown, but probably involves interaction with some cofactor(s) [Kessler 1987]. The cofactors might, for example, cause an increase in the rate of integration of the HPV into the cell or failure of the immune system. Several possible cofactors are currently under investigation.

Permissiveness of the individual cell may be a factor. For example, HPV 11 proliferates better in foreskin and cervix than in other epithelia [Kreider 1987].

Immunocompetency: Altered immune status is known to be important in at least some cases of cervical neoplasia [Laverty 1978]. The idea that an immune deficiency is important in cervical carcinogenesis is attractive because it could allow infection in the first place as well as escape of abnormal cells from immune surveillance. Support for this theory comes from several sources. First, cervical carcinoma cells are known to be antigenic, expressing tumor associated antigens [McCoy 1981]. In addition, immunosuppressed patients (eg, renal transplant [Alloub 1989, Busnach 1993, V Schneider 1983] and patients suffering from Hodgkin's disease [R Katz 1987] and other immunosuppressive diseases [Shokri-Tabibzadeh 1981]) are more frequently affected by condyloma, and when they are, the condylomas tend to be larger and more numerous. These condylomas are also refractory to therapy [Krebs 1986] and there is an increased progression to ordinary cervical intraepithelial neoplasia [V Schneider 1983]. Moreover, immunosuppressed patients have an increased risk of developing malignancies in general [Porreco 1975]. There is also a strong association between human immunodeficiency virus (HIV) positivity and development of an abnormal Pap smear, after seroconversion, with a highly significant increase in HPV infection and cervical neoplasia [Adachi 1993, Henry-Stanley 1993b, Maiman 1990,1991, Petry 1994, Provencher 1988]. This finding is thought to reflect depressed cellular immunity.

At the cellular level, there is depletion of intraepithelial Langerhans' (antigen presenting) cells, which may be the first line of host defense [Barton 1989a, Koutsky 1988]. Also, there is a lower percentage of $T4^{+}$ helper lymphocytes and a higher percentage of $T8^{+}$ suppressor cells, resulting in a lower $T4^{+}/T8^{+}$ ratio [Koutsky 1988, Tay 1987a]. In addition, there is increased macrophage [Tay 1987c] and natural killer cell [Tay 1987b] infiltration in patients with HPV and cervical intraepithelial neoplasia.

Trauma: Condyloma, dysplasia, and cancer all commonly arise in the anterior cervix, a site exposed to trauma during childbirth and during intercourse. Trauma could facilitate inoculation of a virus.

Pregnancy: Pregnancy is associated with altered immune status and change in lymphoid cell function necessary for fetal allograph survival [Petrucco 1976]. Condylomas and cervical intraepithelial neoplasia are more frequent during pregnancy [Oriel 1971, A Schneider 1987a], but have a high postpartum regression rate [Benedet 1987, Hellberg 1987, Kiguchi 1981]. However, an increase in risk of cervical cancer, in direct proportion to the number of pregnancies, has been reported, possibly related to trauma, hormones, or immunodeficiency [Brinton 1989a].

Steroid Hormones: Dysplasia usually occurs in an estrogenic environment. An increased occurrence of dysplasia has been reported in diethylstilbestrol-exposed women [Robboy 1984] as well as in long-term birth control pill users [Harris 1980, Swan 1982]. Estrogen [Mitrani-Rosenbaum 1989] and glucocorticoids [Gloss 1987] have been shown to increase HPV transcription. Glucocorticoids may also be important in activation of oncogenes by HPV 16 [Pater 1988].

Venereal Infections: There may be a synergistic relation between herpes simplex and HPV [Fenoglio 1982, zur Hausen 1982]. Herpes increases HPV transcription [Gius 1989]. Cytomegalovirus infection may also be associated in some way with development of cervical intraepithelial neoplasia [Koutsky 1992]. Other kinds of organisms, eg, *Chlamydia* [Cevenini 1981, Hare 1982, Koutsky 1992, Syrjänen 1986b] or multiple infections, may also be important in development of cervical cancer. Venereal infections in general may increase the risk of acquiring HPV by causing inflammation, ulceration, or squamous metaplasia [Koutsky 1988,1992].

Smoking: Numerous cancers, particularly lung cancer, but also cervical cancer [Greenberg 1985, LaVecchia 1986a], have been associated with cigarette smoking. The risk is dose dependent [E Clarke 1982]. Products of cigarette smoke are concentrated in the cervical mucus of women who smoke [Hellberg 1988, Sasson 1985], resulting in "mutagenic mucus" [Holly 1986]. Smoking leads to increased modification and damage to DNA in cervical epithelium, providing biochemical evidence that smoking is a cause of cervical cancer [Simons 1993,1994]. Smoking has also been shown to affect immunocompetent cells, both locally in the cervix [Barton 1988] and systemically [L Miller 1982, Phillips 1985].

Diet: Various vitamin deficiencies may be related to development of cervical cancer [Ziegler 1990].

Vitamin A: Carotenoid and to a lesser extent, retinoids may help prevent development of squamous cell carcinomas not only in the genital tract, but also in the head and neck and other sites [LaVecchia 1984b, Romney 1981]. Vitamin A has a significant influence on epithelial differentiation [DeLuca 1972]; deficiency leads to squamous metaplasia [A Bernstein 1984].

Vitamin B: Folate is involved in DNA synthesis, repair, and methylation. Folate deficiency may cause megaloblastosis and chromosomal damage [Yunis 1984]. Birth control pill use is associated with (reversible) folate deficiency, which is more marked in patients with dysplasia [Butterworth 1982, Harper 1994]. Although folate deficiency may be involved as a cocarcinogen during initiation of dysplasia, folic acid supplements apparently do not alter the course of established disease [Butterworth 1992].

Vitamin C: There is a strong association of hypovitaminosis C with cervical dysplasia and carcinoma in situ [Romney 1985, Wassertheil-Smoller 1981].

Genetic Susceptibility: Patients with the rare autosomal recessive disease, epidermodysplasia verruciformis, have a defect in epithelial maturation and cellular immunity. In these patients, specific HPV types produce multiple wart-like lesions, which are followed, in about one third of cases, by invasive cancers on sun-exposed skin, after many years. This pattern (HPV infection, precursor lesion, cofactor[s], and time) is similar to the multistep development of cervical cancer [T Wright 1990], providing not only a model of the disease, but also suggesting that genetic predisposition may be a cofactor in its development, at least in some cases.

Summary: HPV infection seems to be a necessary, but not sufficient, condition for the development of cervical cancer [Reid 1989]. HPV infection, if not ubiquitous, is very common, even in women with negative Pap smear findings [Anon 1987, Bauer 1991, Bevan 1989, de Villiers 1992, M Johnson 1990, Koss 1993a, Pasetto 1992, Schiffman 1991, A Schneider 1992, Tidy 1989a, L Young 1989]. Yet, the lifetime probability that an average-risk woman in the United States will develop invasive cervical cancer is less than 1% (0.7% in 1985) [Eddy 1990]. Therefore, some other unknown factor(s) must be involved in carcinogenesis. An analogous situation exists with other virally associated tumors. For example, many people have evidence of past Epstein-Barr virus or hepatitis B virus infection, but few develop the associated tumors (Burkitt's lymphoma and nasopharyngeal carcinoma, or hepatocellular carcinoma) [zur Hausen 1986]. (Of further interest is that the cervix frequently harbors Epstein-Barr virus; its role, if any, in cervical carcinogenesis remains to be elucidated [Y Taylor 1994].)

Prognosis

Unfortunately, the key question the clinician wants answered—which lesions will progress, and which will not—cannot be predicted for individual patients. Although on average the behavior of dysplasia is predictable from the morphology, the grades of dysplasia/carcinoma in situ do not necessarily reflect the true biologic potential of a particular lesion [Koss 1978]. To put this problem into clinical perspective, at least 10–20 million women, possibly substantially more, are infected with HPV, and at least 2.5 million women are diagnosed with squamous intraepithelial lesions each year in the United States alone [Koutsky 1988, Kurman 1994]. Yet, far less than 1% (~15,800) of those infected develop cervical cancer annually and fewer still die of the disease (~4,800) [Wingo 1995]. It would be extremely useful to be able to accurately predict which patients with HPV infection or squamous intraepithelial lesions would develop cancer if untreated, because the alternative of having to treat everyone with these lesions is tremendously expensive [Herbst 1990]. New insights into the physical state and type of HPV as well as DNA ploidy provide some additional prognostic information, but to date still cannot answer the key clinical question precisely.

Physical State, Viral Typing, and Prognosis: The physical state of the virus in the cell (ie, episomal or integrated) is important in the clinical outcome. When the viral DNA is free in the nucleus (extrachromosomal or episomal), full viral expression and productive infection can ensue: ie, complete virions are produced in association with koilocyte formation (condyloma). As previously discussed, the morphology (flat, warty) depends on the degree of maturation of the infected epithelium; koilocytosis and complete virus production require mature cells—the lesions are well differentiated.

When the viral DNA is integrated into the host's genome (into the "immortal" basal/reserve cell), the viral DNA is not fully expressed, although it remains present, perhaps for the life of the patient (latent infection). In advanced dysplasia, with little squamous maturation, the lesion is poorly differentiated, koilocytes are not formed, and complete virions are not produced (nonproductive infection). Thus, the development of high-grade cervical intraepithelial neoplasia is, for the virus, a biologic dead end.

There are scores (at least 70) of HPV types known, of which less than two dozen infect the female genital tract and only a few cause high-grade lesions [T6.24]. Certain viral types, eg, HPV 16 and 18 (also 31, 33, 35, 52, 56, and rarely 39 and 45 [Nelson 1989, zur Hausen 1987]) are more likely to integrate into the host genome and be associated with high-grade dysplasia and cancer (high-risk virus), while others, eg, 6 and 11, are unlikely to integrate or be associated with cancer (low-risk virus).

T6.24 **Female Genital Tract Lesions**

HPV Type	L SIL	H SIL	SCC
6, 11	70%-90% exophytic condyloma 15% CIN I	Few	Rare
16	20%	40% CIN II 60% CIN III	50%
18	Few	Few	20%
31	15%	15%	5%
Other*	15%	15%	20%

[Willett 1989]
* HPV type 33, 35, etc.

Any of the nearly two dozen HPVs that infect the female genital tract can cause low-grade squamous intraepithelial lesions. High-grade squamous intraepithelial lesions are usually associated with a half dozen viral types (16, 31, 35, etc, but rarely 18), while squamous cell carcinoma is usually associated with HPV 16 or 18. HPV 18 seems to short circuit the sequence of progressive dysplasia and may invade directly from low-grade lesions (ie, mild dysplasia) [Arends 1993, Beaudenon 1986, Bergeron 1987, Brescia 1986, Fuchs 1988, Gissman 1983, Kadish 1992, Koutsky 1988, Kurman 1988, Lorincz 1987a,b,1992, Lutzner 1983, Park 1991, Reid 1987, Wilczynski 1988a, Willett 1989, T Wright 1990].

Low-risk virus produces low-grade squamous intraepithelial lesions, which tend to regress, even without therapy, and usually do not recur. Low-risk viruses have little malignant potential and are seldom found in cancers (but can be found in verrucous carcinoma, and sometimes others) [T Wright 1990]. High-risk virus tends to cause lesions that persist or progress, rarely regress, and are associated with a relatively high risk of developing neoplasia. It is important to emphasize, however, that low-risk virus by no means completely excludes the possibility of clinical progression to carcinoma in situ and invasive carcinoma [Syrjänen 1988]. Conversely, by no means do all patients with high-risk virus progress to carcinoma in situ or carcinoma [F6.19].

HPV 18 seems to "short circuit" the process of intraepithelial neoplasia [Arends 1993]. There are very few HPV 18–associated intraepithelial lesions, yet HPV 18 is found in at least 20% of invasive carcinomas. Thus, HPV 18 lesions may invade directly from low-grade squamous intraepithelial lesions [Kurman 1988]. As previously discussed, rapidly progressive cervical cancers probably occur, and these more aggressive cancers may be associated with HPV 18 [Barnes 1988,1990]. The patients tend to be young, may have had a normal Pap smear finding within the preceding 3 years, and have rapidly advancing, widely disseminated, poorly differentiated cancers, with more frequent recurrences [Hadjimichael 1989, Schwartz 1988, J Walker 1989]. HPV 18 is also associated with small cell neuroendocrine carcinoma [Stoler 1991] and endocervical adenocarcinoma [Wilczynski 1988a,b].

DNA Ploidy and Prognosis: The evidence suggests that dysplasia/carcinoma in situ is truly a neoplastic process (hence, cervical intraepithelial *neoplasia)*. Furthermore, not only do the cells seem to be neoplastic but they may actually be *malignant* from the inception. Aneuploid DNA patterns, a feature usually associated with malignancy, can be found in any grade of dysplasia, including at least some cases of mild dysplasia [Bibbo 1989b, Fu 1981,1983, Wilbanks 1967]. Lesion ploidy has been found to be a reasonably accurate statistical predictor of biologic behavior. The great majority (90%) of diploid and polyploid lesions do not progress, while aneuploid lesions, regardless of grade, seldom regress (7%), often persist (45%), and may progress to more advanced dysplasia (36%) or cancer (12%) [Fu 1981].

Most CIN I and classic, well-differentiated condylomas (ie, low-grade squamous intraepithelial lesions) have been reported to be diploid or polyploid (however, see below). When high-risk virus integrates into the genome, it may cause the cell to become aneuploid [Waggoner 1990]. Aneuploidy is probably secondary to disordered mitosis [Richart 1973] and abnormal mitotic figures are a marker for aneuploidy [Winkler 1984]. More than 60% of CIN II and more than 75% of CIN III lesions are aneuploid [Reid 1984].

In summary, most high-grade dysplasias (high-grade squamous intraepithelial lesions) are caused by high-risk HPV and are aneuploid, while many, but not all, low-grade dysplasias (low-grade squamous intraepithelial lesions) are caused by low-risk HPV and may be diploid/polyploid [Fu 1981, Willett 1989].

Implications for Pap Smear Diagnosis—Morphology and Prognosis: Due to research demonstrating the importance of high- and low-risk viruses and DNA ploidy states, the question arises

F6.19 **Morphology of Squamous Intraepithelial Lesion, Viral Type, and Risk**

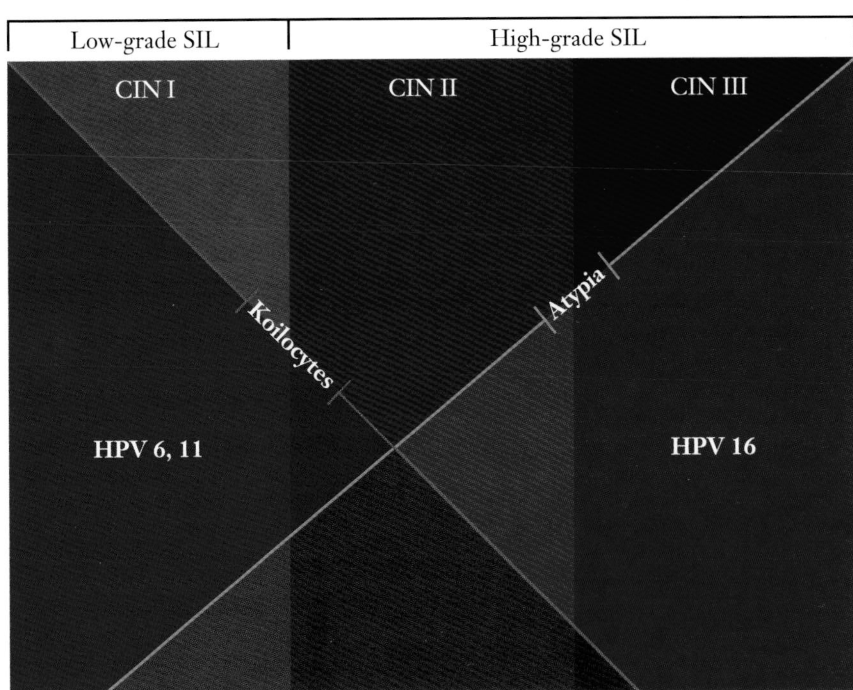

CIN I = low, but definite risk; CIN II = intermediate risk; CIN III = high risk.
Note: Up to 25% of low-grade SILs are associated with high-risk viral types, but few high-grade SILs are associated with low-risk viral types [Franquemont 1989, Willett 1989].

as to whether patients with abnormal Pap smears should be routinely viral typed and DNA analyzed, and indeed, whether the Pap smear could be completely replaced with these techniques. Unfortunately, even with these newer diagnostic methods, there is still no way to predict which *individual* lesions will progress to cancer (the small minority) and which will not (the great majority).

For example, low-risk viruses are not without risk, while few high-risk virus infections actually result in cancer. Moreover, *any* of the HPVs that infect the female genital tract can cause mild basal cell hyperplasia, mild cytologic atypia, and koilocytosis, ie, mild dysplasia (CIN I) and condyloma (now grouped as low-grade squamous intraepithelial lesions) [Ambros 1990]. Although high-grade lesions are usually associated with high-risk virus, a substantial minority of cases of low-grade squamous intraepithelial lesions (roughly 25%) also contain high-risk viral types [Franquemont 1989, Willett 1989]. Furthermore, high-risk HPV is frequently found in the genital tract of apparently normal women with normal Pap smears [Meanwell 1987, Murdoch 1988, Tidy 1989a, L Young 1989]. Multiple HPVs, including mixtures of both high- and low-risk types, have been found within a single neoplasm [Griffin 1990], and even invasive cancers can sometimes be associated with low-risk virus. Therefore, viral type is not by itself completely predictive of biologic behavior. In fact, these findings have cast doubt upon the direct causal role of HPV in cervical cancer, and have increased the presumed importance of various cofactors. Thus, the type of HPV should not influence therapy.

The critical event in carcinogenesis may be integration of the viral DNA into the host genome, which appears to induce aneuploidy. This is accompanied by a morphologic change from low- to high-grade cervical intraepithelial neoplasia with increasing cytologic atypia, disorganization, and abnormal mitotic figures [Richart 1990]. However, using highly sensitive techniques (combination of Feulgen microspectrophotometry and flow cytometry), 100% (!) of CIN I lesions (and 0% of normal controls, 68% of HPV, as well as 83% of reactive atypia) contained aneuploid cells by one or both methods [Watts 1987]. Thus, the idea that "ploidy" is predictive of behavior may have to be revised to specify the degree or extent of aneuploidy—and this may correlate with the morphology.

Any agent that can induce a high-grade lesion has the proven ability to induce cellular anaplasia. Since most cancers arise from the most advanced lesions, predominantly carcinoma in situ, CIN III is a high-risk lesion. However, the average cell of carcinoma in situ may be *too* abnormal to cause invasive cancer, since the invasive malignant clone must be able to divide relatively normally in order to proliferate. Thus, while aneuploidy is the rule in carcinoma in situ, invasive cancers can be diploid [J Davis 1989]. (Note that diploidy does not necessarily mean the genes are normal, only that the chromosomes are diploid.) Again, "ploidy" is not by itself completely predictive of biologic behavior.

Although the viral type cannot be determined by the morphology of the lesion, currently it is not clinically important even to know *if* virus is present, let alone its *type*, since the accepted approach to cervical intraepithelial neoplasia is to destroy the lesion [Sedlacek 1991]. Unfortunately, if there is no lesion to destroy, currently there is little that can be done for the HPV-positive patient—even if she has an oncogenic virus. On the other hand, most physicians would not withhold treatment for high-grade dysplasias, no matter how "diploid" they were [Crum 1989b]. Furthermore, viral typing and DNA analysis are generally applied to lesions that have already been detected by screening. In fact, patients with high-risk viruses are more likely than patients with low-risk viruses to have an abnormal Pap smear in the first place [Nuovo 1991].

The morphologic features that suggest a low-risk lesion (ie, the presence of low-risk virus and diploid/polyploidy) include the presence of many well-formed koilocytes, few mitoses, undifferentiated cells confined to the lower third of the epithelium, little or no pleomorphism, and few or no abnormal mitoses [Fu 1981,1988]. These features indicate mild dysplasia (CIN I) and condyloma, or low-grade squamous intraepithelial lesion.

High-risk lesions (ie, presence of high-risk virus and aneuploidy) are suggested morphologically by the presence of few or no koilocytes, many mitoses, undifferentiated cells in the upper third of the epithelium, and marked nuclear pleomorphism [Fu 1981,1988]. Most aneuploid cases have numerous, markedly abnormal mitoses as a major histologic feature. These findings indicate high-grade dysplasia or carcinoma in situ (CIN III). The diagnosis is based upon the "worst cells" detected. T6.25 summarizes prognostic features related to low- and high-risk lesions.

Although modern viral testing and DNA ploidy studies have been very helpful in understanding the biology of cervical neoplasia, in practice, classical morphology remains a more important factor in management of precancerous lesions. Low-grade lesions are low-risk lesions, and high-grade lesions are high-risk lesions. Unfortunately, the morphology still cannot

T6.25 **Summary of Prognostic Features**

Low-Risk Lesion	High-Risk Lesion
Morphology	
Well differentiated	Poorly differentiated
L SIL (CIN I, condyloma)	H SIL (or SCC)
Many, well-formed koilocytes	Few or no koilocytes
Abnormal mitoses rare	Abnormal mitoses frequent
Molecular Biology	
Low-risk virus (eg, HPV 6, 11)	High-risk virus (eg, HPV 16, 18)
Episomal	May integrate
Diploid/Polyploid	Aneuploid
Behavior	
Few progress	More progress
Little malignant potential	Greater malignant potential

predict the outcome of a given lesion in an individual patient. Therefore, colposcopy is the key to the proper and complete evaluation of this spectrum of diseases, and the gynecologist must share responsibility for diagnosis of these lesions.

More Epithelial Changes ("Atypias")

There are a wide variety of epithelial changes (or "atypias") that are distinct from dysplasia, but they sometimes mimic dysplasia almost perfectly. (Use of the *unqualified* word "atypia" is discouraged because it could be used to describe virtually any abnormality, including cancer.) Distinguishing benign "atypia" from truly neoplastic cells can sometimes be very difficult. Remember, the key is the nucleus: the nucleus reveals the state of health of a cell. Most nondysplastic epithelial changes are associated with one or more of the following: inflammation, repair/regeneration, vitamin deficiency (B_{12}, folate), atypia of atrophy (maturity), radiation/chemotherapy, intrauterine devices.

Inflammation and Inflammatory Change

Pruritus and leukorrhea (itching and discharge) are among the most common reasons that a woman seeks medical advice from her gynecologist. Leukorrhea usually indicates an infection, but occasionally may signify a neoplasm. Women with sexually transmitted diseases are at increased risk of developing squamous intraepithelial lesions. Although the Pap smear can be useful in identifying specific infectious agents, it should not be used in lieu of more effective diagnostic tests [Roongpisuthipong 1987]. Because many things can cause inflammation, the mere presence of inflammatory change on Pap smear is a poor indicator of the presence of infection [Parsons 1993]. As noted, inflammatory change ("inflammatory atypia") can mimic dysplasia. But keep in mind that patients with inflammatory change, particularly if persistent, are at high risk for a bona fide squamous abnormality (ie, cervical intraepithelial neoplasia/ squamous intraepithelial lesion). Most inflammation is associated with endocervical glandular or atrophic squamous epithelium, since a mature stratified squamous epithelium provides a good defense against most assaults. Thus, inflammatory change is less common in women with hysterectomies, as long as they have a mature epithelium.

Causes of Inflammatory Changes

Infection: Viral, bacterial, fungal, protozoal
Physical: IUD, tampon, diaphragm, pessary, polyps, trauma, including childbirth
Hormonal: Birth control pills, atrophy, lactation
Chemical: Douches, gels, foams
Malignancy and cancer therapy (radiation, chemotherapy)
Nonspecific, idiopathic

Normal Flora and Cytolysis: The normal flora of the female genital tract form a polymicrobial, dynamic ecosystem (including lactobacilli, peptococci, bacteroides, staphylococcus epidermidis, corynebacteria, peptostreptococci, and eubacteria) in which anaerobes usually predominate [Bartlett 1977]. The vaginal flora maintain the normal, acid pH and help fight infection.

The bacterial infection or inflammation can result in destruction of cells. Even components of the normal flora, *Bacillus vaginalis* (the Döderlein bacilli, a heterogeneous group of large, rod-shaped lactobacilli and *Leptothrix*) can cause cellular changes. *B vaginalis* often causes lysis of the cell membrane—cytolysis—as it attacks the cell (usually intermediate cells) for glycogen, leaving normal-appearing nuclei floating in cytoplasmic debris [80 I6.46]. This is especially frequent in pregnancy, during the second half of the menstrual cycle, and in diabetes mellitus. The differential diagnosis of cytolysis includes endocervical mucus, which also contains naked (endocervical) nuclei, but the nuclei float in pools of mucus rather than cytoplasmic fragments. Cytolysis seldom involves dysplastic cells, due to their low glycogen content (the basis of the Schiller iodine test) and the dense, immature nature of the cytoplasm.

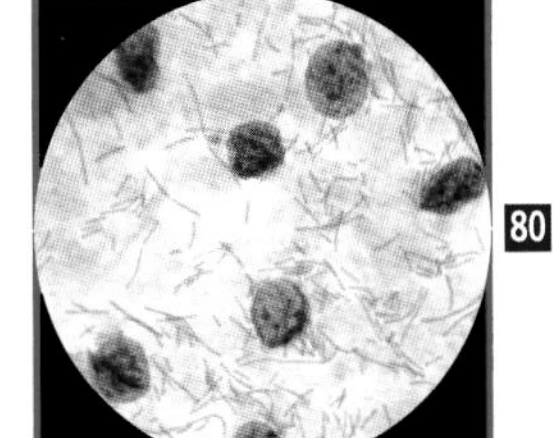
80

When other bioagents grow in the female genital tract, they inhibit the normal Döderlein bacilli responsible for cytolysis. Inflammation can also cause nonhormonal maturation to superficial cells, which do not contain significant glycogen and rarely undergo cytolysis. Therefore, cytolysis is less frequently seen in such cases with inflammation. However, enzymes released from degenerating inflammatory cells can damage epithelial cells leading to degenerative catalysis. This results not only in lysis of the cell membrane but also nuclear damage, in contrast with cytolysis, where only the cytoplasm is damaged.

Inflammatory Change ("Inflammatory Atypia"): Rather than completely destroying cells, inflammation more commonly merely alters them [Kiviat 1985]. For example, in some cases, inflamed cells imbibe water, resulting in nuclear and cytoplasmic enlargement [T6.26]. The intensity of nuclear staining decreases as a result of dilution by water (chromatolysis). Therefore, chromolytic nuclei, although enlarged, appear bland and hypochromatic (ie, the nuclei are big but not dark), and are unlikely to be mistaken for dysplasia. Unfortunately, in other cases, nuclear and cytoplasmic changes associated with inflammation can closely mimic dysplasia. *The differential diagnosis between inflammatory change and dysplasia is a common, everyday problem in Pap smear diagnosis.* As a general rule, the difference between inflammatory change and dysplasia is a matter of degree: the nuclei of dysplasia are more enlarged, more pleomorphic, more irregular, with more extensive chromatin abnormalities, and the cell arrange-

Differential Diagnosis of Dysplasia vs Inflammatory Change

Inflamed nuclei:
Big, but not dark; or dark, but not big
Red nuclei indicate inflammation
Dysplastic nuclei:
Big and dark
Blue nuclei indicate true dysplasia
Dysplasia vs inflammation: Matter of degree
More pleomorphic, larger nuclei
More irregular nuclear outline
More abnormal chromatin: Crisp and distinct
More cellular disorder
Halos: Inflammatory vs koilocytotic

T6.26 **Summary of Findings in Inflammatory Change**

Cytoplasm
- Vacuolization
- Perinuclear halo
- Pale stain
- Polychromatic
- Eosinophilic/Pseudokeratinized
- Frayed, ragged edges
- Engulfed PMNs
- Enlarged, irregular shape

Nucleus
- Enlargement (usually <2x intermediate nucleus)
- Vacuolization
- Chromatin: Either hypochromatic, bland (chromatolysis) or hyperchromatic, clumped (degeneration)
- Karyopyknosis, -rhexis, -lysis
- Bi- or multinucleated

Background
- "Dirty"
- Inflammatory
- Mimics tumor diathesis

ments are more disorderly. Of note is that inflammatory change usually mimics low-grade, rather than high-grade, dysplasia.

Nuclear Features: Inflamed cells can have enlarged, hyperchromatic—big, dark—nuclei, and increased N/C ratios, mimicking dysplasia. However, inflamed nuclei are usually less than twice the area of an intermediate cell nucleus (ie, not too big), and inflamed nuclei usually have paler, finer chromatin (ie, not too dark—pale, in fact), while dysplastic nuclei are characterized by darker, coarser chromatin. Therefore, most characteristically, inflamed nuclei are big, but not dark [81 I6.41, I6.42]. However, inflamed nuclei can sometimes be dark (but not too big), eg, in *Trichomonas* infection. (Remember: if it's big *and* it's dark, it's dysplasia.)

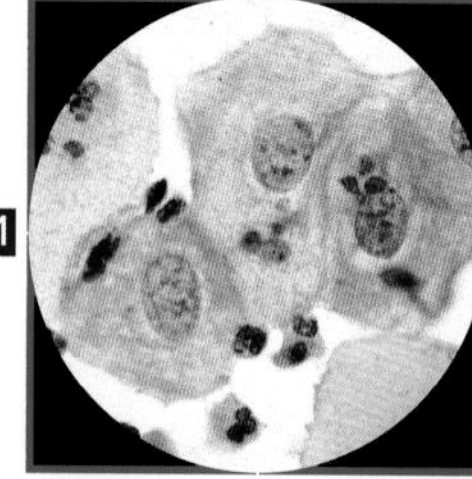
81

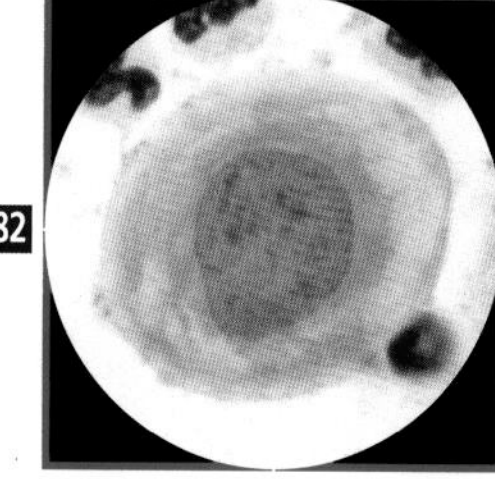
82

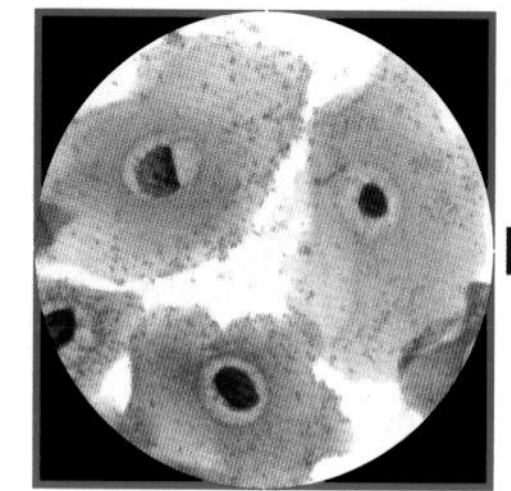
83

The chromatin of inflamed cells typically appears smudgy, rather than crisp and distinct as in dysplasia. Although the chromatin of inflamed cells may clump, it is a degenerative rather than neoplastic change. Inflammatory degeneration commonly results in karyopyknosis, karyorrhexis, or karyolysis. The clumped chromatin particles of degenerated nuclei tend to be rounded, like beads of mercury, while those in dysplasia tend to be angular, like shards of pottery. In short, the nuclei of inflammatory change do not have the chromatin of dysplasia.

The presence of nucleoli favors a reactive process [Patten 1978]. Nevertheless, irregular small nucleoli can be seen in dysplasia [Meisels 1976a]. It is reasonable to assume that dysplastic cells are not immune to inflammation and can show secondary inflammatory alterations.

One peculiar but potentially helpful diagnostic feature is the tendency of some inflamed nuclei to "shine red" (and be hypochromatic) compared with dysplastic nuclei, which stain dark blue [82 I6.43]. Cells that have increased N/C ratios, as seen in dysplasia, but with reddish chromatin, should serve as a warning to the cytologist to be cautious in making a diagnosis of dysplasia. Binucleation or multinucleation is a frequent feature of inflamed cells, but it can also be seen in dysplasia or condyloma.

Cytoplasmic Features: The cytoplasm often stains polychromatically ("two–toned"), or with decreased intensity as a result of inflammation. Commonly, however, especially in *Trichomonas* infection, the cytoplasm becomes eosinophilic or orangeophilic. This pseudokeratinized cytoplasm, together with a somewhat enlarged, dark nucleus (also common with *Trichomonas* infection), can mimic low-grade keratinizing dysplasia.

There is often a small, clear space around the nucleus of inflamed squamous cells, known as the perinuclear halo. These halos are common in (but not limited to) *Trichomonas* infection, in which case they are known as "trich halos" (they can trick the unwary into a diagnosis of condyloma by suggesting the presence of koilocytes) [83 I6.50]. In inflammation, the width of the space between the nucleus and the edge of the vacuole is usually less than the diameter of an intermediate cell nucleus and the outline of the halo is somewhat hazy. Such inflammatory perinuclear halos are generally not a prominent feature of dysplastic cells. However, bona fide koilocytes are commonly seen in dysplasia, but their halos are usually much larger and more sharply defined, and associated with "dysplastic" nuclei.

Both the nucleus and the cytoplasm can become vacuolated as a result of inflammatory change. Vacuolar cytoplasmic degeneration is particularly common in metaplastic cells, sometimes giving them a soap bubble appearance. The cytoplasmic vacuoles frequently contain ingested neutrophils. The combination of vacuolated cytoplasm and atypical nuclei may suggest glandular cancer. In practice, highly vacuolated cells are more likely to be benign metaplasia than adenocarcinoma, particularly in the presence of inflammation [I6.59, I6.143](see "IUD Effect").

Background Features: When inflammation is severe, a protein-rich exudate, with deposition of fibrin and finely granular precipitate, may occur. In addition, mucus, bacteria, inflammatory cells, and lysed cells may cause the "dirty background" of inflammation to closely resemble a tumor diathesis. Although a tumor diathesis can rarely occur in the absence of identifiable tumor cells, careful search for the presence of cancer cells is the key to the correct diagnosis.

Management of Patients With Inflammatory Change: When the lesion is apparently inflammatory, but there is some question as to its true nature, the patient can be treated appropriately for any specific infection and the smear repeated in a short period of time ("treat and repeat"). If no specific infectious agent can be identified in the Pap smear, sometimes a Betadine® douche or broad-spectrum antibiotics will be effective in clearing a nonspecific inflammatory process. In cases where there is no doubt that the epithelial changes are completely benign and inflammatory in nature, a quick repeated Pap smear may not be necessary, and the next regularly scheduled examination may be sufficient for cancer surveillance. Of great importance, however, is that patients with merely inflammatory smears, particularly when persistent, may be at significant risk (up to ~25%) of having high-grade squamous intraepithelial lesions [Busseniers 1991, Cecchini 1990a, Frisch 1990, McLachlan 1994, Pearlstone 1992, J Wilson 1990]. Patients with Pap smears that are suspicious for cervical neoplasia should be considered for immediate colposcopy.

Something to keep in mind is that dysplasia can, and frequently does, coexist with inflammation [Reagan 1956]. If the cells *look* dysplastic, they probably *are*. Some authorities advocate performing colposcopy on all patients having any degree of dysplasia, or even ASCUS, despite the presence of inflammation. However, others advise that on the first diagnosis of low-grade dysplasia, and in the presence of significant inflammation, the smear can be repeated after appropriate therapy ("treat and repeat"). If the change does not regress with therapy, it must be assumed to be genuine dysplasia, and colposcopy is indicated. If the dysplastic changes go away after medical therapy, however, this does not prove that the lesion was only inflammatory in nature. Dysplasia may have been present, but subsequently regressed. Moreover, there is a high false-negative diagnostic rate on quickly repeated Pap smears. Therefore, careful follow-up is warranted. Finally, for a diagnosis of moderate dysplasia, or worse (ie, high-grade squamous intraepithelial lesion), *or* repeated diagnoses of ASCUS or low-grade squamous intraepithelial lesion, colposcopy is recommended.

T6.27 Pap Smear Features Associated With *Trichomonas*

"Cannonballs" indicate polymorphonuclear neutrophils or *Trichomonas* agglomerated onto squamous cells [I6.49]. However, polymorphonuclear neutrophil cannonballs are nonspecific.
Cytoplasm
- Pseudokeratinization (ie, eosinophilia/orangeophilia)
- Bubbly, degenerated
- Autolysis
- Anucleate squames common (not heavily keratinized)

Nucleus
- Binucleation
- Slight nuclear enlargement
- Nuclear hyperchromasia
- Variable chromatin clumping
- Pyknosis, karyorrhexis
- A few naked nuclei

Perinuclear halos (differential diagnosis: koilocytes) [I6.50]
Dirty, granular background common; may resemble diathesis
Cocci or *Gardnerella* are often present
Leptothrix may be present
Can culture or identify in wet mount
Differential diagnosis
- Mild* keratinizing dysplasia (with enlarged dark nuclei and eosinophilic/orangeophilic cells); when uncertain, treat and repeat
- Condyloma (koilocyte vs inflammatory halos)

* Never mimics advanced dysplasia, carcinoma in situ, or cancer.

Specific Infections

Multiple infections are the rule, not the exception. Gonorrhea, syphilis, staphylococcus, and streptococcus infections can all cause inflammation, and the changes in the Pap smear are usually nonspecific. However, some agents produce more or less characteristic epithelial changes. Interestingly, some infections, such as *Trichomonas* and *Candida*, may show some seasonal variation in prevalence [Sodhani 1994].

Trichomonas vaginalis

This is an oval or pear-shaped organism that varies from 8 to 30 µm (ie, ranges in size from intermediate nucleus to parabasal cell) [84 I6.47]. There may be an inverse relation between the size of the organism and the severity of the infection [Winston 1974]. The trichomonad nucleus (thin, elliptical) *must* be identified to diagnose this infection (differentiates from cytoplasmic fragments, other debris). Red granules in cytoplasm may be seen. Flagella are never seen in the Pap smear [T6.27].

Infection $\rightarrow$ Nonhormonal Maturation: This is demonstrated by superficial cells, generalized eosinophilia, and pseudokeratinization. Slightly enlarged, dark nuclei and perinuclear halos [I6.50] are common, mimicking low grade dysplasia.

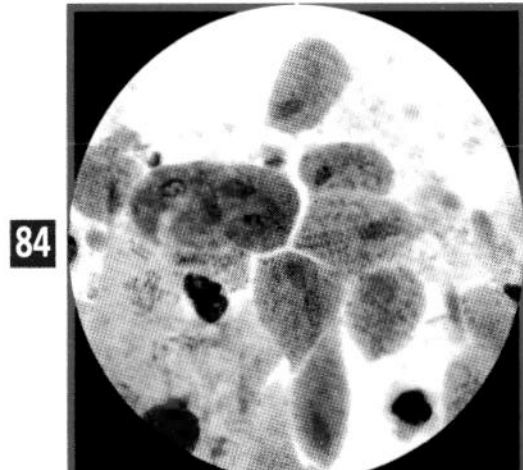
84

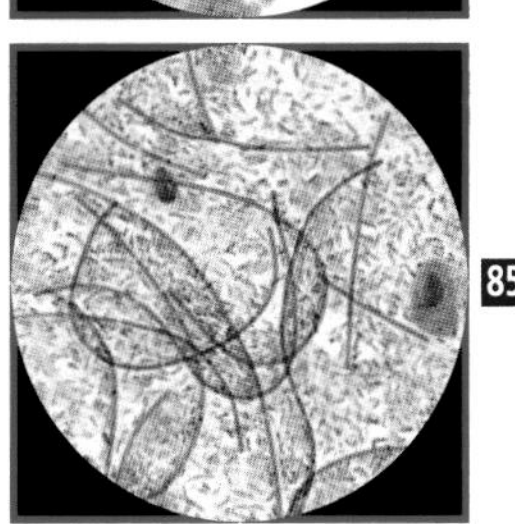
85

Infection vs Infestation: Infection is associated with itching, foul-smelling yellow-green discharge, clinically, and evidence of inflammation, including increased lymphocytes [Kiviat 1985], cytologically.

Leptothrix

Leptothrix is mixed lactobacilli or *Actinomyces* [85 I6.48]. The organisms are long, thin (less than half as thick as *Candida*), and flexible. It looks like limp spaghetti. If *Leptothrix* is present, *Trichomonas* is usually also present ("spaghetti and meatballs"), but the reverse is not true, ie, *Trichomonas* is often present without *Leptothrix*.

Candida *Species*

Candida [I6.51] is associated with a change in vaginal glycogen, flora, or pH. For example: Pregnancy, late luteal phase of cycle [Kalo-Klein 1989]; diabetes mellitus, immunosuppression; debilitating disease; steroids (birth control pills, corticoids); broad-spectrum antibiotics, chemotherapy are associated with *Candida* infection. Clinical findings include itching and discharge (thin, watery, or

Candida Effect on Pap Smear

Nuclear enlargement: Mild, generalized [Kiviat 1985] (differential diagnosis: dysplasia, but chromatin not dark or coarse)
Hyperkeratosis, usually slight
Neutrophil lysis, occasionally extensive; hyphae may appear to have impaled squamous cells (paper spindle effect)

characteristic white cottage cheese–like). Patients can also be asymptomatic.

Candida cannot be speciated based on morphology; a culture needs to be performed. Pap smear sensitivity is approximately 80% [Siapco 1986]. Both pseudohyphae (sticks) and yeast (stones) [86 I6.51]. If hyphae alone are seen, consider *Geotrichum*; if yeast alone is seen, consider *Torulopsis* (*Candida glabrata*) [Boquet-Jimenez 1978].

Actinomyces

Actinomyces [87 I6.53] is associated with IUD use; rarely, it is associated with other foreign objects (eg, tampons, pessaries). The patient may be asymptomatic or have pain (pelvic, menstrual, dyspareunia). Pain suggests significant infection or pelvic inflammatory disease (rare). Cytologic examination finds colonies of variably gram-positive, long, thin, filamentous bacteria that are reddish, branch, are irregularly beaded, and radiate from a central area. *Actinomyces* is associated with fuzzy masses of bacteria ("dust bunnies"). Therapy is controversial; however, removal of the IUD and antibiotic therapy are recommended if there are signs of pelvic inflammatory disease [Dybdahl 1991].

Herpes

Herpes [88 I6.54] can be asymptomatic or present as blisters, which can ulcerate and be painful. Genital herpes is associated with neonatal morbidity and mortality; therefore, it is very important to make the diagnosis in a pregnant patient. However, there is a high false-negative rate. Herpes simplex types I and II are morphologically indistinguishable. The most characteristic cells are multinucleated and the nuclei mold each other. The nuclei are enlarged and the chromatin marginates, resulting in a ground glass appearance [Coleman 1982, Naib 1966, Stowell 1994]. There may be red nuclear inclusions (said to be more characteristic of secondary infection [Ng 1970]).

The 3 M's of Herpes Diagnosis

Multinucleation
Molding (of nuclei)
Margination ("ground glass" chromatin)
± nuclear inclusions

Late changes are characteristic and diagnostic. Early changes (mononucleated cells with high N/C ratios, abnormal chromatin) can mimic CIN III: CIN III has granular, clumped chromatin, irregular nuclear membranes, and accompanying lower-grade dysplasia, while herpes has ground glass chromatin and accompanying cells with classic herpetic changes. Note: Patients with herpes infection are in the high-risk group for CIN/SIL.

Reactive changes in endocervical cells obtained by the endocervical brush can mimic herpes virus effect (multinucleation, molding): ground glass chromatin and (if present) inclusions are helpful in the differential diagnosis [Stowell 1994].

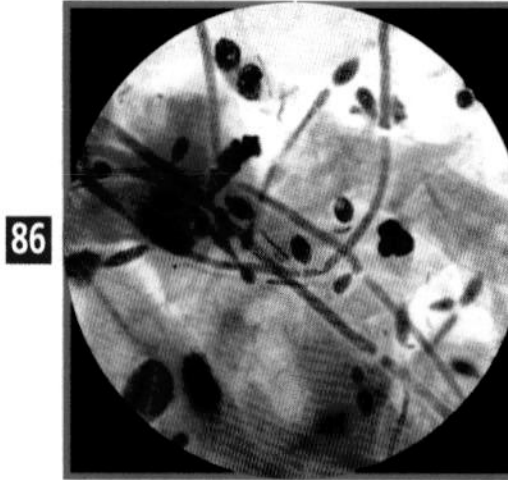
86

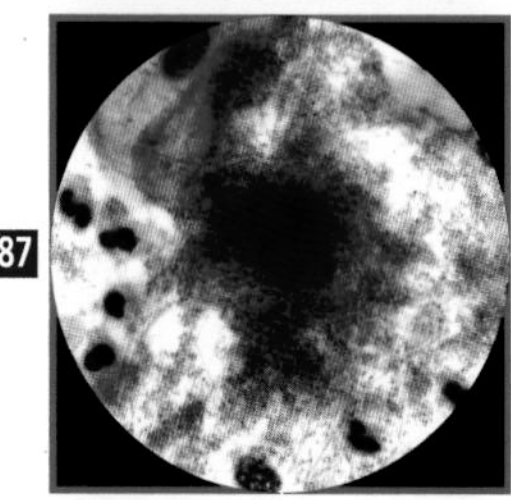
87

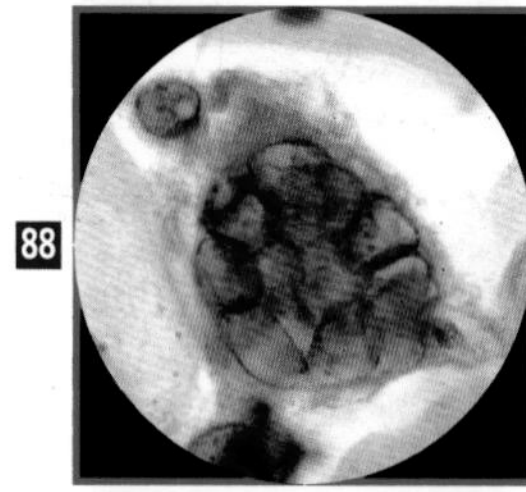
88

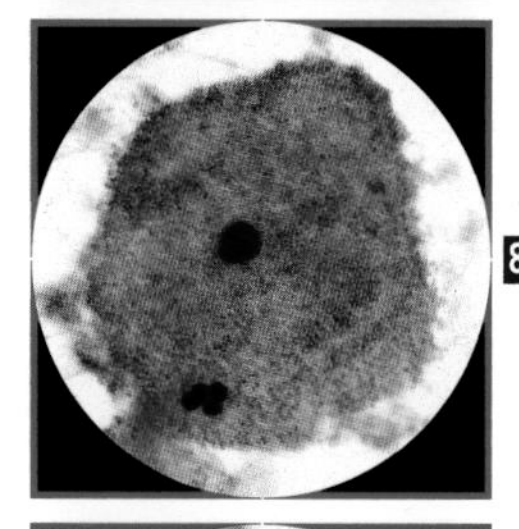
89

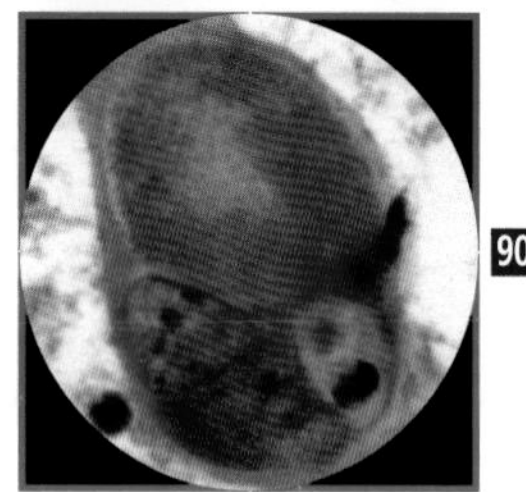
90

Cytomegalovirus

This is a member of the herpes virus family that has also been reported in the Pap smear [Coleman 1982, Gideon 1991, Henry-Stanley 1993a, Huang 1993, Mulford 1991, Naib 1966, Sickel 1991].

Gonorrhea

In gonorrhea, intracytoplasmic diplococci may be seen but are not diagnostic. There is abundant purulent exudate. Culture must be performed to reliably diagnose gonorrhea.

Gardnerella vaginalis *and Nonspecific Bacterial Vaginosis*

Gardnerella (Hæmophilus) vaginalis [89 I6.52] can be cultured from 30% to 40% of apparently normal women, but is found in approximately 90% of patients with nonspecific bacterial vaginosis. Nonspecific bacterial vaginosis is a clinical, rather than a pathologic, entity. It is characterized by profuse, foul-smelling (fishy due to anime release with potassium hydroxide, the "whiff" test), yellow-gray discharge, with itching and burning. Bacterial vaginosis is a polymicrobial process involving several different types of obligate and facultative anaerobic bacteria, usually including but not limited to *Gardnerella, Mobiluncus,* and *Bacteroides* [Giacomini 1992]. A shift from the normal *Lactobacillus* dominated vaginal flora to a predominance of coccobacilli provides supportive evidence of a clinical diagnosis of bacterial vaginosis [NCI 1993a,b].

Gardnerella is a gram-negative, comma-shaped coccobacillus. The bacteria tend to agglomerate onto squamous cells (ie, "clue cells") [89 I6.52]. The clue cells have a velvety surface, obscured cell edges, and are covered by small coccobacilli. Note: Other bacteria can adhere to cells. Smears usually show a characteristic granular blue background of small coccobacilli, but the background is otherwise clean, often accompanied by slight parakeratosis. Lactobacilli and inflammation are conspicuously absent [Schnadig 1989].

A shift in vaginal flora is indicated by mixed coccobacilli, with or without clue cells. Associated findings include slight parakeratosis and a clean background; *B vaginalis* is absent. These changes are not specific and can be seen in the absence of clinical symptoms. Therefore, according to the Bethesda System, the findings should be reported as "bacteria morphologically consistent with shift in vaginal flora." Note that patients can have bacterial vaginosis in the absence of *Gardnerella* or clue cells.

Chlamydia trachomatis

Chlamydia trachomatis [90 I6.56] is an obligate intracellular bacterium that is associated with granular cytoplasmic inclusions. It is the most common cause of nongonococcal urethritis/

cervicitis. It may cause 20% to 25% of cases of pelvic inflammatory disease, which can result in infertility and ectopic pregnancy. *Chlamydia trachomatis* is frequently asymptomatic.

Metaplastic and endocervical cells are affected, as are young reparative cells. Nuclear changes are nonspecific but can mimic dysplasia. There may be nuclear enlargement, increased N/C ratio, hyperchromasia, and multinucleation. Nucleoli are rare or absent. Granular cytoplasmic inclusions may be seen, but their diagnostic significance is controversial. *Chlamydia trachomatis* can also cause cellular enlargement (20–100 μm). *Chlamydia trachomatis* may be associated with intense acute inflammation or follicular cervicitis [Kiviat 1985].

The value of the Pap smear in diagnosing *Chlamydia* is uncertain [Bernal 1989, R Clark 1985, Geerling 1985, Ghirardini 1991, Gupta 1988, Kiviat 1985, Lindner 1985, Pandit 1993, T Quinn 1987, Roongpisuthipong 1987, Shafer 1985]. Controversial targetoid cytoplasmic inclusions are probably not diagnostic [91 I6.55]. At least some of these inclusions are mucin vacuoles [R Clark 1985]. Fine vacuolization of metaplastic cells (having a "moth eaten" appearance) may correlate with high risk of infection [Gupta 1988]. Nebular bodies [Shiina 1985], though rare and difficult to see, may be more specific [Waters 1991]. Nebular bodies do not displace the nucleus and their cytoplasm is not distended. The inclusion is finely granular, and has a thin wall [T6.28] [Shiina 1985]. Note: *Chlamydia* changes can mimic low-grade dysplasia.

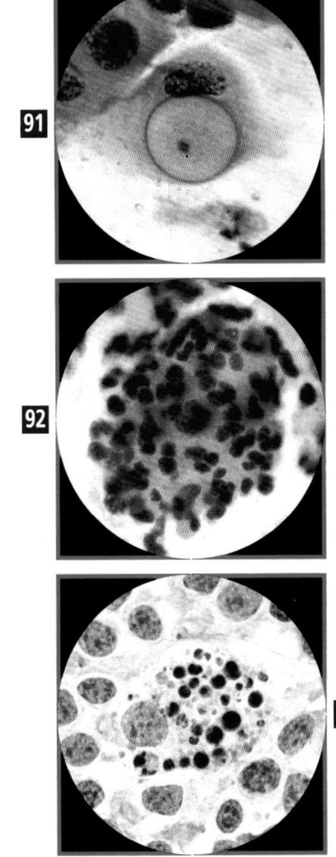
91
92
93

Other Manifestations of Inflammation

The delicate, single layer of columnar cells of the endocervix affords little protection from infection and inflammation. Inflammatory cells easily traverse the endocervical epithelium and are commonly present in Pap smears. In patients who have had a hysterectomy, the background of inflammatory cells often clears, even though the patient may be subjected to the same physical, chemical, or microbiologic assaults as before surgery.

Neutrophils: In most sites, neutrophils indicate acute inflammation or infection. However, polymorphonuclear lymphocytes (PMNs) are a common, physiologic accompaniment of the premenstrual and menstrual phases of the normal cycle. Therefore, the presence of neutrophils does not necessarily indicate acute inflammation. However, numerous neutrophils, other than related to the menses, suggest acute inflammation. PMNs adherent to squamous cells are sometimes referred to as "cannonball" cells [92 I6.49]. Cannonball cells are associated with *Trichomonas* infection, but are not specific. Sometimes neutrophils are so numerous that they obscure the epithelial cells. A specimen with excess exudate may be unsatisfactory for evaluation, and repeating the Pap smear after therapy may be indicated for proper cancer surveillance.

Eosinophils: Increased numbers of eosinophils may mean that the patient has an allergic vaginitis/cervicitis due to bacteria, chemical, drugs, powders, or even sperm (a possible cause of infertility). Allergic vaginitis is frequently unrecognized or misdiagnosed clinically, resulting in inappropriate therapy. Therefore, it may be worthwhile to report the presence of eosinophils in a Pap smear. Some cancers are associated with eosinophils (eg, glassy cell adenosquamous carcinoma).

Lymphocytes, Plasma Cells, and Follicular Cervicitis: Lymphocytes and plasma cells are characteristic of chronic inflammation. Mild chronic inflammation of the cervix (ie, mild chronic cervicitis) is so common—in tissue—as to be considered essentially normal. However, lymphocytes and plasma cells are seldom found in normal Pap smears; their presence usually indicates significant inflammation.

Occasionally lymphoid follicles, complete with germinal center formation, occur in the cervix. This condition is called follicular cervicitis. It is sometimes associated with *Chlamydia* infection [Hare 1982]. Follicular cervicitis can occur at any age, but is both more common and more likely to be detected in Pap smears in postmenopausal patients who have a thin, atrophic overlying epithelium, than in women with a thick, mature overlying epithelium [Roberts 1975].

The cytologic appearance of follicular cervicitis is identical to a smear of a germinal center of a lymph node [93 I6.45] [Eisenstein 1965]. The two main diagnostic features are: range of maturation of the lymphoid cells (mature and immature lymphocytes in varying stages of differentiation) and presence of tingible body macrophages. Capillaries can also be seen.

Lymphoid cells lie singly, have high N/C ratios, do not form groups, and show no significant nuclear molding. The majority of the lymphoid cells are small, mature lymphocytes with coarse, dark chromatin, smooth nuclear membranes, no visible nucleoli, and very little cytoplasm. The immature lymphocytes (follicular center cells) vary in size, but are larger than mature lymphocytes. Immature lymphocytes have more open chromatin and somewhat more cytoplasm, and may have irregular nuclear membranes or prominent nucleoli. Plasma cells may also be found.

Tingible body macrophages contain cellular debris in their cytoplasm, which is visualized microscopically as tingible (ie, stainable) bodies. The debris is the result of cell turnover in the germinal center (necrobiosis).

Pleomorphic (lymphoid) cells with coarse chromatin and nucleoli may appear quite alarming and could be mistaken for carcinoma in situ, small cell carcinoma, endometrial carcinoma, or malignant lymphoma. In contrast with epithelial neoplasia, all of the cells are single in follicular cervicitis. There is little or no molding, nor are there epithelial groupings, such as syncytia,

T6.28 **Comparison of Features in Nebular Bodies and Nonspecific Inclusions**

	Nebular Bodies	Nonspecific Inclusions
Nucleus	Not displaced	Displaced
Cytoplasm	Not distended	Distended
Inclusion	Thin wall, finely granular	Thick wall, coarsely granular

sheets, or glands, in follicular cervicitis. Although patients with follicular cervicitis are in the high-risk group for developing cervical dysplasia, dysplasia does not necessarily accompany follicular cervicitis. In contrast, carcinoma in situ is usually accompanied by dysplasia.

The differential diagnosis of follicular cervicitis also includes malignant lymphoma. Malignant lymphoma of the cervix is very rare, and such patients usually have a history of the disease. Also, lymphoma is associated with gross abnormality of the cervix. Follicular cervicitis is common by comparison and does not produce a grossly abnormal cervix. Follicular cervicitis presents a polytypic lymphoid population ("range of maturation") and tingible body macrophages, indicative of germinal center formation and a benign reactive lymphoid process. Malignant lymphoma, on the other hand, is characterized by a block in maturation of the lymphoid cells. The classic cytologic appearance of lymphoma is a monotypic population of cells, often lacking tingible body macrophages (except when high grade).

Histiocytes: Histiocytes, like neutrophils, can be either physiologically or pathologically present [94 I6.22]. They are a normal component of the Pap smear just before and after the menses. Histiocytes (along with glandular endometrial cells) are present in such large numbers between days 5 and 11 of the menstrual cycle that this part of the cycle was referred to as "exodus" by Papanicolaou [Papanicolaou 1953]. Morphologically similar cells originate from the superficial endometrial stroma, may be of müllerian origin, and are recognized by their tendency to form loose aggregates ("sticky histiocytes") (see "Endometrial Stromal Cells," p 123).

Histiocytes can be seen in early or late pregnancy, following abortion, or postpartum. If numerous histiocytes are present after menopause or in the second half of the menstrual cycle, they may be associated with hyperplasia or neoplasia of the endometrium. Histiocytes are also seen with foreign bodies, sutures, IUD, chronic inflammation, including ulcers, and after radiation, biopsy, or cryotherapy. Very rarely, histiocytes containing characteristic intracytoplasmic Michaelis-Gutmann bodies are seen in malacoplakia [Stewart 1991].

Histiocytes are classified as being small, large (often associated with phagocytosis), or giant (multinucleated) [94 I6.22, 95 I6.23]. Typical histiocytes are present singly and do not form tightly cohesive sheets or molded groups. The histiocyte nucleus varies in size and is eccentrically located. It ranges from round to oval, or most characteristically, bean shaped. However, only a minority have the classic bean-shaped nucleus. The chromatin is usually fine and pale, but may have a "salt-and-pepper" pattern. One or more small nucleoli may be present.

The cytoplasm is typically delicate and vacuolar with indistinct cell borders. Sometimes, the histiocyte's cytoplasm becomes surprisingly dense, almost like a squamous cell. However, instead of the glassy appearance of squamous cytoplasm (sometimes with keratin rings), the cytoplasm of the histiocytes has a foamy or granular texture.

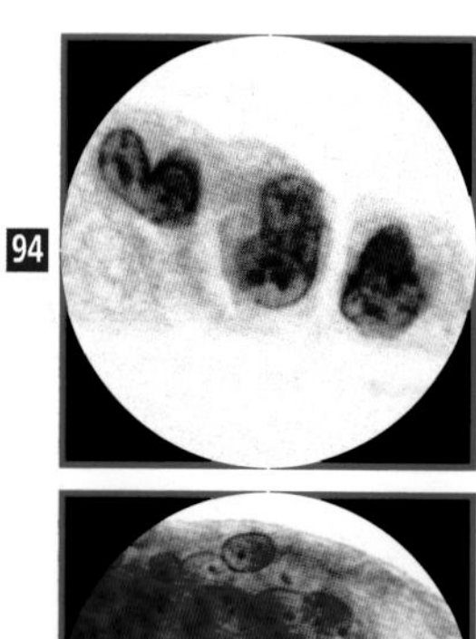
94

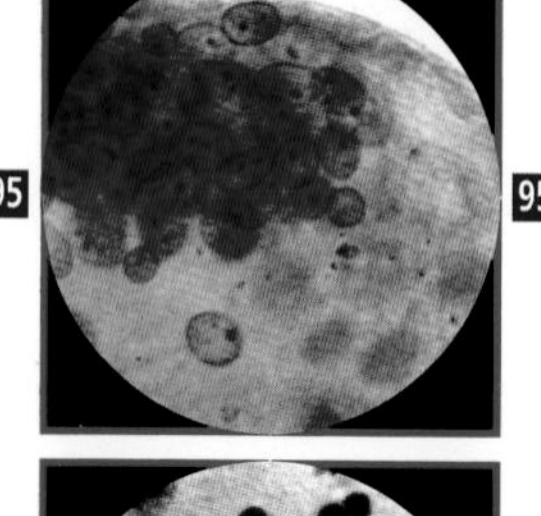
95

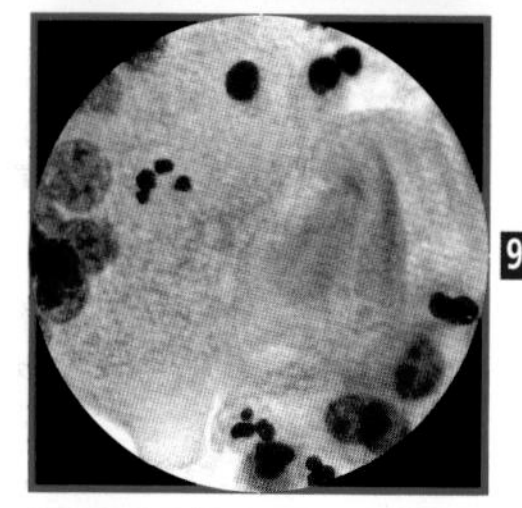
96

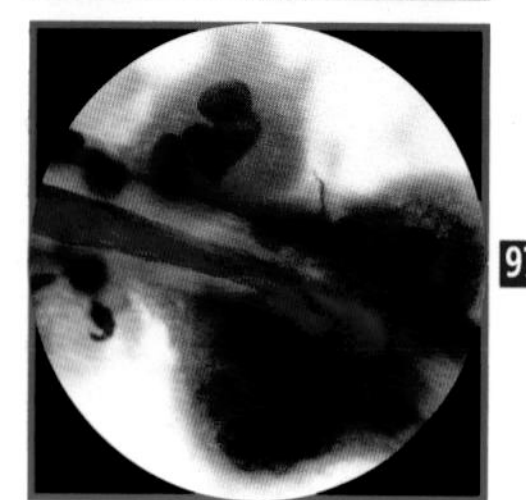
97

Histiocytes are great impersonators. They can mimic many other cell types, eg, squamous, endocervical, endometrial, reserve, even dysplasia or cancer. A good clue to the histiocyte's true identity is its characteristic nuclear chromatin structure, described above. Also, the nucleus is typically eccentric, but not compressed by secretory vacuoles, and there is no perinuclear halo. Histiocytes are usually single, or at most loosely aggregated, with spaces between cells and no nuclear molding. They do not form true tissue aggregates. Mitoses are frequent in histiocytes.

Large histiocytes often have phagocytosed debris in their cytoplasm (bacteria, white blood cells, red blood cells, etc). If the cytoplasm contains lipid or hemosiderin, particularly after menopause, there is an increased risk of endometrial hyperplasia/neoplasia, because such cells may indicate tissue destruction (lipophages) or old bleeding (hemosiderin-laden macrophages), respectively. Look for diagnostic epithelial cells.

Multinucleated giant cell histiocytes are common in postmenopausal women or after radiation therapy or surgery [C Evans 1984, Murad 1985, Tweeddale 1968]. They are also common postpartum [95 I6.23]. Characteristically, the multiple histiocytic nuclei are not exactly identical but do closely resemble each other as siblings do ("sibling nuclei"). The nuclear chromatin and characteristic cytoplasm identifies the cells as histiocytic. Other differential diagnostic possibilities include "syncytial" parabasal cells seen in longstanding atrophy (with squamous cytoplasm) and syncytiotrophoblastic cells (central, degenerated nuclei, dense cytoplasm with tails; see "Cytology of Pregnancy," p133).

Granulomatous Cervicitis

- *Tuberculosis (mimics SCC grossly)*
- *Foreign body (eg, suture, inclusion cyst)*
- *Posttherapy reaction (radiation, surgery)*
- *Schistosomiasis*
- *Granuloma inguinale (Donovan bodies)*
- *Lymphogranuloma venereum*
- *Syphilis (gumma)*
- *Chlamydia (?)*

Granulomatous cervicitis, eg, tuberculosis, can be another explanation for finding giant cells [Kutteh 1992]. Tuberculous cervicitis, which is rare, can mimic squamous cell carcinoma of the cervix grossly. A variety of other organisms can also cause granulomatous inflammation of the cervix [Christie 1980]. The presence of epithelioid histiocytes in a nodular collection is diagnostic for granuloma. Foreign body granulomatous reactions are *commonly* observed after radiation therapy (reaction to squamous cells or altered ground substance) or after surgery (suture granuloma) [96 I6.66, 97 I6.67]] [Bardales 1993]. In foreign body reactions, the giant cells tend to surround and ingest the foreign material. Granulomas can also be seen as a response to infiltrating squamous cell carcinoma.

Granulation Tissue—Capillaries and Myofibroblasts: Granulation tissue is sometimes sampled in the Pap smear, particularly if there is an ulcer. Granulation tissue forms in reaction to severe inflammation, including surgery or radiation [Montanari 1968].

The Pap smear is characterized by an inflammatory background, mononucleated and multinucleated histiocytes, repair, and blood. The diagnostic finding is small blood vessels surrounded by histiocytes. Capillaries or venules are small tubular structures, sometimes with red blood cells in the lumen. The endothelial cells may be reactive and therefore, appear atypical. When single, reactive endothelial cells resemble small endocervical cells or small histiocytes with eccentric nuclei. A longitudinal groove is often present in the nuclear membrane. The chromatin is very fine and pale, and regularly distributed. A small, but distinct, nucleolus may also be present. There may be a pale zone in the perinuclear cytoplasm. The cytoplasm is very delicate, with indistinct cell boundaries.

In addition, reactive myofibroblasts may be obtained from the ulcer bed. Myofibroblasts produce collagen and have a role in scar contraction. They are spindle to stellate in shape. A characteristic feature of these cells is the presence of thin little "rootlets" extending from the main cytoplasmic mass. The nuclei are pleomorphic and active in appearance, with large, prominent nucleoli, but pale chromatin. Myofibroblasts can appear particularly large and pleomorphic in radiation-induced ulcers, possibly suggesting a sarcoma. However, the atypical cells are relatively sparse and there is a history of radiation [98 I6.64].

98

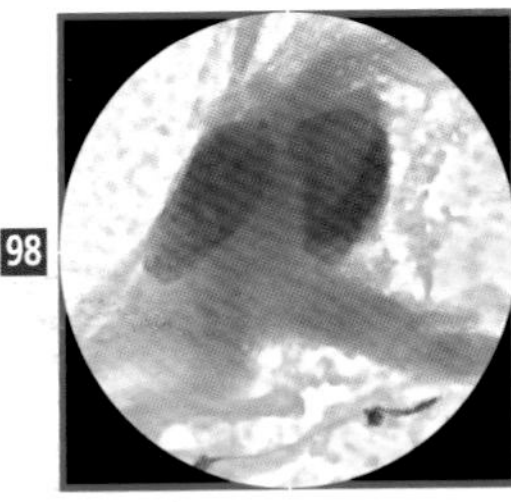

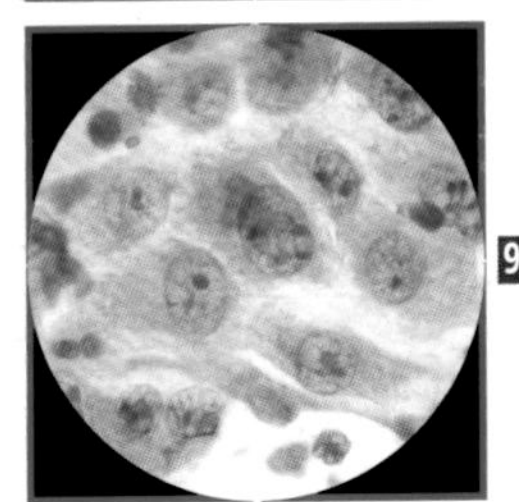

99

Repair/Regeneration

When the mucosa is denuded, the epithelial cells at the periphery begin to proliferate to repair the defect. As the cells begin to grow and make various cellular products, they become mitotically active, somewhat pleomorphic, and develop prominent nucleoli (features indicative of active protein synthesis and cellular regeneration). These benign cellular changes can mimic neoplasia. Distinguishing regeneration/repair from carcinoma can be a difficult diagnostic dilemma. Although repair is most common in younger patients, no age is spared. For example, repair is frequent in older patients after radiation therapy. Repair/regeneration is the result of an extremely heterogeneous group of injuries, and can also be seemingly idiopathic, associated only with normal vaginal flora. Behçet's disease is a rare cause of repair, which can be very atypical [Wilbur 1993].

Causes of Regeneration/Repair

Severe inflammation, eg, *Trichomonas*
Cautery, cryotherapy, or laser therapy
Biopsy, surgery
Delivery
Radiation
Spontaneous, idiopathic

Reparative cells can resemble squamous, glandular, or metaplastic epithelium. Benign reparative cells usually exfoliate in cohesive sheets, and may have a swirling tissue culture–like appearance. Nuclear "atypia" ranges from mild to severe, and may suggest malignancy. Cell boundaries vary from well to poorly defined, or "syncytial."

There are a few key diagnostic points regarding regeneration/repair [Bibbo 1971b, Geirsson 1977]. Because it is a benign process, repair maintains a high degree of orderliness. The cells line up in fairly orderly ranks and files. Each cell has adequate cytoplasm; therefore, the N/C ratio is relatively normal or only somewhat increased. The rows of nuclei ("nuclear streaming") show little or no overlap or crowding [99 I6.44].

Sheets of reparative cells are very cohesive. Single cells are usually sparse or absent in repair, in contrast with cancer, in which single cells are usually prominent. When single cells are present in repair, they are usually found in proximity to a group. Unfortunately, single reparative cells are more common in the most atypical reparative processes—cases that are cytologically more difficult to distinguish from cancer.

Although reparative nuclei can be pleomorphic and enlarged (usually no more than two to three times the size of an intermediate cell nucleus), the chromatin is normochromatic or, frequently, pale and hypochromatic. Cancer is associated with distinctly abnormal, generally hyperchromatic, coarse chromatin. Normal mitotic figures are commonly seen in repair. Perhaps surprisingly, nucleoli can sometimes be more prominent in repair than cancer. Irregular contours of the nucleoli can also be seen in benign repair. Thus, mitotic figures (unless abnormal), and macronucleoli or even irregular nucleoli are not diagnostic of cancer.

The cytoplasm of repair is relatively abundant, usually stains blue, sometimes pink, or commonly, both (polychromatic), but does not keratinize. Cytoplasmic vacuolization may be seen. Cancer is associated with a tumor diathesis, while repair has a clean or inflammatory background, in which inflammatory cells may be present. Neutrophils in the cytoplasm of the atypical cells favor a diagnosis of repair. However, occasionally it can be difficult to distinguish a "dirty" background of inflammation from a tumor diathesis, and cancers are not immune to becoming inflamed.

In summary, in repair there is a disparity between the abnormal appearing, pleomorphic nuclei with prominent nucleoli versus the orderliness of the cells with bland chromatin. In cancer, all of the abnormal cellular features point to malignancy. This disparity of cytologic features is an important clue to the proper diagnosis of repair [T6.29]. With repair/regeneration, treat any identifiable infection/inflammation as specifically as possible, and repeat the smear immediately. If cervical neoplasia cannot be ruled out, refer to colposcopy. Patients who have a reparative process are statistically at high risk of having or developing cervical dysplasia (squamous intraepithelial lesion) and should be monitored more closely.

Differential Diagnosis of Repair

Endocervical Adenocarcinoma
- Single cells, tall columnar shape, ± mucin
- Crowding, rosettes
- Coarse, dark, irregular chromatin
- Diathesis

Squamous Cell Carcinoma
- Single cells, may be keratinized
- Abnormal, hyperchromatic, irregular chromatin
- Variable nucleoli (not same in every cell)
- Diathesis

Sarcoma
- (May have elongated cells, enlarged nuclei and nucleoli, and pale chromatin)
- Single cells
- Considerable nucleolar variation among cells (number, size, shape)

T6.29 **Comparative Features of Repair and Cancer**

	Repair/Regeneration	Cancer
Background	Clean, with inflammatory cells	Diathesis
Cells	More cohesive Few single cells	Less cohesive Many single cells
Cytoplasm	Adequate No keratinization Ingested PMNs common Polychromasia	High nuclear/cytoplasmic ratio ± Keratinization PMNs unusual Monochromasia
Nucleus	Hypochromatic, pale Fine, even chromatin	Hyperchromatic, dark Coarse, irregular chromatin
Nucleoli	Macronucleoli, every cell ± Irregular shapes	Variable among cells ± Irregular shapes
Summary	Order Disparity of features	Disorder Parity of features

Atypical Repair

Occasional cases of repair are particularly atypical in appearance [I6.63, 100 I6.147]. Atypical repair presents as tissue fragments of immature squamous or glandular cells, resembling ordinary repair but showing significant cellular abnormalities, such as crowding and piling up, nuclear enlargement and pleomorphism, and irregularities of nuclear outline and chromatin that exceed those of typical repair. Single cells may also be present. These cells, exhibiting cytologic features of both repair and dysplasia, could be difficult to distinguish from true neoplasia. Some forms of atypical repair may actually represent a reparative process occurring in a dysplastic epithelium. *If dysplasia or cancer cannot be ruled out, refer the patient for colposcopy*. Patients with atypical repair are high-risk patients.

Vitamin Deficiency States

In the face of either folate or B_{12} vitamin deficiency, cellular changes may occur that are similar to those seen due to radiotherapy. Folate and B_{12} are coenzymes in DNA synthesis (B_{12}–methyl deficiency leads to thymine deficiency, which mimics radiation DNA injury). Folate deficiency is relatively common in late pregnancy, postmenopause, and with use of some birth control pills [Kitay 1969, Whitehead 1973]. The epithelial changes may antedate megaloblastic changes in the bone marrow by several weeks.

The characteristic cytologic changes are primarily nuclear and cytoplasmic enlargement with the formation of macrocytes. Macrocytes can also be seen in radiation or chemotherapy (particularly if treatment is with folate antagonists, eg, methotrexate and cyclophosphamide) and in condyloma [101 I6.77]. Similar cells can rarely be seen in other viral infections such as measles [Heimann 1992].

Macrocytes

Cell: Large to giant
Cytoplasm: Polychromatic, vacuolization (often with PMNs, other cells)
Nucleus: Enlarged (nuclear/cytoplasmic ratio about normal), ± multiple
Seen in: Vitamin deficiency (folate, B_{12}), radiation/chemotherapy, condyloma

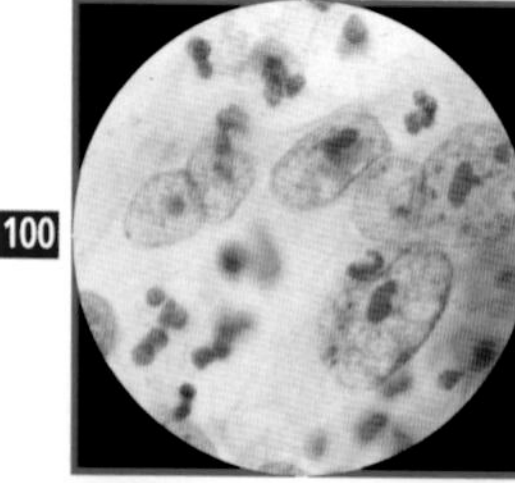
100

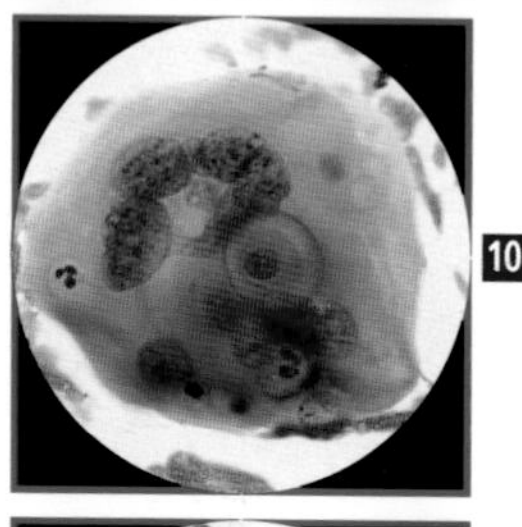
101

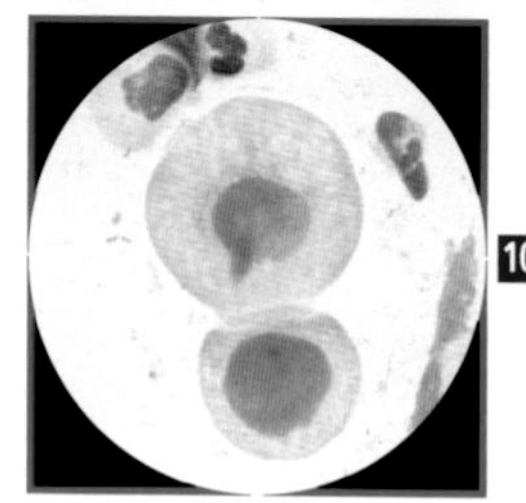
102

Cells with enlarged nuclei may be essentially indistinguishable from dysplasia usually of mild degree (low-grade squamous intraepithelial lesion) [Kitay 1969]. A course of vitamin therapy and disappearance of the change on repeated Pap smear supports a diagnosis of vitamin effect, but patients should probably be considered for colposcopy.

Atypia of Atrophy and Maturity

The great majority of patients with condyloma or dysplasia, perhaps as many as 90%, are younger than 35 years of age [Binder 1985, Carson 1993, Reid 1986]. Therefore, it could be stated with some degree of accuracy that dysplasia is not a disease of old women. Keeping this simple fact in mind will help prevent a great deal of difficulty in diagnosis of atrophic smears. Furthermore, when dysplasia is present in older women, it is usually associated with increased maturation, rather than atrophy [Patten 1978]. Although a postmenopausal woman will seldom have dysplasia or condyloma, she may have carcinoma in situ or invasive carcinoma. In women in their 20s, dysplasia is two to three times as common as in situ or invasive carcinoma, whereas in women older than 60, in situ or invasive carcinoma is two to three times as common as dysplasia [F6.20] [Binder 1985, Carson 1993, L Johnson 1968, Reid 1986, Stern 1963].

Since the transition zone is often high in the endocervical canal and lesions tend to mature distally, a true squamous dysplasia seen in a Pap smear from a postmenopausal patient may be only the "tip of the iceberg" of a more significant lesion, possibly including invasive carcinoma, occurring higher up in the endocervix. Therefore, it may be worthwhile to evaluate all postmenopausal dysplasias colposcopically.

Atypia of Atrophy: Some atrophic smears, although benign, can be quite alarming microscopically, mimicking dysplasia, carcinoma in situ, or even cancer. This benign change is known as atypia of atrophy; screening such a smear can be challenging. The atypical cells are parabasal- or basal-sized (ie, atrophic) [102 I6.139]. They are usually poorly preserved and often appear dried and degenerated. The nuclei can be pleomorphic, hyperchromatic, and enlarged into the range seen in dysplasia, with high N/C ratios. The cytoplasm is usually blue-gray, sometimes pink, but may also be orangeophilic due to degeneration (ie, pseudokeratinized). Syncytia-like aggregates of atypical parabasal/basal cells form hyperchromatic crowded groups (HCGs) that may be difficult to distinguish from carcinoma in situ or even invasive cancer. (Conversely, malignant tissue fragments may be difficult to distinguish from benign atrophy [Koike 1994].) In severe atrophy there is frequently a dirty background, with degenerated cells, debris, granular precipitate, fresh/old blood, and inflammatory cells, including neutrophils and histiocytes ("atrophy with inflammation"). This granular background can resemble a tumor diathesis.

F6.20 **Relative Proportions of Dysplasia vs Carcinoma In Situ/Cancer by Age**

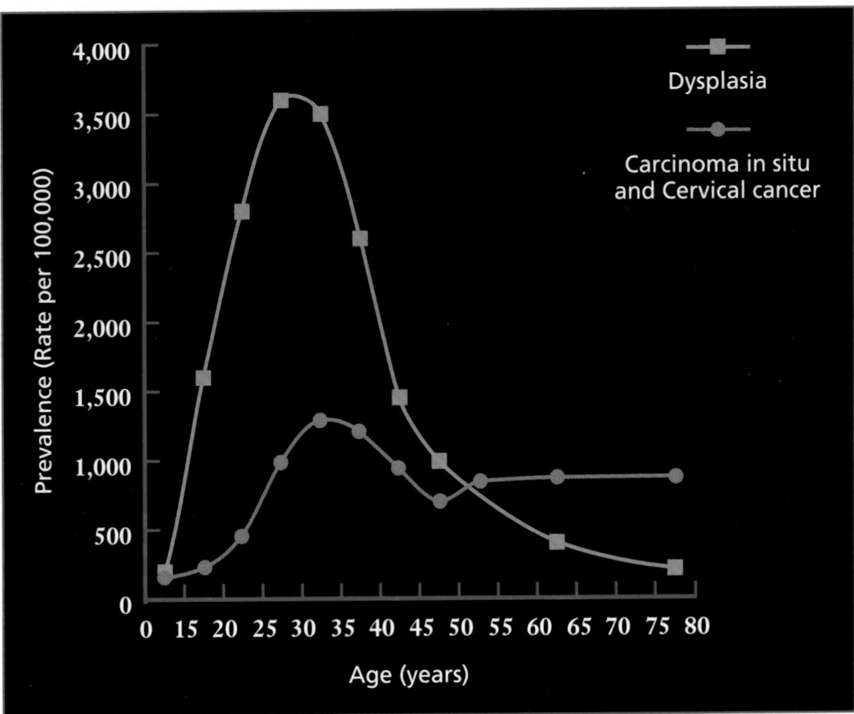

[Reid 1986]

The key differential diagnostic feature between atypia of atrophy and actual cervical neoplasia is the quality of the chromatin. Dysplasia and cancer have a *crisp* and distinct chromatin pattern: the chromatin particles are usually well preserved and may seem to "sparkle" in the light of the microscope. Moreover, in cancer, the chromatin is often irregularly arranged and tends to vary in quality from cell to cell. In contrast, the chromatin of atypia of atrophy is usually poorly preserved, and indistinct or *smudgy*. When it is well preserved, the chromatin is fine and even, and although it may be hyperchromatic, it is not coarse, distinct, or irregular. Compare the chromatin of the cell in question with that of a normal parabasal or intermediate cell: if it is similar, it is probably benign atrophy; if coarser and darker, consider cervical neoplasia.

Mitoses are not usually found in an atrophic epithelium; therefore, when seen in this setting, the presence of mitotic figures suggests neoplasia, if a reactive/reparative process can be excluded [Buckley 1994]. Conversely, however, neoplastic lesions in older women may have a paucity of mitotic figures; therefore, the absence of mitotic figures does not completely exclude a neoplastic process. Abnormal arrangements of the cells (chaotic architecture) favors a neoplastic process. An accompanying bona fide squamous dysplasia supports a diagnosis of carcinoma in situ or cancer; however, particularly in older women, carcinoma in situ may occur as a pure lesion, without an associated dysplasia.

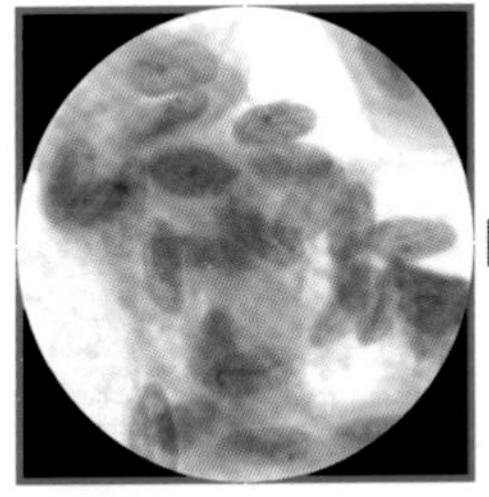
103

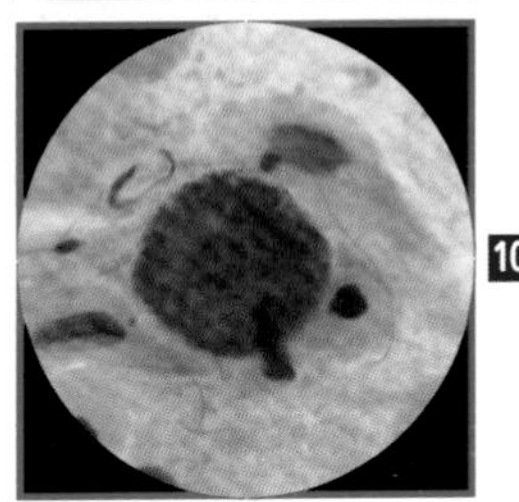
104

Transitional, or urothelial, metaplasia of the cervix also enters into differential diagnosis of high-grade dysplasia or carcinoma in situ [Ambros 1990]. It usually occurs on the ectocervix, but occasionally also in the transformation zone [Lawrence 1991], of perimenopausal or postmenopausal women [103 I6.8]. It is characterized by relatively monotonous sheets of bland, parabasal-like cells with high N/C ratios and elongated or spindle-shaped nuclei, often with a prominent groove in the nuclear membrane. In contrast with cervical neoplasia, mitotic figures and nuclear atypia are absent.

If, after careful evaluation, differentiating atypia of atrophy from a neoplastic lesion still cannot be achieved, there are three things that can be done. One is the estrogen test [Keebler 1974]. The underlying theory of the estrogen test is that if the atypical cells are simply atrophic, a trial of estrogen will cause them to mature, revealing their benign nature. On the other hand, malignant cells will remain abnormal, thus contrasting sharply with the benign cells. Note that if the lesion is already mature, eg, keratinizing dysplasia or keratinizing squamous cell carcinoma, no additional information will be gained by performing an estrogen test. Also, the test does not help diagnose adenocarcinoma or other kinds of neoplasms, such as sarcomas.

Another diagnostic choice is to simply repeat the Pap smear (without estrogen administration). Sometimes, the mechanical stimulation of the first speculum examination will cause enough maturation (by stimulating blood flow?) to allow atypical atrophic cells to transform into recognizably benign cells. However, colposcopy may be the safest course of action, since Pap smears repeated in a relatively short time have a high false-negative rate. Although the prevalence of human papilloma virus diminishes in older women [de Villiers 1992, Ley 1991, Melkert 1993], older patients who are human papilloma virus positive may be at increased risk of having bona fide neoplastic lesions [Mandelblatt 1992].

In some atrophic smears, "blue blobs" may be encountered, which can be alarming because they look rather like naked nuclei from some horrible malignancy [104 I6.10] [Ziabowski 1976]. Blue blobs vividly reinforce a principle: never render an unequivocal malignant diagnosis based only on naked nuclei. On careful inspection, blue blobs lack nuclear chromatinic structure. Sometimes a small nucleus can be seen in the center of a blue blob, which may mimic a large nucleolus. Blue blobs have been variously ascribed to inspissated mucin or dystrophic calcification, but special stains are negative for both mucin and calcium [Carson 1990]. Apparently, blue blobs result from unusual precipitation of the hematoxylin stain on mummified atrophic squamous cells.

At times, the atrophic cells undergo coagulative necrosis. The cytoplasm becomes orangeophilic and the nuclei become small, dark, and pyknotic (pseudokeratosis) [Buckley 1994]. These small, orange, atrophic cells resemble parakeratosis ("pseudo-pseudoparakeratosis"), except that the cell outlines are rounded rather than polygonal, and the cells are scattered randomly throughout the smear. (Pseudoparakeratosis affects endocervical glandular cells.)

Atypia of Maturity: In older women, who have a mature epithelium, occasional nuclei may show some degree of enlargement, into the range of squamous atypia (minimal dysplasia, ASCUS) [105 I6.140]. Unless the nuclei are also hyperchromatic (compared with an intermediate cell nucleus), this effect is probably not true minimal dysplasia. Follow-up of older patients with so-called squamous atypia shows that the great majority, as many as 85% to 95% or more, have negative colposcopy or biopsy findings, and that of the few abnormalities found, most correspond to low-grade squamous intraepithelial lesions [Cunnane 1993, Kaminski 1989b, Saminathan 1994, Symmans 1992]. The nuclear alterations seem to be an accumulation of benign change in the nuclei of the cells occurring with age. The nuclear changes may be related to a defect in DNA metabolism, perhaps akin to folate deficiency [Patten 1978], although many will respond to estrogen therapy [Kaminski 1989b]. Note, however, that older patients with atypical squamous cells of undetermined significance (ASCUS) on Pap smear have a small, but real, risk of having bona fide cervical or vaginal dysplasia [Cunnane 1993, Saminathan 1994]. And, as previously mentioned, dysplasia on Pap smear in older patients may only be the "tip of the iceberg" of a more serious lesion [Saminathan 1994].

105

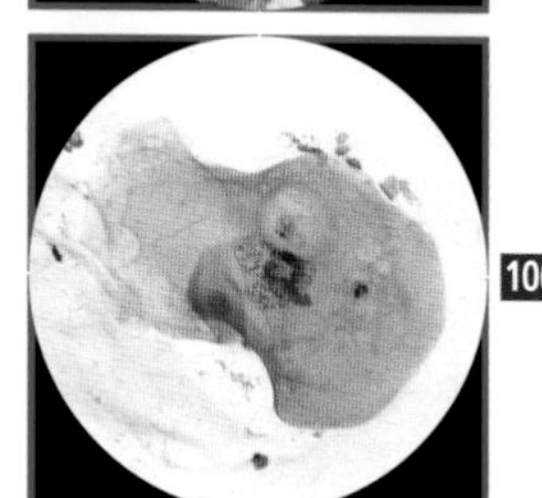

106

Radiation Cytology

Radiation is often used in the therapy of various kinds of genital cancer, particularly squamous cell carcinoma of the cervix. Radiation can be very effective in destroying tumor cells. However, it also affects the native epithelium and can damage the genetic code of the basal, mitotically active, germinative cells. Radiation results in a change of the epithelium, which can be transitory (acute) or may persist (chronic), sometimes for the life of the patient [Koss 1961]. Some forms of systemic chemotherapy can also cause cytologic changes, similar to radiation change or mimicking a precancerous state [Doss 1995, Koss 1965].

Cytology is one of the most useful methods to detect persistence or recurrence of tumor in patients who have had cervical carcinoma. Cytology can also detect the development of postradiation dysplasia, a new lesion that, particularly if it occurs within 3 years of radiation, may be very serious and have a poor prognosis [Murad 1985, Wentz 1970]. Because radiation can induce striking cellular changes in benign cells, the most common diagnostic error is interpreting benign radiation changes as neoplastic, resulting in a false-positive diagnosis. On the other hand, false-negative diagnoses may result from interpreting residual carcinoma as benign radiation effect.

A variety of radiation sensitivity tests have been proposed to try to predict which patients will respond well to radiation therapy. None is currently thought to be clinically useful. The most important clinical predictors of radiation effectiveness are the histologic type of the tumor and its extent. The qualitative changes due to radiation are independent of type of radiation and method of administration. However, the quantitative change is dependent on several variables.

Cells are most sensitive to radiation when they are approaching the phase of DNA synthesis in the cell cycle [F6.21]. Cells are resistant to radiation during DNA synthesis and moderately resistant after DNA synthesis is complete.

Cells with a high rate of turnover, like those in small cell squamous carcinoma, are the most sensitive to radiation since they spend relatively more time in the vulnerable phases. However, while small cell carcinoma is among the most radiosensitive of the cervical cancers, it is one of the least radiocurable [Wentz 1965].

Radiation Effect: Radiation causes sometimes bizarre changes in the epithelial (and mesenchymal) cells, which can mimic those seen in condyloma, dysplasia, or carcinoma (or even sarcoma). Nevertheless, cytology is a valuable tool for detection of locally recurrent cervical cancer [Shield 1992]. The cytologic effects are divided into acute and chronic changes, which are basically similar [Murad 1985]. Cytomegaly and polychromasia are particularly characteristic features of radiation change [106 I6.61, I6.64]. Chemotherapy can also affect the epithelium and cause certain changes that are not as well defined as those due to radiation effect [I6.65] [Doss 1995, Koss 1965].

Acute Radiation Change: When radiation is first administered, it induces a severe inflammatory reaction with a "diathesis" consisting of white blood cells, histiocytes (including giant cells), debris, necrosis, and evidence of epithe-

***F6.21* DNA Synthesis in a Cell Cycle**

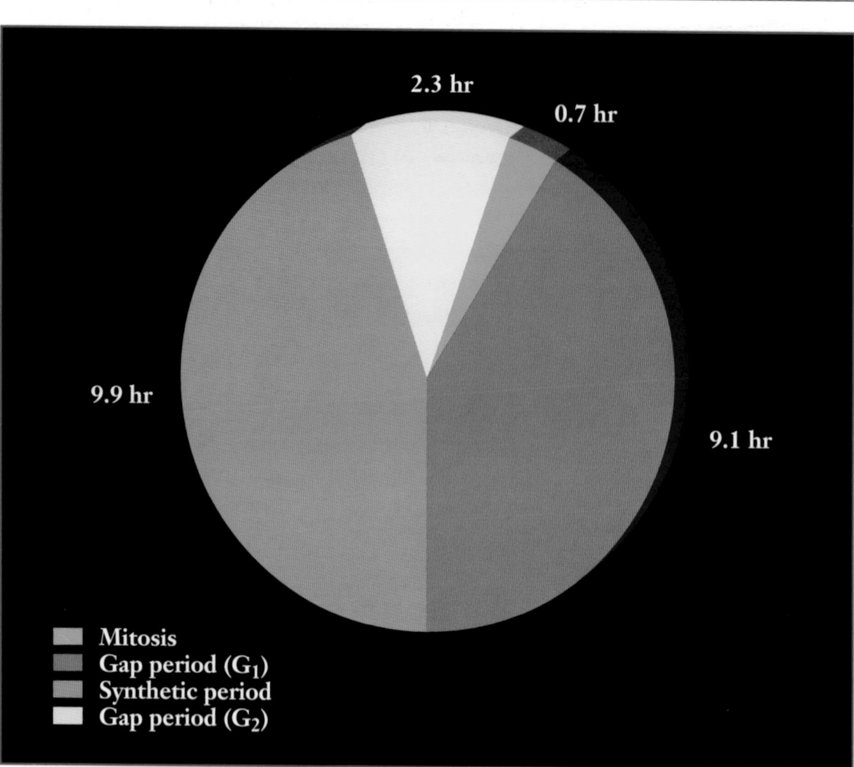

lial regeneration and repair. In this background, degenerated as well as viable appearing tumor cells are expected for a period of 4 to 8 weeks after therapy. Therefore, during this acute phase, smears are unsatisfactory in evaluation of the presence of persistent or recurrent carcinoma. The tumor cells then clear relatively rapidly and the maturation pattern may become atrophic (if the ovaries were sterilized). At about 6 to 8 weeks after radiation treatment, a baseline Pap smear can be assessed for the presence of tumor cells as well as for the presence of a radiation reaction. The absence of a good radiation reaction at this time may be a poor prognostic factor.

The most characteristic radiation-induced change in squamous epithelial cells consists primarily of cytomegaly (ie, the formation of macrocytes) [107 I6.61]. The nuclei and the cytoplasm enlarge in concert, so that the N/C ratio remains about normal or only slightly increased. Nuclei may be multiple; nucleoli may be prominent. The chromatin varies from granular to smudged. Nuclear degeneration, including chromatolysis or vacuolization, may occur [T6.30].

The cytoplasm often stains both pink and blue (polychromasia, or "two-tone" staining). However, heavy keratinization (dense orangeophilia) suggests malignancy. Cytoplasmic vacuolization is a common and early change, and therefore is particularly characteristic of acute radiation change. The vacuoles may contain ingested neutrophils, other cells, or debris. The cell shape may become somewhat irregular or abnormal or even bizarre.

Similar macrocytes may also be seen in chemotherapy, condyloma, and vitamin deficiency (folate or B_{12}). Evidence of inflammation and necrosis is frequently seen in the background of the smear. A histiocytic reaction, including giant and multinucleated histiocytes, some with prominent nucleoli, may also be found.

In response to radiation and some forms of chemotherapy [108 I6.65], the glandular cells of the endocervix and endometrium can also show vacuolization, macrocytosis, macrokaryosis or polykaryosis, hyperchromasia, prominent nucleoli, and irregular shapes. As with radiated squamous cells, the N/C ratio usually remains within normal limits [Doss 1995, Frierson 1990]. Since similar changes may occur in nonirradiated glandular cells, radiation changes are better appreciated in squamous cells.

107 108
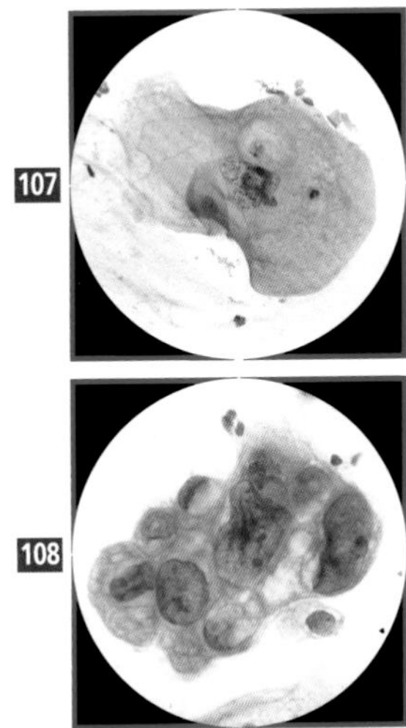

109
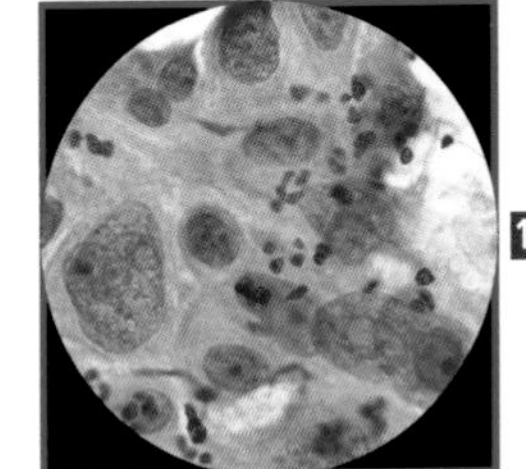

One of the most strikingly abnormal, but benign, changes that can be seen in a Pap smear is radiated repair. It can look wild, with the atypia of radiation superimposed upon the atypia of repair [I6.62, 109 I6.63]. Radiated repair retains the usual features of benign repair (eg, cohesive groups, relatively orderly arrangements) but also shows radiation change (eg, bountiful and colorful cytoplasm together with enlarged, often multiple, nuclei).

Chronic Radiation Change: Administration of radiation affects growing cells, including not only cancer cells but also benign mitotically active cells. Since radiation injures the cell's DNA, if the cell is not killed outright, many of these radiation changes can persist for years, even for the rest of the life of the woman. This is chronic radiation change. Chronic radiation change is similar to acute radiation change, and is primarily represented by the persistence of macrocytes. Pleomorphic cell shapes and polychromasia are also characteristic of chronic radiation change. Inflammation and repair generally disappear, and the epithelium remains atrophic, unless the ovaries are functional or the patient is on hormone replacement.

Persistent vs Recurrent Carcinoma: Usually, the Pap smear clears up fairly rapidly after radiation and most of the tumor cells disappear. However, some tumor cells may persist with acute radiation changes for 4 to 8 weeks after therapy. These tumor cells are not biologically active, and have no effect on survival.

After this grace period, the Pap smear can be used to evaluate the presence of persistent or recurrent carcinoma. Radiation causes changes in malignant cells similar to those seen in benign cells. Therefore, radiated benign cells must be differentiated from radiated malignant cells. Radiated malignant cells have typical malignant features, eg, coarse, irregular chromatin, thick appearing nuclear membranes, and hyperchromasia, with crisp, sharply defined chromatin granules [Koss 1961]. The nuclei of benign radiation change may be slightly hyperchromatic, but the chromatin usually appears somewhat smudgy or indistinct. The N/C ratio is significantly increased in radiated malignant cells, but is relatively normal in benign radiated cells. Enlarged or irregular nucleoli are not necessarily indicative of cancer, as they may also be seen in benign repair. However, cells with bizarre, irregular configurations, particularly if keratinized, suggest cancer.

If malignant tumor cells with radiation effect are found after the 8-week grace period, this suggests that they were present when the radiation was administered and, therefore, is consistent with *persistent* tumor. While these radiated tumor cells may not be biologically active, they are a very worrisome finding. However, if mitoses are seen in these malignant appearing cells, this proves it is viable tumor.

***T6.30* Radiation Effect: Macrocytic Features**

Nucleus
- Enlargement
- Binucleation/Multinucleation
- Irregular shape
- Macronucleoli
- Degeneration (chromatolysis, vacuolization, karyorrhexis, pyknosis)
- Inflammation and necrobiosis are predominant early
- Histiocytosis, also includes giant and multinucleated histiocytes, prominent nucleoli

Cytoplasm
- Increased amount
- Nuclear/cytoplasmic ratio about normal
- Vacuolization,* phagocytosis
- Small perinuclear space
- Irregular, abnormal shape†
- Polychromasia/Amphophilia

* Particularly characteristic of acute radiation change.
† Particularly characteristic of chronic radiation change.

On the other hand, if malignant tumor cells without radiation effect are seen after 8 weeks, this suggests that the tumor regrew after cessation of radiotherapy. This is consistent with *recurrent* cancer. (Note, however, that proof of tumor recurrence, as opposed to persistence, requires clinical or biopsy evidence of a disease-free interval.)

Cancer After Radiation

(>8 weeks after radiation)
Persistent tumor
  Tumor with radiation effect
  Mitoses → viability
Recurrent tumor
  Tumor without radiation effect
  Viable ± mitoses

The Pap smear is not a very sensitive test for diagnosis of tumor persistence or recurrence, but it is highly specific [Shield 1991]. Finding tumor cells in the Pap smear after therapy (beyond the 4–8 week grace period) is a poor prognostic sign, proof that the cancer has not been cured. Further therapy is indicated without waiting for clinical symptoms of relapse. Negative cytology at the end of treatment does not guarantee cure, but most tumors that recur do so in less than 3 years. Clinical stage is more important in the case of negative cytology; the number of cytologically negative patients who die is directly related to the clinical stage of the disease [Campos 1970].

Postradiation Dysplasia: Unfortunately, a number of patients (up to 25%) treated with radiation, usually for squamous cell carcinoma of the cervix, who have apparently been cured, will develop a new lesion of dysplasia, from 6 months to many years (or even decades) after therapy [Davey 1992a, Friedell 1961, Koss 1961, Patten 1963, Wentz 1970]. Postradiation dysplasia is a significant predictor of poor prognosis, particularly if the dysplasia develops within 3 years after radiation [Wentz 1970]. The development of postradiation dysplasia is apparently not directly related to human papilloma virus but rather to the ionizing radiation.

Postradiation dysplasia progresses to cancer in a much higher proportion of cases than ordinary dysplasia (30%–50% vs <15%) [Patten 1978]. The associated cancers tend to grow rapidly and metastasize early. In addition, postradiation dysplasia predicts the presence of residual carcinoma, which usually is not in continuity with the dysplasia but rather is found in a distant site, eg, pelvic (parametrial) or lymph node metastases [Patten 1963]. There is no correlation between the degree of the dysplasia and the presence of residual cancer. However, aneuploid postradiation dysplasia may forecast clinical recurrence within 2 years [Okagaki 1974].

Cytologically, postradiation dysplasia usually looks like ordinary dysplasia, often keratinizing type, occurring in a background of radiation effect [Koss 1961, Patten 1963]. Like ordinary dysplasia, postradiation dysplasia usually occurs in a mature (nonatrophic) epithelium. The N/C ratio is increased, the nuclei are enlarged and hyperchromatic, and the chromatin is coarse and distinct. In contrast, benign acute radiation change is characterized by macrocytes with relatively normal N/C ratios, polychromasia, cytoplasmic vacuolization, phagocytosis, fine or smudgy chromatin, and occasionally, macronucleoli. However, it can be particularly difficult to distinguish mild postradiation dysplasia (or low-grade squamous intraepithelial lesion) from benign radiation effect.

A small cell type of postradiation dysplasia, more reminiscent of CIN III, also occurs, particularly in an atrophic background [Patten 1963]. The cells are small, have high N/C ratios, and hyperchromatic, distinct chromatin. The large cell (mature, dysplastic) type is more common in younger women, while the small cell (carcinoma in situ–like) type is more common in an older age group [Patten 1963].

The persistence of maturation after radiotherapy, which in practice means the formation of superficial cells, indicates that the patient has the milieu in which postradiation dysplasia or residual disease may occur [Rubio 1966]. Close cytologic follow-up of all postradiation patients, but particularly those with increased maturation, is indicated, looking for evidence of postradiation dysplasia or persistent/recurrent carcinoma. It can be difficult to distinguish benign radiation changes from postradiation dysplasia or even recurrent carcinoma in some cases. DNA analysis can be useful; aneuploidy is rarely, if ever, seen in benign radiation changes [Davey 1992a].

Postradiation dysplasia, of any grade, is a potentially serious lesion, particularly when occurring within 3 years of therapy. Patients should undergo colposcopy. A careful pelvic examination and appropriate tests, possibly including pelvic FNA biopsy, should be conducted in an effort to detect residual carcinoma. Postradiation dysplasia developing after 3 years does not guarantee the patient is completely safe from recurrence, but the risk is reduced.

II. Cytology of the Glandular Epithelium

The glandular epithelium of the female genital tract includes the lining of the endocervix, endometrium, and fallopian tube. These structures are of müllerian origin. Cytology of glandular epithelium of the female genital tract is of increasing interest and importance. Adenocarcinomas are currently the most common invasive malignancies of the female genital tract. Unfortunately, the Pap smear is not nearly as good a screening test for glandular lesions as it is for squamous lesions [J Burk 1974, Kim 1991, Mitchell 1993a]. Diagnostic problems can arise because of paucity or degeneration of the glandular cells, particularly of endometrial origin. Conversely, an abundance of well-preserved glandular cells, often in large, cellular groups, may be obtained with an endocervical brush, which can show a spectrum of benign and malignant changes that can be difficult to interpret. Reactive glandular cells can possibly result in overdiagnosis of both glandular and squamous abnormalities [Chakrabarti 1994, Lickrish 1993]. Even normal endocervical cells can show a multitude of cytomorphologic features.

Endocervical Cells

The endocervix does not form true tubular or acinar glands; there is no organization into a glandular unit with neck, body, and fundus [110 I6.2] [Fluhmann 1957]. Instead, the endocervix is a series of grooves or clefts, ie, deep infoldings that may tunnel into the endocervical stroma forming crypts that give the histologic appearance of compound, racemose glands, but are not. The mucosal folds, known as plicae palmatae, are lined by a single layer of endocervical columnar cells. Knowledge of the normal histology becomes critically important in diagnosis of endocervical glandular neoplasia.

The presence of endocervical cells is one measure of the adequacy of a Pap smear, indicating that the transformation zone has been sampled. Endocervical (or metaplastic) cells seen in a direct vaginal scrape (as opposed to a cervical smear or vaginal pool) are suggestive of vaginal adenosis. Adenosis is most common in women who were exposed to diethylstilbestrol in utero, but also occurs in patients who were not exposed to diethylstilbestrol [Kurman 1974, Robboy 1986, Vooijs 1973]. (Since this drug has not been given during pregnancy for more than two decades, the diseases associated with its use, vaginal adenosis and clear cell carcinoma, are on the decline.)

Endocervical cells are tall and columnar, and can be secretory or ciliated [111 I6.11, 112 I6.12, 113 I6.13]. "Pencil-thin" endocervical cells are elongated and slender, sometimes resembling smooth muscle cells, and are thought to result from application of Lugol's iodine solution (which is extremely hypertonic) to the cervix at the time of colposcopy or cone biopsy before taking the Pap smear [I6.14] [Benda 1987]. Intercalated cells also occur, but are rarely specifically recognizable in Pap smears.

Endocervical Cell Features

- Columnar cells
- Secretory and ciliated
  - Sheets, honeycomb
  - Strips, palisade
  - Single, polar
  - Naked nuclei in mucus
- Presence → transformation zone sampled

Secretory endocervical cells have relatively abundant cytoplasm that contains either multiple fine vacuoles or one large one. These cells may be particularly "plump and juicy" in pregnancy, in response to some birth control pills, and in endocervical polyps.

Ciliated endocervical cells are similar in appearance to ciliated respiratory ("bronchial") cells [I6.13]. They have a somewhat denser cytoplasm than the secretory endocervical cells

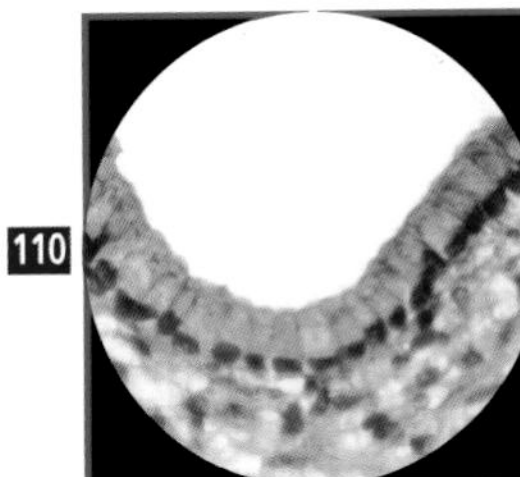
110

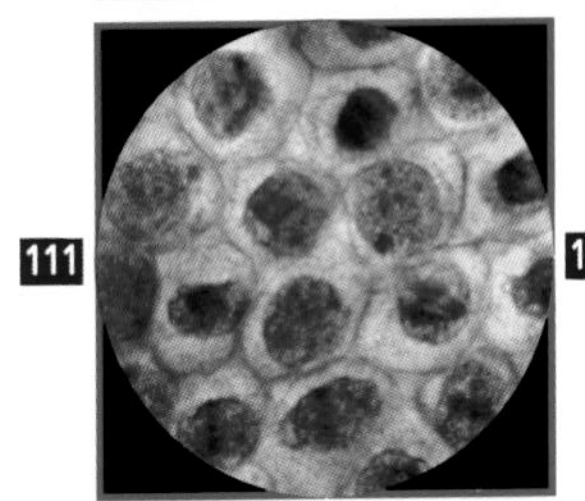
111

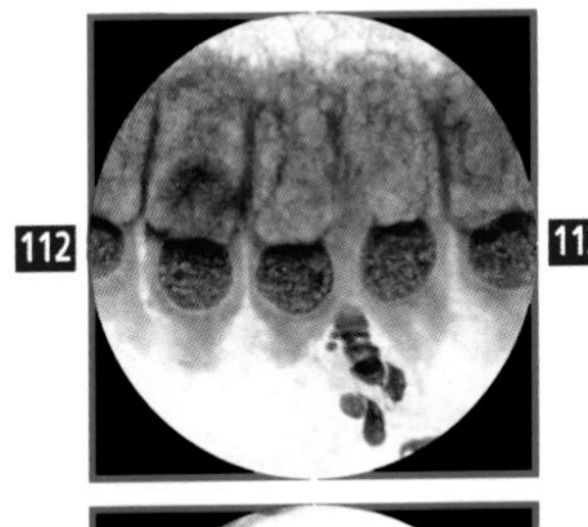
112

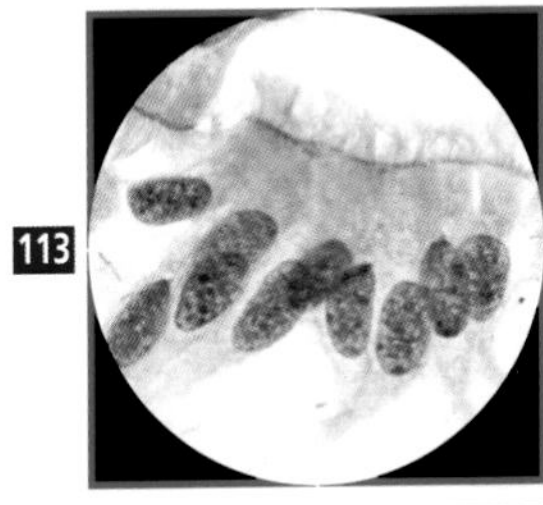
113

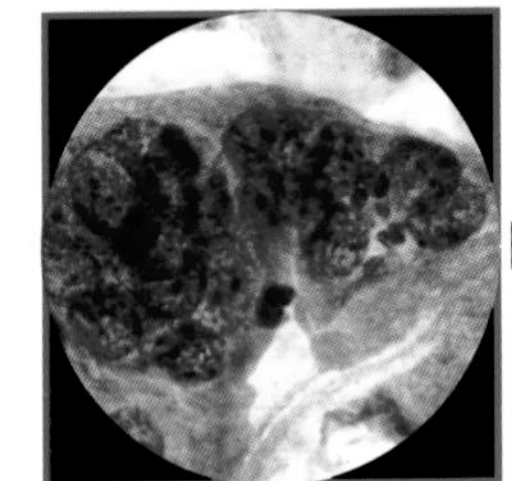
114

and, of course, a terminal bar and cilia. The cilia stain red in an optimal Pap stain. Ciliated endocervical cells are less commonly present in Pap smears than secretory cells. However, they may be more common in the first half or estrogenic part of the cycle. As in the lung, ciliated cells may have a role in propelling mucus. Rarely, the ciliated tops detach from the cells (ciliocytophthoria); these free little red "wigs" should not be mistaken for protozoa [Ashfaq-Drewett 1990]. Ciliated cells are also associated with tubal metaplasia.

Endocervical cells can be seen singly or in strips or sheets. Two dimensional sheets, seen en face, form a regular, orderly rank and file of uniform cells [111 I6.11]. Each cell lines up in a row and they all look alike—like a "print" with a repeating pattern. There may be a slight prominence of the cell membranes where the cells join one another, causing a "honeycomb" appearance—the classic finding in benign glandular epithelium in any site. Malignancies rarely have this orderly arrangement; malignant cells usually overlap and crowd one another in disorderly arrangements.

Strips of cells, viewed from the side, line up—like pickets in a fence—forming a "palisade" of uniform, orderly cells. Single cells have a columnar configuration, with "basal" nuclei and "apical" cytoplasm [112 I6.12]. This nucleocytoplasmic polarity is characteristic of glandular differentiation. (The terms "honeycomb," "picket fence arrangement," and "palisade" are buzzwords that usually imply a benign process.)

The nucleus of the endocervical cell is round to oval, with open, vesicular chromatin. It resembles the nucleus of a normal intermediate cell, although it is slightly larger (about 55 μm² vs 35 μm²), about the size of the nucleus of a parabasal or immature metaplastic cell (~50 μm²) [Patten 1978]. Endocervical nuclei are usually single, but occasionally binucleation or multinucleation occurs, particularly in reactive conditions. The chromatin is usually delicate and evenly distributed. One or more micronucleoli may be seen.

The cytoplasm of endocervical cells is delicate and often lyses. When this occurs, stripped, naked nuclei lying in delicate finely granular or wispy blue clouds of the degenerated cytoplasm and mucus may be seen (so-called endocervical mucus). Naked nuclei can sometimes appear quite atypical, so—as always—caution is urged in interpretation of naked nuclei.

Reactive Endocervical Cells: Reactive changes are common in endocervical cells [114 I6.16, I6.17]. Reactive endocervical cells may occur due to hormonally induced hyperplasia or endocervicitis.

In reactive conditions, the endocervical nuclei enlarge, occasionally several times normal, and can become hyperchromatic, occasionally markedly so, and may have prominent or macronucleoli, and even mitotic figures [Bose 1994, Nasu 1993]. These features may suggest neoplasia. Multinucleation can also occur and should not be mistaken for viral effect or neoplasia [Stowell 1994]. The nuclei maintain their round to oval outlines, the membranes are smooth, or only minimally irregular, the chromatin is fine, the N/C ratios are not significantly increased, and there is only minimal nuclear crowding or overlap—ie, the cells "lay flat." Markedly crowded clusters with feathery edges or microacinar structures (rosettes) are associated with neoplasia. Moreover, the reactive cells maintain their columnar shape, with eccentric nuclei and moderate amounts of well-defined, cyanophilic cytoplasm with rare mucous vacuoles [Bose 1994]. Inflammatory cells are usually present in the background [Bose 1994]. Although not regarded as a preneoplastic lesion, as many as half of patients with reactive endocervical cells on Pap smear have *squamous* intraepithelial lesions on biopsy [Goff 1992, Nasu 1993]. Mitotic figures can sometimes be seen in reactive endocervical cells, but when present, must be evaluated carefully, because they raise the specter of endocervical adenocarcinoma. Marked crowding, rosettes, coarse chromatin, and elongated, hyperchromatic nuclei suggest endocervical glandular neoplasia.

Reactive Endocervical Cells

- Nuclear enlargement and hyperchromasia
- Smooth nuclear membranes
- Prominent nucleoli
- Mitotic figures possible*
- Nuclear/cytoplasmic ratio within normal limits
- Minimal nuclear crowding or overlap, ie, the cells "lay flat"
- Often associated with squamous intraepithelial lesions
- Differential diagnosis: Cancer—crowding, rosettes, chromatin

* Evaluate carefully when mitotic figures are present.

Atypical Endocervical Cells: These are being seen with increased frequency in samples obtained with the endocervical brush. In some cases, the nuclei are enlarged, pleomorphic, and hyperchromatic, possibly reflecting polyploidy ("brush atypia") [115 I6.18]. Also, endocervical cells obtained high in the endocervical canal, which may be sampled using an endocervical brush, are normally more crowded, with higher N/C ratios, than those obtained with an ordinary spatula [116 I6.15]. The high endocervical cells can form hyperchromatic crowded groups (HCGs) mimicking neoplasia, resulting in false-positive diagnoses [Hoffman 1993]. However, the nuclei are bland and round, and resemble other endocervical nuclei. No mitotic figures are present. Also, in women who have undergone cone biopsy, endometrial cells from the lower uterine segment grow into the endocervix, where they may be directly sampled [Lee 1993]. These endometrial cells may show reactive/regenerative changes and exfoliate hyperchromatic crowded groups mimicking neoplasia (cone biopsy artifact) [Lee 1993]. There are a variety of other explanations for atypical endocervical cells, ranging from tubal metaplasia to Arias-Stella reaction to endocervical glandular neoplasia.

115

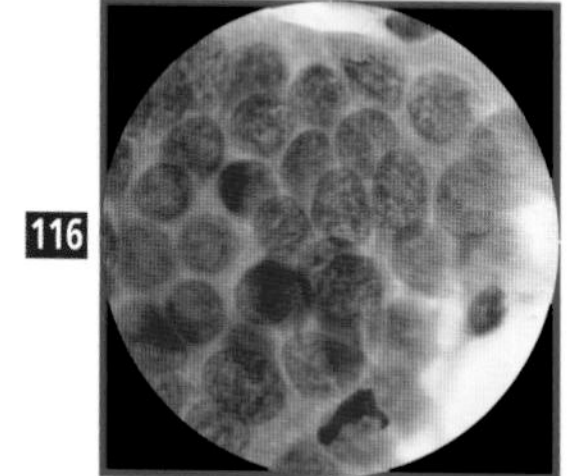

116

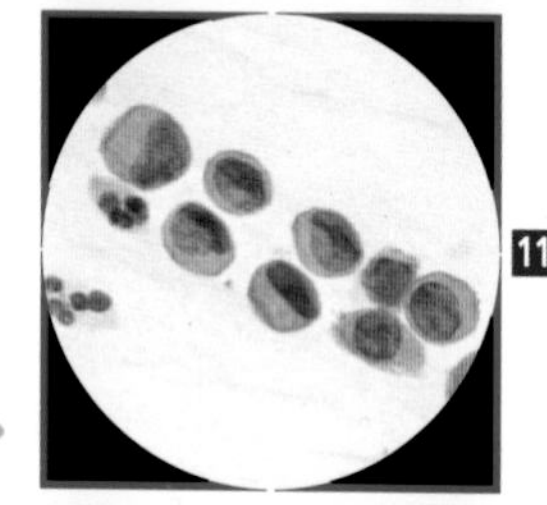

117

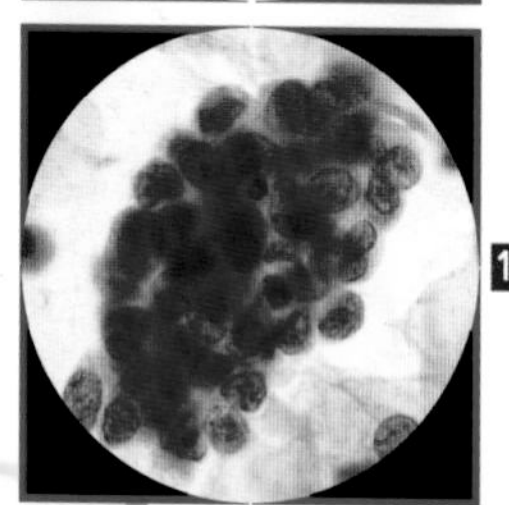

118

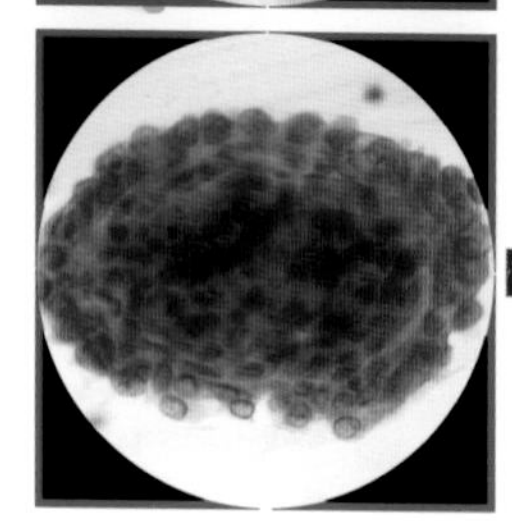

119

Microglandular Endocervical Hyperplasia

Microglandular hyperplasia is a benign, nonneoplastic proliferation of endocervical glands and stroma. It usually occurs in women of reproductive age, but can be seen after menopause. Microglandular hyperplasia is often associated with hormonal therapy, usually birth control pills, or pregnancy, although sometimes there is no such history [Chumas 1985, TS Kline 1970, Leslie 1984, R Young 1989]. Usually both estrogen and progesterone are being taken, although microglandular hyperplasia can be seen in women taking only one of these. For example, in postmenopausal women, microglandular hyperplasia may be associated with estrogen alone. Human papilloma virus DNA is absent from these lesions [Okagaki 1989, Tase 1989b].

Cytologically, masses of single, degenerated endocervical cells are usually seen, frequently in linear arrays [117 I6.40]. The cells typically have pyknotic nuclei and orangeophilic cytoplasm, due to coagulative necrosis. These degenerated cells resemble squamous parakeratosis and, therefore, are also known as pseudoparakeratosis [M Clarke 1993, Patten 1978, Valente 1994b]. Orangeophilia, however, is a staining artifact related to degeneration and not required for diagnosis. Recognizable endocervical cells are also usually present in the vicinity, which aids in the proper identification. Also, in contrast to true parakeratosis, the degenerated endocervical cells have a finely vacuolated or granular cytoplasm. Microglandular hyperplasia may be accompanied by plasma cells or other inflammatory cells.

Some cases show reactive or reparative type endocervical cells, without specific features diagnostic of microglandular hyperplasia [Yahr 1991]. Hyperchromatic crowded groups (nuclear overlap, crowding, and loss of polarity) and cytologic atypia, including nuclear enlargement, hyperchromasia, nucleoli, and mitotic figures may be seen, which may suggest endocervical glandular neoplasia or high-grade squamous intraepithelial lesions [Nichols 1971, Rizzo 1989, Valente 1994b, Yahr 1991]. Absence of coarse chromatin and "feathery" edges and presence of cells with cilia or terminal bars point to a benign diagnosis [Valente 1994b].

Endometrial Cells

(Note: This section on endometrial cytology pertains primarily to *spontaneously* exfoliated cells, *not* direct sampling of the endometrium.)

Endometrial Glandular Cells: Glandular endometrial cells, like endocervical cells, may be either ciliated or nonciliated, and occur singly or in groups [118 I6.24, 119 I6.25]. Ciliated endometrial cells may indicate (fallopian) tubal metaplasia of the surface of the endometrium, which is associated with unopposed estrogen stimulation. Therefore, ciliated endometrial cells would be more likely at midcycle or associated with endometrial hyperplasia or neoplasia, but are rarely observed in the Pap smear. Nonciliated endometrial cells can be either secretory or proliferative.

Spontaneously exfoliated endometrial cells are normally present only in the first half of the menstrual cycle (ie, up to day 14), but can be inadvertently obtained at any time using an endocervical brush. Spontaneously exfoliated endometrial cells are usually degenerated due to ischemia associated with menstrual shedding as well as the fact that they must transit the endocervix, and often float in the vaginal pool before being sampled. Although the vaginal pool may be a good source of endometrial cells, they are better preserved in endocervical samples.

Normal endometrial cells are round to oval, and smaller than endocervical cells. They resemble lymphocytes or histiocytes, but usually appear degenerated. The cytoplasm is variable in amount, but generally scant and ill defined. It usually stains basophilic or amphophilic and may be finely vacuolated. In contrast with endocervical or metaplastic cells, distinct vacuoles are infrequent and, if present, rarely contain neutrophils.

The nuclei are round to oval and usually eccentrically located in the cell. When well preserved, the chromatin is fine and evenly dispersed, but it is usually degenerated. Small chromocenters may be present, but nucleoli are rare in normal endometrial cells. The nucleus is about the size of an intermediate cell nucleus (35–40 µm²): when larger, suspect endometrial hyperplasia or neoplasia. In contrast with endocervical cells, binucleation or multinucleation in endometrial cells is rare.

Spontaneously exfoliated endometrial cells seldom form honeycomb sheets or palisades. Instead, endometrial cells usually exfoliate in crowded, three-dimensional groups, most characteristically forming "double-contour" cell balls, with darkly staining stroma inside and lighter staining epithelium outside [120 I6.25]. Double-contoured endometrial cell balls are particularly common during "exodus," days 6 to 10 of the cycle, but can be seen during menses as well as in patients with benign polyps and hyperplasia.

Endometrial cells can also form three-dimensional clusters of glandular cells, without central stroma. The cells are small and crowded, and the nuclei are usually degenerated and hyperchromatic, ie, they form hyperchromatic crowded groups (HCGs) that can mimic carcinoma in situ [121 I6.24, I6.134]. Possible clues to endometrial origin include the time of the menstrual cycle and presence of nearby endometrial stroma.

A common, everyday problem in Pap smear diagnosis is distinguishing endometrial cells from endocervical cells [T6.31]. This can be important, since shedding of endometrial cells is abnormal in the second half of the menstrual cycle (especially past 40 years of age) or any time in postmenopausal women. Abnormal shedding of endometrial cells carries with it an increased risk of endometrial hyperplasia or neoplasia.

Endocervical cells never form the double contour cell balls characteristic of endometrial cells. Crowding (ie, the way the endometrial cells are "packed together"), degeneration, and smaller cell size point to endometrial origin. Honeycomb sheets, binucleation or multinucleation, more abundant cytoplasm, and distinct cytoplasmic vacuoles point to endocervical origin.

120
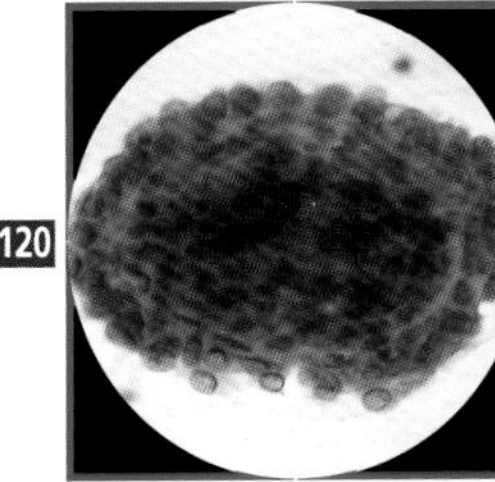

121
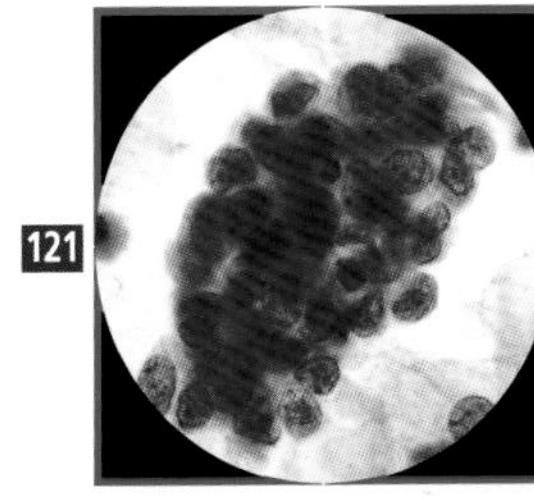

122
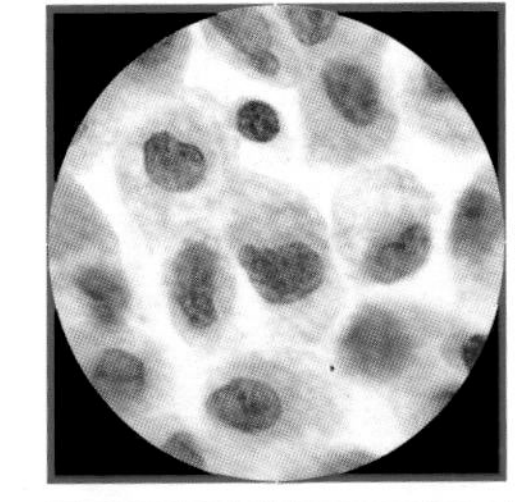

123
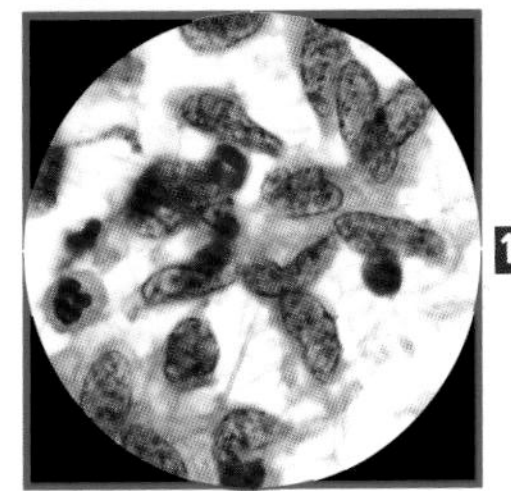

T6.31 **Differential Diagnosis of Benign Glandular Cells**

Endocervix	Endometrium
Larger	Smaller
More variable	More uniform
Loose two-dimensional arrangement	Crowded three-dimensional clusters
Honeycomb sheets	Double contoured balls
Multinucleation relatively common	Multinucleation rare
Finer, paler chromatin	Coarser, darker chromatin
Abundant cytoplasm	Scant cytoplasm
Better preservation	Degeneration

Helpful hint: Compare the cells in question with similar appearing glandular cells that can be clearly identified.

Clusters of naked parabasal nuclei can be seen in atrophic smears, which can mimic endometrial cells [I6.7]. Correct identification is important because the presence of endometrial cells in a postmenopausal patient is abnormal and may be associated with endometrial hyperplasia or neoplasia. Clues to the proper diagnosis are the lack of cytoplasm and the similarity of the naked nuclei to those of "syncytial" aggregates of atrophic cells.

Endometrial Stromal Cells: There are two types of endometrial stromal cells: superficial and deep. Superficial stromal cells derive from the compacta layer of the endometrium. These cells are also the source of decidua. Individual superficial stromal cells are indistinguishable from small histiocytes [122 I6.26]. However, stromal cells tend to form loose aggregates ("sticky histiocytes") and are exclusively small. Superficial stromal cells have a moderate amount of cytoplasm that is poorly stained and ill defined, with fine vacuolization. The nuclei are round to oval, or bean shaped, and often eccentrically located in the cell. In contrast, ordinary histiocytes can range from small to large, or even giant, tend to be single, and may have phagocytosed debris in their cytoplasm.

Deep stromal cells are less mature and arise from the spongiosa layer of the endometrium [123 I6.27]. They are slightly smaller than superficial stromal cells and typically have spindle or stellate shapes, with scant cytoplasm. The nuclei are oval to spindle-shaped, and frequently have a longitudinal groove in the nuclear membrane. The chromatin structure of deep stromal cells is similar to that of histiocytes.

Endometrial stromal cells, like endometrial glandular cells, are normally present only in the first half of the menstrual cycle. During "exodus" (days 6–10), endometrial cell balls, histiocytes, and stromal cells are prominent in the Pap smear [Papanicolaou 1953]. During the secretory phase, only 2% of smears contain endometrial cells; the percentage again rises in the premenstrual phase (after day 25) [Liu 1963, Vooijs 1987b].

Presence of Normal Endometrial Cells (Glandular or Stromal)

First half of cycle
→ Physiologic
Second half of cycle, postmenopause
→ Abnormal shedding
Presence of abnormal endometrial cells is always abnormal

Abnormal Shedding of Endometrial Cells: Other than during the first half of the menstrual cycle, the presence of spontaneously exfoliated endometrial cells in the Pap smear is abnormal. The preferred cutoff day for abnormal shedding ranges from day 10 to 14, according to different authorities. Using an earlier cutoff day theoretically increases the sensitivity of the test, but makes an already fairly nonspecific test even less specific. In fact, the Bethesda System does not currently report abnormal shedding of endometrial cells at all in premenopausal women because of the low incidence of malignancy found on investigation of otherwise asymptomatic women. Note, however, that spontaneous shedding of endometrial cells in postmenopausal women is a significant finding that should always be reported. Also, note that endometrial cells can be obtained inadvertently at any time when using an endocervical brush.

A vaginal pool sample, obtained from the posterior vaginal fornix, is a good source for finding endometrial cells, and can increase detection of occult endometrial carcinoma by one third compared with a routine Pap smear [Koss 1984]. Days 15 to 24 are the most opportune time to detect endometrial lesions in premenopausal women. Cervical, as opposed to vaginal or endocervical, smears do not contribute significantly to diagnosis of endometrial disease [Koss 1981]. Most causes of abnormal shedding of endometrial cells are benign. However, there is a risk of endometrial cancer, even if the cells look normal. Before 40 years of age, the risk is low, but it steadily increases thereafter [Cherkis 1988, Gondos 1977, Ng 1974b]. Estrogen replacement therapy is a fairly common cause of postmenopausal shedding of endometrial cells. However, a history of estrogen replacement therapy should not exclude patients from further evaluation, since a significant number are found to have endometrial disease [Yancy 1990].

Causes of Abnormal Shedding of Endometrial Cells*

- Endometriosis
- Endometritis
- Submucosal myoma
- Early pregnancy
- Postpartum
- Abortion
- IUD
- Instrumentation
- Hormonal therapy (birth control pills, estrogen replacement therapy‡)
- Abnormal or dysfunctional uterine bleeding
- Endometrial polyp
- Endometrial hyperplasia
- Endometrial neoplasia†

* Most cases have an idiopathic or negative history.
† The risk for adenocarcinoma steadily increases after age 40 years.
‡ Commonly causes abnormal shedding, but does not rule out endometrial disease.

In premenopausal women, 1 of 4 cases of abnormal shedding is associated with endometrial pathology (ie, polyps, hyperplasia, or cancer). In postmenopausal women, 1 of 2 cases is associated with endometrial pathology and the risk of malignancy is higher [Ng 1974b]. Some hyperplasias (~10%) and cancers (~5%) shed only endometrial stromal cells, if they shed any endometrial cells at all [Ng 1974b].

Atypical Endometrial Cells (Atypical Glandular Cells of Undetermined Significance): The shedding of abnormal appearing endometrial cells is always abnormal, although not necessarily malignant, regardless of the relationship to the menses. Atypical glandular (endometrial) cells of undetermined significance (AGUS) includes endometrial cells with nuclear enlargement, hyperchromasia, irregular chromatin, and nucleoli. Mild atypia includes nuclear enlargement (larger than intermediate nucleus) and increased N/C ratio; moderate atypia includes hyperchromasia with abnormalities of the chromatin, and marked atypia includes presence of nucleoli.

Abnormality of the endometrial cells may be difficult to appreciate due to degeneration, but endometrial nuclei larger than an intermediate cell nucleus and the presence of nucleoli are suspicious findings. The endometrial cells are usually found in a background of high maturation. A diathesis favors a frankly malignant diagnosis. Nuclear atypia correlates with the risk of malignancy. The risk of cancer also increases with age. More than half of patients over 59 years of age shedding markedly atypical endometrial cells will have endometrial cancer [Cherkis 1987].

Other Cytologic Risk Factors for Endometrial Pathology: Abnormal shedding of endometrial cells is the most reliable indicator of endometrial pathology in the Pap smear [F6.22] [Zucker 1985]. Unfortunately, endometrial carcinoma may not shed diagnostic cells at all, or only intermittently, and when shed, the diagnostic cells may be sparse. Endometrial cells are frequently small and degenerated, making critical assessment difficult or impossible; even malignant endometrial cells may be cytologically indistinguishable from normal. Moreover, the cell morphology is influenced by a variety of hormones.

Because of these diagnostic problems, other parameters have been investigated to try to predict those patients at risk.

F6.22 **Abnormal Shedding of Normal-Appearing Endometrial Cells**

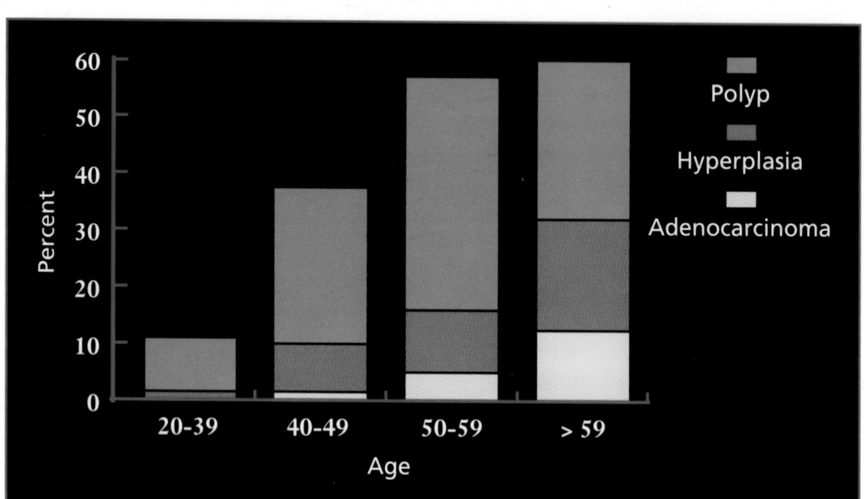

Adenocarcinoma is rare in patients less than 40 years of age, but is found in 2.1% of patients in their 40s, 4.2% of patients in their 50s, and 13.2% of patients in their 60s and older with abnormal shedding [Ng 1974a,b].

Unfortunately, short of finding diagnostic cancer cells, none of these features are specific.

Histiocytes, in moderate or heavy numbers (increased histiocytic activity), particularly with cytoplasmic hemosiderin (evidence of old bleeding) or lipid (evidence of tissue destruction), necrosis, and old (not fresh) blood, are associated with increased risk of endometrial carcinoma in postmenopausal women. Foam cells, which are large and polygonal with voluminous, pale, finely vacuolated cytoplasm (contains fat, not mucin or glycogen) and small central nuclei, are a marker for endometrial malignancy [Dawagne 1982], but can also be seen in benign disease (ie, adenomatous hyperplasia). Foam cells derive from endometrial stroma [Fechner 1979]. Multinucleated histiocytes, on the other hand, are of no consequence in the diagnosis of endometrial carcinoma [Koss 1962]. Since endometrial hyperplasia/neoplasia is often associated with unopposed estrogen stimulation, evidence of increased maturation of the squamous epithelium (>20% superficial cells) in a postmenopausal woman is often considered another risk factor [Cassano 1986, Y Chang 1963, Efstratiades 1982, Gronroos 1986, Liu 1970, Ritchie 1965]. However, an atrophic background by no means excludes the possibility of endometrial cancer [Y Chang 1963, Liu 1970]. Inflammation or infection can also cause pseudomaturation [Lin 1972].

Using the presence of histiocytes to suggest endometrial carcinoma may increase the diagnostic sensitivity of the Pap smear, but at the expense of decreased specificity [Blumenfeld 1985]. Histiocytes can also be seen in various forms of endometritis or pyometra, and can also arise from the cervix, or rarely vagina, so their usefulness in detecting endometrial cancer is questionable [T Hall 1982]. Necrosis, bleeding, and increased maturation are also nonspecific.

Cytological Risk Factors for Endometrial Hyperplasia/Neoplasia

Abnormal shedding (glandular > stromal), particularly of abnormal cells
Histiocytes (increased histiocytic activity)—hemosiderin, lipid
Necrosis
Blood (old)
Increased maturation

By obtaining vaginal pool and endocervical aspiration samples, more endometrial cancers could be detected [Blumenfeld 1985, Creasman 1976, McGowan 1974, Vuopala 1977]. Although endometrial aspiration could further increase the yield, the sample must be obtained under sterile conditions and it is uncomfortable for the patient (few women will submit to it more than once or twice). Endometrial aspirations are also difficult to interpret cytologically; therefore, most pathologists prefer histologic processing.

In summary, *the Pap smear is not a reliable screening procedure for detection of endometrial disease* [J Burk 1974]. Detection of endometrial cancer using the Pap smear increases with stage and grade of the tumor [Kim 1991, Lozowski 1986, M Schneider 1986]. Patients with malignant cytology are at markedly increased risk of having advanced stage disease, including pelvic and para-aortic lymph node metastases [D Larson 1994]. Few cases of endometrial carcinoma are discovered only by the Pap smear, although this can occur [Cherkis 1988, Koss 1962, Ng 1974b]. Finding asymptomatic patients by Pap smear may improve the prognosis by virtue of early detection [Koss 1962]. However, most patients with endometrial malignancy are symptomatic at the time of diagnosis, eg, abnormal bleeding (postcoital, intermenstrual, postmenopausal). Although most cases of postmenopausal bleeding are associated with anovulation or an atrophic endometrium, rather than cancer [Choo 1985], abnormal bleeding must always be investigated. Endometrial biopsy or formal dilatation and curettage are required for definitive diagnosis.

Endometrial Adenocarcinoma

Although endometrial cancer is on the wane, it is the most common (invasive) gynecologic malignancy. The absolute incidence of endometrial adenocarcinoma, which peaked in the mid-1970s, has fallen again to 1950s levels [Gusberg 1989]. The rise and fall of endometrial cancer has closely paralleled the prescription of unopposed estrogens. Endometrial carcinoma currently accounts for about two thirds of uterine cancer, with about 32,800 new cases, and 5,900 deaths, expected in 1995 [Wingo 1995].

Two clinical groups of patients with endometrial carcinoma have been recognized, one associated with endometrial hyperplasia (classical, type I) and the other apparently arising de novo (type II) [T6.32] [Bokhman 1983, Koss 1984].

Type I cancers seem to be the product of endometrial hyperplasia and abnormal proliferation. Estrogen induces hyperplasia and apparently acts as a promoter of endometrial cancer. Risk factors for type I, classical endometrial carcinoma, include diabetes mellitus (or abnormal glucose tolerance), obesity, hypertension, signs of hyperestrinism, nulliparity, and late menopause [MacMahon 1974].

The patients tend to be premenopausal or perimenopausal. Their cancers are usually low to intermediate grade,

***T6.32* Two Endometrial Cancers**

Type I (Classic)	Type II
2/3 cases, decreasing incidence	1/3 cases, slight increase in incidence
Classic: Obesity, diabetes, hypertension, hyperestrinism	Thin, lack classic features
Younger, premenopausal/perimenopausal	Older, postmenopausal
Low-/Moderate-grade adenocarcinoma associated with hyperplasia	High-grade adenocarcinoma
	Atrophic endometrium
Favorable prognosis	Unfavorable prognosis
Response to hormones	Aggressive

[Bokhman 1983]

associated with endometrial hyperplasia, respond to hormones, and have a favorable prognosis.

Type II patients tend to be thin and lack the risk factors classically associated with endometrial cancer, described above. Patients are usually older and postmenopausal. These cancers seem to arise spontaneously, without being preceded by endometrial hyperplasia, apparently arising from true carcinoma in situ, characterized by markedly atypical glandular cells [Sherman 1992b, Spiegel 1995]. They are typically high grade, associated with an atrophic endometrium, and are aggressive. While the incidence of hormonally associated, group I cancers is on the wane, the incidence of the more aggressive group II cancers may be increasing [Bokhman 1983].

F6.23 **Evolution of Type I (Classic) Endometrial Carcinomas [also de novo]**

Proliferation	Adenomatous hyperplasia	Atypical hyperplasia	Adeno-carcinoma

Cytology of Endometrial Hyperplasia and Neoplasia

The majority of endometrial carcinomas (ie, type I, or classic type) apparently evolve through adenomatous hyperplasia, atypical hyperplasia, and finally, invasive adenocarcinoma [I6.17–I6.19; F6.23]. The cytodiagnostic features are summarized in T6.33.

Another entity, cystic hyperplasia, carries little or no increased risk of developing carcinoma, in contrast with adenomatous or particularly atypical hyperplasia. Cystic hyperplasia is related to anovulation and unopposed estrogen effect. (Another classification recognizes simple and complex hyperplasia, with or without cytologic atypia [Kurman 1985].)

In well-preserved material obtained by endocervical or endometrial aspiration, it may be possible to cytologically suggest hyperplasia, atypical hyperplasia, and carcinoma. However, in a routine Pap smear, exfoliation of cells is inconsistent and cells are frequently poorly preserved, often precluding specific diagnosis.

For practical purposes, endometrial cells in a Pap smear can be divided into three groups: normal [124 I6.24], atypical [I6.117, 125 I6.118], or malignant appearing [126 I6.119, I6.120]. The endometrial cells are usually found in a background of high maturation. Remember that even cancer can shed normal-appearing endometrial cells in a Pap smear. A diathesis favors a malignant diagnosis. Endometrial biopsy or dilatation and curettage are required for definitive diagnosis.

124

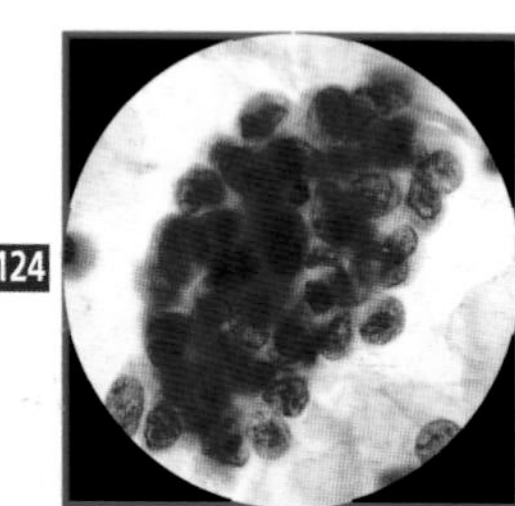

125

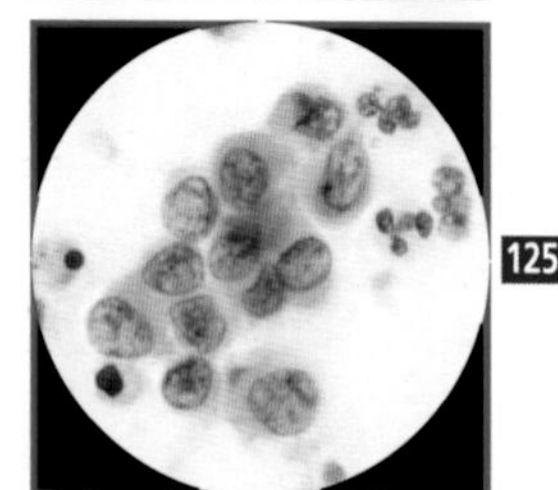

126

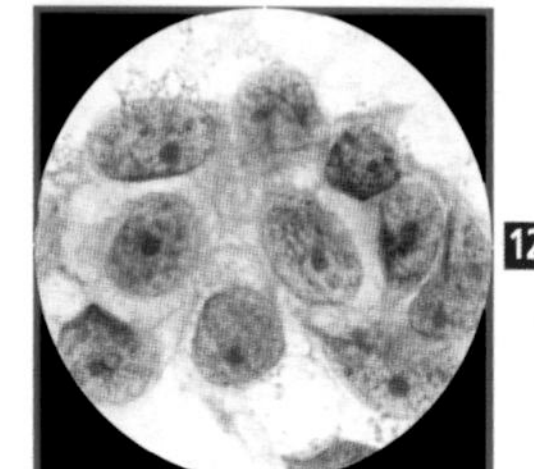

The cytology of endometrial carcinoma depends on the grade of the tumor [I6.118-I6.120]. The malignant cells are usually larger than normal endometrial cells and cellular exfoliation increases with tumor grade. A characteristic clinical feature is a watery vaginal discharge, which is seen in the Pap smear as a finely granular, basophilic diathesis (watery diathesis [I6.120] compared with the coarsely granular, necrotic diathesis characteristic of invasive squamous cell carcinoma). Neutrophils are commonly present in the cytoplasm of the malignant cells [Berg 1958].

Well-differentiated endometrial adenocarcinoma resembles normal or hyperplastic endometrial cells, but the nuclei are larger (mean nuclear area of grade I adenocarcinoma is approximately 60 μm² vs 35 μm² for both normal endometrial and intermediate squamous cell nuclei [F6.24] [Reagan 1973]). The chromatin is abnormal and tends to aggregate irregularly, resulting in areas of chromatin clearing. In low-grade endometrial adenocarcinoma, the nuclei stain less intensely than either normal or hyperplastic endometrial cell nuclei. Nucleolar enlargement is slight in low-grade adenocarcinoma, but increases with grade of the tumor.

With increasing grade, the tumor sheds more and "uglier" cells. The cells have larger nuclei as well as multiple, macronucleoli, or irregular nucleoli. The chromatin becomes more abnormal and more hyperchromatic. Loose cell clusters are characteristic of low-grade adenocarcinoma. With increasing grade, tighter cell balls, reminiscent of those seen with menses, may be seen.

Poorly differentiated endometrial adenocarcinoma tends to occur in older patients without a history of endometrial hyperplasia. The smears typically show an atrophic background, often with marked inflammation and necrosis, ie, a tumor diathesis. Poorly differentiated adenocarcinoma may shed sheets of tumor cells, which can suggest nonkeratinizing squamous cell carcinoma. Squamous cell carcinoma tends to have denser cytoplasm, better defined cell borders, coarser chromatin, and less prominent nucleoli. Note, also, that adenocarcinoma with squamous differentiation is relatively common in the endometrium [Berg 1958].

T6.33 **Cytodiagnostic Features of Endometrial Carcinomas**

	Hyperplasia	Atypical Hyperplasia	Well-Differentiated Adenocarcinoma
	Number of cells progressively increases Cell and nuclear size progressively enlarges		
Nuclear area	45μm²	55μm²	60μm²
Hyperchromasia	(++)	(++)	(+)
Irregular chromatin distribution	(±)	(+)	(+++)
Nucleoli	(±)	(+)	(+++)
Diathesis	(–)	(±)	(+++)

[Ng 1973]

F6.24 **Differential Diagnostic Nuclear Features of Endometrial Cells**

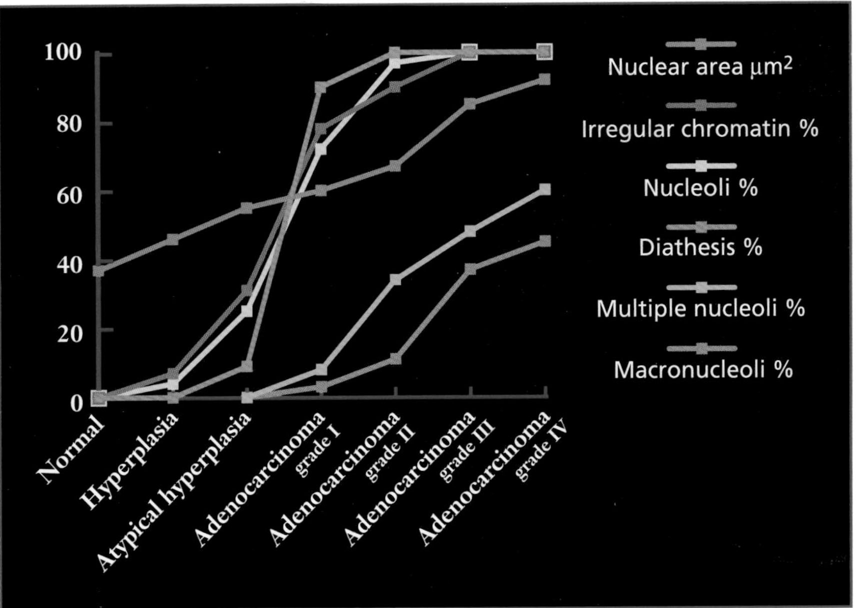

[Ng 1973,1974a]

Endometritis can also shed atypical glandular cells (AGUS), consisting of crowded groups of cells with nuclear enlargement, prominent nucleoli, and cytoplasmic neutrophils suggesting adenocarcinoma. However, the benign cells are cohesive and have uniform nuclei, with smooth nuclear membranes, and regular chromatin. Endometrial polyps, endometrial hyperplasia, and intrauterine contraceptive devices can all be associated with abnormal shedding of atypical endometrial cells. The differential diagnosis also includes endocervical and metastatic adenocarcinomas.

Adenocarcinoma With Squamous Differentiation: The squamous element can have a bland, benign appearance ("adenoacanthoma") or a clearly malignant appearance ("adenosquamous carcinoma"). Squamous differentiation apparently has no effect on prognosis when the tumors are compared grade by grade and stage by stage.

Secretory Adenocarcinoma: Well-differentiated tumor with delicate, glycogen-positive cytoplasm and uniform nuclei [I6.127] [Kusuyama 1989].

Clear Cell Adenocarcinoma: Poorly differentiated tumor with delicate cytoplasm, prominent nucleoli, and naked nuclei [127 I6.124]. The cytoplasm may contain glycogen.

Mucinous Adenocarcinoma: Usually well-differentiated, intestinal-type adenocarcinoma with mucin-positive cells, occasionally signet rings, and mucin in background. Neutrophils may be present in the cytoplasm.

Papillary Serous Adenocarcinoma: High-grade tumor, with prominent nucleoli, numerous papillary groups and occasional psammoma bodies [Kuebler 1989]. Similar to high grade papillary serous adenocarcinoma of ovary [128 I6.122].

127

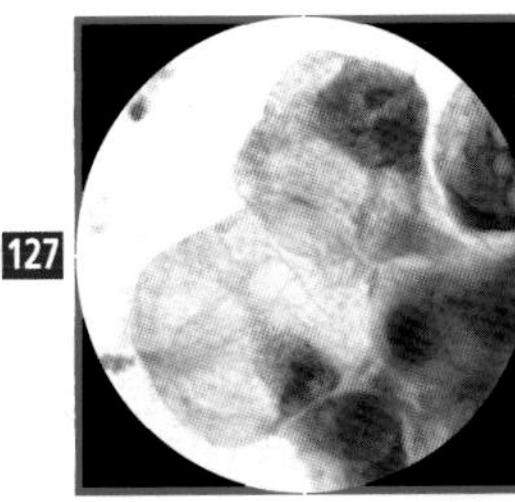

128

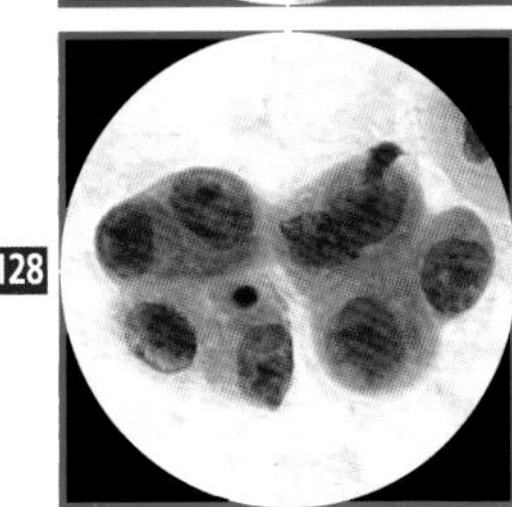

Endocervical Carcinoma

As the incidence of invasive squamous cell carcinoma decreased, the incidence of adenocarcinoma of the cervix increased (though it may now have plateaued) [Devesa 1989]; endocervical adenocarcinoma now accounts for up to one third of all invasive cervical cancers [Berek 1985, Brand 1988, J Davis 1975, Goodman 1989, Greer 1989, Horowitz 1988, Mayer 1976, B Miller 1993, R Peters 1986, Shingleton 1981, Tamimi 1982, Vesterinen 1989, R Weiss 1986]. The cell of origin is thought to be the reserve cell, the same cell implicated in squamous abnormalities (dysplasia, carcinoma) [Boon 1981, Christopherson 1979]. In fact, endocervical glandular neoplasia is frequently associated with squamous intraepithelial lesions [Maier 1980]. At least half the cases of adenocarcinoma in situ will show concurrent squamous dysplasia or carcinoma in situ [Fu 1987, Gloor 1982, Qizilbash 1975]. There is also a strong association with human papilloma virus (HPV), although not as high as for squamous lesions (~70% vs ~90% for squamous lesions) [Griffin 1991]. Also, HPV 18 is more commonly encountered in glandular cancers than HPV 16 [Okagaki 1989, Smotkin 1986]. However, endocervical adenocarcinoma is not as strongly associated with venereal transmission, early age of first intercourse, sexual activity, or smoking as squamous carcinoma, and the patients tend to be of higher socioeconomic class [Brand 1988, Horowitz 1988, Parazzini 1990]. Endocervical glandular neoplasia may share risk factors classically associated with endometrial cancer (eg, nulliparity, overweight, possibly hypertension, and diabetes) [Parazzini 1990]. Endocervical glandular neoplasia may also be associated with progesterone, especially in birth control pills [H Taylor 1967], but this is controversial. These findings suggest there might be two origins of endocervical adenocarcinoma, one associated with HPV and sexual transmission, like squamous lesions, and the other associated with hormones, like many endometrial abnormalities.

Most in situ and invasive endocervical adenocarcinomas occur in women over 30 years of age, on average a slightly older age group than patients with comparable squamous lesions. However, there is a wide age range—adenocarcinoma can even occur in teenagers [Pollack 1947]—and the mean age at diagnosis may be falling [B Miller 1993]. Endocervical adenocarcinoma may have a worse prognosis than cervical squamous cell carcinoma [Fu 1982].

Clinically, the majority of patients with invasive endocervical adenocarcinoma present with abnormal bleeding. However, 15% to 20% of patients are asymptomatic, and about one third have a grossly normal appearing cervix [Brand 1988]. Unfortunately, *the Pap smear is not reliable in detecting endocervical glandular neoplasia*, particularly in women past the age of 35 [Boon 1987, B Miller 1993]. A false-negative rate as high as 50% occurs even in patients with grossly identifiable lesions (as high as 80% if there is no gross lesion) [Hurt 1977]. Although colposcopy has not been fully evaluated in investigation of this disease, it is probably not as reliable as for squamous lesions [Lickrish 1993, Teshima 1985].

Endocervical adenocarcinoma actually occurs more commonly on the ectocervix than in the endocervix [Reagan 1973]. Adenocarcinoma arises in the glandular epithelium adjacent to the squamocolumnar junction, unless there is an associated squamous lesion, in which case it arises in the transformation zone [Jaworski 1988]. As the transformation zone recedes into the endocervical canal with age, early detection by ectocervical scraping and colposcopy becomes more difficult [Fu 1987]. Also, the deep glands tend to be more involved than the surface, which can affect both cytologic and histologic sampling [Jaworski 1988]. Moreover, the lesions can be very focal, particularly when in situ [I6.116] [Jaworski 1988].

If the Pap smear directly samples the lesion, finding an *abundance* of (atypical) endocervical cells in the smear may be the first clue to the diagnosis of endocervical adenocarcinoma. Most characteristically, particularly in low-grade tumors, the cells are tall columnar and the nuclei are elongated with coarse, dark chromatin [Boon 1981]. The malignant cells are usually, but not always, larger than normal endocervical cells, with enlarged, irregular nuclei and increased N/C ratios. The cytoplasm is usually acidophilic and granular with decreased mucin content. Multiple fine vacuoles can also be present, especially in low-grade adenocarcinoma. *Nuclear crowding* and *abnormal glandular arrangements* are important in diagnosis [129 I6.111, 130 I6.112, 131 I6.113, 132 I6.114]. Single cells are of lesser diagnostic importance, but their presence suggests invasion.

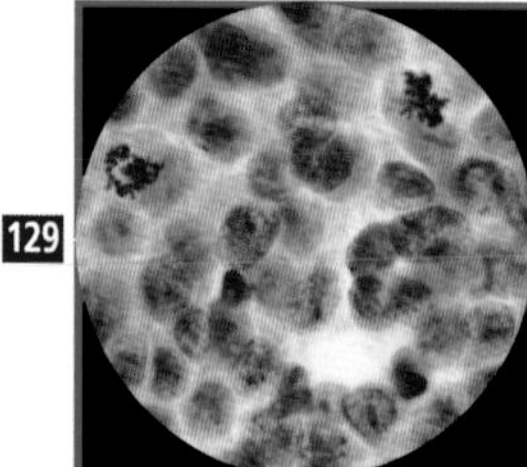
129

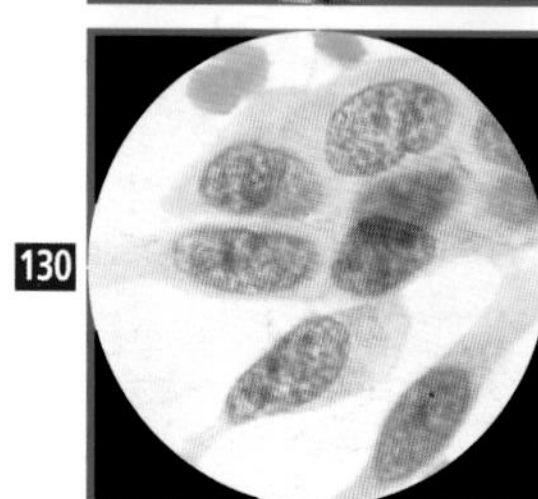
130

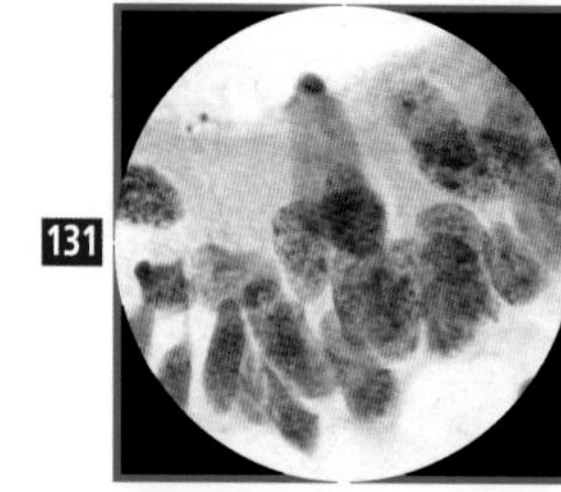
131

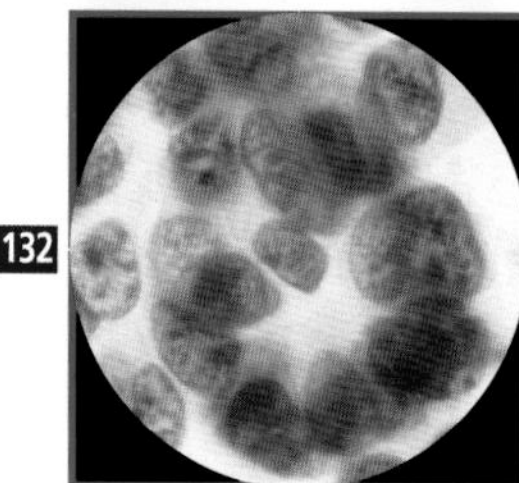
132

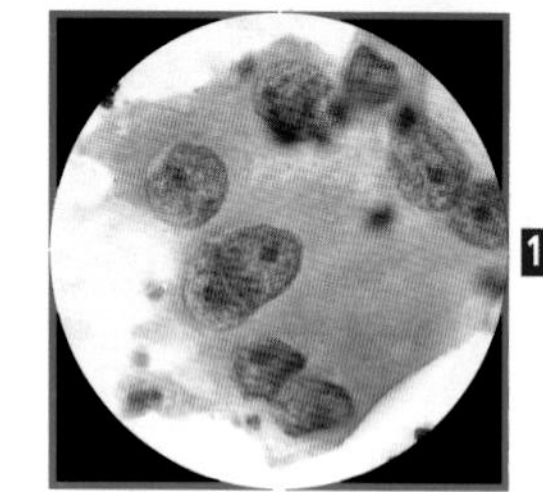
133

Nuclear crowding is often marked, particularly in better differentiated and in situ lesions. Strips of cells have irregularly stratified, hyperchromatic nuclei, reminiscent of the histology. Sheets of cells also show marked nuclear crowding and irregular overlapping. Although reactive endocervical cells can also be pleomorphic and hyperchromatic, they usually form more or less orderly palisades and honeycomb sheets, with little or no crowding or piling up (ie, the cells tend to "lie flat"). Poorly differentiated endocervical adenocarcinomas, however, do not show the marked crowding of nuclei characteristic of better differentiated tumors.

Abnormal glandular arrangements include rosette-like structures or secondary gland openings in sheets of endocervical cells [Krumins 1977]. Recall that there are no true glands in the endocervix, only mucosal folds. Therefore, sheets of endocervical cells with well formed glandular lumens are the equivalent of the "gland-in-gland" pattern characteristic of adenocarcinomas in general. Occasionally, however, sheets of malignant endocervical cells are unexpectedly orderly, even in high-grade cancer, and rarely, rosettes and glandular openings can be seen in benign endocervical cells.

The crowded groups of cells often have irregular, or "feathery," edges [Ayer 1987,1991, Bose 1994]. Feathering refers to the protrusion of nuclei, with scant cytoplasm, from the edges of crowded cell groups. Feathery edges are rarely, if ever, seen in benign endocervical cells [Lee 1991]. The tumors can also exfoliate three-dimensional cell balls and papillae [I6.115]. Syncytial-like aggregates are sometimes seen, but are more closely associated with adenocarcinoma in situ. These "syncytia" can be difficult to distinguish from squamous carcinoma in situ.

Well-differentiated tumors occasionally have nuclei smaller than the normal endocervical nuclei. With increasing grade, the nuclei increase in size (range, 73–165 μm² [Reagan 1973]), resulting in high N/C ratios. In better-differentiated tumors, the nuclei are typically hyperchromatic with coarse chromatin. As the grade increases, nucleoli may become more prominent and multiple, but usually remain round. In high-grade cancer, the chromatin may become paler, finer, and irregularly distributed. Also, with increasing grade, the cells tend to lose their well-formed columnar shape and cell borders become indistinct. Granularity of the cytoplasm becomes more apparent, and vacuolization diminishes. A diathesis is usually present in the background [Bose 1994]. Accompanying squamous intraepithelial lesions are found in a number of patients [Nguyen 1993].

Mixed Adenosquamous Carcinoma: On careful search, up to one third of cases of cervical adenocarcinomas are mixed adenosquamous carcinomas [Benda 1985, Nguyen 1993]. The squamous elements can range from bland to malignant appearing, keratinizing, nonkeratinizing, or small cell (poorly differentiated squamous cell carcinoma). Eosinophils may be prominent. Endocervical adenosquamous carcinoma may be more aggressive than either pure squamous or adenocarcinoma, and responds poorly to radiotherapy [Fu 1987].

Glassy Cell Carcinoma: This tumor is a poorly differentiated variant of adenosquamous carcinoma with abundant, finely granular ("ground glass") cytoplasm, large nuclei, and prominent nucleoli [133 I6.121] [Nguyen 1993, Nunez 1985, Pak 1983, R Young 1990, Zaino 1982]. The cells contain glycogen. Eosinophils may be present. The prognosis is poor.

Endometrioid Endocervical Carcinoma: This variant of endocervical carcinoma is morphologically indistinguishable from endometrial carcinoma, and is a relatively common differential diagnostic problem.

Clear Cell Carcinoma: This is a tumor of müllerian origin, often in diethylstilbestrol-exposed, young patients. Finely vacuolated, delicate, fragile, glycogen-containing cytoplasm of variable, but often abundant amount is characteristic. Nuclei are pale, irregular, with prominent nucleoli. Naked nuclei are common [Nguyen 1993, Taft 1974, Q Young 1978].

Intestinal (Mucinous) Carcinoma: Resembling colorectal carcinoma, the tumor displays goblet cells and "terminal bar-like" apical cytoplasmic densities.

Adenoma Malignum: The tumor is rare and very well differentiated, hence, difficult to diagnose [R Young 1990]. It is characterized by numerous sheets of large cells with abundant, clear, mucinous cytoplasm, and relatively bland nuclei [Fukazawa 1992, Nguyen 1993]. The cells maintain their columnar shape and form loose sheets, with gland openings, crowding, and single cells. The chromatin varies from fine to granular, and tends to be slightly hyperchromatic. Macronucleoli may be present in some cases [Kudo 1987]. Variable numbers of mitotic figures may be seen [Szyfelbein 1984]. The cytology may be reminiscent of repair.

Adenoma malignum is a treacherous malignancy. Because it is so difficult to diagnose, even in tissue, the patient is often left untreated until the clinical signs and symptoms of carcinoma are overwhelming and the diagnosis is finally made. The Pap smear can sometimes aid in its recognition [Silverberg 1975].

Papillary Serous Carcinoma: Resembles similar ovarian or endometrial tumor, with high-grade tumor cells [I6.122].

Mesonephric Carcinoma: This is a very rare, glycogen-negative, clear cell tumor; it should not be confused with more common glycogen-positive clear cell carcinoma. Gland lumens typically contain hyaline material [134 I6.132] [R Young 1990].

Adenoid Cystic Carcinoma: This is a very rare, very aggressive cervical tumor that resembles similar salivary gland tumor [Grafton 1976].

Adenoid Basal Carcinoma: This rare invasive tumor, which resembles squamous carcinoma in situ, differs chiefly in the presence of columnar cells and small gland openings. It may be associated with squamous dysplasia and squamous cell carcinoma [135 I6.152] [Powers 1994, R Young 1990].

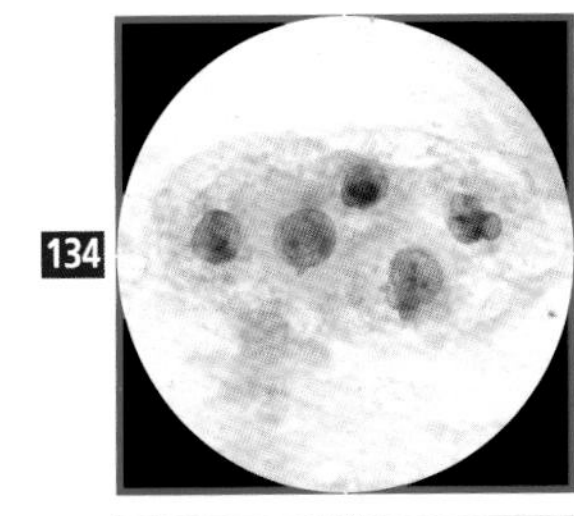

134

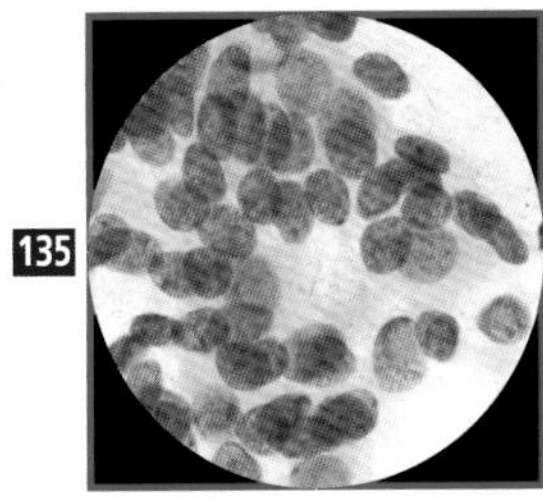

135

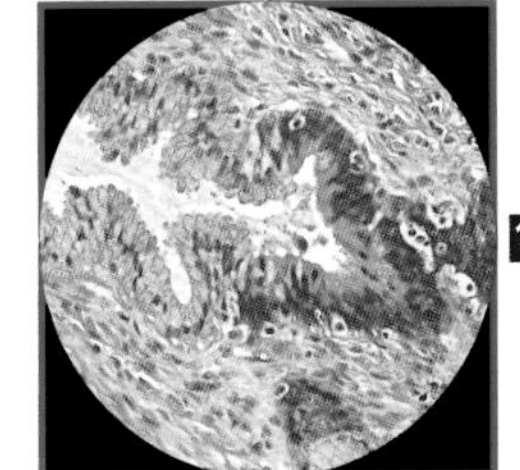

136

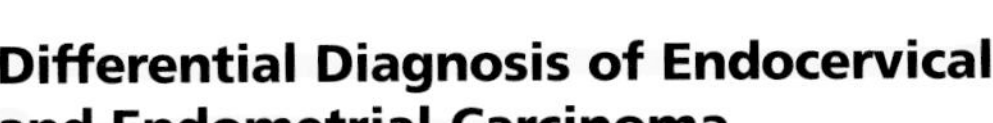

Differential Diagnosis of Endocervical and Endometrial Carcinoma

A common problem is differentiating endocervical from endometrial carcinoma [T6.34]. Many of the morphologic differences between the two are due to the manner in which the cells find their way into the Pap smear. Cells from endocervical adenocarcinoma may be directly scraped, while those of endometrial carcinoma are usually spontaneously exfoliated. Therefore, endocervical adenocarcinoma is usually characterized by the presence of an abundance of well-preserved cells (there may be several orders of magnitude more cells than from endometrial adenocarcinoma). The cells tend to maintain their columnar shape, an important clue to endocervical origin [Nasu 1993]. Endometrial carcinoma is represented by fewer cells, which tend to round up and degenerate, unless the tumor has invaded the endocervix.

T6.34 **Differentiating Endocervical From Endometrial Carcinoma**

	Endocervical	Endometrial
Cellularity	More (orders of magnitude)	Less
Cells	Larger	Smaller
	Columnar, tall	Round, plump
	Preserved	Degenerated
Groups	Rosettes	Balls
	Crowded sheets with holes	Molded groups
Cytoplasm	Granular	Vacuolar
	More acidophilic	More basophilic
	PMNs rare	PMNs relatively common
Nuclei	Larger (~75–165 μm^2)	Smaller (~60–90 μm^2)
	~2–5x intermediate nucleus	<2.5x intermediate nucleus
	Multinucleation common	Multinucleation rare
	More hyperchromatic	Less hyperchromatic
Nucleoli	Often multiple	Usually single
	Larger	Smaller
Associations	Squamous CIN	Clinical risk factors
Diathesis*	Yes	Yes
Immunocytochemistry	CEA	Vimentin

[Reagan 1973]
* Differential diagnosis with metastasis (usually no diathesis).

Endocervical adenocarcinoma typically forms two-dimensional rosettes of cells or sheets with secondary gland openings, while endometrial carcinoma tends to form three-dimensional cell balls. The individual cells of endocervical cancer usually have elongated, dark nuclei, and may have prominent, multiple nucleoli. Multinucleation is common in endocervical carcinoma, but not in endometrial carcinoma [Reagan 1973].

Endometrial carcinoma, on the other hand, has cells that are rounded, with smaller, rounder nuclei, finer chromatin, and (typically) a conspicuous central nucleolus. The cytoplasm of endometrial carcinoma cells is usually vacuolated, while the cytoplasm of malignant endocervical cells is usually granular. Cells from endocervical carcinoma tend to be more acidophilic, while cells of endometrial adenocarcinoma tend to be more basophilic, depending on the stain. Neutrophils are more commonly seen in the cytoplasm of malignant endometrial cells.

Endocervical adenocarcinoma is frequently associated with squamous dysplasia/carcinoma in situ. Endometrial carcinoma may be associated with classic risk factors. Endometrial adenocarcinoma is negative for human papilloma virus DNA, and this may help in distinguishing it from endocervical adenocarcinoma [A Nielsen 1990]. Carcinoembryonic antigen expression favors endocervical origin, but can be seen in endometrial carcinoma. Vimentin expression favors endometrial origin.

Endometrioid endocervical adenocarcinoma is morphologically identical to endometrial carcinoma, but arises in the endocervix. Endometrial carcinoma extends into the endocervix in about 10% of cases [Reagan 1973], in which case several diagnostic features will be shared by endometrial carcinoma.

Early Endocervical Glandular Neoplasia

Endocervical dysplasia, carcinoma in situ, and microinvasive adenocarcinoma are thought to be intermediate steps in the development of frankly invasive endocervical adenocarcinoma [Alva 1975]. However, early glandular neoplasia, particularly microinvasive adenocarcinoma, is not as well defined as the squamous counterparts. Histologic confirmation of these diagnoses is required.

Endocervical Adenocarcinoma In Situ: Endocervical adenocarcinoma in situ was first described, histologically, in 1953 by Friedell and McKay [136 I6.109, I6.110] [Friedell 1953]. The typical patient with endocervical adenocarcinoma in situ is young, white, and asymptomatic [137 I6.110] [Betsill 1986]. Because endocervical adenocarcinoma in situ is asymptomatic and the lesion is usually invisible at colposcopy, cytology is critical in detection of this disease. Endocervical sampling devices such as the endocervical brush are important in obtaining a diagnostic cytologic specimen.

There is usually a moderate number of neoplastic endocervical cells, associated with normal or reactive endocervical cells. Abnormalities of the nucleus and architectural groupings of the cells are the primary diagnostic features [Bousfield 1980, Lickrish 1993, Nasu 1993]. The cells are characteristically found in hyperchromatic crowded groups; there are few single abnormal cells. The groups take three forms: rosettes [138 I6.107, 139 I6.108], stratified strips [140 I6.106], and three-dimensional, syncytial-like aggregates [141 I6.105]. The aggregates typically have "feathery" edges, as seen in invasive endocervical adenocarcinoma. Secondary gland openings can also be seen in sheets of endocervical cells.

Adenocarcinoma In Situ

Groups: Very crowded, few single
- Stratified strips
- Rosettes
- Syncytia with "feathery" edges

Nuclei
- High nuclear/cytoplasmic ratio
- Oval to elongated or irregular
- Marked hyperchromasia
- Coarse chromatin
- Nucleoli typically inconspicuous

No diathesis

Frequently associated with squamous lesions

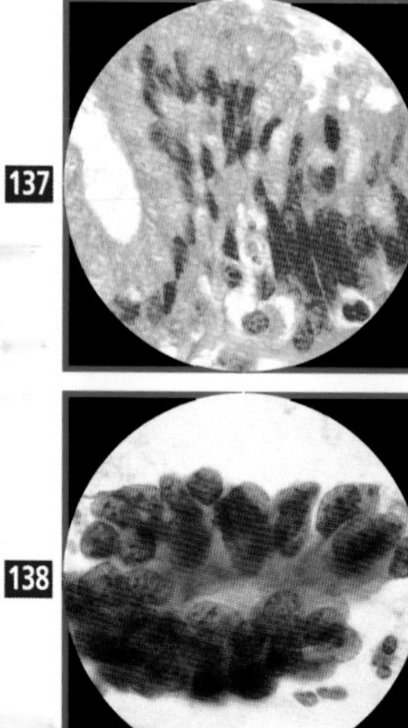

137

138

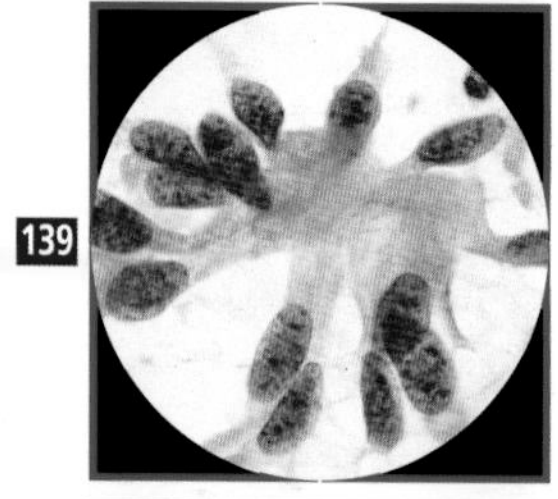

139

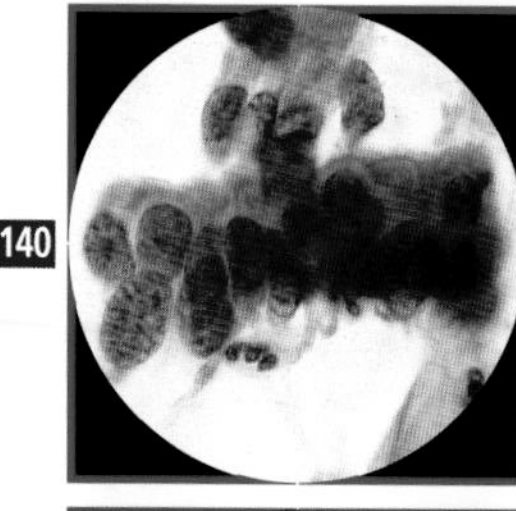

140

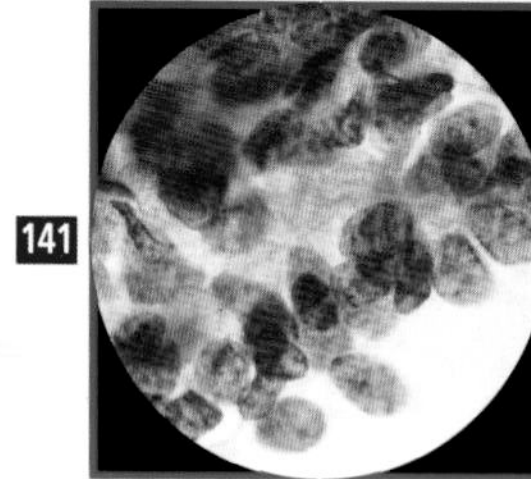

141

The nuclei are characteristically oval to elongated or irregular. The cells have high N/C ratios. The chromatin is markedly hyperchromatic and moderately coarse, similar to squamous carcinoma in situ [A Clark 1986, Lee 1991]. As is also true of squamous intraepithelial lesions, there is usually a paucity of nucleoli, although micronucleoli may be seen in a minority of cells. Macronucleoli are usually rare or absent. The cytoplasm is delicate and cell borders ill defined. Occasional cases have an endometrioid (less cytoplasm, lacks mucin), intestinal (goblet cell, sialomucin), clear cell, or mixed pattern [Nasu 1993].

An inflammatory background is common, but a tumor diathesis is absent. Adenocarcinoma in situ is frequently associated with squamous dysplasia or carcinoma in situ.

There is also a poorly differentiated variant of adenocarcinoma in situ that has more cytoplasm and larger, rounder nuclei, with vesicular chromatin, and prominent nucleoli or macronucleoli. These features can also be seen in invasive adenocarcinoma [Kudo 1991, Lee 1991].

It is not always possible to distinguish in situ from invasive endocervical adenocarcinoma. Invasive adenocarcinoma may have features indistinguishable from the usual form of in situ adenocarcinoma, and the poorly differentiated variant of in situ adenocarcinoma variant may be indistinguishable from invasive adenocarcinoma. However, in general, invasive adenocarcinomas usually show more cytologic atypia, single cells, and a tumor diathesis. Note in particular, that although prominent or macronucleoli suggest invasion, they can be seen in in situ lesions.

Endocervical Glandular Dysplasia: Endocervical glandular dysplasia may be a cause of atypical endocervical cells or AGUS. Dysplasia of the endocervical cells shows changes similar to, but less marked than, endocervical adenocarcinoma in situ. There tend to be fewer atypical cells, and not every cell in a group is necessarily atypical. The atypical cells are columnar, and the nuclei are somewhat enlarged and round to oval in shape. There is loss of polarity, occasional rosettes, and some crowding, but not as marked as in adenocarcinoma in situ. The chromatin is hyperchromatic and granular, but not coarse. Occasional mitotic figures may be seen. Nucleoli are usually inconspicuous. Endocervical glandular dysplasia can have aneuploid DNA patterns similar to that of squamous dysplasia [Alva 1975].

Microinvasive Endocervical Adenocarcinoma: Microinvasive endocervical adenocarcinoma is extremely rare, being present in only about 1 of every 50,000 Pap smears [Ayer 1988]. Even in the most experienced hands, the differential diagnosis between microinvasive adenocarcinoma and adenocarcinoma in situ vs fully invasive adenocarcinoma in a Pap smear is a coin toss (~50% accurate) [Ayer 1988]. Microinvasive adenocarcinoma is not well defined either microscopically or by its clinical behavior. *Microinvasive adenocarcinoma has a low, but definite, risk of pelvic lymph node metastasis* [Berek 1985, Buscema 1984, Fu 1987]. Like microinvasive squamous cell carcinoma, this lesion requires thorough histologic evaluation before the diagnosis is accepted. This is particularly important because microinvasive adenocarcinoma, in comparison with its squamous counterpart, is more often multifocal and has skip areas [Buscema 1984]. Even after thorough evaluation, the clinical behavior may still be unpredictable.

The cytologic features are intermediate between in situ and fully invasive adenocarcinoma. In addition to the features of adenocarcinoma in situ described above, significant numbers of single atypical cells are present [Ayer 1988]. Papillary fragments and squamoid cytoplasm may also be seen [Ayer 1988]. The individual cells of microinvasive adenocarcinoma and adenocarcinoma in situ are quite similar [Betsill 1986, Nguyen 1984b], although the nuclei of microinvasive adenocarcinoma tend to be more round (than oval) and prominent nucleoli, including macronucleoli in some cells, are more frequently seen [Kudo 1991]. A diathesis may begin to make its appearance in the background.

Differential Diagnosis of Early Endocervical Glandular Neoplasia: Reactive endocervical cells, repair, tubal metaplasia, squamous carcinoma in situ, brush artifact, and invasive endocervical adenocarcinoma are all included in the differential diagnosis of early glandular neoplasia [T6.35].

The major diagnostic features of endocervical adenocarcinoma in situ are similar to those of invasive endocervical adenocarcinoma, consisting of tightly crowded sheets of columnar cells with hyperchromatic, oval to elongated nuclei and high N/C ratios (ie, hyperchromatic crowded groups) [Boon 1991, Lee 1991]. Rosettes, secondary gland openings, and feathery edges are also features shared with invasive endocervical adenocarci-

T6.35 **Differential Diagnosis of Reactive Endocervical Cells, Adenocarcinoma In Situ, and Invasive Adenocarcinoma**

	Reactive	AdCIS	Invasive AdCA
Crowding	±	+++	++
Feathering	0	+++	++
Rosettes/Gland openings	±	+++	++
Cilia	±	0	0
Mitoses	±	++	++
Nuclear irregularity	0	+	+++
Irregular chromatin	0	±	+++
High nuclear/cytoplasmic ratio	±	+++	++
Nucleoli	Variable	0 or Micronucleoli	Macronucleoli
Normal endocervical cells	+++	++	+
Background	Clean/Inflammatory	Inflammatory/Clean	Diathesis

noma [Ayer 1987]. However, invasive adenocarcinoma characteristically shows more atypical cells, more single cells, more pleomorphism, more abnormal chromatin patterns, more frequent and larger nucleoli, and the presence of a tumor diathesis. Compared with in situ adenocarcinoma, the cell groups tend to be looser, three-dimensional syncytial-like aggregates are uncommon, and the N/C ratios are lower in invasive adenocarcinoma. The absence of a diathesis does not exclude infiltrating carcinoma [Lee 1991]. On the other hand, the presence of nucleoli does not necessarily indicate invasion.

An important practical problem is to differentiate the wide range of reactive changes that can be seen in benign endocervical cells from changes seen in malignancy [Nasu 1993]. Reactive endocervical cells can be more pleomorphic than those of endocervical adenocarcinoma. Reactive nuclei are large and dark, but tend to be more rounded and often have prominent nucleoli, compared with more elongated shapes of in situ or low-grade malignant nuclei, in which nucleoli are usually inconspicuous or absent. Marked crowding is seen in malignancy, but benign cells tend to "lay flat." Ciliated cells are virtually always benign. (Reported cases of ciliated cells in adenocarcinoma in situ [Betsill 1986, Lee 1991] probably represent misinterpretation of tubal metaplasia [Pacey 1988a,b].) On the other hand, the mere presence of ciliated cells in a smear does not exclude endocervical glandular neoplasia. If the endocervical cells crowd, stratify, "feather," or form rosettes or gland openings, a diagnosis of endocervical glandular neoplasia should be considered.

Reactive changes in endocervical cells, including multinucleation, pleomorphism, and hyperchromasia, are common, while endocervical adenocarcinoma in situ is a relatively rare disease. Macronucleoli in every cell suggest endocervical repair. Endocervical glandular neoplasia can be associated with squamous atypia, dysplasia, or carcinoma in situ [Bose 1994, L Brown 1986, Goff 1992, Kohan 1985, Nasu 1993]. Squamous carcinoma in situ has more single cells (rare in adenocarcinoma in situ), scanty, undifferentiated cytoplasm (vs tall columnar cells with cytoplasmic differentiation), and rounder nuclei (vs oval to elongated nuclei in adenocarcinoma in situ) and is usually associated with squamous dysplasia.

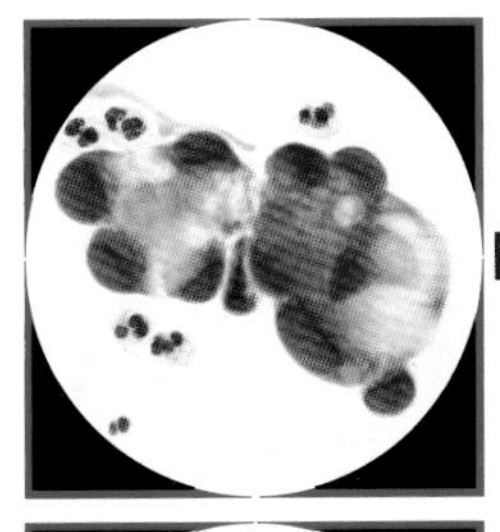
142

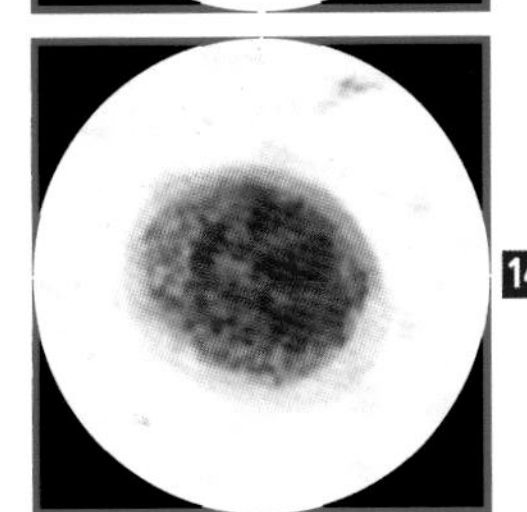
143

IUD Changes

Intrauterine (contraceptive) devices (IUDs) had practically been eliminated from the market due to litigation. However, many women still have them, and recently new IUDs have been introduced. IUDs may be associated with infections or cellular alterations [Gupta 1982]. Since the IUD has a body that sits in the endometrial cavity with a tail in the endocervical canal, an IUD may result in cytologic atypia of endometrial, metaplastic, and endocervical cells. Immediately after insertion, reactive endometrial cells and increased numbers of neutrophils and histiocytes are seen in a few patients. Whether patients are at increased risk of squamous intraepithelial lesions, and if so, why, remain matters of controversy [Misra 1991].

Patients with an IUD can shed endometrial cells at any time during the menstrual cycle. Moreover, any patient using an IUD can also shed atypical glandular cells [142 I6.59, 143 I6.60]. The atypical cells may persist for months after removing the device. There are three types of atypical cells associated with IUDs: hypervacuolated endocervical cells, vacuolated metaplastic cells, and endometrial cells, either in groups or single. *Actinomyces* or *Amoeba*, if present, supports the diagnosis of IUD effect.

Endocervical Cells: The endocervical cells appear as clusters of large, hypervacuolated, columnar cells, often with phagocytosed neutrophils in their cytoplasm. The vacuoles are degenerative in nature [142 I6.59]. The nuclei are enlarged and hyperchromatic and vary moderately in size. In adenocarcinoma the nuclear membranes are irregular, and the chromatin is abnormal and irregularly distributed. Prominent nucleoli can be seen in either cell type.

Metaplastic Cells: In response to irritation, including IUDs, the cytoplasm of immature squamous metaplasia may become distended with degenerative vacuoles and push the nuclei to the periphery, mimicking glandular cells. This finding, together with atypical nuclei, could also be mistaken for adenocarcinoma. However, the bland chromatin, the clear, nonsecretory nature of the vacuoles, and the absence of a tumor diathesis help determine the true nature of the reactive metaplastic cells. Evidence of repair and inflammation (including neutrophils in the vacuoles) is also common.

Endometrial Cells: Endometrial cells may shed singly [143 I6.60] or in clusters. The endometrial cells usually have scant cytoplasm, uniform nuclear size and shape, and at most, only slight hyperchromasia. The cells may be degenerated, occasionally with large cytoplasmic vacuoles and some chromatin clumping, with evidence of inflammation (endometritis) in the background. The glandular cells may be accompanied by endometrial stroma. Although endometrial adenocarcinoma may show only subtle abnormalities in the Pap smear, in general, adenocarcinoma has malignant nuclear features (pleomorphism, abnormal chromatin, prominent nucleoli) and a tumor diathesis. Finally, single, atypical endometrial cells are small, with very high N/C ratios and hyperchromatic nuclei [I6.60]. The cells resemble single cells of carcinoma in situ, but do not form syncytia. Also, these "IUD cells" have bland, fine or dark chromatin with a finely undulating nuclear membrane, rather than the coarse chromatin and deeply folded membranes characteristic of carcinoma in situ. Prominent nucleoli and multinucleation are not seen in this type of IUD cell. Furthermore, in contrast to carcinoma in situ, IUD cells are few in number, exclusively single, and only coincidentally associated with dysplasia.

Differential Diagnosis of IUD Changes

Actinomyces supports diagnosis of IUD change
Differential diagnosis: Adenocarcinoma
- Lack of malignant nuclear features
- No diathesis with IUD

Differential diagnosis: Carcinoma in situ
- Few atypical cells (CIS—many cells)
- Undulating, not deeply folded, nuclear membrane
- Bland, dark chromatin
- No prominent nucleoli (either CIS or IUD)
- No multinucleation, no prominent nucleoli, no syncytia, usually no dysplasia

Some patients wearing an IUD for extended periods of time harbor actinomyces. Usually, the organism merely represents an infestation or superficial infection, rather than a deeply invasive infection. Treatment of actinomyces associated with IUD use is controversial. Some advocate both removal of the IUD and antibiotic therapy, while others recommend only one or the other. Rarely, true clinical pelvic actinomycosis develops, in which case more aggressive therapy is indicated. Very rarely, amebae similar in appearance to *Entamoeba gingivalis* are present in the smears of patients wearing an IUD. Unlike *Entamoeba histolytica*, they do not contain red blood cells.

Differential Diagnosis of Atypical Glandular (Endocervical) Cells

Occasionally, groups of atypical cells, apparently glandular in origin, with crowding, nuclear enlargement, and hyperchromasia, are encountered that are not readily classifiable as reactive or neoplastic in nature. These atypical endocervical cells are also known as atypical glandular cells of undetermined significance (AGUS) in the Bethesda System. The differential diagnosis includes both glandular and squamous lesions [Betsill 1986, Fiorella 1994, Gloor 1982, Lee 1988, Pacey 1988a,b]. Note, however, that squamous and glandular lesions commonly coexist. Criteria for separating reactive from neoplastic atypical endometrial cells are not well defined.

Neoplastic endocervical cells are tall columnar cells, with enlarged, oval to elongated, hyperchromatic nuclei, coarse chromatin, marked crowding, rosettes, and feathery edges [I6.106-I6.116].

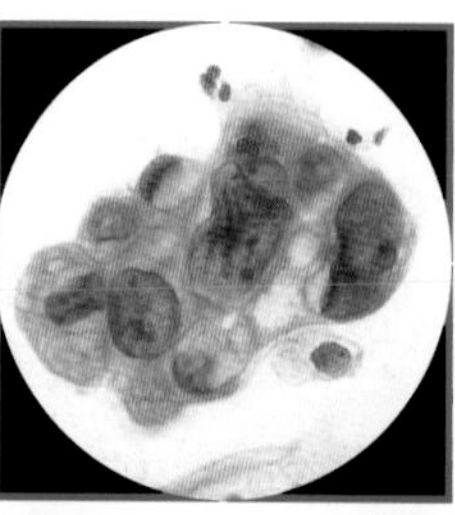
144

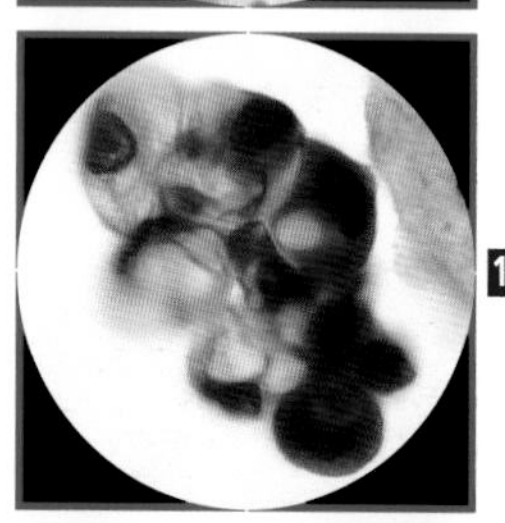
145

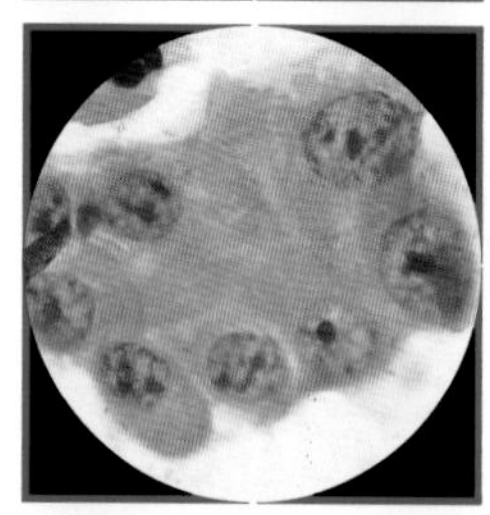
146

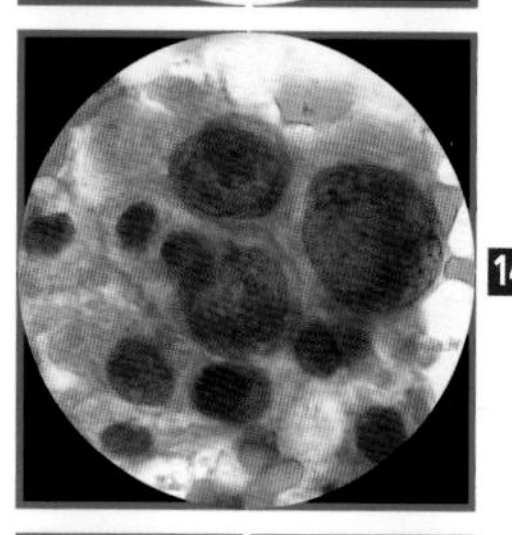
147

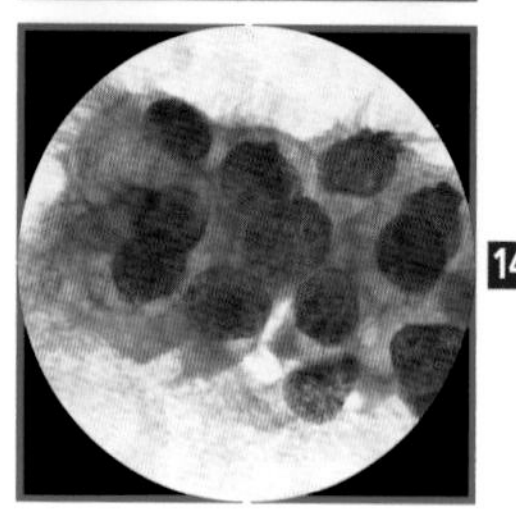
148

Differental Diagnosis of Atypical Endocervical Cells

Endocervical glandular neoplasia
- Dysplasia → adenocarcinoma in situ → invasive carcinoma

Reactive/reparative endocervical cells
Endometrium and endometriosis
Cone biopsy artifact
Tubal metaplasia
Endocervical brush artifacts
Cone biopsy artifact
Arias-Stella reaction
Endocervical microglandular hyperplasia
IUD changes
Squamous carcinoma, in situ and invasive
Metastatic carcinoma

Reactive endocervical cells may be slightly, but not markedly, crowded, with nuclear enlargement, pleomorphism, prominent nucleoli, hyperchromasia, and possibly polyploidy. Reactive endocervical cells may be associated with a variety of conditions, including endocervicitis, polyps, birth control pills, intrauterine contraceptive devices, and radiation/chemotherapy effects [144 I6.65] [Doss 1995, Frierson 1990]. Differential diagnosis also includes vacuolated metaplastic cells [145 I6.143].

Endocervical repair features macronucleoli in every cell, with pale chromatin and plenty of cytoplasm. Stratified strips, marked crowding, rosettes, and secondary gland openings [146 I6.17] favor neoplasia.

Endometrium and endometriosis both feature hyperchromatic crowded groups of endometrial cells with high N/C ratios, possibly secondary gland openings, and mitotic figures. Such cells can mimic endocervical neoplasia, but the cells have a uniform, benign appearance and may be associated with endometrial stromal cells. Endometrial cells may be obtained, at any time during the cycle, with an endocervical brush (which can obtain cells directly from the lower uterine segment or even the endometrial cavity itself), in patients with cervical endometriosis (gland, stroma, hemosiderin), or in patients who have undergone cone biopsy (in whom the endocervical canal is shortened) [Lee 1993].

Tubal metaplasia features crowded columnar cells, which can have enlarged, somewhat pleomorphic nuclei, elevated N/C ratios, and moderate hyperchromasia that may suggest endocervical glandular neoplasia, particularly adenocarcinoma in situ [Lee 1991, Novotny 1992, Pacey 1988a]. Small, discrete, clear cytoplasmic vacuoles are common, and terminal bars and cilia are characteristic. For practical purposes, the presence of cilia excludes malignancy [Ducatman 1993, Hirschowitz 1994, Novotny 1992, Van Le 1991]. Unfortunately, the cilia may degenerate or be difficult to visualize [148 I6.20, I6.21, I6.144, I6.145].

Endocervical brush artifacts include an increased number of cells, with increased thickness and crowding of groups (sheets, strips) [Fiorella 1994]. Also, large, dark, possibly polyploid nuclei may be seen. Benign endocervical cells may show gland openings and rosettes rarely, but the nuclei are not abnormal [147 I6.18].

Cone biopsy artifact may be associated with hyperchromatic crowded groups of atypical glandular cells; however, there are fewer abnormal cells, and they are less crowded than in neoplasia. They are part of a morphologic spectrum that includes clearly benign cells, which may appear of endometrial or endocervical origin. Nuclei are smaller with finer chromatin, and mitotic figures are rare. Ciliated cells are benign, but often not present [Lee 1991,1993, Pacey 1988a].

Arias-Stella reaction shows marked atypia (nuclear enlargement, hyperchromasia, and pleomorphism) but abundant cytoplasm. No stratification or crowding occurs [149 I6.19]. Similar cells can be seen in cases of chemotherapy effect [I6.65] [Doss 1995] (see "Cytology of Pregnancy," below).

Microglandular hyperplasia is indicated by pseudoparakeratosis (linear arrays of degenerated endocervical cells with cytoplasmic orangeophilia and pyknotic nuclei) and reactive endocervical cells. It is more common in patients taking birth control pills [150 I6.40].

IUD effect displays clusters of reactive glandular cells of either endocervical or endometrial origin, and clusters of vacuolated metaplastic cells, which can mimic adenocarcinoma. Also, single endometrial cells will be found, which can mimic squamous carcinoma in situ. *Actinomyces*, if present, and a history of IUD use support this diagnosis [151 I6.59, I6.60].

Squamous Carcinoma In Situ: Both squamous and glandular carcinoma in situ are associated with hyperchromatic crowded groups. Squamous and glandular carcinoma in situ have similar nuclei (coarse, dark regular chromatin) and cytoplasm (delicate, nonsquamous). Both squamous and glandular lesions are thought to arise from the reserve cell and frequently coexist [Lauchlan 1967]. Interestingly, squamous carcinoma in situ frequently shows rudimentary gland formation (ie, microacinar structures) that can mimic endocervical glandular neoplasia [Selvaggi 1994]. Presence of well-formed glandular structures, of course, points to glandular origin. Glandular lesions tend to have more oval to elongated nuclei than the rounder nuclei associated with squamous lesions, and the edges of glandular groups tend to feather. In some cases, this problem may have to be resolved by tissue biopsy, but even then the differential diagnosis can sometimes be difficult [152 I6.156].

Invasive squamous cell carcinoma shows a denser cytoplasm and more central nuclei than adenocarcinoma. Keratinization does not occur in pure endocervical adenocarcinoma; however, squamous cell carcinoma and adenocarcinoma may coexist as adenosquamous carcinoma.

Metastatic adenocarcinoma reveals clusters of malignant-appearing cells, but no diathesis. Usually, there is a known history of cancer [153 I6.122, 6.128-I6.131].

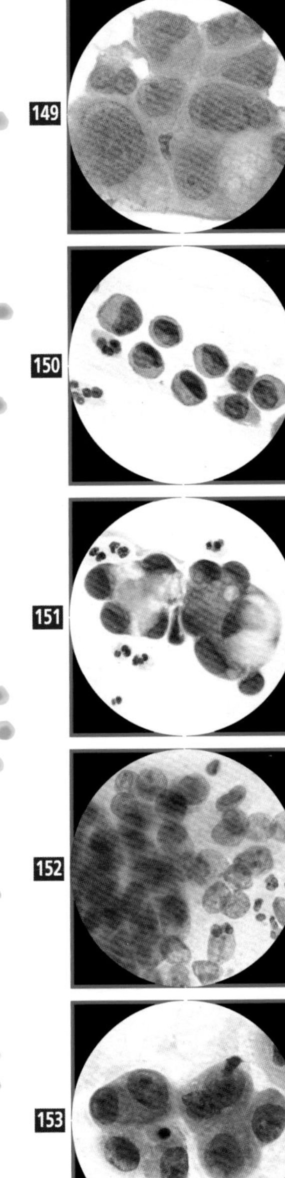

III. Cytology of Pregnancy

Pregnancy cannot be reliably diagnosed by the Pap smear [Meisels 1966b, Van Haam 1961]. Fortunately, there are far more accurate ways to establish that a woman is pregnant. Nevertheless, there are characteristic cellular alterations, and some diagnostic pitfalls, that accompany pregnancy. We will also consider the diagnosis of cervical neoplasia during pregnancy. In addition, a variety of complications of pregnancy can be diagnosed or suspected by cytology (including amniotic fluid cytology [Cohen 1987], which is beyond the scope of this discussion). These include infection, abortions, fetal malformations, and amniotic fluid embolism during pregnancy.

Hormonal Cytology of Pregnancy

During pregnancy, as the corpus luteum (and later the placenta) gear up to manufacture progesterone, the maturation index of the cervical epithelium shifts to intermediate predominance pattern ("shift to the middle" of the maturation index) [Bercovici 1973, Meisels 1966b, 1968, Ortner 1977, Sen 1972]. The intermediate cells are characteristically heavily glycogenated, causing many of the cells to assume an elongated, angular boat shape (navicular cells). Cytolysis may be extensive.

The placenta uses fetal adrenal hormones as building blocks for placental hormones, including progesterone. Thus, an atrophic pattern occurring during pregnancy may indicate intrauterine fetal demise. However, extensive immature squamous metaplasia or dysplasia must be distinguished from parabasal cells of an atrophic smear. At the other extreme, a superficial predominant pattern occurring after the first trimester may suggest intrauterine fetal distress. With decreased fetal adrenal function, decreased progesterone production may result in relative maternal estrogen excess. However, far more commonly, inflammation/infection causes pseudomaturation.

During the postpartum period, with the fall in hormone levels, the mucosa atrophies to varying degrees. Atrophy occurs in one third of nonlactating and two thirds of lactating mothers (parabasal-predominant maturation pattern). The mucosa matures again within 10 days to a month or so, unless the woman is breast-feeding. If the maturation is not normal by 1 year, there may be a serious endocrine problem.

The Cells of Pregnancy

Glycogenated intermediate cells (navicular cells), as mentioned, are characteristic of pregnancy. Increased numbers of histiocytes also characteristically appear, especially early and late in pregnancy. Also, during pregnancy, the endocervical cells tend to grow out onto the ectocervix (ectropion), where they may be more easily sampled. The endocervical cells may become reactive ("plump and juicy") during pregnancy, and remain so postpartum, possibly resulting in a diagnosis of atypical endocervical cells (AGUS). These "atypical" changes, as well as noninfectious inflammatory changes, take up to 8 weeks to regress postpartum [Rarick 1994].

In addition to these cells, there are three cell types specifically associated with pregnancy: decidual cells, Arias-Stella reaction, and trophoblast. These atypical pregnancy-associated cells can be a source of diagnostic errors [Danos 1967,1968, Frank 1991, Hilrich 1955, Kobayashi 1980, Murad 1981, Naib 1961, Soloway 1969, Youseff 1963].

Decidual Cells

Infrequently, decidual cells are identified in the Pap smear of pregnant or postpartum women [Fiorella 1993a, Gladwell 1974, Kobayashi 1980, Murad 1981, V Schneider 1981b, Soloway 1969] (and rarely in patients taking birth control pills) [154 I6.28]. Their presence usually indicates decidualization of the cervical stroma, which is more common in late pregnancy. Decidual cells are usually present singly or in small clusters. The cells are fairly large, about the size of parabasal or low intermediate cells, and have large, but bland, pale nuclei. Prominent nucleoli may be present. The cytoplasm is abundant, delicate, and transparent, but the cell borders are distinct. Occasionally, the cytoplasm is somewhat vacuolated or fibrillar in character. Decidual cells may resemble cells in high-grade squamous intraepithelial lesion, particularly moderate dysplasia in intermediate-type cells (mature metaplastic dysplasia), but the differential diagnosis also includes repair, carcinoma, and sarcoma [Danos 1967].

Differential Diagnosis of Decidual Cells

- Dysplasia
  - Coarse chromatin
  - Increased nuclear/cytoplasmic ratio
  - (–) Nucleoli
- Repair
  - Tighter clusters
  - Few single cells
  - Mitoses
- Carcinoma
  - Crowded groups
  - Abnormal chromatin
  - ± Mucin secretion
- Sarcoma
  - Single cells
  - Often spindle or pleomorphic cells
  - Abnormal chromatin

154
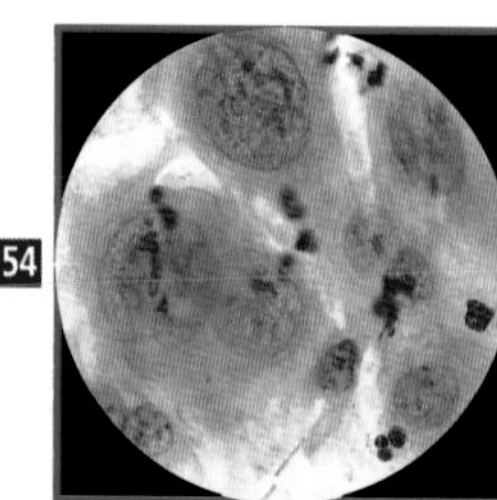

155
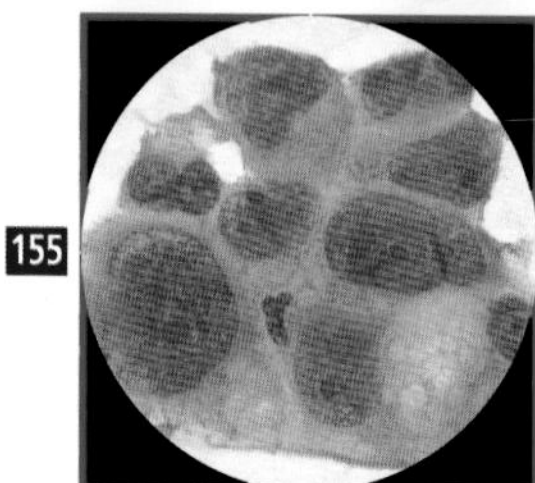

156
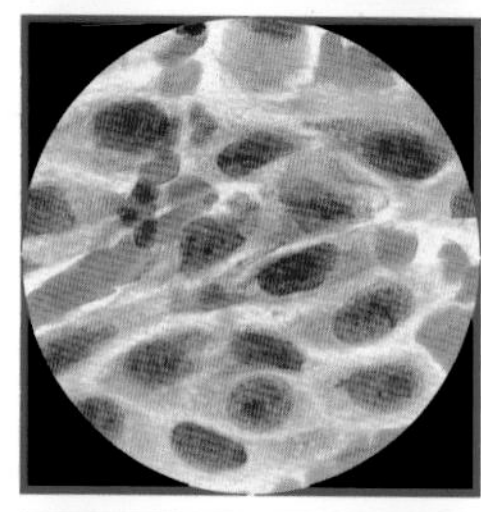

157
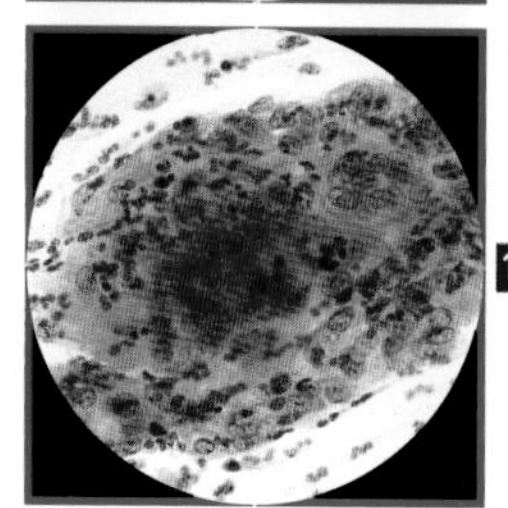

Arias-Stella Reaction

Arias-Stella reaction of glandular epithelium is uncommonly seen in Pap smears [155 I6.19]. Arias-Stella reaction usually affects glandular cells of the endometrium, but it may also affect cells of the endocervix and fallopian tube [Cove 1979, Rhatigan 1992]. Rarely, Arias-Stella reaction is also caused by birth control pills, ovulation-inducing drugs, or other hormonal therapy. Similar cells can be seen in chemotherapy effect [Doss 1995].

In response to high levels of human chorionic gonadotropin and prolonged progesterone stimulation, proliferative and secretory activity occur together, resulting in large, pleomorphic cells with large, hyperchromatic nuclei and prominent nucleoli. The cytoplasm is voluminous and pale, fine to coarsely vacuolated, and PAS-positive [Albukerk 1974,1977, Kobayashi 1980,1983]. The nuclei are enlarged, eccentrically located, have fine to granular, hyperchromatic chromatin and variable nucleoli, which can be prominent and occasionally multiple [Shrago 1977]. Arias-Stella cells are polyploid (but not aneuploid) [Kobayashi 1983]. Occasional bizarre epithelial cells with irregular, giant nuclei may be present [Mulvany 1994]. Mitotic figures [Albukerk 1977] and intranuclear cytoplasmic invaginations [Mulvany 1994, V Schneider 1981a] may be seen.

The pleomorphic, atypical cells may suggest adenocarcinoma, particularly clear cell type. As a practical point, adenocarcinoma should be diagnosed cautiously during pregnancy.

Trophoblasts

Trophoblastic cells are rarely found in Pap smears, but can sometimes be seen in late pregnancy or following delivery [Fiorella 1993a]. If numerous, or abnormal appearing, suspect trophoblastic disease. Although they have been described in the setting of threatened abortion [Holmquist 1967a, Kobayashi 1980, Naib 1961, Wagner 1968], their presence is not a reliable indicator of impending abortion [Fiorella 1993a].

Cytotrophoblasts

These cells occur singly or in small clusters [156 I6.30]. The cells have atypical nuclei and high N/C ratios, which may suggest a high-grade squamous intraepithelial lesion or poorly differentiated carcinoma [Frank 1991]. The cytoplasm is dense, bluish, and may be vacuolated. The nucleus is enlarged, irregular, and hyperchromatic, with a conspicuous nucleolus [Kobayashi 1980].

Syncytiotrophoblasts

These are multinucleated giant cells that characteristically have an extension, or tail, from their cytoplasm where they broke off the placenta [157 I6.29]. Syncytiotrophoblasts resemble multinucleated histiocytes, except that the nuclei are tightly packed and typically concentrated in the center of the cell but do not mold one another. When well preserved, the nuclei have finely granular chromatin and the cytoplasm stains basophilic or eosinophilic [Fiorella 1993a]. However, degenerative changes of both nucleus and cytoplasm are common. With degeneration, the cytoplasm characteristically stains red-orange and, together with degenerated, dark, central nuclei, the syncytiotrophoblast may look like a pomegranate.

After an abortion, syncytiotrophoblasts can be somewhat atypical and should not be mistaken for choriocarcinoma.

Multinucleated Giant Cells in Pregnancy

Syncytiotrophoblast
- Nuclei: Central, multiple
- Chromatin: Dense, often degenerated
- Cytoplasm: Blue to orange with tail
- Evidence of cellular degeneration

Multinucleated giant cell histiocytes
- Nuclei more dispersed than syncytiotrophoblast
  - Sometimes peripheral: Langhans'
- Chromatin: Vesicular or salt and pepper
- Cytoplasm: Rounded contour, without tail
- Usually better preservation

Herpes
- 3 M's: Multinucleation (ground glass), molding, margination
- ± Inclusions
- Very important diagnosis during pregnancy

Tumor
- Malignant nuclei

Dysplasia/Condyloma
- Macrocytes with abnormal nuclei and squamous cytoplasm

Cockleburrs

"Cockleburrs" (radiate crystalline arrays), possibly related to the Splendore-Hoeppli phenomenon, are radiate arrays of golden, refractile crystalline material, usually surrounded by histiocytes [158 I6.58]. Cockleburrs typically measure about 50 to 100 µm in diameter and are composed of somewhat thick, club-shaped spokes. As a rule (>80% of cases), cockleburrs are found in Pap smears in association with pregnancy and are more prevalent in the second half of the term [Capaldo 1983, Hollander 1974, Zaharopoulos 1985b]. Cockleburrs are found in less than 5% of pregnant patients [Capaldo 1983]. Their presence apparently has no effect on maternal or fetal prognosis [Capaldo 1983, Minassian 1993]. However, the question of a possible association with squamous intraepithelial lesions has been raised [Minassian 1993].

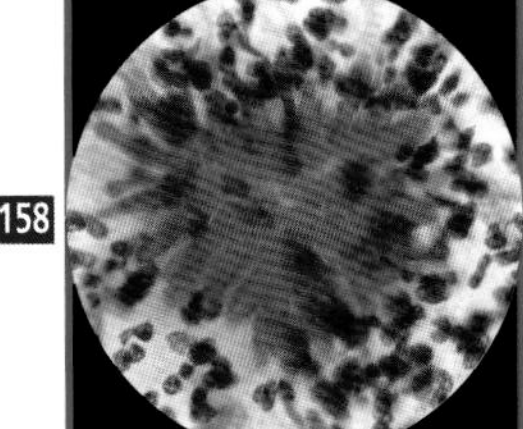
158

Cockleburrs can also be found in nonpregnant patients, usually in association with birth control pills or IUD use [Minassian 1993]. Sometimes no obvious association is appreciated. Similar or identical crystalline bodies, related to the Splendore-Hoeppli phenomenon, can also be found in nongenital sites, where they are most commonly formed around microorganisms, particularly actinomyces ("sulfur granules") or foreign bodies. However, Splendore-Hoeppli phenomenon is thought to be an antigen-antibody reaction, and contains immunoglobulin, in contrast with cockleburrs, which contain neither actinomyces nor immunoglobulins.

In the female genital tract, cockleburrs apparently form in stagnating secretions from products of degenerating cells, which surround microorganisms or biologically inert substances [Zaharopoulos 1985b]. Cockleburrs are composed of nonimmune glycoprotein, lipid, and calcium and do not contain immunoglobulin, glycogen, or mucin [Bhagavan 1982]. In contrast with actinomycotic sulfur granules, genital cockleburrs do not have visible central filaments.

The cockleburrs under discussion should not be mistaken for hematoidin radiate crystals, which are also sometimes known as cockleburrs or chestnut burrs. Hematoidin is an iron-free, bile-like pigment formed in hypoxic tissue from hemoglobin and usually indicates old bleeding. Hematoidin crystals are much less common in Pap smears than the cockleburrs under discussion. Hematoidin crystals are found not only as radiate forms, but also as spherules, rhomboids, or irregular shapes, and are usually much smaller than cockleburrs. However, the primary difference is that the crystalline rays of hematoidin burrs are much finer than those of cockleburrs [Zaharopoulos 1985a].

Puerperal Endometritis

Puerperal endometritis, due to bacterial infection, can occur after abortion or delivery. Before the age of antibiotics, this was a dreaded complication of pregnancy but is now rare. Retained products of conception can be a source of bleeding. A Pap smear might show reactive trophoblastic elements (irregularly distributed chromatin, molding, prominent nucleoli), fresh and old blood, neutrophils, histiocytes, fragmentation of nucleus and cytoplasm, or foreign body giant cells.

Vitamin Deficiency

Folate deficiency usually occurs in postmenopausal women. However, it may be seen in pregnancy, preeclampsia, and dietary deficiency [Kitay 1969]. The cytologic effects are exactly as in folate deficiency in nonpregnant women, and consist mostly of formation of macrocytes.

Cervical Neoplasia During Pregnancy

Pregnancy represents an ideal opportunity for Pap smear screening, since most women seek health care at this time. Women in their reproductive years are also the primary age group at risk for developing cervical intraepithelial neoplasia/squamous intraepithelial lesion, so dysplasia occurring during pregnancy is common [Bouttselis 1972, DePetrillo 1975, Kashimura 1991, M Smith 1968]. In fact, if anything, dysplasia is more common during pregnancy, possibly due to change in a woman's immune status

[Oriel 1971, A Schneider 1987a]. Moreover, cervical cancer is the most common malignancy diagnosed during pregnancy [Haas 1984].

There are no differences in the diagnostic features of dysplasia (or cancer) between pregnant and nonpregnant women: dysplasia is dysplasia. Cytodiagnosis is reasonably accurate during pregnancy [Bertini-Oliveira 1982, Fowler 1980, Kashimura 1991, LaPolla 1988, Reagan 1961, Richart 1963b, Rutledge 1962, Yoonessi 1982]. However, inflammatory changes and increased activity of the various cells can mimic dysplasia, sometimes resulting in a difficult differential diagnosis. On the other hand, the endocervix is shorter and slightly dilated, so the squamocolumnar transformation zone may be more accessible, making it easier to obtain abnormal cells. The cytobrush is safe to use during pregnancy, although minimal traumatic bleeding may occur [Orr 1992]. An important thing to keep in mind is that not all dysplasias progress, in fact, the minority do. Of particular note, many dysplasias regress postpartum, perhaps related to trauma during delivery or change in immune status after delivery [Benedet 1987, Hellberg 1987]. Note, however, that cervical intraepithelial neoplasia may recur in a significant number of cases [Hellberg 1987].

Management of Cervical Neoplasia During Pregnancy: While the morphologic features of dysplasia do not change in pregnancy, the therapy may be very different. *The primary goal is to rule out invasive cancer.* If a noninvasive lesion is detected, it should be followed by careful, repeated colposcopy, cytology, and possibly directed biopsies [Economos 1993, Hellberg 1987, Kirkup 1980, Kohan 1980, LaPolla 1988, Lundvall 1989, McDonnell 1981, Yoonessi 1982]. Cone biopsy and cryotherapy should be avoided if at all possible. If microinvasive squamous cell carcinoma is suspected, the abnormal area should be excised to exclude frankly invasive cancer. If microinvasive disease is confirmed, definitive therapy can be delayed until after delivery [Giuntoli 1991, Sivanesaratnam 1993]. However, if invasive cancer is found or strongly suspected, it must be definitively treated, which usually means terminating the pregnancy (abortion or early delivery). A short delay in cancer therapy may be carefully considered if the fetus is near viability. Finally, the Pap smear diagnosis of trophoblastic disease and choriocarcinoma is unreliable. These diseases occur at some distance from the cervix and the cells do not consistently shed in the Pap smear.

IV. Cytology of Rare Tumors, Metastases, and Miscellaneous Findings

Small Cell Cervical Cancers

Small cell carcinomas are a rare, but aggressive, "mixed bag" of tumors that include not only the poorly differentiated, nonkeratinizing squamous cell carcinoma described previously, but also neuroendocrine carcinomas, including carcinoids [Albores-Saavedra 1976] and small "oat" cell carcinoma (poorly differentiated neuroendocrine carcinoma), as well as poorly differentiated adenocarcinomas and adenoid-basal cell carcinoma. The differential diagnosis is important, because the prognosis may vary. As has been observed in lung cancer, some of these tumors contain mixtures of cell types. Small cell carcinomas may occur in patients with recently normal Pap smears [A Walker 1988].

Small cell carcinomas usually show evidence of epithelial differentiation. Neuroendocrine differentiation can also be detected in at least one third of cases [R Barrett 1987, van Nagell 1988]. Argyrophilia, eg, using the Grimelius stain, is one of the easiest tests to perform to detect the presence of neurosecretory granules. Unfortunately, it is not highly sensitive and may show nonspecific staining. Electron microscopy is relatively sensitive and highly specific, but not always applicable [Ueda 1989]. Immunocytochemistry can be employed, using neuron-specific enolase, chromogranin, and synaptophysin to detect neuroendocrine differentiation. Epithelial membrane antigen and cytokeratin are epithelial markers [R Joseph 1992, Kamiya 1993].

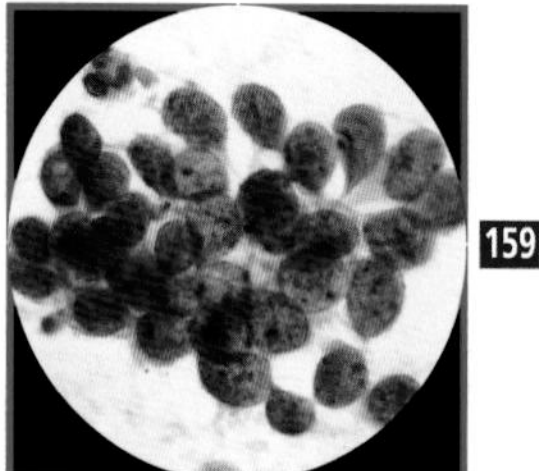
159

Small cell carcinomas of the neuroendocrine type are usually poorly differentiated in the cervix and resemble small oat cell carcinoma of the lung [Fujii 1986, Gersell 1988, Groben 1985, R Joseph 1992, Kamiya 1993] cytologically [159 I6.138]. Like small cell lung cancer, these neuroendocrine carcinomas show fine chromatin, inconspicuous or absent nucleoli, delicate cytoplasm, and prominent nuclear molding. This contrasts with small cell squamous carcinoma, which shows somewhat more cytoplasm, more cytoplasmic density, better defined cell borders, and less crush artifact. Coarse chromatin with parachromatin clearing, more conspicuous nucleoli, and little nuclear molding also favor squamous origin. Abnormal keratinized cells favor small cell squamous carcinoma, but do not completely exclude small cell neuroendocrine carcinoma (which can be associated with a squamous intraepithelial lesion). Either type may have spindle cells.

General Diagnostic Features of Sarcoma

- Cells
  - Single
  - Spindle, small, or pleomorphic
  - Mixed population common
- Nuclei
  - Multinucleation common (uncommon in usual genital carcinomas)
  - Chromatin may appear bland, pale (or coarse)
  - Macronucleoli
- Cytoplasm
  - Glassy, fibrillar, or granular
  - Often stains blue-green
- Background
  - Diathesis
- Differential diagnosis
  - Decidual reaction, repair, metaplastic dysplasia, squamous cell carcinoma

Sarcomas

Sarcomas are usually easy to diagnose as malignant, but may be difficult to classify. Genital sarcomas can arise from the vagina, cervix, uterus (corpus), ovary, and fallopian tube. Sarcomas can be pure (eg, leiomyosarcoma, endometrial stromal sarcoma, rhabdomyosarcoma, fibrosarcoma) or mixed with epithelial elements, which can be either benign-appearing (adenosarcoma) [Hidvegi 1982] or malignant (malignant mixed müllerian tumor).

Endometrial Stromal Sarcoma: Resembles endometrial stromal cells, occurring mostly singly or in small groups. The cells are small, round, uniform, or rarely spindle-shaped. They have scant cytoplasm and high N/C ratios. The nucleus is small, with coarse, hyperchromatic chromatin and micronucleoli. The tumor cells may be difficult to distinguish from benign stromal cells.

Leiomyosarcoma: Usually a smear reveals few cells; either single or in small groups. The tumor cells are spindle-shaped but vary (from case to case) from uniform and small to pleomorphic and giant. Cytoplasm is ill defined, transparent, or fibrillar. Nuclei are usually oval, with finely granular, irregular chromatin. Nucleoli vary from small and round to very irregular [160 I6.153].

Rhabdomyosarcoma: Spindle and strap cells (ie, rhabdomyoblasts). Cross striations are diagnostic of skeletal muscle differentiation, but rarely observed. Multinucleated tumor giant cells are common.

Malignant Mixed Müllerian Mesodermal Tumor: This rare, but highly aggressive, mixed carcinosarcoma, often presents as a fungating uterine mass, which may protrude from the cervical os [161 I6.125, 162 I6.126]. The epithelial element is usually endometrial carcinoma, which can vary from well differentiated to anaplastic. Other types of carcinoma, including squamous, papillary, clear cell or undifferentiated, can also occur. The stromal elements either can be composed of cells native to the uterus (ie, homologous elements), most commonly smooth muscle or stroma (leiomyosarcoma, stromal sarcoma), or can also be striated muscle, cartilage, or bone (rhabdomyosarcoma, chondrosarcoma, osteosarcoma) (ie, heterologous elements). However, all elements are probably of epithelial (metaplastic) origin [Bitterman 1990, Silverberg 1990]. The smears are often bloody and necrotic and the cells may be sparse and degenerated. Look for atypical spindle cells or bizarre tumor cells in addition to adenocarcinoma. However, the sarcomatous component may shed few cells [An-Foraker 1985, Costa 1992, Massoni 1984].

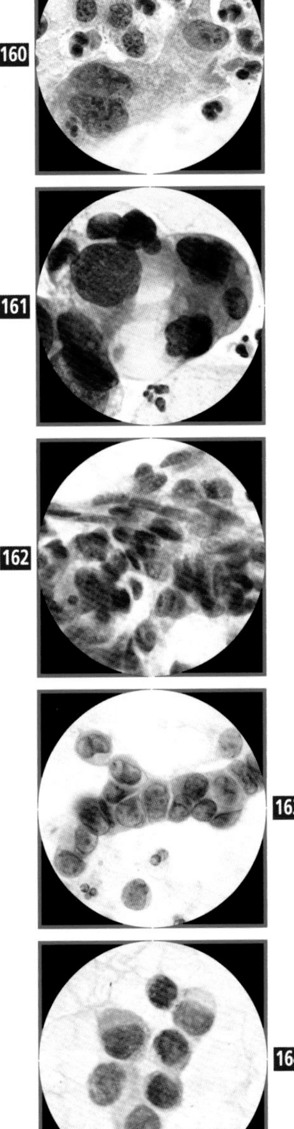

Melanoma

Five to ten percent of malignant melanomas in females arise in the genital tract (vulva, vagina), although primary melanoma of the cervix is very rare [Fleming 1994]. Metastatic melanoma is relatively more common. The Pap smear in the case of melanoma is characterized by dissociated cells with hyperchromatic, irregular nuclei, prominent nucleoli, and cytoplasmic melanin pigment [Fleming 1994, D Hall 1980, Holmquist 1988, H Jones 1971, Krishnamoorthy 1986, Mudge 1981, Podczaski 1990, Yu 1987].

Metastases

Metastatic malignancies can be easy to diagnose. First, the patient usually has a known history of cancer; rarely is the Pap smear the first place an extrauterine cancer is detected. However, occasionally, the Pap smear does lead to a diagnosis of primary cancer elsewhere in the body [McGill 1990]. Many patients will also have a history of ascites. Ovarian cancer is the most common source of metastasis. The most common sources of nongenital metastatic cancers include GI tract, pancreas, breast [163 I6.130], urinary tract, and lung, as well as mesothelioma and melanoma [I6.128-I6.130, 164 I6.131]. Rarely, other malignancies, such as germ cell tumors, metastasize to the cervix, where they may shed cells picked up in the Pap smear [Chong 1994].

Metastatic Malignancy in Pap Smear

- Can be easy diagnosis
- Known history of cancer (usual)
  - Pap smear rarely first place an extrauterine carcinoma is diagnosed
- Many patients also have ascites
- Ovarian cancer most common source
- Nongenital sources:
  - GI tract, pancreas, breast, urinary tract, lung, mesothelium, melanoma
- Most are adenocarcinomas, often
  - poorly differentiated
    - Papillary groups, psammoma bodies are suggestive, not diagnostic, of primary ovarian cancer
- Characteristic features: Absence of diathesis; looks like "floater"

Most metastatic malignancies are adenocarcinomas, often poorly differentiated [Ng 1974c]. A signet ring pattern suggests a metastasis [Fiorella 1993b]. Papillary groups and/or psammoma bodies suggest ovarian origin, but neither finding is specific [Ng 1974c, Takashina 1988]. A characteristic feature of metastatic carcinoma is that it typically (~80%) lacks a tumor diathesis, unless the metastasis becomes locally invasive. The metastatic tumor cells often look foreign to the smear, and a contaminant "floater" may be considered in the differential diagnosis.

Some Miscellaneous Findings in the Pap Smear

Fallopian Tube Cells

These normal cells are benign but rarely observed in the Pap smear. More commonly, such cells indicate tubal metaplasia of the endometrium or endocervix. The cells may be fairly atypical—cilia provide a benign clue. Fallopian tube cells may appear similar to normal or reactive ciliated endocervical cells (see findings in patients who have undergone hysterectomy, below).

Very rarely fallopian tube adenocarcinoma may shed cells in a Pap smear [165 I6.123]. Most patients are postmenopausal, many are nulliparous. Patients may suffer the characteristic syndrome of crampy lower abdominal pain and profuse watery discharge. In patients whose Pap smears indicate adenocarcinoma or adenosquamous carcinoma, but who have (1) negative cone biopsy findings (rules out endocervical adenocarcinoma), (2) negative dilatation and curettage findings (rules out endometrial adenocarcinoma), and (3) no known primary tumor, consider fallopian tube adenocarcinoma [P Benson 1974, Hirai 1987, Takashina 1985].

Benign Glandular Cells in Post-hysterectomy Patients

This finding may be explained by any of the following:

1. The history is wrong. For example, either no hysterectomy or a subtotal hysterectomy was performed. Radiation shrinks the cervix, making it difficult to visualize clinically, giving the impression that a hysterectomy was done.
2. The "glandular" cells are actually atrophic parabasal cells, which can have delicate (gland-like) cytoplasm and orderly arrangement (mimicking honeycomb). Look for intracytoplasmic mucin.
3. The cells are fallopian tube cells. The fallopian tube may granulate (prolapse) into the vaginal apex [Hellen 1993, Silverberg 1974] or may be implanted during hysterectomy for vaginal support. Occasional ciliated cells may be a clue.
4. The cells are goblet-like cells, which are relatively common in atrophy (~20% of cases). These are single, oval cells in parabasal "syncytia." They are mucin positive [Bewtra 1992, Koike 1990,1993]. For purposes of specimen adequacy, these cells are not considered endocervical cells.
5. Other: Vaginal adenosis, endometriosis, mesonephric remnants, Bartholin glands, rectovaginal fistula.

Note: Rule out well-differentiated metastatic or recurrent cancer; although these cells are not benign, they may be bland.

Ferning of the Cervical Mucus

First described by Papanicolaou, the cervical mucus tends to crystallize in an arborizing pattern, resembling ferns or palm leaves, near the time of ovulation [166 I6.149] [Papanicolaou 1946]. This is apparently associated with a peak in estrogen. Estrogen treatment may induce ferning, while progestational agents inhibit it. A direct relationship exists between the optimal time of sperm penetration and the degree of ferning [Zaneveld 1975].

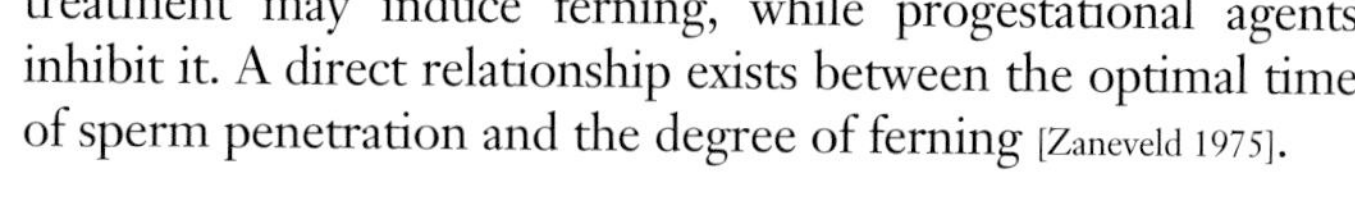

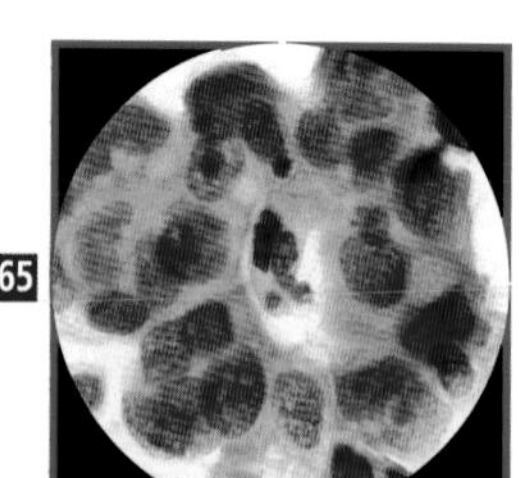

165

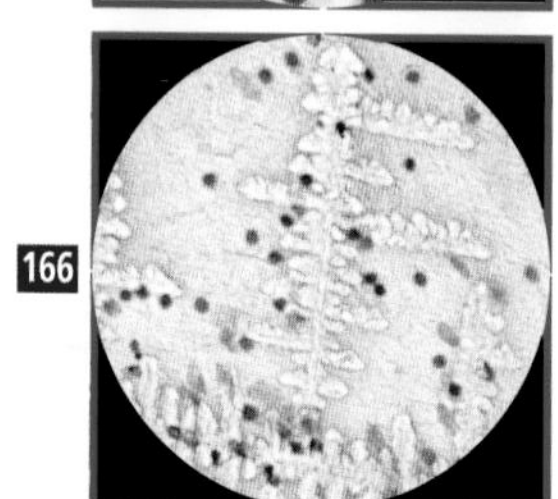

166

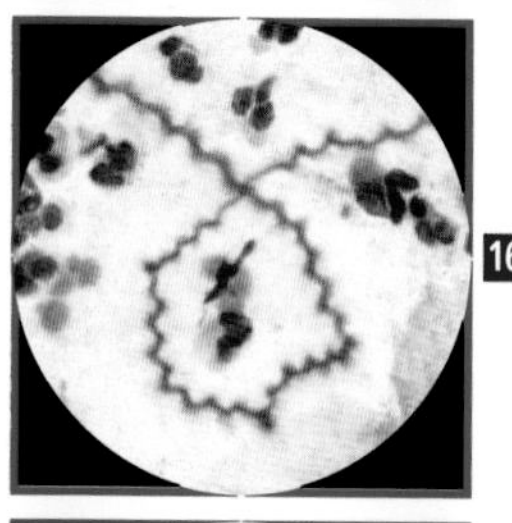

167

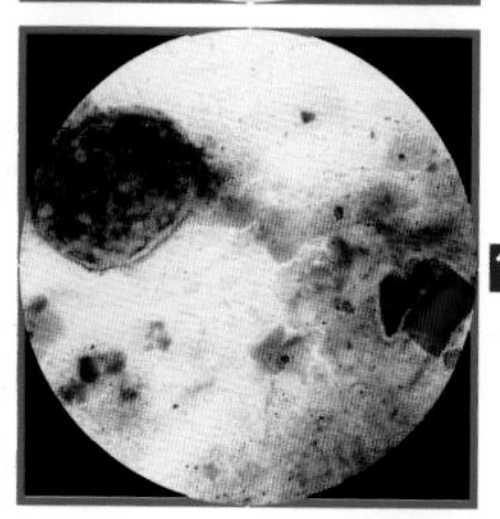

168

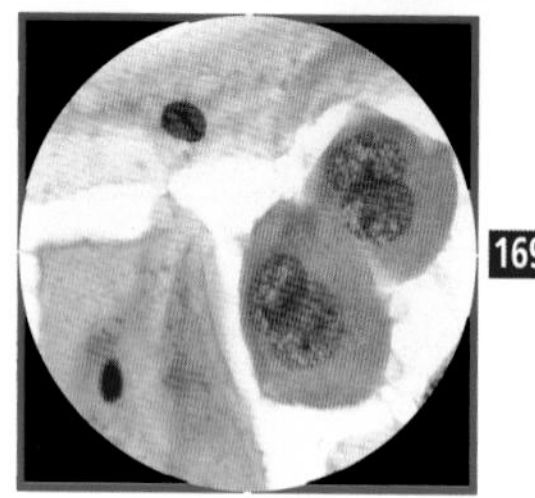

169

Curschmann's Spirals

Although much more commonly found in sputum, Curschmann's spirals occur, rarely, in the Pap smear [167 I6.150]. Their formation seems to be an intrinsic property of the endocervical mucus itself, rather than a foreign contaminant of the female genital tract, and is not related to cigarette smoking [Bornstein 1987, Novak 1984].

Fistulae

Rectovaginal fistula [168 I6.69] is associated with tall, columnar colorectal cells, which may be reactive. Look for evidence of debris, bacteria (especially *Escherichia coli*), digested food, etc, in the background [Angeles 1994]. (Note: Benign reactive cells may be "overdiagnosed" as carcinoma.)

Vesicovaginal fistula [169 I6.70] is associated with umbrella and other transitional cells. There may be watery discharge.

Neovagina

Sections of colon or skin grafts are sometimes used in constructing a vagina in patients with congenital absence or surgical removal, or in male-to-female transsexuals. The cytologic features after skin graft operation show a strong resemblance to the normal vaginal epithelium [Lelle 1990], but after colonic graft, colonic epithelium is seen [I6.68]. Rarely, "colitis" or neoplasia (squamous or glandular, depending on the type of graft) can occur in the graft [Munkarah 1994, Toolenaar 1993]. Thus, regular cytologic examinations are suggested.

Seminal Vesicle Cells and Sperm

Seminal Vesicle Cells: These are large "ugly" cells, with big, hyperchromatic (polyploid) nuclei that can mimic high-grade malignancy such as poorly differentiated adenocarcinoma. Cytoplasmic pigment may suggest metastatic melanoma. The cells are often degenerated or

Clues to Proper Diagnosis of Seminal Vesicle Cells

Clinical: Older male partner
Cells: Often degenerated, necrotic
Cytoplasm: Lipochrome pigment*; differential diagnosis is melanoma
Nuclei: Often smudgy chromatin
Background: Sperm,* corpora amylacea

[Meisels 1976b]
* Best clues.

necrotic. The presence of cytoplasmic lipochrome pigment and sperm in the vicinity are the two best clues to benign diagnosis [170 I6.146].

Sperm: Spermatozoa [171 I6.148] decrease in number over a period of a few days after intercourse, are found irregularly after the seventh day, and rarely after the tenth postcoital day, although they may remain for more than 3 weeks, perhaps even a few months, in rare cases. Sperm can be detected in roughly half the cases within 3 days of coitus (range, 28%–56%) [Costa 1991c, Randall 1987, Silverman 1978]. The percentage of sperm with tails does not correlate significantly with time. Douching, pregnancy, oral contraceptives, coitus interruptus, condoms, and vasectomy are associated with reduced prevalence of spermatozoa in smears [Silverman 1978]. Cytologic study can add to the criminal investigation of rape cases by detecting spermatozoa [Costa 1991c].

Psammoma Bodies

These are rarely found in the Pap smear: estimated at approximately 1 in 30,000 cases [172 I6.57] [Kern 1991a]. Psammoma bodies can be associated with either benign or malignant conditions, in a proportion of roughly one to two [Kern 1991a]. Associated benign conditions include intrauterine contraceptive device [Barter 1987, Gupta 1982, Highman 1971], ovarian inclusion cysts, tuberculous endometritis [Jenkins 1977], tubo-ovarian adhesions, endosalpingiosis [Hallman 1991], birth control pills [Valicenti 1977], and other benign endometrial and ovarian lesions [Kanbour 1980, Luzzatto 1981, Picoff 1970]. Associated malignant conditions include ovarian carcinoma (particularly papillary serous carcinoma) [Beyer-Boon 1974, Differding 1967, Fujimoto 1982, Jenkins 1977], endometrial malignancies [Fujimoto 1982, Hidvegi 1982, Spjut 1964], neuroendocrine carcinoma of the cervix, fallopian tube carcinoma, and metastases [Fugimoto 1982, Kern 1991a].

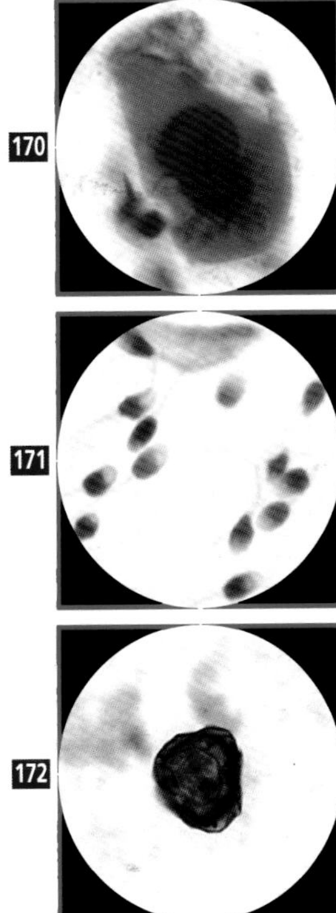
170
171
172

V. Clinical Considerations

The Pap smear is an imperfect test. Yet, because it has the ability to detect treatable precursor lesions, introduction of the Pap smear into clinical practice has correlated with a remarkable reduction in the morbidity and mortality of squamous cell carcinoma of the uterine cervix [Christopherson 1970a,1970b,1976,1977b, J Dunn 1981, Koss 1989a]. Precursor lesions, as previously discussed, are increasing in incidence: millions of women have squamous intraepithelial lesions, but relatively few develop cervical cancer. Colposcopy and therapy are already costing billions of dollars in the United States alone [Herbst 1992, Kurman 1994]. So, there is a real dilemma: the risk of not treating all lesions vs the cost and morbidity of such therapy for all patients. Recently, the management of precursor lesions has been complicated by new diagnostic terminology (ie, the Bethesda System), new outpatient therapeutic and screening procedures (such as loop electrosurgical excision procedure, viral testing, and cervicography), and recognition of human papilloma virus as a significant risk factor for cervical neoplasia [Kurman 1994].

Clinical Management

Under ideal conditions, there are four steps to clinical management of dysplasia (ie, cervical intraepithelial neoplasia/squamous intraepithelial lesion), which can be summarized as the four D's: detect, delineate, diagnose, and destroy. The prime objective is to rule out the presence of invasive disease [Creasman 1981]. Once this has been accomplished, the remaining objectives are to determine the grade and distribution of the intraepithelial lesion [ACOG 1993].

4 D's of Clinical Management of Dysplasia

- Detect (cytology)
- Delineate (colposcopy)
- Diagnose (histology)
- Destroy (cryosurgery, laser, etc)

Detection

The first step is detection of the precursor lesion, which is identified by the cytologist in the Pap smear. Of fundamental importance is procuring an adequate sample of well-preserved cells. Cytology provides little or no information about the exact location or extent of the disease (although with the use of the "VCE" slide [Wied 1959], some guidance may be given). Once a precursor lesion has been detected by cytology, the next step is delineation of the extent of the lesion by colposcopic examination of the cervix [Benedet 1992]. Note that Pap smears repeated at the time of colposcopy have a significant false-negative rate [Beeby 1993].

Delineation

The stromal changes, often neglected in microscopy, are of primary importance in colposcopy. In concert with the epithelial changes, angiogenesis occurs in the stroma. These new blood vessels produce punctation (vessels grow vertically toward surface), mosaicism (vascular proliferation and interconnections), and abnormal vessels (neovascularization, associated with invasive cancer), which are important diagnostic features that can be seen with the colposcope. The vessels supply oxygen and nutrients for neoplastic growth. The stroma probably produces the basement membrane and definitely the vessels. White epithelium corresponds to surface keratosis and hypergranulosis (spiegelosis [173 I6.34]).

The goal is outpatient treatment, avoiding hospitalization, if possible. If the *entire* lesion can be seen at colposcopy *and* there is no cytologic or colposcopic evidence of invasion *and* this is confirmed by tissue biopsy (ie, diagnosed), then the lesion can be destroyed on an outpatient basis by cryotherapy, laser ablation, or even by a thorough biopsy resection. Ablation without histologic confirmation of the diagnosis is considered unacceptable [Kurman 1994].

Histologic biopsies include colposcopically directed biopsy, endocervical curettage, and conization biopsy. Using directed biopsy, samples of abnormal areas are obtained under direct visualization during colposcopy. Endocervical curettage is used to detect disease in the endocervical canal, but may inadvertently pick up a lesion on the ectocervix, near the external os, resulting in a false-positive curettage. Some clinicians view a good cytologic sample of the endocervix using an endocervical brush as an alternative to curettage. Cone biopsy can be obtained by surgery (so-called cold knife cone) or laser; more recently, loop electrocautery has become popular. The loop procedure (aka LEEP, for loop electrosurgical excision procedure, or LLETZ for large loop excision transformation zone) can be performed on an outpatient basis to destroy and diagnose cervical abnormalities detected by Pap smear. With this procedure, the abnormal area is entirely excised (if possible) under colposcopic guidance, and the diagnosis is subsequently rendered on the removed tissue. The disadvantages include "cautery artifact," which interferes with histologic interpretation. Also, there is a fear that this procedure will be overutilized because of its simplicity. Routine electroexcision of the transformation zone or of nonstaining areas to evaluate an abnormal Pap smear diagnosed as low-grade squamous intraepithelial lesion or atypical squamous cells of undetermined significance is not recommended [Kurman 1994]. Colposcopy has reduced the incidence of conization to about 5% to 20% of patients with abnormal cytology [ACOG 1993]. However, if the colposcopy is inadequate, a cone biopsy will likely be required [Richart 1981b]. On the other hand, since many low-grade squamous intraepithelial lesions will spontaneously regress, close follow-up, without cone biopsy, may be appropriate for reliable patients [Kurman 1994].

Indications for Cone Biopsy

Inadequate colposcopy
- No lesion seen
- Lesion seen, but limits not seen
- Entire transformation zone not visualized

Marked disparity between cytology and histology, particularly if cytology suggests invasion and histology does not confirm

Marked disparity between colposcopy and histology; colposcopy suggests invasion, histology does not confirm

Biopsy suggests microinvasion; perform cone biopsy to confirm

Endocervical curettage shows SIL or microinvasive carcinoma

Cytologic or histologic evidence of glandular lesion

Patient unreliable

173

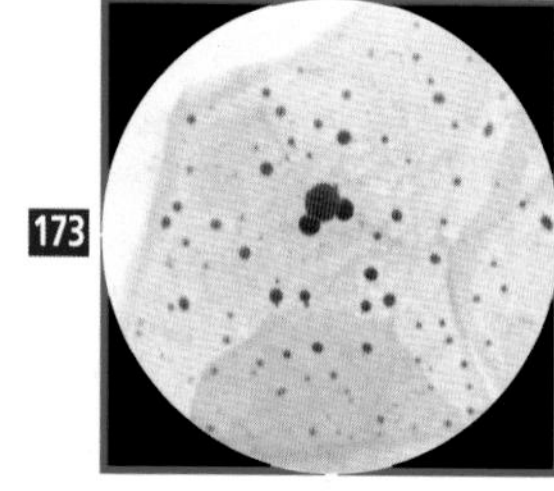

The chances of missing an invasive cancer during colposcopy are more importantly related to the size and complexity of the lesion than the lesion's grade. Similarly, the therapeutic failure rate may be more closely related to the size of the lesion than its grade [Richart 1980]. Some believe that a large CIN I may be more significant than a small CIN III (this being part of the reason for the introduction of the CIN terminology). However, the lesion's size and its grade are usually directly related (ie, large lesions tend to be high grade and small lesions tend to be low grade). The rate of recurrence of adequately treated cervical intraepithelial neoplasia is similar to the incidence rate in a high-risk population [Richart 1980].

Screening

Lack of Pap smear screening is a significant risk factor for the development of cervical cancer [Acs 1989, Brinton 1987, Christopherson 1976, Herrero 1992, CJ Jones 1990, LaVecchia 1987]. With screening, the lifetime risk of developing cervical cancer is about 0.7%; without screening it is 2.5% [Eddy 1990]. Women without a recent Pap smear (more than 10 years) may have up to a 12-fold increase in the risk of developing cervical cancer compared with regularly screened women [Shy 1989].

While the need for Pap smear screening is undisputed, the interval between screenings has been controversial [Foltz 1978, Green 1978, Marx 1979, Walton 1976,1982]. Traditionally, an annual Pap smear has been the standard of practice. However, recently, increasing the interval to 2 or even 3 years has been recommended, largely from a cost-effectiveness point of view. There are several problems with this recommendation. First of all, rapid onset cancers probably occur. Also, Pap smears have unknown, but probably high, false-negative rates, including both sampling and interpretation errors, which are very variable among providers [Eddy 1990, Koss 1989a, Richart 1981a]. Thus, some patients who actually have cervical lesions will be falsely reassured by "negative" Pap smears, and possibly lost to follow-up for a significant time. Furthermore, a key element not to be overlooked is that the lengthened interval between screenings should only be considered for low-risk patients. Because sexual histories are notoriously unreliable and difficult to obtain, it may cost more in terms of time and money to do an in-depth interview to get this history than to simply take a Pap smear [T6.36].

Low-risk patients are virgins, patients with hysterectomies, or patients in a long-term monogamous relationship with a long history of negative Pap smears. Patients considered to be *at risk* (or moderate risk) include sexually active women, who began having intercourse after 20 years of age and have had no more than two partners. *High-risk* patients are defined as women who began having intercourse before 20 years of age or who have had more than two partners (in a lifetime) [Richart 1981a]. Another consideration is the number of coital partners of the male [Brinton 1989b]. With the "sexual revolution," there may be relatively few

T6.36 **Procedure for Taking a Pap Smear**

Smear should be taken before the bimanual examination and before other tests, eg, for gonococcus and *Chlamydia*.

1. Instruct patient not to douche or use any type of lubricant, and refrain from intercourse for 24 hours prior to obtaining the smear.
2. Use speculum lubricated only with warm water.
3. Cervix and adjacent vagina should be well visualized.
4. Sample endocervix and ectocervix separately.
   A. Cervix: Rotate spatula with good pressure over entire ectocervix.
   B. Endocervix: Recommend endocervical brush, rotate 1/4 to 1/2 turn (can substitute cervical "broom" for A and B)
5. Spread material thinly, but rapidly, on labeled glass slide(s) and fix immediately (<10 seconds) either by immersion (95% ethanol) or with a commercial spray fixative (held at least 10 inches from slide to prevent cellular distortion). Rapid fixation is crucial to providing an adequate specimen for proper evaluation of the Pap smear.
6. Particularly in older women, some method of detecting endometrial disease, such as vaginal pool specimen or cervical canal aspiration, should be included.

[ACOG 1993, Lundberg 1989]

women who are not at risk or at high risk [Noller 1987]. Other important risk factors include history of atypical squamous cells of undetermined significance/squamous intraepithelial lesions, sexually transmitted diseases including human papilloma virus infection, immunosuppression including human immunodeficiency virus infection, and smoking.

The current recommendation is for all women who have been sexually active or have reached 18 years of age to have an annual Pap test. After a woman has had three or more consecutive, satisfactory, normal annual examinations, the test may be performed less frequently at the discretion of her physician.

This recommendation is endorsed by the American Cancer Society, the American College of Obstetricians and Gynecologists, the American Cancer Society, and the American Medical Association, as well as a number of other medical societies [ACOG 1993, Averette 1993, Mettlin 1991]. Patients at high risk should be screened more often. Annual examinations should be considered for all women past 65 years of age.

Most doctors will probably continue to recommend annual Pap smears. Even when annual examinations are recommended, as few as 25% return for a repeat smear in the second year [Wied 1981]. The yearly Pap smear is a major stimulus for women to have an annual physical examination, including other important procedures (eg, breast examination). Thus, an extra benefit of screening is increased detection of other cancers, including nongenital sites [Koss 1984]. Also, the Pap smear is capable of diagnosing a wide range of conditions beyond dysplasia, eg, facilitating the diagnosis of various infections. The false-negative rate has now been widely publicized and, since some cancers possibly develop rapidly, there is the threat of litigation by a patient who develops a cancer when an increased interval was recommended to her. Combining cytology and colposcopy helps reduce the problem of false-negative results [Lozowski 1982]. And finally, with regard to increasing the time interval between smears, there is a feeling among many that "if it ain't broke, don't fix it." It could, of course, take years to see the negative impact of tampering with the Pap smear interval.

Failure of the Pap Smear

No other test ever invented has been as successful as the Pap smear in eradicating cancer. Yet, in the past few years, the Pap smear has gotten a lot of bad press—some deserved, some not [Bedrossian 1994, Bogdanich 1987a,b, Koss 1989a, Wang 1994]. Because of its outstanding success in cancer prevention, expectations regarding the Pap smear's ability to detect premalignant lesions have now been raised so high that any result short of perfection is likely to be considered malpractice (and in an ominous development, possibly even reckless homicide) [Austin 1994b, Carr 1994, Koss 1978,1993a, P Martin 1972, Robb 1993]. Unfortunately, *the Pap smear is not a perfect test.*

In theory, cervical carcinoma is preceded by a long prodrome of preinvasive disease that can be detected and treated, which should make it possible to prevent this cancer [Briggs 1979, Walton 1976,1982]. In practice, although a remarkable reduction in cervical cancer has in fact occurred, this disease has never been completely eradicated in any population ever reported, even in the most thoroughly screened communities [J Carmichael 1984, J Dunn 1981, Fidler 1968, Koss 1989a,1993a, P Martin 1972, Rylander 1976, Walton 1982]. In the United States, despite half a century of screening, with an estimated 50,000,000 Pap smears now performed yearly [Austin 1993], 15,800 women are still expected to get cervical cancer, and 4,800 die of it, annually [Wingo 1995]. Moreover, cervical carcinoma remains a leading cause of cancer-related deaths in many countries [Parkin 1988]. Thus, in the real world, the goal of completely conquering cervical carcinoma is probably impossible to achieve through Pap smear screening. Why?

There is a chain of events that cannot be broken in order for the screening process to work in cancer prevention. First, the patient must come in for the test. Then, the clinician must take an adequate, representative, well-prepared Pap smear. Next, the cytologist must correctly identify any neoplastic lesion in the Pap smear. Then, the results must go back to the clinician, who must act appropriately on the results. And finally, the patient must present herself either for therapy or her next Pap smear.

Although the Pap smear can fail at many levels, ironically, the single most important error is failure of women to get Pap smears in the first place [P Martin 1972, Mitchell 1993b, Slater 1994]. This can be because a woman—for whatever reason—fails to visit a health care provider or because the provider fails to obtain a Pap smear. Unfortunately, other clinical errors, such as failure to follow up abnormal results, failure to perform a biopsy of suspicious lesions, and failure to investigate the patient's symptoms, are also important factors in failure of prevention of cervical cancer morbidity and mortality. In addition, some cancers may progress so rapidly that they develop between screenings.

Of course, problems in diagnosis also occur (discussed in more detail below). However, many, if not most, diagnostic problems relate to sampling errors, ie, few or no abnormal cells present on the glass slide, rather than errors of interpretation ("no cells, no diagnosis") [Dehner 1993, DiBonito 1993, Dodd 1993, Gay 1985, Husain 1974, M Joseph 1991, Joste 1995, Kristensen 1991, Lundberg 1989, Mobiüs 1993, Rohr 1990, Vooijs 1985]. Given that a woman has a serious lesion, the Pap smear can detect it in 90% to 95% of cases. If we were to grade this test, it would get an "A." Nevertheless, it should be clearly understood, by clinicians and the general public alike, that no cytology laboratory is completely free of diagnostic errors, the most important being false-negative results. False-negative results occur at a low, but well-documented and probably irreducible rate of at least 5% to 10%, ie, at least 1 in 10 to 20 positive cases will be missed in routine screening, even in the finest laboratories [Austin 1994a,b, Beilby 1982, Bonfiglio 1993, Boon 1993, Bosch 1992, J Carmichael 1984, Cecchini 1985, D Collins 1986, Coppleson 1974, Davey 1993, J Davis 1981, Davison 1994, Dehner 1993, Derman 1981, Fidler 1968, Gay 1985, Grosskopf 1978, Husain 1974, Janerich 1995, B Jones 1993, S Jordan 1981, Kierkegaard 1994, Klinkhamer 1988, Koss 1989a,b,1993a,b, Krieger 1994, Mitchell 1988, Plott 1987, Richart 1964a,1965b, Robb 1993, Sedlis 1974, Seybolt 1971, Shingleton 1975, Shulman 1974, Soost 1991, Syrjänen 1992, Tabbara 1993, Tuncer 1967, van der Graaf 1987b, Wied 1981, Yobs 1985, Yule 1972]. Simultaneously obtained, duplicate smears indicate a false-negative rate of at least 20%, including sampling and interpretation errors [Beilby 1982, J Davis 1981, Luthy 1978, Sedlis 1974, Shulman 1975]. Even when patients are part of a study group, and the smears are taken with great care and thoroughness and screened with exceptional attention, false-negative results still occur [Richart 1964a]. When the prior "negative" Pap smears are reviewed following a "positive" diagnosis, abnormal cells are in fact present, on average, in nearly half of cases [T6.37] [Allen 1994, Attwood 1985, Berkeley 1980, Berkowitz 1979, DiBonito 1993, Dodd 1993, Gay 1985, Hatem 1993, Husain 1974, Koss 1993a, Kristensen 1991, Liu 1967, LiVolsi 1984, Lundberg 1989, Macgregor 1993, Mitchell 1990b, Morell 1982, Pairwuti 1991, Paterson 1984, R Peters 1988, Richart 1964a, J Robertson 1993,1994, Rylander 1976,1977, Sherman 1992a, Slater 1994, van der Graaf 1987a,b, Wain 1992, Walker 1983]. In many cases, the mistakes may seem to be obvious errors on review in the "retrospectoscope" [Bosch 1992, J Robertson 1993,1994]. However, most patients with false-negative results only appear to have "negative" smears, when in reality many specimens were of limited adequacy (transformation zone not sampled, obscured by exudate, etc) or entirely unsatisfactory for evaluation [Fetherston 1983, Mitchell 1990b, Sherman 1992a].

Although the false-negative *rate* (false negatives compared with all positives, basically a quality assurance statistic [Lundberg 1989]) may seem alarmingly high, patients should be reassured that the vast majority of *all* negative results are truly negative [Anderson 1987, Austin 1994b, Lundberg 1989]. No one ever died of cervical dysplasia or carcinoma in situ. Even invasive carcinoma is rarely lethal when caught early (especially when microinvasive). Of clinical importance is that as many as 9 of 10 patients with a false-negative Pap smear have a history of abnormal Pap smears, although multiple or recent "negatives" do not completely exclude a serious lesion [Figge 1970, Hatem 1993, Hopkins 1991, Mitchell 1990b, Paterson 1984, Sherman 1992a, Shulman 1974, Wain 1992]. In addition, most patients have well-defined risk factors, and those with frank cancer are frequently symptomatic or have visible cervical lesions; yet too often, appropriate follow-up is not undertaken [Fetherston 1983, Frable 1994, Liu 1967, P Martin 1972, Pretorius 1991, Schwartz 1988, Tuncer 1967].

T6.37* False-Negative Results in the Pap Smear

Study	Interval Preceding Positive Diagnosis	No. of Negative Smears Reviewed	No. (%) Reclassified as Abnormal
Tuncer 1967	Unknown	7	6 (85.7%)
P Martin 1972	Within 1 yr	13	10 (76.9%)
Hatem 1993	Averaged 9.3 mo	17	13 (76.5%)
Attwood 1985	Within 5 yr	28	20 (71.4%)
J Robertson 1993	Up to 12 yr	139	92 (66.2%)
Rylander 1977	4 to 5 yr	56	35 (62.5%)
Berkowitz 1979	Within 2 yr	13	8 (61.5%)
Pairwuti 1991	Unknown	70	43 (61.4%)
Paterson 1984	Within 10 yr	58	34 (58.6%)
Mitchell 1990b	Within 36 mo	136	75 (55.1%)
van der Graaf 1987b	3 yr	226	121 (53.5%)
Wain 1992	Within 2 yr	30	16 (53.3%)
Sherman 1992a	Median 93.5 mo	123	65 (52.8%)
LiVolsi 1984	Within 1 yr	10	5 (50.0%)
Kristensen 1991	Within 3 yr	96	39 (40.6%)
Gay 1985	Within 1 yr	63	24 (38.1%)
Husain 1974	3 mn	25	9 (36.0%)
Dodd 1993	Unknown	153	55 (35.9%)
DiBonito 1993	Unknown	59	21 (35.6%)
R Peters 1988	Within 3 yr	32	10 (31.3%)
Walker 1983	Within 5 yr	11	3 (27.3%)
Schwartz 1988†	6 to 17 mo	22	5 (22.7%)
Slater 1994	1 to 8 yr	17	3 (17.6%)
Allen 1994	75% within 2 yr	80	12 (15.0%)
Morell 1982	Within 3 yr	36	2 (5.6%)
Liu 1967	3.4 yr	16	0 (0.0%)
Richart 1964a	Unknown	9	0 (0.0%)
Total		1545	726 (47.0%)

* On average, nearly half of cases (47%) actually had abnormal cells on review. Many of the other cases were actually unsatisfactory or limited, rather than negative. A few cases may represent rapidly progressive cancers.
† Includes 10 cases from a previous report [Berkeley 1980].

Clinically, many patients have a lapse in screening of 2 or more years [Sherman 1992a]. False-negative results may be more common in younger patients [Paterson 1984, Rylander 1977] and with more serious lesions [Benoit 1984, Berkeley 1980, Berkowitz 1979, Richart 1965b, Rubio 1981b, Tuncer 1967, van der Graaf 1987b].

False-positive results also occur, but are of less concern because abnormal Pap smear results should always be confirmed histologically before therapy (ablation, major surgery, radiation, etc) is undertaken [Koss 1989a,1993b, Kurman 1994]. The false-positive rate for a diagnosis of invasive carcinoma or high-grade dysplasia is probably on the order of 1% to 10%, respectively [Eddy 1990, Yobs 1987]. True false-positive results are usually due to interpretation errors, eg, overinterpretation of changes due to radiation, inflammation, repair, degeneration, florid squamous metaplasia, etc [Davey 1993, Dodd 1993, Koss 1993b, Sidawy 1994]. However, apparent false-positive results can also occur, ie, "false false positives." For example, a false false positive could occur if the Pap smear correctly identifies a lesion, but it subsequently regresses before colposcopic or biopsy confirmation [Eddy 1990, Husain 1974]. The spontaneous regression rate for dysplasia diagnosed cytologically is significant: as high as 60% [Campion 1986, Eddy 1990, Fox 1967, Macgregor 1978, Richart 1969, J Robertson 1988]. False false positive cytology could also represent sampling error on the part of the biopsy; this is more likely if the biopsy is scant or the lesion is small or inaccessible [Frost 1969, Husain 1974, Nichols 1968, Sidawy 1994]. Squamous precursor lesions of the cervix, especially when high grade (CIN III), can be easily wiped off, inadvertently, in sterile preparation of the biopsy site, dilatation and curettage preceding biopsy, or rough handling of the excised tissue [Frost 1969]. Rarely, even the minimal trauma of taking the Pap smear itself can remove the dysplastic epithelium [Berner 1980]. Also, an apparent overinterpretation or "false positive" of the Pap smear may actually represent underinterpretation or misdiagnosis of the histology [Dodd 1993, Hellberg 1994, P Martin 1972, Seybolt 1971]. Colposcopy, too, has a significant false-negative rate, which could result in an apparently false-positive Pap smear [Hellberg 1994]. Of clinical importance is that a substantial number of patients with apparently false-positive Pap smears will eventually show significant lesions on further follow-up [Dodd 1993].

Factors Related to Failure of Pap Smear Screening

Reasons for failure of the Pap smear in cervical cancer prevention are discussed in more detail below. In a way, the Pap smear has been a victim of its own success, ie, because the prevalence of cervical cancer has fallen so precipitously, the predictive value is diminished, irrespective of the sensitivity and specificity of the test itself.

Factors related to failure of the Pap smear in cervical cancer prevention can be divided into five groups: (1) patient, (2) clinician, (3) instrument and smear, (4) cytopreparation and diagnosis, and (5) the lesion. These factors are, of course, interrelated.

Patient-Related Errors

The largest group of problems related to failure of Pap smear screening are patient-related errors, including failure of women to get an annual Pap examination or even to get any health examination at all [J Carmichael 1984, Janerich 1995, Koss 1989a, Macgregor 1993, P Martin 1972, Wied 1981, S Wilson 1992]. Twenty-five percent of all women 18 years of age and older, with an intact cervix, have not had a Pap smear in the past 3 years, and 10% have never had a Pap smear [Pretorius 1991, USHHS]. These figures are even higher among poor, poorly educated, or older women [USHHS]. Failure to get Pap smears can be due to a wide variety of reasons, ranging from inability to pay to distrust of doctors [P Martin 1972]. Some women are unaware of the importance of the Pap smear and 1 in 25 has never even heard of the test [NCHS 1987, USHHS]. In some cases, patients simply refuse a Pap smear, even when it is offered to them [P Martin 1972]. (Clinicians may also fail to offer the test—read on.)

In an unpublished study from the University of Chicago, of 500 patients with squamous cell carcinoma of the cervix, 387 had not had a Pap smear within the previous 10 years and an additional 63 had not had one in the previous 5 years (total = 450/500 cancer patients without a Pap smear in at least 5 years) [Wied 1995]. Of the remaining 50 patients, 42 had "positive" Pap smears, but did not return for therapy. Therefore, 492 of the 500 (>98%) cases of invasive carcinoma could be considered patient-related errors. Of the remaining 8 patients, 3 had been treated for cervical intraepithelial neoplasia but developed invasive carcinoma later. In contrast, of another 500 patients with squamous cell carcinoma detected by the Pap smear, 453 were still alive at 10 years and only 3 had died of disease (the remaining 44 were lost to follow-up). Finally, of 1 million patients, about one half did not return at all during the 27 years of the study. And only 3% had more than six smears in the same period.

Other patient-related factors occur. For example, douching or coitus may mechanically remove the superficial cell layers that the Pap smear samples, resulting in false-negative smears due to sampling error [Rubio 1975b,1981b,1994]. Patients may also delay seeking medical attention even when they have symptoms that they know are suspicious, such as abnormal vaginal bleeding [P Martin 1972]. In addition, many things known to be important risk factors for cervical cancer (not to mention other diseases) are under the patient's control, such as smoking, age at first intercourse, number of sexual partners, and method of contraception [Averette 1993, Devesa 1989]. In fact, some evidence suggests that the risk of cervical cancer may be more closely related to sexual practices than to differences in screening [Kjaer 1989].

Clinical Errors

The next largest group of errors, unfortunately, comes from those who should "know better," the health care providers or clinicians [P Martin 1972]. Among the most common errors are failure to take a Pap smear at all [Koss 1989a, P Martin 1972, Mobius 1993, Slater 1994] or failure to take an adequate Pap smear (ie, a thinly spread, well-fixed smear containing an endocervical component when appropriate) [Attwood 1985, Mobius 1993, Rubio 1981b]. Obtaining a Pap smear is more complex than many health care providers appreciate [Koss 1989a, Nasca 1991]. The smear must be taken under direct visualization, with considerable pressure [Koss 1989a]. The speculum should not be lubricated with anything other than water [Fetherston 1983]. Rubbing, swabbing, or "cleaning" the cervix before taking the smear can remove the diagnostic cells, resulting in false-negative results [Rubio 1975b]. Well-trained health care providers take better smears; thus, false-negative results may be higher when students or untrained physicians take the smears [Brink 1989, Frost 1969, Husain 1974, Koss 1989a, Macgregor 1993, von Haam 1962]. Failure of the clinician to provide pertinent clinical data may compromise cytologic interpretation of the Pap smear [Koss 1993a, Wain 1992].

Other common clinical errors include failure to follow up abnormal Pap smear results, failure to perform a biopsy of suspicious lesions, and failure to investigate suspicious clinical symptoms [J Carmichael 1984, Koss 1989a, P Martin 1972, Mobius 1993, E Walker 1983]. Unfortunately, it also seems likely that some clinicians accept a negative report at face value, disregarding statements of specimen adequacy [Attwood 1985]. Miscellaneous problems, such as clerical errors, also occur [Attwood 1985, P Martin 1972].

Instrument and Smear Errors

The instrument used to obtain the Pap smear can also be a source of errors related to sampling [Rubio 1994]. It has been known for quite some time that the original Papanicolaou method of vaginal pool aspiration is much less efficient in obtaining cervicovaginal cells than the direct scrape method of Ayre [Ayre 1947, Richart 1965b, Wied 1955]. However, vaginal pool smears are more useful in detecting cancer cells from the endometrium, tubes, and ovaries, cancers which become increasingly common in women past 50 [Husain 1974, Koss 1984,1989a, Lundberg 1989]. An endocervical smear can be obtained by scrape, aspiration, or brush. The endocervical brush may be more sensitive, but less specific, than formal endocervical curettage for diagnosis [Hoffman 1993, Weitzman 1988].

The shape of the sampling device is important for obtaining an adequate sample, particularly of the endocervix. The material from which the sampling device is made is also important. Cotton swabs and wooden spatulas tend to trap cells so they never reach the slides [L Katz 1979, Rubio 1977a]. Smears taken by cotton swabs or with plastic spatulas render fewer atypical cells than do endocervical brushes [Rubio 1980a,b,c].

The manner in which the slides are made is also important, including the smearing technique (zigzag, back and forth, circular, etc) [Frost 1969, Rubio 1981c] and the pressure exerted while smearing [Rubio 1983]. In addition, once on the slide, the cells—"floaters"—may become detached during processing (possibly resulting in a false-negative result) and can even reattach to the wrong slide (possibly resulting in a false-positive result) [Rubio 1975a].

Sufficient numbers of cells must be collected and the sample must be representative, including the transformation zone. The smear must be thinly spread and immediately and properly fixed [Frost 1969]. Hair spray is not an acceptable fixative [Holm 1988]. Thick smears hamper or prevent microscopic examination, which may result in false-negative findings [Gay 1985, Rubio 1981b]. Air drying due to delayed fixation causes cellular artifacts that may make it impossible to recognize atypical cells [Frost 1969, Gay 1985, Husain 1974, Koss 1974, Richart 1964a, Rubio 1981b].

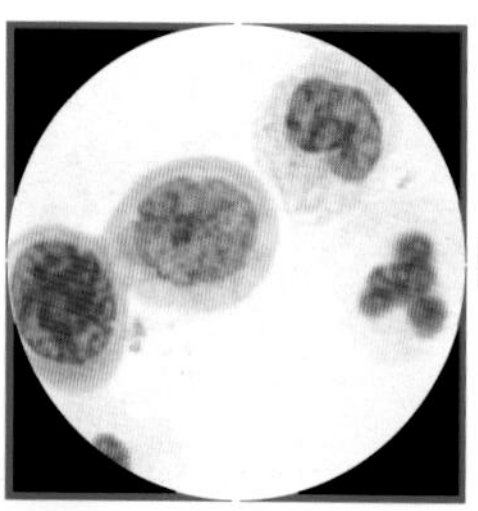
174

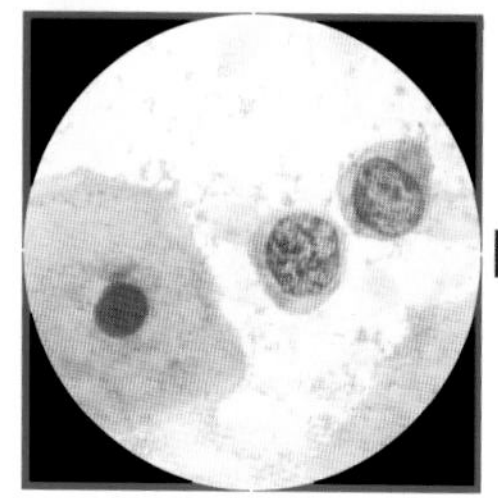
175

Cytopreparation and Diagnostic Errors

Errors in diagnosis can occur in relation to cytopreparation, screening, or interpretation, as well as to general laboratory problems, such as mislabeling slides [Morell 1982, Rubio 1975a]. The Papanicolaou stain must be carefully monitored to prevent staining artifacts that can make interpretation difficult or impossible. Also, as previously mentioned, stains can become contaminated with "floaters," which can lead to false diagnoses [Husain 1974, Rubio 1975a]. Therefore, fresh preparation or frequent filtration of the stains is necessary [Koss 1989a, Rubio 1981b]. Pap smears should be stained separately from nongynecologic specimens [Lundberg 1989].

There are several points to be considered in assessing screening errors, ie, failure to detect abnormal cells that are present on the slide. Three of the most important diagnostic problems relate to the presence of *few* abnormal cells, *small* abnormal cells, and *bland* abnormal cells [**174** I6.141, **175** I6.142] [Bosch 1992, Dressel 1992, Fetherston 1983, Hatem 1993, Koss 1978,1989a,1993a, Liu 1967, Pairwuti 1991, J Robertson 1993, Sherman 1992a, van der Graaf 1987a].

A Pap smear can have up to 500,000 cells. When abnormal cells are extremely sparse, they may be very difficult to detect by routine screening. In fact, the presence of fewer than 100 abnormal cells has been shown to be an important factor in false-negative diagnoses [Bosch 1992, Hatem 1993, Sherman 1992a]. Therefore, it may be that 100 abnormal cells represents a threshold below which detection is possible, but not reliable, by routine screening.

Paradoxically, low-grade lesions can be easier to detect than high-grade, serious lesions in the Pap smear. Low-grade lesions tend to occur on the portio vaginalis, where they are readily sampled, and have the biggest, "ugliest" nuclei, which are found in the largest (most mature) cells. Therefore, these low-grade abnormal cells tend to be not only numerous but conspicuous in the Pap smear. Most of these low-grade lesions are insignificant, and many of them will disappear on their own, even without treatment [Brown 1985, Montz 1992, Nasiell 1986, Patten 1978]. On the other hand, high-grade dysplasias are significant lesions that are more likely to progress to invasive cancer if undetected. Unfortunately, high-grade dysplasias tend to be hidden in the endocervical canal, where they may be difficult to sample and may be represented only by tiny cells with subtle cytologic abnormalities. Consequently, the small, bland cells may be sparse and difficult to detect in the first place, and then difficult to diagnose once detected [Bosch 1992, Hatem 1993, J Robertson 1993, Sherman 1992a]. These small cells have high N/C ratios and minimal chromatin abnormality, and may resemble ordinary immature metaplasia or even histiocytes [176 I6.87, 177 I6.141] [Bosch 1992, Dressel 1992, Hatem 1993, J Robertson 1993, Sherman 1992a]. A clue to the correct diagnosis is that high-grade dysplasia usually has irregular nuclear membranes, resulting in characteristic "raisinoid" nuclei. Another factor in misdiagnosis is that high-grade lesions are usually accompanied by a low-grade component in the smear. Thus, the large and conspicuous but low-grade cells may dominate the smear and obscure a smaller but more serious high-grade component [Jarmulowicz 1989]. In fact, 20% to 30% of cases suggestive of a low-grade lesion on Pap smear will show a high-grade lesion on biopsy [S Hall 1994, Jarmulowicz 1989, Koss 1993b, Montz 1992, J Robertson 1988, Rohr 1990, Soutter 1986, Tay 1987d, Tidbury 1992, E Walker 1986].

As with precancerous lesions, cancerous lesions can also exfoliate cells with bland cytologic features, making recognition difficult [178 I6.142] [Koss 1989a, Seybolt 1971]. At the other end of the diagnostic spectrum, accurately and reproducibly interpreting "atypical" smears may be impossible [Koss 1993b, Robb 1994, Seybolt 1971]. Unfortunately, in some cases, atypical squamous cells of undetermined significance may be the only identifiable cytologic abnormality during the early development of high-grade squamous intraepithelial lesions [Sherman 1992a].

Tissue fragments or hyperchromatic crowded groups (HCGs), as has been emphasized throughout the chapter, can also present difficult diagnostic problems, and are also documented sources of false diagnoses [Boon 1991, J Robertson 1993, Sherman 1992a]. Although hyperchromatic crowded groups are usually benign and include such entities as endometrial cells and severe atrophy [179 I6.133], they can also represent a variety of serious lesions, eg, carcinoma in situ [180 I6.137]. Look for disorderly arrangements of the cells ("loss of nuclear polarity," chaotic architecture [Boon 1993]), coarse, dark chromatin, and mitotic figures—features that suggest carcinoma. Another diagnostic clue: squamous carcinoma in situ is usually accompanied by squamous dysplasia. Other lesions, besides carcinoma in situ, that can present as hyperchromatic crowded groups include invasive squamous cell carcinoma and endocervical adenocarcinoma, in situ or invasive [Boon 1991]. At high-power magnification, hyperchromatic crowded groups of endocervical glandular neoplasia resemble hyperchromatic crowded groups of squamous carcinoma in situ, but have so-called feathery edges, well-defined microacini, and elongated, oval nuclei with coarse, dark chromatin.

Other problems in interpretation include inflammatory changes, regeneration/repair, radiation effect, and atrophy [J Robertson 1993, Seybolt 1971]. Another diagnostic error is rendering a negative diagnosis on unsatisfactory material [Berkowitz 1979, Gay 1985, P Martin 1972, Paterson 1984, Schwartz 1988, Slater 1994, van der Graaf 1987b, Wain 1992]. This problem is specifically addressed in the Bethesda System by requiring a statement, in every case, regarding specimen adequacy. Inadequate clinical information can also compromise cytologic interpretation [Koss 1993a, Wain 1992].

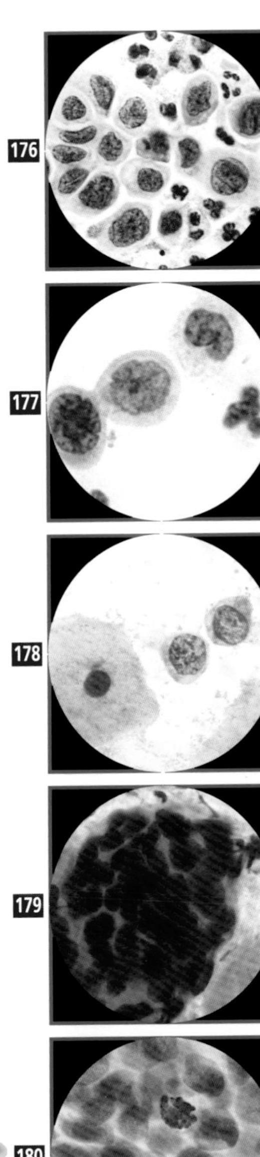

However, probably the single most important source of error in cytologic diagnosis is loss of concentration due to screener fatigue, rather than inability to diagnose abnormal cells [Husain 1974, Koss 1993a, Pairwuti 1991, J Robertson 1993]. Screening is like looking for a needle in a haystack. It is an extremely tedious and mentally demanding chore [Husain 1974, Koss 1989a]. Compounding the tedium of screening is that most smears have no abnormal cells (most haystacks have no needles). Sustaining attention (maintaining vigilance) is difficult, particularly when the screener expects relatively few abnormalities to be present [Fowkes 1986]. Screeners should have regular, short breaks, and it is best if they do not spend the entire day screening: it is better if they can spend part of the day on other duties [Husain 1974]. Screening has also been compared to proofreading, with misspelled words being analogous to abnormal cells. Most slides have on the order of 50,000 to 300,000 cells [Koss 1989a]. Imagine reading up to 100 books a day, each averaging more than 100,000 words, looking for a few spelling errors in an occasional manuscript.

There is also a class of cells that have been designated "litigation cells" [Austin 1994b, Frable 1994]. (And with the filing of criminal charges in cases of Pap smear misdiagnoses, these cells may well become known as "jail cells.") Litigation cells are important sources of false diagnoses, including both false-positive and false-negative readings [Frable 1994]. The clinical significance of litigation cells ranges from completely benign to frankly malignant. They can be found singly or in groups, including sheets or clusters. They are small, medium, or large cells, with low, intermediate, or high N/C ratios, smooth or irregular nuclear membranes, fine to coarse chromatin, which can range from pale to dark, and have inconspicuous to prominent nucleoli. The cytoplasm varies from squamoid to glandular, with smooth or irregular contours. The cells can be few or numerous, well preserved or degenerated, and obvious or obscured in the smear. Litigation cells can be mistaken for normal, reactive, or neoplastic cells, including, but not limited to, metaplasia, parakeratosis, repair, human papilloma virus effect, dysplasia, endometrial cells, tubal metaplasia, and squamous or adenocarcinoma. They are expensive cells [Frable 1994]. Found *prospectively*, they may lead to overdiagnosis in order to prevent false-negative results and potential litigation, or even criminal prosecution. Such defensive medicine often results in unnecessary colposcopy, biopsy, conization, and even hysterectomy—all at enormous expense [Frable 1994, TJ Kline 1994]. These procedures are already costing over a billion dollars annually [Herbst 1992]. Found *retrospectively*, in patients with "bad outcomes," litigation cells can cost as much as $750,000 *each* in malpractice judgments [Frable 1994]. When smears are reviewed for malpractice cases, experts cannot always agree on exactly which cells are abnormal, even though the same experts may testify that abnormal cells were present [Austin 1994b]. Ultimately, the idea that every cell in every Pap smear can always be accurately identified is just plain wrong.

Finally, to detemine that a cytologic diagnosis is false-negative, it is usually compared against the "gold standard" of histologic diagnosis. However, as we have seen, histologic examination is not error-free [DiBonito 1993, J Dunn 1981, Richart 1965b]. Few studies have examined the "gold standard" itself when evaluating apparant cytodiagnostic errors. One study that did, however, changed the histologic diagnosis in one of four cases [Dodd 1993]. Moreover, there is a body of evidence that competant pathologists cannot agree with each other—or even with themselves from day to day—on the classification of the tissue biopsies, let alone the smears [Cocker 1968, Holmquist 1967b, Husain 1974, Ismail 1989,1990, Koss 1978,1989a, Mitchell 1993b, Rohr 1990, Seybolt 1971, Siegler 1956, Willcox 1987, N Young 1994b].

How good a screener are you? There are three spelling errors in the preceding paragraph. Did you find all of them on the first reading? If you have to go back to look for them, it is akin to the "special case" kind of rescreening that is equivalent to proficiency testing or legal case review. A test in the normal screening (reading) environment is completely different from a test in which one has been previously alerted. In the normal screening situation, abnormal cells (or spelling errors) are more commonly missed than in a known testing situation. This is why one should be skeptical of the value (or honesty) of rescreening smears for proficiency testing (or legal reasons) [Bosch 1992, TJ Kline 1994]. Moreover, when cases are reviewed under such conditions, although the false-negative cases may be "caught," the false-positive rates and screening times soar, which seriously compromises laboratory efficiency and cannot help but increase health care costs [Bosch 1992].

Lesion-Related Errors

Certain problems in diagnosis relate to the lesion itself, some of which have been discussed in the previous section. For various reasons, some lesions fail to exfoliate cells in numbers sufficient for diagnosis [Husain 1974, P Martin 1972, R Peters 1988, Richart 1964a]. Small or inaccessible lesions (eg, high in the endocervix) may be difficult to sample adequately [P Martin 1972, Morell 1982, J Robertson 1993, Rylander 1977, Sherman 1992a]. False-negative cytology is more common with smaller lesions [Barton 1989b, Giles 1988, Jarmulowicz 1989]. Interestingly, the shape of the cell [Rubio 1981c] and the quality of the cervical mucus also affect the smear [Rubio 1983]. Unfortunately, smears are more often inadequate in patients with severe epithelial abnormalities [Benoit 1984, Berkeley 1980, Berkowitz 1979, Richart 1965b, Rubio 1981b, Tuncer 1967, van der Graaf 1987b]. Necrosis, inflammation, or bleeding may obscure, alter, or dilute the abnormal cells, making diagnosis difficult [Gay 1985, Husain 1974, Koss 1989a, Pairwuti 1991, J Robertson 1993, Rubio 1977b, Seybolt 1974, van der Graaf 1987a]. Consequently, the Pap smear may be less efficient in diagnosis of invasive carcinoma than of preinvasive disease, being falsely negative in up to 75% of cases of squamous cell carcinoma (average, ~50%) [Benoit 1984, Gay 1985, Gondos 1972, Husain 1974, Jafari 1978, Konikov 1969, Koss 1989b,1993a, Pairwuti 1991, Richart 1964a, Rubio 1981b, van der Graaf 1987a,b]. Certain types of tumors are known to be more difficult to detect or diagnose in the Pap smear, eg, adenocarcinoma, adenosquamous carcinoma, lymphoma, and sarcoma, leading to increased false-negative rates for these tumors [Benoit 1984, Bosch 1992, J Carmichael 1984, Gay 1985, Jafari 1978, Kristensen 1991, Liu 1967, P Martin 1972, Mitchell 1988,1993a, Rylander 1977, Schwartz 1988, Wain 1992]. Some tumors (eg, verrucous carcinoma, adenoma malignum) are composed of normal, or nearly normal-appearing cells, making interpretation problematic.

Cytologic Factors in False-Negative Diagnosis

Few cells: <100 abnormal cells
Small cells: Difficult to spot ("no-see-ums")
Bland cells: Difficult to interpret (differential diagnosis: immature metaplasia, histiocytes)
Hyperchromatic crowded groups (HCGs): Atrophy, glandular cells, etc, vs tumor
Certain tumor types: Adenocarcinoma, lymphoma, sarcoma, etc
Obscuration of smear: Excess exudate, blood, air drying, degeneration, etc
Inadequate patient information

Pap smears repeated within a short time (up to several weeks) have a particularly high false-negative rate, up to 60%, even when carefully obtained at the time of colposcopy [D Jones 1987, Koss 1989a, Nyirjesy 1972, Wheelock 1989]. Apparently it takes the lesion a relatively long time to regenerate sufficient diagnostic cells for the smear. A "negative" following a "positive" diagnosis can mislead the clinician into thinking the lesion has regressed or the previous positive report was wrong. It is also possible that some tumors progress so rapidly that they develop in between Pap smear screenings [Adcock 1982, Albert 1981, Ashley 1966a,b, Bain 1983, Bamford 1983, Benoit 1984, Berkeley 1980, J Dunn 1967,1981, Fetherston 1983, Fidler 1968, Figge 1970, Fox 1968, Hadjimichael 1989, Hammond 1968, M Jordan 1964, Laskey 1979, Liu 1967, LiVolsi 1984, Macgregor 1982, P Martin 1972, Mitchell 1990b, Paterson 1984, Pedersen 1971, R Peters 1988, Prendiville 1980, Sandmire 1976, Schwartz 1988].

Toward a Practice Standard

A zero screening error is an impossible standard of practice. It is both unreasonable and unachievable [Austin 1994b, Bosch 1992, Carr 1994, Koss 1989a, Robb 1993,1994, Valente 1994a]. Unfortunately, however, acceptable practice standards have not been well defined in cytology [Dehner 1993]. Therefore, the following proposal is made. A screening error rate (false-negative fraction) of 5% to 10% may be an admirable goal and below 15% to 20% a possible standard for Pap smear accuracy [Austin 1994b, J Carmichael 1984, Koss 1993a, Krieger 1994]. Errors must be judged not as individual cases but in the context of overall laboratory performance. The definition of an acceptable screening error rate is not meant to condone sloppy work or incompetence, but rather to acknowledge the reality of significant errors by competent, conscientious cytologists [Carr 1994].

Although it is a common assumption that screening errors are usually the result of professional incompetence, poor supervision, inadequate continuing education, or excessive number of smears, this is not the case in most accredited laboratories. *Most diagnostic errors occur because screeners are human and humans make mistakes*. This fact cannot be remedied by rules and regulations. Moreover, the ability of the Pap smear to prevent cervical cancer is inversely related to its cost [Austin 1994b, Helfand 1992]. Quality assurance measures, including automated screening systems [Boon 1993, Koss 1994, Ouwerkerk-Noordam 1994], take time and cost money [Austin 1991, Davila 1994, Koss 1993a]. Therefore, paradoxically, well-intentioned efforts by the "cytobureaucracy" to reduce the false-negative rate might actually *increase* the number of invasive cancers by reducing access to this lifesaving test for the very women (low-income, high-risk) who are most likely to benefit from it [Austin 1994a]. More women develop cervical cancer related to failure to get regular Pap smears than to errors in cytodiagnosis [Attwood 1985, J Carmichael 1984, E Clarke 1979, Janerich 1995, P Martin 1972, Mobius 1993, Morell 1982, Nasca 1991, Paterson 1984, M Quinn 1989, Tuncer 1967, E Walker 1983, S Wilson 1992]. It may be that keeping the price of the Pap smear low, encouraging more frequent Pap smears, casting the screening net wider to encompass as many women at risk as possible, and/or public education regarding the importance of the Pap smear are more cost-effective than some of the other quality assurance measures [Bachner 1991, Benedet 1992, Helfand 1992, Holland 1993, Sherlaw-Johnson 1994, M Quinn 1989]. The value of regulatory proficiency testing in particular has been questioned [Austin 1994a, Bachner 1991, Bosch 1992, CL Collins 1994]. In fact, some evidence suggests that such regulations cause more harm than good [Austin 1991,1994a]. Because regulatory policies directly affect health care, perhaps they should be subjected to the same standards required of medical tests and pharmaceuticals, such as proof of efficacy, safety, etc [Helfand 1992].

Summary and Conclusions

The Pap smear is only a screening test [Robb 1993]. Although the Pap smear is a critical component in cancer detection, it is not the only important component [Koss 1989a]. Clinicians must guard against a false sense of security generated by negative Pap smear results [Ashley 1966a, Berkowitz 1979, Koss 1989a, P Martin 1972, Schwartz 1988, Sherman 1992a]. A "negative" report does not guarantee the absence of cervical cancer [Hadjimichael 1989, P Martin 1972, Schwartz 1988]. The Pap smear is not a replacement for careful clinical evaluation [Berkowitz 1979]. The clinician must decide whether to follow or treat the patient according to the clinical findings and level of risk for disease [Robb 1993]. A biopsy must be taken of suspicious visible lesions, and clinical symptoms cannot be ignored, even if the Pap smear is completely normal. The Pap smear is not nearly as good a screening test for glandular cancers of the female genital tract, which are increasingly common [Kim 1991, Mitchell 1993a].

WARNING

The Pap smear is only a screening test for cervical cancer; it has a low, but significant, diagnostic error rate.

In summary, the Pap smear has been remarkably effective in reducing cervical cancer mortality. In fact, it bears repeating, no other test ever invented has been so successful in eradicating cancer. But this must be tempered by realizing that the Pap smear is not perfect. It is virtually impossible to avoid all false-negative reporting [Bosch 1992]. It is thought that at least 10% of cervical cancers are just not preventable [P Martin 1972]. Therefore, unfortunately, some women will develop cervical cancer in spite of appropriate screening [Kurman 1994, P Martin 1972]. But most women who develop cervical cancer have not been adequately screened, rather than misdiagnosed cytologically [Attwood 1985, J Carmichael 1984, E Clarke 1979, Janerich 1995, P Martin 1972, Mobius 1993, Morell 1982, Nasca 1991, M Quinn 1989, Tuncer 1967, E Walker 1983, S Wilson 1992].

There are some important steps that can be taken to help prevent a tragic outcome [Koss 1989a]. First and foremost, women should get regular Pap smears, even if they have a long history of "normals" [R Peters 1988, Sandmire 1976, Sherman 1992a]. Women should also be informed of the fallibility of the test [Bosch 1992]. They should have at least three consecutive, satisfactory negative smears before being reassured. Close surveillance of high-risk patients, including those with multiple infections and heavy inflammation, is important [Pairwuti 1991, Sherman 1992a]. All abnormal Pap smear results should be followed up, even if the abnormality is "only" atypical squamous cells of undetermined significance [J Carmichael 1984, Sherman 1992a]. And, of great importance, suspicious lesions should be biopsied and suspicious symptoms investigated, even when the Pap smear is negative [Berkeley 1980, Koss 1989a].

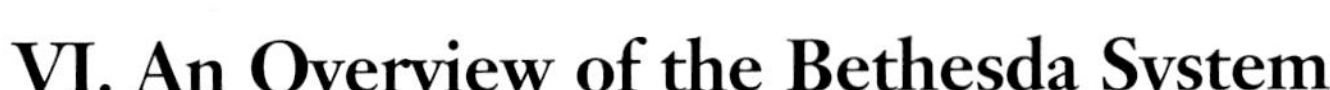

VI. An Overview of the Bethesda System

In 1988, with revisions in 1991, a National Cancer Institute workshop proposed the Bethesda System of Nomenclature for Reporting Cervical/Vaginal Cytologic Diagnoses [T6.38]

T6.38 **The 1991 Bethesda System**

Adequacy of the Specimen
- Satisfactory for evaluation
- Satisfactory for evaluation but limited by … [specify reason]
- Unsatisfactory for evaluation … [specify reason]

General Categorization (Optional)
- Within normal limits
- Benign cellular changes: See Descriptive Diagnosis
- Epithelial cell abnormality: See Descriptive Diagnosis

Descriptive Diagnosis
- Benign Cellular Changes
  - Infection
    - *Trichomonas vaginalis*
    - Fungal organisms morphologically consistent with *Candida* species
    - Predominance of coccobacilli consistent with shift in vaginal flora
    - Bacteria morphologically consistent with *Actinomyces* species
    - Cellular changes associated with herpes simplex virus
    - Other*
- Reactive Changes
  - Reactive cellular changes associated with:
    - Inflammation (includes typical repair)
    - Atrophy with inflammation ("atrophic vaginitis")
    - Radiation
    - Intrauterine contraceptive device (IUD)
    - Other

Epithelial Cell Abnormalities
- Squamous Cell
  - Atypical squamous cells of undetermined significance: [Qualify†]
  - Low-grade squamous intraepithelial lesion encompassing:
    - HPV* mild dysplasia/CIN I
  - High-grade squamous intraepithelial lesion encompassing:
    - Moderate and severe dysplasia, CIS/CIN II and CIN III
  - Squamous cell carcinoma
- Glandular Cell
  - Endometrial cells, cytologically benign, in a postmenopausal woman
  - Atypical glandular cells of undetermined significance: [Qualify†]
  - Endocervical adenocarcinoma
  - Endometrial adenocarcinoma
  - Extrauterine adenocarcinoma
  - Adenocarcinoma, not otherwise specified

Other Malignant Neoplasms: [Specify]

Hormonal Evaluation (applies to vaginal smears only)
- Hormonal pattern compatible with age and history
- Hormonal pattern incompatible with age and history: [Specify]
- Hormonal evaluation not possible: [Specify]

* Cellular changes of human papillomavirus (HPV) previously termed koilocytosis, koilocytotic atypia, or condylomatous atypia are included in the category of low-grade squamous intraepithelial lesion.
† Atypical squamous or glandular cells of undetermined significance should be further qualified, if possible, as to whether a reactive or a premalignant/malignant process is favored.

[NCI 1989a,b,c,1992,1993a,b]. The Bethesda System is the work of a large committee (with representatives from many different groups interested in cervical cancer) reaching a consensus opinion. Since its introduction, the Bethesda System has received widespread [Davey 1992b] but not universal support [Herbst 1990, Kühler-Obbarius 1994a, Syrjänen 1992,1994].

The goal of the Bethesda System is to provide a uniform system of cytopathology reporting. Effective communication between the pathologist and the clinician is essential for patient care, and the basis for this is a report that clearly conveys the significant morphologic findings. The irreproducible Papanicolaou system was discarded, as were loosely defined terms such a "atypia." Communication is a two-way street, however, and the clinician is expected to provide relevant patient information to the pathologist.

The Bethesda System is a complete diagnostic system that recognized the cytopathology report as a medical consultation. The Bethesda System addresses four points: (1) the need for a standardized system of nomenclature so that results are comparable among various laboratories; (2) a clear statement of specimen adequacy (satisfactory, or limited, or unsatisfactory); (3) a general categorization for triage; and (4) the appropriateness of making recommendations for further evaluation if clinically indicated.

Specimen Adequacy

One of the most important contributions of the Bethesda System is the requirement of a statement, in every case, regarding the adequacy of the specimen, including a positive statement of "Satisfactory," when appropriate, and an explanation for "Satisfactory, but limited by (specify)" or "Unsatisfactory" specimens. A "limited" specimen is intended to indicate that a diagnostic interpretation may be given; however, the interpretation may be compromised for the reason(s) stated [NCI 1993a,b].

The goal of reporting specimen adequacy is to obtain better samples by providing feedback to the clinician regarding the quality of the specimen [M Nielsen 1993]. Thus, the statement of adequacy is perhaps the single most important feature of the Bethesda System for quality improvement. There is generally good reproducibility of the Bethesda criteria for adequacy, particularly in designating a specimen "satisfactory" [Spires 1995]. Most laboratories are now reporting specimen adequacy [Davey 1992b].

Four important factors to consider in evaluation of specimen adequacy are (1) patient and specimen identification, (2) pertinent clinical information, (3) technical interpretability (eg,

Four Elements of Adequacy

1. Proper identification
   Patient
   Specimen
2. Clinical history
3. Technical factors
   Air drying
   Obscuration
4. Cellular composition
   Includes transformation zone sample

Note: Specimens with abnormal cells are not unsatisfactory.

adequate fixation without air drying), and (4) cellular composition and sampling of the T zone (eg, presence of squamous and endocervical cells in the Pap smear) [NCI 1993a,b]. All four elements must be satisfactory for a specimen to be entirely satisfactory. In order to reliably fulfill its role, appropriate clinical history *must* be provided by the clinician (including age, pregnancy and menstrual history, usage of birth control pills or other hormones or drugs, use of intrauterine contraceptive device, previous abnormal cytology or histology, history of neoplasia, therapy, smoking, and any other pertinent information). Specimens received without pertinent clinical information may be placed in the "Satisfactory but limited" category. In cases in which a smear is "limited," it is the responsibility of the clinician to correlate the findings from the individual patient to determine whether the Pap smear should be repeated immediately or at the next regular examination.

A specimen may be considered entirely unsatisfactory for evaluation if (1) there is lack of patient identification or no requisition form, (2) the slide is technically unacceptable (eg, irreparably broken, inadequate preservation), or (3) there is scant cellularity, eg, 75% or more of the cells are obscured (excess blood, exudate, thick smears, etc). An unsatisfactory specimen is unreliable for interpretation. However, if abnormal cells are present, the specimen should not be categorized as unsatisfactory [NCI 1993a,b].

Cellular composition, which in the Pap smear encompasses endocervical and squamous cells, is influenced by many factors. The smear must include an adequate number of cells that are representative of the anatomic site. Well-preserved and well-visualized squamous cells should be spread over more than 10% of the slide surface [NCI 1993a,b]. Most Pap smears have on the order of 50,000 to 300,000 cells [Koss 1989a]. It is suggested that at least 5,000 cells be present for an adequate Pap smear, with less than 1,000 being unsatisfactory, and between 1,000 and 5,000 being "limited."

The clinician must obtain a good sample of the transformation zone, which is the key area (if present), since this is the site where most precursor lesions arise. An endocervical component is considered a necessary, but not sufficient, condition for the adequacy of a Pap smear in patients with a cervix, since its presence suggests the critical zone was sampled. Numerous studies have shown the importance of an endocervical component in the detection of cervical lesions (higher frequency, higher grade) [Alons-van Kordelaar 1988, Boon 1986,1989a, Elias 1983, Frost 1969, Killough 1988, Mauney 1990, Mitchell 1992, NCI 1993a,b, Richart 1965b, J Robertson 1993, Vooijs 1985,1986, Wied 1955, Woodman 1989]. In contrast, however, a few studies have shown no significant difference in detection rates for epithelial abnormalities between smears with and without endocervical cells [Beilby 1982, Hislop 1994, Kivlahan 1986, Szarewski 1990,1993]. Also, short-term longitudinal studies, to date, show little or no difference in rates of dysplasia or cancer in women without an endocervical component [Kivlahan 1986, Mitchell 1991, NCI 1993a,b, Vooijs 1985]. Moreover, the presence of endocervical cells may not be reported consistently [Klinkhamer 1989, Mitchell 1994].

The Bethesda System accepts both actual endocervical cells and squamous metaplastic cells as being indicative of a transformation zone component. Endocervical mucus is insufficient evidence of an endocervical sample. At least two clusters of well-preserved endocervical or metaplastic cells, with each cluster composed of at least five cells, must be present. The absence of an endocervical component usually indicates a "limited," but not necessarily entirely unsatisfactory, specimen. The definition applies to both premenopausal and postmenopausal women with a cervix. However, parabasal cells in severe atrophy can closely resemble metaplastic or endocervical cells. Therefore, the absence of an identifiable transformation zone component in the setting of severe atrophy does not affect the specimen adequacy [NCI 1993a,b].

The presence of endocervical cells is related not only to method of collection but also to the patient's age, day of the cycle, pregnancy, parity, method of contraception, and cervical disease, among other factors [Vooijs 1987a]. The transformation zone recedes with age, making it more difficult to obtain endocervical cells [Gondos 1972, Mauney 1990]. Patients who have had a cone biopsy or previous smear with an inadequate endocervical component are more likely to have a repeat smear with an inadequate endocervical component [Sherman 1993]. A smear composed exclusively of endocervical cells, without squamous cells, is unsatisfactory for evaluation. Note that the mere presence of endocervical or metaplastic cells does not guarantee adequate sampling of the transformation zone or that the smear is necessarily adequate (it could be air dried, too thick, etc). Furthermore, the presence of transformation zone cells in a "negative" smear does not completely exclude the possibility of an epithelial abnormality [Gilbert 1974, Koss 1974]. On the other hand, abnormal cells can be present, even though endocervical cells are absent [Koss 1974]. Such specimens should not be considered unsatisfactory, and the abnormality should be reported.

Factors Influencing Cellularity and Presence of Endocervical Cells

Age
Menstrual history
Pregnancy
Radiation
Chemotherapy
Exogenous hormones (including birth control pills)
Cervical disease (eg, inflammation)
Anatomy
Collection methods
Prior surgery (including cone biopsy)
Slide preparation
Douching, lubricants, etc
Method of contraception

The sampling device may have a great deal of influence over the ultimate composition of the smear [Boon 1989a, Kristensen 1989a,b]. Among the most commonly used devices today are the Ayre spatula (or a variation), cotton swab, endocervical brush, and the endocervical "broom" (Cervex Brush®) [T6.39]. Endocervical aspiration is recommended, but seldom performed, to

T6.39 **Advantages and Disadvantages of Sampling Devices**

Advantages	Disadvantages
Ayre Spatula	
Very inexpensive (~1¢) Good yield Minimal discomfort	May cause trauma May not sample transformation zone
Cotton Swab	
Very inexpensive (~1¢) Minimal discomfort	Low yield of endocervical cells Two slide cases
Endocervical Brush	
Relatively inexpensive (~25¢) High endocervical yield	Trauma* Not for pregnant patients Two slide cases
Endocervical Broom	
Minimal trauma Good endocervical/ectocervical sample One slide case	Different technique, requires training† Occasional low cell yield Relatively more expensive (~50¢)

* Discomfort and bleeding are relatively common, but may result from overvigorous brushing. The brush need only be rotated one quarter to one half of a turn (ie, 90°–180°) in the endocervical canal.
† The broom should be rotated through four complete turns (ie, 1440°), then "painted" on the slide, first with one side of the broom, then the other. Smearing is easy, thereby reducing the chance of air drying before fixation.

obtain a good endocervical sampling. The use of a saline moistened cotton swab may be adequate, but is not recommended due to low yield of endocervical cells. The nylon endocervical brush is much better, not only to increase the rate of recovery of endocervical cells [Boon 1986, Kawaguchi 1987, Kristensen 1989a,b, P Taylor 1987], but more to the point, to increase the rate of detection of dysplasia, especially the more significant advanced lesions that typically occur in the endocervical canal [Alons-van Kordelaar 1988]. The endocervical brush is more sensitive, but less specific, than endocervical curettage in evaluating the endocervical canal [Hoffman 1993, Weitzman 1988]. The brush or the swab should be used with another sampling device, usually an Ayre spatula, to obtain an ectocervical specimen.

The Ayre spatula, with or without a cotton swab, is probably the most commonly used technique; the endocervical brush together with the Ayre spatula may be the best sampling combination; and the endocervical broom seems to hold promise as a good sampling device—it is easy to use and reduces technical artifacts, including air drying [Cannon 1993, German 1994, Hutchinson 1991, Laverty 1989, Reissman 1988]. Although the brush or the broom are relatively more expensive than an Ayre spatula or cotton swab, the expense is more than offset by the increased yield of satisfactory specimens, thereby reducing the need for repeat examinations [Brink 1989, Harrison 1993]. New sampling devices continue to be developed [Longfield 1993]. Note that the smears should be taken before application of acetic acid of Lugol's solution (used for colposcopy) and before biopsy [Griffiths 1989].

Technical interpretability can usually be determined by a quick scan at low power. Limiting factors can be divided into three groups: cellularity, distortion (eg, air drying, spray fixative artifact, extensive cytolysis), and obscuration (eg, excess exudate, foreign material). The Pap smear itself must be adequately prepared. This means an abundance of representative ectocervical and endocervical cells must be forcefully scraped (not gently swabbed), thinly smeared on a properly labeled slide (or slides), and immediately fixed (<10 seconds), either by immersion in 95% ethanol or with commercial spray fixative. For proper evaluation, there should not be an excess of blood or exudate diluting or obscuring the cells. Paired smears may help increase sensitivity [Beilby 1982, J Davis 1981, Luthy 1978, Sedlis 1974, Shulman 1975, Tabbara 1994].

The presence of air drying, excess blood or exudate, thick smears, marked degeneration, poor stain, extraneous material, or other artifacts should be visually assessed. For a satisfactory specimen, at least 50% of the slide should be well visualized and well preserved. If more than 75% of the slide is obscured or distorted, the specimen may be unsatisfactory (with 50% to 75% obscuration being classified as "limited"). However, even an apparently unsatisfactory slide should be carefully scrutinized for diagnostic cells. For example, a few indubitable cancer cells may be found in blood or inflammation [Costa 1991b]. Such smears may be diagnostic rather than unsatisfactory.

A specimen reported as "unsatisfactory" should be repeated. However, "limited" specimens do not necessarily require an immediately repeated smear. Patient factors, such as location of the transformation zone, age, pregnancy, and previous therapy, may limit the clinician's ability to obtain an endocervical sample. *Ultimately, the clinician must determine what is "adequate sampling" for an individual patient, based on integrating information from the clinical history, visual inspection of the cervix, and the cytopathology report* [NCI 1993a,b].

General Categorization

The Bethesda System also provides for a general categorization of the specimen: (1) within normal limits, (2) benign cellular changes, and (3) epithelial cell abnormality. The general categorization is included as an aid to busy clinics as a clerical device for triage of patients as well as for use in compiling statistics. Although "within normal limits" can be used as a diagnosis without further explanation, the general categorization is *not* to be used as a substitute for a descriptive diagnosis. Benign cellular changes provides a category for infection and reactive changes. The final category, "abnormal," is for potentially premalignant or malignant lesions (including "suspicious," "dysplastic," or "positive" cases).

Descriptive Diagnosis

The Bethesda System includes four categories under descriptive diagnosis: benign cellular changes, epithelial cell abnormalities, other malignant neoplasms, and hormonal evaluation [NCI 1993a,b]. A new terminology of squamous intraepithelial lesion, low and high grade (encompassing dysplasia/carcinoma in situ or cervical intraepithelial neoplasia, as previously discussed), has been introduced. For other diagnoses, the Bethesda System incorporates previously existing terminology.

Benign Cellular Changes

Benign cellular changes incorporates two subheadings: infection and reactive changes [Luff 1994, N Young 1994a].

Infection

Infection provides for the diagnosis of organisms that can be identified cytologically with reasonable reliability. Certain cytologic features are considered diagnostic of specific agents, eg, *Trichomonas vaginalis*. However, because there are limitations to microscopic identification of pathogens, most findings are qualified by such statements as "consistent with" to remind clinicians that cytologic diagnosis is not the definitive method of microbiologic identification [NCI 1993a,b]. "Predominance of coccobacilli consistent with shift in vaginal flora" is used to designate a smear pattern consistent with bacterial vaginosis. Because cytologic detection of *Chlamydia* is inaccurate, reference to its diagnosis has been deleted from the Bethesda System lexicon [NCI 1993a,b]. Other cytologic diagnoses are neither as specific nor as sensitive as culture or immunoassay, thus qualifying phases, eg, "consistent with" or "suggestive of," are used.

Infection

- Trichomonas vaginalis
- Fungal organisms morphologically consistent with Candida species
- Predominance of coccobacilli consistent with shift in vaginal flora
- Bacteria morphologically consistent with Actinomyces species
- Cellular changes associated with herpes simplex virus
- Other

Evidence of human papilloma virus is not included in the category of infection, but rather is under the category of epithelial cell abnormality.

Reactive Changes

Reactive changes include benign cellular alterations that are reactive in response to such factors as inflammation, radiation, or an intrauterine device (IUD). This category includes benign reparative changes, or "typical repair" [NCI 1993a,b]. However, when significant atypia is present that raises the concern

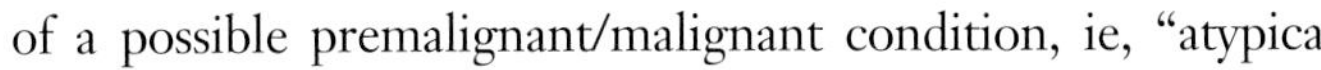

of a possible premalignant/malignant condition, ie, "atypical repair," the lesion should be categorized under atypical squamous (or glandular) cells of uncertain significance (ASCUS, AGUS) [NCI 1993a,b].

Certain miscellaneous changes included in this category require clinical correlation, eg, radiation or IUD effect. Changes due to chemotherapy can also be included in this category, in the proper clinical setting, under the catchall phrase of "other." However, premalignant or noninflammatory squamous atypia, dysplasia, etc, are not included in this category, but instead are placed under epithelial cell abnormality.

Reactive Changes

Reactive cellular changes associated with:
- Inflammation (includes typical repair)
- Atrophy with inflammation ("atrophic vaginitis")
- Radiation
- Intrauterine contraceptive device (IUD)
- Other

Epithelial Cell Abnormalities

Epithelial cell abnormalities are divided into three groups—squamous, glandular, and other—that are then further subdivided. Squamous cell abnormalities include squamous intraepithelial lesions and squamous cell carcinoma. Low-grade squamous intraepithelial lesion includes both mild dysplasia (CIN I) and cellular changes associated with human papilloma virus (HPV). High-grade squamous intraepithelial lesion includes moderate dysplasia (CIN II) as well as severe dysplasia and carcinoma in situ (which together constitute CIN III).

In the Bethesda System, the use of word "atypia" is discouraged unless specifically defined. In the past, the word atypia has been used to describe everything from completely benign to frankly malignant cells. Moreover, "atypia," according to the dictionary, also means "abnormal" and therefore, medicolegally, may be construed as *requiring* significant medical intervention. Changes that are purely reactive in nature should not be classified as "atypical." For example, use of the terms "radiation atypia" or "inflammatory atypia" is discouraged; they should be replaced with radiation effect or inflammatory change, or the like. For cellular alterations that are less than diagnostic of a squamous intraepithelial lesion but thought to be noninflammatory in nature (eg, squamous atypia or minimal dysplasia), the terminology of "atypical squamous cells of undetermined significance" (ASCUS) can be used. This terminology can also be used for other squamous cell changes that are less than diagnostic or of uncertain nature, in each case qualifying as best as possible the nature of the change, to aid the clinician in patient management. Hyperkeratosis and parakeratosis are not included in the category of ASCUS, although atypical parakeratosis or dyskeratocytes may be categorized as ASCUS or squamous intraepithelial lesion, depending on the degree of nuclear abnormality [NCI 1993a,b]. A diagnosis of ASCUS is expected for about 5% of patients in most popula-

tions. However, in high-risk populations, with a high prevalence of squamous intraepithelial lesion, there will be a correspondingly higher prevalence of ASCUS (about two to three times the rate of squamous intraepithelial lesions) [Kurman 1994].

"Koilocytosis" is a descriptive not a diagnostic term. When present, bona fide koilocytes are diagnostic of condyloma and HPV infection. However, overdiagnosis of cellular changes of HPV has been a problem due to the incorrect interpretation of any cytoplasmic halo as koilocytosis or use of "non-classic" signs of condyloma [NCI 1993a,b].

One of the most controversial aspects of the Bethesda System is the inclusion of mild dysplasia (CIN I) and HPV effect (condyloma) in the same category, low-grade squamous intraepithelial lesion. Some experts maintain that there is a difference between these two entities. One—dysplasia—represents a precursor lesion and the other—condyloma—mere infection. However, as previously discussed, CIN I and HPV have been grouped because the lesions are difficult to reliably distinguish by light microscopy, by progression rate, or by HPV virology. Therefore, specific comments regarding the presence of cellular changes of HPV are no longer included in the Bethesda System, but may be mentioned in the report according to individual preferences [NCI 1993a,b]. Squamous intraepithelial lesions should be graded according to the degree of abnormality of the nucleus as well as the immaturity of the cell, regardless of whether HPV is thought to be present or not.

For the purposes of the Bethesda System, squamous cell carcinoma can be used without further qualification. However, at the discretion of the cytologist, this category can be further specified, eg, nonkeratinizing, keratinizing, or small cell squamous cell carcinoma, or microinvasive squamous cell carcinoma.

Squamous Cell Abnormalities

- Atypical squamous cells of undetermined significance [qualify]
- Squamous intraepithelial lesion (SIL)
  - Low-grade SIL, encompassing
    - Mild dysplasia (CIN I)
    - HPV effect (condyloma)
  - High-grade SIL, encompassing
    - Moderate dysplasia (CIN II)
    - Severe dysplasia (CIN III)
    - Carcinoma in situ (CIN III)
- Squamous cell carcinoma

It is thought that the squamous intraepithelial lesion terminology will allow for more reproducible and less subjective grading of premalignant cervical disease, which has been a problem in the past [Duca 1988, Hicklin 1984, Klinkhamer 1988,1989, Lambourne 1973, Seybolt 1971, Yobs 1987]. By reducing the number of diagnostic categories, the Bethesda System, in theory, should reduce observer variation in diagnosis of intraepithelial lesions [Mitchell 1993b, Sherman 1992c]. However, in practice, the very common problem of distinguishing mild dysplasia, CIN I (ie, *low*-grade squamous intraepithelial lesion), from moderate dysplasia, CIN II (ie, *high*-grade squamous intraepithelial lesion), is among the most irreproducible diagnoses, yet is now the most important, in fact, in some sense, the *only* distinction for noninvasive neoplasia. It is also doubtful that the grouping of all "high-grade" lesions into one category will further our understanding of the pathology of these diseases. However, the Bethesda System does allow continued use of standard diagnostic terms, ie, cervical intraepithelial neoplasia or dysplasia/carcinoma in situ. It is to be hoped that most cytologists will continue to use established, well-recognized terminology in conjunction with the Bethesda System's squamous intraepithelial lesion. However, it is also expected that guidelines will be published for management of low- and high-grade squamous intraepithelial lesions [Kurman 1994].

Glandular cell abnormalities also encompass a spectrum of lesions, ranging from the presence of cytologically benign endometrial cells found in a smear from a postmenopausal woman to adenocarcinoma. In cases of adenocarcinoma, an attempt should be made to classify by site. The Bethesda System does not report cytologically benign endometrial cells occurring out-of-phase in a premenopausal woman. There are two reasons: first, there is a low yield of pathologic abnormalities in these patients, and second, endometrial cells may be inadvertently obtained at any time of the cycle when using an endocervical brush. Still, many experts believe the presence of spontaneously exfoliated endometrial cells out-of-cycle may be significant, particularly after 40 years of age. Of course, *atypical* endometrial cells are always abnormal, regardless of menstrual status.

Glandular Cell Abnormalities

- Endometrial cells, cytologically benign, in a postmenopausal woman
- Atypical glandular cells of uncertain significance [qualify]
- Adenocarcinoma
  - Endocervical
  - Endometrial
  - Extrauterine
  - Not otherwise specified

A category of atypical glandular cells of uncertain significance (AGUS) is also included. AGUS demonstrates changes beyond ordinary reactive change but less than diagnostic of invasive adenocarcinoma. If possible, the diagnosis should indicate whether the cells are endocervical or endometrial in origin. For atypical endocervical cells of undetermined significance, an attempt should be made to specify as best as possible whether a reactive or neoplastic process is favored. It is important to note that many patients with endocervical glandular atypia have a coexisting squamous atypia or dysplasia [Bose 1994, L Brown 1986, Goff 1992, Kohan 1985, Nasu 1993]. Criteria for separating reactive from neoplastic endometrial AGUS are not well defined, and the category is not further subdivided [NCI 1993a,b]. Finally, a diagnosis of adenocarcinoma indicates a probably invasive glandular tumor. The origin should be specified, if possible [NCI 1993a,b].

Other Malignant Neoplasms

Other malignant neoplasms have a separate category in recognition of the fact that not all lesions are epithelial in origin. If possible, the tumor should be specifically diagnosed.

Hormonal Evaluation

Hormonal evaluation (vaginal smears only) indicates simply whether the hormonal pattern is compatible or incompatible (reason specified) with the patient's age and provided history, or that such a determination is not possible, the reason to be specified.

Recommendations

Recommendations should generally be provided only as a guide to further *diagnostic*, as opposed to *therapeutic*, management of the patient, and should generally include the phrase "if clinically indicated" [T6.40]. Be aware that making specific recommendations may essentially force clinicians to do procedures that are not actually indicated or go to great lengths to document why they were not performed, due to the possible medicolegal consequences of not following recommendations. However, many clinicians, particularly nongynecologists, appreciate having specific recommendations for further evaluation of the patient. The recommendations in T6.40 are guidelines only; patients must be managed individually, based on the clinical impression, degree of risk, etc.

Note: Some inflammatory changes closely mimic dysplasia. Treat the inflammation as specifically as possible and immediately repeat the Pap smear. With other inflammatory changes that do not mimic dysplasia it may not be necessary to immediately repeat the Pap smear after therapy. The routine follow-up may be adequate. However, patients whose Pap smears show repeated inflammatory changes are at high risk for significant dysplasia.

Key clinical points on management:

1. *Biopsy any visible suspicious lesion*
2. *Investigate any suspicious signs or symptoms (Despite negative Pap smear)*

Follow-up of a diagnosis of cervical intraepithelial neoplasia/squamous intraepithelial lesion is controversial. University and other tertiary care hospitals often have a dysplasia clinic in which they perform colposcopy on every patient with a diagnosis of low-grade squamous intraepithelial lesion or even ASCUS. This approach is favored because a cytologic diagnosis of low-grade squamous intraepithelial lesion (mild dysplasia, condyloma) may be inaccurate in a significant number of patients, ie, the actual lesion may be a high-grade squamous intraepithelial lesion, or, rarely, even cancer [Koss 1993a]. A more conservative approach to low-grade dysplasia is to treat any inflammation as specifically as possible, then repeat the smear. Unfortunately, Pap smears repeated in a relatively short time (weeks) may have a very high false-negative rate, as high as 60% [D Jones 1987, Koss 1989a, Nyirjesy 1972, Wheelock 1989]. However, it is usually agreed that if there are repeated diagnoses of low-grade squamous intraepithelial lesion or ASCUS (ie, more than one, possibly two), or a single diagnosis of a high-grade squamous intraepithelial lesion, immediate colposcopy is warranted [Lyall 1995]. Suspected lack of patient compliance for return visits is another consideration in justifying immediate colposcopy after the first diagnosis of squamous atypia (ASCUS) or mild dysplasia (low-grade squamous intraepithelial lesion). Also, HIV-positive patients must be managed aggressively [M Fink 1994, Korn 1994]. Finally, ablative therapy without histologic confirmation is considered unacceptable.

T6.40* Suggested Guidelines for Patient Management

Diagnosis	Recommendation
Within normal limits, negative	Routine follow-up
Severe inflammation	Treat and repeat
Reserve cell hyperplasia	Routine follow-up
Squamous metaplasia	Routine follow-up
Hyperkeratosis, parakeratosis	
Slight	Routine follow-up
Extensive	Repeat Pap smear; if persists, possibly colposcopy
ASCUS / L SIL	Individualized follow-up / High-risk patient†
H SIL	Immediate colposcopy/possible biopsy
Condyloma	See L SIL
Squamous cell carcinoma	Biopsy confirmation
Atypical repair	See ASCUS, AGUS (endocervical)
Postradiation dysplasia	Colposcopy minimum
Atypia of atrophy	Consider estrogen test
Reactive endocervical cells	Treat and repeat
Atypical glandular cells (AGUS)	
Endocervical	
Favor reactive	Careful follow-up, possible colposcopy High-risk patient for SIL
Favor neoplastic	Endocervical curettage, cone biopsy Patient may have ordinary SIL
Endometrial	Endometrial biopsy or dilatation and curettage
Adenocarcinoma	Note: Rule out extrauterine adenocarcinoma
Endocervix	Cone biopsy
Endometrial	Endometrial biopsy or dilatation and curettage
Pregnancy	
SIL	Frequent Pap smears, colposcopy/biopsy as indicated by Pap smear
Microinvasive SCC	Excise area to rule out frank SCC; if microinvasive SCC confirmed, can postpone treatment until after delivery
Invasive SCC	Definitive treatment usually required
Inadequate sample (no endocervical sample, scant, excess blood or exudate, air dried, etc)	Immediately repeat, especially in high-risk patient

[ACOG 1993, Bibbo 1989a, Patten 1978]
* Viral testing and typing are not currently recommended.
† Treat inflammation, repeat smear every 4–6 months; if abnormality persists, perform colposcopy/biopsy. After three consecutive, satisfactory, negative smears, revert to routine screening. However, some studies recommend colposcopy/biopsy immediately on first diagnosis of any degree of dysplasia, or even ASCUS.

Synopsis of Diagnostic Criteria for the Bethesda System

The following represents the "official" criteria as defined in *The Bethesda System for Reporting Cervical/Vaginal Cytologic Diagnoses: Definitions, Criteria, and Explanatory Notes for Terminology and Specimen Adequacy* [Kurman 1994]. Note that diagnostic terminology and criteria defined in the preceding text may differ somewhat from those of the Bethesda System.

Reactive Changes

Reactive changes are defined as reactive cellular changes that are benign in nature, associated with inflammation (including typical repair, atrophy with inflammation, radiation, IUD, other nonspecific causes) [T6.41].

Reparative changes can involve squamous, metaplastic, or columnar cells. Nuclear enlargement and prominent nucleoli may suggest a more significant lesion; however, monolayered sheets with streaming and absence of similar single cells are associated with repair.

Atrophy can also be associated with intermediate cells with nuclear enlargement (3–5 times normal atrophic nucleus) but bland chromatin (normochromatic or mildly hyperchromatic), and monolayers of basaloid cells with slightly enlarged nuclei, which may be elongated and hyperchromatic. Air drying, which is common in atrophic smears, can also cause nuclear enlargement.

Radiation changes may be accompanied by repair (resulting in cells with prominent single or multiple nucleoli). Radiation changes usually regress several weeks after therapy, but may persist for the life of the patient. Certain chemotherapeutic agents may produce similar changes.

Patients who use IUDs may also shed single cells with nuclear enlargement and high N/C ratios that mimic cells seen

T6.41 Reactive Changes

Reactive Cellular Changes Associated With Inflammation

Nuclei
- Minimal enlargement* (usually <2x an intermediate nucleus)
- Occasional binucleation or multinucleation
- Smooth nuclear membranes
- Mild hyperchromasia possible, but chromatin remains fine and uniform
- Degeneration may result in pyknosis or karyorrhexis
- Nucleoli, single or multiple, can be prominent

Cytoplasm may show:
- Polychromasia
- Vacuolization
- Perinuclear halos (without peripheral thickening)

Typical Repair

Cytologic changes as above, but cells in flat, monolayered sheets
- No loss of nuclear polarity
- → "Streaming"

Typical mitotic figures may be seen
Single reparative cells are usually absent

Reactive Cellular Changes Associated With Atrophy—With or Without Inflammation

[Predominance of basal/parabasal cells]
Generalized nuclear enlargement
- Without significant hyperchromasia
- Nuclear membranes, chromatin remain uniform

± Naked nuclei (due to autolysis)
± Cellular degeneration (→ shrunken cells mimicking parakeratosis)
- Nuclear pyknosis
- Cytoplasmic eosinophilia/orangeophilia
- ["Pseudo-pseudoparakeratosis"]

± Abundant inflammation
± Granular basophilic background [benign diathesis]
± Blue blobs

Reactive Cellular Changes Associated With Radiation

Cells
- Markedly enlarged [macrocytes] without substantial increase in nuclear/cytoplasmic ratio
- Bizarre shapes possible

Nuclei
- May be enlarged†
- Binucleation or multinucleation common
- ± Some hyperchromasia
- Degenerative changes frequent (eg, pale or hyperchromatic, smudgy chromatin, wrinkling, vacuolization)

Cytoplasm
- Vacuolization, polychromasia may be seen

Reactive Cellular Changes Associated With IUD

Cells‡
- Small clusters of glandular cells (usually 5–15 cells)

Nuclei
- Degeneration frequent
- Nucleoli may be prominent

Cytoplasm
- Variable in amount
- Large vacuoles frequent (may → "signet rings")

Background
- Clean, no diathesis
- Psammoma body-like calcifications may be present

* Reactive endocervical cells can show greater nuclear enlargement.
† May see both normal sized and enlarged nuclei in same group.
‡ May mimic adenocarcinoma; diagnose adenocarcinoma cautiously in a patient using an IUD.
Note: Author's comments in brackets.

in high-grade squamous intraepithelial lesions, but the spectrum of accompanying abnormalities is absent.

Epithelial Cell Abnormalities

Squamous Cell

Atypical Squamous Cells of Undetermined Significance (ASCUS): ASCUS is defined as cellular abnormalities that are more marked than those seen in reactive change, but quantitatively or qualitatively fall short of a definitive diagnosis of a squamous intraepithelial lesion [T6.42].

Sparsity of abnormal cells or artifacts, such as air drying, may contribute to the diagnostic difficulty, resulting in a diagnosis of ASCUS. The diagnosis can be qualified as to whether a reactive process or squamous intraepithelial lesion is favored. Diagnostic rate of ASCUS should not exceed two to three times the rate of squamous intraepithelial lesions.

T6.42 ASCUS

Nuclei
- 2-1/2 to 3 times size of intermediate nucleus or 1-1/2 to 2 times size of metaplastic nucleus
- Slightly increased nuclear/cytoplasmic ratio
- Variation in size/shape may occur
- Binucleation may occur
- Membrane smooth, or very limited irregularity
- Normochromatic or mildly hyperchromatic
- Chromatin evenly distributed without granularity

Cytoplasm
- Usually mature, superficial/intermediate type [ie, squamous atypia]
- Can also be metaplastic ("atypical [squamous] metaplasia")

Atypical Repair (ASCUS, AGUS)
- Marked cellular changes in tissue fragments or sheets, with
  - Nuclear piling up
  - Significant anisonucleosis
  - Irregular chromatin distribution
  - Nucleolar pleomorphism (size, shape)

  } Exceeding typical repair
- Differential diagnosis is exuberant repair vs carcinoma
  - Repair lacks both tumor diathesis and numerous single abnormal cells

ASCUS Associated With Atrophy [Atypia of Atrophy]
- Consider diagnosis for any of following:
  - Nuclear enlargement (>2x normal) and significant hyperchromasia
  - Irregularity of nuclear contour or chromatin distribution
  - Marked pleomorphism (tadpole, spindle cells)
- Differential diagnosis: H SIL or SCC; estrogen test may be helpful

[Atypical Parakeratosis*]
- Parakeratotic-type cells [ie, miniature superficial cells] demonstrating any or all of the following:
  - Cellular pleomorphism (caudate, elongate shapes)
  - Increased nuclear size
  - Hyperchromasia
- Single or in clusters

* The terms hyperkeratosis, parakeratosis, atypical parakeratosis, and dyskeratosis are not used in the Bethesda System. The changes described above should be categorized as ASCUS or SIL, depending on the degree of cellular abnormality.
Note: Author's comments in brackets.

T6.43 Squamous Intraepithelial Lesions

Low-Grade Squamous Intraepithelial Lesion (L SIL)

Cells
- Single, or in sheets
- Usually, mature type [ie, intermediate, superficial]
- Polygonal cell borders

Nuclei
- At least 3x area of intermediate nucleus
- Increased nuclear/cytoplasmic ratio
- Moderate variation size/shape
- Binucleation or multinucleation frequent
- Nuclear membranes slightly irregular
- Hyperchromasia with uniform chromatin distribution
  - Or chromatin degeneration, smudging (if associated with HPV)
- Nucleoli rare; inconspicuous if present

Cytoplasm
- Distinct cell borders
- May have well-defined, perinuclear clearing [ie, koilocytotic halo]
  - Requires peripheral dense rim of cytoplasm and nuclear abnormality to be diagnostic

High-Grade Squamous Intraepithelial Lesion (H SIL)

Cells
- Single, sheets, syncytial-like aggregates
- Usually immature, rounded cell borders
- Overall cell size smaller than L SIL

Nuclei
- Enlarged in range of L SIL,* but diminished amount of cytoplasm
  - → marked increase in nuclear/cytoplasmic ratio
- Nuclear membranes are irregular
- Hyperchromasia; fine to coarse, evenly distributed chromatin
- Nucleoli generally absent

Cytoplasm
- Lacy and delicate [~carcinoma in situ], or
- Dense, metaplastic [~metaplastic dysplasia], or
- Occasionally, densely keratinized [~keratinizing dysplasia]

* Cells with very high nuclear/cytoplasmic ratios may have smaller nuclei than L SIL.
Note: Author's comments in brackets.

Squamous Intraepithelial Lesion: Squamous intraepithelial lesion (SIL) encompasses a spectrum of noninvasive epithelial abnormalities traditionally classified as flat condyloma, dysplasia/carcinoma in situ, and cervical intraepithelial neoplasia (CIN) [T6.43]. SILs are divided into low and high grades. Low-grade SIL encompasses condyloma (including "koilocytotic atypia"), mild dysplasia, and CIN I. High-grade SIL encompasses moderate dysplasia, severe dysplasia, carcinoma in situ, and CIN II, III.

Features favoring high-grade SIL over low-grade SIL include increased numbers of abnormal cells, higher N/C ratios, greater nuclear membrane irregularities, and coarsening and clumping of chromatin. Low-grade SIL typically occurs in mature type cells (intermediate/superficial). High-grade SIL occurs in immature cells with lacy, delicate cytoplasm, or dense,

T6.44 **Squamous Cell Carcinoma**
Nonkeratinizing SCC
Cells
Single, or syncytial-like aggregates
Cellular features of H SIL plus
Prominent macronucleoli
Markedly irregular chromatin, including
Coarse chromatin clumping
Parachromatin clearing
Tumor diathesis (necrotic debris, old blood) often present
Keratinizing SCC
Cells
Single, less commonly in aggregates
Marked variation size/shape, including
Caudate and spindle cells
Nuclei
Marked variation size/configuration
Numerous dense, opaque forms
Chromatin (when discernible)
Coarsely granular
Irregularly distributed
Parachromatin clearing
Macronucleoli less common than in nonkeratinizing SCC
Cytoplasm
Frequently dense and orangeophilic
Background
Tumor diathesis may be present

metaplastic cytoplasm, or abnormally keratinized cytoplasm. Overall cell size is smaller in high-grade SIL than in low-grade SIL. When it is not possible to grade an SIL, a diagnosis of "squamous intraepithelial lesion, grade cannot be determined" is appropriate.

The treatment of patients with low-grade SIL may include follow-up with smears or directed biopsy. Patients with high-grade SIL should be evaluated by colposcopy and directed biopsy. The goal is to prevent invasive cancer by the most conservative means possible.

Some high-grade SILs [keratinizing dysplasia, pleomorphic dysplasia, atypical condyloma] are composed of cells with more abundant, but abnormally keratinized, cytoplasm. These cells may shed singly or in dense clusters. The cells are pleomorphic in shape (including elongate/spindle cells and caudate/tadpole cells). The nuclei are elongated, with variation in nuclear size, and often have smudgy chromatin. In contrast with invasive carcinoma, nucleoli and a tumor diathesis are lacking. However, these keratinized lesions may be indistinguishable from invasive carcinoma in some cases, particularly if there are relatively few abnormal cells.

Squamous Cell Carcinoma: This is a malignant invasive tumor composed of squamous cells. Although the Bethesda System does not subdivide SCC, it is listed separately for descriptive purposes [T6.44].

Small Cell Carcinoma: This is a heterogeneous group of neoplasms, including poorly differentiated squamous cell carcinoma, as well as neuroendocrine carcinomas. In the Bethesda System, poorly differentiated carcinomas with squamous features are included in the squamous cell carcinoma category. Undifferentiated carcinomas or neuroendocrine carcinomas are classified under "other malignant neoplasms."

Glandular Cell

Endometrial Cells, Cytologically Benign, in a Postmenopausal Woman: The presence of endometrial cells—whether epithelial or stromal, and even when normal in appearance—in a postmenopausal woman not taking hormonal therapy must be explained. Possible explanations include vigorous sampling of the lower uterine segment, endometrial polyps, hormonal therapy, IUD, endometrial hyperplasia, or endometrial carcinoma [T6.45].

Atypical Glandular Cells of Undetermined Significance (AGUS): These cells show either endometrial or endocervical differentiation, displaying nuclear atypia that exceeds obvious reactive or reparative changes, but they lack unequivocal features of invasive adenocarcinoma [T6.46].

The diagnosis of AGUS should be qualified, if possible, to indicate whether the cells are thought to be of endometrial or endocervical origin. Atypical endocervical cells should be further classified, if possible, as to whether a reactive or neoplastic process is favored.

A spectrum of conditions can be associated with atypical endocervical cells, including atypical reactive processes, microglandular hyperplasia, Arias-Stella reaction, tubal metaplasia, and adenocarcinoma in situ. Atypical endocervical cells may coexist with squamous intraepithelial lesions.

T6.45 **Endometrial Cells**
Benign Endometrial Epithelial Cells
Cells
Small clusters, and less commonly, single cells
Sheets when directly obtained
Nuclei
Small, round
~ Size of intermediate cell nucleus
Nucleoli: Typically small, inconspicuous
Cytoplasm
Scant, basophilic, sometimes vacuolated
Ill-defined cell borders
Double contoured cell masses, with stroma inside and epithelium outside, appear days 6 to 10 [exodus].
Benign Endometrial Stromal Cells
Deep stromal cells
Vary from round to spindle shaped, with small, oval nuclei and scant cytoplasm
Superficial stromal cells with decidual changes
The cells have abundant foamy cytoplasm and may be difficult to distinguish from endometrial epithelial cells and histiocytes

T6.46 Atypical Glandular Cells of Undetermined Significance

Atypical Endometrial Cells of Undetermined Significance
Cells
  Small groups (usually 5–10 cells)
Nuclei
  Slightly enlarged
  Slight hyperchromasia may be seen
  Small nucleoli may be present
Cytoplasm
  Scant (compared with endocervical cells)
  Occasionally vacuolated
  Indistinct cell borders

Atypical Endocervical Cells, Favor Reactive
Cells
  Sheets and strips, with minor nuclear overlap
Nuclei
  May be enlarged, up to 3–5x normal endocervical nucleus
  Mild variation size/shape
  Slight hyperchromasia frequent
  Nucleoli often present
Cytoplasm
  Abundant
  Distinct cell borders often seen

Atypical Endocervical Cells, Probably Neoplastic
(Note: This category includes cases thought to represent endocervical adenocarcinoma in situ.)
Cells
  Crowded sheets, strips, rosettes
  Sheets
    Honeycomb pattern lost
    Feathery edges
  Strips
    Palisading of nuclei
Nuclei
  Crowded, overlapped
  Enlargement, elongation, stratification in most cases
  Variation size/shape
  Hyperchromasia
    Fine to moderately coarse chromatin
  Nucleoli: Small or inconspicuous
  Mitotic figures may be seen
Cytoplasm
  Diminished
  Ill-defined cell borders

Similar criteria for reactive vs neoplastic endometrial cells are not well defined; therefore, the category of atypical endometrial cells is not further subdivided. Nuclear size is the primary criterion on which atypicality is based. Like their bland counterparts, atypical endometrial cells can be associated with a spectrum of conditions ranging from inflammation to cancer.

Typical reactive/reparative processes in glandular cells are not included in AGUS. (Benign reactive endocervical nuclei may be enlarged to several times normal, multinucleated, slightly hyperchromatic, and have nucleoli, but they maintain honeycomb arrangements, abundant cytoplasm, well-defined cell borders, and have round to oval nuclei with minimal overlap, smooth or slightly irregular contour, and finely granular chromatin.)

Tubal metaplasia (pseudostratified columnar cells with nuclear enlargement and hyperchromasia) may resemble in situ or invasive adenocarcinoma. In tubal metaplasia, the nuclei tend to be round to oval and have more finely granular, evenly dispersed chromatin, while feathered edges, rosettes, and mitoses are uncommon. However, the most helpful criterion of tubal metaplasia is the presence of cilia.

Endocervical Adenocarcinoma: This is a malignant invasive neoplasm composed of endocervical-type cells. Diagnostic criteria include those outlined for atypical endocervical cells, probably neoplastic (ie, adenocarcinoma in situ) [T6.47].

It may be difficult to distinguish in situ from invasive endocervical adenocarcinoma. Irregular clearing, uneven chromatin distribution, and macronucleoli strongly suggest invasion. However, a diathesis and macronucleoli may be absent in well-differentiated, early cancers. Subtypes, including endometrioid, intestinal, clear cell, and serous neoplasms, are recognized. Abnormal squamous cells may also be present: either as coexisting squamous lesion or squamous differentiation in adenocarcinoma.

Endometrial Adenocarcinoma: This is a malignant invasive neoplasm of endometrial-type cells. The cytologic appearance varies with the degree of differentiation (and tumor subtype). Criteria listed are for the endometrioid subtype [T6.47]. Well-differentiated adenocarcinoma typically sheds few cells with subtle nuclear alterations, making diagnosis difficult. Compared with endocervical adenocarcinoma, endometrial adeno-

T6.47 Adenocarcinoma

Endocervical Adenocarcinoma
Cells
  Single, flat sheets, or clusters
  Columnar shape may be retained
Nuclei
  Enlarged
  Irregular chromatin, parachromatin clearing
  Macronucleoli may be present
Cytoplasm
  Eosinophilic or cyanophilic
Background
  Tumor diathesis may be evident

Endometrial Adenocarcinoma
Cells
  Typically single or small, loose clusters
Nuclei
  Size, chromasia, nucleoli increase with grade of tumor
  Variation in size
  Loss of polarity
  Irregular chromatin distribution, parachromatin clearing.
    Particularly higher-grade tumors
Cytoplasm
  Scant, cyanophilic (typical)
  Often vacuolated
Background
  Watery (finely granular) tumor diathesis

carcinoma sheds fewer and smaller cells, with less prominent nucleoli, and a watery rather than necrotic diathesis.

Extrauterine Adenocarcinoma: This appears as adenocarcinoma cells in a clean background or has an unusual morphology suggesting extrauterine origin.

Other Malignant Neoplasms

A wide variety of other malignant neoplasms can be identified in the Pap smear, including small cell (neuroendocrine) carcinoma. A specific diagnosis should be provided, if possible.

I6.1
Cervix (tissue). Normal, nonkeratinizing stratified squamous epithelium is shown; note normal "basket weave" pattern due to glycogenation of squamous cells. Glycogen does not stain in H&E.

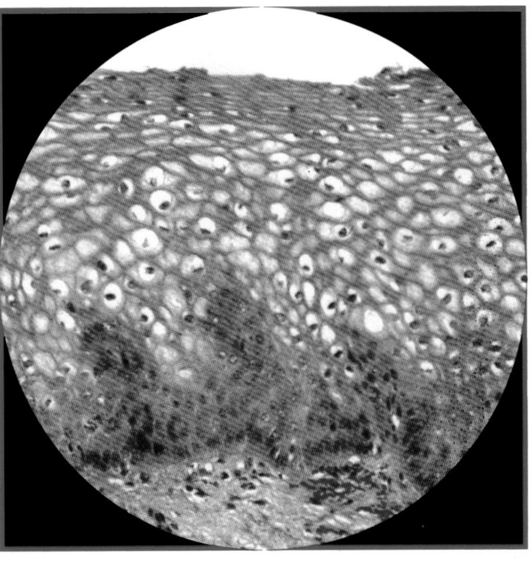

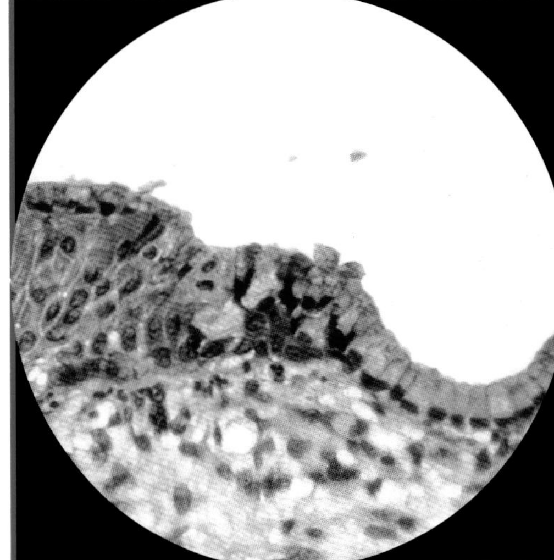

I6.2
Cervix (tissue). Transformation zone is shown; note transition from simple columnar epithelium of endocervix into squamous metaplasia. This area is of particular interest because it is where most neoplastic lesions of the cervix arise.

I6.3
Superficial cells are normally the largest squamous cells in a Pap smear. Note voluminous, thin cytoplasm and pyknotic (ink-dot) nucleus. Superficial cell predominance is associated with estrogen and reaches its peak in midcycle.

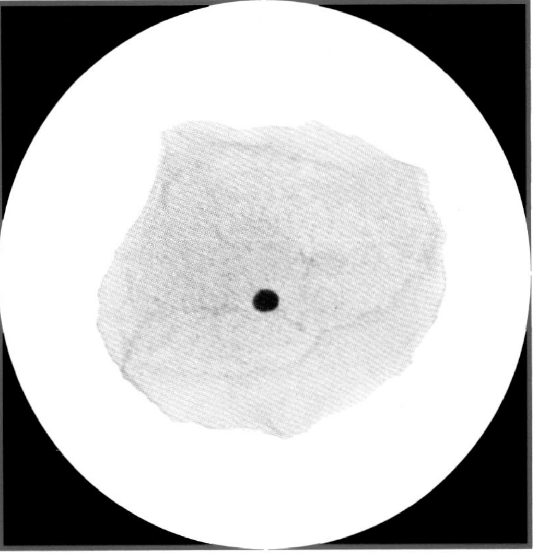

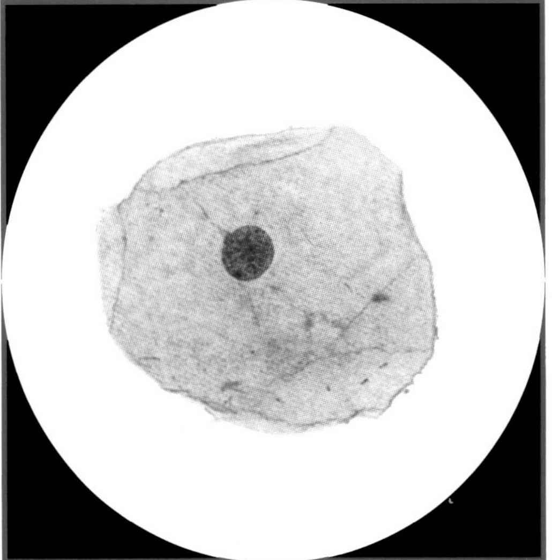

I6.4
Intermediate cells range from parabasal to superficial in overall cell size. Intermediate cell predominance is associated with progesterone and is characteristic of the second half of the menstrual cycle as well as pregnancy. Remember this: the intermediate cell nucleus is a key reference for size (35 μm^2) and chromatin quality (staining, texture). Dysplastic nuclei are "big and dark" compared with the intermediate nucleus.

I6.5
Navicular cells. Glycogenated intermediate cells are particularly associated with pregnancy. Androgenic atrophy, ie, glycogenated parabasal cells, which can be seen postpartum, during lactation, or associated with androgens, has a similar appearance.

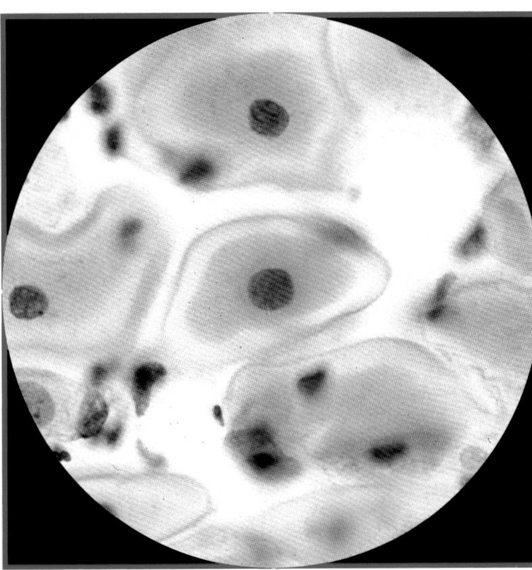

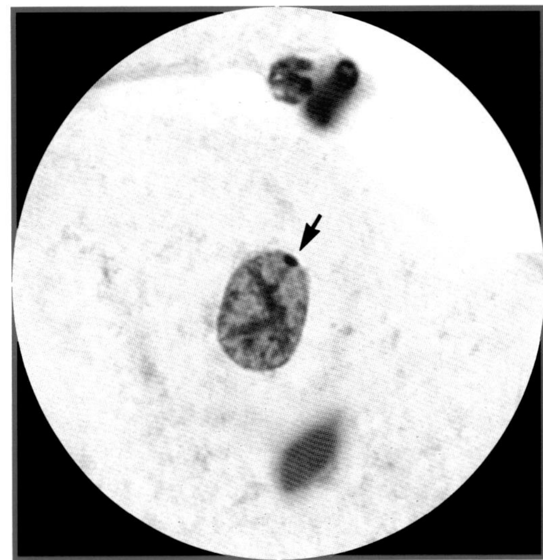

I6.6
Barr body (arrow). An extra X chromosome and a condensed bit of heterochromatin are seen along the inner nuclear membrane. (Oil)

I6.7
Parabasal cells are associated with atrophy, which may be seen postmenopause and postpartum. Naked nuclei are commonly present due to the delicate nature of cytoplasm. Clusters of these naked parabasal nuclei can mimic endometrial cells.

I6.8
Spindle parabasal cells may be seen in atrophy, possibly representing transitional metaplasia. Note longitudinal folds in some of the nuclear membranes.

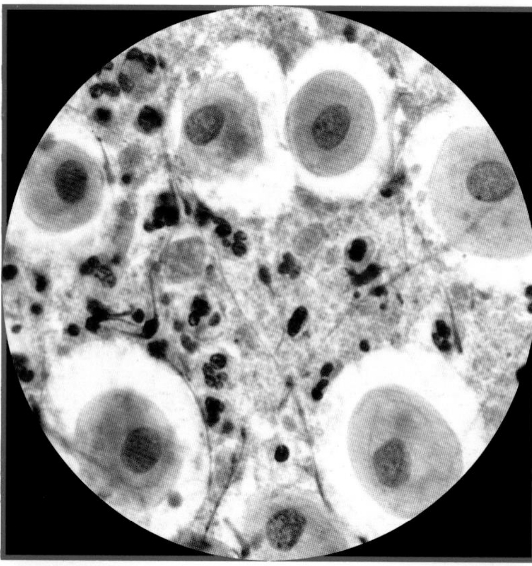

I6.9
Atrophy with inflammation ("atrophic vaginitis"). Generalized nuclear enlargement, without significant hyperchromasia, and inflammatory exudate are shown. Granular background mimics a necrotic tumor diathesis.

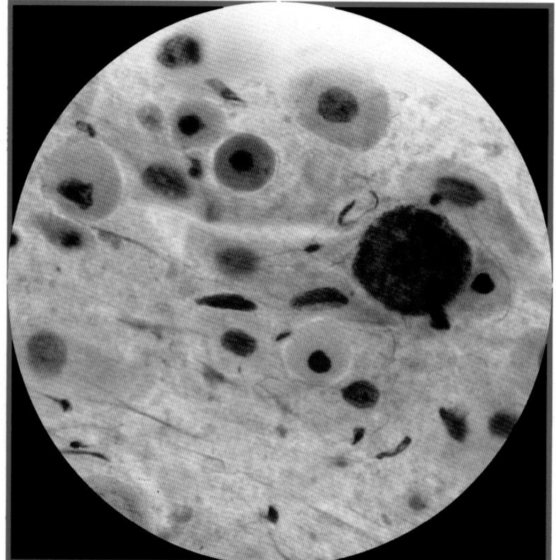

I6.10
"Blue blobs" seen in severe atrophy. Their exact nature is disputed, variously described as inspissated mucus and dystrophic calcification, but they are probably mummified parabasal cells. Note darker staining spot near center—apparently a nucleus. Also note "benign diathesis" in background and pseudokeratinized parabasal cell.

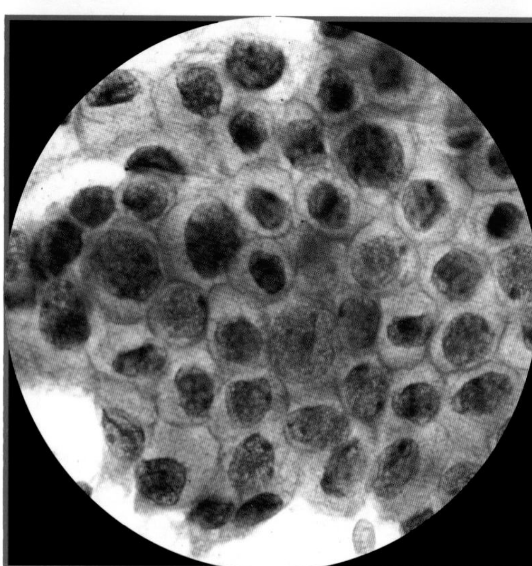

I6.11
Endocervical cells. Note uniformity of cells: seen en face in orderly ranks and files. Prominent cell borders—a benign feature of endocervical cells—results in characteristic "honeycomb" appearance. Nuclei are round to oval with smooth outlines. This is the classic cytologic appearance of benign glandular epithelium from virtually any site.

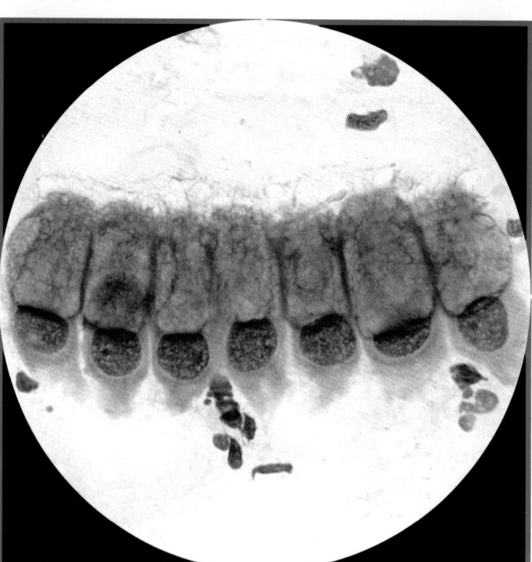

I6.12
Endocervical cells. Seen from the side in orderly "palisades." Note how the nuclei are uniform, basal, and do not stratify (compare with in situ and invasive endocervical adenocarcinoma).

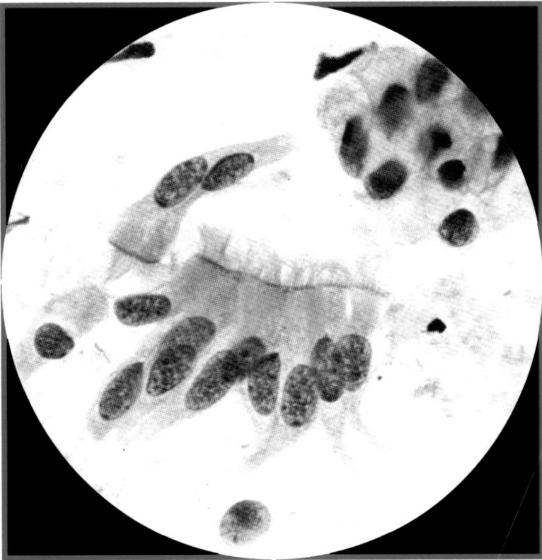

I6.13
Ciliated endocervical cells with terminal bars and cilia.

I6.14
Pencil-thin endocervical cells. Elongated endocervical cells are thought to be caused by application of Lugol's solution (at time of colposcopy) prior to obtaining the Pap Smear.

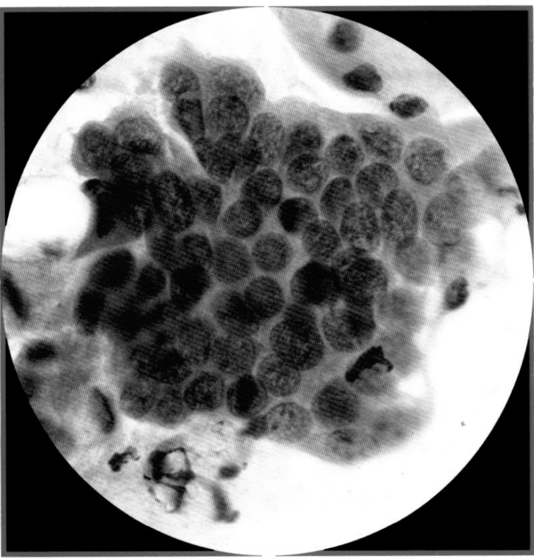

I6.15
Endocervical cells. Cells obtained by an endocervical brush, from high in the endocervical canal, are crowded and hyperchromatic compared with the endocervical cells usually obtained with an Ayre spatula.

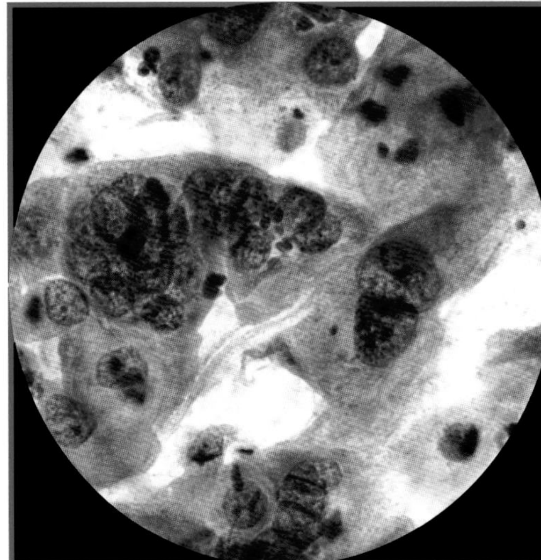

I6.16
Reactive endocervical cells. Note mild hyperchromasia, pleomorphism, multinucleation, and prominent nucleoli in some cells. Multinucleation should not be mistaken for viral effect (lacks characteristic ground glass chromatin of herpes).

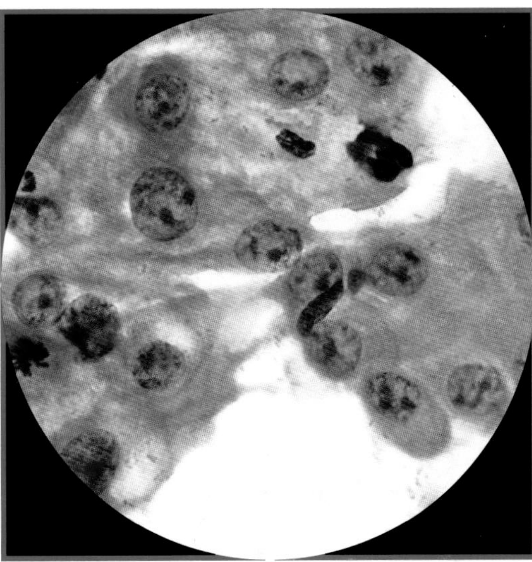

I6.17
Reactive/reparative endocervical cells. Reparative process is characterized by nuclear "atypia" (enlargement, prominent nucleoli, pleomorphism), but distinguished from cancer by orderly, cohesive groupings, pale chromatin, and lack of tumor diathesis. Mitotic figures, generally a worrisome feature in endocervical cells, can be seen in repair.

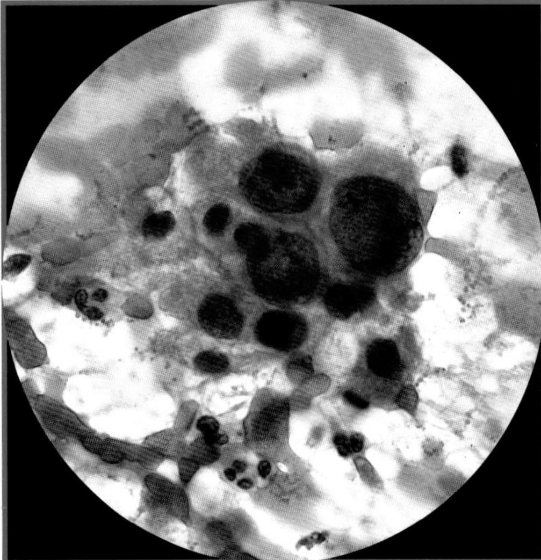

I6.18
Endocervical brush artifact. Occasionally, endocervical cells with large, dark, possibly polyploid nuclei are obtained with the endocervical brush. In contrast with features seen in endocervical glandular neoplasia, marked crowding, rosettes, or feathery edges are not seen, and the benign cells tend to "lay flat."

I6.19
Arias-Stella reaction in endocervical cells. Markedly atypical, hypersecretory endocervical cells are pleomorphic with prominent nucleoli. Note that despite atypia, the cells remain fairly orderly, lie flat, and do not crowd. Although the cells usually remain fairly cohesive, this case also had a few single atypical cells, a generally worrisome feature. (Case courtesy of Marshall Austin, MD, Charleston, SC.)

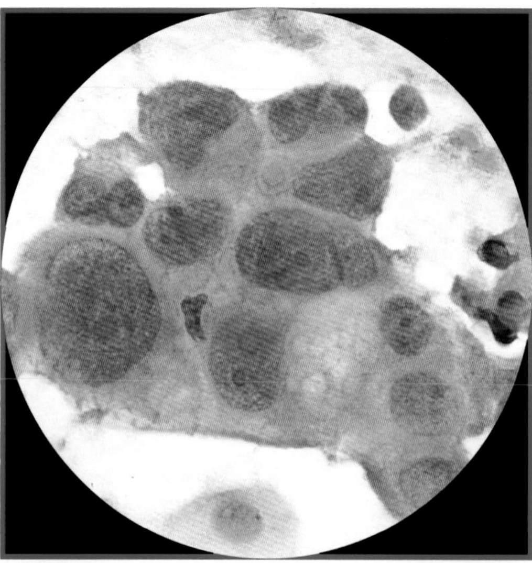

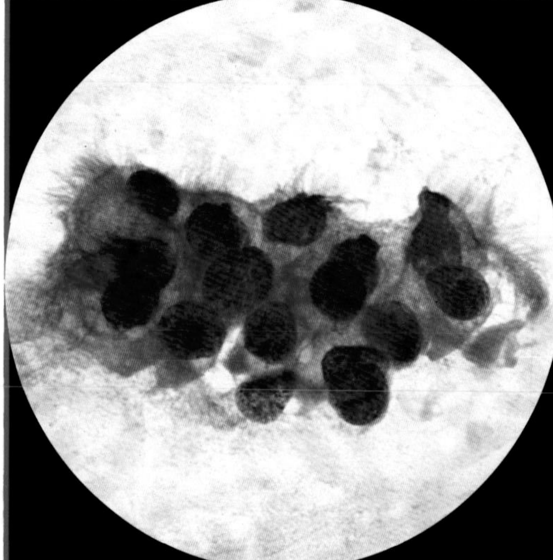

I6.20
Tubal metaplasia is characterized by hyperchromatic, pleomorphic, crowded cells suggesting the possibility of endocervical glandular neoplasia. The nuclei tend to be round or oval with finely granular, evenly distributed chromatin. Feathery edges, rosettes, and mitotic figures are uncommon. The best clue to the proper diagnosis is the presence of cilia (visible along one side of the group).

I6.21
Tubal metaplasia of endocervix (tissue). Note stratification and cilia.

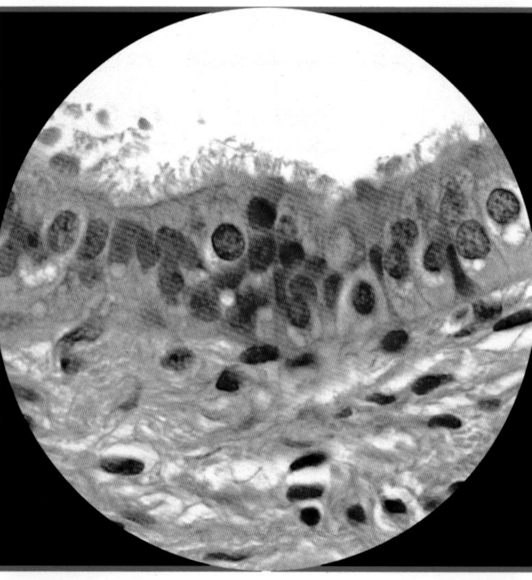

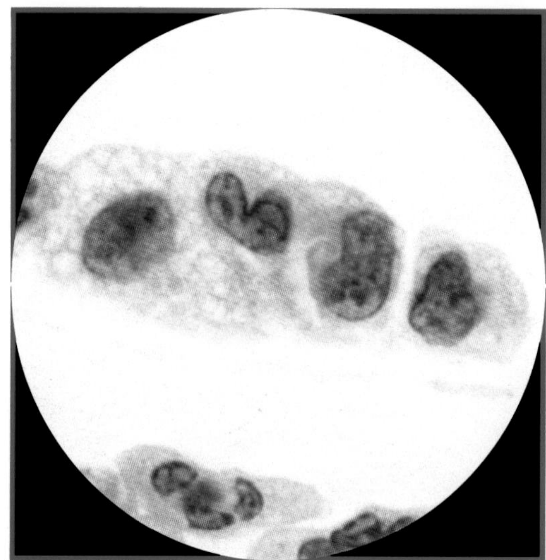

I6.22
Histiocytes are a common finding in the Pap smear (eg, associated with menses, pregnancy, foreign bodies, inflammation). These large histiocytes have characteristic bean-shaped nuclei; however, not all histiocytes have reniform nuclei. Also note foamy cytoplasm. (Oil)

I6.23
Giant cell histiocytes are common postpartum, postmenopausally, and after surgery or radiation.

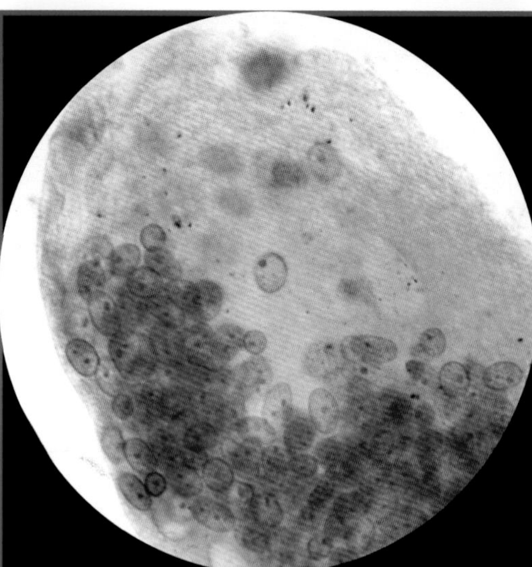

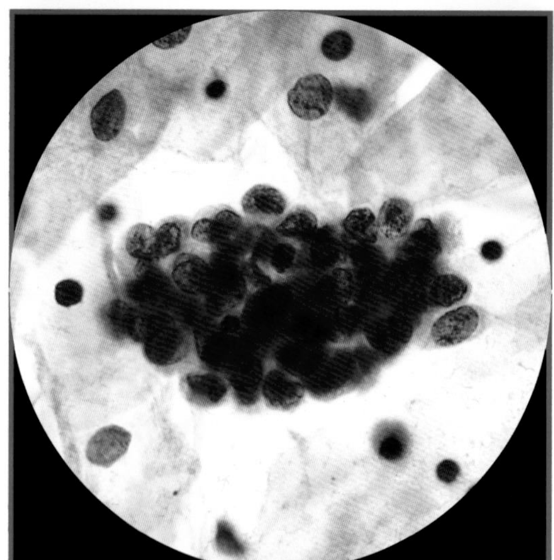

I6.24
Endometrial cells. In contrast with usually flat lying, well-preserved endocervical cells, endometrial cells tend to be "packed together" and degenerated. Note that the normal endometrial cell nucleus is approximately the size of the intermediate squamous cell nucleus.

I6.25
Endometrial cells. Classic "double contour" arrangement (stroma in center surrounded by epithelium) is associated with "exodus" (days 6 to 10).

I6.26
Superficial endometrial stromal cells ("sticky histiocytes"). Individual superficial stromal cells are indistinguishable from small histiocytes, but form loose aggregates.

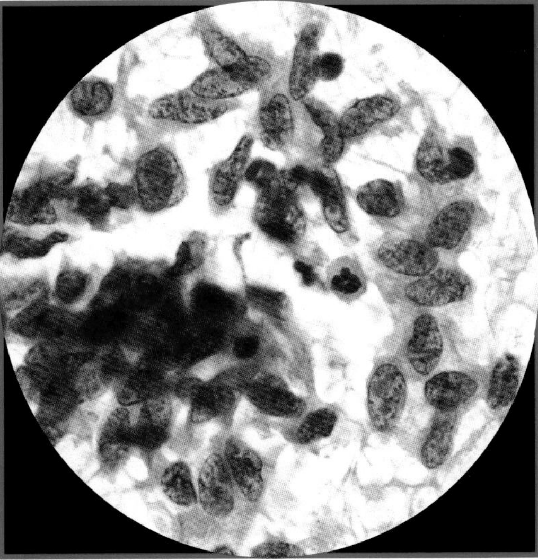

I6.27
Deep endometrial stromal cells vary from round to characteristic spindle-shaped cells, with small, oval nuclei and scant cytoplasm.

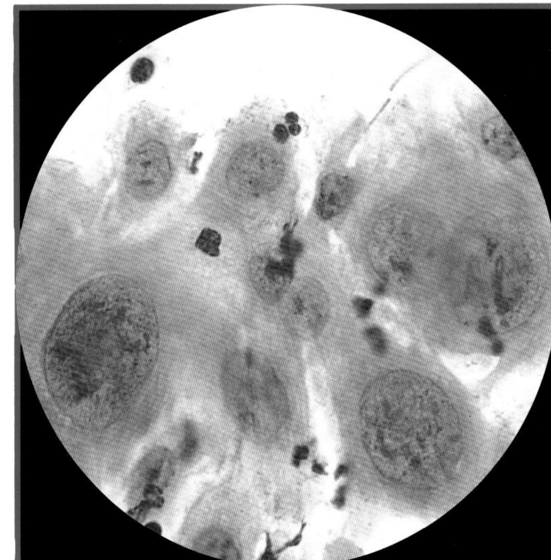

I6.28
Decidual cells indicate decidualization of the cervical stroma, more common in late pregnancy. Could be mistaken for moderate dysplasia or atypical repair.

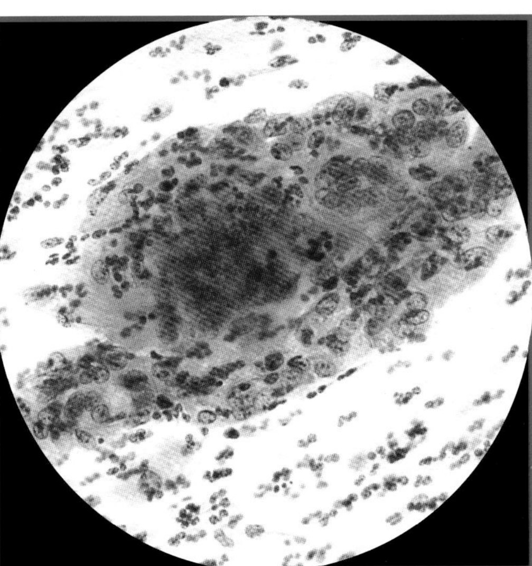

I6.29
Syncytiotrophoblast. Multinucleated giant cells surrounded by mononucleated cytotrophoblasts from a patient who recently had an abortion.

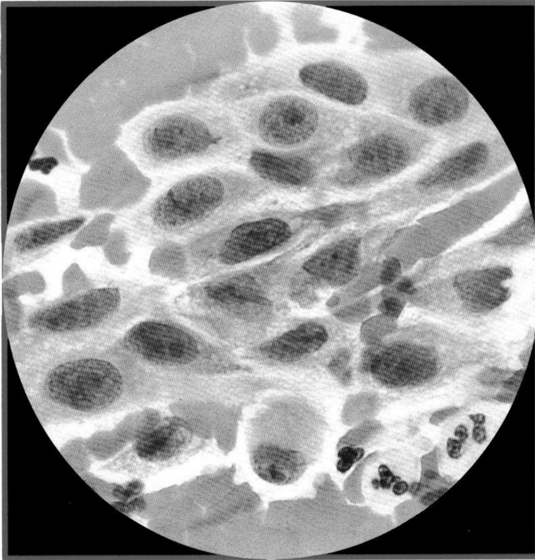

I6.30
Cytotrophoblasts (proliferating). These are from a Pap smear of a patient with trophoblastic proliferation.

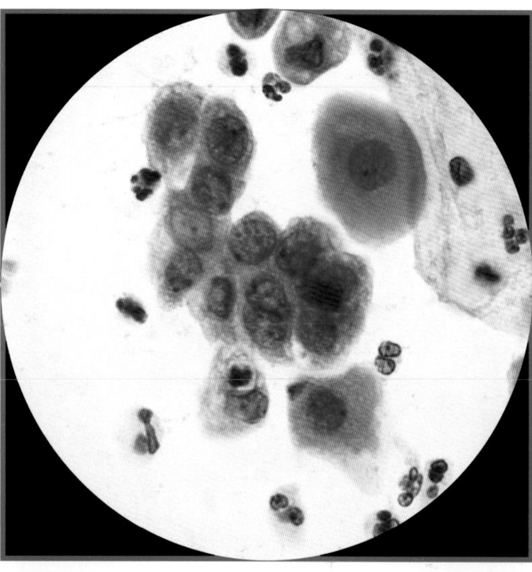

I6.31
Reserve cell hyperplasia. Reserve cells are small and basaloid, with high nuclear/cytoplasmic ratios, and delicate, undifferentiated cytoplasm. Common in tissue, but rarely recognized in cytology, particularly when present as single cells. Clue to diagnosis is associated endocervical cells or immature metaplasia.

I6.32
Immature squamous metaplasia. Parabasal-sized cells, in cobblestone arrangement, with thick, dense cytoplasm that looks like it has been cut out of cardboard. Also note endo/ectoplasmic rim, a common feature of immature metaplastic cells.

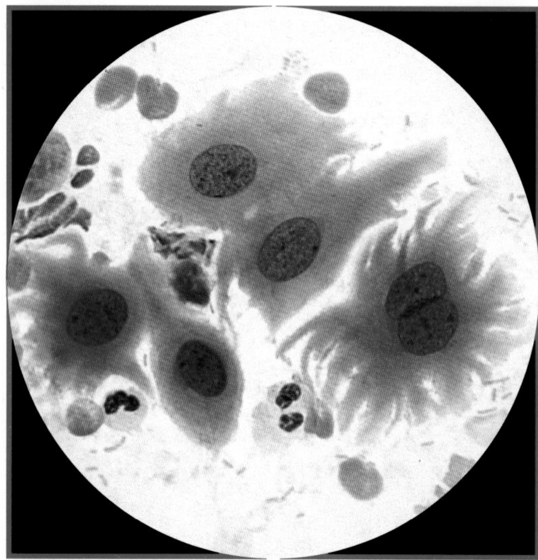

I6.33
Spider cells are immature squamous metaplastic cells forcibly scraped from the mucosal surface; they are characterized by thin, spidery legs extending from the main cytoplasmic body.

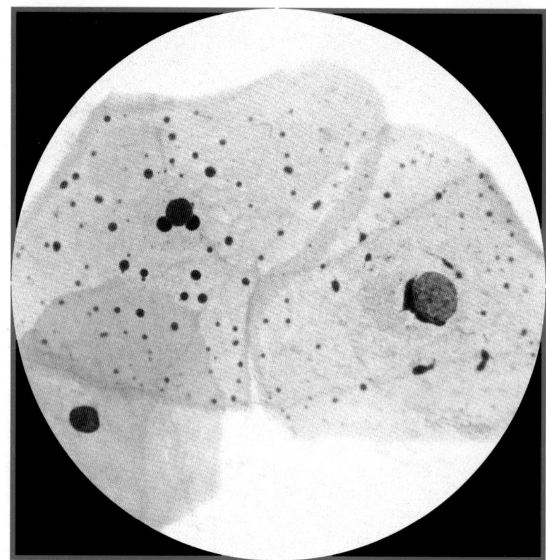

I6.34
Spiegelosis aka hypergranulosis. Mature type squamous cells with dark keratohyaline granules indicate formation of granular cell layer in tissue. Compare with "cornflakes" artifact, I6.151.

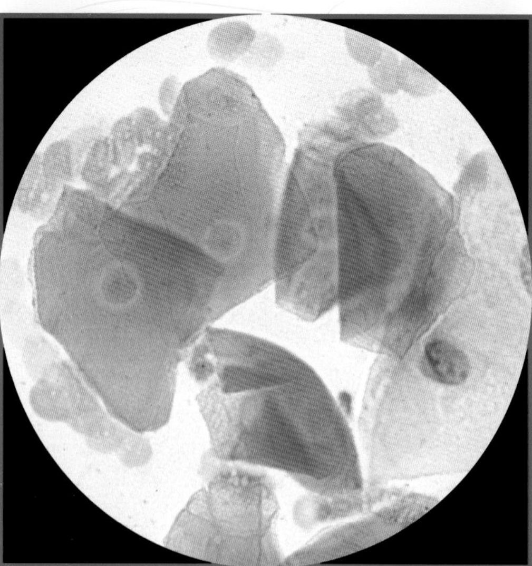

I6.35
Hyperkeratosis. Formation of stratum corneum in tissue is characterized by presence of anucleate squames in cytology. Note nuclear ghosts.

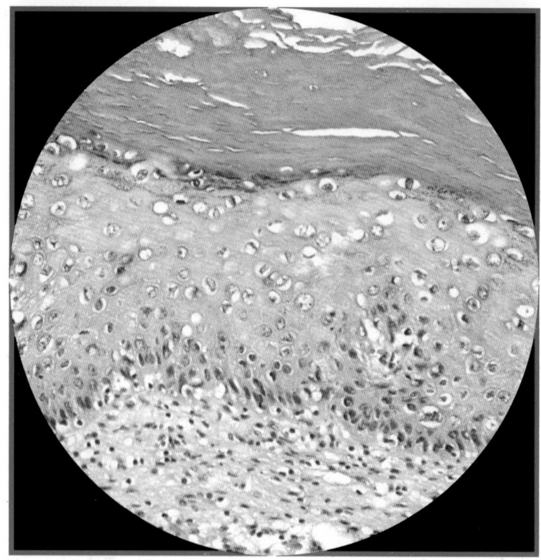

I6.36
Hyperkeratosis (tissue). Sometimes, surface keratotic reactions cover and mask an underlying dysplasia, as in this example.

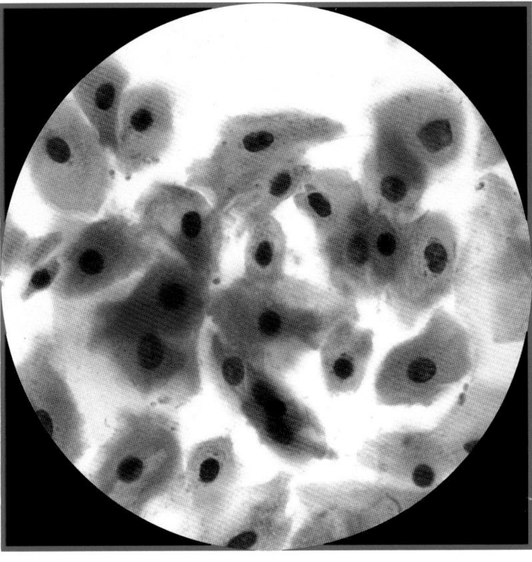

I6.37
Parakeratosis. The surface keratotic reaction is similar to that seen in hyperkeratosis. The diagnostic feature is the presence of miniature superficial cells (small polygonal cells with pyknotic nuclei). Although orangeophilia is classic, some examples stain blue. Single parakeratotic cells are shown.

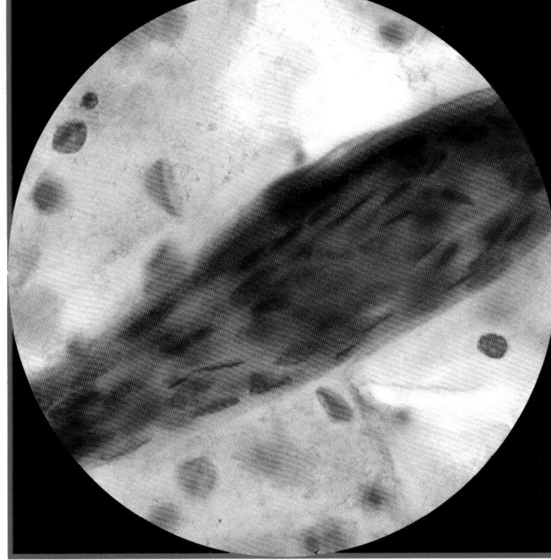

I6.38
Parakeratosis. Linear strips of miniature superficial cells are shown.

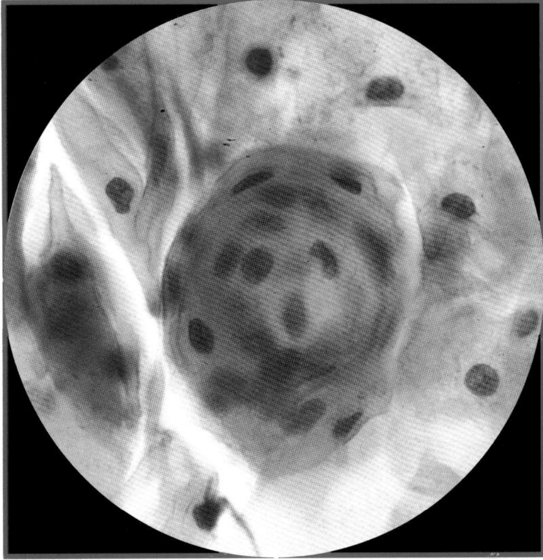

I6.39
Parakeratosis. A pearl of miniature superficial cells is shown.

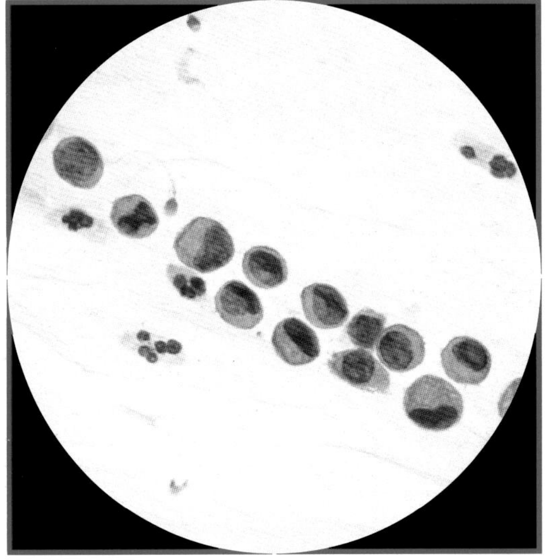

I6.40
Pseudoparakeratosis. Degenerated endocervical cells, with cytoplasmic orangeophilia and nuclear pyknosis, mimic parakeratosis. This probably represents microglandular endocervical hyperplasia, which is usually associated with hormone therapy, particularly birth control pills. The cells are seen in the classic linear arrangement.

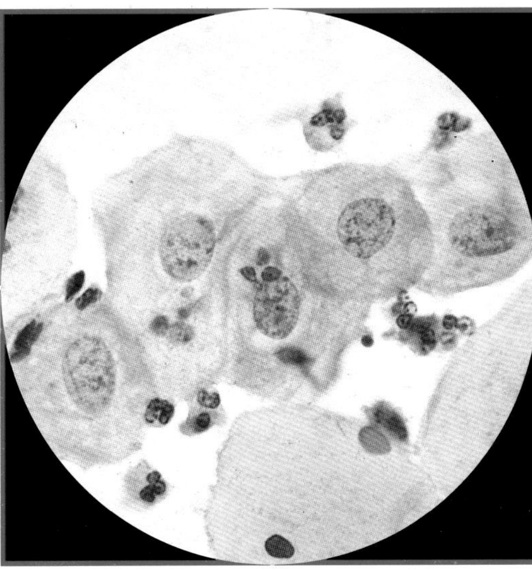

I6.41
Inflammatory change. There is nuclear enlargement but pale chromatin (ie, big but not dark nuclei). In contrast, dysplasia has nuclei that are *both* big *and* dark compared with the intermediate cell nucleus.

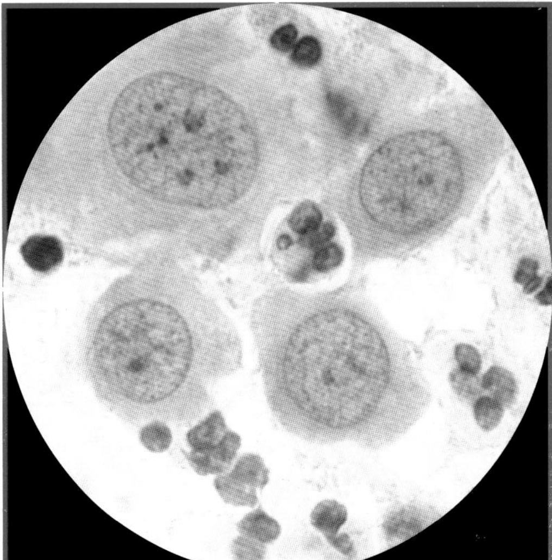

I6.42
Inflammatory change. Nuclear enlargement is usually minimal, ie, less than two times the intermediate cell nucleus. Note that the nuclear membranes are smooth and the chromatin is pale, fine and evenly distributed. Nucleoli may be prominent. (Oil)

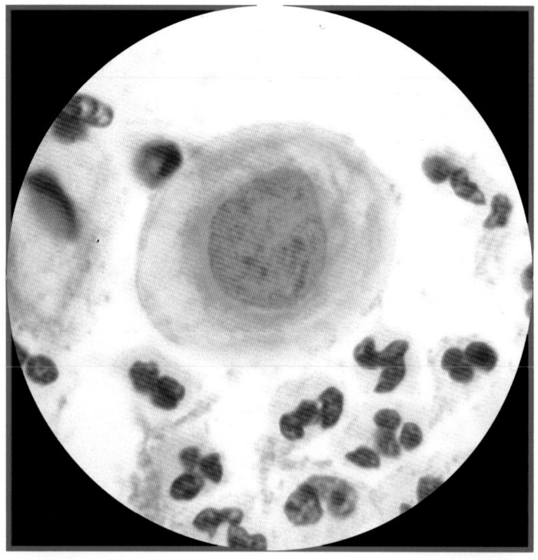

I6.43
Inflammatory change. A peculiar feature associated with inflammation is the way the inflamed chromatin sometimes "shines red." Unfortunately, this diagnostic clue to inflammatory change is not consistently present. (Oil)

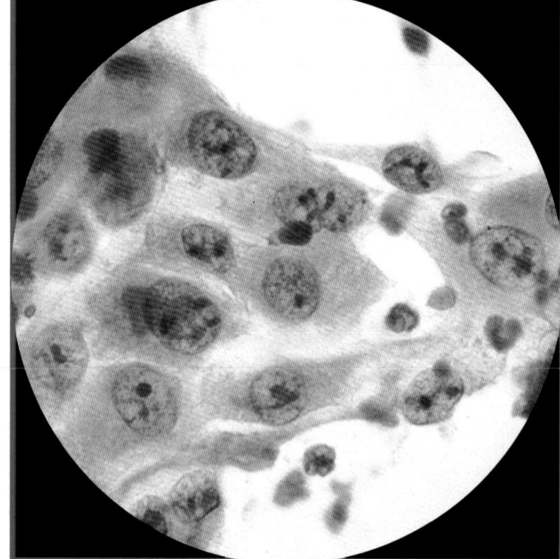

I6.44
Repair. Although the nuclei are "atypical" (enlarged, pleomorphic, prominent nucleoli, typical mitotic figures), the groups remain cohesive and orderly without loss of nuclear polarity ("streaming"). Note fine chromatin and smooth nuclear membranes. (See also endocervical repair I6.17, atypical repair I6.147.)

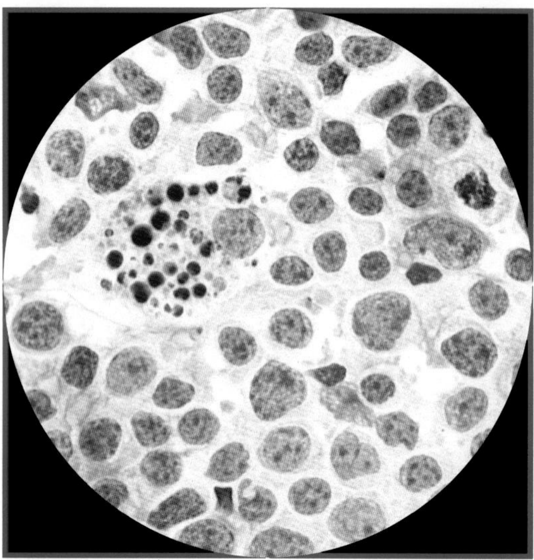

I6.45
Follicular cervicitis. This looks like the touch preparation of a reactive lymph node. It is characterized by predominance of small "mature" lymphocytes with admixture of "immature" lymphocytes and presence of tingible body macrophages.

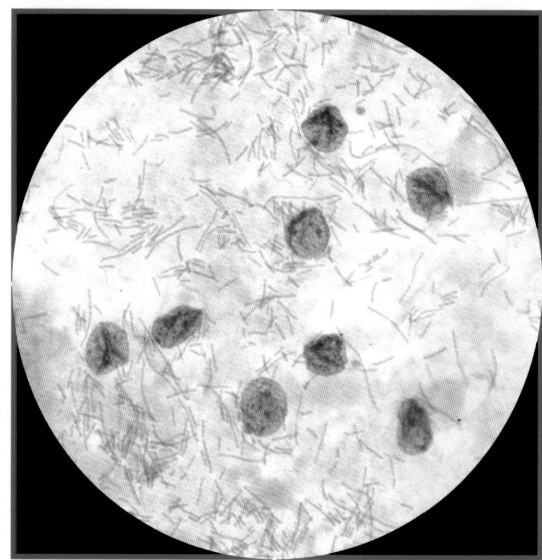

I6.46
Cytolysis. Lactobacilli, aka Döderlein bacilli and *Bacillus vaginalis*, are a diverse group of rod-like bacteria that compose the normal vaginal flora. The action of these bacteria may cause the cells to lyse ("cytolysis"), leaving naked nuclei stripped of their cytoplasm strewn in the background of the smear. Cytolysis is more or less limited to intermediate cells.

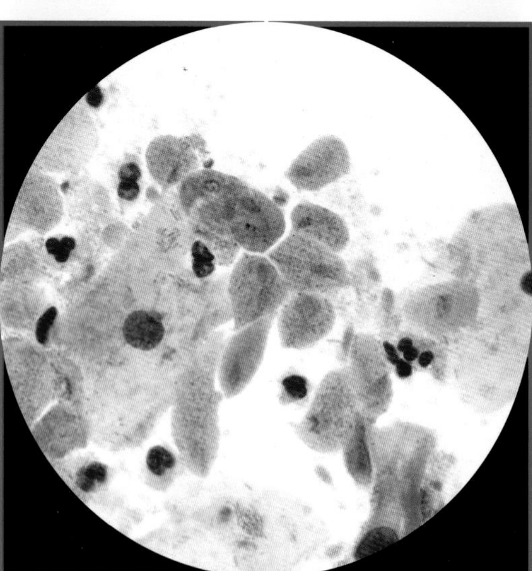

I6.47
Trichomonas vaginalis is represented by pear-shaped organisms that can range in size from 15 to 30 µm. *Must see* the nucleus (eccentrically located, elliptical) for diagnosis (to distinguish from mere cytoplasmic fragments, etc). *May see* red cytoplasmic granules. *Never* see flagella in the Pap smear.

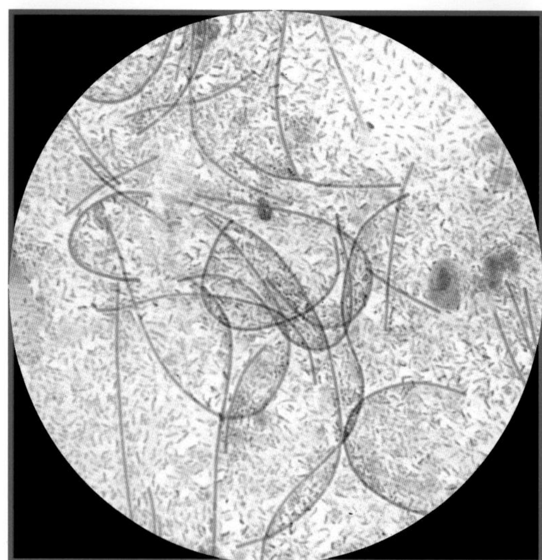

I6.48
Leptothrix are long, filamentous bacteria (like limp spaghetti). Where *Leptothrix* goes, can *Trichomonas* be far behind? The presence of *Leptothrix* usually implies the presence of *Trichomonas*, but *Trichomonas* can be present in the absence of *Leptothrix*.

I6.49
Cannonballs are neutrophils agglomerated onto the surface of the squamous cell, and are associated with *Trichomonas* infection but not specifically.

I6.50
Inflammatory ("Trich") halos are also associated with *Trichomonas* infection, but not specifically. Do not be tricked into thinking such halos indicate condyloma. Koilocyte halos are larger, and much more distinct, with peripheral condensation of the cytoplasm, and the nuclei appear dysplastic.

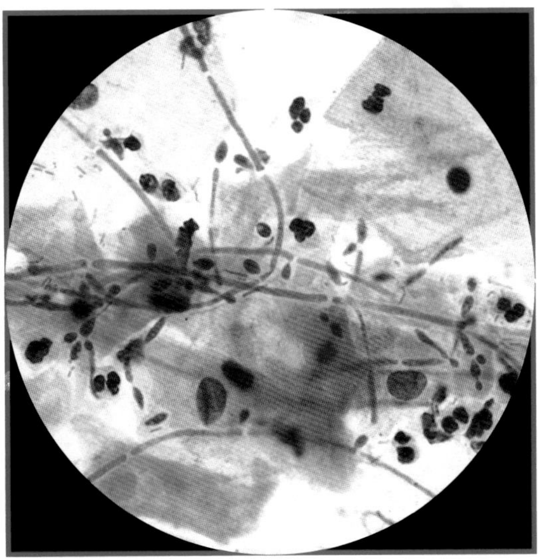

I6.51
Candida species. Budding yeasts (3–7 μm) and pseudohyphae (elongated budding) occur. They are often associated with neutrophil lysis, slight hyperkeratosis, and mild enlargement of squamous nuclei (inflammatory change).

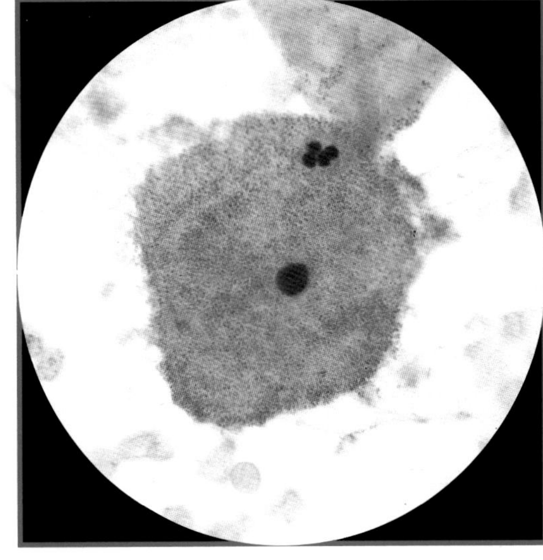

I6.52
Clue cell and "shift in vaginal flora." Clue cells are a velvety coating of random squamous cells with small coccobacilli; they provide a clue to presence of *Gardnerella vaginalis*, which can be normal. A diffuse background of coccobacilli, with or without clue cells, in the absence of lactobacilli, is "consistent with a shift in vaginal flora." This diagnosis provides supportive evidence of a clinical diagnosis of bacterial vaginosis.

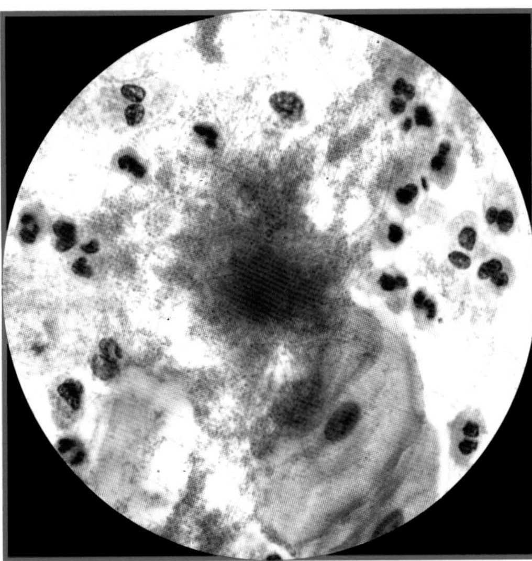

I6.53
Actinomyces is represented by clusters of branching, filamentous organisms, which tend to stain red and have associated bacteria (blue) forming "dust bunnies." Usually they are found in patients using an IUD.

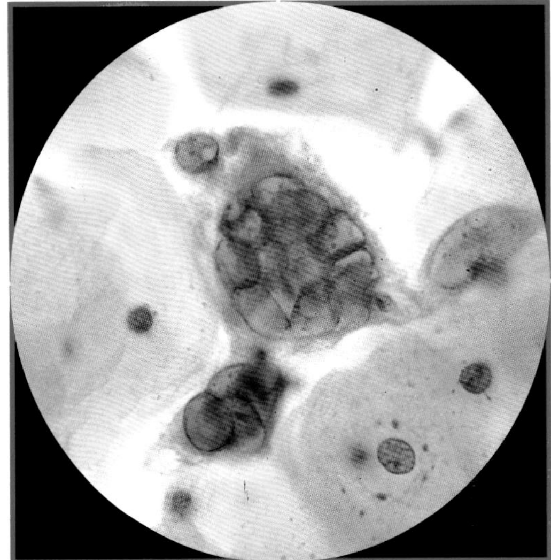

I6.54
Herpes is represented by multinucleation, molding, ground glass chromatin, and a "thickened nuclear membrane." Smaller mononucleated infected cells, which can mimic a high-grade squamous intraepithelial lesion, may also be present. Intranuclear inclusions, if present, suggest secondary infection.

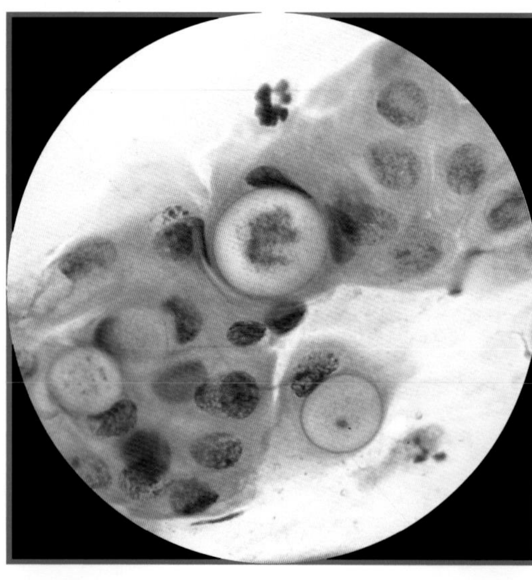

I6.55
Faux *Chlamydia*. Targetoid cytoplasmic vacuoles, with thick walls and coarse granules, which distend the cytoplasm and displace the nucleus, are not diagnostic of *Chlamydia*. Such vacuoles may contain mucin—a not completely unexpected finding in immature metaplastic cells.

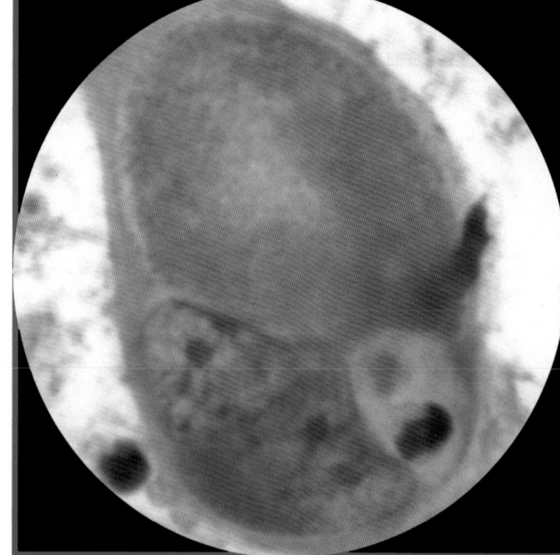

I6.56
Bona fide *Chlamydia*. Inclusions like the one illustrated are more specific but extremely rare (very low sensitivity). This case is the real McCoy—proven by McCoy Cell Culture. (Case courtesy of Denise Hidvegi, MD, Northwestern University.)

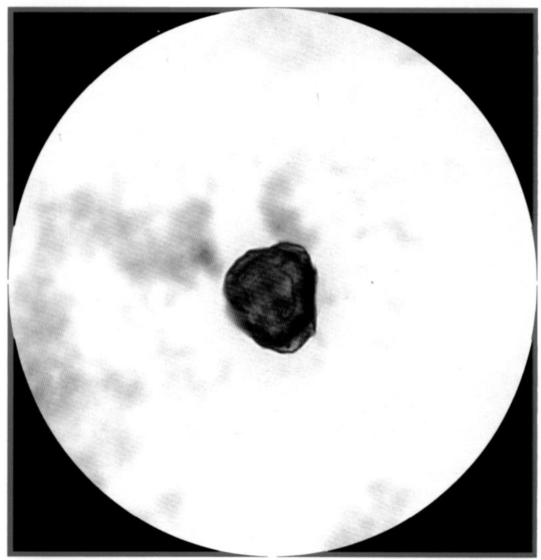

I6.57
Psammoma body or calcospherite. This is a rare finding in a Pap smear, and is not necessarily associated with malignancy. Note concentric laminations.

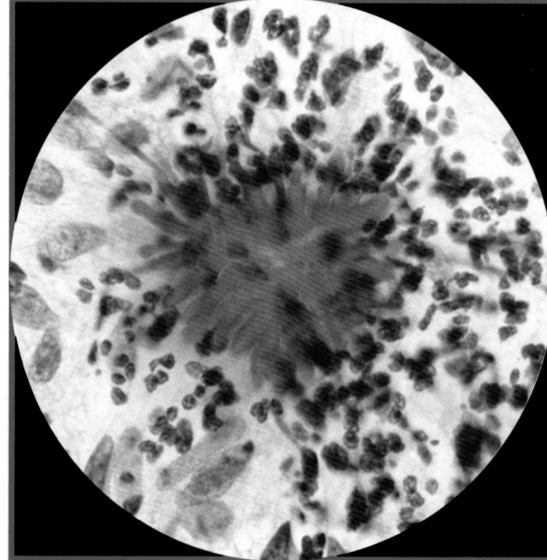

I6.58
Cockleburrs are radiate crystalline arrays surrounded by histiocytes. They are usually associated with pregnancy. They are not hematoidin crystals as formerly believed, nor do they contain immunoglobulin. They probably represent products of cellular degeneration.

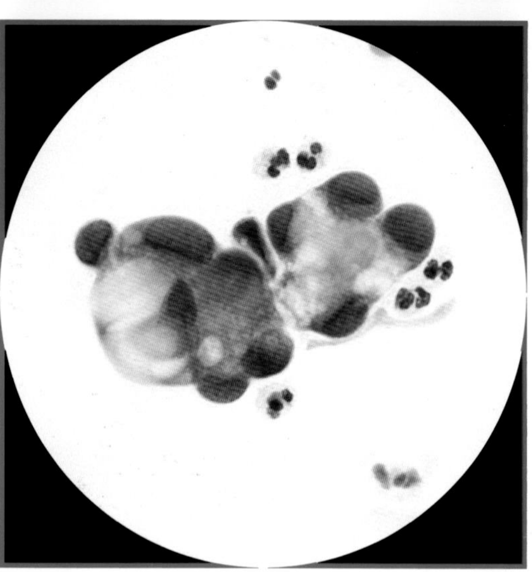

I6.59
IUD cells. A three-dimensional cluster of hypervacuolated endocervical cells, mimicking adenocarcinoma, from a patient using an intrauterine contraceptive device is shown. Nuclear degeneration is common; nucleoli may be prominent. Be careful when diagnosing adenocarcinoma in patients wearing an IUD. Note that IUD cells can persist for months after removal of the device.

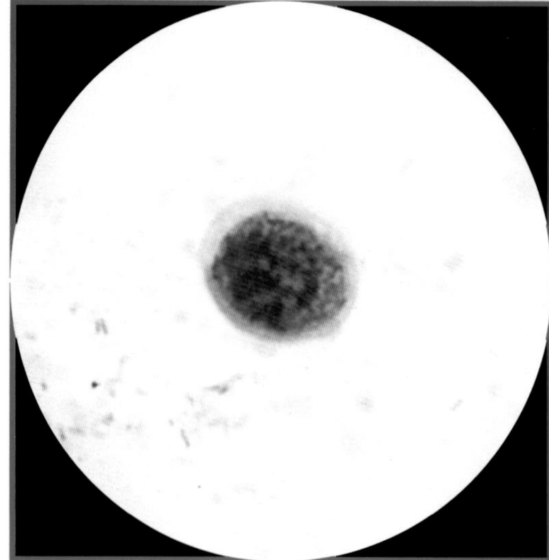

I6.60
IUD cell. "Dings" are single endometrial cells that mimic single cells of carcinoma in situ. However, in contrast with CIS, "dings" are sparse and exclusively single (no syncytia), are usually not associated with dysplasia (as CIS usually is), have finely undulating, rather than deeply folded, nuclear membranes, and may have conspicuous nucleoli. (Oil)

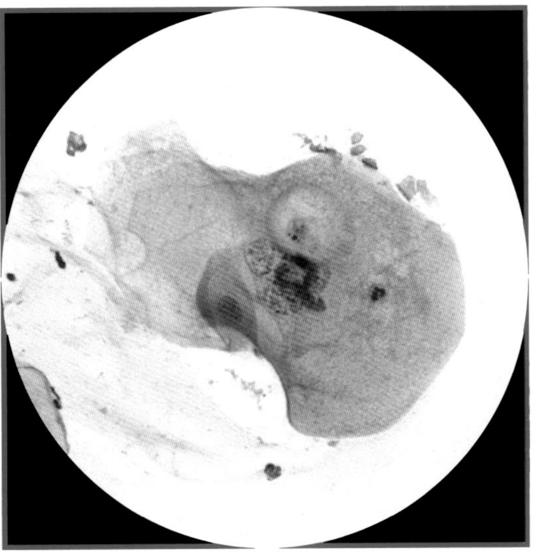

I6.61
Radiation effect (macrocyte). Radiation change is characterized primarily by cytomegaly, ie, macrocytes. Macrocytes also occur in condyloma and vitamin deficiency (folate, B_{12}). The nuclei, which may be multiple, enlarge in concert with the cytoplasm, without a significant increase in the nuclear/cytoplasmic ratio. Two-tone staining of cytoplasm (polychromasia) is common, and cytoplasmic vacuolization, which may contain neutrophils, can also be seen.

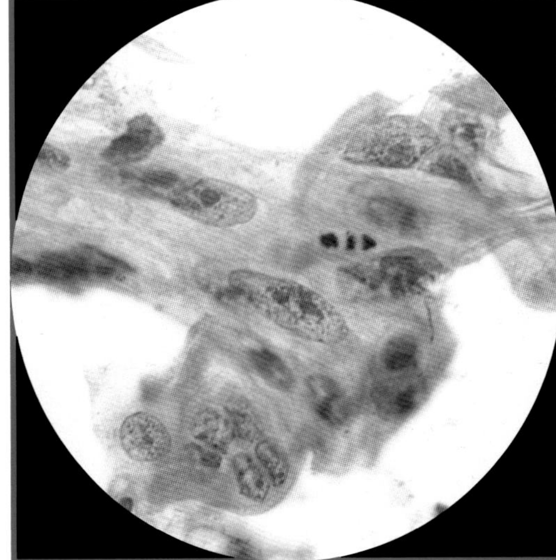

I6.62
Postradiation repair combines "atypia" of repair with "atypia" of radiation, sometimes giving rather spectacular appearing cells in the Pap smear. Note high degree of cohesion and order, and pale chromatin.

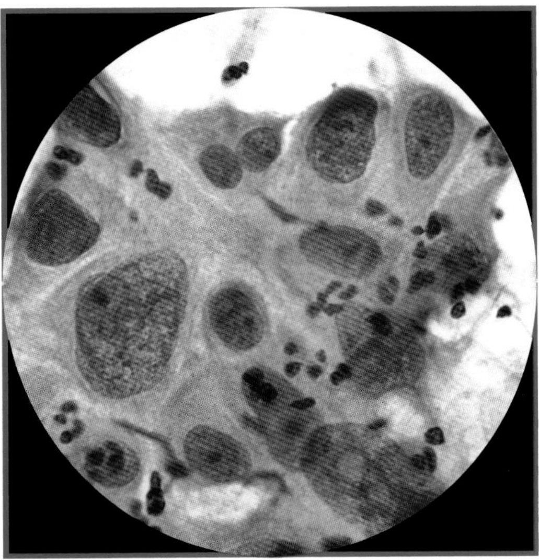

I6.63
Postradiation repair. Nuclei are more crowded, atypical, and hyperchromatic compared with I6.62. A diagnosis of atypical repair, a form of ASCUS, could be considered.

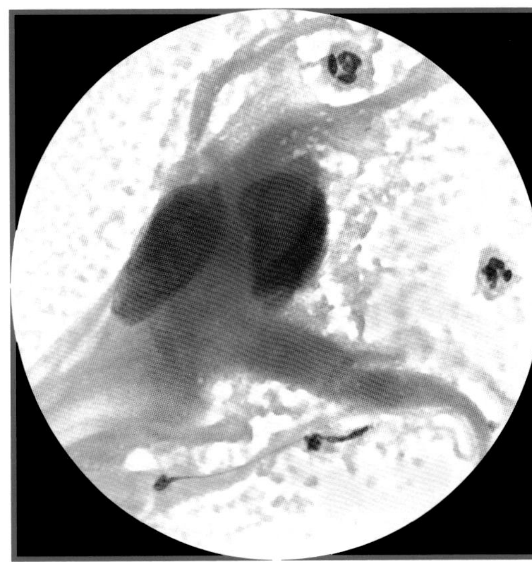

I6.64
Radiated mesenchymal cells are commonly observed in irradiated patients with an ulcer. Changes are similar to those seen in irradiated epithelial cells (ie, cytomegaly). Note the characteristic slender arms (or rootlets) in this octopus-like example.

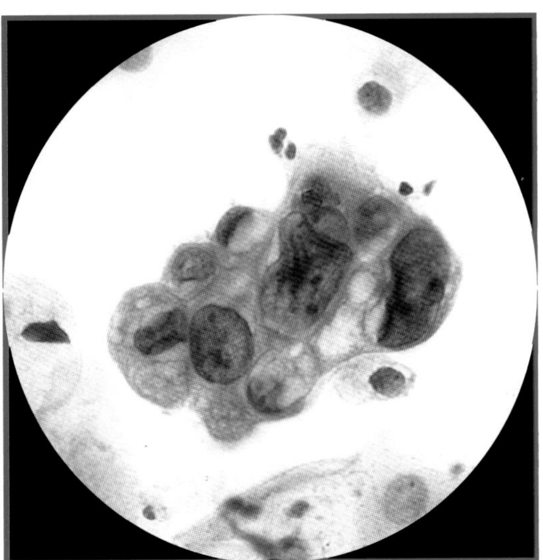

I6.65
Chemotherapy effect. Antineoplastic drugs may have an effect on the cells, which varies according to the type of drug. This is an example of atypical endocervical cells (AGUS, favor reactive) from a patient who had undergone a bone marrow transplant.

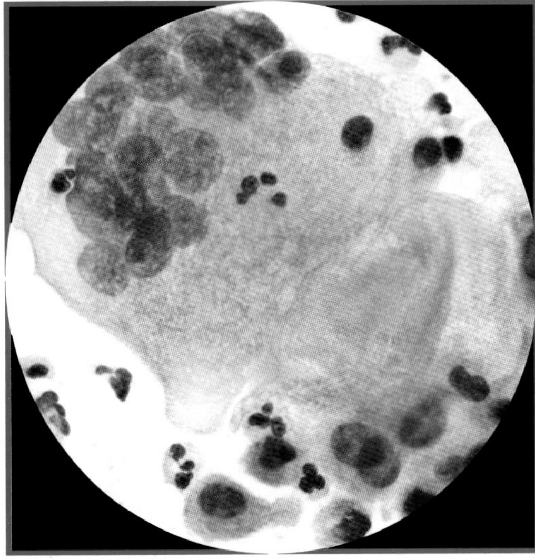

I6.66
Posttherapy foreign body reaction. Giant cell reactions, often to squamous debris, are common after surgery or radiation. Note ingested squame in the cytoplasm of the giant cell histiocyte.

I6.67
Suture granuloma. Foreign body reaction to suture material after surgery is shown.

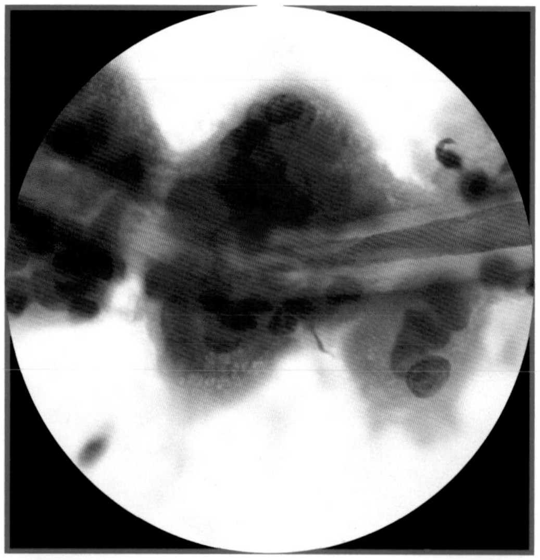

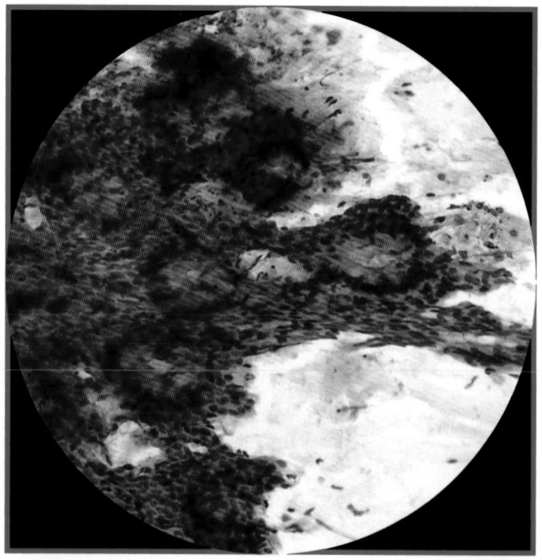

I6.68
Colonic neovagina. Most of the Pap smear consisted of mucus containing markedly degenerated epithelial cells. However, a few fragments of colonic-type mucosa were also present. Note the normal, well defined gland openings, which would be an abnormal feature in endocervical glandular cells, suggesting neoplasia.

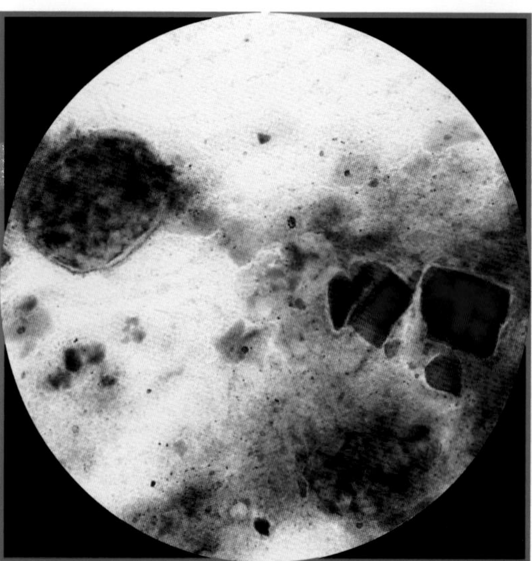

I6.69
Rectovaginal fistula. Note the presence of degenerated cells, meat (skeletal muscle fibers), vegetable matter (with cell walls), and abundant bacteria.

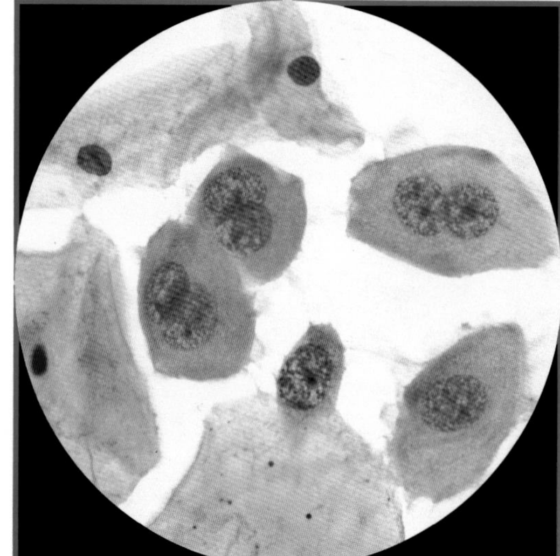

I6.70
Vesicovaginal fistula. Note the presence of both squamous and transitional (urothelial) cells. The transitional cells have dense blue-gray cytoplasm and scalloped cell borders (reminiscent of bladder wash).

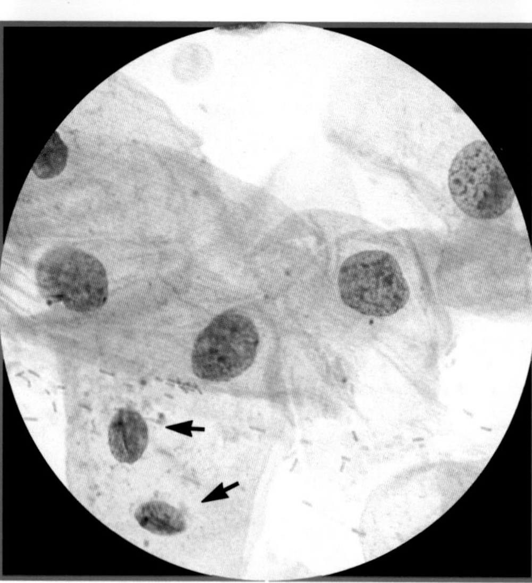

I6.71
Squamous atypia (ASCUS). Compare the atypical cells with the normal intermediate cells in the field (arrows). The atypical nuclei are enlarged (~2 to 3 or more times the size of the normal intermediate nucleus) and usually slightly hyperchromatic. The nuclear membranes are smooth or minimally irregular, and the chromatin is fine and evenly distributed, without granularity. Note that the cytoplasm of the atypical cells tends to be thin and delicate, like normal mature cells.

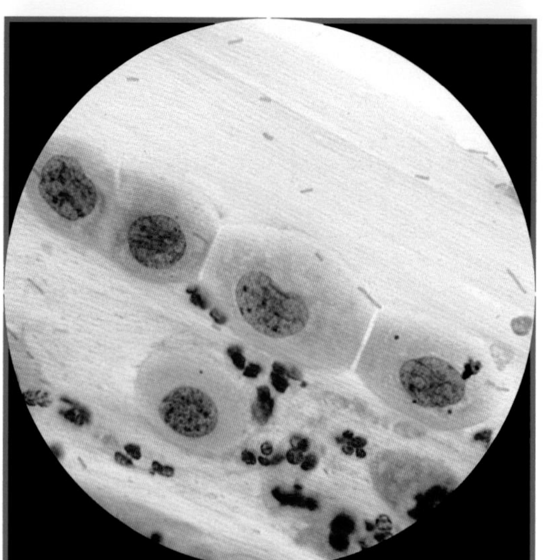

I6.72
Atypical squamous metaplasia (ASM) (ASCUS). ASM is a difficult diagnosis: the nuclei are very subtly abnormal, less abnormal than even mild (immature) metaplastic dysplasia. As in squamous atypia, the nuclei are enlarged into the range of 70–120 μm^2. The nuclear membranes are smooth or only slightly irregular, and the chromatin is fine and evenly distributed, without granularity.

I6.73
Koilocytes. Koilocytes are pathognomonic of condyloma and HPV infection, which is recognized by the Bethesda System as a low-grade squamous intraepithelial lesion. To be a diagnostic koilocyte, the cytoplasmic vacuole must be clear and extremely well defined, with condensation of the peripheral cytoplasm. In addition, the nucleus must appear abnormal (enlarged and dark, ie, "dysplastic"). Binucleation is common.

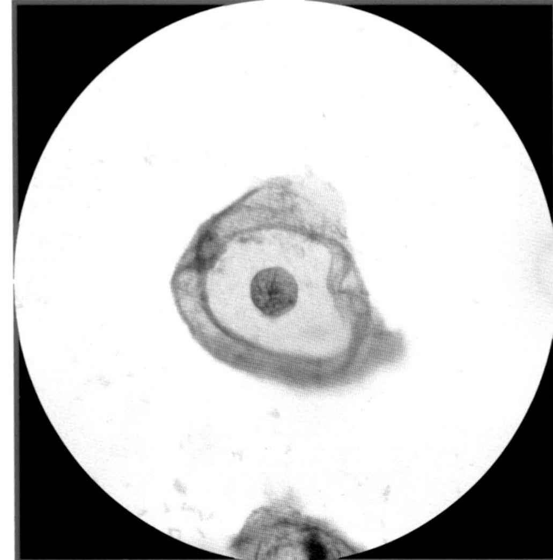

I6.74
Pseudokoilocytes. This is a glycogenated intermediate cell, not a koilocyte. Although this particular example has a relatively well-defined vacuole, note that the nucleus is not abnormal. Slight yellow staining of the vacuole suggests glycogen.

I6.75
Dyskeratocytes (keratinizing dysplasia). Dyskeratocytes are similar to, or identical with, atypical parakeratosis and/or keratinizing dysplasia. Although some observers contend that such cells are diagnostic of condyloma, most require koilocytes to make the diagnosis. This example illustrates keratinizing dysplasia (note similarity to superficial cell, but with "big, dark" nuclei).

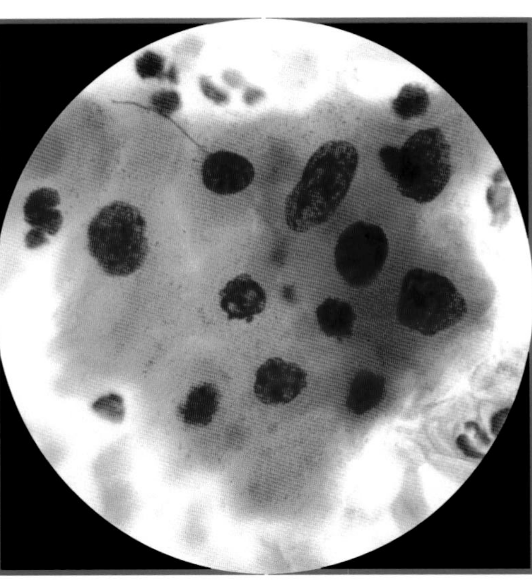

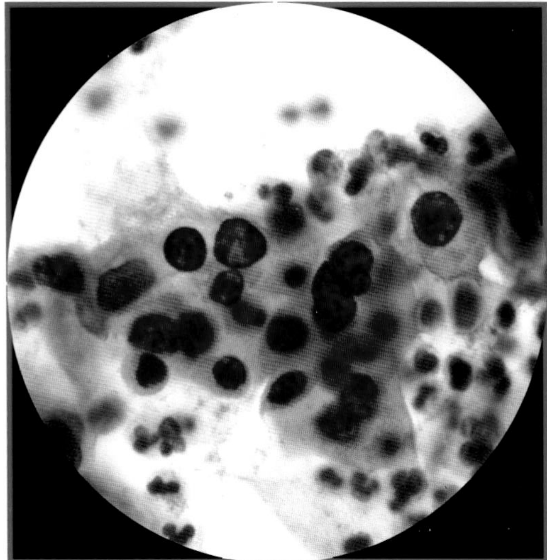

I6.76
Dyskeratocytes (atypical parakeratosis). The cytologic findings are similar to keratinizing dysplasia, except they occur in miniature superficial cells.

I6.77
Macrocytes. This is a rather spectacular example of a macrocyte. Macrocytes need not be anything more than very large intermediate or superficial cells. Macrocytes are very commonly observed in condyloma. However, similar macrocytes can also be seen in radiation/chemotherapy effect or vitamin deficiency (folate, B_{12}).

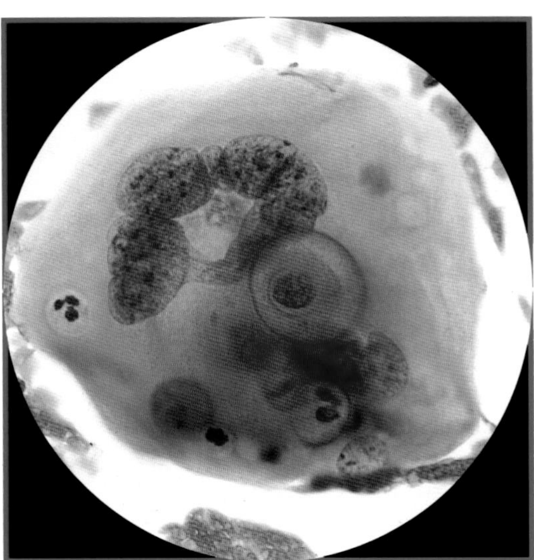

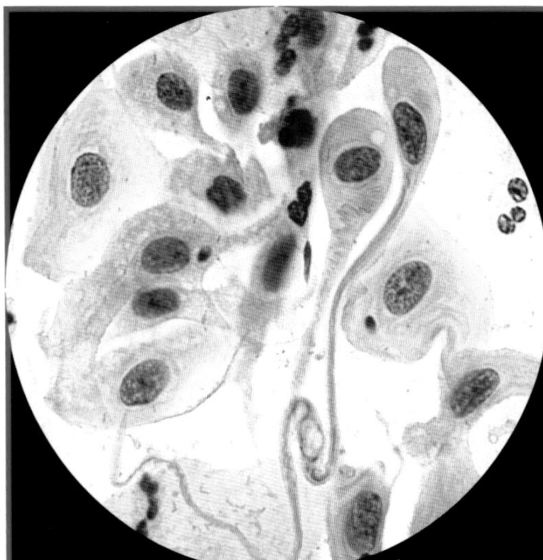

I6.78
Kite cells have long cytoplasmic processes. These cells are minor criteria in diagnosis of condyloma. When such cells are spotted, the slide should be scrutinized for more diagnostic findings of low-grade SIL.

I6.79
Balloon cells look like adipocytes, with large, clear cytoplasm and a peripheral nucleus. These cells are minor criteria in diagnosis of condyloma. When such cells are spotted, the slide should be scrutinized for more diagnostic findings of low-grade SIL. (Image courtesy of Denise Hidvegi, MD, Northwestern University.)

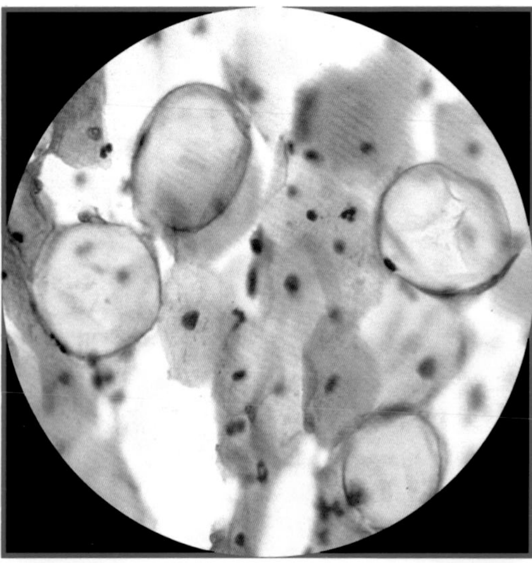

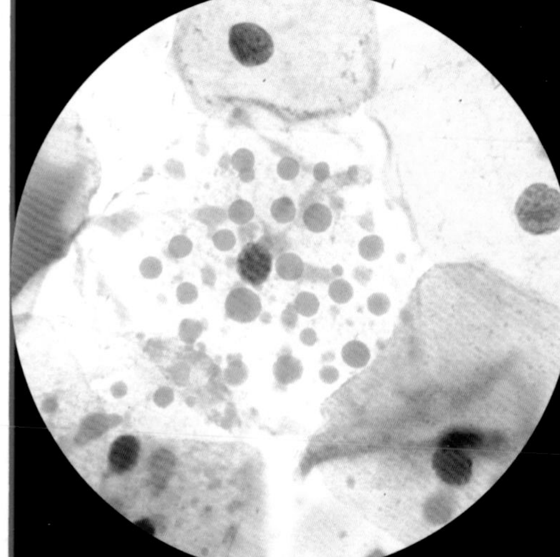

I6.80
Polka dot cells. Cytoplasmic degeneration can lead to presence of hyaline globules. These cells are also a very common finding in condyloma, a minor criterion in diagnosis. Minor criteria of condyloma are merely suggestive, not diagnostic. However, their presence should elicit a search for more diagnostic features of low-grade SIL.

I6.81
Flat condyloma (tissue). Note well-defined cytoplasmic vacuoles and nuclear atypia of the koilocytes. The nuclear atypia helps distinguish the vacuoles of koilocytes from glycogen vacuoles of normal cells. Koilocytes tend to be most prominent in the intermediate cell layers. Compare with I6.1.

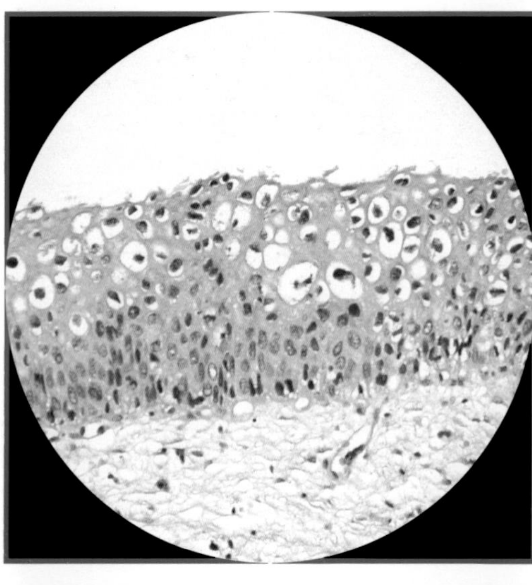

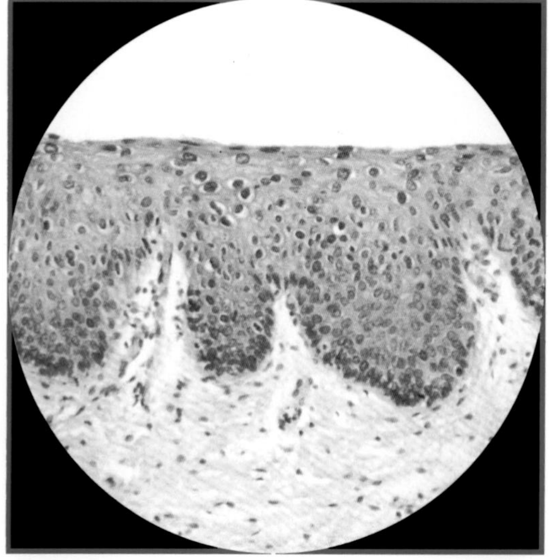

I6.82
Low-grade squamous intraepithelial lesion (tissue). In mild dysplasia, the basal cell proliferation is limited to the bottom one third of the epithelium. Note, however, that abnormal but differentiated cells are present through the full thickness of the epithelium—as they must be in order for the Pap smear to sample them at the surface.

I6.83
High-grade squamous intraepithelial lesion (tissue). In moderate dysplasia, the basal layer rises above the bottom third of the epithelium. In severe dysplasia, the basal proliferation reaches the top third, but there is still some squamous differentiation at the surface.

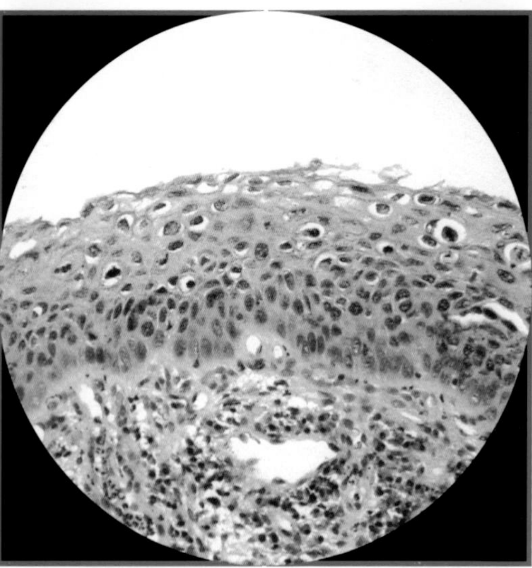

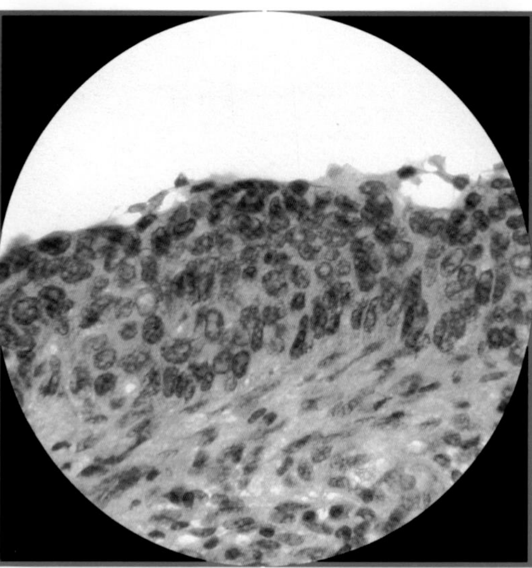

I6.84
High-grade squamous intraepithelial lesion (tissue). In carcinoma in situ, the epithelium is completely replaced with undifferentiated cells.

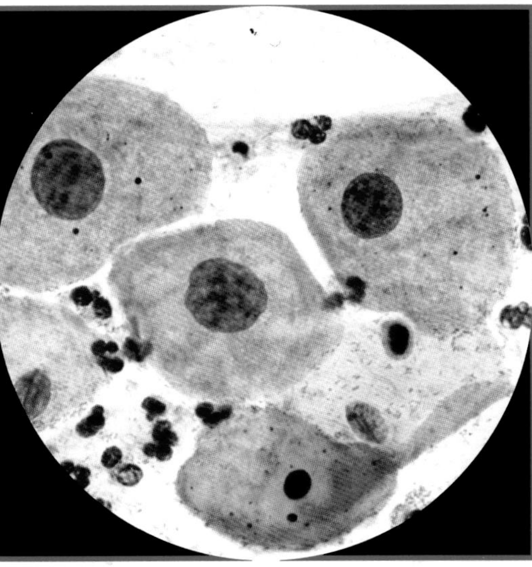

I6.85
Low-grade squamous intraepithelial lesion: mild dysplasia, mature metaplastic type (aka large cell, nonkeratinizing dysplasia). Note resemblance to normal intermediate cells, although the cytoplasm is slightly thick and dense. However, the nuclei are "big and dark," ranging from 120 to 210 μm² (compared with 35μm² for the normal intermediate nucleus).

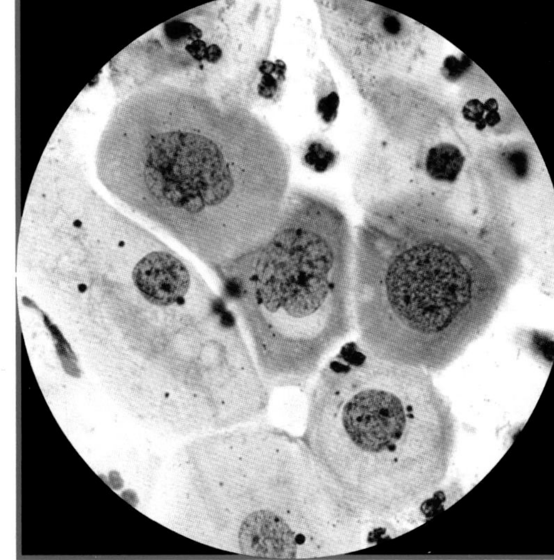

I6.86
High-grade squamous intraepithelial lesion: moderate dysplasia, immature metaplastic (or simply metaplastic) type. Note resemblance to ordinary immature squamous metaplasia (parabasal-sized cells) except that the nuclei are "big and dark" (120 to 210 μm² compared with 50 μm² of normal metaplastic nucleus).

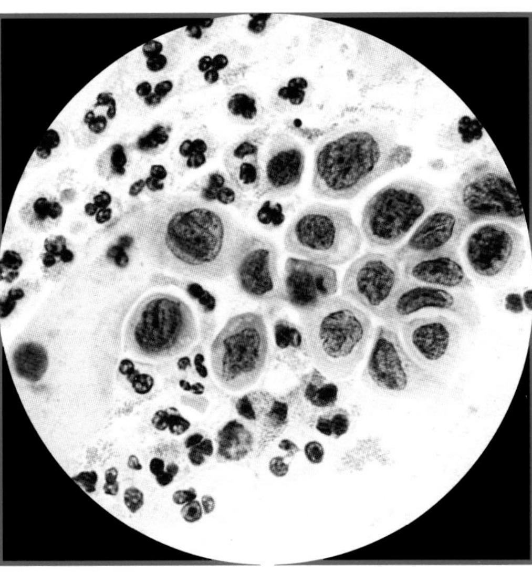

I6.87
High-grade squamous intraepithelial lesion: severe dysplasia, (very immature) metaplastic type. This is represented by small cells with high nuclear/cytoplasmic ratios and irregular, "raisinoid" nuclei. Note thin rim of dense cytoplasm (compare with carcinoma in situ).

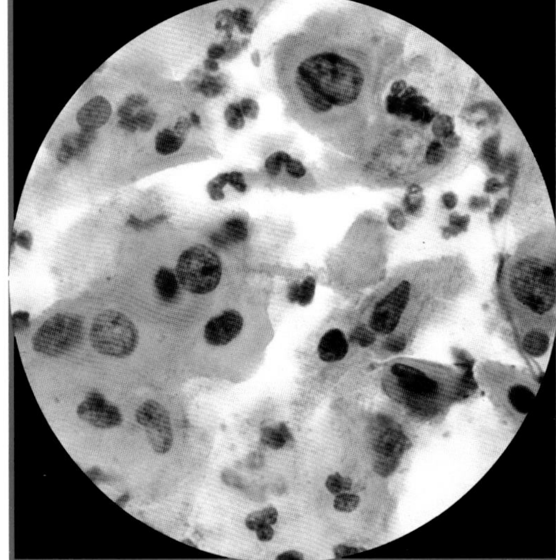

I6.88
High-grade squamous intraepithelial lesion: keratinizing dysplasia, aka pleomorphic dysplasia—a good descriptive term for higher grade keratinizing lesions. (See also I6.75, I6.76.)

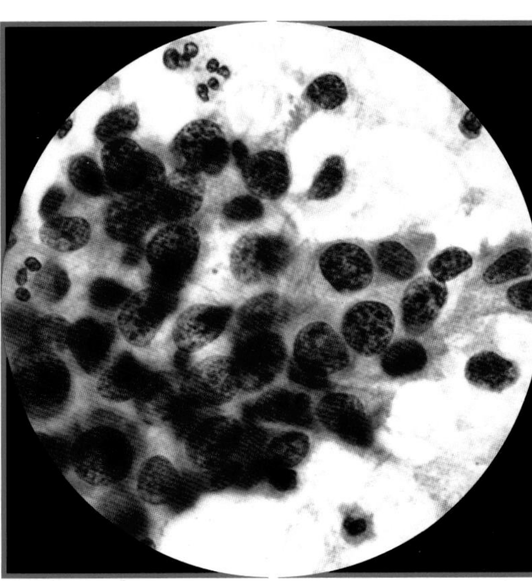

I6.89
High-grade squamous intraepithelial lesion: carcinoma in situ. The most characteristic feature of CIS is the presence of three-dimensional syncytial aggregates of cells with scant, delicate cytoplasm, loss of nuclear polarity, and abnormal nuclei. Syncytial aggregates of CIS are important forms of "hyperchromatic crowded groups."

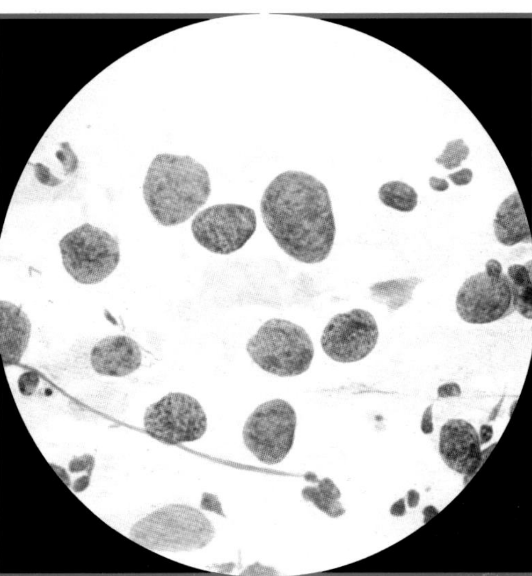

I6.90
High-grade squamous intraepithelial lesion: carcinoma in situ. Because of the delicate nature of the undifferentiated cytoplasm, numerous atypical naked nuclei may be present. Note, however, that naked nuclei are not diagnostic in themselves of CIS.

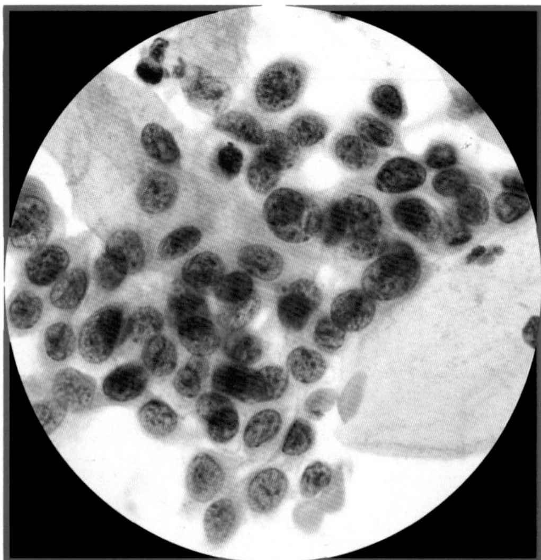

I6.91
High-grade squamous intraepithelial lesion: carcinoma in situ, small cell type. Note the small size of the nuclei—compare with normal intermediate cell nuclei.

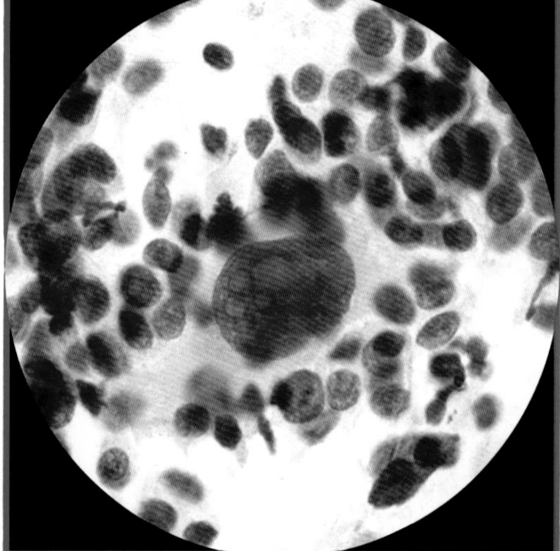

I6.92
High-grade squamous intraepithelial lesion: carcinoma in situ, Bowenoid type. This type has an occasional enormous nucleus.

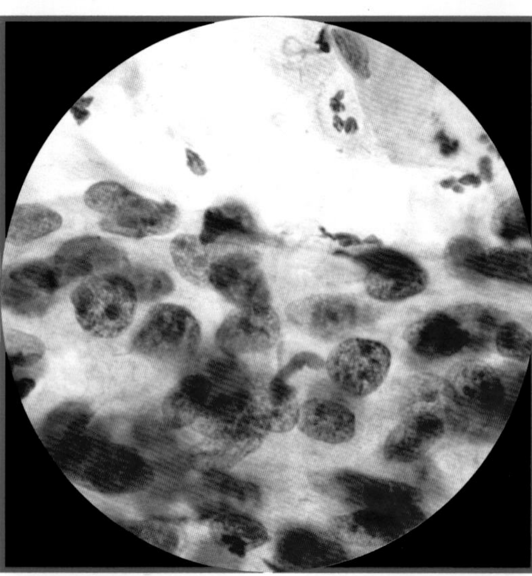

I6.93
Microinvasive squamous cell carcinoma. Note presence of prominent nucleoli and irregular chromatin distribution. Prominent nucleoli, in syncytial aggregates otherwise characteristic of CIS, are a sensitive, but not specific, feature of microinvasive carcinoma; irregular chromatin distribution is the earliest truly malignant feature.

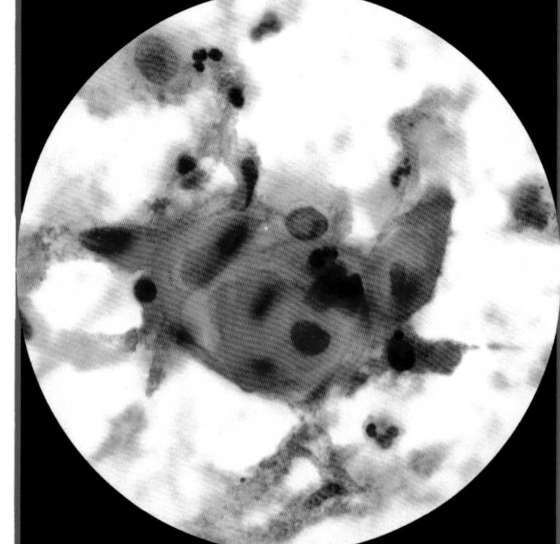

I6.94
Microinvasive squamous cell carcinoma. Abnormal squamous differentiation and sometimes a tumor diathesis (as illustrated), are two more features that can be seen in microinvasive SCC. However, a necrotic tumor diathesis is a worrisome feature suggestive of frankly invasive carcinoma. Ultimately, microinvasive SCC is a histologic, not a cytologic, diagnosis.

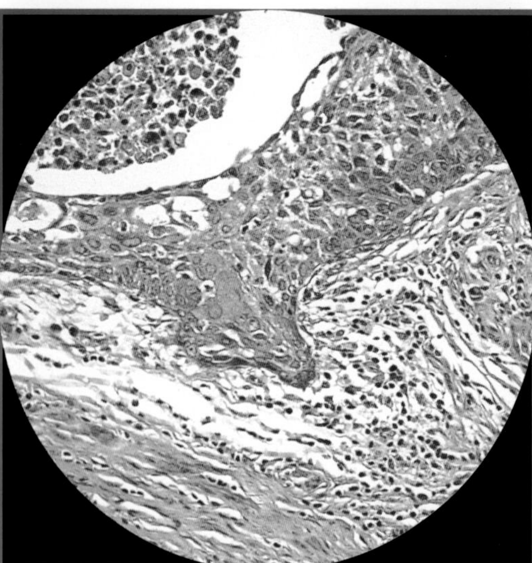

I6.95
Microinvasive squamous cell carcinoma (tissue). In tissue, the cells "redifferentiate" in the invasive tongues, and the stroma shows a desmoplastic response, including edema and chronic inflammation.

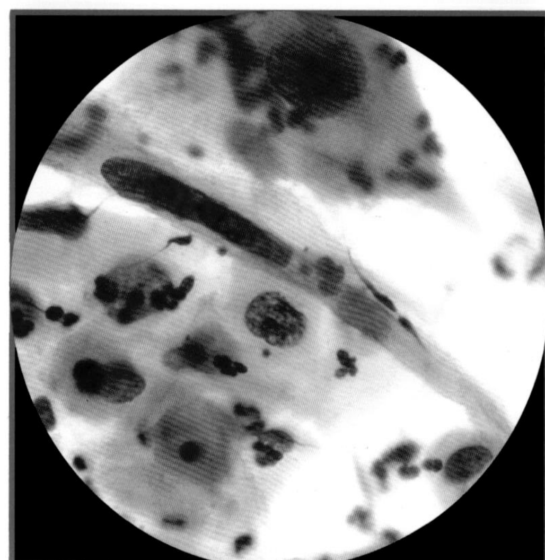

I6.96
Keratinizing squamous cell carcinoma. Markedly pleomorphic or bizarre shaped, heavily keratinized tumor cells, and marked hyperchromasia are characteristic. Cells tend to occur singly.

I6.97
Keratinizing squamous cell carcinoma. The differential diagnosis with keratinizing dysplasia may be difficult in some cases. Also, a tumor diathesis may not be prominent in exophytically growing keratinized squamous cancers. However, when a smear is dominated by dysplastic, keratinized cells, such as these, strongly suspect frank cancer.

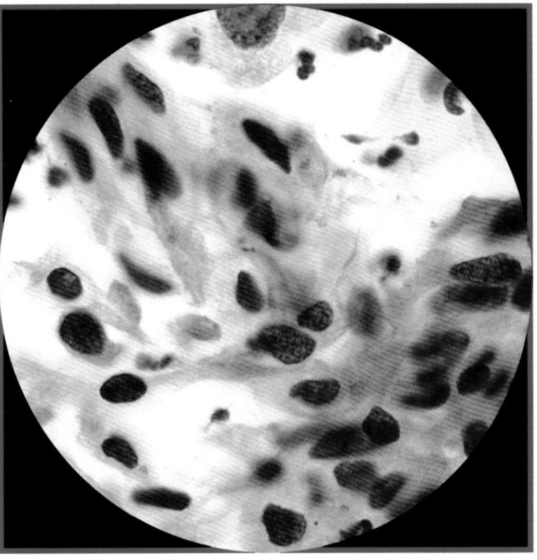

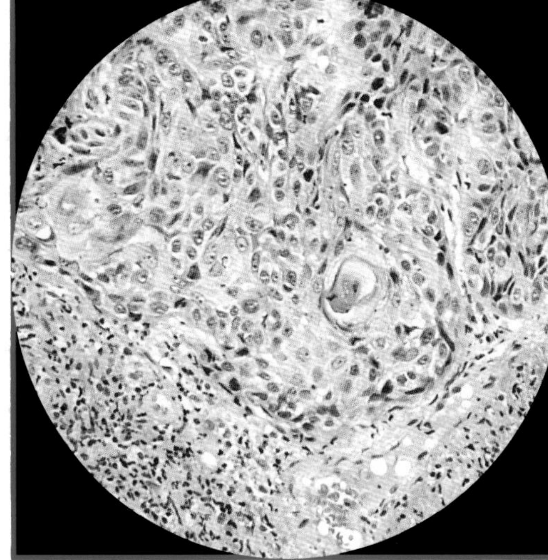

I6.98
Keratinizing squamous cell carcinoma (tissue). Note squamous pearl (aka squamous eddy): pearls are pathognomonic of keratinization.

I6.99
Nonkeratinized squamous cell carcinoma. Compared with keratinizing SCC, the cells of nonkeratinizing SCC are more uniform and more often occur in aggregates. Nuclear abnormalities are usually easier to appreciate in nonkeratinizing SCC.

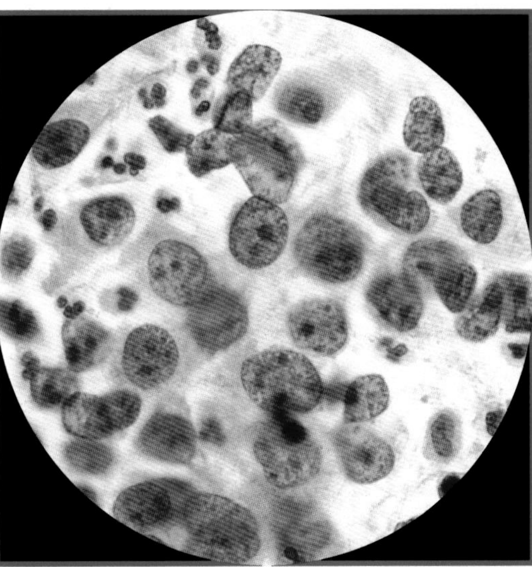

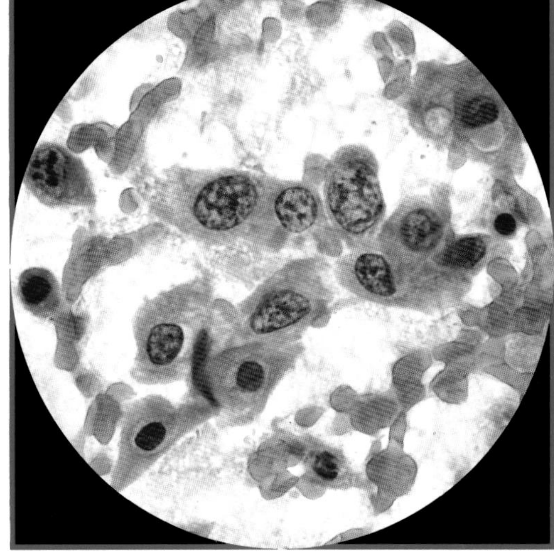

I6.100
Nonkeratinized squamous cell carcinoma. Note irregular chromatin distribution (with clumping and clearing) and prominent nucleoli. A tumor diathesis is commonly present. It consists of fibrin, fresh and old blood, and necrotic debris, and represents the host response to the invading tumor. The presence of occasional keratinized cells (dyskeratosis) does exclude nonkeratinized SCC, but pearls are not seen.

I6.101
Nonkeratinized squamous cell carcinoma (corresponding tissue).

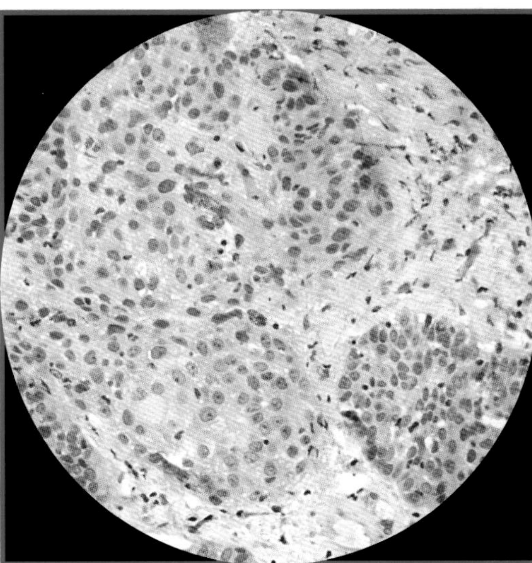

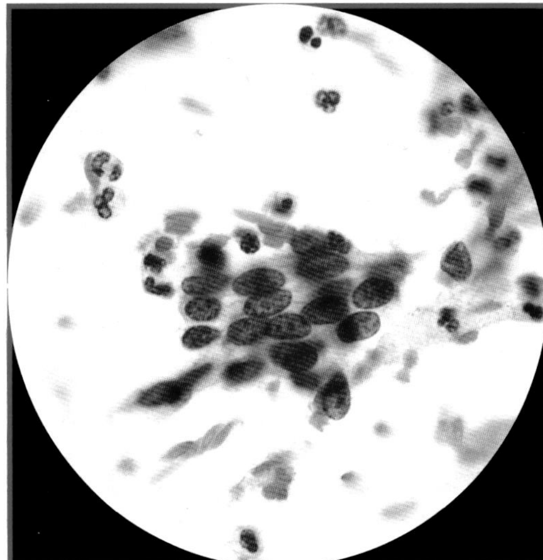

I6.102
Small cell squamous carcinoma. The cells are small, with very hyperchromatic, oval to spindle-shaped nuclei, which average about 1 to 2 times the size (area) of an intermediate cell nucleus. This is not to be confused with small cell neuroendocrine carcinoma, which does occur rarely in the cervix, but is far more common in the lung (see I6.138).

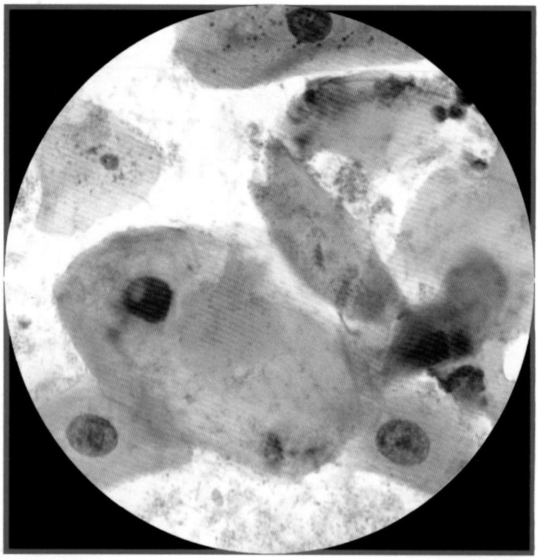

I6.103
Verrucous squamous carcinoma is represented by papillary growth, infiltrates by rete peg expansion, and is extremely well differentiated. Cytology may suggest only low-grade keratinizing dysplasia. Koilocytes are absent or few.

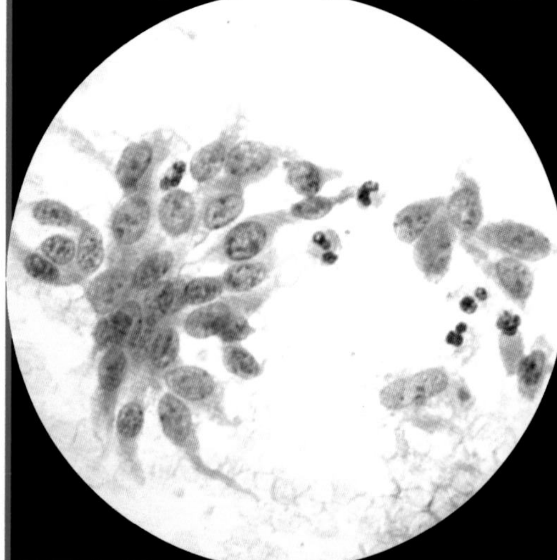

I6.104
Spindle squamous carcinoma is represented by spindly, nonkeratinized, malignant squamous cells that may suggest a sarcoma ("pseudosarcoma").

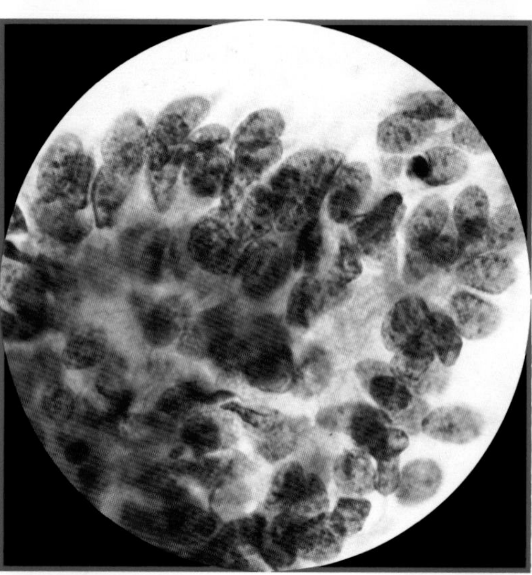

I6.105
Endocervical adenocarcinoma in situ. Crowded syncytial-like aggregates of cells with high nuclear/cytoplasmic ratios, indistinct cell borders, and irregular "feathery" edges (hyperchromatic crowded groups). The nuclei are oval, with moderately coarse, dark chromatin, and, like squamous CIS, usually lack nucleoli. Mitotic figures may be present.

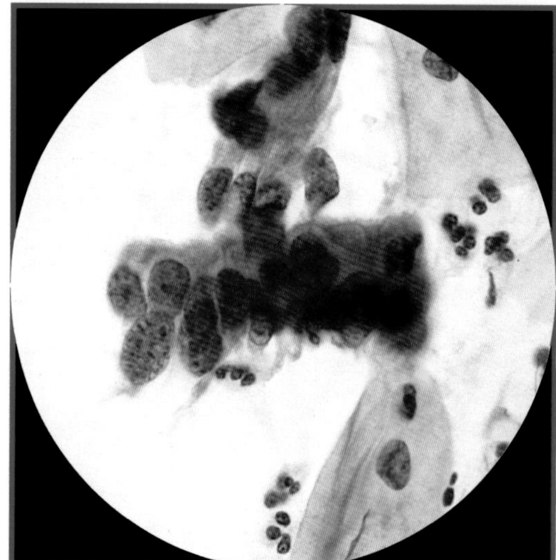

I6.106
Endocervical adenocarcinoma in situ. Crowded, stratified strips (compare with strips of normal endocervical cells, I6.12) are shown.

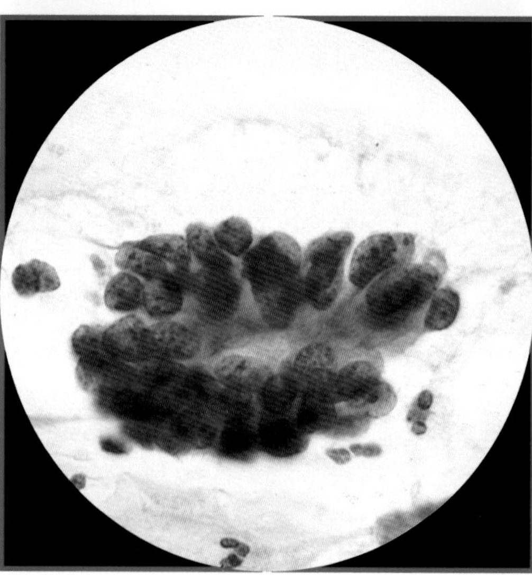

I6.107
Endocervical adenocarcinoma in situ. Crowded rosette. Benign endocervical cells rarely form rosettes.

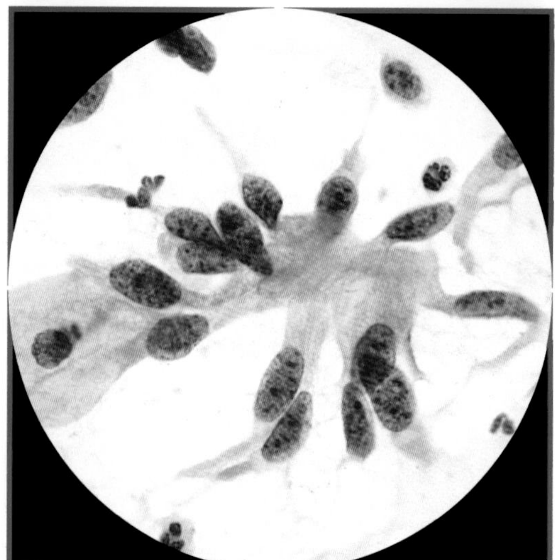

I6.108
Endocervical adenocarcinoma in situ. Rosette of atypical endocervical cells with elongated, hyperchromatic nuclei. Note characteristic columnar shape is maintained. In the Bethesda System, the diagnosis for adenocarcinoma in situ is "atypical glandular cells of undetermined significance, favor neoplastic."

I6.109
Endocervical adenocarcinoma in situ (tissue). Note abrupt transition from normal to adenocarcinoma in situ.

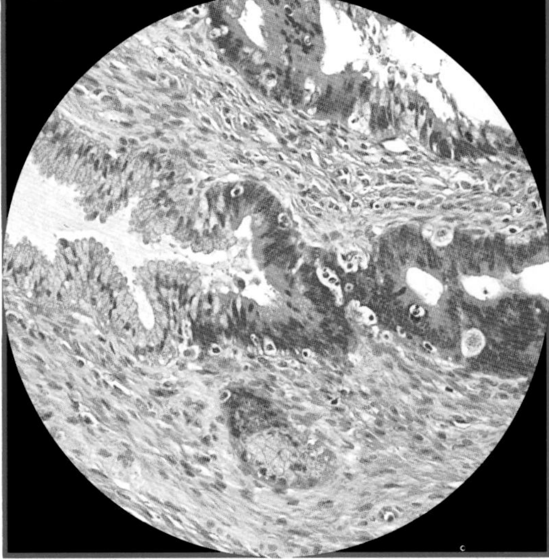

I6.110
Endocervical adenocarcinoma in situ (tissue). Compare normal endocervical cells, which have uniform, round, basal nuclei, with neoplastic endocervical cells, which have stratified, oval to elongated, hyperchromatic nuclei.

I6.111
Endocervical adenocarcinoma (invasive). Findings may be similar to the in situ lesion, including crowded sheets of cells as seen here. However, prominent nucleoli and, particularly, a tumor diathesis are associated with invasion. Note the presence of mitotic figures: mitotic figures are abnormal in (nonreparative) endocervical cells and strongly suggest malignancy.

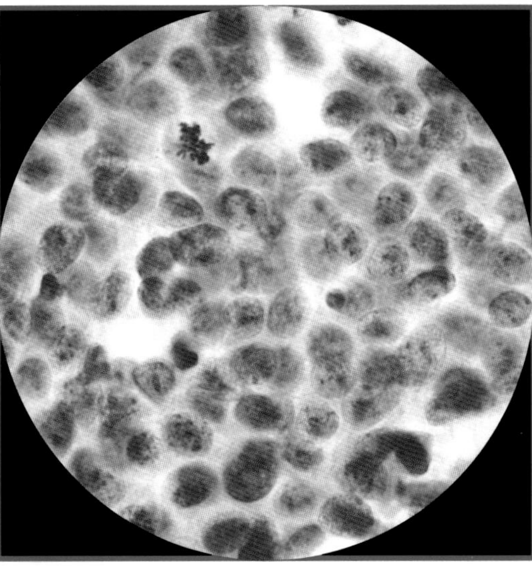

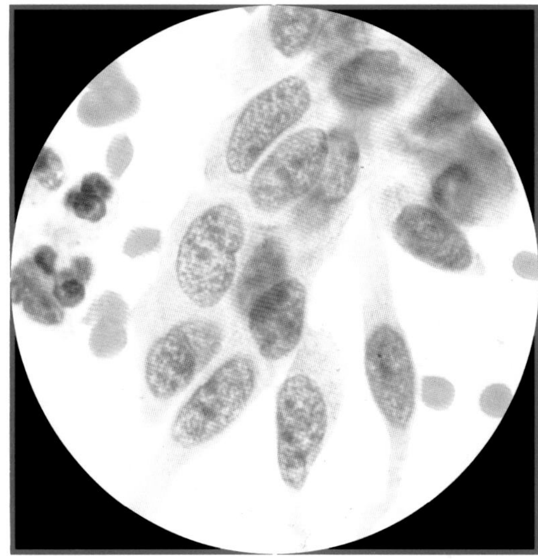

I6.112
Endocervical adenocarcinoma. The malignant cells tend to retain their columnar shape.

I6.113
Endocervical adenocarcinoma. Stratified strips of malignant endocervical cells. The nuclei are enlarged, hyperchromatic, and have coarse chromatin (compare with endometrial adenocarcinoma).

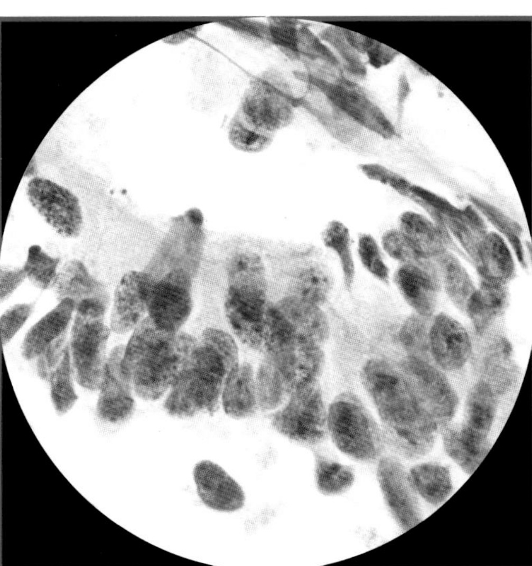

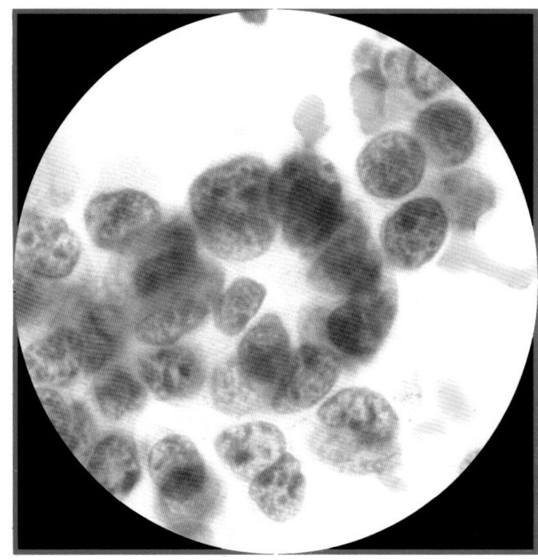

I6.114
Endocervical adenocarcinoma is represented by a rosette-like arrangement of malignant endocervical cells. Note prominent nucleoli.

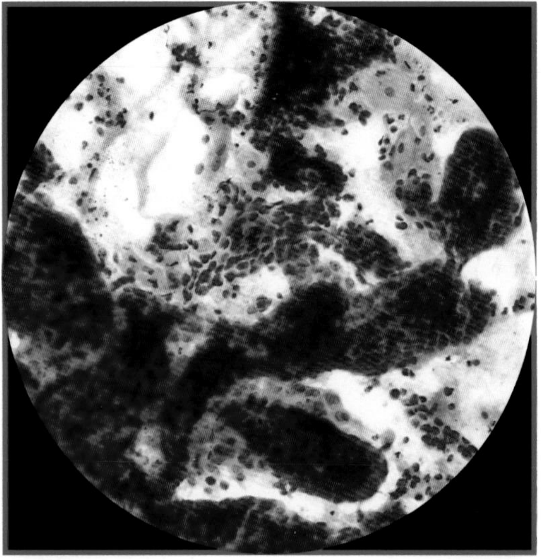

I6.115
Endocervical adenocarcinoma. Occasional cases have a papillary configuration.

I6.116
Endocervical adenocarcinoma (tissue). Note classic gland-in-gland pattern of adenocarcinoma. The tumor cells are reminiscent of benign endocervical cells, but have abnormal nuclei.

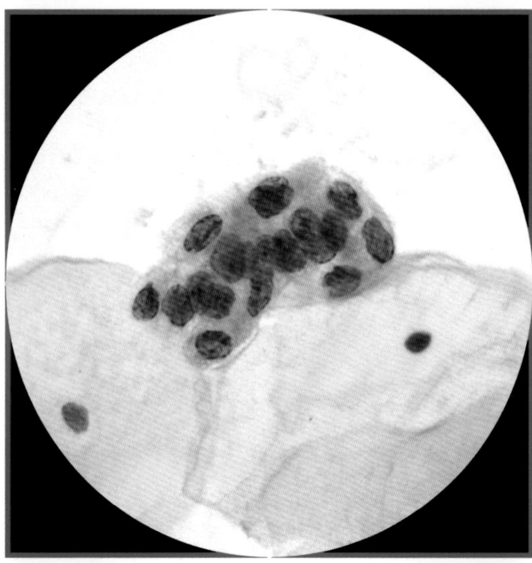

I6.117
Atypical endometrial cells (AGUS). The significance of these cells was eventually determined to be endometrial hyperplasia. Note that the nuclei are larger than intermediate cell nuclei. The nuclei are hyperchromatic and an occasional nucleolus is noted, but a tumor diathesis is absent.

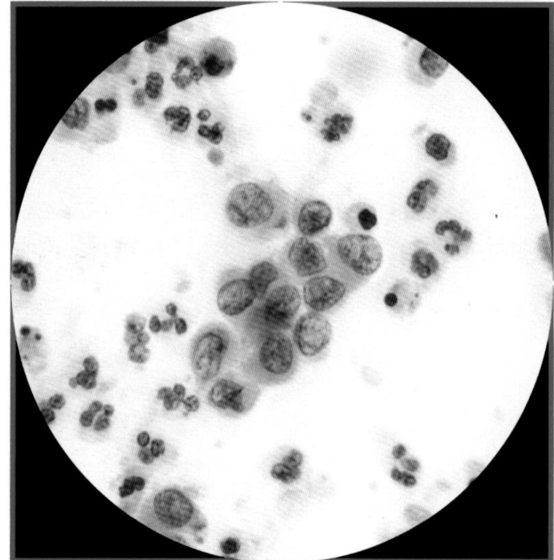

I6.118
Atypical endometrial cells (AGUS). This patient had a well-differentiated endometrial adenocarcinoma. The nuclei are larger than those of hyperplasia, and prominent nucleoli are noted in most, but the chromatin is not as dark.

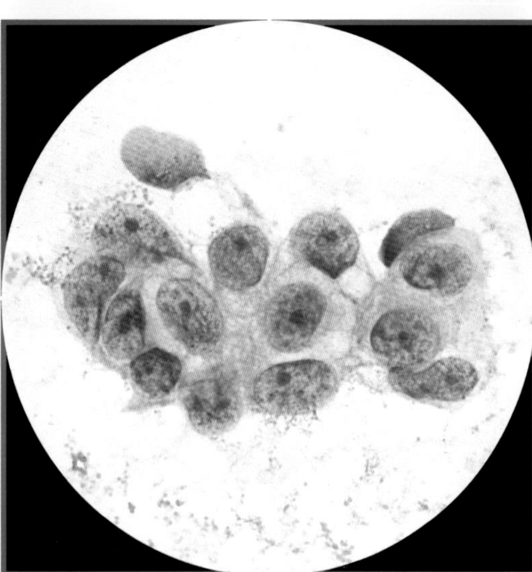

I6.119
Endometrial adenocarcinoma. Compare the rounded configuration of malignant endometrial cells to the columnar shape characteristic of endocervical adenocarcinoma (I6.112).

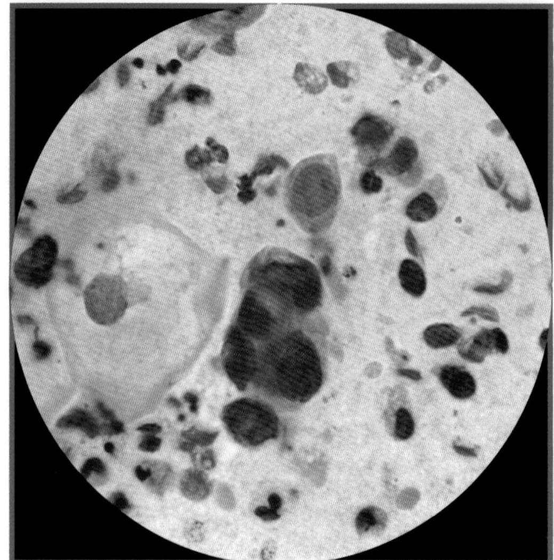

I6.120
Endometrial adenocarcinoma is represented by malignant endometrial cells in characteristic "watery" tumor diathesis (ie, finely granular rather than coarsely necrotic background).

I6.121
Glassy cell carcinoma. A poorly differentiated adenosquamous carcinoma with abundant "glassy" cytoplasm that contains PAS-positive glycogen is shown.

I6.122
Metastatic papillary serous carcinoma (ovary). Note papillary configuration and clean background.

I6.123
Carcinoma of the fallopian tube. Primary malignancies at this site are rare. Adenocarcinomas and adenosquamous carcinomas are the most common types.

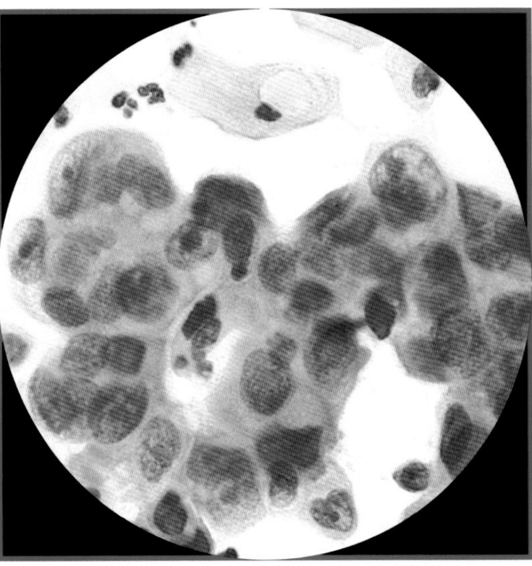

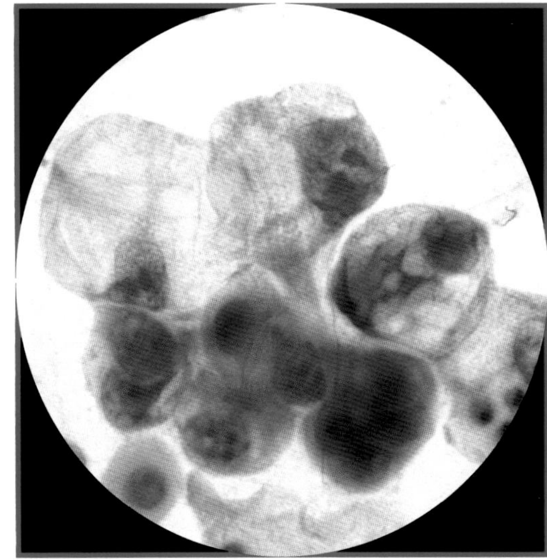

I6.124
Clear cell carcinoma (endometrium). Similar tumors can occur in the vagina associated with intrauterine DES exposure.

I6.125
Malignant mixed mesodermal (müllerian) tumor or carcinosarcoma. Often, only the malignant epithelial component (adenocarcinoma, illustrated) is seen in the Pap smear. The adenocarcinoma can range from well differentiated to poorly differentiated.

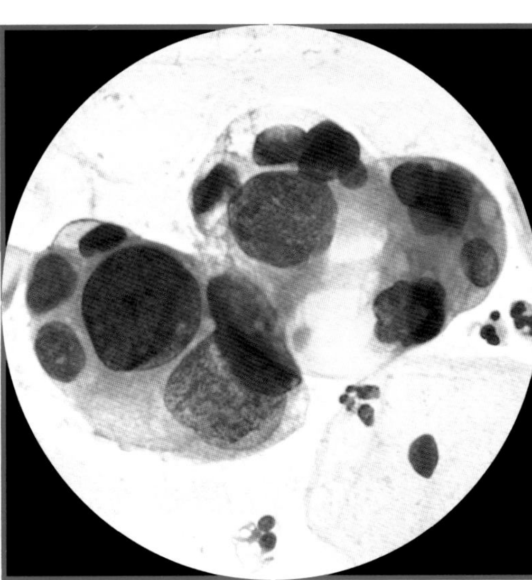

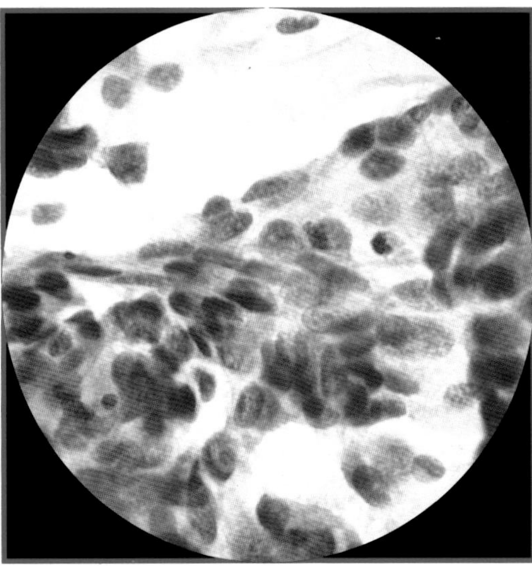

I6.126
Carcinosarcoma: metaplastic spindle cell carcinoma.

I6.127
Secretory endometrial adenocarcinoma. Well-differentiated carcinoma with delicate, glycogen positive cytoplasm and bland, uniform nuclei is shown.

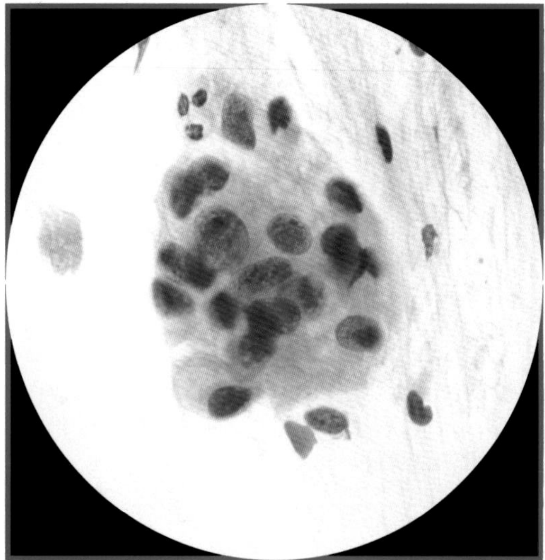

I6.128
Metastatic gastric carcinoma. Note clean background, characteristic of metastatic carcinomas in the Pap smear.

I6.129
Rectal carcinoma more often represents direct extension than actual metastasis. Note nuclear palisading and well-defined apical cytoplasmic border.

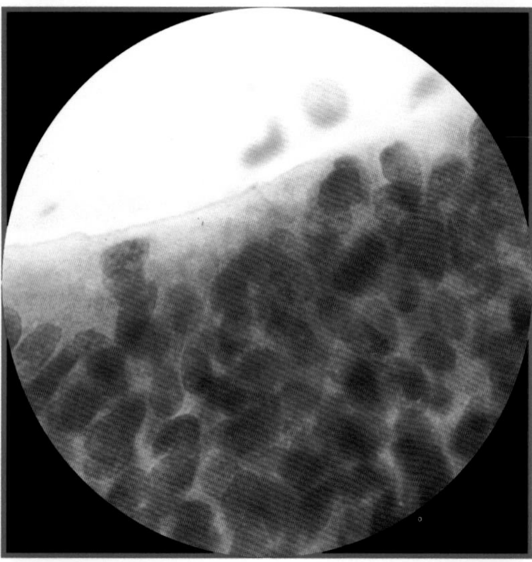

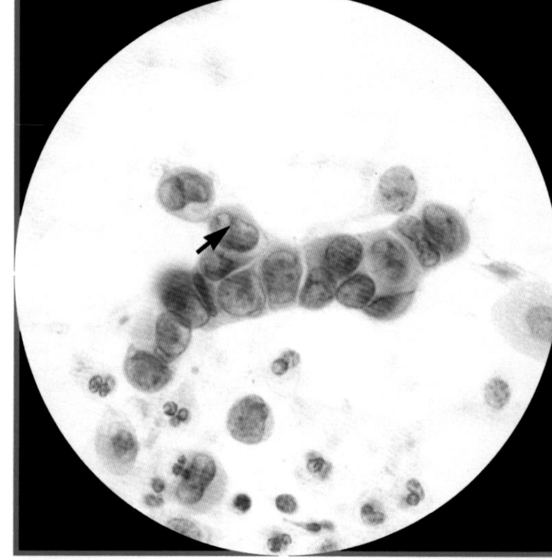

I6.130
Metastatic breast carcinoma. Note clean background and "Indian file" arrangement, a characteristic, but not specific feature. Intracytoplasmic lumen (arrow) also suggests breast origin.

I6.131
Metastatic melanoma is frequently amelanotic in metastases, and can mimic a wide variety of other tumors. It would be easy to mistake this example for metastatic adenocarcinoma. History can be critical.

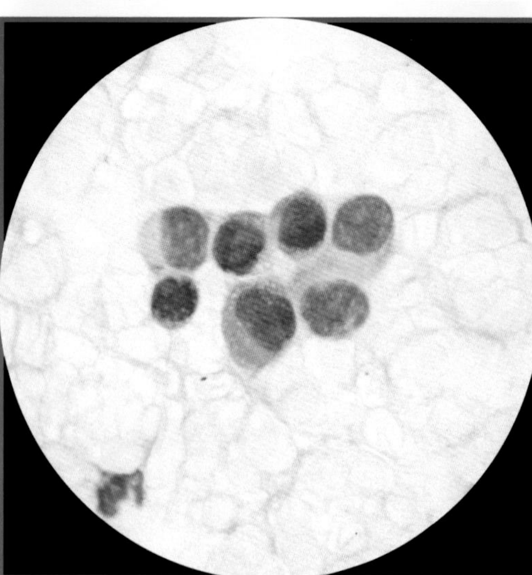

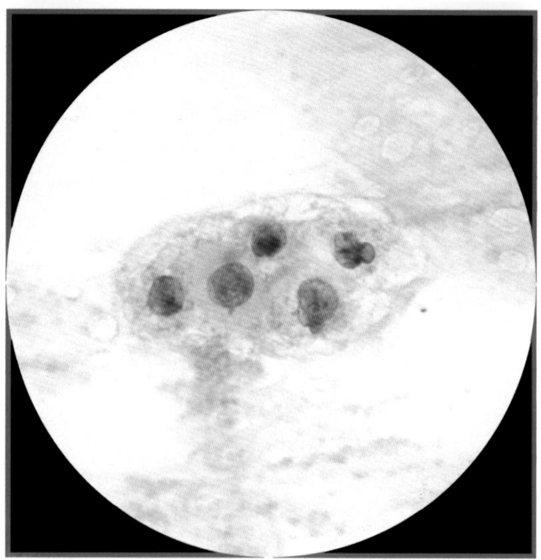

I6.132
Clear cell mesonephric carcinoma. This is a putative example of a very rare tumor arising from mesonephric duct remnants.

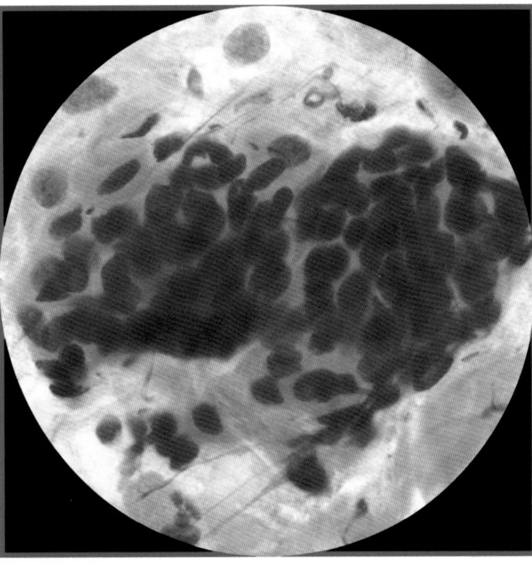

I6.133
Hyperchromatic crowded group (atrophy). In extreme atrophy, the basal cells form three-dimensional, crowded aggregates of small, hyperchromatic cells with high nuclear/cytoplasmic ratios, which may mimic squamous carcinoma in situ. However, the nuclei are uniform, with smooth nuclear membranes, fine chromatin, and no mitotic figures. The cells may differentiate into parabasal cells along the edge.

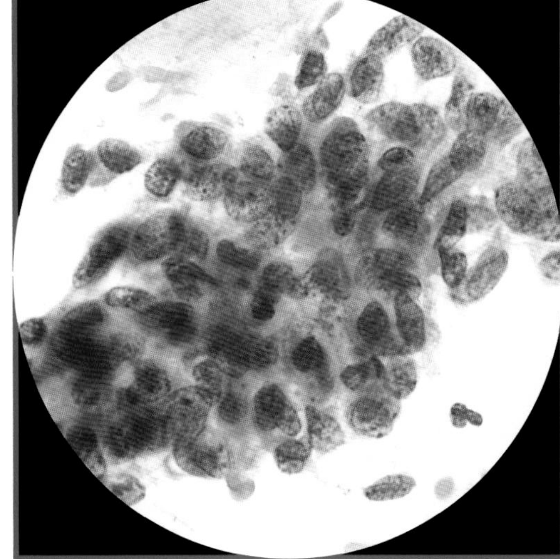

I6.134
Hyperchromatic crowded group (endometrial cells). Endometrial glandular cells can also be responsible for the presence of HCGs in the Pap smear. The cells are commonly degenerated, but have uniform nuclei, and may be associated with stromal cells.

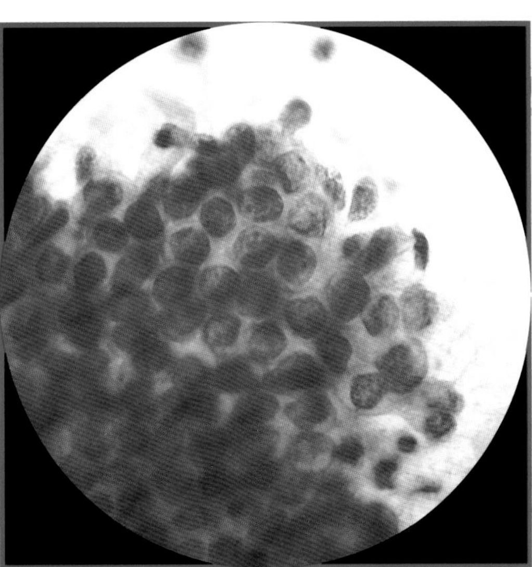

I6.135
Hyperchromatic crowded group (endocervical cells). Endocervical cells deriving from high in the endocervix are commonly crowded and hyperchromatic. Note overall uniformity of the nuclei and resemblance to other, more obvious, endocervical cells. No mitotic figures are present.

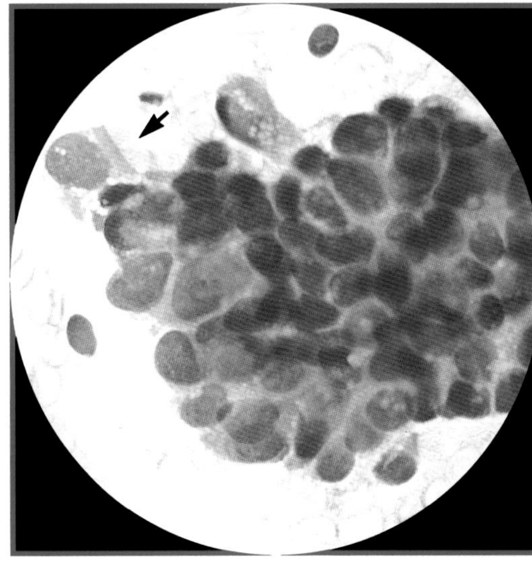

I6.136
Hyperchromatic crowded group (tubal metaplasia). Cells deriving from tubal metaplasia also present as "hyperchromatic crowded groups." Look for presence of cilia (arrow) to confirm benign diagnosis. Unfortunately, however, the cilia can degenerate, making the differential diagnosis more difficult. No mitotic figures are present.

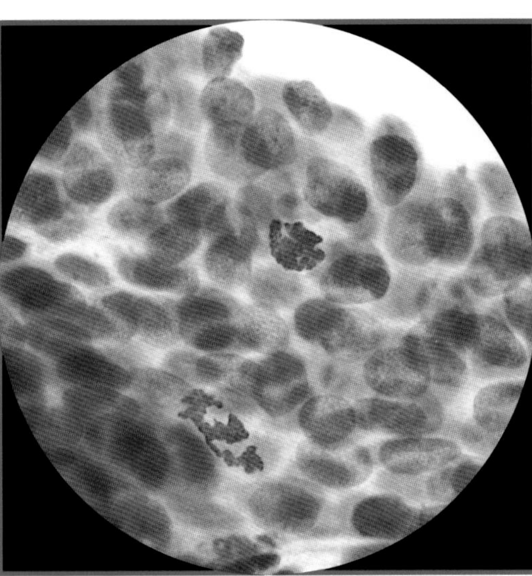

I6.137
Hyperchromatic crowded group (squamous carcinoma in situ). Possibility of a neoplastic lesion is the reason to carefully evaluate all HCGs in the Pap smear. CIS is usually characterized by abnormal cells with irregular nuclear membranes and an associated squamous dysplasia. However, some cases have unexpectedly bland appearing cells and no accompanying dysplasia (more likely in older women). Mitotic figures in HCGs strongly suggest a neoplastic lesion.

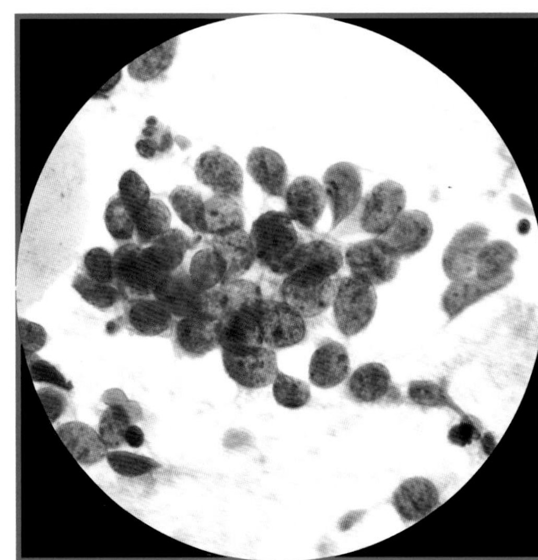

I6.138
Small cell neuroendocrine carcinoma. A rare cause of HCGs, small cell neuroendocrine carcinoma is cytologically similar to the far more common small "oat" cell carcinoma that occurs in the lung. Note high nuclear/cytoplasmic ratios, fine, dark chromatin, and inconspicuous nucleoli. There is an attempt at rosette formation by the cells in this field.

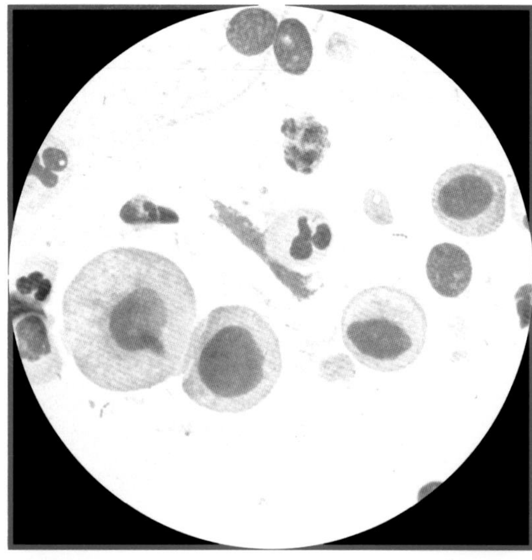

I6.139
Atypia of atrophy. High nuclear/cytoplasmic ratio suggests high-grade dysplasia. The atypical cells completely disappeared (ie, matured) after estrogen therapy.

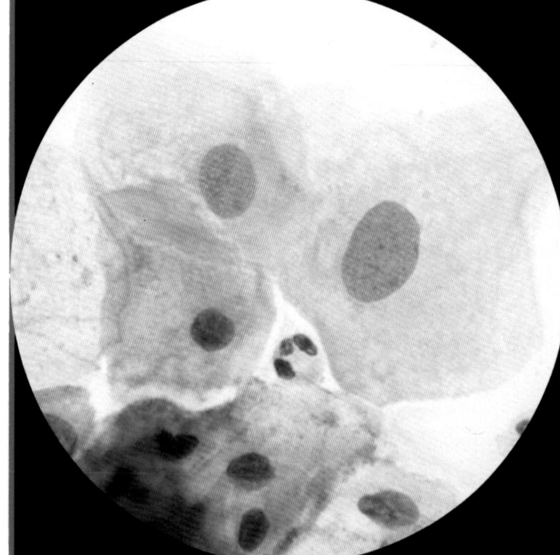

I6.140
Atypia of maturity. In older women, nuclear enlargement in mature cells may suggest squamous atypia or low-grade dysplasia. However, unless the enlarged nuclei are also at least slightly hyperchromatic (compare with intermediate cell nuclei, also in field), it is unlikely that this change is related to dysplasia or HPV.

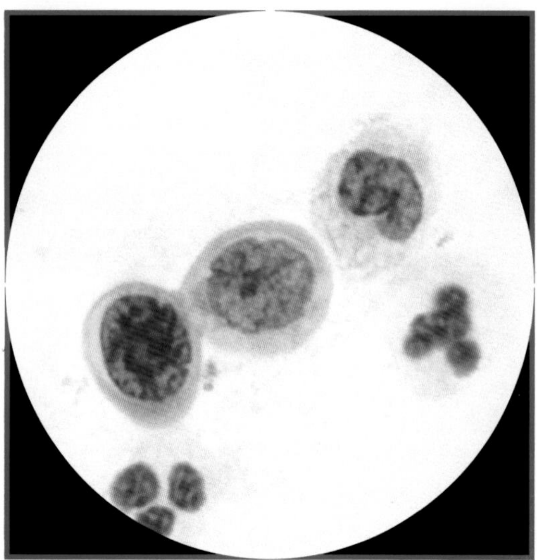

I6.141
Small, bland, severely dysplastic cells indicate very immature metaplastic dysplasia. These small cells (compare with neutrophil), indicative of severe dysplasia (CIN III, high-grade SIL), can be difficult to spot and difficult to distinguish from benign immature metaplasia or even histiocytes. Note irregular, "raisinoid" nuclei. (Oil)

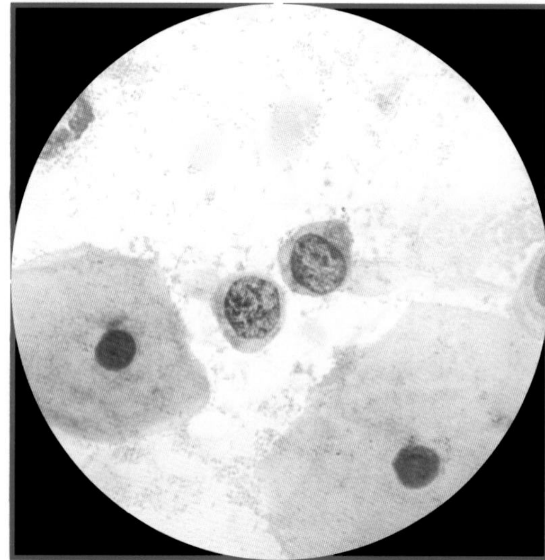

I6.142
Small, bland, malignant cells. Despite the fairly bland chromatin and smooth nuclear membranes, these are fully malignant cells from a biopsy proven invasive squamous cell carcinoma of identical morphology. They would be easy to overlook in screening (a possible example of litigation cells).

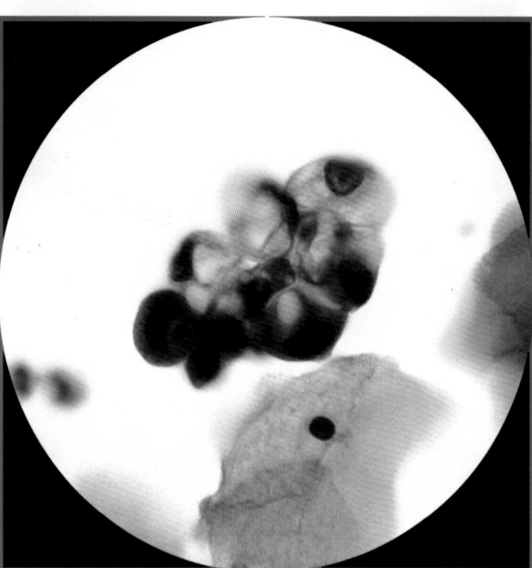

I6.143
Vacuolated metaplastic cells. Hydropic degeneration of metaplastic cells is a common phenomenon; the cells often have active nuclei and can mimic adenocarcinoma. Sometimes the vacuoles contain neutrophils or debris. Secretory vacuoles containing mucin can also occur in metaplastic cells (see I6.55).

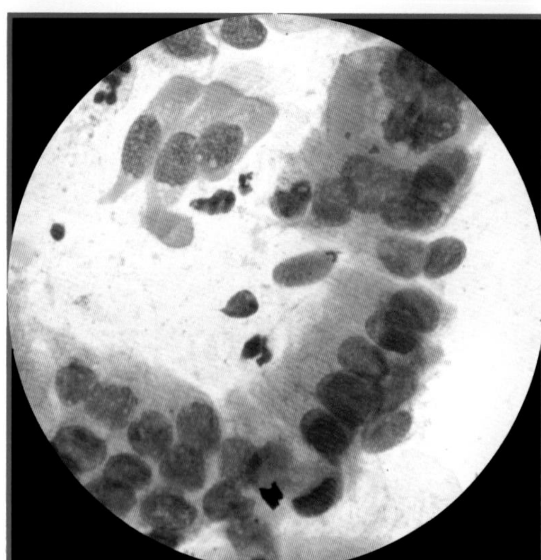

I6.144
AGUS (atypical endocervical cells). These endocervical cells are somewhat hyperchromatic, crowded, and stratified, features that may suggest endocervical glandular neoplasia. However, these cells represent tubal metaplasia. Note round, rather than elongated, nuclei and bland, rather than coarse, chromatin. Also note ciliated cells.

I6.145
AGUS (atypical endocervical cells). These endocervical cells are forming a microacinar structure, a feature that may suggest endocervical glandular neoplasia. However, these cells also represent tubal metaplasia, with bland, round nuclei. (Same case as I6.144.)

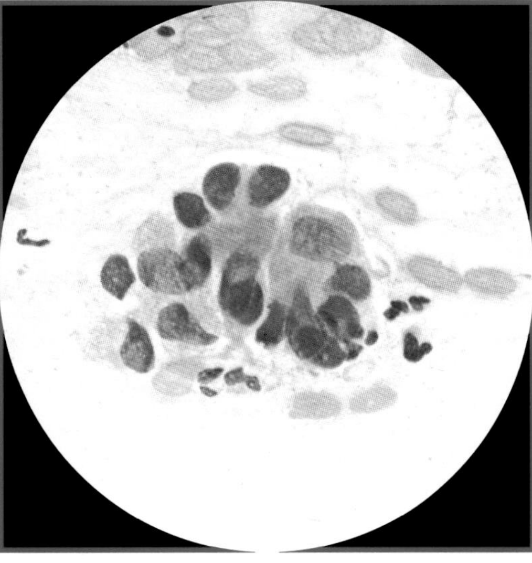

I6.146
Seminal vesicle cell. Large, "ugly" pigmented cell, may suggest melanoma or high-grade malignancy. However, note degenerated, smudgy appearance of the chromatin and sperm in the background. Cytoplasmic pigment is lipochrome, and is also a good clue to the correct diagnosis.

I6.147
Atypical repair. Tissue fragment resembles ordinary repair, but shows significant cellular abnormalities that exceed those usually seen in a regenerative/reparative process, including marked pleomorphism, crowding, and abnormalities of the nucleus. Note fine chromatin and good intercellular cohesion.

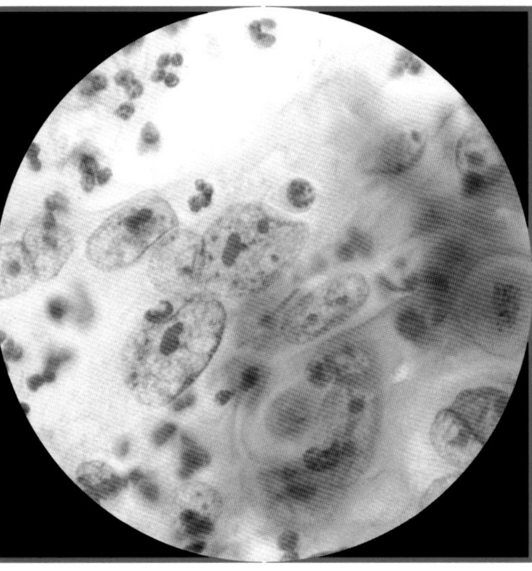

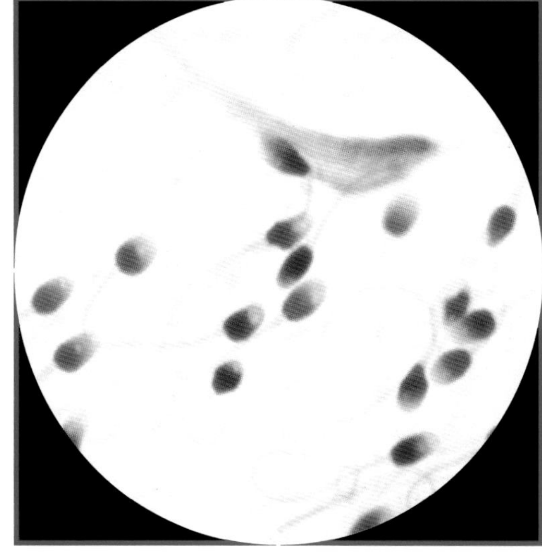

I6.148
Sperm. Tails degenerate rapidly and may not be present. For identification without tails, note that the basal portion of the head is thicker and darker than the apical portion.

I6.149
Ferning of cervical mucus. This is associated with ovulation.

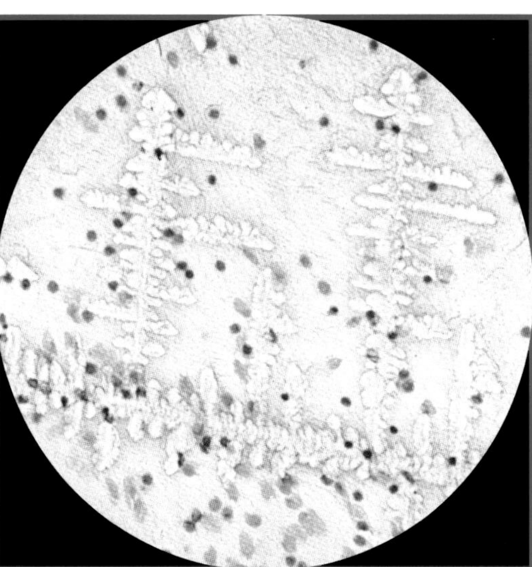

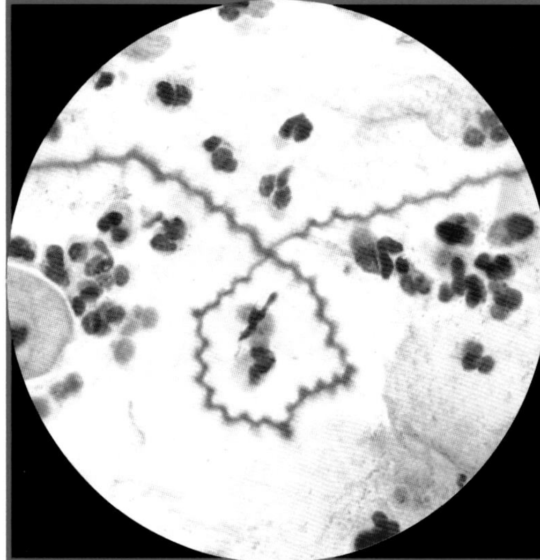

I6.150
Curschmann's spirals are similar to those more commonly observed in sputum, and apparently represent an intrinsic property of mucus that leads to coiling.

I6.151
Cornflakes. Tiny air bubbles trapped on top of squamous cell give the appearance of a brown cornflake. When severe, this artifact interferes with proper evaluation of the slide.

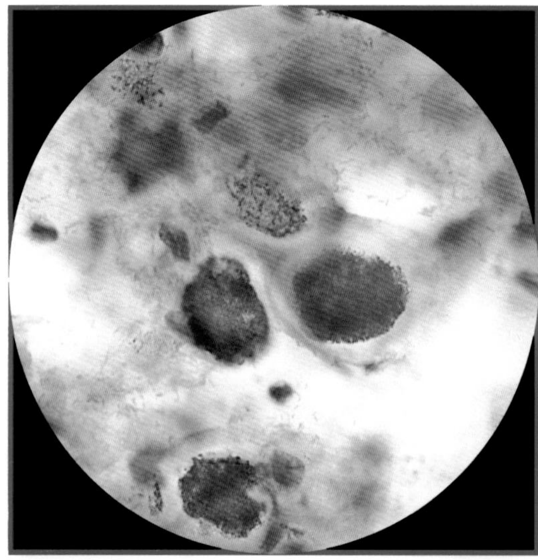

I6.152
Adenoid basal cell carcinoma is a very rare invasive tumor that resembles squamous carcinoma in situ, but with columnar cells and small gland openings. It is associated with squamous dysplasia and SCC.

I6.153
Sarcoma. This is an example of a high grade leiomyosarcoma. Note the characteristic spindle to stellate shaped, pleomorphic cells with fibrillar to granular cytoplasm and oval, malignant appearing nuclei.

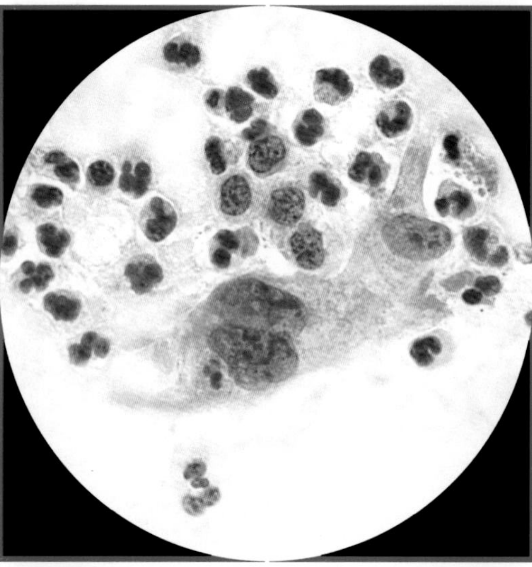

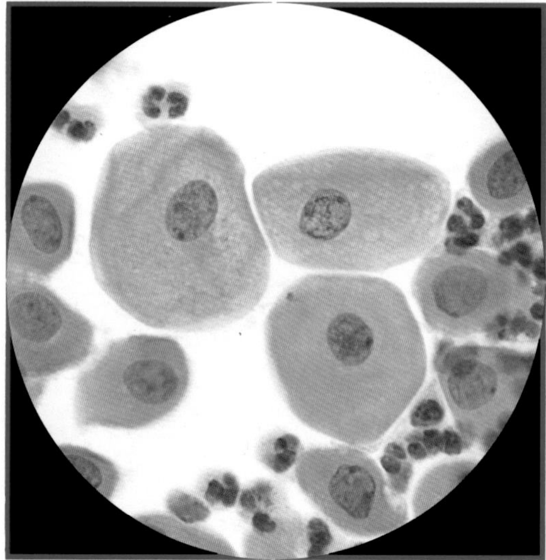

I6.154
Mature squamous metaplasia. The cells resemble normal intermediate cells, except that their cell outlines may be a little more rounded than polygonal, and the cytoplasm may be slightly denser than mature intermediate cells. Remnants of a cobblestone arrangement of the cells may be seen cytologically. Eventually, the squamous metaplasia matures completely and becomes cytologically indistinguishable from the native squamous epithelium, including the presence of cyclic hormonal changes.

I6.155
Large cell CIS. Like other kinds of classical carcinoma in situ, large cell CIS lacks features of squamous differentiation. Although the N/C ratio is elevated, these cells may have somewhat more abundant cytoplasm and may not appear as crowded as other forms of CIS.

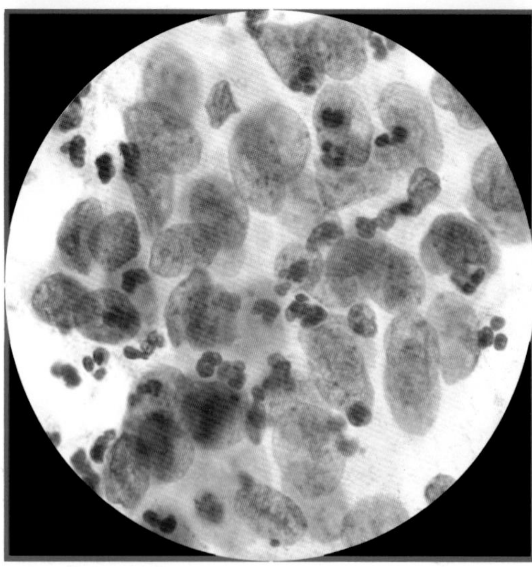

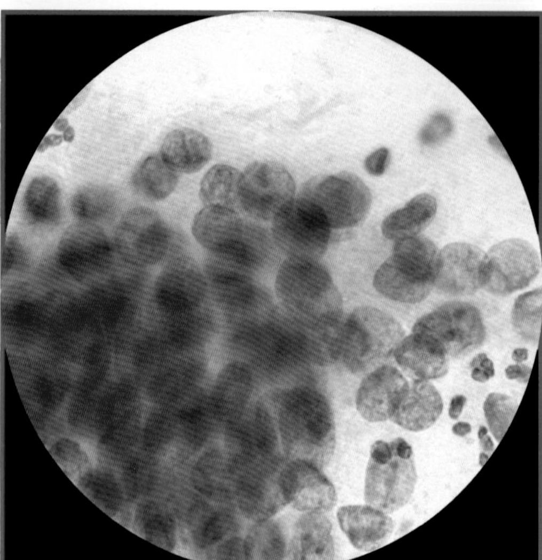

I6.156
Carcinoma in situ. Rudimentary glandular differentiation (ie, microacini) can also be seen in the syncytial-like aggregates of carcinoma in situ, a feature which has been associated with endocervical glandular extension, but may reflect the dual nature of the reserve cell.

References

ACOG Technical Bulletin: Cervical Cytology: Evaluation and Management of Abnormalities. 183: 1–8, 1993.

Acs J, Hildesheim A, Reeves WC, et al: Regional Distribution of Human Papillomavirus DNA and Other Risk Factors for Invasive Cervical Cancer in Panama. *Cancer Res* 49: 5725–5729, 1989.

Adachi A, Fleming I, Burk RD, et al: Women With Human Immunodeficiency Virus Infection and Abnormal Papanicolaou Smears: A Prospective Study of Colposcopy and Clinical Outcome. *Obstet Gynecol* 81: 372–377, 1993.

Adami H-O, Ponten J, Sparen P, et al: Survival Trend After Invasive Cervical Cancer Diagnosis in Sweden Before and After Cytologic Screening. 1960–1984. *Cancer* 73: 140–147, 1994.

Adcock LL, Julian TM, Okagaki T, et al: Carcinoma of the Uterine Cervix FIGO Stage I-B. *Gynecol Oncol* 14: 199–208, 1982.

Affandi MZ, Dun T, Mantuano V, et al: Epidemiology of Cervical Carcinoma in Brunei Darussalam. Analysis of Data on 27,208 Women Screened With Cytologic Examinations. *Acta Cytol* 37: 175–180, 1993.

Aitken-Swan J, Baird D: Cancer of the Uterine Cervix in Aberdeenshire. Aetiological Aspects. *Br J Cancer* 20: 642–659, 1966.

Albert A: Estimated Cervical Cancer Disease State and Incidence and Transition Rates. *J Natl Cancer Inst* 67: 571–576, 1981.

Albores-Saavedra J, Larraza O, Poucell S, et al: Carcinoid of the Uterine Cervix, Additional Observations on a New Tumor Entity. *Cancer* 38: 2328–2342, 1976.

Albukerk J: False-Positive Cytology in Ectopic Pregnancy. *N Engl J Med* 291: 1142, 1974.

Albukerk JN, Gnecco CA: Atypical Cytology in Tubal Pregnancy. *J Reprod Med* 19: 273–276, 1977.

Allen KA, Zaleski S, Cohen MB: Review of Negative Papanicolaou Tests. Is the Retrospective 5-Year Review Necessary? *Am J Clin Pathol* 101: 19–21, 1994.

Alloub MI, Barr BBB, McLaren KM, et al: Human Papillomavirus Infection and Cervical Intraepithelial Neoplasia in Women With Renal Allografts. *Br Med J* 298: 153–156, 1989.

Alons-van Kordelaar JJM, Boon ME: Diagnostic Accuracy of Squamous Cervical Lesions Studied in Spatula-Cytobrush Smears. *Acta Cytol* 32: 801–804, 1988.

Alva J, Lauchlan SC: The Histogenesis of Mixed Cervical Carcinomas: The Concept of Endocervical Columnar-Cell Dysplasia. *Am J Clin Pathol* 64: 20–25, 1975.

Ambros RA, Kurman RJ: Current Concepts in the Relationship of Human Papillomavirus Infection to the Pathogenesis and Classification of Precancerous Squamous Lesions of the Uterine Cervix. *Semin Diagn Pathol* 7: 158–172, 1990.

Anderson GH, Flynn KJ, Hickey LA, et al: A Comprehensive Internal Quality Control System for a Large Cytology Laboratory. *Acta Cytol* 31: 895–899. 1987.

Andrews S, Hernandez E, Miyazawa K: Paired Papanicolaou Smears in the Evaluation of Atypical Squamous Cells. *Obstet Gynecol* 73: 747–750, 1989a.

Andrews S, Miyazawa K: The Significance of a Negative Papanicolaou Smear With Hyperkeratosis or Parakeratosis. *Obstet Gynecol* 73: 751–753, 1989b.

Anello C, Lao C: U.S. Trends in Mortality From Carcinoma of Cervix. *Lancet* (i): 1038, 1979.

An-Foraker SH, Kawada CY: Cytodiagnosis of Endometrial Malignant Mixed Mesodermal Tumor. *Acta Cytol* 29: 137–141, 1985.

Angeles MA, Saigo PE: Cytologic Findings in Rectovaginal Fistulae. *Acta Cytol* 38: 373–376, 1994.

Anonymous: Human Papillomaviruses and Cervical Cancer: A Fresh Look at the Evidence. *Lancet* (i): 725–726, 1987.

Anonymous: Human Papillomaviruses and the Polymerase Chain Reaction. *Lancet* (i): 1051–1052, 1989.

Arends MJ, Donaldson YK, Duvall E, et al: Human Papillomavirus Type 18 Associates With More Advanced Cervical Neoplasia Than Human Papillomavirus Type 16. *Hum Pathol* 24: 432–437, 1993.

Armstrong B, Holman D: Increasing Mortality From Cancer of the Cervix in Young Australian Women. *Med J Aust* 1: 460–462, 1981.

Armstrong, BK: The Falling, Rising Incidence of Invasive Cancer of the Cervix. *Med J Aust* 1: 147–148, 1983.

Ashfaq-Drewett R, Allen C, Harrison, RL: Detached Ciliary Tufts: Comparison With Intestinal Protozoa and a Review of the Literature. *Am J Clin Pathol* 93: 541–545, 1990.

Ashley DJB: The Biological Status of Carcinoma In-Situ of the Uterine Cervix. *J Obstet Gynaecol Br Cwlth* 73: 372–381, 1966a.

Ashley DJB: Evidence for the Existence of Two Forms of Cervical Carcinoma. *J Obstet Gynaecol Br Cwlth* 73: 382–389, 1966b.

Athanassiadou PP, Kyrkou KA, Antoniades LG, et al: Cytological Evaluation of the Effect of Tamoxifen in Premenopausal and Post-Menopausal Women With Primary Breast Cancer by Analysis of the Karyopyknotic Indices of Vaginal Smears. *Cytopathology* 3: 203–208, 1992.

Attwood ME, Woodman CBJ, Luesley D, et al: Previous Cytology in Patients With Invasive Carcinoma of the Cervix. *Acta Cytol* 29: 108–110, 1985.

August N: Cervicography for Evaluating the "Atypical" Papanicolaou Smear. *J Reprod Med* 36: 89–94, 1991.

Austin RM: Why CLIA '88 Will Increase Cervical Cancer Deaths. *CAP Today* 5: 15–18, 1991.

Austin RM: The Future of Cytology: Prospects for the Nonprofit Hospital Cytology Laboratory. *Diagn Cytopathol* 9: 130–132, 1993.

Austin RM: Can Regulatory Proficiency Testing by the Cytobureaucracy Decrease Both False Negatives and Cervical Cancer Deaths? *Diagn Cytopathol* 11: 109–112, 1994a.

Austin RM: In Search of a "Reasonable Person Standard" for Gynecologic Cytologists. *Diagn Cytopathol* 11: 216–218, 1994b.

Averette HE, Steren A, Nguyen HN: Screening in Gynecologic Cancers. *Cancer* 72: 1043–1049, 1993.

Ayer B, Pacey F, Greenberg M, Bousfield L: The Cytologic Diagnosis of Adenocarcinoma In Situ of the Cervix Uteri and Related Lesions: I. Adenocarcinoma In Situ. *Acta Cytol* 31: 397–411, 1987.

Ayer B, Pacey F, Greenberg M: The Cytologic Diagnosis of Adenocarcinoma In Situ of the Cervix Uteri and Related Lesions: II. Microinvasive Adenocarcinoma. *Acta Cytol* 32: 318–324, 1988.

Ayer BS, Pacey FN, Greenberg ML: The Cytological Features of Invasive Adenocarcinoma of the Cervix Uteri. *Cytopathology* 2: 181–191, 1991.

Ayre JE: Vaginal and Cervical Cytology in Uterine Cancer Diagnosis. *Am J Obstet Gynecol* 51: 743–750, 1946.

Ayre JE: Selective Cytology Smear for Diagnosis of Cancer. *Am J Obstet Gynecol* 53: 609–617, 1947.

Ayre JE: Cervical Cytology in the Diagnosis of Early Cancer. *JAMA* 136: 513–517, 1948.

Ayre JE: The Vaginal Smear. "Precancer" Cell Studies Using A Modified Technique. *Am J Obstet Gynecol* 58: 1205–1219, 1949.

Ayre JE: Role of the Halo Cell in Cervical Cancerigenesis: A Virus Manifestation in Premalignancy? *Obstet Gynecol* 15: 481–491, 1960.

Babès A: Diagnostic du Cancer du Col Utérin par les Frottis. *La Presse Medicale* 36: 451–454, 1928.

Babès A: Sur le Cancer Superficiel du Col Utérin. *Gynecologie et Obstetrique* 23: 417–433, 1931.

Bachner P: Can Cytology Proficiency Testing Programs Discriminate Between Competent and Incompetent Practitioners? *Qual Rev Bull* 17: 150–151, 1991.

Bain RW, Crocker DW: Rapid Onset of Cervical Cancer in an Upper Socioeconomic Group. *Am J Obstet Gynecol* 146: 366–371, 1983.

Bajardi F, Gompel CM, Tsanov K, et al: European Comment on Statement of Caution in Reference to Human Papillomavirus Infection. *Acta Cytol* 30: 445–446, 1986.

Bamford PN, Beilby JOW, Steele SJ, et al: The Natural History of Cervical Intraepithelial Neoplasia as Determined by Cytology and Colposcopic Biopsy. *Acta Cytol* 27: 482– 484, 1983.

Bardales RH, Valente PT, Stanley MW: Cytology of Suture Granulomas in Posthysterectomy Vaginal Smears. *Acta Cytol* 37: 777, 1993.

Barnes W, Delgado G, Kurman RJ, et al: Possible Prognostic Significance of Human Papillomavirus Type in Cervical Cancer. *Gynecol Oncol* 29: 267–273, 1988.

Barnes W, Woodworth C, Waggoner S, et al: Rapid Dysplastic Transformation of Human Genital Cells by Human Papillomavirus Type 18. *Gynecol Oncol* 38: 343–346, 1990.

Barr ML, Bertram EG: A Morphological Distinction Between Neurones of the Male and Female, and the Behaviour of the Nucleolar Satellite During Accelerated Nucleoprotein Synthesis. *Nature* 163: 676–677, 1949.

Barrasso R, De Brux J, Croissant O, et al: High Prevalence of Papillomavirus-Associated Penile Intraepithelial Neoplasia in Sexual Partners of Women With Cervical Intraepithelial Neoplasia. *N Engl J Med* 317: 916–923, 1987.

Barrett RJ II, Davos I, Leuchter RS, et al: Neuroendocrine Features in Poorly Differentiated and Undifferentiated Carcinomas of the Cervix. *Cancer* 60: 2325–2330, 1987.

Barrett TJ, Silbar JD: Genital Warts—A Venereal Disease. *JAMA* 154: 333–334, 1954.

Barron BA, Richart RM: A Statistical Model of the Natural History of Cervical Carcinoma Based on a Prospective Study of 557 Cases. *J Nat Cancer Inst* 41: 1343–1353, 1968.

Barron BA, Richart RM: An Epidemiologic Study of Cervical Neoplastic Disease: Based on a Self-Selected Sample of 7,000 Women in Barbados, West Indies. *Cancer* 27: 978–986, 1971.

Barron BA, Cahill MC, Richart RM: A Statistical Model of the Natural History of Cervical Neoplastic Disease: The Duration of Carcinoma In Situ. *Gynecol Oncol* 6: 196–205, 1978.

Barter JF, Orr JW, Holloway RW, et al: Psammoma Bodies in a Cervicovaginal Smear Associated With an Intrauterine Device. *J Reprod Med* 32: 147, 1987.

Barter JF: The Life and Contributions of Doctor George Nicholas Papanicolaou. *Surg Gynecol Obstet* 174: 530–532, 1992.

Bartlett JG, Onderdonk AB, Drude E, et al: Quantitative Bacteriology of the Vaginal Flora. *J Infect Dis* 136: 271–277, 1977.

Barton SE, Jenkins D, Cuzick J, et al: Effect of Cigarette Smoking on Cervical Epithelial Immunity: A Mechanism for Neoplastic Change? *Lancet* (ii): 652–654, 1988.

Barton SE, Hollingsworth A, Maddox PH, et al: Possible Cofactors in the Etiology of Cervical Intraepithelial Neoplasia: An Immunopathologic Study. *J Reprod Med* 34: 613–616, 1989a.

Barton SE, Jenkins D, Hollingsworth A, et al: An Explanation for the Problem of False Negative Cervical Smears. *Br J Obstet Gynaecol* 96: 482–485, 1989b.

Barua R, Matthews CD: Verrucous Carcinoma of the Uterine Cervix: A Case Report. *Acta Cytol* 27: 540–542, 1983.

Bauer HM, Ting Y, Greer CE, et al: Genital Human Papillomavirus Infection in Female University Students as Determined by a PCR-Based Method. *JAMA* 265: 472–477, 1991.

Beaudenon S, Kremsdorf D, Croissant O, et al: A Novel Type of Human Papillomavirus Associated With Genital Neoplasias. *Nature* 321: 246–249, 1986.

Bedrossian CWM, Gupta PK: Cytology in the Headlines. *Diagn Cytopathol* 11: 1–3, 1994.

Beeby AR, Wadehra V, Keating PJ, et al: A Retrospective Analysis of 94 Patients with CIN and False Negative Cervical Smears Taken at Colposcopy. *Cytopathology* 4: 331–337, 1993.

Beilby JOW, Bourne R, Guillebaud J, et al: Paired Cervical Smears: A Method of Reducing the False-Negative Rate in Population Screening. *Obstet Gynecol* 60: 46–48, 1982.

Benda JA, Platz CE, Buchsbaum H, et al: Mucin Production in Defining Mixed Carcinoma of the Uterine Cervix: A Clinicopathologic Study. *Int J Gynecol Pathol* 4: 314–327, 1985.

Benda JA, Lamoreaux J, Johnson SR: Artifact Associated With the Use of Strong Iodine Solution (Lugol's) in Cone Biopsies. *Am J Surg Pathol* 11: 367–374, 1987.

Benedet JL, Selke PA, Nickerson KG: Colposcopic Evaluation of Abnormal Papanicolaou Smears in Pregnancy. *Am J Obstet Gynecol* 157: 932–937, 1987.

Benedet JL, Anderson GH, Matisic JP: A Comprehensive Program for Cervical Cancer Detection and Management. *Am J Obstet Gynecol* 166: 1254–1259, 1992.

Benoit AG, Krepart GV, Lotocki RJ: Results of Prior Cytologic Screening in Patients With a Diagnosis of Stage I Carcinoma of the Cervix. *Am J Obstet Gynecol* 148: 690–694, 1984.

Benson PA: Cytologic Diagnosis in Primary Carcinoma of Fallopian Tube: Case Report and Review. *Acta Cytol* 18: 429–434, 1974.

Benson WL, Norris HJ: A Critical Review of the Frequency of Lymph Node Metastasis and Death From Microinvasive Carcinoma of the Cervix. *Obstet Gynecol* 49: 632–638, 1977.

Beral V: Cancer of the Cervix: A Sexually Transmitted Infection? *Lancet* (i): 1037–1040, 1974.

Beral V, Booth M: Predictions of Cervical Cancer Incidence and Mortality in England and Wales. *Lancet* (i): 495, 1986.

Bercovici B, Diamant Y, Polishuk WZ: A Simplified Evaluation of Vaginal Cytology in Third Trimester Pregnancy Complications. *Acta Cytol* 17: 67–72, 1973.

Berek JS, Hacker NF, Fu Y-S, et al: Adenocarcinoma of the Uterine Cervix: Histologic Variables Associated With Lymph Node Metastasis and Survival. *Obstet Gynecol* 65: 46–52, 1985.

Berg JW, Durfee GR: The Cytological Presentation of Endometrial Carcinoma. *Cancer* 11: 158–172, 1958.

Bergeron C, Ferenczy A, Shah KV, et al: Multicentric Human Papillomavirus Infections of the Female Genital Tract: Correlation of Viral Types With Abnormal Mitotic Figures, Colposcopic Presentation, and Location. *Obstet Gynecol* 69: 736–742, 1987.

Berkeley AS, LiVolsi VA, Schwartz PE: Advanced Squamous Cell Carcinoma of the Cervix with Recent Normal Papanicolaou Tests. *Lancet* (ii): 375–376, 1980.

Berkowitz RS, Ehrmann RL, Lavizzo-Mourey R, et al: Invasive Cervical Carcinoma in Young Women. *Gynecol Oncol* 8: 311–316, 1979.

Bernal JN, Martinez MA, Dabancens A: Evaluation of Proposed Cytomorphologic Criteria for the Diagnosis of *Chlamydia trachomatis* in Papanicolaou Smears. *Acta Cytol* 33: 309–313, 1989.

Berner A, Hoeg K, Oppedal BR: Smear Biopsies. A Cause of Negative Follow-up Biopsies in Patients with Premalignant Conditions of the Uterine Cervix. *Diagn Gynecol Obstet* 2: 99–102, 1980.

Bernstein A, Harris B: The Relationship of Dietary and Serum Vitamin A to the Occurrence of Cervical Intraepithelial Neoplasia in Sexually Active Women. *Am J Obstet Gynecol* 148: 309–312, 1984.

Bernstein SG, Voet RL, Guzick DS, et al: Prevalence of Papillomavirus Infection in Colposcopically Directed Cervical Biopsy Specimens in 1972 and 1982. *Am J Obstet Gynecol* 151: 577–581, 1985.

Bertini-Oliveira AM, Keppler MM, Luisi A, et al: Comparative Evaluation of Abnormal Cytology, Colposcopy and Histopathology in Preclinical Cervical Malignancy During Pregnancy. *Acta Cytol* 26: 636–644, 1982.

Betsill WL Jr, Clark AH: Early Endocervical Glandular Neoplasia: I. Histomorphology and Cytomorphology. *Acta Cytol* 30: 115–126, 1986.

Bevan IS, Blomfield PI, Johnson MA, et al: Oncogenic Viruses and Cervical Cancer. *Lancet* (i): 907–908, 1989.

Bewtra C: Columnar Cells in Posthysterectomy Vaginal Smears. *Diagn Cytopathol* 8: 342–345, 1992.

Beyer-Boon ME: Psammoma Bodies in Cervicovaginal Smears: An Indicator of the Presence of Ovarian Carcinoma. *Acta Cytol* 18: 41–44, 1974.

Bhagavan BS, Ruffier J, Shinn B: Pseudoactinomycotic Radiate Granules in the Lower Female Genital Tract: Relationship to the Splendore-Hoeppli Phenomenon. *Hum Pathol* 13: 898–904, 1982.

Bibbo M, Keebler CM, Wied GL: Prevalence And Incidence Rates of Cervical Atypia: A Computerized File Analysis on 148,735 Patients. *J Reprod Med* 6: 184–188, 1971a.

Bibbo M, Keebler CM, Wied GL: The Cytologic Diagnosis of Tissue Repair in the Female Genital Tract. *Acta Cytol* 15: 133–137, 1971b.

Bibbo M: What You Should Know About Papanicolaou Smears. *Diagn Cytopathol* 5: 104–107, 1989a.

Bibbo M, Dytch HE, Alenghat E, et al: DNA Ploidy Profiles as Prognostic Indicators in CIN Lesions. *Am J Clin Pathol* 92: 261–265, 1989b.

Binder MA, Cates GW, Emson HE, et al: The Changing Concepts of Condyloma: A Retrospective Study of Colposcopically Directed Cervical Biopsies. *Am J Obstet Gynecol* 151: 213–219, 1985.

Bitterman P, Chun B, Kurman RJ: The Significance of Epithelial Differentiation in Mixed Mesodermal Tumors of the Uterus. A Clinicopathologic and Immunohistochemical Study. *Am J Surg Pathol* 14: 317–328, 1990.

Blumenfeld W, Holly EA, Mansur DL, et al: Histiocytes and the Detection of Endometrial Adenocarcinoma. *Acta Cytol* 29: 317–322, 1985.

Bogdanich W: The Pap Test Misses Much Cervical Cancer Through Lab's Errors. *The Wall Street Journal* 88: 1,20, November 2, 1987a.

Bogdanich W: Physician's Carelessness With Pap Tests Is Cited in Procedure's High Failure Rate. *The Wall Street Journal* 88: 17, December 29, 1987b.

Bokhman JV: Two Pathogenetic Types of Endometrial Carcinoma. *Gynecol Oncol* 15: 10–17, 1983.

Bonfiglio TR, cited by Voelker R. Cytology Proficiency Testing Has Stumped the Experts. *JAMA* 270: 2779–2780, 1993.

Boon ME, Kirk RS, Rietveld-Scheffers PEM: The Morphogenesis of Adenocarcinoma of the Cervix—A Complex Pathological Entity. *Histopathology* 5: 565–577, 1981.

Boon ME, Alons-van Kordelaar JJM, Rietveld-Scheffers PEM: Consequences of the Introduction of Combined Spatula and Cytobrush Sampling for Cervical Cytology: Improvements in Smear Quality and Detection Rates. *Acta Cytol* 30: 264–270, 1986.

Boon ME, DeGraaf Guilloud JC, Kob LP, et al: Efficacy of Screening for Cervical Squamous and Adenocarcinoma: The Dutch Experience. *Cancer* 59: 862–866, 1987.

Boon ME, Schneider A, Hogewoning CJA, et al: Penile Studies and Heterosexual Partners: Peniscopy, Cytology, Histology, and Immunocytochemistry. *Cancer* 61: 1652–1659, 1988.

Boon ME, de Graaff Guilloud JC, Rietveld WJ: Analysis of Five Sampling Methods for the Preparation of Cervical Smears. *Acta Cytol* 33: 843–848, 1989a.

Boon ME, Susanti I, Tasche MJA, et al: Human Papillomavirus (HPV)-Associated Male and Female Genital Carcinomas in a Hindu Population. *Cancer* 64: 559–565, 1989b.

Boon ME, Zeppa P, Ouwerkerk-Noordam E, et al: Exploiting the "Toothpick Effect" of the Cytobrush by Plastic Embedding of Cervical Samples. *Acta Cytol* 35: 57–63, 1991.

Boon ME, Kok LP: Neural Network Processing Can Provide Means to Catch Errors That Slip Through Human Screening of Pap Smears. *Diagn Cytopathol* 9: 411–416, 1993.

Boquet-Jiménez E, San Cristóbal AA: Cytologic and Microbiologic Aspects of Vaginal Torulopsis. *Acta Cytol* 22: 331–334, 1978.

Boras VF, Duggan MA: Cervical Dyskeratotic Cells as Predictors of Condylomatous Changes on Biopsy. *Acta Cytol* 33: 223–227, 1989.

Boring C, Silverberg SG: Annual Cancer Statistics. *CA-Cancer J Clin.* Volumes 20 to 44: 1970–1994.

Bornstein J, Stinson-Carter T, Kaufman RH: Curschmann's Spiral in an Endocervical Brushing. *Acta Cytol* 31: 530–531, 1987.

Borst M, Butterworth CE, Baker V, et al: Human Papillomavirus Screening for Women with Atypical Papanicolaou Smears. *J Reprod Med* 36: 95–99, 1991.

Bosch MMC, Rietveld-Scheffers PEM, Boon ME: Characteristics of False-Negative Smears Tested in the Normal Screening Situation. *Acta Cytol* 36: 711–716, 1992.

Bose S, Kannan V, Kline TS: Abnormal Endocervical Cells. Really Abnormal? Really Endocervical? *Am J Clin Pathol* 101: 708–713, 1994.

Bottles K, Reiter RC, Steiner AL, et al: Problems Encountered With the Bethesda System: The University of Iowa Experience. *Obstet Gynecol* 78: 410–414, 1991.

Bourne RG, Grove WD: Invasive Carcinoma of the Cervix in Queensland: Change in Incidence and Mortality, 1959-1980. *Med J Aust* 1: 156–158, 1983.

Bousfield L, Pacey F, Young Q, et al: Expanded Cytologic Criteria for the Diagnosis of Adenocarcinoma In Situ of the Cervix and Related Lesions. *Acta Cytol* 24: 283–296, 1980.

Bouttselis JG: Intraepithelial Carcinoma of the Cervix Associated With Pregnancy. *Obstet Gynecol* 40: 657–666, 1972.

Boyd JT, Doll R: A Study of the Aetiology of Carcinoma of the Cervix Uteri. *Br J Cancer* 18: 419–434, 1964.

Brand E, Berek JS, Hacker NF: Controversies in the Management of Cervical Adenocarcinoma. *Obstet Gynecol* 71: 261–269, 1988.

Breathnach CS: Biographical Sketches No. 29—Papanicolaou. *Irish Med J* 76: 220, 1983.

Brescia RJ, Jenson AB, Lancaster WD, et al: Progress in Pathology: The Role of Human Papillomaviruses in the Pathogenesis and Histologic Classification of Precancerous Lesions of the Cervix. *Hum Pathol* 17: 552–559, 1986.

Briggs RM: Dysplasia and Early Neoplasia of the Uterine Cervix. A Review. *Obstet Gynecol Surv* 34: 70–99, 1979.

Brink A, DuToit JP, Deale CJC: In Search of More Representative Cervical Cytology. A Preliminary Prospective Study. *S Afr Med J* 76: 55–57, 1989.

Brinton LA, Huggins GR, Lehman HF, et al: Long-Term Use of Oral Contraceptives and Risk of Invasive Cervical Cancer. *Int J Cancer* 38: 339–344, 1986a.

Brinton LA, Schairer C, Haenszel W, et al: Cigarette Smoking and Invasive Cervical Cancer. *JAMA* 255: 3265–3269, 1986b.

Brinton LA, Hamman RF, Huggins GR, et al: Sexual and Reproductive Risk Factors for Invasive Squamous Cell Cervical Cancer. *J Natl Cancer Inst* 79: 23–30, 1987.

Brinton LA, Reeves WC, Brenes MM, et al: Parity as a Risk Factor for Cervical Cancer. *Am J Epidemiol* 130: 486–496, 1989a.

Brinton LA, Reeves WC, Brenes MM, et al: The Male Factor in the Etiology of Cervical Cancer Among Sexually Monogamous Women. *Int J Cancer* 44: 199–203, 1989b.

Britsch CJ, Azar HA: Estrogen Effect in Exfoliated Vaginal Cells Following Treatment With Digitalis: A Case Report With Experimental Observations in Mice. *Am J Obstet Gynecol* 85: 989–993, 1963.

Broders AC: Carcinoma In Situ Contrasted With Benign Penetrating Epithelium. *JAMA* 99: 1670–1674, 1932.

Brown LJR, Wells M: Cervical Glandular Atypia Associated With Squamous Intraepithelial Neoplasia: A Premalignant Lesion? *J Clin Pathol* 39: 22–28, 1986.

Brown MS, Phillips GL Jr: Management of the Mildly Abnormal Pap Smear: A Conservative Approach. *Gynecol Oncol* 22: 149–153, 1985.

Buckley CH, Herbert A, Johnson J, et al: Borderline Nuclear Changes in Cervical Smears: Guidelines on Their Recognition and Management. *J Clin Pathol* 47: 481–492, 1994.

Burghardt E, Östör AG: Site and Origin of Squamous Cervical Cancer: A Histomorphologic Study. *Obstet Gynecol* 62: 117–127, 1983.

Burghardt E, Girardi F, Lahousen M, et al: Microinvasive Carcinoma of the Uterine Cervix (International Federation of Gynecology and Obstetrics IA). *Cancer* 67: 1037–1045, 1991.

Burk JR, Lehman HF, Wolf FS: Inadequacy of Papanicolaou Smears in the Detection of Endometrial Cancer. *N Engl J Med* 291: 191–192, 1974.

Burk RD, Kadish AS, Calderin S, Romney SL: Human Papillomavirus Infection of the Cervix Detected by Cervicovaginal Lavage and Molecular Hybridization: Correlation With Biopsy Results and Papanicolaou Smear. *Am J Obstet Gynecol* 154: 982–989, 1986.

Buscema J, Woodruff JD: Significance of Neoplastic Atypicalities in Endocervical Epithelium. *Gynecol Oncol* 17: 356–362, 1984.

Busnach G, Civati G, Brando B, et al: Viral and Neoplastic Changes of the Lower Genital Tract in Women With Renal Allografts. *Transplant Proc* 25: 1389–1390, 1993.

Busseniers AE, Sidawy MK: Inflammatory Atypia on Cervical Smears: A Diagnostic Dilemma for the Gynecologist. *J Reprod Med* 36: 85–88, 1991.

Butterworth CE Jr, Hatch KD, Gore H, et al: Improvement in Cervical Dysplasia Associated With Folic Acid Therapy in Users of Oral Contraceptives. *Am J Clin Nutr* 35: 73–82, 1982.

Butterworth CE Jr, Hatch KD, Soong S-J, et al: Oral Folic Acid Supplementation for Cervical Dysplasia: A Clinical Intervention Trial. *Am J Obstet Gynecol* 166: 803–809, 1992.

Campion MJ, Singer A, Clarkson PK, et al: Increased Risk of Cervical Neoplasia in Consorts of Men With Penile Condylomata Acuminata. *Lancet* (i): 943–946, 1985.

Campion MJ, Cuzick J, McCance DJ, Singer A: Progressive Potential of Mild Cervical Atypia: Prospective Cytological, Colposcopic, and Virological Study. *Lancet* (ii): 237–240, 1986.

Campion MJ, McCance DJ, Mitchell HS, et al: Subclinical Penile Human Papillomavirus Infection and Dysplasia in Consorts of Women With Cervical Neoplasia. *Genitourin Med* 64: 90–99, 1988.

Campos R, De CJ: Persistent Tumor Cells in the Vaginal Smears and Prognosis of Cancer of the Radiated Cervix. *Acta Cytol* 14: 519–522, 1970.

Cannon JM, Blythe JG: Comparison of the Cytobrush Plus Plastic Spatula With the Cervex Brush for Obtaining Endocervical Cells. *Obstet Gynecol* 82: 569–572, 1993.

Capaldo G, LeGolvan DP, Dramczyk JE: Hematoidin Crystals in Cervicovaginal Smears: Review of 27 Cases Seen in One Year. *Acta Cytol* 27: 237–240, 1983.

Carmichael E: Dr. Papanicolaou and the Pap Smear. *Alabama J Med Sci* 21: 101–104, 1984.

Carmichael JA, Jeffrey JF, Steele HD, et al: The Cytologic History of 245 Patients Developing Invasive Cervical Carcinoma. *Am J Obstet Gynecol* 148: 685–690, 1984.

Carmichael JA, Clarke DH, Moher D, et al: Cervical Carcinoma in Women Aged 34 and Younger. *Am J Obstet Gynecol* 154: 264–269, 1986.

Carr RF: Response to Editorial on the Pap Smear as a Cancer Screening Test. *Diagn Cytopathol* 10: 95, 1994.

Carson HJ: Unpublished observations. 1990.

Carson HJ, DeMay RM.: The Mode Ages of Women With Cervical Dysplasia. *Obstet Gynecol* 82: 430–434, 1993.

Casas-Cordero M, Morin C, Roy M, et al: Origin of the Koilocyte in Condylomata of the Human Cervix: Ultrastructural Study. *Acta Cytol* 25: 383–392, 1981.

Cassano PA, Saigo PE, Hajdu SI: Comparison of Cytohormonal Status of Postmenopausal Women With Cancer to Age-Matched Controls. *Acta Cytol* 30: 93–98, 1986.

CDC: Condyloma Acuminatum—United States, 1966-1981. *MMWR* 32: 306–308, 1983.

CDC: Black-White Differences in Cervical Cancer Mortality—United States, 1980-1987. *MMWR* 39: 245–248, 1990.

Cecchini S, Palli D, Casini A: Cervical Intraepithelial Neoplasia III. An Estimate of Screening Error Rates and Optimal Screening Interval. *Acta Cytol* 29: 329–333, 1985.

Cecchini S, Iossa A, Ciatto S: Routine Colposcopic Survey of Patients With Squamous Atypia: A Method for Identifying Cases With False-Negative Smears. *Acta Cytol* 34: 778–780, 1990a.

Cecchini S, Confortini M, Bonardi L, et al: "Nonclassic" Cytologic Signs of Cervical Condyloma: A Case-Control Study. *Acta Cytol* 34: 781–784, 1990b.

Cecchini S, Iossa A, Ciatto S, et al: Colposcopic Survey of Papanicolaou Test-Negative Cases With Hyperkeratosis or Parakeratosis. *Obstet Gynecol* 76: 857–859, 1990c.

Cevenini R, Costa R, Rumpianesi F, et al: Cytological and Histopathological Abnormalities of the Cervix in Genital *Chlamydia trachomatis* Infections. *Br J Vener Dis* 57: 334–337, 1981.

Chakrabarti S, Guijon FB, Paraskevas M: Brush vs Spatula for Cervical Smears. Histologic Correlation With Concurrent Biopsies. *Acta Cytol* 38: 315–318, 1994.

Chang AR: Health Screening: An Analysis of Abnormal Cervical Smears at Dunedin Hospital 1963–82. *N Z Med J* 98: 104–107, 1985.

Chang F: Role of Papillomaviruses. *J Clin Pathol* 43: 269–276, 1990.

Chang YC, Craig JM: Vaginal-Smear Assessment of Estrogen Activity in Endometrial Carcinoma. *Obstet Gynecol* 21: 170–174, 1963.

Chapman GW Jr, Abreo F, Thompson HE: Carcinoma of the Cervix in Young Females (35 Years, and Younger). *Gynecol Oncol* 31: 430–434, 1988.

Cherkis RC, Patten SF Jr, Dickinson JC, et al: Significance of Atypical Endometrial Cells Detected by Cervical Cytology. *Obstet Gynecol* 69: 786–789, 1987.

Cherkis RC, Patten SF Jr, Andrews TJ, et al: Significance of Normal Endometrial Cells Detected by Cervical Cytology. *Obstet Gynecol* 71: 242–244, 1988.

Chong S-M, Wee A, Yeoh S-C, et al: Retroperitoneal Endodermal Sinus Tumor. Report of a Case With an Abnormal Cervicovaginal Smear. *Acta Cytol* 38: 562–567, 1994.

Choo YC, Mak KC, Hsu C, et al: Postmenopausal Uterine Bleeding of Nonorganic Cause. *Obstet Gynecol* 66: 225–228, 1985.

Christie AJ, Krieger HA: Indolent Necrotizing Granulomas of the Uterine Cervix, Possibly Related to Chlamydial Infection. *Am J Obstet Gynecol* 136: 958–960, 1980.

Christopherson WM, Mendez WM, Ahuja EM, et al: Cervix Cancer Control in Louisville, Kentucky. *Cancer* 26: 29–38, 1970a.

Christopherson WM, Parker JE, Mendez WM, et al: Cervix Cancer Death Rates and Mass Cytologic Screening. *Cancer* 26: 808–811, 1970b.

Christopherson WM, Lundin FE Jr, Mendez WM, et al: Cervical Cancer Control: A Study of Morbidity and Mortality Trends Over A Twenty-One-Year Period. *Cancer* 38: 1357–1366, 1976.

Christopherson WM: Dysplasia, Carcinoma In Situ, and Microinvasive Carcinoma of the Uterine Cervix. *Hum Pathol* 8: 489–501, 1977a.

Christopherson WM, Scott MA: Trends in Mortality from Uterine Cancer in Relation to Mass Screening. *Acta Cytol* 21: 5–9, 1977b.

Christopherson WM, Nealon N, Gray LA Sr: Noninvasive Precursor Lesions of Adenocarcinoma and Mixed Adenosquamous Carcinoma of the Cervix Uteri. *Cancer* 44: 975–983, 1979.

Chu J, White E: Decreasing Incidence of Invasive Cervical Cancer in Young Women. *Am J Obstet Gynecol* 157: 1105–1107, 1987.

Chumas JC, Nelson B, Mann WJ, et al: Microglandular Hyperplasia of the Uterine Cervix. *Obstet Gynecol* 66: 406–409, 1985.

Chung HR, Riccio JA Jr, Gerstung RA, et al: Discovery Rate of Dysplasia and Carcinoma of the Uterine Cervix in an Urban Medical Center Serving Patients at High Risk. *Int J Gynaecol Obstet* 20: 449–454, 1982.

Clark AH, Betsill WL Jr: Early Endocervical Glandular Neoplasia: II. Morphometric Analysis of the Cells. *Acta Cytol* 30: 127–134, 1986.

Clark RB, Schneider V, Gentile FG, et al: Cervical Chlamydial Infections: Diagnostic Accuracy of the Papanicolaou Smear. *South Med J* 78: 1301–1303, 1985.

Clarke EA, Anderson TW: Does Screening by "Pap" Smears Help Prevent Cervical Cancer? A Case-Control Study. *Lancet* (ii): 1–4, 1979.

Clarke EA, Morgan RW, Newman AM: Smoking as a Risk Factor in Cancer of the Cervix: Additional Evidence From a Case-Control Study. *Am J Epidemiol* 115: 59–66, 1982.

Clarke MC, DeMay RM, Spiegel GW: Pseudoparakeratosis in Uterine Endocervical Pap Smears (Abstract). *Mod Pathol* 6: 28A, 1993.

Cocker J, Fox H, Langley FA: Consistency in the Histological Diagnosis of Epithelial Abnormalities of the Uterine Cervix. *J Clin Pathol* 21: 67–70, 1968.

Cohen ML, Ducatman BS, Stock RJ: Differential Staining Techniques in Amniotic Fluid Cytology of Neural Tube Defects: A Prospective Study of 129 Pregnancies. *Diagn Cytopathol* 3: 271–277, 1987.

Coleman DV: Cytological Diagnosis of Virus-Infected Cells in Cervical Smears. *Diagn Gynecol Obstet* 4: 363–373, 1982.

Collins C, Dhurandhan: Cervical Biopsy Findings in Women With Benign Cellular Atypia on a Routine Pap Smear. *Am J Clin Pathol* 97: 442, 1992.

Collins CL: The Challenge of Cytology Proficiency Testing. *Lab Med* 25: 219–220, 1994.

Collins DN, Patacsil DP: Proficiency Testing in Cytology in New York: Analysis of a 14-Year State Program. *Acta Cytol* 30: 633–642, 1986.

Coppleson LW, Brown B: Estimation of the Screening Error Rate From the Observed Detection Rates in Repeated Cervical Cytology. *Am J Obstet Gynecol* 119: 953–958, 1974.

Costa MJ, Grimes C, Tackett E, Naib ZM: Cervicovaginal Cytology in an Indigent Population: Comparison of Results for 1964, 1981 and 1989. *Acta Cytol* 35: 51–56, 1991a.

Costa MJ, Kenny MB, Naib ZM: Cervicovaginal Cytology in Uterine Adenocarcinoma and Adenosquamous Carcinoma: Comparison of Cytologic and Histologic Findings. *Acta Cytol* 35: 127–134, 1991b.

Costa MJ, Tadros T, Tackett E, et al: Vaginocervical Cytology in Victims of Sexual Assault. *Diagn Cytopathol* 7: 337–340, 1991c.

Costa MJ, Tidd C, Willis D: Cervicovaginal Cytology in Carcinosarcoma (Malignant Mixed Müllerian [Mesodermal] Tumor) of the Uterus. *Diagn Cytopathol* 8: 33–40, 1992.

Cove H: The Arias-Stella Reaction Occurring in the Endocervix in Pregnancy: Recognition and Comparison With an Adenocarcinoma of the Endocervix. *Am J Surg Pathol* 3: 567–568, 1979.

Covell JL, Frierson HF: Intraepithelial Neoplasia Mimicking Microinvasive Squamous-Cell Carcinoma in Endocervical Brushings. *Diagn Cytopathol* 8: 18–22, 1992.

Cramer DW: The Role of Cervical Cytology in the Declining Morbidity and Mortality of Cervical Cancer. *Cancer* 34: 2018–2027, 1974.

Creasman WT, Parker RT: Management of Early Cervical Neoplasia. *Clin Obstet Gynecol* 18: 233–245, 1975.

Creasman WT, Weed JC Jr: Screening Techniques in Endometrial Cancer. *Cancer* 38: 436–440, 1976.

Creasman WT, Clarke-Pearson DL, Ashe C, et all: The Abnormal Pap Smear—What to Do Next? *Cancer* 48: 515–522, 1981.

Creasman WT, Fetter BF, Clarke-Pearson DL, et al: Management of Stage IA Carcinoma of the Cervix. *Am J Obstet Gynecol* 153: 164–172, 1985.

Crum CP, Egawa K, Barron B, et al: Human Papilloma Virus Infection (Condyloma) of the Cervix and Cervical Intraepithelial Neoplasia: A Histopathologic and Statistical Analysis. *Gynecol Oncol* 15: 88–94, 1983a.

Crum CP, Egawa K, Fu Y-S, et al: Atypical Immature Metaplasia (AIM): A Subset of Human Papilloma Virus Infection of the Cervix. *Cancer* 51: 2214–2219, 1983b.

Crum CP, Levine RU: Human Papillomavirus Infection and Cervical Neoplasia: New Perspectives. *Int J Gynecol Pathol* 3: 376–388, 1984.

Crum CP, Mitao M, Levin RU, et al: Cervical Papillomaviruses Segregate Within Morphologically Distinct Precancerous Lesions. *J Virol* 54: 675–681, 1985.

Crum CP, Fu Y-S, Kurman RJ, et al: Editorial Board Symposium: Practical Approach to Cervical Human Papillomavirus—Related Intraepithelial Lesions. *Int J Gynecol Pathol* 8: 388–399, 1989a.

Crum CP: Identifying High-Risk Precursors of Cervical Cancer: How and Why. *Am J Clin Pathol* 92: 379–382, 1989b.

Cunnane MF, Rothblat IP: Atypical Squamous Cells of Uncertain Significance: Histologic Correlation. *Acta Cytol* 36: 630, 1992.

Cunnane MF, Rothblat IP: Atypical Squamous Cells in Women Over 50: Histologic Correlations. *Acta Cytol* 37: 784, 1993.

Cuzick J. Terry G, Ho L, et al: Type-Specific Human Papillomavirus DNA in Abnormal Smears as a Predictor of High-Grade Cervical Intraepithelial Neoplasia. *Br J Cancer* 69: 167–171, 1994.

Daling JR, Sherman KJ, Weiss NS: Risk Factors for Condyloma Acuminatum in Women. *Sex Transmit Dis* 13: 16–18, 1986.

Danos M, Holmquist ND: Cytologic Evaluation of Decidual Cells: A Report of Two Cases With False Abnormal Cytology. *Acta Cytol* 11: 325–330, 1967.

Danos ML: Post Partum Cytology: Observations Over a Four Year Period. *Acta Cytol* 12: 309–312, 1968.

Davey DD, Gallion H, Jennings CD: DNA Cytometry in Postirradiation Cervical-Vaginal Smears. *Hum Pathol* 23: 1027–1031, 1992a.

Davey DD, Nielsen ML, Rosenstock W, et al: Terminology and Specimen Adequacy in Cervicovaginal Cytology. The College of American Pathologists Interlaboratory Comparison Program Experience. *Arch Pathol Lab Med* 116: 903–907, 1992b.

Davey DD, Nielsen ML, Frable WJ, et al: Improving Accuracy in Gynecologic Cytology: Results of the College of American Pathologists Interlaboratory Comparison Program in Cervicovaginal Cytology. *Arch Pathol Lab Med* 117: 1193–1198, 1993.

Davey DD, Naryshkin S, Nielsen ML, et al: Atypical Squamous Cells of Undetermined Significance: Interlaboratory Comparison and Quality Assurance Monitors. *Diagn Cytopathol* 11: 390–396, 1994.

Davila RM: Cervicovaginal Smear, True or False? *Am J Clin Pathol* 102: 1–2, 1994.

Davis GL, Hernandez E, Davis JL, et al: Atypical Squamous Cells in Papanicolaou Smears. *Obstet Gynecol* 69: 43–46, 1987.

Davis JR, Moon LB: Increased Incidence of Adenocarcinoma of Uterine Cervix. *Obstet Gynecol* 45: 79–83, 1975.

Davis JR, Hindman WM, Paplanus SH, et al: Value of Duplicate Smears in Cervical Cytology. *Acta Cytol* 25: 533–538, 1981.

Davis JR, Aristizabal S, Way DL, et al: DNA Ploidy, Grade, and Stage in Prognosis of Uterine Cervical Cancer. *Gynecol Oncol* 32: 4–7, 1989.

Davison JM, Marty JJ: Detecting Premalignant Cervical Lesions. Contributions of Screening Colposcopy to Cytology. *J Reprod Med* 39: 388–392, 1994.

Dawagne MP, Silverberg SG: Foam Cells in Endometrial Carcinoma—A Clinicopathologic Study. *Gynecol Oncol* 13: 67–75, 1982.

de Borges RJ, Garcia-Tamayo J, Zaitzman M. Cytologic and Ultrastructural Findings of a Peculiar Alteration in Cervical Cells From Patients With Human Papillomavirus Infections. *Acta Cytol* 33: 314–318, 1989.

Dehner LP: Cervicovaginal Cytology, False-Negative Results, and Standards of Practice. *Am J Clin Pathol* 99: 45–47, 1993.

De Luca L, Maestri N, Bonanni F, Nelson D: Maintenance of Epithelial Cell Differentiation: The Mode of Action of Vitamin A. *Cancer* 30: 1326–1331, 1972.

DePetrillo AD, Townsend DE, Morrow CP, et al: Colposcopic Evaluation of the Abnormal Papanicolaou Test in Pregnancy. *Am J Obstet Gynecol* 121: 441–445, 1975.

Derman H, Koss LG, Hyman MP, et al: Cervical Cytopathology I: Peers Compare Performance. *Pathologist* 35: 317–325, 1981.

de Roda Husman A-M, Walboomers JMM, Meijer CJLM, et al: Analysis of Cytomorphologically Abnormal Cervical Scrapes for the Presence of 27 Mucosotropic Human Papillomavirus Genotypes, Using Polymerase Chain Reaction. *Int J Cancer* 56: 802–806, 1994.

DeTorres EF, Mora A: Verrucous Carcinoma of the Cervix Uteri: Report of a Case. *Acta Cytol* 25: 307–309, 1981.

Devesa SS, Silverman DT, Young JL Jr, et al: Cancer Incidence and Mortality Trends Among Whites in the United States, 1947-1984. *J Natl Cancer Inst* 79: 701–770, 1987.

Devesa SS, Young JL, Brinton LA, et al: Recent Trends in Cervix Uteri Cancer. *Cancer* 64: 2184–2190, 1989.

de Villiers E-M, Schneider A, Miklaw H, et al: Human Papillomavirus Infections in Women With and Without Abnormal Cervical Cytology. *Lancet* (ii): 703–706, 1987.

de Villiers E-M, Wagner D, Schneider A, et al: Human Papillomavirus DNA in Women Without and With Cytological Abnormalities: Results of a 5-Year Follow-up Study. *Gynecol Oncol* 44: 33–39, 1992.

DiBonito L, Falconieri G, Tomasic G, et al: Cervical Cytopathology: An Evaluation of Its Accuracy Based on Cytohistologic Comparison. *Cancer* 72: 3002–3006, 1993.

Differding JT: Psammoma Bodies in a Vaginal Smear. *Acta Cytol* 11: 199–201, 1967.

Dodd LG, Sneige N, Villarreal Y, et al: Quality-Assurance Study of Simultaneously Sampled, Non-correlating Cervical Cytology and Biopsies. *Diagn Cytopathol* 9: 138–144, 1993.

Douglass LE: A Further Comment on the Contributions of Aurel Babes to Cytology and Pathology. *Acta Cytol* 11: 217–224, 1967.

Doss BJ, DeMay RM, Larson RA, et al: Chemotherapy Induced Epithelial Atypia in the Female Lower Genital Tract. (Abstract in press, *Mod Pathol*, 1995.)

Drake M: Nomenclature of Precancerous Lesions of the Uterine Cervix: A Position Paper. *Acta Cytol* 28: 527–534, 1984.

Draper GJ, Cook GA: Changing Patterns of Cervical Cancer Rates. *Br Med J* 287: 510–512, 1983.

Dressel DM, Wilber DC: Atypical Immature Squamous Metaplastic Cells in Cervical Smears: Association With High Grade Squamous Intraepithelial Lesions and Carcinoma of the Cervix (Abstract). *Acta Cytol* 36: 630, 1992.

Duca P, Braga M, Chiappa L, et al: Intralaboratory Reproducibility of Interpretation of Pap Smears: Results of an Experiment. *Tumori* 74: 737–744, 1988.

Ducatman BS, Wang HH, Jonasson JG, et al: Tubal Metaplasia: A Cytologic Study With Comparison to Other Neoplastic and Non-neoplastic Conditions of the Endocervix. *Diagn Cytopathol* 9: 98–105, 1993.

Dunn AEG, Ogilvie MM: Intranuclear Virus Particles in Human Genital Wart Tissue: Observations on the Ultrastructure of the Epidermal Layer. *J Ultrastruct Res* 22: 282–295, 1968.

Dunn JE Jr, Martin PL: Morphogenesis of Cervical Cancer. Findings From San Diego County Cytology Registry. *Cancer* 20: 1899–1906, 1967.

Dunn JE Jr, Schweitzer V: The Relationship of Cervical Cytology to the Incidence of Invasive Cervical Cancer and Mortality in Alameda County, California, 1960 to 1974. *Am J Obstet Gynecol* 139: 868–876, 1981.

Dürst M, Gissmann L, Ikenberg H, et al: A Papillomavirus DNA From a Cervical Carcinoma and Its Prevalence in Cancer Biopsy Samples From Different Geographic Regions. *Proc Natl Acad Sci* 80: 3812–3815, 1983.

Dürst M, Kleinheinz A, Hotz M, et al: The Physical State of Human Papillomavirus Type 16 DNA in Benign and Malignant Genital Tumours. *J Gen Virol* 66: 1515–1522, 1985.

Dürst M, Croce CM, Gissmann L, et al: Papillomavirus Sequences Integrate Near Cellular Oncogenes in Some Cervical Carcinomas. *Proc Natl Acad Sci* 84: 1070–1074, 1987.

Dybdahl H, Hastrup J, Baandrup U: The Clinical Significance of Actinomyces Colonization as Seen in Cervical Smears. *Acta Cytol* 35: 142–143, 1991.

Dyson N, Howley PM, Münger K, et al: The Human Papilloma Virus-16 E7 Oncoprotein Is Able to Bind to the Retinoblastoma Gene Product. *Science* 243: 934–937, 1989.

Economos K, Veridiano NP, Delke I, et al: Abnormal Cervical Cytology in Pregnancy: A 17-Year Experience. *Obstet Gynecol* 81: 915–918, 1993.

Eddy DM: Screening for Cervical Cancer. *Ann Intern Med* 113: 214–226, 1990.

Edebiri AA: Cervical Intraepithelial Neoplasia: The Role of Age at First Coitus in Its Etiology. *J Reprod Med* 35: 256–259, 1990.

Eells TP, Alpern HD, Grzywacz C, et al: The Effect of Tamoxifen on Cervical Squamous Maturation in Papanicolaou Stained Cervical Smears of Post-Menopausal Women. *Cytopathology* 1: 263–268, 1990.

Efstratiades M, Tamvakopoulou E, Papatheodorou B, et al: Postmenopausal Vaginal Cytohormonal Pattern in 597 Healthy Women and 301 Patients With Genital Cancer. *Acta Cytol* 26: 126–130, 1982.

Eisenstein R, Battifora H: Lymph Follicles in Cervical Smears. *Acta Cytol* 9: 344–346, 1965.

Elias A, Linthorst G, Bekker B, et al: The Significance of Endocervical Cells in the Diagnosis of Cervical Epithelial Changes. *Acta Cytol* 27: 225–229, 1983.

Elliott PM, Tattersall MHN, Coppleson M, et al: Changing Character of Cervical Cancer in Young Women. *Br Med J* 298: 288–290, 1989.

Evans AS, Monaghan JM: Spontaneous Resolution of Cervical Warty Atypia: The Relevance of Clinical and Nuclear DNA Features: A Prospective Study. *Br J Obstet Gynaecol* 92: 165–169, 1985.

Evans CS, Klein HZ, Goldman R, et al: Necrobiotic Granulomas of the Uterine Cervix: A Probably Postoperative Reaction. *Am J Surg Pathol* 8: 841–844, 1984.

Evans DMD, Hudson EA, Brown CL, et al: Terminology in Gynaecological Cytopathology: Report of the Working Party of The British Society for Clinical Cytology. *J Clin Pathol* 39: 933–944, 1986.

Fechner RE, Bossart MI, Spjut HJ: Ultrastructure of Endometrial Stromal Foam Cells. *Am J Clin Pathol* 72: 628–633, 1979.

Feldman MJ, Linzey EM, Srebnik E, et al: Abnormal Cervical Cytology in the Teen-ager: A Continuing Problem. *Am J Obstet Gynecol* 126: 418–421, 1976.

Fenoglio CM: Viruses in the Pathogenesis of Cervical Neoplasia: An Update. *Hum Pathol* 13: 785–787, 1982.

Ferenczy A, Richart RM, Okagaki T: Endometrial Involvement by Cervical Carcinoma In Situ. *Am J Obstet Gynecol* 110: 590–592, 1971.

Ferenczy A, Braun L, Shah KV: Human Papillomavirus (HPV) in Condylomatous Lesions of Cervix: A Comparative Ultrastructural and Immunohistochemical Study. *Am J Surg Pathol* 5: 661–670, 1981.

Ferguson JH: Positive Cancer Smears in Teenage Girls. *JAMA* 178: 365–368, 1961.

Fetherston WC: False-Negative Cytology in Invasive Cancer of the Cervix. *Clin Obstet Gynecol* 26: 929–937, 1983.

Fidler HK, Boyes DA, Worth AJ: Cervical Cancer Detection in British Columbia. A Progress Report. *J Obstet Gynaecol Br Cwlth* 75: 392–404, 1968.

Figge DC, Bennington JL, Schweid AI: Cervical Cancer After Initial Negative and Atypical Vaginal Cytology. *Am J Obstet Gynecol* 108: 422–428, 1970.

FIGO Cancer Committee: Staging Announcement. *Gynecol Oncol* 25: 383–385, 1986.

Fink DJ: Change in American Cancer Society Checkup Guidelines for Detection of Cervical Cancer. *CA Cancer J Clin* 38: 127–128, 1988.

Fink MJ, Fruchter RG, Maiman M, et al: The Adequacy of Cytology and Colposcopy in Diagnosing Cervical Neoplasia in HIV-Seropositive Women. *Gynecol Oncol* 55: 133–137, 1994.

Fiorella RM, Cheng J, Kragel PJ: Papanicolaou Smears in Pregnancy. Positivity of Exfoliated Cells for Human Chorionic Gonadotropin and Human Placental Lactogen. *Acta Cytol* 37: 451–456, 1993a.

Fiorella RM, Beckwith LG, Miller LK, et al: Metastatic Signet Ring Carcinoma of the Breast as a Source of Positive Cervicovaginal Cytology. A Case Report. *Acta Cytol* 37: 948–952, 1993b.

Fiorella RM, Casafrancisco D, Yokota S, et al: Artifactual Endocervical Atypia Induced by Endocervical Brush Collection. *Diagn Cytopathol* 11: 79–84, 1994.

Fleming H, Mein P: Primary Melanoma of the Cervix. A Case Report. *Acta Cytol* 38: 65–69, 1994.

Fletcher S: Histopathology of Papilloma Virus Infection of the Cervix Uteri: The History, Taxonomy, Nomenclature and Reporting of Koilocytic Dysplasias. *J Clin Pathol* 36: 616–624, 1983.

Fluhmann CF: The Nature and Development of the So-called Glands of the Cervix Uteri. *Am J Obstet Gynecol* 74: 753–768, 1957.

Foltz AM, Kelsey JL: The Annual Pap Test: A Dubious Policy Success. *Milbank Memorial Fund Quarterly—Health and Society* 56: 426–462, 1978.

Foote FW, Li K: Smear Diagnosis of In Situ Carcinoma of the Cervix. *Am J Obstet Gynecol* 56: 335–339, 1948.

Fowkes FGR: Diagnostic Vigilance. *Lancet* (i): 493–494, 1986.

Fowler WC Jr, Walton LA, Edelman DA: Cervical Intraepithelial Neoplasia During Pregnancy. *South Med J* 73: 1180–1185, 1980.

Fox CH: Biologic Behavior of Dysplasia and Carcinoma In Situ. *Am J Obstet Gynecol* 99: 960–974, 1967.

Fox CH: Time Necessary for Conversion of Normal to Dysplastic Cervical Epithelium. *Obstet Gynecol* 31: 749–754, 1968.

Frable WJ: Litigation Cells: Definition and Observations on a Cell Type in Cervical Vaginal Smears Not Addressed by the Bethesda System. *Diagn Cytopathol* 11: 213–215, 1994.

Frank TS, Bhat N, Noumoff JS, et al: Residual Trophoblastic Tissue as a Source of Highly Atypical Cells in the Postpartum Cervicovaginal Smear. *Acta Cytol* 35: 105–108, 1991.

Frankel K: Formal Proposal to Combine the Papanicolaou Numerical System With Bethesda Terminology for Reporting Cervical/Vaginal Cytologic Diagnoses. *Diagn Cytopathol* 10: 395–396, 1994.

Franquemont DW, Ward BE, Andersen WA, et al: Prediction of 'High-Risk' Cervical Papillomavirus Infection by Biopsy Morphology. *Am J Clin Pathol* 92: 577–582, 1989.

Fremont-Smith M, Graham RM, Meigs JV: Vaginal Smears as an Aid in the Diagnosis of Early Carcinoma of the Cervix. *N Engl J Med* 237: 302–304, 1947.

Friedell GH, McKay DG: Adenocarcinoma In Situ of the Endocervix. *Cancer* 6: 887–897, 1953.

Friedell GH, Parsons L: Late Manifestation of Cancer of the Cervix After Irradiation Therapy: Report of Two Cases. *Obstet Gynecol* 17: 582–586, 1961.

Frierson HF Jr, Covell JL, Anderson WA: Radiation Changes in Endocervical Cells in Brush Specimens. *Diagn Cytopathol* 6: 243–247, 1990.

Frisch LE: Inflammatory Atypia: An Apparent Link With Subsequent Cervical Intraepithelial Neoplasia Explained by Cytologic Underreading. *Acta Cytol* 31: 869–872, 1987a.

Frisch LE: Inflammatory Atypia and the False-Negative Smear in Cervical Intraepithelial Neoplasia. *Acta Cytol* 31: 873–877, 1987b.

Frisch LE, Parmar H, Buckley LD, et al: Colposcopy of Patients With Cytologic Inflammatory Epithelial Changes. *Acta Cytol* 34: 133–135, 1990.

Frost JK: Diagnostic Accuracy of "Cervical Smears." *Obstet Gynecol Surv* 24: 893–908, 1969.

Fry R, Linder AM: The Value of Exfoliative Cytology During Pregnancy. *South Afr Med J* 43: 1231–1232, 1969.

Fu YS, Reagan JW, Richart RM: Definition of Precursors. *Gynecol Oncol* 12: S220–S231, 1981.

Fu YS, Reagan JW, Hsiu JG, et al: Adenocarcinoma and Mixed Carcinoma of the Uterine Cervix: I. A Clinicopathologic Study. *Cancer* 49: 2560–2570, 1982.

Fu YS, Braun L, Shah KV, et al: Histologic, Nuclear DNA, and Human Papillomavirus Studies of Cervical Condylomas. *Cancer* 52: 1705–1711, 1983.

Fu YS, Berek JS, Hilborne LH: Diagnostic Problems of In Situ and Invasive Adenocarcinomas of the Uterine Cervix. *Appl Pathol* 5: 47–56, 1987.

Fu YS, Huang I, Beaudenon S, et al: Correlative Study of Human Papillomavirus DNA, Histopathology, and Morphometry in Cervical Condyloma and Intraepithelial Neoplasia. *Int J Gynecol Pathol* 7: 297–307, 1988.

Fuchs PG, Girardi F, Pfister H: Human Papillomavirus DNA in Normal, Metaplastic, Preneoplastic and Neoplastic Epithelia of the Cervix Uteri. *Int J Cancer* 41: 41–45, 1988.

Fugimoto I, Masubuchi S, Miwa H, et al: Psammoma Bodies Found in Cervicovaginal and/or Endometrial Smears. *Acta Cytol* 26: 317–322, 1982.

Fujii S, Konishi I, Ferenczy A, et al: Small Cell Undifferentiated Carcinoma of the Uterine Cervix: Histology, Ultrastructure, and Immunohistochemistry of Two Cases. *Ultrastruct Pathol* 10: 337–346, 1986.

Fukazawa I, Iwasaki H, Endo N, et al: A Case Report of Adenoma Malignum of the Uterine Cervix. *Acta Cytol* 36: 780, 1992.

Gardner JW, Lyon JL: Cancer of the Cervix: A Sexually Transmitted Infection? *Lancet* (ii): 470–471, 1974.

Gardner JW, Schuman KL, Slattery ML, et al: Is Vaginal Douching Related to Cervical Carcinoma? *Am J Epidemiol* 133: 368–375, 1991.

Gay JD, Donaldson LD, Goellner JR: False-Negative Results in Cervical Cytologic Studies. *Acta Cytol* 29: 1043–1046, 1985.

Geerling S, Nettum JA, Lindner LE, et al: Sensitivity and Specificity of the Papanicolaou-Stained Cervical Smear in the Diagnosis of *Chlamydia trachomatis* Infection. *Acta Cytol* 29: 671–675, 1985.

Geirsson G, Woodworth FE, Patten SF Jr, et al: Epithelial Repair and Regeneration in the Uterine Cervix I: An Analysis of the Cells. *Acta Cytol* 21: 371–378, 1977.

Genadry R, Olson J, Parmley T, et al: The Morphology of the Earliest Invasive Cell in Low Genital Tract Epidermoid Neoplasia. *Obstet Gynecol* 51: 718–722, 1978.

German M, Heaton R, Erickson D, et al: A Comparison of the Three Most Common Papanicolaou Smear Collection Techniques. *Obstet Gynecol* 84: 168–173, 1994.

Gersell DJ, Mazoujian G, Mutch DG, et al: Small-Cell Undifferentiated Carcinoma of the Cervix: A Clinicopathologic, Ultrastructural, and Immunocytochemical Study of 15 Cases. *Am J Surg Pathol* 12: 684–698, 1988.

Ghirardini C, Ghinosi P, Raisi O, et al: Detection of *Chlamydia trachomatis* in Papanicolaou-Stained Cervical Smears: Control Study by In Situ Hybridization. *Diagn Cytopathol* 7: 211–214, 1991.

Giacomini G, Simi U: CIN or not CIN. *Acta Cytol* 27: 543–545, 1983.

Giacomini G, Simi U: Nomenclature for the Cytodiagnosis of Cervical Intraepithelial Lesions. *Acta Cytol* 35: 657–658, 1991.

Giacomini G, Schnadig VJ: The Cervical Papanicolaou Smear: Bacterial Infection and the Bethesda System. *Acta Cytol* 36: 109–110, 1992.

Gideon K, Zaharopoulos P: Cytomegalovirus Endocervicitis Diagnosed by Cervical Smear. *Diagn Cytopathol* 7: 625–627, 1991.

Gilbert FE, Hicklin MD, Inhorn SL, et al: Standards of Adequacy of Cytologic Examination of the Female Genital Tract. *Am J Clin Pathol* 61: 285–286, 1974.

Giles JA, Hudson E, Crow J, et al: Colposcopic Assessment of the Accuracy of Cervical Cytology Screening. *Br Med J* 296: 1099–1102, 1988.

Gissmann L, zur Hausen H: Partial Characterization of Viral DNA From Human Genital Warts (Condylomata Acuminata). *Int J Cancer* 25: 605–609, 1980.

Gissmann L, De Villiers E-M, zur Hausen H: Analysis of Human Genital Warts (Condylomata Acuminata) and other Genital Tumors for Human Papillomavirus Type 6 DNA. *Int J Cancer* 29: 143–146, 1982.

Gissmann L, Wolnik L, Ikenberg H, et al: Human Papillomavirus Types 6 and 11 DNA Sequences in Genital and Laryngeal Papillomas and in Some Cervical Cancers. *Proc Natl Acad Sci* 80: 560–563, 1983.

Gitsch G, Kainz C, Reinthaller A, et al: Cervical Neoplasia and Human Papillomavirus Infection in Prostitutes. *Genitourin Med* 67: 478–480, 1991.

Giuntoli R, Yeh IT, Bhuett N, et al: Conservative Management of Cervical Intraepithelial Neoplasia During Pregnancy. *Gynecol Oncol* 42: 68–73, 1991.

Gius D, Laimins LA: Activation of Human Papillomavirus Type 18 Gene Expression by Herpes Simplex Virus Type 1 Viral Transactivators and a Phorbol Ester. *J Virol* 63: 555–563, 1989.

Gladwell P, Duncan P, Barham K, et al: Amnioscopy of Late Pregnancy With Fetal Membrane and Decidual Cytology. *Acta Cytol* 18: 333–337, 1974.

Gloor E, Ruzicka J: Morphology of Adenocarcinoma In Situ of the Uterine Cervix: A Study of 14 Cases. *Cancer* 49: 294–302, 1982.

Gloss B, Bernard HU, Seedorf K, et al: The Upstream Regulatory Region of the Human Papilloma Virus-16 Contains an E2 Protein-Independent Enhancer Which Is Specific for Cervical Carcinoma Cells and Regulated by Glucocorticoid Hormones. *EMBO J* 6: 3735–3743, 1987.

Goff BA, Atanasoff P, Brown E, et al: Endocervical Glandular Atypia in Papanicolaou Smears. *Obstet Gynecol* 79: 101–104, 1992.

Goff BA, Muntz HG, Bell DA, et al: Human Papillomavirus Typing in Patients With Papanicolaou Smears Showing Squamous Atypia. *Gynecol Oncol* 48: 384–388, 1993.

Gondos B, Marshall D, Ostergard DR: Endocervical Cells in Cervical Smears. *Am J Obstet Gynecol* 114: 833–834, 1972.

Gondos B, King EB: Significance of Endometrial Cells in Cervicovaginal Smears. *Ann Clin Lab Sci* 7: 486–490, 1977.

Goodman HM, Buttlar CA, Niloff JM, et al: Adenocarcinoma of the Uterine Cervix: Prognostic Factors and Patterns of Recurrence. *Gynecol Oncol* 33: 241–247, 1989.

Grafton WD, Kamm RC, Cowley LH: Cytologic Characteristics of Adenoid Cystic Carcinoma of the Uterine Cervix. *Acta Cytol* 20: 164–166, 1976.

Graham S, Priore R, Graham M, et al: Genital Cancer in Wives of Penile Cancer Patients. *Cancer* 44: 1870–1874, 1979a.

Graham S, Schotz W: Epidemiology of Cancer of the Cervix in Buffalo, New York. *J Natl Cancer Inst* 63: 23–27, 1979b.

Green GH: Cervical Cancer and Cytology Screening in New Zealand. *Br J Obstet Gynaecol* 85: 881–886, 1978.

Green GH: Rising Cervical Cancer Mortality in Young New Zealand Women. *NZ Med J* 89: 89–91, 1979.

Greenberg ER, Vessey M, McPherson K, et al: Cigarette Smoking and Cancer of the Uterine Cervix. *Br J Cancer* 51: 139–141, 1985.

Greer BE, Figge DC, Tamimi HK, et al: Stage 1B Adenocarcinoma of the Cervix Treated by Radical Hysterectomy and Pelvic Lymph Node Dissection. *Am J Obstet Gynecol* 160: 1509–1514, 1989.

Griffin NR, Bevan IS, Lewis FA, et al: Demonstration of Multiple HPV Types in Normal Cervix and in Cervical Squamous Cell Carcinoma Using the Polymerase Chain Reaction on Paraffin Wax Embedded Material. *J Clin Pathol* 43: 52–56, 1990.

Griffin NR, Dockey D, Lewis FA, et al: Demonstration of Low Frequency of Human Papillomavirus DNA in Cervical Adenocarcinoma and Adenocarcinoma In Situ by Polymerase Chain Reaction and In Situ Hybridization. *Int J Gynecol Pathol* 10: 36–43, 1991.

Griffiths M, Turner MJ, Partington CK, et al: Should Smears in a Colposcopy Clinic Be Taken After the Application of Acetic Acid? *Acta Cytol* 33: 324–326, 1989.

Griffiths M: "Nuns, Virgins, and Spinsters." Rigoni-Stern and Cervical Cancer Revisited. *Br J Obstet Gynaecol* 98: 797–802, 1991.

Groben P, Reddick R, Askin F: The Pathologic Spectrum of Small Cell Carcinoma of the Cervix. *Int J Gynecol Pathol* 4: 42–57. 1985.

Gronroos M, Tyrkko J, Siiteri PK, et al: Cytolysis and Karyopyknosis in Postmenopausal Vaginal Smears as Markers of Endometrial Cancer, Diabetes and Obesity. Studies Based on a Ten-Year Follow-up. *Acta Cytol* 30: 628–632, 1986.

Grosskopf SK: Cytopathology: Past, Present, and Future. *JAMWA* 33: 415–418, 1978.

Gupta PK: Intrauterine Contraceptive Devices: Vaginal Cytology, Pathologic Changes and Clinical Implications. *Acta Cytol* 26: 571–613, 1982.

Gupta PK, Shurbaji MS, Mintor LJ, et al: Cytopathologic Detection of *Chlamydia trachomatis* in Vaginopancervical (Fast) Smears. *Diagn Cytopathol* 4: 224–229, 1988.

Gusberg SB: The Rise and Fall of Endometrial Cancer. *Gynecol Oncol* 35: 124, 1989.

Haas JF: Pregnancy in Association With a Newly Diagnosed Cancer: A Population-Based Epidemiologic Assessment. *Int J Cancer* 34: 229–235, 1984.

Hadjimichael O, Janerich D, Lowell DM, et al: Histologic and Clinical Characteristics Associated With Rapidly Progressive Invasive Cervical Cancer: A Preliminary Report From the Yale Cancer Control Research Unit. *Yale J Biol Med* 62: 345–350, 1989.

Hall DJ, Schneider V, Goplerud DR: Primary Malignant Melanoma of the Uterine Cervix. *Obstet Gynecol* 56: 525–529, 1980.

Hall JE, Walton L: Dysplasia of the Cervix: A Prospective Study of 206 Cases. *Am J Obstet Gynecol* 100: 662–671, 1968.

Hall S, Wu TC, Soudi N, et al: Low-Grade Squamous Intraepithelial Lesions: Cytologic Predictors of Biopsy Confirmation. *Diagn Cytopathol* 10: 3–9, 1994.

Hall TE, Stapleton JJ, McCance JM: The Isolated Finding of Histiocytes in Papanicolaou Smears From Postmenopausal Women. *J Reprod Med* 27: 647–650, 1982.

Hallman KB, Nahhas WA, Connelly PJ: Endosalpingiosis as a Source of Psammoma Bodies in a Papanicolaou Smear. Report of a Case. *J Reprod Med* 36: 675–678, 1991.

Hammond EC, Burns EL, Seidman H, et al: Detection of Uterine Cancer. High and Low Risk Groups. *Cancer* 22: 1096–1107, 1968.

Hare MJ, Taylor-Robinson D, Cooper P: Evidence for an Association Between *Chlamydia trachomatis* and Cervical Intraepithelial Neoplasia. *Br J Obstet Gynaecol* 89: 489–492, 1982.

Harper JM, Levine AJ, Rosenthal DL, et al: Erythrocyte Folate Levels, Oral Contraceptive Use and Abnormal Cervical Cytology. *Acta Cytol* 38: 324–330, 1994.

Harris RWC, Brinton LA, Cowdell RH, et al: Characteristics of Women With Dysplasia or Carcinoma In Situ of the Cervix Uteri. *Br J Cancer* 42: 359–369, 1980.

Harrison DD, Hernandez E, Dunton CJ: Endocervical Brush Versus Cotton Swab for Obtaining Cervical Smears at a Clinic. A Cost Comparison. *J Reprod Med* 38: 285–288, 1993.

Hatem F, Wilbur D: High-Grade Cervical Lesions Following Negative Pap Smears: False-Negatives or Rapid Progression? (Abstract) *Mod Pathol* 6: 30A, 1993.

Heimann A, Scanlon R, Gentile J, et al: Measles Cervicitis. Report of a Case With Cytologic and Molecular Biologic Analysis. *Acta Cytol* 36: 727–730, 1992.

Hein K, Schreiber K, Cohen MI, et al: Cervical Cytology: The Need for Routine Screening in the Sexually Active Adolescent. *J Pediatr* 91: 123–126, 1977.

Helfand M, O'Connor GY, Zimmer-Gembec M, et al: Effect of Clinical Laboratory Improvement Amendments of 1988 (CLIA 88) on the Incidence of Invasive Cervical Cancer. *Med Care* 30: 1067–1082, 1992.

Hellberg D, Axelsson O, Gad A, et al: Conservative Management of the Abnormal Smear During Pregnancy. A Long-Term Follow-Up. *Acta Obstet Gynaecol Scand* 66: 195–199, 1987.

Hellberg D, Nilsson S, Haley NJ, et al: Smoking and Cervical Intraepithelial Neoplasia: Nicotine and Cotinine in Serum and Cervical Mucus in Smokers and Nonsmokers. *Am J Obstet Gynecol* 158: 910–913, 1988.

Hellberg D, Nilsson S, Valentin J: Positive Cervical Smear With Subsequent Normal Colposcopy and Histology—Frequency of CIN in a Long-Term Follow-up. *Gynecol Oncol* 53: 148–151, 1994.

Hellen EA, Coghill SB, Clark JV: Prolapsed Fallopian Tube After Abdominal Hysterectomy: A Report of the Cytological Findings. *Cytopathology* 4: 181–185, 1993.

Henry-Stanley MJ, Stanley MW, Burton LG, et al: Cytologic Diagnosis of Cytomegalovirus in Cervical Smears. *Diagn Cytopathol* 9: 364–365, 1993a.

Henry-Stanley MJ, Simpson M, Stanley MW: Cervical Cytology Findings in Women Infected With the Human Immunodeficiency Virus. *Diagn Cytopathol* 9: 508–509, 1993b.

Herbst AL: The Bethesda System for Cervical/Vaginal Cytologic Diagnoses: A Note of Caution. *Obstet Gynecol* 76: 449–450, 1990.

Herbst AL: The Bethesda System for Cervical/Vaginal Cytologic Diagnoses. *Clin Obstet Gynecol* 35: 22–27, 1992.

Herrero R, Brinton LA, Reeves WC, et al: Sexual Behavior, Venereal Diseases, Hygiene Practices, and Invasive Cervical Cancer in a High-Risk Population. *Cancer* 65: 380–386, 1990.

Herrero R, Brinton LA, Reeves WC, et al: Screening for Cervical Cancer in Latin America: A Case-Control Study. *Int J Epidemiol* 21: 1050–1056, 1992.

Hicklin MD, Watts JC, Plott AE, et al: Retrospective Evaluation of Gynecologic Cytodiagnosis. I. Reproducibility Using an Experimental Diagnostic Scale. *Acta Cytol* 28: 58–71, 1984.

Hidvegi DF, DeMay RM, Sorensen K: Uterine Müllerian Adenosarcoma With Psammoma Bodies. Cytologic, Histologic and Ultrastructural Studies of a Case. *Acta Cytol* 26: 323–326, 1982.

Highman WJ: Calcified Bodies and the Intrauterine Device. *Acta Cytol* 15: 473–475, 1971.

Hilrich NM, Hipke MM: Endometrial and Cytologic Atypism in the Postabortal State. *Obstet Gynecol* 6: 452–454, 1955.

Hinsey JC: George Nicholas Papanicolaou, M.D., Ph.D., D.Sc.: May 13, 1883-February 19, 1962. *Acta Cytol* 6: 483–486, 1962.

Hirai Y, Chen J-T, Hamada T, et al: Clinical and Cytologic Aspects of Primary Fallopian Tube Carcinoma: A Report of Ten Cases. *Acta Cytol* 31: 834–840, 1987.

Hirochika H, Broker TR, Chow LT: Enhancers and Trans-Acting E2 Transcriptional Factors of Papillomaviruses. *J Virol* 61: 2599–2606, 1987.

Hirschowitz L, Raffle AE, Mackenzie EFD, et al: Long Term Follow Up of Women with Borderline Cervical Smear Test Results: Effects of Age and Viral Infections on Progression to High Grade Dyskaryosis. *BMJ* 304: 1209–1212, 1992.

Hirschowitz L, Eckford SD, Phillpotts B, et al: Cytological Changes Associated With Tubo-Endometrioid Metaplasia of the Uterine Cervix. *Cytopathology* 5: 1–8, 1994.

Hislop TG, Band PR, Deschamps M, et al: Cervical Cancer Screening in Canadian Native Women. Adequacy of the Papanicolaou Smear. *Acta Cytol* 38: 29–32, 1994.

Hoffman MS, Sterghos S Jr, Gordy LW, et al: Evaluation of the Cervical Canal With the Endocervical Brush. *Obstet Gynecol* 82: 573–577, 1993.

Holland BK, Foster JD, Louria DB: Cervical Cancer and Health Care Resources in Newark, New Jersey, 1970 to 1988. *Am J Public Health* 83: 45–48, 1993.

Hollander DH, Gupta PK: Hematoidin Cockleburrs in Cervico-Vaginal Smears. *Acta Cytol* 18: 268–269, 1974.

Holloway RW, Farrell MP, Castellano C, et al: Identification of Human Papillomavirus Type 16 in Primary and Recurrent Cervical Cancer Following Radiation Therapy. *Gynecol Oncol* 41: 123–128, 1991.

Holly EA, Petrakis NL, Friend NF, et al: Mutagenic Mucus in the Cervix of Smokers. *J Natl Cancer Inst* 76: 983–986, 1986.

Holm K, Grinsted P, Poulsen EF, et al: Can Hairspray Be Used as a Smear Fixative? A Comparison Between Two Types of Coating Fixatives. *Acta Cytol* 32: 422–424, 1988.

Holmquist ND, Danos M: The Cytology of Early Abortion. *Acta Cytol* 11: 262–266, 1967a.

Holmquist ND, McMahan CA, Williams OD: Variability in Classification of Carcinoma In Situ of the Uterine Cervix. *Arch Pathol* 84: 334–345, 1967b.

Holmquist ND, Torres J: Malignant Melanoma of the Cervix: A Report of a Case. *Acta Cytol* 32: 252–2567, 1988.

Hopkins MP, Morley GW: Stage IB Squamous Cell Cancer of the Cervix: Clinicopathologic Features Related to Survival. *Am J Obstet Gynecol* 164: 1520–1529, 1991.

Horowitz IR, Jacobson LP, Zucker PK, et al: Epidemiology of Adenocarcinoma of the Cervix. *Gynecol Oncol* 31: 25–41, 1988.

Howard L Jr, Erickson CC, Stoddard LD: Study of Incidence and Histogenesis of Endocervical Metaplasia and Intraepithelial Carcinoma. Observations of 400 Uteri Removed for Noncervical Disease. *Cancer* 4: 1210–1223, 1951.

Howell LP, Davis RL: Follow-up of Papanicolaou Smears Diagnosed as Atypical Squamous Cells of Undetermined Significance. *Acta Cytol* 37: 783, 1993.

Huang JC, Naylor B: Cytomegalovirus Infection of the Cervix Detected by Cytology and Histology: A Report of Five Cases. *Cytopathology* 4: 237–241, 1993.

Hudock J, Hanau CA, Hawthorne C, et al: Predictors of Human Papilloma Virus in Patients With Keratinization. *Diagn Cytopathol* 12: 28–31, 1995.

Hulka BS: Cytologic and Histologic Outcome Following an Atypical Cancer Smear. *Am J Obstet Gynecol* 101: 190–199, 1968.

Hunt JM, Irwig LM, Towler BP: The Management of Women With Initial Minor Pap Smear Abnormalities. *Med J Aust* 160: 558–563, 1994.

Hurt WG, Silverberg SG, Frable WJ, et al: Adenocarcinoma of the Cervix: Histopathologic and Clinical Features. *Am J Obstet Gynecol* 129: 304–315, 1977.

Husain OAN, Butler EB, Evans DMD, et al: Quality Control in Cervical Cytology. *J Clin Pathol* 27: 935–944, 1974.

Hutchinson M, Fertitta L, Goldbaum B, et al: Cervex-Brush and Cytobrush. Comparison of Their Ability to Sample Abnormal Cells for Cervical Smears. *J Reprod Med* 36: 581–586, 1991.

Inaba N, Fukazawa I, Iwasaki H, et al: Cervical Verrucous Carcinoma: A Case Report. *Acta Cytol* 36: 790, 1992.

Ismail SM, Colclough AB, Dinnen JS, et al: Observer Variation in Histopathological Diagnosis and Grading of Cervical Intraepithelial Neoplasia. *Br Med J* 298: 707–710, 1989.

Ismail SM, Colclough AB, Dinnen JS, et al: Reporting Cervical Intra-epithelial Neoplasia (CIN): Intra- and Interpathologist Variation and Factors Associated With Disagreement. *Histopathology* 16: 371–376, 1990.

Jafari K: False-Positive Pap Smear in Uterine Malignancy. *Gynecol Oncol* 6: 76–82, 1978.

Janerich DT, Hadjimichael O, Schwartz P, et al: The Screening Histories of Women With Invasive Cancer, Connecticut. *Am J Public Health* 85: 791–794, 1995.

Jarmulowicz MR, Jenkins D, Bartons SE, et al: Cytological Status and Lesion Size: A Further Dimension in Cervical Intraepithelial Neoplasia. *Br J Obstet Gynaecol* 96: 1061–1066, 1989.

Jaworski RC, Pacey NF, Greenberg ML, et al: The Histologic Diagnosis of Adenocarcinoma In Situ and Related Lesions of the Cervix Uteri: Adenocarcinoma In Situ. *Cancer* 61: 1171–1181, 1988.

Jenkins DM, Goulden R: Psammoma Bodies in Cervical Cytology Smears. *Acta Cytol* 21: 112–113, 1977.

Jenkins D, Tay SK, McCance DJ, et al: Histological and Immunocytochemical Study of Cervical Intraepithelial Neoplasia (CIN) With Associated HPV 6 and HPV 16 Infections. *J Clin Pathol* 39: 1177–1180, 1986.

Johnson LD, Nickerson RJ, Easterday CL, et al: Epidemiologic Evidence for the Spectrum of Change From Dysplasia Through Carcinoma In Situ to Invasive Cancer. *Cancer* 22: 901–914, 1968.

Johnson MA, Blomfield PI, Bevan IS, et al: Analysis of Human Papillomavirus Type 16 E6-E7 Transcription in Cervical Carcinomas and Normal Cervical Epithelium Using the Polymerase Chain Reaction. *J Gen Virol* 71: 1473–1479, 1990.

Johnson TL, Joseph CLM, Caison-Sorey TJ, et al: Prevalence of HPV 16 and 18 DNA Sequences in CIN III Lesions of Adults and Adolescents. *Diagn Cytopathol* 10: 276–283, 1994.

Johnston M, Benrubi GI, Nuss RC, et al: Age and Cervical Dysplasia. *South Med J* 81: 1458–1459, 1988.

Johnston WW, Myers B, Creasman WT, et al: Cytopathology and the Management of Early Invasive Cancer of the Uterine Cervix. *Obstet Gynecol* 60: 350–353, 1982.

Jones BA, Heard NV: Pap Smear Rescreening Data Analysis and Critique. *College of American Pathologists Q-Probe Study* 3: 1–16, 1993.

Jones CA, Neustaedter T, Mackenzie LL: The Value of Vaginal Smears in the Diagnosis of Early Malignancy. *Am J Obstet Gynecol* 49: 159–168, 1945.

Jones CJ, Brinton LA, Hamman RF, et al: Risk Factors for In Situ Cervical Cancer: Results From a Case-Control Study. *Cancer Res* 50: 3657–3662, 1990.

Jones DED, Creasman WT, Dombroski RA, et al: Evaluation of the Atypical Pap Smear. *Am J Obstet Gynecol* 157: 544–549, 1987.

Jones EG, MacDonald I, Breslow L: A Study of Epidemiologic Factors in Carcinoma of the Uterine Cervix. *Am J Obstet Gynecol* 76: 1–10, 1958.

Jones HW, Droegemueller W, Makowski EL: A Primary Melanocarcinoma of the Cervix. *Am J Obstet Gynecol* 111: 959–963, 1971.

Jones WB, Saigo PE: The "Atypical" Papanicolaou Smear. *CA Cancer J Clin* 36: 237–242, 1986.

Jordan MJ, Bader GM, Day E: Carcinoma In Situ of the Cervix and Related Lesions. An 11 Year Prospective Study. *Am J Obstet Gynecol* 89: 160–182, 1964.

Jordan SW, Smith NL, Dike LS: The Significance of Cervical Cytologic Dysplasia. *Acta Cytol* 25: 237–244, 1981.

Joseph MG, Cragg F, Wright VC, et al: Cyto-Histological Correlates in a Colposcopic Clinic: A 1-Year Prospective Study. *Diagn Cytopathol* 7: 477–481, 1991.

Joseph RE, Enghardt MH, Doering DL, et al: Small Cell Neuroendocrine Carcinoma of the Vagina. *Cancer* 70: 784–789, 1992.

Joste NE, Crum CP, Cibas ES: Cytologic/Histologic Correlation for Quality Control in Cervicovaginal Cytology. *Am J Clin Pathol* 103: 32–34, 1995.

Kadish AS, Burk RD, Kress Y, et al: Human Papillomaviruses of Different Types in Precancerous Lesions of the Uterine Cervix: Histologic, Immunocytochemical and Ultrastructural Studies. *Hum Pathol* 17: 384–392, 1986.

Kadish AS, Hagan RJ, Ritter DB, et al: Biologic Characteristics of Specific Human Papillomavirus Types Predicted From Morphology of Squamous Lesions. *Hum Pathol* 23: 1262–1269, 1992.

Kalo-Klein A, Witkin SS: *Candida albicans*: Cellular Immune System Interactions During Different Stages of Menstrual Cycle. *Am J Obstet Gynecol* 161: 1132–1136, 1989.

Kaminski PF, Stevens CW Jr, Wheelock JB: Squamous Atypia on Cytology: The Influence of Age. *J Reprod Med* 34: 617–620, 1989a.

Kaminski PF, Sorosky JI, Wheelock JB, et al: The Significance of Atypical Cervical Cytology in an Older Population. *Obstet Gynecol* 73: 13–15, 1989b.

Kaminski PF, Lyon DS, Soroky JI, et al: Significance of Atypical Cervical Cytology in Pregnancy. *Am J Perinatol* 9: 340–343, 1992.

Kamiya M, Uei Y, Higo Y, et al: Immunocytochemical Diagnosis of Small Cell Undifferentiated Carcinoma of the Cervix. *Acta Cytol* 37: 131–134, 1993.

Kanbour AI, Stock RJ: Squamous Cell Carcinoma In Situ of the Endometrium and Fallopian Tube as Superficial Extension of Invasive Cervical Carcinoma. *Cancer* 42: 570–580, 1978.

Kanbour A, Doshi N: Psammoma Bodies and Detached Ciliary Tufts in a Cervicovaginal Smear Associated With Benign Ovarian Cystadenofibroma. *Acta Cytol* 24: 549–552, 1980.

Kashimura M, Matsuura Y, Shinohara M, et al: Comparative Study of Cytology and Punch Biopsy in Cervical Intraepithelial Neoplasia During Pregnancy. A Preliminary Report. Acta Cytol 35: 100–104, 1991.

Kataja V, Syrjänen K, Mäntyjärvi R, et al: Prospective Follow-up of Cervical HPV Infections: Life-Table Analysis of Histopathological, Cytological and Colposcopic Data. *Eur J Epidemiol* 8: 1–7, 1989.

Katz L, Hinberg I, Weber F: False-Negative Smears in Gynaecological Cytology. *Lancet* (i): 562, 1979.

Katz RL, Veanattukalathil S, Weiss KM: Human Papillomavirus Infection and Neoplasia of the Cervix and Anogenital Region in Women With Hodgkin's Disease. *Acta Cytol* 31: 845–854, 1987.

Kaufman RH, Burmeister RE, Spjut HJ: Cervical Cytology in the Teen-age Patient. *Am J Obstet Gynecol* 108: 515–519, 1970.

Kaufman R, Koss LG, Kurman RJ, et al: Statement of Caution in the Interpretation of Papillomavirus-Associated Lesions of the Epithelium of the Uterine Cervix. *Acta Cytol* 27: 107–108, 1983a.

Kaufman R, Koss LG, Kurman RJ, et al: Statement of Caution in the Interpretation of Papillomavirus-Associated Lesions of the Epithelium of Uterine Cervix. *Am J Obstet Gynecol* 146: 125, 1983b.

Kaur P, McDougall JK, Cone R: Immortalization of Primary Human Epithelial Cells by Cloned Cervical Carcinoma DNA Containing Human Papillomavirus Type 16 E6/E7 Open Reading Frames. *J Gen Virol* 70: 1261–1266, 1989.

Kawaguchi K, Nogi M, Ohya M, et al: The Value of the Cytobrush for Obtaining Cells From the Uterine Cervix. *Diagn Cytopathol* 3: 262–267, 1987.

Kaye KS, Dhurandhar NR: Atypical Cells of Undetermined Significance: Follow-up Biopsy and Pap Smear Findings: *Am J Clin Pathol* 99: 332, 1993.

Keebler CM, Wied GL: The Estrogen Test: An Aid in Differential Cytodiagnosis. *Acta Cytol* 18: 482–493, 1974.

Kern SB: Prevalence of Psammoma Bodies in Papanicolaou-Stained Cervicovaginal Smears. *Acta Cytol* 35: 81–88, 1991a.

Kern SB: Significance of Anucleated Squames in Papanicolaou-Stained Cervicovaginal Smears. *Acta Cytol* 35: 89–93, 1991b.

Kessler II, Kulcar Z, Zimolo A, et al: Cervical Cancer in Yugoslavia. II. Epidemiologic Factors of Possible Etiologic Significance. *J Natl Cancer Inst* 53: 51–60, 1974.

Kessler II: Human Cervical Cancer as a Venereal Disease. *Cancer Res* 36: 783–791, 1976.

Kessler II: Etiological Concepts in Cervical Carcinogenesis. *Gynecol Oncol* 12: S7–S24, 1981.

Kessler II: Etiological Concepts in Cervical Carcinogenesis. *Appl Pathol* 5: 57–75, 1987.

Kierkegaard O, Byrjalsen C, Frandsen KH, et al: Diagnostic Accuracy of Cytology and Colposcopy in Cervical Squamous Intraepithelial Lesions. *Acta Obstet Gynecol Scand* 73: 648–651, 1994.

Kiguchi K, Bibbo M, Hasegawa T, et al: Dysplasia During Pregnancy: A Cytologic Follow-up Study. *J Reprod Med* 26: 66–72, 1981.

Killough BV, Clark AH, Garvin J: Correlation Between Cytodiagnosis and the Presence of Endocervical or Squamous Metaplastic Cells in Gynecologic Smears. *Acta Cytol* 32: 758, 1988.

Kim H-S, Underwood D: Adenocarcinoma in the Cervicovaginal Papanicolaou Smear: Analysis of a 12 Year Experience. *Diagn Cytopathol* 7: 119–124, 1991.

Kirkup W, Singer A: Colposcopy in the Management of the Pregnant Patient With Abnormal Cervical Cytology. *Br J Obstet Gynaecol* 87: 322–325, 1980.

Kitay DZ, Wentz WB: Cervical Cytology in Folic Acid Deficiency of Pregnancy. *Am J Obstet Gynecol* 104: 931–938, 1969.

Kiviat NB, Paavonen JA, Brockway J, et al: Cytologic Manifestations of Cervical and Vaginal Infections. I. Epithelial and Inflammatory Cellular Changes. *JAMA* 253: 989–996, 1985.

Kiviat NB, Koutsky LA, Paavonen JA, et al: Prevalence of Genital Papillomavirus Infection Among Women Attending a College Student Health Clinic or a Sexually Transmitted Disease Clinic. *J Infect Dis* 159: 293–302, 1989.

Kivlahan C, Ingram E: Papanicolaou Smears Without Endocervical Cells: Are They Inadequate? *Acta Cytol* 30: 258–260, 1986.

Kjaer SK, de Villiers E-M, Haugaard BJ, et al: Human Papillomavirus, Herpes Simplex Virus and Cervical Cancer Incidence in Greenland and Denmark. A Population-Based Cross-Sectional Study. *Int J Cancer* 41: 518–524, 1988.

Kjaer SK, Teisen C, Haugaard BJ, et al: Risk Factors for Cervical Cancer in Greenland and Denmark: A Population-Based Cross-Sectional Study. *Int J Cancer* 44: 40–47, 1989.

Kjaer SK, Engholm G, Teisen C, et al: Risk Factors for Cervical Human Papillomavirus and Herpes Simplex Virus Infections in Greenland and Denmark: A Population-Based Study. *Am J Epidemiol* 131: 669–682, 1990.

Kline TJ: Cytopathology: Negligence and a Lawyer's Opinion. *Diagn Cytopathol* 11: 219, 1994.

Kline TS, Holland M, Wemple D: Atypical Cytology With Contraceptive Hormone Medication. *Am J Clin Pathol* 53: 215–222, 1970.

Kling TG, Buchsbaum HJ: Cervical Carcinoma in Women Under Twenty-One Years of Age. *Obstet Gynecol* 42: 205– 207, 1973.

Klinkhamer PJJM, Vooijs GP, de Haan AFJ: Intraobserver and Interobserver Variability in the Diagnosis of Epithelial Abnormalities in Cervical Smears. *Acta Cytol* 32: 794–800, 1988.

Klinkhamer PJJM, Vooijs GP, de Haan AFJ: Intraobserver and Interobserver Variability in the Quality Assessment of Cervical Smears. *Acta Cytol* 33: 215–218, 1989.

Knebel Doeberitz MV, Oltersdorf T, Schwarz E, et al: Correlation of Modified Human Papilloma Virus Early Gene Expression With Altered Growth Properties in C4-1 Cervical Carcinoma Cells. *Cancer Res* 48: 3780–3786, 1988.

Kobayashi TK, Yuasa M, Fujimoto T, et al: Cytologic Findings in Postpartum and Postabortal Smears. *Acta Cytol* 24: 328–334, 1980.

Kobayashi TK, Fujimoto T, Okamoto H, et al: Cytologic Evaluation of Atypical Cells in Cervicovaginal Smears From Women With Tubal Pregnancies. *Acta Cytol* 27: 28–32, 1983.

Kohan S, Beckman EM, Bigelow B, et al: The Role of Colposcopy in the Management of Cervical Intraepithelial Neoplasia During Pregnancy and Postpartum. *J Reprod Med* 25: 279–284, 1980.

Kohan S, Noumoff J, Beckman EM, et al: Colposcopic Screening of Women With Atypical Papanicolaou Smears. *J Reprod Med* 30: 383–387, 1985.

Koike N, Higuchi T, Sakai Y: Goblet-Like Cells in Atrophic Vaginal Smears and Their Histologic Correlation: Possible Confusion With Endocervical Cells. *Acta Cytol* 34: 785–788, 1990.

Koike N, Kobayashi TK: Appearance of Goblet Cells in Atrophic Vaginal Smears. *Diagn Cytopathol* 9: 475–476, 1993.

Koike N, Kasamatsu T: Efficacy of the Cytobrush Method in Aged Patients. *Diagn Cytopathol* 10: 311–314, 1994.

Kolstad P: Follow-up Study of 232 Patients With Stage Ia1 and 411 Patients With Stage Ia2 Squamous Cell Carcinoma of the Cervix (Microinvasive Carcinoma). *Gynecol Oncol* 33: 265–272, 1989.

Konikov NF, Kempson RL, Piskie V: Cytohistologic Correlation in Dysplasia, Carcinoma In Situ, and Invasive Carcinoma of the Uterine Cervix. *Am J Clin Pathol* 51: 463–469, 1969.

Koprowska I: Early Use of the Vaginal Smear for Cervical Cancer Detection. *Acta Cytol* 25: 202, 1981.

Koprowska I: Concurrent Discoveries of the Value of Vaginal Smears for Diagnosis of Uterine Cancer. *Diagn Cytopathol* 1: 245–248, 1985.

Korn AP, Autry M, DeRemer PA, et al: Sensitivity of the Papanicolaou Smear in Human Immunodeficiency Virus–Infected Women. *Obstet Gynecol* 83: 401–404, 1994.

Koss LG, Durfee GR: Unusual Patterns of Squamous Epithelium of the Uterine Cervix: Cytologic and Pathologic Study of Koilocytotic Atypia. *Ann NY Acad Sci* 63: 1245–1261, 1956.

Koss LG, Melamed MR, Daniel WW: In Situ Epidermoid Carcinoma of the Cervix and Vagina Following Radiotherapy for Cervical Cancer. *Cancer* 14: 353–360, 1961.

Koss LG, Durfee GR: Cytologic Diagnosis of Endometrial Carcinoma. Result of Ten Years of Experience. *Acta Cytol* 6: 519–531, 1962.

Koss LG, Stewart FW, Foote FW, et al: Some Histological Aspects of Behavior of Epidermoid Carcinoma In Situ and Related Lesions of the Uterine Cervix: A Long-Term Prospective Study. *Cancer* 16: 1160–1211, 1963.

Koss LG, Melamed MR, Mayer K: The Effect of Busulfan on Human Epithelia. *Am J Clin Pathol* 44: 385–397, 1965.

Koss LG, Hicklin MD: Standards of Adequacy of Cytologic Examination of the Female Genital Tract. Conclusions of Study Group on Cytology. *Obstet Gynecol* 43: 792–793, 1974.

Koss LG: Dysplasia: A Real Concept or a Misnomer? *Obstet Gynecol* 57: 374–379, 1978.

Koss LG, Schreiber K, Oberlander SG, et al: Screening of Asymtomatic Women for Endometrial Cancer. *Obstet Gynecol* 57: 681–691, 1981.

Koss LG, Schreiber K, Oberlander SG, et al: Detection of Endometrial Carcinoma and Hyperplasia in Asymptomatic Women. *Obstet Gynecol* 64: 1–11, 1984.

Koss LG: Current Concepts of Intraepithelial Neoplasia in the Uterine Cervix (CIN). *Appl Pathol* 5: 7–18, 1987a.

Koss LG: Cytologic and Histologic Manifestations of Human Papillomavirus Infection of the Female Genital Tract and Their Clinical Significance. *Cancer* 60: 1942–1950, 1987b.

Koss LG: The Papanicolaou Test for Cervical Cancer Detection. A Triumph and a Tragedy. *JAMA* 261: 737–743, 1989a.

Koss LG: Cytology. Accuracy of Diagnosis. *Cancer* 64 (Suppl): 249–252, 1989b.

Koss LG: Cervical (Pap) Smear: New Directions. *Cancer* 71: 1406–1412, 1993a.

Koss LG: Diagnostic Accuracy in Cervicovaginal Cytology. *Arch Pathol Lab Med* 117: 1240–1242, 1993b.

Koss LG, Lin E, Schreiber K, et al: Evaluation of the PAPNET™ Cytologic Screening System for Quality Control of Cervical Smears. *Am J Clin Pathol* 101: 220–229, 1994.

Koutsky LA, Galloway DA, Holmes KK: Epidemiology of Genital Human Papillomavirus Infection. *Epidemiol Rev* 10: 122–163, 1988.

Koutsky LA, Holmes KK, Critchlow CW, et al: A Cohort Study of the Risk of Cervical Intraepithelial Neoplasia Grade 2 or 3 in Relation to Papillomavirus Infection. *New Engl J Med* 327: 1272–1278, 1992.

Kovi J, Tillman L, Lee SM: Malignant Transformation of Condyloma Acuminatum. A Light Microscopic and Ultrastructural Study. *Am J Clin Pathol* 61: 702–710, 1974.

Krebs H-B, Schneider V, Hurt WG, et al: Genital Condylomas in Immunosuppressed Women: A Therapeutic Challenge. *South Med J* 79: 183–187, 1986.

Krebs H-B, Helmkamp BF: Treatment Failure of Genital Condylomata Acuminata in Women: Role of the Male Sexual Partner. *Am J Obstet Gynecol* 165: 337–340, 1991.

Kreider JW, Howett MK, Stoler MH, et al: Susceptibility of Various Human Tissues to Transformation In Vivo With Human Papillomavirus Type 11. *Int J Cancer* 39: 459–465, 1987.

Krieger P, Naryshkin S: Random Rescreening of Cytologic Smears: A Practical and Effective Component of Quality Assurance in Both Large and Small Cytology Laboratories. *Acta Cytol* 38: 291–298, 1994.

Krishnamoorthy A, De Sai M, Simanowitz M: Primary Malignant Melanoma of the Cervix. Case Report. *Br J Obstet Gynaecol* 93: 84–86, 1986.

Kristensen GB, Jensen LK, Ejersbo D, et al: The Efficiency of the Cytobrush and Cotton Swab in Obtaining Endocervical Cells in Smears Taken After Conization of the Cervix. *Arch Gynecol Obstet* 246: 207–210, 1989a.

Kristensen GB, Holund B, Grinsted P: Efficacy of the Cytobrush Versus the Cotton Swab in the Collection of Endocervical Cells. *Acta Cytol* 33: 849–851, 1989b.

Kristensen GB, Skyggebjerg K-D, Holund B, et al: Analysis of Cervical Smears Obtained Within Three Years of the Diagnosis of Invasive Cervical Cancer. *Acta Cytol* 35: 47–50, 1991.

Krumins I, Young Q, Pacey F, et al: The Cytologic Diagnosis of Adenocarcinoma In Situ of the Cervix Uteri. *Acta Cytol* 21: 320–329, 1977.

Kudo R, Sagae S, Hayakawa O, et al: The Cytological Features and DNA Content of Cervical Adenocarcinoma. *Diagn Cytopathol* 3: 191–197, 1987.

Kudo R, Sagae S, Hayakawa O, et al: Morphology of Adenocarcinoma In Situ and Microinvasive Adenocarcinoma of the Uterine Cervix: A Cytologic and Ultrastructural Study. *Acta Cytol* 35: 109–116, 1991.

Kuebler DL, Nikrui N, Bell DA: Cytologic Features of Endometrial Papillary Serous Carcinoma. *Acta Cytol* 33: 120–126, 1989.

Kühler-Obbarius C, Milde-Langosch K, Löning T, et al: Polymerase Chain Reaction—Assisted Evaluation of Low and High Grade Squamous Intraepithelial Lesion Cytology and Reappraisal of the Bethesda System. *Acta Cytol* 38: 681–686, 1994a.

Kühler-Obbarius C, Milde-Langosch K, Helling-Giese G, et al: Polymerase Chain Reaction–Assisted Papillomavirus Detection in Cervicovaginal Smears: Stratification by Clinical Risk and Cytology Reports. *Virchows Arch* 425: 157–163, 1994b.

Kurman RJ, Scully RE: The Incidence and Histogenesis of Vaginal Adenosis. An Autopsy Study. *Hum Pathol* 5: 265–276, 1974.

Kurman RJ, Shah KH, Lancaster WD, et al: Immunoperoxidase Localization of Papillomavirus Antigens in Cervical Dysplasia and Vulvar Condylomas. *Am J Obstet Gynecol* 140: 931–935, 1981.

Kurman RJ, Jenson AB, Lancaster WD: Papillomavirus Infection of the Cervix. II: Relationship to Intraepithelial Neoplasia Based on the Presence of Specific Viral Structural Proteins. *Am J Surg Pathol* 7: 39–52, 1983.

Kurman RJ, Kaminski PF, Norris HJ: The Behavior of Endometrial Hyperplasia: A Long-Term Study of "Untreated Hyperplasia" in 170 Patients. *Cancer* 56: 403–412, 1985.

Kurman RJ, Schiffman MH, Lancaster WD, et al: Analysis of Individual Human Papillomavirus Types in Cervical Neoplasia: A Possible Role for Type 18 in Rapid Progression. *Am J Obstet Gynecol* 159: 293–296, 1988.

Kurman RJ, Malkasian GD, Sedlis A, et al: Clinical Commentary: From Papanicolaou to Bethesda: The Rationale for a New Cervical Cytologic Classification. *Obstet Gynecol* 77: 779–782, 1991.

Kurman RJ, et al: Interim Guidelines for Management of Abnormal Cervical Cytology. *JAMA* 271: 1866–1869, 1994.

Kusuyama Y, Yoshida M, Imai H, et al: Secretory Carcinoma of the Endometrium. *Acta Cytol* 33: 127–130, 1989.

Kutteh WH, Hatch KD: Case Report: Primary Vaginal Tuberculosis After Vaginal Carcinoma. *Gynecol Oncol* 44: 113–115, 1992.

Kyle RA, Shampo MA: [Philatelic Vignette] *JAMA* 238: 1636, 1977.

Kyriakos M, Kempson RL, Perez CA: Carcinoma of the Cervix in Young Women: I. Invasive Carcinoma. *Obstet Gynecol* 38: 930–944, 1971.

Lambert PF, Spalholz BA, Howley PM: A Transcriptional Repressor Encoded by BPV-1 Shares a Common Carboxy-Terminal Domain with the E2 Transactivator. *Cell* 50: 69–78, 1987.

Lambourne A, Lederer H: Effects of Observer Variation in Population Screening for Cervical Carcinoma. *J Clin Pathol* 26: 564–569, 1973.

Lancaster WD, Castellano C, Santos C, et al: Human Papillomavirus Deoxyribonucleic Acid in Cervical Carcinoma From Primary and Metastatic Sites. *Am J Obstet Gynecol* 154: 115–119, 1986.

LaPolla JP, O'Neill C, Wetrich D: Colposcopic Management of Abnormal Cervical Cytology in Pregnancy. *J Reprod Med* 33: 301–306, 1988.

Larson DM, Johnson KK, Reyes CN, et al: Prognostic Significance of Malignant Cervical Cytology in Patients With Endometrial Cancer. *Obstet Gynecol* 84: 399–403, 1994.

Larson NS: Invasive Cervical Cancer Rising in Young White Females. *J Natl Cancer Inst* 86: 6–7, 1994.

Larsson G, Alm P, Gullberg B, et al: Prognostic Factors in Early Invasive Carcinoma of the Uterine Cervix: A Clinical, Histopathologic, and Statistical Analysis of 343 Cases. *Am J Obstet Gynecol* 146: 145–153, 1983.

Laskey PW, Meigs JW, Flannery JT: Uterine Cervical Carcinoma in Connecticut, 1935-1973: Evidence for Two Classes of Invasive Disease. *J Natl Cancer Inst* 57: 1037–1043, 1979.

Lauchlan SC, Penner DW: Simultaneous Adenocarcinoma In Situ and Epidermoid Carcinoma In Situ: Report of Two Cases. *Cancer* 20: 2250–2254, 1967.

La Vecchia C, Franceschi S, DeCarli A, et al: Invasive Cervical Cancer in Young Women. *Br J Obstet Gynaecol* 91: 1149–1155, 1984a.

La Vecchia C, Franceschi S, DeCarli A, et al: Dietary Vitamin A and the Risk of Invasive Cervical Cancer. *Int J Cancer* 34: 319–322, 1984b.

La Vecchia C, Franceschi S, DeCarli A, et al: Cigarette Smoking and the Risk of Cervical Neoplasia. *Am J Epidemiol* 123: 22–29, 1986a.

La Vecchia C, Franceschi S, DeCarli A, et al: Sexual Factors, Venereal Diseases, and the Risk of Intraepithelial and Invasive Cervical Neoplasia. *Cancer* 58: 935–941, 1986b.

La Vecchia C, DeCarli A, Gallus G: Epidemiological Data on Cervical Carcinoma Relevant to Cytopathology. *Appl Pathol* 5: 25–32, 1987.

Laverty CR, Russell P, Hills E, et al: The Significance of Noncondylomatous Wart Virus Infection of the Cervical Transformation Zone: A Review With Discussion of Two Illustrative Cases. *Acta Cytol* 22: 195–201, 1978.

Laverty CR, Farnsworth A, Thurloe JK, et al: The Importance of the Cell Sample in Cervical Cytology: A Controlled Trial of a New Sampling Device. *Med J Aust* 150: 432–436, 1989.

Lawley TB, Lee RB, Kapela R: The Significance of Moderate and Severe Inflammation on Class I Papanicolaou Smear. *Obstet Gynecol* 76: 997–999, 1990.

Lawrence WD: Advances in the Pathology of the Uterine Cervix. *Hum Pathol* 22: 792–806, 1991.

Lee KR, Ayer B: False-Positive Diagnosis of Adenocarcinoma In Situ of the Cervix. *Acta Cytol* 32: 276–277, 1988.

Lee KR, Manna EA, Jones MA: Comparative Cytologic Features of Adenocarcinoma In Situ of the Uterine Cervix. *Acta Cytol* 35: 117–126, 1991.

Lee KR: Atypical Glandular Cells in Cervical Smears From Women Who Have Undergone Cone Biopsy. A Potential Diagnostic Pitfall. *Acta Cytol* 37: 705–709, 1993.

Lehn H, Krieg P, Sauer G: Papillomavirus Genomes in Human Cervical Tumors: Analysis of Their Transcriptional Activity. *Proc Natl Acad Sci* 82: 5540–5544, 1985.

Lehn H, Villa LL, Marziona F, et al: Physical State and Biological Activity of Human Papillomavirus Genomes in Precancerous Lesions of the Female Genital Tract. *J Gen Virol* 69: 187–196, 1988.

Lelle RJ, Heidenreich W, Schneider J: Cytologic Findings After Construction of a Neovagina Using Two Surgical Procedures. *Surg Gynecol Obstet* 170: 21–24, 1990.

Leslie KO, Silverberg SG: Microglandular Hyperplasia of the Cervix: Unusual Clinical and Pathological Presentations and Their Differential Diagnosis. *Prog Surg Pathol* 5: 95–114, 1984.

Leung K-M, Chan W-Y, Hui P-K: Invasive Squamous Cell Carcinoma and Cervical Intraepithelial Neoplasia III of the Uterine Cervix. Morphologic Differences Other Than Stromal Invasion. *Am J Clin Pathol* 101: 508–513, 1994.

Levin ML, Kress LC, Goldstein H: Syphilis and Cancer. Reported Syphilis Prevalence Among 7,761 Cancer Patients. *NY State J Med* 42: 1737–1745, 1942.

Levine AJ, Harper J, Hilborne L, et al: HPV DNA and the Risk of Squamous Intraepithelial Lesions of the Uterine Cervix in Young Women. *Am J Clin Pathol* 100: 6–11, 1993.

Ley C, Bauer HM, Reingold A, et al: Determinants of Genital Human Papillomavirus Infection in Young Women. *J Natl Cancer Inst* 83: 997–1003, 1991.

Li J-Y, Li FP, Blot WJ, et al: Correlation Between Cancers of the Uterine Cervix and Penis in China. *J Natl Cancer Inst* 69: 1063–1065, 1982.

Lickrish GM, Colgan TJ, Wright VC: Colposcopy of Adenocarcinoma In Situ and Invasive Adenocarcinoma of the Cervix. *Obstet Gynecol Clin North Am* 20: 111–122, 1993.

Lin TJ, So-Bosita JL: Pitfalls in the Interpretation of Estrogenic Effect in Postmenopausal women. *Am J Obstet Gynecol* 114: 929–931, 1972.

Lindheim SR, Smith-Nguyen G: Aggressive Evaluation for Atypical Squamous Cells in Papanicolaou Smears. *J Reprod Med* 35: 971–973, 1990.

Lindner LE, Geerling S, Nettum JA, et al: The Cytologic Features of Chlamydial Cervicitis. *Acta Cytol* 29: 676–682, 1985.

Liu W, Barrow MJ, Spitler MF, et al: Normal Exfoliation of Endometrial Cells in Premenopausal Women. *Acta Cytol* 7: 211–214, 1963.

Liu W: Positive Smears in Previously Screened Patients (Certain Cytologic Findings of Public Health Importance). *Acta Cytol* 11: 193–198, 1967.

Liu W: Hypoestrogenism and Endometrial Carcinoma. *Acta Cytol* 14: 583–585, 1970.

LiVolsi VA: Cytologic Screening Intervals. *Am J Obstet Gynecol* 148: 833, 1984.

Long SR, Cohen MB: Classics in Cytology: IV. Traut and the "Pap Smear." *Acta Cytol* 35: 140–142, 1991.

Longfield JC, Grimshaw RN, Monaghan JM: Simultaneous Sampling of the Endocervix and Ectocervix Using the Profile Brush. *Acta Cytol* 37: 472–476, 1993.

Lörincz AT, Temple GF, Patterson JA, et al: Correlation of Cellular Atypia and Human Papillomavirus Deoxyribonucleic Acid Sequences in Exfoliated Cells of the Uterine Cervix. *Obstet Gynecol* 68: 508–512, 1986.

Lörincz AT, Temple GF, Kurman RJ, et al: Oncogenic Association of Specific Human Papillomavirus Types With Cervical Neoplasia. *J Natl Cancer Inst* 79: 671–677, 1987a.

Lörincz AT, Quinn AP, Lancaster WD, et al: A New Type of Papillomavirus Associated With Cancer of the Uterine Cervix. *Virology* 159: 187–190, 1987b.

Lörincz AT, Reid R, Jenson AB, et al: Human Papillomavirus Infection of the Cervix: Relative Risk Associations of 15 Common Anogenital Types. *Obstet Gynecol* 79: 328–337, 1992.

Lowry S, Harte R, Atkinson R: Cervical Cancer Deaths in Young Women. *Lancet* (i): 784, 1989.

Lozowski MS, Mishriki Y, Talebian F, et al: The Combined Use of Cytology and Colposcopy in Enhancing Diagnostic Accuracy in Preclinical Lesions of the Uterine Cervix. *Acta Cytol* 26: 285–291, 1982.

Lozowski MS, Mishriki Y, Solitare GB: Factors Determining the Degree of Endometrial Exfoliation and Their Diagnostic Implications in Endometrial Adenocarcinoma. *Acta Cytol* 30: 623–627, 1986.

Luesley D, Blomfield P, Dunn J, et al: Cigarette Smoking and Histological Outcome in Women With Mildly Dyskaryotic Cervical Smears. *Br J Obstet Gynecol* 101: 49–52, 1994.

Luff RD: Benign Cellular Changes: Have We Inadvertently Reinvented the Class II Cytology Sign-Out? *Diagn Cytopathol* 10: 309–310, 1994.

Lundberg GD: Quality Assurance in Cervical Cytology: The Papanicolaou Smear. *JAMA* 262: 1672–1679, 1989.

Lundvall L: Comparison Between Abnormal Cytology, Colposcopy and Histopathology During Pregnancy. *Acta Obstet Gynecol Scand* 68: 447–452, 1989.

Luthy DA, Briggs RM, Buyco A, et al: Cervical Cytology. Increased Sensitivity With a Second Cervical Smear. *Obstet Gynecol* 51: 713–717, 1978.

Lutzner MA: The Human Papillomaviruses: A Review. *Arch Dermatol* 119: 631–635, 1983.

Luzzatto R, Brucker N: Benign Inclusion Cysts of the Ovary Associated With Psammoma Bodies in Vaginal Smears. *Acta Cytol* 25: 282–284, 1981.

Lyall H, Duncan ID: Inaccuracy of Cytologic Diagnosis of High Grade Squamous Intraepithelial Lesions (CIN 3). *Acta Cytol* 39: 50–54, 1995.

Macgregor JE, Teper S: Uterine Cervical Cytology and Young Women. *Lancet* (i): 1029–1031, 1978.

Macgregor JE: Rapid Onset Cancer of the Cervix. *Br Med J* 284: 441, 1982.

Macgregor JE: False Negative Cervical Smears. *Br J Obstet and Gynaecol* 100: 801–802, 1993.

MacMahon B: Risk Factors for Endometrial Cancer. *Gynecol Oncol* 2: 122–129, 1974.

Maguire NC: Current Use of the Papanicolaou Class System in Gynecologic Cytology. *Diagn Cytopathol* 4: 169–176, 1988.

Maier RC, Norris HJ: Coexistence of Cervical Intraepithelial Neoplasia With Primary Adenocarcinoma of the Endocervix. *Obstet Gynecol* 56: 361–364, 1980.

Maier RC, Schultenover SJ: Evaluation of the Atypical Squamous Cell Papanicolaou Smear. *Int J Gynecol Pathol* 5: 242–248, 1986.

Maiman M, Fruchter RG, Serur E, et al: Human Immunodeficiency Virus Infection and Cervical Neoplasia. *Gynecol Oncol* 38: 377–382, 1990.

Maiman M, Tarricone N, Vieira J, et al: Colposcopic Evaluation of Human Immunodeficiency Virus-Seropositive Women. *Obstet Gynecol* 78: 84–88, 1991.

Mandelblatt J, Richart R, Thomas L, et al: Is Human Papillomavirus Associated With Cervical Neoplasia in the Elderly? *Gynecol Oncol* 46: 6–12, 1992.

Martin CE: II. Marital and Coital Factors in Cervical Cancer. *Am J Public Health* 57: 803–814, 1967.

Martin HE, Ellis EB: Biopsy by Needle Puncture and Aspiration. *Ann Surg* 92: 169–181, 1930.

Martin PL: How Preventable Is Invasive Cervical Cancer? A Community Study of Preventable Factors. *Am J Obstet Gynecol* 113: 541–548, 1972.

Marx JL: The Annual Pap Smear: An Idea Whose Time Has Gone? *Science* 205: 177–178, 1979.

Massoni EA, Hajdu SI: Cytology of Primary and Metastatic Uterine Sarcomas. *Acta Cytol* 28: 93–100, 1984.

Mauney M, Eide D, Sotham J: Rates of Condyloma and Dysplasia in Papanicolaou Smears With and Without Endocervical Cells. *Diagn Cytopathol* 6: 18–21, 1990.

Mayelo V, Garaud P, Renjard L, et al: Cell Abnormalities Associated With Human Papillomavirus-Induced Squamous Intraepithelial Cervical Lesions. Multivariate Data Analysis. *Am J Clin Pathol* 101: 13–18, 1994.

Mayer EG, Galindo J, Davis J, et al: Adenocarcinoma of the Uterine Cervix: Incidence and the Role of Radiation Therapy. *Radiology* 121: 725–729, 1976.

Mazur MT, Cloud GA: The Koilocyte and Cervical Intraepithelial Neoplasia: Time-Trend Analysis of a Recent Decade. *Am J Obstet Gynecol* 150: 354–358, 1984.

McCoy JP Jr, Haines HG: The Antigenicity and Immunology of Human Cervical Squamous Cell Carcinoma: A Review. *Am J Obstet Gynecol* 140: 329–336, 1981.

McDonnell JM, Mylotte MJ, Gustafson RC: Colposcopy in Pregnancy. A Twelve Year Review. *Br J Obstet Gynaecol* 88: 414–420, 1981.

McGill F, Adachi A, Karimi N, et al: Abnormal Cervical Cytology Leading to the Diagnosis of Gastric Cancer. *Gynecol Oncol* 36: 101–105, 1990.

McGowan L: Cytologic Methods for the Detection of Endometrial Cancer. *Gynecol Oncol* 2: 272–278, 1974.

McIndoe WA, McLean MR, Jones RW, et al: The Invasive Potential of Carcinoma In Situ of the Cervix. *Obstet Gynecol* 64: 451–458, 1984.

McKay DG, Terjanian B, Poschyachinda D, et al: Clinical and Pathologic Significance of Anaplasia (Atypical Hyperplasia) of the Cervix Uteri. *Obstet Gynecol* 13: 2–21, 1959.

McLachlan N, Patwardhan JR, Ayer B, et al: Management of Suboptimal Cytologic Smears. Persistent Inflammatory Atypia. *Acta Cytol* 38: 531–536, 1994.

Meanwell CA, Blackledge G, Cox MF, Maitland NJ: HPV 16 DNA in Normal and Malignant Cervical Epithelium: Implications for the Aetiology and Behaviour of Cervical Neoplasia. *Lancet* 1: 703–707, 1987.

Meanwell CA, Kelly KA, Wilson S, et al: Young Age as a Prognostic Factor in Cervical Cancer: Analysis of Population Based Data From 10022 Cases. *Br Med J* 296: 386–391, 1988.

Meisels A: The Menopause: A Cytohormonal Study. *Acta Cytol* 10: 49–55, 1966a.

Meisels A: Hormonal Cytology During Pregnancy. *Acta Cytol* 10: 376–382, 1966b.

Meisels A: Hormonal Cytology of Pregnancy. *Clin Obstet Gynecol* 11: 1121–1142, 1968.

Meisels A, Fortin R: Condylomatous Lesions of the Cervix and Vagina I. Cytologic Patterns. *Acta Cytol* 20: 505–509, 1976a.

Meisels A, Ayotte D: Cells From the Seminal Vesicles: Contaminants of the V-C-E- Smear. *Acta Cytol* 20: 211–219, 1976b.

Meisels A, Bégun R, Schneider V: Dysplasias of Uterine Cervix Epidemiological Aspects: Role of Age at First Coitus and Use of Oral Contraceptives. *Cancer* 40: 3076–3081, 1977a.

Meisels A, Fortin R, Roy M: Condylomatous Lesions of the Cervix II. Cytologic, Colposcopic and Histopathologic Study. *Acta Cytol* 21: 379–390, 1977b.

Meisels A, Morin C: Human Papillomavirus and Cancer of the Uterine Cervix. *Gynecol Oncol* 12: S111–S123, 1981a.

Meisels A, Roy M, Fortier M, et al: Human Papillomavirus Infection of the Cervix: The Atypical Condyloma. *Acta Cytol* 25: 7–16, 1981b.

Meisels A: The Story of a Cell: The George N. Papanicolaou Award Lecture. *Acta Cytol* 27: 584–596, 1983.

Meisels A: Cytologic Diagnosis of Human Papillomavirus. Influence of Age and Pregnancy Stage. *Acta Cytol* 36: 480–482, 1992.

Melamed MR, Flehinger BJ: Non-Diagnostic Squamous Atypia in Cervico-Vaginal Cytology as a Risk Factor for Early Neoplasia. *Acta Cytol* 20: 108–110, 1976.

Melkert PWJ, Hopman E, van den Brule AJC, et al: Prevalence of HPV in Cytomorphologically Normal Cervical Smears, as Determined by the Polymerase Chain Reaction, Is Age Dependent. *Int J Cancer* 53: 919–923, 1993.

Mettlin C, Dodd GD: The American Cancer Society Guidelines for the Cancer-Related Checkup: An Update. *CA Cancer J Clin* 41: 279–282, 1991.

Miller BE, Flax SD, Arheart K, et al: The Presentation of Adenocarcinoma of the Uterine Cervix. *Cancer* 72: 1281–1285, 1993.

Miller LG, Goldstein G, Murphy M, et al: Reversible Alterations in Immunoregulatory T Cells in Smoking: Analysis by Monoclonal Antibodies and Flow Cytometry. *Chest* 82: 526–529, 1982.

Minassian H, Schinella R, Reilly JC: Crystalline Bodies in Cervical Smears: Clinicopathologic Correlation. *Acta Cytol* 37: 149–152, 1993.

Misra JS, Engineer AD, Das K, et al: Cervical Carcinogenesis and Contraception. *Diagn Cytopathol* 7: 346–352, 1991.

Mitao M, Nagai N, Levine RU, et al: Human Papillomavirus Type 16 Infection: A Morphological Spectrum With Evidence for Late Gene Expression. *Int J Gynecol Pathol* 5: 287–296, 1986.

Mitchell H, Drake M, Medley G: Prospective Evaluation of Risk of Cervical Cancer After Cytological Evidence of Human Papillomavirus Infection. *Lancet* (i): 573–575, 1986.

Mitchell H, Medley G, Drake M: Quality Control Measures for Cervical Cytology Laboratories. *Acta Cytol* 32: 288–292, 1988.

Mitchell H, Medley G: Age and Time Trends in the Prevalence of Cervical Intraepithelial Neoplasia on Papanicolaou Smear Tests, 1970-1988. *Med J Aust* 152: 252–255, 1990a.

Mitchell H, Medley G, Giles G: Cervical Cancers Diagnosed After Negative Results on Cervical Cytology in the 1980s. *BMJ* 300: 1622–1626, 1990b.

Mitchell H, Medley G: Longitudinal Study of Women With Negative Cervical Smears According to Endocervical Status. *Lancet* 337: 265–267, 1991.

Mitchell H, Medley G: Influence 6f Endocervical Status on the Cytologic Prediction of Cervical Intraepithelial Neoplasia. *Acta Cytol* 36: 875–880, 1992.

Mitchell H, Giles G, Medley G: Accuracy and Survival Benefit of Cytological Prediction of Endometrial Carcinoma on Routine Cervical Smears. *Int J Gynecol Pathol* 12: 34–40, 1993a.

Mitchell H: Improving Consistency in Cervical Cytology Reporting. *J Natl Cancer Inst* 85: 1592–1596, 1993b.

Mitchell H: Consistency of Reporting Endocervical Cells. An Intralaboratory and Interlaboratory Assessment. *Acta Cytol* 38: 310–314, 1994.

Mitrani-Rosenbaum S, Tsvieli R, Tur-Kaspa R: Oestrogen Stimulates Differential Transcription of Human Papillomavirus Type 16 in SiHa Cervical Carcinoma Cells. *J Gen Virol* 70: 2227–2232, 1989.

Mobiüs G: Cytological Early Detection of Cervical Carcinoma: Possibilities and Limitations. Analysis of Failures. *J Cancer Res Clin Oncol* 119: 513–521, 1993.

Montanari GD, Marconato A, Montanari GR, et al: Granulation Tissue on the Vault of the Vagina After Hysterectomy for Cancer: Diagnostic Problems. *Acta Cytol* 12: 25–29, 1968.

Montz FJ, Monk BJ, Fowler JM, et al: Natural History of the Minimally Abnormal Papanicolaou Smear. *Obstet Gynecol* 80: 385–388, 1992.

Morell ND, Taylor JR, Snyder RN, et al: False-Negative Cytology Rates in Patients in Whom Invasive Cervical Cancer Subsequently Developed. *Obstet Gynecol* 60: 41–45, 1982.

Morrison BW, Erickson ER, Doshi N, et al: The Significance of Atypical Cervical Smears. *J Reprod Med* 33: 809–812, 1988.

Moscicki A-B, Palefsky JM, Gonzales J, et al: The Association Between Human Papillomavirus Deoxyribonucleic Acid Status and the Results of Cytologic Rescreening Tests in Young, Sexually Active Women. *Am J Obstet Gynecol* 165: 67–71, 1991.

Mudge TJ, Johnson J, MacFarlane A: Primary Malignant Melanoma of the Cervix: A Case Report. *Br J Obstet Gynaecol* 88: 1257–1259, 1981.

Mulford D, Rutkowski M, Sickel J: Unusual Cytologic Manifestations in Human Immunodeficiency Virus-Infected Patients: A Pot-Pourri of Cases. *Acta Cytol* 35: 630, 1991.

Mulvany NJ, Khan A, Ostor A: Arias-Stella Reaction Associated With Cervical Pregnancy. Report of a Case With a Cytologic Presentation. *Acta Cytol* 38: 218–222, 1994.

Münger K, Werness BA, Dyson N, et al: Complex Formation of Human Papillomavirus E7 Proteins With the Retinoblastoma Tumor Suppressor Gene Product. *EMBO J* 8: 4099–4105, 1989.

Munkarah A, Malone JM Jr, Budev HD, et al: Mucinous Adenocarcinoma Arising in a Neovagina. *Gynecol Oncol* 52: 272–275, 1994.

Muñoz N, Bosch X, Kaldor JM: Does Human Papillomavirus Cause Cervical Cancer? The State of the Epidemiological Evidence. *Br J Cancer* 57: 1–5, 1988.

Muñoz N, Bosch FX, de Sanjose S, et al: The Role of HPV in the Etiology of Cervical Cancer. *Mutation Research* 305: 293–301, 1994.

Murad TM, Terhart K, Flint A: Atypical Cells in Pregnancy and Postpartum Smears. *Acta Cytol* 25: 623–630, 1981.

Murad TM, August C: Radiation-Induced Atypia: A Review. *Diagn Cytopathol* 1: 137–152, 1985.

Murdoch JB, Cassidy LJ, Fletcher K, et al: Histological and Cytological Evidence of Viral Infection and Human Papillomavirus Type 16 DNA Sequences in Cervical Intraepithelial Neoplasia and Normal Tissue in the West of Scotland: Evaluation of Treatment Policy. *Br Med J* 296: 381–385, 1988.

Nagai N, Nuovo G, Friedman D, et al: Review Article: Detection of Papillomavirus Nucleic Acids in Genital Precancers With the In Situ Hybridization Technique. *Int J Gynecol Pathol* 6: 366–379, 1987.

Naib ZM: Single Trophoblastic Cells as a Source of Error in the Interpretation of Routine Vaginal Smears. *Cancer* 14: 1183–1185, 1961.

Naib ZM: Exfoliative Cytology of Viral Cervico-Vaginitis. *Acta Cytol* 10: 126–129, 1966.

Nasca PC, Ellish N, Caputo TA, et al: An Epidemiologic Study of Pap Screening Histories in Women With Invasive Carcinomas of the Uterine Cervix. *N Y State J Med* 91: 152–156, 1991.

Nash JD, Burke TW, Hoskins WJ: Biologic Course of Cervical Human Papillomavirus Infection. *Obstet Gynecol* 69: 160–162, 1987.

Nasiell K, Nasiell M, Vaclavinkova: Behavior of Moderate Cervical Dysplasia During Long-Term Follow-up. *Obstet Gynecol* 61: 609–614, 1983.

Nasiell K, Roger V, Nasiell M: Behavior of Mild Cervical Dysplasia During Long-Term Follow-up. *Obstet Gynecol* 67: 665–669, 1986.

Nasu I, Meurer W, Fu YS: Endocervical Glandular Atypia and Adenocarcinoma: A Correlation of Cytology and Histology. *Int J Gynecol Pathol* 12: 208–218, 1993.

National Cancer Institute: The 1988 Bethesda System for Reporting Cervical/Vaginal Cytologic Diagnoses. *Acta Cytol* 33: 567–574, 1989a.

National Cancer Institute: The 1988 Bethesda System for Reporting Cervical/Vaginal Cytologic Diagnoses. *Diagn Cytopathol* 5: 331–334, 1989b.

National Cancer Institute: The 1988 Bethesda System for Reporting Cervical/Vaginal Cytological Diagnoses. *JAMA* 262: 931–934, 1989c.

National Cancer Institute: The Revised Bethesda System for Reporting Cervical/Vaginal Cytologic Diagnoses: Report of the 1991 Bethesda Workshop. *Acta Cytol* 36: 273–276, 1992.

National Cancer Institute: The Bethesda System for Reporting Cervical/Vaginal Cytologic Diagnoses. *Acta Cytol* 37: 115–124, 1993a.

National Cancer Institute: The Bethesda System for Reporting Cervical/Vaginal Cytologic Diagnoses. *Diagn Cytopathol* 9: 235–243, 1993b.

Nauth HF, Boon ME: Significance of the Morphology of Anucleated Squames in the Cytologic Diagnosis of Vulvar Lesions. A New Approach in Diagnostic Cytology. *Acta Cytol* 27: 230–236, 1983.

Navab A, Koss LG, LaDue JS: Estrogen-like Activity of Digitalis: Its Effect on the Squamous Epithelium of the Female Genital Tract. *JAMA* 194: 142–144, 1965.

NCHS: National Center for Health Statistics. National Health Interview Survey: United States 1987. *Vital Health Statistics* 10: 118, 1987.

Nelson JH Jr, Averette HE, Richart RM: Cervical Intraepithelial Neoplasia (Dysplasia and Carcinoma In Situ) and Early Invasive Cervical Carcinoma. *CA Cancer J Clin* 39: 157–178, 1989.

Ng ABP, Reagan JW: Microinvasive Carcinoma of the Uterine Cervix. *Am J Clin Pathol* 52: 511–529, 1969.

Ng ABP, Reagan JW, Lindner EA: The Cellular Manifestations of Primary and Recurrent Herpes Genitalis. *Acta Cytol* 14: 124–129, 1970.

Ng ABP, Reagan JW, Lindner EA: The Cellular Manifestation of Microinvasive Squamous Cell Carcinoma of the Uterine Cervix. *Acta Cytol* 16: 5–13, 1972.

Ng ABP, Reagan JW, Cechner RL: The Precursors of Endometrial Cancer: A Study of Their Cellular Manifestations. *Acta Cytol* 17: 439–448, 1973.

Ng ABP: The Cellular Detection of Endometrial Carcinoma and Its Precursors. *Gynecol Oncol* 2: 162–179, 1974a.

Ng ABP, Reagan JW, Hawliczek S, Wentz BW: Significance of Endometrial Cells in the Detection of Endometrial Carcinoma and Its Precursors. *Acta Cytol* 18: 356–361, 1974b.

Ng ABP, Teeple D, Linder EA, et al: The Cellular Manifestations of Extrauterine Cancer. *Acta Cytol* 18: 108–117, 1974c.

Nguyen G-K: Exfoliative Cytology of Microinvasive Squamous-Cell Carcinoma of the Uterine Cervix: A Retrospective Study of 42 Cases. *Acta Cytol* 28: 457–460, 1984a.

Nguyen G-K, Jeannot AB: Exfoliative Cytology of In Situ and Microinvasive Adenocarcinoma of the Uterine Cervix. *Acta Cytol* 28: 461–467, 1984b.

Nguyen G-K, Daya DE: Cervical Adenocarcinoma and Related Lesions. Cytodiagnostic Criteria and Pitfalls. *Pathol Annu* 28(2):53–75, 1993.

Nichols TM, Boyes DA, Fidler HK: Advantages of Routine Step Serial Sectioning of Cervical Cone Biopsies. *Am J Clin Pathol* 49: 342–346, 1968.

Nichols TM, Fidler HK: Microglandular Hyperplasia in Cervical Cone Biopsies Taken for Suspicious and Positive Cytology. *Am J Clin Pathol* 56: 424–429, 1971.

Nielsen AL: Human Papillomavirus Type 16/18 in Uterine Cervical Adenocarcinoma In Situ and Adenocarcinoma: A Study by In Situ Hybridization With Biotinylated DNA Probes. *Cancer* 65: 2588–2593, 1990.

Nielsen ML, Davey DD, Kline TS: Specimen Adequacy Evaluation in Gynecologic Cytopathology: Current Laboratory Practice in the College of American Pathologists Interlaboratory Comparison Program and Tentative Guidelines for Future Practice. *Diagn Cytopathol* 9: 394–403, 1993.

Noller KL, O'Brien PC, Melton LJ III, et al: Coital Risk Factors for Cervical Cancer: Sexual Activity Among White Middle Class Women. *Am J Clin Oncol* 10: 222–226, 1987.

Noumoff JS: Atypia in Cervical Cytology as a Risk Factor for Intraepithelial Neoplasia. *Am J Obstet Gynecol* 156: 628–631, 1987.

Novak PM, Kumar NB, Naylor B: Curschmann's Spirals in Cervicovaginal Smears: Prevalence, Morphology, Significance and Origin. *Acta Cytol* 28: 5–8, 1984.

Novotny DB, Maygarden SJ, Johnson DE, et al: Tubal Metaplasia: A Frequent Potential Pitfall in the Cytologic Diagnosis of Endocervical Glandular Dysplasia on Cervical Smears. *Acta Cytol* 36: 1–10, 1992.

Nunez C, Abdul-Karim FW, Somrak TM: Glassy-Cell Carcinoma of the Cervix: Cytopathologic and Histopathologic Study of Five Cases. *Acta Cytol* 29: 303–309, 1985.

Nuovo GJ, Walsh LL, Gentile JL, et al: Correlation of the Papanicolaou Smear and Human Papillomavirus Type in Women with Biopsy-Proven Cervical Squamous Intraepithelial Lesions. *Am J Clin Pathol* 96: 544–548, 1991.

Nyirjesy I: Atypical or Suspicious Cervical Smears: An Aggressive Diagnostic Approach. *JAMA* 222: 691–693, 1972.

Okagaki T, Lerch V, Younge PA, et al: Diagnosis of Anaplasia and Carcinoma In Situ by Differential Cell Counts. *Acta Cytol* 6: 343–347, 1962.

Okagaki T, Meyer AA, Sciarra JJ: Prognosis of Irradiated Carcinoma of Cervix Uteri and Nuclear DNA in Cytologic Postirradiation Dysplasia. *Cancer* 33: 647–652, 1974.

Okagaki TR, Tase T, Twiggs LB, et al: Histogenesis of Cervical Adenocarcinoma With Reference to Human Papillomavirus-18 as a Carcinogen. *J Reprod Med* 34: 639–644, 1989.

Okagaki T: Impact of Human Papillomavirus Research on the Histopathologic Concepts of Genital Neoplasms. *Curr Topics Pathol* 85: 273–307, 1992.

Oriel JD: Natural History of Genital Warts. *Br J Vener Dis* 47: 1–13, 1971.

Orr JW Jr, Barrett JM, Orr PF, et al: The Efficacy and Safety of the Cytobrush During Pregnancy. *Gynecol Oncol* 44: 260–262, 1992.

Ortner A, Klammer J, Geir W: Cytology at the End of Pregnancy: Significance of Determinations of the Eosinophilic and Karyopyknotic Indices. *Acta Cytol* 21: 429–431, 1977.

Ostor AG: Natural History of Cervical Intraepithelial Neoplasia: A Critical Review. *Int J Gynecol Pathol* 12: 186– 192, 1993a.

Ostor AG: Studies on 200 Cases of Early Squamous Cell Carcinoma of the Cervix. *Int J Gynecol Pathol* 12: 193–207, 1993b.

Ouwerkerk-Noordam E, Boon ME, Beck S: Computer-Assisted Primary Screening of Cervical Smears Using the PAPNET Method: Comparison With Conventional Screening and Evaluation of the Role of the Cytologist. *Cytopathology* 5: 211–218, 1994.

Paavonen J, Kiviat NB, Wölner-Hanssen P, et al: Significance of Mild Cervical Cytologic Atypia in a Sexually Transmitted Disease Clinic Population. *Acta Cytol* 33: 831–838, 1989.

Pacey F, Ayer B, Greenberg M: The Cytologic Diagnosis of Adenocarcinoma In Situ of the Cervix Uteri and Related Lesions: III. Pitfalls in Diagnosis. *Acta Cytol* 33: 325–330, 1988a.

Pacey F: The Histologic Diagnosis of Adenocarcinoma In Situ and Related Lesions of the Cervix Uteri: Adenocarcinoma In Situ. *Cancer* 61: 1171–1181, 1988b.

Pairwuti S: False Negative Papanicolaou Smears From Women With Cancerous and Precancerous Lesions of the Uterine Cervix. *Acta Cytol* 35: 40–46, 1991.

Pak HY, Yokota SB, Paladugu, et al: Glassy Cell Carcinoma of the Cervix: Cytologic and Clinicopathologic Analysis. *Cancer* 52: 307–312, 1983.

Pandit AA, Klhilnani PH, Powar HS, et al: Value of Papanicolaou Smear in Detection of *Chlamydia trachomatis* Infection. *Diagn Cytopathol* 9: 164–167, 1993.

Papanicolaou GN: New Cancer Diagnosis. *Proceedings of the Third Race Betterment Conference.* pp 528–534. Battle Creek, Michigan, 1928.

Papanicolaou GN, Traut HF: The Diagnostic Value of Vaginal Smears in Carcinoma of the Uterus. *Am J Obstet Gynecol* 42: 193–206, 1941.

Papanicolaou GN, Traut HF: *Diagnosis of Uterine Cancer by the Vaginal Smear.* New York. The Commonwealth Fund, 1943.

Papanicolaou GN: A General Survey of the Vaginal Smear and Its Use in Research and Diagnosis. *Am J Obstet Gynecol* 51: 316–328, 1946.

Papanicolaou GN: Observations on the Origin and Specific Function of the Histiocytes in the Female Genital Tract. *Fertil Steril* 4: 472–478, 1953.

Papanicolaou G: *Atlas of Exfoliative Cytology*. The Commonwealth Fund by Harvard University Press, Cambridge, MA 1954.

Paraskevaidis E, Kitchener HC, Miller ID, et al: A Population-Based Study of Microinvasive Disease of the Cervix—A Colposcopic and Cytologic Analysis. *Gynecol Oncol* 45: 9–12, 1992.

Parazzini F, La Vecchia C: Epidemiology of Adenocarcinoma of the Cervix. *Gynecol Oncol* 39: 40–46, 1990.

Park JS, Namkoong SE, Lee HY, et al: Detection of Human Papillomavirus Genotypes in Cervical Neoplasia from Korean Women Using Polymerase Chain Reaction. *Gynecol Oncol* 41: 129–134, 1991.

Parkin DM, Läärä E, Muir CS: Estimates of the Worldwide Frequency of Sixteen Major Cancers in 1980. *Int J Cancer* 41: 184–197, 1988.

Parsons WL, Godwin M, Robbins C, et al: Prevalence of Cervical Pathogens in Women With and Without Inflammatory Changes on Smear Testing. *BMJ* 306: 1173–1174, 1993.

Pasetto N, Sesti F, De Santis L, et al: The Prevalence of HPV16 DNA in Normal and Pathological Cervical Scrapes Using the Polymerase Chain Reaction. *Gynecol Oncol* 46: 33–36, 1992.

Pater MM, Hughes GA, Hyslop DE, et al: Glucocorticoid-Dependent Oncogenic Transformation by Type 16 but not Type 11 Human Papilloma Virus DNA. *Nature* 335: 832–835, 1988.

Paterson MEL, Peel KR, Joslin CAF: Cervical Smear Histories of 500 Women With Invasive Cervical Cancer in Yorkshire. *Br Med J* 289: 896–898, 1984.

Patten SF Jr, Reagan JW, Obenauf M, et al: Postirradiation Dysplasia of Uterine Cervix and Vagina: An Analytical Study of the Cells. *Cancer* 16: 173–182, 1963.

Patten SF Jr: *Diagnostic Cytopathology of the Uterine Cervix*. 2nd, revised edition. *Monographs in Clinical Cytology*, Vol 3, Edited by GL Wied. Basel, S. Karger, 1978.

Paul C: The New Zealand Cervical Cancer Study: Could It Happen Again? *BMJ* 297: 533–539, 1988.

Pearlstone AC, Grigsby PW, Mutch DG: High Rates of Atypical Cervical Cytology: Occurrence and Clinical Significance. *Obstet Gynecol* 80: 191–195, 1992.

Pedersen E, Hoeg K, Kolstad P: Mass Screening for Cancer of the Uterine Cervix in Ostfold County, Norway: An Experiment—Second Report of the Norwegian Cancer Society. *Acta Obstet Gynecol Scand* 11 (Suppl): 5–18, 1971.

Peters AAW, Trimbos JB: The Absence of Human Papilloma Virus (HPV) Related Parameters in Sexually Non-Active Women. *Eur J Gynaecol Oncol* 15: 43–45, 1994.

Peters RK, Chao A, Mack TM, et al: Increased Frequency of Adenocarcinoma of the Uterine Cervix in Young Women in Los Angeles County. *J Natl Clin Inst* 76: 423–428, 1986.

Peters RK, Thomas D, Skultin G, et al: Invasive Squamous Cell Carcinoma of the Cervix After Recent Negative Cytologic Test Results—A Distinct Subgroup? *Am J Obstet Gynecol* 158: 926–935, 1988.

Petersen O: Precancerous Changes of the Cervical Epithelium in Relation to Manifest Cervical Carcinoma. Clinical and Histological Aspects. *Acta Radiol* 127(Suppl): 1–163, 1955.

Petrucco OM, Seamark RF, Holmes K, et al: Changes in Lymphocyte Function During Pregnancy. *Br J Obstet Gynaecol* 83: 245–250, 1976.

Petry KU, Scheffel D, Bode U, et al: Cellular Immunodeficiency Enhances the Progression of Human Papillomavirus-Associated Cervical Lesions. *Int J Cancer* 57: 836–840, 1994.

Phelps WC, Yee CL, Münger K, et al: The Human Papillomavirus Type 16 E7 Gene Encodes Transactivation and Transformation Functions Similar to Those of Adenovirus E1A. *Cell* 53: 539–547, 1988.

Phillips B, Marshall ME, Brown S, et al: Effect of Smoking on Human Natural Killer Cell Activity. *Cancer* 56: 2789–2792, 1985.

Picoff RC, Meeker CI: Psammoma Bodies in the Cervicovaginal Smear in Association With Benign Papillary Structures of the Ovary. *Acta Cytol* 14: 45–47, 1970.

Pisani P, Parkin DM, Ferlay J: Estimates of the Worldwide Mortality From Eighteen Major Cancers in 1985. Implications for Prevention and Projections of Future Burden. *Int J Cancer* 55: 89–903, 1993.

Plott AE, Martin FJ, Cheek SW, et al: Measuring Screening Skills in Gynecologic Cytology. Results of Voluntary Self-Assessment. *Acta Cytol* 31: 911–923, 1987.

Podczaski E, Abt A, Kaminski P, et al: Case Report: A Patient With Multiple Malignant Melanomas of the Lower Genital Tract. *Gynecol Oncol* 37: 422–426, 1990.

Pollack RS, Taylor HC Jr: Carcinoma of the Cervix During the First Two Decades of Life. *Am J Obstet Gynecol* 53: 135–141, 1947.

Porreco R, Penn I, Droegemueller W, et al: Gynecologic Malignancies in Immunosuppressed Organ Homograft Recipients. *Obstet Gynecol* 45: 339–364, 1975.

Powers CN, Stastny JF, Frable WJ: Adenoid Basal Cell Carcinoma of the Cervix: A Potential Pitfall in Cervico-Vaginal Cytology (Abstract). *Acta Cytol* 38: 820, 1994.

Prempree T, Patanaphan V, Sewchand W, et al: The Influence of Patients' Age and Tumor Grade on the Prognosis of Carcinoma of the Cervix. *Cancer* 51: 1764–1771, 1983.

Prendiville W, Guillebaud J, Bamford P, et al: Carcinoma of Cervix with Recent Normal Papanicolaou Tests. *Lancet* (ii): 853–854, 1980.

Pretorius R, Semrad N, Watring W, et al: Presentation of Cervical Cancer. *Gynecol Oncol* 42: 48–53, 1991.

Pridan H, Lilienfeld AM: Carcinoma of the Cervix in Jewish Women in Israel, 1960-67: An Epidemiological Study. *Israel J Med Sci* 7: 1465–1470, 1971.

Provencher D, Valme B, Averette HE, et al: HIV Status and Positive Papanicolau [sic] Screening: Identification of a High-Risk Population. *Gynecol Oncol* 31: 184–188, 1988.

Pund ER, Niebrugs HE, Nettles JB, et al: Preinvasive Carcinoma of the Cervix Uteri. Seven Cases in Which It Was Detected by Examination of Routine Endocervical Smears. *Arch Pathol* 44: 571–577, 1947.

Purola E, Savia E: Cytology of Gynecologic Condyloma Acuminatum. *Acta Cytol* 21: 26–31, 1977.

Qizilbash AH: In-Situ and Microinvasive Adenocarcinoma of the Uterine Cervix: A Clinical, Cytologic and Histologic Study of 14 Cases. *Am J Clin Pathol* 64: 155–170, 1975.

Quinn MA: Screening for Cervical Cancer—Where Are We Going Wrong? *Med J Aust* 150: 414–415, 1989.

Quinn TC, Gupta PK, Burkman RT, et al: Detection of *Chlamydia trachomatis* Cervical Infection: A Comparison of Papanicolaou and Immunofluorescent Staining With Cell Culture. *Am J Obstet Gynecol* 157: 394–399, 1987.

Rader JS, Rosenzweig BA, Spirtas R, et al: Atypical Squamous Cells: A Case-Series Study of the Association Between Papanicolaou Smear Results and Human Papillomavirus DNA Genotype. *J Reprod Med* 36: 291–297, 1991.

Rakoff AE: Hormonal Cytology in Gynecology. *Clin Obstet Gynecol* 4: 1045–1061, 1961a.

Rakoff, AE: The Vaginal Cytology of Gynecologic Endocrinopathies. *Acta Cytol* 5: 153–167, 1961b.

Randall B: Persistence of Vaginal Spermatozoa as Assessed by Routine Cervicovaginal (Pap) Smears. *J Forensic Sci* 32: 678–683, 1987.

Rarick TL, Tchabo J-G: Timing of the Postpartum Papanicolaou Smear. *Obstet Gynecol* 83: 761–765, 1994.

Raymond CA: Cervical Dysplasia Upturn Worries Gynecologists, Health Officials. *JAMA* 257: 2397–2398, 1987a.

Raymond CA: For Women Infected With Papillomavirus, Close Watch Counseled. *JAMA* 257: 2398–2399, 1987b.

Rayter Z, Gazet J-C, Trott PA, et al: Gynaecological Cytology and Pelvic Ultrasonography in Patients With Breast Cancer Taking Tamoxifen Compared With Controls. *Eur J Surg Oncol* 20: 134–140, 1994.

Reagan JW, Seidemann IL, Saracusa Y: The Cellular Morphology of Carcinoma In Situ and Dysplasia or Atypical Hyperplasia of the Uterine Cervix. *Cancer* 6: 224–235, 1953.

Reagan JW, Hamonic MJ: Part IV. The Cytology of Early Cancer: Dysplasia of the Uterine Cervix. *Ann NY Acad Sci* 63: 1236–1244, 1956.

Reagan JW, Bell BA, Neuman JL, et al. Dysplasia in the Uterine Cervix During Pregnancy: An Analytical Study of the Cells. *Acta Cytol* 5: 17–29, 1961.

Reagan JW, Patten SF Jr: Dysplasia: A Basic Reaction to Injury in the Uterine Cervix. *Ann NY Acad Sci* 97: 662–682, 1962.

Reagan JW: Presidential Address. *Acta Cytol* 9: 265–267, 1965.

Reagan JW, Wentz WB: Genesis of Carcinoma of the Uterine Cervix. *Clin Obstet Gynecol* 10: 883–921, 1967.

Reagan JW, Ng ABP: *The Cells of Uterine Adenocarcinoma*. 2nd, revised edition. *Monographs in Clinical Cytology*, Vol 1, Edited by GL Wied. Basel, S. Karger, 1973.

Reeves WC, Brinton LA, Brenes MM, et al: Case Control Study of Cervical Cancer in Herrera Province, Republic of Panama. *Int J Cancer* 36: 55–60, 1985.

Reeves WC, Brinton LA, García M, et al: Human Papillomavirus Infection and Cervical Cancer in Latin America. *N Engl J Med* 320: 1437–1441, 1989.

Reid R, Fu YS, Herschman BR, et al: Genital Warts and Cervical Cancer: IV. The Relationship between Aneuploid and Polyploid Cervical Lesions. *Am J Obstet Gynecol* 150: 189–199, 1984.

Reid R, Fu YS: In *Banbury Report 21: Viral Etiology of Cervical Cancer*, Edited by R Peto. Cold Spring Harbor, NY, 1986.

Reid R, Greenberg M, Jenson AB, et al: Sexually Transmitted Papillomaviral Infections: I. The Anatomic Distribution and Pathologic Grade of Neoplastic Lesions Associated With Different Viral Types. *Am J Obstet Gynecol* 156: 212–222, 1987.

Reid R, Campion MJ: HPV-Associated Lesions of the Cervix: Biology and Colposcopic Features. *Clin Obstet Gynecol* 32: 157–179, 1989.

Reissman SE: Comparison of Two Papanicolaou Smear Techniques in a Family Practice Setting. *J Fam Pract* 26: 525– 529, 1988.

Reiter RC: Management of Initial Atypical Cervical Cytology: A Randomized Prospective Study. *Obstet Gynecol* 68: 237–240, 1986.

Rhatigan RM: Endocervical Gland Atypia Secondary to Arias-Stella Change. *Arch Pathol Lab Med* 116: 943–946, 1992.

Richardson AC, Lyon JB: The Effect of Condom Use on Squamous Cell Cervical Intraepithelial Neoplasia. *Am J Obstet Gynecol* 140: 909–913, 1981.

Richart RM: A Radioautographic Analysis of Cellular Proliferation in Dysplasia and Carcinoma In Situ of the Uterine Cervix. *Am J Obstet Gynecol* 86: 925–930, 1963a.

Richart RM: Cervical Neoplasia in Pregnancy. *Am J Obstet Gynecol* 87: 474–477, 1963b.

Richart RM: Evaluation of the True False Negative Rate in Cytology. *Am J Obstet Gynecol* 89: 724–726, 1964a.

Richart RM: The Correlation of Schiller-Positive Areas on the Exposed Portion of the Cervix With Intraepithelial Neoplasia. *Am J Obstet Gynecol* 90: 697–701, 1964b.

Richart RM: Colpomicroscopic Studies of the Distribution of Dysplasia and Carcinoma In Situ on the Exposed Portion of the Human Uterine Cervix. *Cancer* 18: 950–954, 1965a.

Richart RM, Vaillant HW: Influence of Cell Collection Techniques Upon Cytological Diagnosis. *Cancer* 18: 1474–1478, 1965b.

Richart RM: Colpomicroscopic Studies of Cervical Intraepithelial Neoplasia. *Cancer* 19: 395–405, 1966a.

Richart RM: Influence of Diagnostic and Therapeutic Procedures on the Distribution of Cervical Intraepithelial Neoplasia. *Cancer* 19: 1635–1638, 1966b.

Richart RM: Natural History of Cervical Intraepithelial Neoplasia. *Clin Obstet Gynecol* 5: 748–784, 1968.

Richart RM, Barron BA: A Follow-up Study of Patients With Cervical Dysplasia. *Am J Obstet Gynecol* 105: 386–393, 1969.

Richart RM: Cervical Intraepithelial Neoplasia. *Pathol Annu* 8: 301–328, 1973.

Richart RM: Current Concepts in Obstetrics and Gynecology: The Patient With an Abnormal Pap Smear—Screening Techniques and Management. *N Engl J Med* 302: 332–334, 1980.

Richart RM: Screening Strategies for Cervical Cancer and Cervical Intraepithelial Neoplasia. *Cancer* 47: 1176–1181, 1981a.

Richart RM, Crum CP, Townsend DE: Workup of the Patient With an Abnormal Papanicolaou Smear. *Gynecol Oncol* 12: S265–S276, 1981b.

Richart RM: Causes and Management of Cervical Intraepithelial Neoplasia. *Cancer* 60: 1951–1959, 1987.

Richart RM: A Modified Terminology for Cervical Intraepithelial Neoplasia. *Obstet Gynecol* 75: 131–133, 1990.

Richart RM, Wright TC: Controversies in the Management of Low-Grade Cervical Intraepithelial Neoplasia. *Cancer* 71: 1413–1421, 1993.

Ridgley R, Hernandez E, Cruz C, et al: Abnormal Papanicolaou Smears After Earlier Smears With Atypical Squamous Cells. *J Reprod Med* 33: 285–288, 1988.

Riou G, Le MG, Le Doussal V, et al: C-*myc* Proto-Oncogene Expression and Prognosis in Early Carcinoma of the Uterine Cervix. *Lancet* (i): 761–763, 1987.

Ritchie DA: The Vaginal Maturation Index and Endometrial Carcinoma. *Am J Obstet Gynecol* 91: 578–579, 1965.

Ritter DB, Kadish AS, Vermund SH, et al: Detection of Human Papillomavirus Deoxyribonucleic Acid in Exfoliated Cervicovaginal Cells as a Predictor of Cervical Neoplasia in a High-Risk Population. *Am J Obstet Gynecol* 159: 1517–1525, 1988.

Rizzo T, Linker G, Schumann GB: Cytologic Pitfalls Associated With Microglandular Hyperplasia. *Acta Cytol* 33: 738, 1989.

Robb J: The Pap Smear Is a Cancer Screening Test: Why Not Put the Screening Error Rate in the Report? *Diagn Cytopathol* 9: 485–486, 1993.

Robb JA: The "ASCUS" Swamp. *Diagn Cytopathol* 11: 319–320, 1994.

Robboy SJ, Truslow GY, Anton J, et al: Role of Hormones Including Diethylstilbestrol (DES) in the Pathogenesis of Cervical and Vaginal Intraepithelial Neoplasia. *Gynecol Oncol* 12: S98–S110, 1981.

Robboy SJ, Noller KL, O'Brien P, et al: Increased Incidence of Cervical and Vaginal Dysplasia in 3,980 Diethylstilbestrol-Exposed Young Women: Experience of the National Collaborative Diethylstilbestrol Adenosis Project. *JAMA* 252: 2979–2983, 1984.

Robboy SJ, Hill EC, Sandberg EC, et al: Vaginal Adenosis in Women Born Prior to the Diethylstilbestrol Era. *Hum Pathol* 17: 488–492, 1986.

Robert ME, Fu YS: Squamous Cell Carcinoma of the Uterine Cervix—A Review With Emphasis on Prognostic Factors and Unusual Variants. *Semin Diagn Pathol* 7: 173–189, 1990.

Roberts TH, Ng ABP: Chronic Lymphocytic Cervicitis: Cytologic and Histopathologic Manifestations. *Acta Cytol* 19: 235–243, 1975.

Robertson AJ: Histopathological Grading of Cervical Intraepithelial Neoplasia (CIN)—Is There a Need for Change? *J Pathol* 159: 273–275, 1989a.

Robertson AJ, Anderson JM, Beck JS, et al: Observer Variability in Histopathological Reporting of Cervical Biopsy Specimens. *J Clin Pathol* 42: 231–238, 1989b.

Robertson JH, Woodend BE, Hutchinson J: Risk of Cervical Cancer Associated With Mild Dyskaryosis. *Br Med J* 297: 18–21, 1988.

Robertson JH, Woodend B: Negative Cytology Preceding Cervical Cancer: Causes and Prevention. *J Clin Pathol* 46: 700–702, 1993.

Robertson JH, Woodend B, Elliott H: Cytological Changes Preceding Cervical Cancer. *J Clin Pathol* 47: 278–279, 1994.

Rogo KO, Linge K: Human Immunodeficiency Virus Seroprevalence Among Cervical Cancer Patients. *Gynecol Oncol* 37: 87–92, 1990.

Rohr LR: Quality Assurance in Gynecologic Cytology. What Is Practical? *Am J Clin Pathol* 94: 754–758, 1990.

Romney SL, Palan PR, Duttagupta C, et al: Retinoids and the Prevention of Cervical Dysplasias. *Am J Obstet Gynecol* 141: 890–894, 1981.

Romney SL, Duttagupta C, Basu J, et al: Plasma Vitamin C and Uterine Cervical Dysplasia. *Am J Obstet Gynecol* 151: 976–980, 1985.

Roongpisuthipong A, Grimes DA, Hadgu A: Is the Papanicolaou Smear Useful for Diagnosing Sexually Transmitted Diseases? *Obstet Gynecol* 69: 820–824, 1987.

Rosenfeld WD, Vermund SH, Wentz SJ, et al: High Prevalence Rate of Human Papillomavirus Infection and Association With Abnormal Papanicolaou Smears in Sexually Active Adolescents. *Am J Dis Child* 143: 1443–1447, 1989.

Rotkin ID: Relation of Adolescent Coitus to Cervical Cancer Risk. *JAMA* 179: 486–491, 1962.

Rotkin ID: Adolescent Coitus and Cervical Cancer: Associations of Related Events With Increased Risk. *Cancer Res* 27: 603–617, 1967a.

Rotkin ID: III. Sexual Characteristics of a Cervical Cancer Population. *Am J Public Health* 5: 815–829, 1967b.

Rotkin ID, Cameron JR: Clusters of Variables Influencing Risk of Cervical Cancer. *Cancer* 21: 663–671, 1968.

Rotkin ID: A Comparison Review of Key Epidemiological Studies in Cervical Cancer Related to Current Searches for Transmissible Agents. *Cancer Res* 33: 1353–1367, 1973.

Rous P, Beard JW: The Progression to Carcinoma of Virus-Induced Rabbit Papillomas (Shope). *J Exp Med* 62: 523–554, 1935.

Rubin IC: The Pathological Diagnosis of Incipient Carcinoma of the Uterus. *Am J Obstet* 62: 668–676, 1910.

Rubio CA: Prognostic Value of the Karyopyknotic Index in Carcinoma of the Cervix. *Obstet Gynecol* 28: 383–393, 1966.

Rubio CA: The False Positive Smear. *Acta Cytol* 19: 212–213, 1975a.

Rubio CA, Lagerlof B: Who Is Responsible for the False Negative Smear? *Acta Cytol* 19: 319, 1975b.

Rubio CA, Kranz I: The Exfoliating Cervical Epithelial Surface in Dysplasia, Carcinoma In Situ and Invasive Squamous Carcinoma: I. Scanning Electron Microscopic Study. *Acta Cytol* 20: 144–150, 1976.

Rubio CA: The False Negative Smear: II. The Trapping Effect of Collecting Instruments. *Obstet Gynecol* 49: 576–580, 1977a.

Rubio CA, Einhorn N: The Exfoliating Epithelial Surface of the Uterine Cervix: IV. Scanning Electron Microscopical Study in Invasive Squamous Carcinoma of Human Subjects. *Beitr Pathol* 161: 72–81, 1977b.

Rubio CA, Kock Y, Berglund K: Studies of the Distribution of Abnormal Cells in Cytologic Preparations. I. Making the Smear With a Wooden Spatula. *Acta Cytol* 24: 49–53, 1980a.

Rubio CA, Kock Y, Berglund K, et al: Studies on the Distribution of Abnormal Cells in Cytological Preparations. II. Making the Smear With the Cotton Swab. *Gynecol Oncol* 9: 127–134, 1980b.

Rubio CA, Berglund K, Kock Y, et al: Studies on the Distribution of Abnormal Cells in Cytologic Preparations. III. Making the Smear With a Plastic Spatula. *Am J Obstet Gynecol* 137: 843–846, 1980c.

Rubio CA: Cellular Changes Preceding Slight Dysplasia of the Uterine Cervix. *Acta Cytol* 25: 193–194, 1981a.

Rubio CA: False Negatives in Cervical Cytology: Can They Be Avoided? *Acta Cytol* 25: 199–202, 1981b.

Rubio CA, Kock Y: Studies on the Distribution of Abnormal Cells in Cytologic Preparations: V. The Gradient of Cell Deposition on Slides. *Obstet Gynecol* 57: 754–758, 1981c.

Rubio CA, Stormby N, Kock Y, et al: Studies on the Distribution of Abnormal Cells in Cytologic Preparations: VI. Pressure Exerted by the Gynecologist While Smearing. *Gynecol Oncol* 15: 391–395, 1983.

Rubio CA: Review of Negative Papanicolaou Tests: Is the Retrospective 5-Year Review Necessary? *Am J Clin Pathol* 102: 266, 1994.

Rutledge CE, Christopherson WM, Parker JE: Cervical Dysplasia and Carcinoma in Pregnancy. *Obstet Gynecol* 19: 351–354, 1962.

Rylander E: Cervical Cancer in Women Belonging to a Cytologically Screened Population. *Acta Obstet Gynecol Scand* 55: 361–366, 1976.

Rylander E: Negative Smears in Women Developing Invasive Cervical Cancer. *Acta Obstet Gynecol Scand* 56: 115–118, 1977.

Sadeghi SB, Hsieh EW, Gunn SW: Prevalence of Cervical Intraepithelial Neoplasia in Sexually Active Teenagers and Young Adults: Results of Data Analysis of Mass Papanicolaou Screening of 796,337 Women in the United States in 1981. *Am J Obstet Gynecol* 148: 726–729, 1984.

Sadeghi SB, Sadeghi A, Robboy SJ: Prevalence of Dysplasia and Cancer of the Cervix in a Nationwide, Planned Parenthood Population. *Cancer* 61: 2359–2361, 1988.

Sadeghi SB, Sadeghi A, Cosby M, et al: Human Papillomavirus Infection: Frequency and Association With Cervical Neoplasia in a Young Population. *Acta Cytol* 33: 319–323, 1989.

Saigo PE: Cytology of Condyloma of the Uterine Cervix. *Semin Diagn Pathol* 3: 204–210, 1986.

Saito K, Saito A, Fu YS, et al: Topographic Study of Cervical Condyloma and Intraepithelial Neoplasia. *Cancer* 59: 2064–2070, 1987.

Saminathan T, Lahoti C, Kannan V, et al: Postmenopausal Squamous-Cell Atypias: A Diagnostic Challenge. *Diagn Cytopathol* 11: 226–230, 1994.

Sand PK, Bowen LW, Blischke SO, Ostergard DR: Evaluation of Male Consorts of Women With Genital Human Papilloma Virus Infection. *Obstet Gynecol* 68: 679–681, 1986.

Sandmire HF, Austin SD, Bechtel RC: Experience with 40,000 Papanicolaou Smears. *Obstet Gynecol* 48: 56–60, 1976.

Sasson IM, Haley NJ, Hoffmann D, et al: Cigarette Smoking and Neoplasia of the Uterine Cervix: Smoke Constituents in Cervical Mucus. *N Engl J Med* 312: 315–316, 1985.

Sato S, Okagaki T, Clark BA, et al: Sensitivity of Koilocytosis, Immunocytochemistry, and Electron Microscopy as Compared to DNA Hybridization in Detecting Human Papillomavirus in Cervical and Vaginal Condyloma and Intraepithelial Neoplasia. *Int J Gynecol Pathol* 5: 297–307, 1987.

Schiffman MH, Bauer HM, Lorincz AT, et al: Comparison of Southern Blot Hybridization and Polymerase Chain Reaction Methods for the Detection of Human Papillomavirus DNA. *J Clin Microbiol* 29: 573–577, 1991.

Schiffman MH, Bauer HM, Hoover RN, et al: Epidemiologic Evidence Showing That Human Papillomavirus Infection Causes Most Cervical Intraepithelial Neoplasia. *J Natl Cancer Inst* 85: 958–964, 1993.

Schiller W: Leucoplakia, Leucokeratosis, and Carcinoma of the Cervix. *Am J Obstet Gynecol* 35: 17–38, 1938.

Schlaen I, Gonzalez Garcia MR, Weismann EA: Predictive Value of Phenotypic Cytologic Characteristics in Early Dysplastic Cervical Lesions. *Acta Cytol* 32: 298–302, 1988.

Schnadig VJ, Davie KD, Shafer SK, et al: The Cytologist and Bacterioses of the Vaginal-Ectocervical Area: Clues, Commas and Confusion. *Acta Cytol* 33: 287–297, 1989.

Schneider A, Hotz M, Gissmann L: Increased Prevalence of Human Papillomaviruses in the Lower Genital Tract of Pregnant Women. *Int J Cancer* 40: 198–201, 1987a.

Schneider A, Meinhardt G, De-Villiers E-M, et al: Sensitivity of the Cytologic Diagnosis of Cervical Condyloma in Comparison With HPV-DNA Hybridization Studies. *Diagn Cytopathol* 3: 250–255, 1987b.

Schneider A, Sawada E, Gissman L, et al: Human Papillomaviruses in Women With a History of Abnormal Papanicolaou Smears and in Their Male Partners. *Obstet Gynecol* 69: 554–562, 1987c.

Schneider A, Kirchmayr R, De Villiers E-M, et al: Subclinical Human Papillomavirus Infections in Male Sexual Partners of Female Carriers. *J Urol* 140: 1431–1434, 1988a.

Schneider A, Sterzik K, Buck G, et al: Colposcopy is Superior to Cytology for the Detection of Early Genital Human Papillomavirus Infection. *Obstet Gynecol* 71: 236– 241, 1988b.

Schneider A: What Are the Various Methods for HPV Detection? *Diagn Cytopathol* 5: 339–341, 1989.

Schneider A, Meinhardt G, Kirchmayr R, et al: Prevalence of Human Papillomavirus Genomes in Tissues From the Lower Genital Tract as Detected by Molecular In Situ Hybridization. *Int J Gynecol Pathol* 10: 1–14, 1991.

Schneider A, Kirchhoff T, Meinhardt G, et al: Repeated Evaluation of Human Papillomavirus 16 Status in Cervical Swabs of Young Women With a History of Normal Pap Smears. *Obstet Gynecol* 79: 683–688, 1992.

Schneider ML, Wortmann, Weigel A: Influence of the Histologic and Cytologic Grade and the Clinical and Postsurgical Stage on the Rate of Endometrial Carcinoma Detection by Cervical Cytology. *Acta Cytol* 30: 616–622, 1986.

Schneider V: Arias-Stella Reaction of the Endocervix: Frequency and Location. *Acta Cytol* 25: 224–228, 1981a.

Schneider V, Barners LA: Ectopic Decidual Reaction of the Uterine Cervix: Frequency and Cytologic Presentation. *Acta Cytol* 25: 616–622, 1981b.

Schneider V, Kay S, Lee HM: Immunosuppression as a High-Risk Factor in the Development of Condyloma Acuminatum and Squamous Neoplasia of the Cervix. *Acta Cytol* 27: 220–224, 1983.

Schneider V: Microscopic Diagnosis of HPV Infection. *Clin Obstet Gynecol* 32: 148–156, 1989.

Schwartz PE, Merino MJ, Curnen MGM: Clinical Management of Patients With Invasive Cervical Cancer Following a Negative Pap Smear. *Yale J Biol Med* 61: 327–338, 1988.

Sedlacek TV, Cunnane M, Carpiniello V: Colposcopy in the Diagnosis of Penile Condyloma. *Am J Obstet Gynecol* 154: 494–496, 1986.

Sedlacek TV, Sedlacek AE, Neff DK, et al: The Clinical Role of Human Papilloma Virus Typing. *Gynecol Oncol* 42: 222–226, 1991.

Sedlis A, Walters AT, Balin H, et al: Evaluation of Two Simultaneously Obtained Cervical Cytological Smears: A Comparison Study. *Acta Cytol* 18: 291–296, 1974.

Selvaggi SM: Cytologic Detection of Condylomas and Cervical Intraepithelial Neoplasia of the Uterine Cervix with Histologic Correlation. *Cancer* 58: 2076–2081, 1986.

Selvaggi SM: Cytologic Features of Squamous Cell Carcinoma In Situ Involving Endocervical Glands in Endocervical Cytobrush Specimens. *Acta Cytol* 38: 687–692, 1994.

Sen DK, Langley FA: Vaginal Cytology as a Monitor of Fetal Wellbeing in Early Pregnancy. *Acta Cytol* 16: 116–119, 1972.

Seski JC, Abell MR, Morley GW: Microinvasive Squamous Carcinoma of the Cervix: Definition, Histologic Analysis, Late Results of Treatment. *Obstet Gynecol* 50: 410–414, 1977.

Seybolt JF, Johnson WD: Cervical Cytodiagnostic Problems—A Survey. Am J Obstet Gynecol 109: 1089–1103, 1971.

Shafer M-A, Chew KL, Kromhout LK, et al: Chlamydial Endocervical Infections and Cytologic Findings in Sexually Active Female Adolescents. *Am J Obstet Gynecol* 151: 765–771, 1985.

Sheils LA, Wilbur DC: The Significance of Atypical Cells of Squamous Type (AS) on Papanicolaou Smears: A Five-Year Follow-up Study. *Acta Cytol* 36: 580, 1992.

Sherlaw-Johnson C, Gallivan S, Jenkins D, et al: Cytological Screening and Management of Abnormalities in Prevention of Cervical Cancer: An Overview With Stochastic Modelling. *J Clin Pathol* 47: 430–435, 1994.

Sherman ME, Kelly D: High-Grade Squamous Intraepithelial Lesions and Invasive Carcinoma Following the Report of Three Negative Papanicolaou Smears: Screening Failures or Rapid Progression? *Mod Pathol* 5: 337–342, 1992a.

Sherman ME, Bitterman P, Rosenshein NB, et al: Uterine Serous Carcinoma. A Morphologically Diverse Neoplasm with Unifying Clinical Features. *Am J Surg Pathol* 16: 600–610, 1992b.

Sherman ME, Schiffman MH, Erozan YS, et al: The Bethesda System. A Proposal for Reporting Abnormal Cervical Smears Based on the Reproducibility of Cytopathologic Diagnoses. *Arch Pathol Lab Med* 116: 1155–1158, 1992c.

Sherman ME, Weinstein M, Sughayer M, et al: The Bethesda System. Impact on Reporting Cervicovaginal Specimens and Reproducibility of Criteria for Assessing Endocervical Sampling. *Acta Cytol* 37: 55–60, 1993.

Shield PW, Wright RG, Free K, et al: The Accuracy of Cervicovaginal Cytology in the Detection of Recurrent Cervical Carcinoma Following Radiotherapy. *Gynecol Oncol* 41: 223–229, 1991.

Shield PW, Daunter B, Wright RG: Post-Irradiation Cytology of Cervical Cancer Patients. *Cytopathology* 3: 167–182, 1992.

Shiina Y: Cytomorphologic and Immunocytochemical Studies of Chlamydial Infections in Cervical Smears. *Acta Cytol* 29: 683–691, 1985.

Shingleton HM, Richart RM, Wiener J, et al: Human Cervical Intraepithelial Neoplasia: Fine Structure of Dysplasia and Carcinoma In Situ. *Cancer Res* 28: 695–706, 1968.

Shingleton HM, Gore H, Straughn JM, et al: The Contribution of Endocervical Smears to Cervical Cancer Detection. *Acta Cytol* 19: 261–264, 1975.

Shingleton HM, Gore H, Bradley DH, et al: Adenocarcinoma of the Cervix: I. Clinical Evaluation and Pathologic Features. *Am J Obstet Gynecol* 139: 799–814, 1981.

Shirasawa H, Tomita Y, Sekiya S, et al: Integration and Transcription of Human Papillomavirus Type 16 and 18 Sequences in Cell Lines Derived From Cervical Carcinomas. *J Gen Virol* 68:583–591, 1987.

Shokri-Tabibzadeh S, Koss LG, Molnar J, et al: Association of Human Papillomavirus With Neoplastic Processes in the Genital Tract of Four Women With Impaired Immunity. *Gynecol Oncol* 12: S129–S140, 1981.

Shrago SS: The Arias Stella Reaction: A Case Report of a Cytologic Presentation. *Acta Cytol* 21: 310–313, 1977.

Shroyer KR, Hosey J, Swanson LE, et al: Cytologic Diagnosis of Human Papillomavirus Infection: Spindled Nuclei. *Diagn Cytopathol* 6: 178–183, 1990.

Shulman JJ, Leyton M, Hamilton R: The Papanicolaou Smear: An Insensitive Case-Finding Procedure. *Am J Obstet Gynecol* 120: 446–451, 1974.

Shulman JJ, Hontz A, Sedlis A, et al: The Pap Smear: Take Two. *Am J Obstet Gynecol* 121: 1024–1028, 1975.

Shy K, Chu J, Mandelson M, et al: Papanicolaou Smear Screening Interval and Risk of Cervical Cancer. *Obstet Gynecol* 74: 838–843, 1989.

Siapco BJ, Kaplan BJ, Bernstein GS, et al: Cytodiagnosis of *Candida* Organisms in Cervical Smears. *Acta Cytol* 30: 477–480, 1986.

Sickel J, Rutkowski M, Bonfiglio T: Cytomegalovirus Inclusions in Routine Cervical Papanicolaou Smears: A Clinicopathologic Study of Three Cases. *Acta Cytol* 35: 646, 1991.

Sidawy MK, Tabbara SO: Reactive Change and Atypical Squamous Cells of Undetermined Significance in Papanicolaou Smears: A Cytohistologic Correlation. *Diagn Cytopathol* 9: 423–429, 1993.

Sidawy MK, Siriaunkgul S, Frost AR: Retrospective Analysis of Non-Correlating Cervical Smears and Colposcopically Directed Biopsies. *Diagn Cytopathol* 11: 343–347, 1994.

Siegler EE: Microdiagnosis of Carcinoma In Situ of the Uterine Cervix: A Comparison Study of Pathologist's Diagnoses. *Cancer* 9: 463–469, 1956.

Silcocks PBS, Moss SM: Rapidly Progressive Cervical Cancer: Is It a Real Problem? *Br J Obstet Gynaecol* 95: 1111–1116, 1988.

Silverberg SG, Frable WJ: Prolapse of Fallopian Tube Into Vaginal Vault After Hysterectomy: Histopathology, Cytopathology, and Differential Diagnosis. *Arch Pathol* 97: 100–103, 1974.

Silverberg SG, Hurt WG: Minimal Deviation Adenocarcinoma ("Adenoma Malignum") of the Cervix: A Reappraisal. *Am J Obstet Gynecol* 121: 971–975, 1975.

Silverberg SG, Major FJ, Blessing JA, et al: Carcinosarcoma (Malignant Mixed Mesodermal Tumor) of the Uterus. A Gynecologic Oncology Group Pathologic Study of 203 Cases. *Int J Gynecol Pathol* 9: 1–19, 1990.

Silverberg SG, Boring C: Annual Cancer Statistics. *CA Cancer J Clin.* Volumes 20 to 43 (No. 1): 1970–1994.

Silverman EM, Silverman AG: Persistence of Spermatozoa in the Lower Genital Tracts of Women. *JAMA* 240: 1875–1877, 1978.

Simons AM, Phillips DH, Coleman DV: Damage to DNA in Cervical Epithelium Related to Tobacco Smoking. *BMJ* 306: 1444–1448, 1993.

Simons AM, Phillips DH, Coleman DV: DNA Adduct Assay in Cervical Epithelium. *Diagn Cytopathol* 10: 284–288, 1994.

Singer A: The Uterine Cervix from Adolescence to the Menopause. *Br J Obstet Gynaecol* 82: 81–99, 1975.

Sivanesaratnam V, Jayalakshmi P, Loo C: Surgical Management of Early Invasive Cancer of the Cervix Associated With Pregnancy. *Gynecol Oncol* 48: 68–75, 1993.

Skrabanek P: Cervical Cancer in Nuns and Prostitutes: A Plea for Scientific Continence. *J Clin Epidemiol* 41: 577–582, 1988.

Slater DN, Milner PC, Radley H: Audit of Deaths From Cervical Cancer: Proposal for an Essential Component of the National Screening Program. *J Clin Pathol* 47: 27–28, 1994.

Slattery ML, Robison LM, Schuman KL, et al: Cigarette Smoking and Exposure to Passive Smoke are Risk Factors for Cervical Cancer. *JAMA* 261: 1593–1598, 1989.

Slawson DC, Bennett JH, Herman JM: Follow-up Papanicolaou Smear for Cervical Atypia: Are We Missing Significant Disease? A HARNET Study. *J Fam Pract* 36: 289–293, 1993.

Smith MR, Figge DC, Bennington JL: The Diagnosis of Cervical Cancer During Pregnancy. *Obstet Gynecol* 31: 193–197, 1968.

Smith JW, Townsend DE, Sparkes RS: Genetic Variants of Glucose-6-Phosphate Dehydrogenase in the Study of Carcinoma of the Cervix. *Cancer* 28: 529–532, 1971.

Smotkin D, Berek JS, Fu YS, et al: Human Papillomavirus Deoxyribonucleic Acid in Adenocarcinoma and Adenosquamous Carcinoma of the Uterine Cervix. *Obstet Gynecol* 68: 241–244, 1986.

Snyder RN, Ortiz Y, Willie S, et al: Dysplasia and Carcinoma In Situ of the Uterine Cervix: Prevalence in Very Young Women (Under Age 22). *Am J Obstet Gynecol* 124: 751–756, 1976.

Sodhani P, Murthy NS, Sardana S, et al: Seasonal Variation in Genital Tract Infections as Detected on Papanicolaou's Smear Examination. *Diagn Cytopathol* 10: 98–99, 1994.

Soloway HB: Vaginal and Cervical Cytology of the Early Puerperium. *Acta Cytol* 13: 136–138, 1969.

Soost H-J, Lange H-J, Lehmacher W, et al: The Validation of Cervical Cytology. Sensitivity, Specificity and Predictive Value. *Acta Cytol* 31: 8–14, 1991.

Sorosky JI, Kaminski PF, Wheelock JB, et al: Clinical Significance of Hyperkeratosis and Parakeratosis in Otherwise Negative Papanicolaou Smears. *Gynecol Oncol* 39: 132–134, 1990.

Southern EM: Detection of Specific Sequences Among DNA Fragments Separated by Gel Electrophoresis. *J Mol Biol* 98: 503–517, 1975.

Soutter WP, Wisdom S, Brough AK, et al: Should Patients with Mild Atypia in a Cervical Smear Be Referred for Colposcopy? *Br J Obstet Gynaecol* 93: 70–74, 1986.

Spanos WJ Jr, King A, Keeney E, et al: Age as a Prognostic Factor in Carcinoma of the Cervix. *Gynecol Oncol* 35: 66–68, 1989.

Spiegel GW: Endometrial Carcinoma In Situ in Postmenopausal Women. *Am J Surg Pathol* 19: 417–432, 1995.

Spires SE, Banks ER, Weeks JA, et al: Assessment of Cervicovaginal Smear Adequacy. The Bethesda System Guidelines and Reproducibility. *Am J Clin Pathol* 102: 354–359, 1995.

Spitzer M, Krumholz BA, Chernys AE, et al: Comparative Utility of Repeat Papanicolaou Smears, Cervicography, and Colposcopy in the Evaluation of Atypical Papanicolaou Smears. *Obstet Gynecol* 69: 731–735, 1987.

Spjut HJ, Kaufman RH, Carrig SS: Psammoma Bodies in the Cervicovaginal Smear. *Acta Cytol* 8: 352–355, 1964.

Spriggs AI, Bowley CE, Cowdell RH: Chromosomes of Precancerous Lesions of the Cervix Uteri: New Data and a Review. *Cancer* 27: 1239–1254, 1971.

Stafl A, Mattingly RF: Colposcopic Diagnosis of Cervical Neoplasia. *Obstet Gynecol* 41: 168–176, 1973.

Stanhope CR, Smith JP, Wharton JT, et al: Carcinoma of the Cervix: The Effect of Age on Survival. *Gynecol Oncol* 10: 188–193, 1980.

Stavola BD: Statistical Facts About Cancers on Which Doctor Rigoni-Stern Based His Contribution to the Surgeons' Subgroup of the IV Congress of the Italian Scientists on 23 September 1842. *Stat Med* 6: 881–884, 1987.

Stern E, Neely PM: Carcinoma and Dysplasia of the Cervix: A Comparison of Rates for New and Returning Populations. *Acta Cytol* 7: 357–361, 1963.

Stern E, Neely PM: Dysplasia of the Uterine Cervix: Incidence of Regression, Recurrence, and Cancer. *Cancer* 17: 508–512, 1964.

Stern E: Epidemiology of Dysplasia. *Obstet Gynecol Surv* 24: 711–723, 1969.

Stewart CJ, Thomas MA: Malacoplakia of the Uterine Cervix and Endometrium. *Cytopathology* 2: 271–275, 1991.

Stewart CJ, Livingstone D, Mutch AF: Borderline Nuclear Abnormality in Cervical Smears: A Cytological Review of 200 Cases With Histological Correlation. *Cytopathology* 4: 339–345, 1993.

Stocks P: Cancer of the Uterine Cervix and Social Conditions. *Br J Cancer* 9: 487–494, 1955.

Stoler MH, Broker TR: In Situ Hybridization Detection of Human Papillomavirus DNAs and Messenger RNAs in Genital Condylomas and a Cervical Carcinoma. *Hum Pathol* 17: 1250–1258, 1986.

Stoler MH, Mills SE, Gersell DJ, et al: Small-Cell Neuroendocrine Carcinoma of the Cervix: A Human Papillomavirus Type 18-Associated Cancer. *Am J Surg Pathol* 15: 28–32, 1991.

Stowell SB, Wiley CM, Powers CN: Herpesvirus Mimics. A Potential Pitfall in Endocervical Brush Specimens. *Acta Cytol* 38: 43–50, 1994.

Sugimori H, Iwasak T, Yoshimura T, Tsukamoto N: Cytology of Microinvasive Squamous-Cell Carcinoma of the Uterine Cervix. *Acta Cytol* 31: 412–416, 1987.

Swan SH, Petitti DB: A Review of Problems of Bias and Confounding in Epidemiologic Studies of Cervical Neoplasia and Oral Contraceptive Use. *Am J Epidemiol* 115: 10–18, 1982.

Swinker M, Cutlip AC, Ogle D: A Comparison of Uterine Cervical Cytology and Biopsy Results: Indications and Outcomes for Colposcopy. *J Fam Pract* 38: 40–44, 1994.

Symmans F, Mechanic L, MacConnell P, et al: Correlation of Cervical Cytology and Human Papillomavirus DNA Detection in Postmenopausal Women. *Int J Gynecol Pathol* 11: 204–209, 1992.

Syrjänen KJ: Morphologic Survey of the Condylomatous Lesions in Dysplastic and Neoplastic Epithelium of the Uterine Cervix. *Arch Gynecol* 227: 153–161, 1979.

Syrjänen KJ: Condylomatous Lesions in Dysplastic and Neoplastic Epithelium of the Uterine Cervix. *Surg Gynecol Obstet* 150: 372–376, 1980.

Syrjänen KJ, Heinonen U-M, Kauraniemi T: Cytologic Evidence of the Association of Condylomatous Lesions With Dysplastic and Neoplastic Changes in the Uterine Cervix. *Acta Cytol* 25: 17–22, 1981.

Syrjänen KJ: Human Papillomavirus Lesions in Association With Cervical Dysplasias and Neoplasias. *Obstet Gynecol* 62: 617–624, 1983.

Syrjänen KJ, Väyrynen M, Castrén O, et al: Sexual Behavior of Women With Human Papillomavirus (HPV) Lesions of the Uterine Cervix. *Br J Vener Dis* 60: 243–248, 1984.

Syrjänen K, Väyrynen M, Saarikoski S, et al: Natural History of Cervical Human Papillomavirus (HPV) Infections Based on Prospective Follow-up. *Br J Obstet Gynaecol* 92: 1086–1092, 1985.

Syrjänen KJ: Human Papillomavirus (HPV) Infections of the Female Genital Tract and Their Associations With Intraepithelial Neoplasia and Squamous Cell Carcinoma. *Pathol Annu* 21: 53–89, 1986a.

Syrjänen K, Mäntyjärvi R, Väyrynen M, et al: Coexistent Chlamydial Infections Related to Natural History of Human Papillomavirus Lesions in Uterine Cervix. *Genitourin Med* 62: 345–351, 1986b.

Syrjänen K, Mäntyjärvi R, Saarikoski S, et al: Factors Associated With Progression of Cervical Human Papillomavirus (HPV) Infections Into Carcinoma In Situ During a Long-Term Prospective Follow-up. *Br J Obstet Gynecol* 95: 1096–1102, 1988.

Syrjänen K, Hakama M, Saarikoski S, et al: Prevalence, Incidence, and Estimated Life-time Risk of Cervical Human Papillomavirus Infections in a Nonselected Finnish Female Population. *Sex Transmit Dis* 17: 15–19, 1990.

Syrjänen K, Kataja V, Yliskoski M, et al: Natural History of Cervical Human Papillomavirus Lesions Does Not Substantiate the Biologic Relevance of the Bethesda System. *Obstet Gynecol* 79: 675–682, 1992.

Syrjänen K: Human Papillomavirus in Genital Carcinogenesis. *Sex Trans Dis* 21(S2): S86–S89, 1994.

Szarewski A, Cuzick J, Nayagam M, et al: A Comparison of Four Cytological Sampling Techniques in a Genitourinary Medicine Clinic. *Genitourin Med* 66: 439–443, 1990.

Szarewski A, Curran G, Edwards R, et al: Comparison of Four Cytologic Sampling Techniques in a Large Family Planning Center. *Acta Cytol* 37: 457–460, 1993.

Szyfelbein WM, Young RH, Scully RE: Adenoma Malignum of the Cervix: Cytologic Findings. *Acta Cytol* 28: 691–698, 1984.

Tabbara S, Saleh AM, Andersen WA, et al: The Bethesda Classification for Squamous Intraepithelial Lesions: Histologic, Cytologic, and Viral Correlates. *Obstet Gynecol* 79: 338–346, 1992.

Tabbara SO, Sidawy MK: Evaluation of the Five-Year Review of Negative Cervical Smears in Patients With High Grade Squamous Intraepithelial Lesions. *Acta Cytol* 37: 767, 1993.

Tabbara SO, Horbach N, Sidawy MK: The Adequacy of the One-Slide Cervical Smear in the Detection of Squamous Intraepithelial Lesions. *Am J Clin Pathol.* 101: 647-650, 1994.

Taft PD, Robboy SJ, Herbst AL, et al: Cytology of Clear-Cell Adenocarcinoma of Genital Tract in Young Females: Review of 95 Cases From the Registry. *Acta Cytol* 18: 279–290, 1974.

Takashina T, Ito E, Kudo R: Cytologic Diagnosis of Primary Tubal Cancer. *Acta Cytol* 29: 367–372, 1985.

Takashina T, Ono M, Kanda Y, et al: Cervicovaginal and Endometrial Cytology in Ovarian Cancer. *Acta Cytol* 32: 159–162, 1988.

Tamimi HK, Figge DC: Adenocarcinoma of the Uterine Cervix. *Gynecol Oncol* 13: 335–344, 1982.

Tanaka H, Chua KL, Lindh E, et al: Patients With Various Types of Human Papillomavirus: Covariation and Diagnostic Relevance of Cytological Findings in Papanicolaou Smears. *Cytopathology* 4: 273–283, 1993.

Tase T, Okagaki T, Clark BA, et al: Human Papillomavirus DNA in Adenocarcinoma In Situ, Microinvasive Adenocarcinoma of the Uterine Cervix, and Coexisting Cervical Squamous Intraepithelial Neoplasia. *Int J Gynecol Pathol* 8: 8–17, 1989a.

Tase T, Okagaki T, Clark BA, et al: Human Papillomavirus DNA in Glandular Dysplasia and Microglandular Hyperplasia: Presumed Precursors of Adenocarcinoma of the Uterine Cervix. *Obstet Gynecol* 73: 1005–1008, 1989b.

Tay SK, Jenkins D, Maddox P, et al: Lymphocyte Phenotypes in Cervical Intraepithelial Neoplasia and Human Papillomavirus Infection. *Br J Obstet Gynaecol* 94: 16–21, 1987a.

Tay SK, Jenkins D, Singer A: Natural Killer Cells in Cervical Intraepithelial Neoplasia and Human Papillomavirus Infection. *Br J Obstet Gynaecol* 94: 901–906, 1987b.

Tay SK, Jenkins D, Maddox P, et al: Tissue Macrophage Response in Human Papillomavirus Infection and Cervical Intraepithelial Neoplasia. *Br J Obstet Gynaecol* 94: 1094–1097, 1987c.

Tay SK, Jenkins D, Singer A: Management of Squamous Atypia (Borderline Nuclear Abnormalities): Repeat Cytology or Colposcopy? *Aust N Z J Obstet Gynaecol* 27: 140–141, 1987d.

Taylor HB, Irey NS, Norris HJ: Atypical Endocervical Hyperplasia in Women Taking Oral Contraceptives. *JAMA* 202: 185–187, 1967.

Taylor PT Jr, Andersen WA, Barber SR, et al: The Screening Papanicolaou Smear: Contribution of the Endocervical Brush. *Obstet Gynecol* 70: 734–738, 1987.

Taylor Y, Melvin WT, Flannelly G, et al: Prevalence of Epstein-Barr Virus in the Cervix. *J Clin Pathol* 47: 92–93, 1994.

Terris M, Wilson F, Nelson JH Jr: Relation of Circumcision to Cancer of the Cervix. *Am J Obstet Gynecol* 117: 1056–1066, 1973.

Terris M, Wilson F, Nelson JH Jr: Comparative Epidemiology of Invasive Carcinoma of the Cervix, Carcinoma In Situ, and Cervical Dysplasia. *Am J Epidemiol* 112: 253–257, 1980.

Teshima S, Shimosato Y, Kishi K, et al: Early Stage Adenocarcinoma of the Uterine Cervix: Histopathologic Analysis With Consideration of Histogenesis. *Cancer* 56: 167–172, 1985.

Tidbury P, Singer A, Jenkins D: CIN 3: The Role of Lesion Size in Invasion. *Br J Obstet Gynaecol* 99: 583–586, 1992.

Tidy JA, Parry GCN, Ward P, et al: High Rate of Human Papillomavirus Type 16 Infection in Cytologically Normal Cervices. *Lancet* (i): 434, 1989a. (Retraction: *Lancet* (ii): 1535, 1989.)

Tidy J, Vousden KH, Mason P, Farrell PJ: A Novel Deletion Within the Upstream Regulatory Region of Episomal Human Papillomavirus Type 16. *J Gen Virol* 70: 999–1004, 1989b.

Toolenaar TA, Freundt I, Huikeshoven FJ, et al: The Occurrence of Diversion Colitis in Patients With a Sigmoid Neovagina. *Hum Pathol* 24: 846–849, 1993.

Toon PG, Arrand JR, Wilson LP, Sharp DS: Human Papillomavirus Infection of the Uterine Cervix of Women Without Cytological Signs of Neoplasia. *Br Med J* 293: 1261–1264, 1986.

Towne JE: Carcinoma of the Cervix in Nulliparous and Celibate Women. *Am J Obstet Gynecol* 69: 606–613, 1955.

Trevathan E, Layde P, Webster LA, et al: Cigarette Smoking and Dysplasia and Carcinoma In Situ of the Uterine Cervix. *JAMA* 250: 499–502, 1983.

Tuncer M, Graham R, Graham J: Diagnostic Efficiency in Invasive Cervical Cancer. *N Y State J Med* 11: 2317–2319, 1967.

Tweeddale DN, Scott RC, Fields MJ, et al: Giant Cells in Cervico-Vaginal Smears. *Acta Cytol* 12: 298–304, 1968.

Tweeddale DN, Langenbach SR, Roddick JW Jr, et al: The Cytopathology of Microinvasive Squamous Cancer of the Cervix Uteri. *Acta Cytol* 13: 447–454, 1969.

Ueda G, Shimizu C, Shimizu H, et al: An Immunohistochemical Study of Small-Cell and Poorly Differentiated Carcinomas of the Cervix Using Neuroendocrine Markers. *Gynecol Oncol* 34: 164–169, 1989.

USHHS: United States Department of Health and Human Services: The National Strategic Plan for the Early Detection and Control of Breast and Cervical Cancers. Public Health Service.

Valente PT: Government Mandated Cytology Proficiency Testing: Time for Reality Testing. *Diagn Cytopathol* 10: 105–106, 1994a.

Valente PT: Cytologic Atypia Associated With Microglandular Hyperplasia. *Diagn Cytopathol* 10: 326–331, 1994b.

Valicenti JF, Priester SK: Psammoma Bodies of Benign Endometrial Origin in Cervicovaginal Cytology. *Acta Cytol* 21: 550–552, 1977.

van der Graaf Y, Vooijs GP: False Negative Rate in Cervical Cytology. *J Clin Pathol* 40: 438–442, 1987a.

van der Graaf Y, Vooijs GP, Gaillard HLJ, et al: Screening Errors in Cervical Cytologic Screening. *Acta Cytol* 31: 434–438, 1987b.

van der Graaf Y, Vooijs GP, Zielhuis GA: Cervical Screening Revisited. *Acta Cytol* 34: 366–372, 1990.

Van Le L, Novotny D, Dotters DJ: Distinguishing Tubal Metaplasia From Endocervical Dysplasia on Cervical Papanicolaou Smears. *Obstet Gynecol* 78: 974–976, 1991.

van Nagell JR Jr, Greenwell N, Powell DF, et al: Microinvasive Carcinoma of the Cervix. *Am J Obstet Gynecol* 145: 981–991, 1983.

van Nagell JR Jr, Powell DE, Gallion HH, et al: Small Cell Carcinoma of the Uterine Cervix. *Cancer* 62: 1586–1593, 1988.

van Oortmarssen GJ, Habbema JDF: Epidemiologic Evidence for Age-Dependent Regression of Pre-Invasive Cervical Cancer. *Br J Cancer* 64: 559–565, 1991.

Varma VA, Sanchez-Lanier M, Unger ER, et al: Association of Human Papillomavirus With Penile Carcinoma: A Study Using Polymerase Chain Reaction and In Situ Hybridization. *Hum Pathol* 22: 908–913, 1991.

Vessey MP, McPherson K, Lawless M, et al: Neoplasia of the Cervix Uteri and Contraception: A Possible Adverse Effect of the Pill. *Lancet* (i): 930–934, 1983.

Vesterinen E, Forss M, Nieminen U. Increase of Cervical Adenocarcinomas: A Report of 520 Cases of Cervical Carcinomas Including 112 Tumors With Glandular Elements. *Gynecol Oncol* 33: 49–53, 1989.

Villa LL, Lopes A: Human Papillomavirus DNA Sequences in Penile Carcinomas in Brazil. *Int J Cancer* 37: 853–855, 1986.

Villa LL, Franco ELF: Epidemiologic Correlates of Cervical Neoplasia and Risk of Human Papillomavirus Infection in Asymptomatic Women in Brazil. *J Natl Cancer Inst* 81: 332–340, 1989.

von Haam E: The Cytology of Pregnancy. *Acta Cytol* 5: 320–329, 1961.

von Haam E: A Comparative Study of the Accuracy of Cancer Cell Detection by Cytological Methods. *Acta Cytol* 6: 508–518, 1962.

Vooijs GP, Ng ABP, Wentz WB: The Detection of Vaginal Adenosis and Clear Cell Carcinoma. *Acta Cytol* 17: 59–63, 1973.

Vooijs GP, Elias A, van der Graaf Y, et al: Relationship Between the Diagnosis of Epithelial Abnormalities and the Composition of Cervical Smears. *Acta Cytol* 29: 323–328, 1985.

Vooijs GP, Elias A, van der Graaf Y, et al: The Influence of Sample Takers on the Cellular Composition of Cervical Smears. *Acta Cytol* 30: 251–257, 1986.

Vooijs GP, van der Graaf Y, Elias AG: Cellular Composition of Cervical Smears in Relation to the Day of the Menstrual Cycle and Method of Contraception. *Acta Cytol* 31: 417–426, 1987a.

Vooijs GP, van der Graaf Y, Vooijs MA: The Presence of Endometrial Cells in Cervical Smears in Relation to the Day of the Menstrual Cycle and the Method of Contraception. *Acta Cytol* 31: 427–433, 1987b.

Vuopala S: Diagnostic Accuracy and Clinical Applicability of Cytological and Histological Methods for Investigating Endometrial Carcinoma. *Acta Obstet Gynecol Scand* 10(Suppl): 1–72, 1977.

Waggoner SE, Woodworth CD, Stoler MH, et al: Human Cervical Cells Immortalized In Vitro With Oncogenic Human Papillomavirus DNA Differentiate Dysplastically In Vivo. *Gynecol Oncol* 38: 407–412, 1990.

Wagner D: Trophoblastic Cells in the Blood Stream in Normal and Abnormal Pregnancy. *Acta Cytol* 12: 137–139, 1968.

Wagner D, Ikenberg H, Boehm N, et al: Identification of Human Papillomavirus in Cervical Swabs by Deoxyribonucleic Acid In Situ Hybridization. *Obstet Gynecol* 64: 767–772, 1984.

Wagner D, de Villiers E-M, Gissmann L: Der Nachweis Verschiedener Papillomvirustypen in Zytologischen Abstrichen Von Präkanzerosen und Karzinomen der Cervix Uteri. *Geburtsh U Frauenheilk* 45: 226–231, 1985.

Wain GV, Farnsworth A, Hacker NF: Cervical Carcinoma After Negative Pap Smears: Evidence Against Rapid-Onset Cancers. *Int J Gynecol Cancer* 2: 318, 1992.

Walker AN, Mills SE, Taylor PT: Cervical Neuroendocrine Carcinoma: A Clinical and Light Microscopic Study of 14 Cases. *Int J Gynecol Pathol* 7: 64–74, 1988.

Walker EM, Hare MJ, Cooper P: A Retrospective Review of Cervical Cytology in Women Developing Invasive Squamous Cell Carcinoma. *Br J Obstet Gynaecol* 90: 1087–1091, 1983.

Walker EM, Dodgson J, Duncan ID: Does Mild Atypia on a Cervical Smear Warrant Further Investigation? *Lancet* (ii): 672–673, 1986.

Walker J, Bloss JD, Liao S-Y, et al: Human Papillomavirus Genotype as a Prognostic Indicator in Carcinoma of the Uterine Cervix. *Obstet Gynecol* 74: 781–785, 1989.

Wallace DL, Slankard JE: Teenage Cervical Carcinoma In Situ. *Obstet Gynecol* 41: 697–700, 1973.

Walton RJ: Cervical Cancer Screening Programs. *Can Med Assoc J* 114: 1003–1033, 1976.

Walton RJ: Cervical Cancer Screening Programs: Summary of the 1982 Canadian Task Force Report. *Can Med Assoc J* 127: 581–589, 1982.

Wang SE: The Consequences of Public Disclosure: An Opinion From Newport Hospital, Newport, Rhode Island. *Diagn Cytopathol* 11: 211–212, 1994.

Ward BE, Burkett B, Petersen C, et al: Cytologic Correlates of Cervical Papillomavirus Infection. *Int J Gynecol Pathol* 9: 297–305, 1990.

Ward BG, Shepherd JH, Monaghan JM: Occult Advanced Cervical Cancer. *Br Med J* 290: 1301–1302, 1985.

Ward P, Parry GN, Yule R, et al: Comparison Between the Polymerase Chain Reaction and Slot Blot Hybridization for the Detection of HPV Sequences in Cervical Scrapes. *Cytopathology* 1: 19–23, 1990.

Wassertheil-Smoller S, Romney SL, Wylie-Rosett J, et al: Dietary Vitamin C and Uterine Cervical Dysplasia. *Am J Epidemiol* 114: 714–724, 1981.

Waters SA, Sterrett GF: Intracytoplasmic Vacuoles in Cervical Smears: Relationship to Chlamydial Inclusions-Morphology, Mucin Histochemistry, and Immunocytochemistry. *Diagn Cytopathol* 7: 252–260, 1991.

Watts KC, Campion MJ, Butler EB, et al: Quantitative Deoxyribonucleic Acid Analysis of Patients With Mild Cervical Atypia: A Potentially Malignant Lesion? *Obstet Gynecol* 70: 205–207, 1987.

Weiss LK, Kau T-Y, Sparks BT, et al: Trends in Cervical Cancer Incidence Among Young Black and White Women in Metropolitan Detroit. *Cancer* 73: 1849–1854, 1994.

Weiss RJ, Lucas WE: Adenocarcinoma of the Uterine Cervix. *Cancer* 57: 1996–2001, 1986.

Weitzman GA, Korhonen MO, Reeves KO, et al: Endocervical Brush Cytology. An Alternative to Endocervical Curettage? *J Reprod Med* 33: 677–683, 1988.

Wentz WB: The Significance of Mucosal Lesions Antedating Mouse Cervical Cancer. *Am J Obstet Gynecol* 84: 1506–1511, 1962.

Wentz WB, Lewis GC: Correlation of Histologic Morphology and Survival in Cervical Cancer Following Radiation Therapy. *Obstet Gynecol* 26: 228–232, 1965.

Wentz WB, Reagan JW: Clinical Significance of Postirradiation Dysplasia of the Uterine Cervix. *Am J Obstet Gynecol* 106: 812–817, 1970.

Werness BA, Levine AJ, Howley PM: Association of Human Papillomavirus Types 16 and 18 E6 Proteins with p53. *Science* 248: 76–79, 1990.

Wheelock JB, Kaminski PF: Value of Repeat Cytology at the Time of Colposcopy for the Evaluation of Cervical Intraepithelial Neoplasia on Papanicolaou Smears. *J Reprod Med* 34: 815–817, 1989.

Whitehead N, Reyner F, Lindenbaum J: Megaloblastic Changes in the Cervical Epithelium: Association With Oral Contraceptive Therapy and Reversal With Folic Acid. *JAMA* 226: 1421–1424, 1973.

Wied GL: Importance of the Site From Which Vaginal Cytologic Smears Are Taken. *Am J Clin Pathol* 25: 742–750, 1955.

Wied GL, Bahr GF: Vaginal, Cervical and Endocervical Cytologic Smears on a Single Slide. *Obstet Gynecol* 14: 362–367, 1959.

Wied GL: An International Agreement on Histological Terminology for Lesions of the Uterine Cervix. *Acta Cytol* 6: 235–236, 1962.

Wied GL: Pap-Test or Babes Method? *Acta Cytol* 8: 173–174, 1964.

Wied GL (moderator): Symposium on Hormonal Cytology. *Acta Cytol* 12: 87–91, 1968.

Wied GL, Bartels PH, Bibbo M, et al: Frequency and Reliability of Diagnostic Cytology of the Female Genital Tract. *Acta Cytol* 25: 543–549, 1981.

Wied GL: Tutorial on Clinical Cytology. Universal City, CA, February 25, 1995.

Wilbanks GD, Richart RM, Terner JY: DNA Content of Cervical Intraepithelial Neoplasia Studied by Two-Wavelength Feulgen Cytophotometry. *Am J Obstet Gynecol* 98: 792–799, 1967.

Wilbur DC, Maurer S, Smith NJ: Behçet's Disease in a Vaginal Smear. Report of a Case with Cytologic Features and Their Distinction From Squamous Cell Carcinoma. *Acta Cytol* 37: 525–530, 1993.

Wilczynski SP, Bergen S, Walker J, et al: Human Papillomaviruses and Cervical Cancer: Analysis of Histopathologic Features Associated With Different Viral Types. *Hum Pathol* 19: 697–704, 1988a.

Wilczynski SP, Walker J, Liao S-Y, et al: Adenocarcinoma of the Cervix Associated With Human Papillomavirus. *Cancer* 62: 1331–1336, 1988b.

Willcox F, de Somer ML, Van Roy J: Classification of Cervical Smears With Discordance Between the Cytologic and/or Histologic Ratings. *Acta Cytol* 31: 883–886, 1987.

Willett GD, Kurman RJ, Reid R, et al: Correlation of the Histologic Appearance of Intraepithelial Neoplasia of the Cervix With Human Papillomavirus Types: Emphasis on Low Grade Lesions Including So-Called Flat Condyloma. *Int J Gynecol Pathol* 8: 18–25, 1989.

Williams AE, Jordan JA, Allen JM, et al: The Surface Ultrastructure of Normal and Metaplastic Cervical Epithelia and of Carcinoma In Situ. *Cancer Res* 33: 504–513, 1973.

Wilson JD, Robinson AJ, Kinghorn SA, et al: Implications of Inflammatory Changes on Cervical Cytology. *Br Med J* 300: 638–640, 1990.

Wilson SH, Johnson J: An Audit of Cervical Cancer Deaths in Nottingham. *Cytopathology* 3: 79–83, 1992.

Wingo PA, Tong T, Bolden S: Cancer Statistics, 1995. *CA Cancer J Clin* 45: 8–30, 1995.

Winkelstein W Jr: Smoking and Cancer of the Uterine Cervix: Hypothesis. *Am J Epidemiol* 106: 257–259, 1977.

Winkelstein W Jr, Shillitoe EJ, Brand R, et al: Further Comments on Cancer of the Uterine Cervix, Smoking, and Herpesvirus Infection. *Am J Epidemiol* 119: 1–8, 1984.

Winkelstein W Jr: Smoking and Cervical Cancer—Current Status: A Review. *Am J Epidemiol* 131: 945–957, 1990.

Winkler B, Crum CP, Fujii T, et al: Koilocytotic Lesions of the Cervix: The Relationship of Mitotic Abnormalities to the Presence of Papillomavirus Antigens and Nuclear DNA Content. *Cancer* 53: 1081–1087, 1984.

Winston RML: The Relation Between Size and Pathogenicity of *Trichomonas vaginalis*. *J Obstet Gynaecol Br Cwlth* 81: 399–404, 1974.

Wolfendale MR, King S, Usherwood MM: Abnormal Cervical Smears: Are We in for an Epidemic? *Br Med J* 287: 526–528, 1983.

Woodman CBJ, Yates M, Ward K, et al: Indicators of Effective Cytological Sampling of the Uterine Cervix. *Lancet* (ii): 88–90, 1989.

Woodruff JD, Peterson WF: Condylomata Acuminata of the Cervix. *Am J Obstet Gynecol* 75: 1354–1362, 1958.

Woodworth CD, Bowden PE, Doniger J, et al: Characterization of Normal Human Exocervical Epithelial Cells Immortalized In Vitro by Papillomavirus Types 16 and 18 DNA. *Cancer Res* 48: 4620–4628, 1988.

Wosnitzer M: Use of Office Colposcope to Diagnose Subclinical Papillomaviral and Other Infections of Male and Female Genitalia. *Urology* 31: 340–341, 1988.

Wright NH, Vessey MP, Kenward B, et al: Neoplasia and Dysplasia of the Cervix Uteri and Contraception: A Possible Protective Effect of the Diaphragm. *Br J Cancer* 38: 273–279, 1978.

Wright TC, Richart RM: Role of Human Papillomavirus in the Pathogenesis of Genital Tract Warts and Cancer. *Gynecol Oncol* 37: 151–164, 1990.

Wright TC, Kurman RJ, Ferenczy A: Precancerous Lesions of the Cervix. In Kurman RJ, ed: *Blaustein's Pathology of the Female Genital Tract.* 4th ed. New York: Springer-Verlag NY Inc, 1994.

Wynder EL. Cornfield J, Schroff PD, et al: A Study of Environmental Factors in Carcinoma of the Cervix. *Am J Obstet Gynecol* 68: 1016–1052, 1954.

Yahr LJ, Lee KR: Cytologic Findings in Microglandular Hyperplasia of the Cervix. *Diagn Cytopathol* 7: 248–251, 1991.

Yancy M, Magelssen D, Demaurez A, et al: Classification of Endometrial Cells on Cervical Cytology. *Obstet Gynecol* 76: 1000–1005, 1990.

Yobs AR, Swanson RA, Lamotte LC: Laboratory Reliability of the Papanicolaou Smear. *Obstet Gynecol* 65: 235–244, 1985.

Yobs AR, Plott AE, Hicklin MD, et al: Retrospective Evaluation of Gynecologic Cytodiagnosis. II. Interlaboratory Reproducibility as Shown in Rescreening Large Consecutive Samples of Reported Cases. *Acta Cytol* 31: 900–910, 1987.

Yoonessi M, Wieckowska W, Mariniello D, et al: Cervical Intra-Epithelial Neoplasia in Pregnancy. *Int J Gynaecol Obstet* 20: 111–118, 1982.

Younes MS: Electron Microscope Observations on Carcinoma In Situ of the Cervix. *Obstet Gynecol Surv* 24: 768–784, 1969.

Young LS, Bevan IS, Johnson MA, et al: The Polymerase Chain Reaction: A New Epidemiological Tool for Investigating Cervical Human Papillomavirus Infection. *Br Med J* 298: 14–18, 1989.

Young NA, Kline TS: Benign Cellular Changes: Allied Ambiguity in CLIA '88 and The Bethesda System. *Diagn Cytopathol* 10: 307–308, 1994a.

Young NA, Naryshkin S, Atkinson BF, et al: Interobserver Variability of Cervical Smears With Squamous-Cell Abnormalities: A Philadelphia Study. *Diagn Cytopathol* 11: 352–357, 1994b.

Young QA, Pacey NF: The Cytologic Diagnosis of Clear Cell Adenocarcinoma of the Cervix Uteri. *Acta Cytol* 22: 3–6, 1978.

Young RH, Scully RE: Atypical Forms of Microglandular Hyperplasia of the Cervix Simulating Carcinoma: A Report of Five Cases and Review of the Literature. *Am J Surg Pathol* 13: 50–56, 1989.

Young RH, Scully RE: Invasive Adenocarcinoma and Related Tumors of the Uterine Cervix. *Semin Diagn Pathol* 7: 205–227, 1990.

Youseff AF, Fayad MM: The Post-Partum Vaginal Smear. *J Obstet Gynaecol Br Cwlth* 70: 32–38, 1963.

Yu HC, Ketabchi M: Detection of Malignant Melanoma of the Uterine Cervix From Papanicolaou Smears: A Case Report. *Acta Cytol* 31: 73–76, 1987.

Yule R: False Negative Cytology in a Randomly Selected Group of Women. *Acta Cytol* 16: 389–390, 1972.

Yule R: Mortality From Carcinoma of the Cervix. *Lancet* (i): 1031–1032, 1978.

Yunis JJ, Soreng AL: Constitutive Fragile Sites and Cancer. *Science* 226: 1199–1204, 1984.

Zaharopoulos P, Wong JY, Keagy N: Hematoidin Crystals in Cervicovaginal Smears: Report of Two Cases. *Acta Cytol* 29: 1029–1034, 1985a.

Zaharopoulos P, Wong JY, Edmonston G, et al: Crystalline Bodies in Cervicovaginal Smears: A Cytochemical and Immunochemical Study. *Acta Cytol* 29: 1035–1042, 1985b.

Zaino RJ, Nahhas WA, Mortel R: Glassy Cell Carcinoma of the Uterine Cervix: An Ultrastructural Study and Review. *Arch Pathol Lab Med* 106: 250–254, 1982.

Zaneveld LJD, Tauber PF, Port C, et al: Scanning Electron Microscopy of Cervical Mucus Crystallization. *Obstet Gynecol* 46: 419–428, 1975.

Ziabkowski TA, Naylor B: Cyanophilic Bodies in Cervico-Vaginal Smears. *Acta Cytol* 20: 340–342, 1976.

Ziegler RG, Brinton LA, Hamman RF, et al: Diet and the Risk of Invasive Cervical Cancer Among White Women in the United States. *Am J Epidemiol* 132: 432–445, 1990.

Zucker PK, Kasdon EJ, Feldstein ML: The Validity of Pap Smear Parameters as Predictors of Endometrial Pathology in Menopausal Women. *Cancer* 56: 2256–2263, 1985.

Zuna RE: Association of Condylomas With Intraepithelial and Microinvasive Cervical Neoplasia: Histopathology of Conization and Hysterectomy Specimens. *Int J Gynecol Pathol* 2: 364–372, 1984.

Zunzunegui MV, King M-C, Coria CF, et al: Male Influences on Cervical Cancer Risk. *Am J Epidemiol* 123: 302– 307, 1986.

zur Hausen H, Meinhof W, Scheiber W, et al: Attempts to Detect Virus-Specific DNA in Human Tumors: I. Nucleic Acid Hybridizations With Complementary RNA of Human Wart Virus. *Int J Cancer* 13: 650–656, 1974.

zur Hausen H, de Villiers E-M, Gissmann L: Papillomavirus Infections and Human Genital Cancer. *Gynecol Oncol* 12: S124–S128, 1981.

zur Hausen H: Human Genital Cancer: Synergism Between Two Virus Infections for Synergism Between a Virus Infection and Initiating Events? *Lancet* (ii): 1370–1372, 1982.

zur Hausen H: Intracellular Surveillance of Persisting Viral Infections: Human Genital Cancer Results From Deficient Cellular Control of Papillomavirus Gene Expression. *Lancet* (ii): 489–491, 1986.

zur Hausen H: Papillomaviruses in Human Cancer. *Appl Pathol* 5: 19–24, 1987.

7

Respiratory Cytology

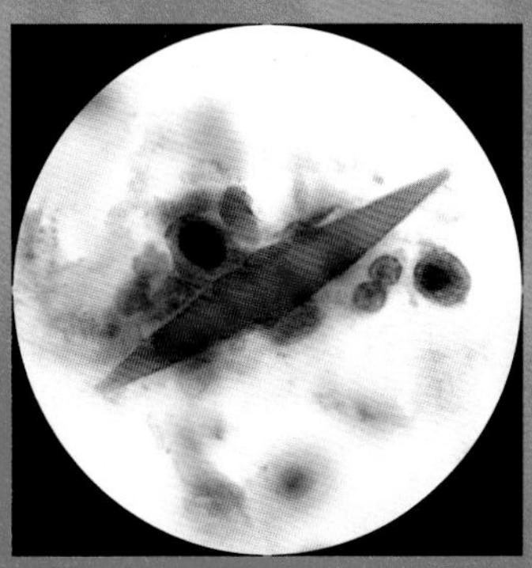

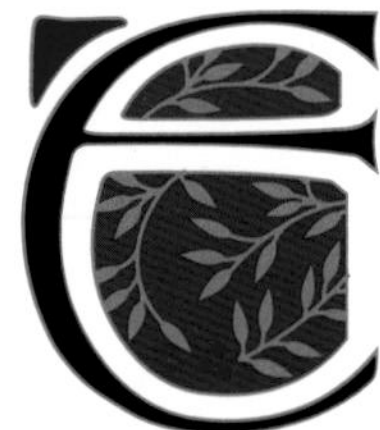

Extending from the nose to the alveoli, the respiratory system is divided into upper and lower portions. The upper respiratory system consists of the nasal cavities, sinuses, mouth, pharynx, and larynx. The lower respiratory system consists of the trachea, bronchi, bronchioles, and alveoli.

There are two basic types of epithelium that line the respiratory system—nonkeratinizing stratified squamous epithelium and respiratory epithelium. The squamous epithelium is essentially identical to that of the uterine cervix. Normal respiratory epithelium is composed primarily of pseudostratified, ciliated columnar cells, each attached to the basement membrane. There is also a variable component of mucous cells and a small component of reserve cells as well as Kulchitsky cells and other rare cell types.

The stratified squamous epithelium lines the anterior nasal cavity, the mouth, the oropharynx, pharynx, epiglottis (upper portion), and the vocal cords. The respiratory epithelium lines most of the nasal cavity, the nasal sinuses, nasopharynx, part of the larynx, and the tracheobronchial tree out to the alveoli (which are lined with their own special cells). Cells from any of these areas can be found in the sputum.

Respiratory cytology is primarily concerned with diseases of the lower respiratory tract. For general diagnostic purposes, the lower respiratory tract is further subdivided into central and peripheral portions. The central portion consists of the trachea and major bronchi (visible through a rigid bronchoscope) and the peripheral portion consists of all the rest (minor bronchi to alveoli).

Exfoliative Respiratory Cytology

Exfoliative respiratory cytology has a long history [Grunze 1960, Johnston 1986]. It includes both sputum and bronchial cytology, but not aspiration biopsy (which is discussed in Chapter 20) [Foot 1952, Herbut 1946, Spjut 1955]. Bronchial cytology includes bronchial brushing and washing. Additional morphologic methods of studying the respiratory tract include bronchoalveolar lavage (BAL) and bronchial biopsy. Exfoliative cytology can also be employed to diagnose lesions of the upper respiratory tract [Druce 1992, Granados 1994, Lee 1993, Lundgren 1981].

Diagnostic Triad

1. Sputum (3 to 5 early morning specimens)
2. Bronchial cytology
   - Bronchial washing
   - Bronchial brushing
3. Postbronchoscopy sputum

Compared with the remarkable success of the Pap smear in detecting and preventing cervical cancer, respiratory cytology (mostly sputum) has been a disappointment as a mass screening test for lung cancer. The problem is not lack of accuracy (sensitivity or specificity), but rather that even in high-risk patients (such as

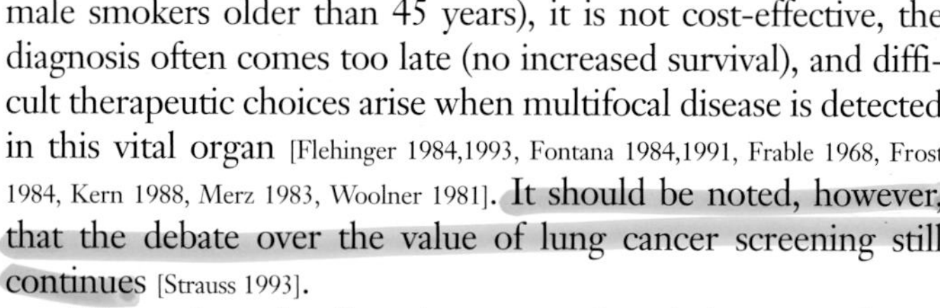

male smokers older than 45 years), it is not cost-effective, the diagnosis often comes too late (no increased survival), and difficult therapeutic choices arise when multifocal disease is detected in this vital organ [Flehinger 1984,1993, Fontana 1984,1991, Frable 1968, Frost 1984, Kern 1988, Merz 1983, Woolner 1981]. It should be noted, however, that the debate over the value of lung cancer screening still continues [Strauss 1993].

The major role of respiratory cytology is in tumor detection, confirmation, and typing of both primary and metastatic disease. It can also be useful in posttherapeutic monitoring of patients with lung cancer [Korfhage 1986], as a complementary procedure to radiologic examinations. In addition, respiratory cytology can be useful in diagnosing a variety of benign diseases, and plays an important role in assessing the presence of opportunistic infections in immunocompromised hosts such as patients with AIDS and transplant recipients [DeFine 1987, Kyriazis 1993, Miles 1990, Selvaggi 1992, Strigle 1989, Walts 1991, Weiss 1991].

The diagnostic sensitivity of respiratory cytology depends on several factors, including time and method of collection, number of samples submitted, and tumor cell type, as well as size and location of the lesion. False-negative results are associated with improper specimen collection, sampling error, peripheral location, small tumor size, misinterpretation, too few specimens, tumor obstruction of bronchus, small cell or metastatic carcinomas, or benign tumors.

Diagnostic specificity is also influenced by various factors, including necrosis, variable differentiation, inflammation, state of preservation [R Gupta 1982], or lack of clinical history. False-positive diagnoses may be associated with atypical squamous metaplasia, cellular repair/regeneration, or atypical glandular cells. Atypical cells mimicking malignancy can be seen in pneumonia, including tuberculosis; pulmonary infarcts; or chronic irritation (eg, bronchiectasis, chronic bronchitis, asthma, abscess, diffuse alveolar damage, interstitial lung disease, vasculitis, radiation and chemotherapy, air pollution, and tracheostomy stomas) [Cahan 1966, Caya 1984,1985, Jay 1980, Johnston 1976,1982,1986, Lukeman 1973, Nunez 1966, Teir 1963, Truong 1985]. Be particularly cautious when diagnosing lung cancer in patients with necrotizing pneumonia—the two diseases seldom coexist [Jay 1980]. Dysplasia and carcinoma in situ may be difficult to distinguish from invasive cancer. Also bear in mind that an apparent "false-positive" result could be due to occult cancer ("false false-positive").

Some Factors Affecting Diagnostic Reliability

Number of Specimens

Three satisfactory sputum specimens will detect, on average, about 60% of cases of lung cancer [Böcking 1992]. Three bronchial cytologic specimens can detect up to 90% of cases [Popp 1992]. Of the tumors that can be diagnosed with routine exfoliative respiratory cytology (ie, sputum and bronchial cytology), roughly half to three quarters of cases will be diagnosed on the first specimen, another 15% to 20% on the second, and about 10% on the third [Johnston 1981a, Popp 1992]. Few additional lung cancers will be detected after five consecutive specimens have been found to be negative [Risse 1985]. Unfortunately, a single specimen is so unreliable in diagnosing even advanced cancer, that as many as every other patient with cancer in a screening program could be given a falsely reassuring benign diagnosis [Grunze 1973]. In summary, the optimum number of respiratory cytology specimens is three to five.

Location of Tumor

Both bronchial and sputum cytology are able to detect central tumors in a high proportion of cases. The more peripheral the tumor, the fewer the diagnostic cells that will be found in the sputum and the more difficult the cells are to obtain bronchoscopically [Böcking 1992]. However, bronchial cytology is generally superior to sputum cytology in the diagnosis of peripheral lesions.

Size of Tumor

There is a rough correlation between the size of the tumor and the number of diagnostic cells—the larger the tumor, the more cells, and therefore, the more likely that the lesion can be diagnosed by cytologic methods [Tanaka 1985]. Similarly, higher-stage (ie, more advanced) tumors are more likely to be diagnosable cytologically [Böcking 1992]. Smaller tumors (eg, T_1) may not exfoliate sufficient numbers of cells to make a diagnosis. Paradoxically, however, sometimes large tumors can actually be more difficult to diagnose than smaller ones. For example, a large tumor can cause obstruction of the bronchus, resulting in a decreased harvest of malignant cells in the sputum or via the bronchoscope. Also, large tumors may yield only necrotic debris. Thus, there may be an optimum tumor size for diagnosis [Pilotti 1982a], roughly between 3 to 6 cm [Koss 1964, Ng 1983a].

Type of Tumor and Degree of Differentiation

Cell type influences both diagnostic sensitivity and specificity [Böcking 1992]. Squamous cell carcinomas, particularly of the well-differentiated or keratinizing type, and small cell carcinomas are the most accurately classified primary lung cancers [Barbazza 1992, Liang 1989, Suprun 1980, Truong 1985]. Bronchioloalveolar carcinoma (BAC) and adenosquamous carcinoma are among the least commonly detected and least accurately classified lung carcinomas, while adenocarcinoma and large cell carcinoma fall in between [Ng 1983a,1983b]. Of major clinical importance, the accuracy of bronchial cytology in distinguishing small cell carcinoma from non–small cell carcinoma approaches 100% [Barbazza 1992]. However, sputum cytology may misclassify a few cases of small cell carcinoma [MacDougall 1992].

In general, sputum cytology is more reliable for squamous cell carcinoma, while bronchial cytology is more reliable for adenocarcinoma. Metastatic cancer is usually diagnosed at a lower rate than primary lung cancer [Hattori 1971, Risse 1985, Truong 1985]. Also, exfoliative respiratory cytology may be unreliable in the diagnosis of benign tumors because of submucosal growth or failure to shed diagnostic cells.

Due to decreased intercellular cohesion, poorly differentiated tumors tend to shed more cells than well-differentiated tumors. Thus, poorly differentiated carcinoma may be more readily detected than well-differentiated cancers, cytologically. There may also be some discrepancies between the cytologic and the histologic grading of a tumor. For example, since exfoliative cytology is primarily surface cytology, better differentiated surface cells may be found cytologically in a tumor whose main mass is less differentiated [Reid 1961]. This is particularly likely in squamous cell carcinoma. On the other hand, a poorly differentiated component of an otherwise well-differentiated tumor may preferentially exfoliate cells, giving a misleading impression of the overall degree of differentiation. Finally, tumors are well known to be inhomogeneous, and sampling can be a problem in any biopsy.

Histology-Cytology Diagnostic Discrepancies

1. Differences in cell cohesion
2. Surface differentiation
3. Deep cells fail to shed
4. Tumor inhomogeneity

Diagnostic Respiratory Cytology

Using strict diagnostic criteria, false-positive cytologic diagnoses are rare. Patients can be treated on the basis of the cytologic diagnosis, without tissue confirmation, *in the appropriate clinical setting* [Caya 1988,1990, Erozan 1970, Hsu 1983, Oswald 1971, Yoneyama 1978]. With satisfactory specimens, the overall sensitivity (tumor finding) and specificity (tumor typing) of sputum and bronchial cytology (brushings, washings) are each about 70% to 80%. Under optimum conditions (increased number of submitted specimens, optimum tumor size, favorable location, etc), the sensitivity and specificity can be as high as 90%, or even better. However, a certain proportion of lung cancers do not yield diagnostic cells and therefore cannot be diagnosed with exfoliative respiratory cytology (in such cases, try fine needle aspiration biopsy).

Sputum and bronchial cytology are complementary; both types of specimens are necessary for maximum diagnostic sensitivity [Erozan 1970, Hsu 1983, Johnston 1981a]. The diagnostic accuracy of bronchial cytology compares favorably with bronchial biopsy [Fry 1970, Kvale 1976, Koss 1964, Naryshkin 1992, Skitarelic 1974]. Combining bronchial biopsy and cytology may pick up additional cases, giving optimal diagnostic sensitivity [Chaudhary 1978, Kvale 1976, Mak 1990, Naryshkin 1992]. However, bronchial biopsy is not without potential hazards, including pneumothorax and hemorrhage [Herf 1978, Meyer 1961]. Cytology can be a helpful adjunct to histology in classification of lung tumors [Gagneten 1976].

Sputum cytology is the most sensitive technique for finding cases of small cell carcinoma, but is the most specific in cytotyping squamous cell carcinoma [T7.1]. Bronchial brushing is most sensitive to the presence of squamous cell carcinoma, but most specific for cytotyping small cell carcinomas and adenocarcinomas. Bronchial washing does not add much sensitivity, but may help in tumor typing (specificity) [Bibbo 1973].

Summary of Conditions for Specimen Adequacy

Sputum
- Numerous alveolar macrophages
- The adequacy of a sputum sample is directly proportional to the number of alveolar macrophages it contains [Greenberg 1983].
- "Bronchial" cells are insufficient evidence of adequacy.

Bronchial washing/brushing
- Numerous bronchial cells

Bronchoalveolar lavage
- Abundant alveolar macrophages
- Squamous cells should be few in bronchial brushing/washing or bronchoalveolar lavage.

Note: The above are necessary, but not sufficient, conditions of specimen adequacy. Of course, the specimen must also be submitted with all relevant clinical history, properly fixed and prepared, etc, to be satisfactory for evaluation.

Sputum

Sputum is composed predominantly of mucus, but also contains a number of cellular and noncellular components [Johnston 1986]. Significant spontaneous sputum production indicates that pulmonary disease is present. Most smokers, as well as many patients with bronchogenic carcinoma, have a cough and can produce sputum. Increased numbers of macrophages, with increased pigmentation and enzymatic activity, neutrophils, Curschmann's spirals, and epithelial cells, including metaplastic and dysplastic cells, have also been found in reaction to smoking and particulate air pollution [Athanassiadou 1995, Mylius 1986, Roby 1991, Swan 1991, Wehle 1988]. Elevations of these cytologic indices may be associated with abnormal lung function [Swan 1994].

Sputum is the most readily accessible specimen for pulmonary cytology [T7.2]. Sputum diagnosis is optimum in patients spontaneously producing sputum, especially when it is bloody [Risse 1987b]. For patients not producing sputum, a sputum sample can be induced (eg, by having patients breath either a nebulized solution of 15% saline, with or without 20% propylene glycol, or plain 3% to 8% saline heated to 115°F) [Sproul 1962]. Cytologic examination of an induced sputum specimen can be effective in the diagnosis of lung cancer [Khajotia 1991]. However, sputum cytology, even with an induced specimen, may not be useful in diagnosing asymptomatic patients, especially those with a peripheral "coin" lesion [Koss 1964]. Screening high-risk patients for cancer using chest x-rays and sputum cytology can detect resectable disease, particularly squamous cell carcinoma [Cortese 1992]. Patients with adenocarcinoma or small cell carcinoma in the sputum have a poor 5-year survival, even when bronchoscopic findings are negative [Miura 1992]. Unfortunately, as previously mentioned, chest radiography and sputum cytology are probably not cost-effective screening procedures for lung cancer. (The truth is, screening cannot overcome the consequences of smoking.)

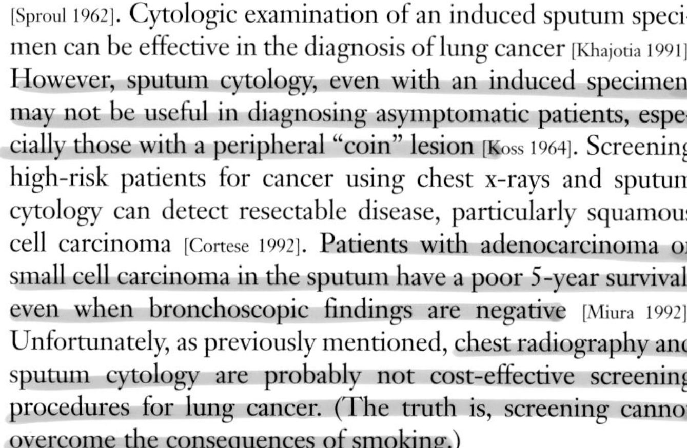

To look for cancer in (spontaneous) sputum specimens, it is best to examine morning pooled secretion. The optimum number of specimens to submit to diagnose cancer is three, and to exclude cancer is five. Using five specimens, the detection rate (sensitivity) can be as high as 90% to 95% [Erozan 1974, Koss 1964]. The sensitivity of the technique depends on the tumor type, ranging from most to least sensitive—squamous cell carcinoma ≥ small cell carcinoma > large cell carcinoma ≥ adenocarcinoma > metastatic carcinoma. Central tumors are more readily detected by sputum cytology [Koss 1964], although not every study has shown a significant difference between central and peripheral tumor location [Jay 1980, Pilotti 1982a]. In cytotyping by sputum cytology, the range from most to least specific is—small cell carcinoma > squamous cell carcinoma > adenocarcinoma > large cell carcinoma.

T7.1 **Sensitivity and Specificity of the Three Diagnostic Cytologic Procedures***

Method	Most Sensitive to	Most Specific for
Sputum	Squamous, small cell carcinomas	Squamous cell carcinomas
Bronchial washing	Squamous cell carcinomas	Squamous, small cell carcinomas
Bronchial brushing	Squamous cell carcinomas	Small cell, adenocarcinoma

* The sensitivity of the three procedures for the diagnosis of adenocarcinoma is about equal. In fact, the overall performance of sputum cytology, bronchial washing, and bronchial brushing are about equal, but complementary.

T7.2 **Sputum Cytology**

Advantages	Disadvantages
Easily obtained, if spontaneous	Difficult to obtain if not spontaneous
Extensive area sampled	Cannot localize lesion
Good for central tumors	Poor for peripheral tumors
Malignant tumors amenable to diagnosis	Benign tumors difficult to diagnose
Accurate diagnosis, especially squamous and small cell carcinomas	Less accurate for adenocarcinoma, metastases, lymphoma
Best screening test	

Saccomanno Blender vs "Pick-and-Smear" Techniques

Whether the Saccomanno or the "pick-and-smear" sputum preparatory method is more sensitive and specific is controversial [Perlman 1989, Rizzo 1990].

For the pick-and-smear technique, fresh specimens are preferred. If a significant delay in processing is unavoidable, 50% to 70% ethanol fixation can be used. However, alcohol does not penetrate mucus well, thus trapped cells may not be well fixed. Also, alcohol coagulates mucus, making it difficult to smear the specimen. Finally, alcohol may cause significant shrinkage of the cells, making cytologic evaluation more difficult. The specimen should be inspected for strands or flecks of dense or bloody material, which is selected for smearing [Chodosh 1970].

The Saccomanno technique collects cells in 50% ethanol and 2% polyethylene glycol (Carbowax). Then, using a blender, the specimen is broken up, centrifuged, and smears prepared. When properly performed, the Saccomanno method also specifies that direct smears should be made of blood-flecked material [Saccomanno 1963]. The Saccomanno method concentrates cells and may yield a higher number of diagnostic cells than the pick-and-smear technique [Rizzo 1990, Saccomanno 1963]. The Saccomanno technique can be particularly useful in diagnosing premalignant lesions [Rizzo 1990]. Small cell carcinoma may be easier to diagnose in the pick-and-smear samples, since the small tumor cells are dispersed by the blender, making them difficult to detect in screening [Perlman 1989]. Tissue fragments, fungal hyphae, and secretory vacuoles may also be disrupted using the Saccomanno technique. In addition, problems with infection of laboratory personnel, due to aerosolization of infectious agents, have occurred with the Saccomanno technique.

Postbronchoscopy Sputum

The postbronchoscopy sputum specimen may have the highest diagnostic rate of any respiratory cytology specimen [Jay 1980]. It may be the only positive specimen when preceding sputum, bronchial washing, or brushing samples are all negative [Bender 1985, Chaudhary 1978, Chopra 1977], although the added sensitivity may in part be a function of submitting an extra specimen [Risse 1987b]. The postbronchoscopy sputum specimen not only has the highest sensitivity, it is also equally sensitive to central and peripheral lesions, and for all tumor cell types [Jay 1980]. (In contrast, ordinary sputum is better for central lesions and squamous cell type [Risse 1987a].) It may be that the cells are loosened up by the bronchoscopic procedure, freeing them to be coughed up. Postbronchoscopy sputum analysis is more likely to be helpful in patients with obstructive ventilatory defects and in patients without a history of prior sputum production [Risse 1987b]. (A word of caution: postbronchoscopy sputum specimens may contain degenerated bronchial cells whose atypia may be mistaken for neoplasia.)

Bronchial Cytology: Bronchial Brushing and Washing

The most frequent indications for bronchoscopy include cough, hemoptysis, tumor on chest x-ray, bronchial obstruction, atelectasis, and localized wheezes. Any of these can be produced by inflammation, foreign bodies, or tumors [Landa 1978]. Particularly ominous are persisting infiltrates, or hilar or parenchymal (especially peripheral) lung mass on chest x-ray, and hemoptysis associated with a lung mass or infiltrate [Janower 1971, Jay 1980].

Patients with abnormal sputum cytology should undergo bronchoscopy. Bronchial cytology is useful for peripheral lung lesions [Chopra 1977, Fennessy 1970]. Bronchoscopy is also useful in diagnosing patients with central lesions and at least three negative sputum specimens, who also have severe diffuse lung disease, evidence of inoperability, or other risk factors precluding surgery [Solomon 1974]. For very peripheral tumors or pleural-based lesions, which may not be reachable by bronchoscopy and in which sputum cytology is negative, fine needle aspiration biopsy may be indicated. Blind sampling in the absence of bronchoscopic findings rarely yields diagnostic material [Pilotti 1982b]. The various diagnostic cytologic procedures are complementary [T7.3, T7.4] [Johnston 1988b].

Bronchial brushing has a higher diagnostic yield (increased sensitivity) than either bronchial washing or sputum cytology for metastatic carcinoma, peripheral tumors, and large, necrotic cancers [Truong 1985]. Bronchial washing may allow typing of some tumors that could not be typed by bronchial brushing (increased cytotyping specificity) [Bibbo 1973]. Although repeated bronchial cytology specimens are rarely submitted by clinicians, when initial bronchial cytologic findings are negative, it is recommended to repeat the bronchial cytology rather than rely on sputum cytology [Solomon 1974]. Overall sensitivity of bronchial brushing is about 70% but depends on tumor cell type, ranging from most to least sensitive—squamous cell carcinoma > large cell carcinoma > small cell carcinoma > adenocarcinoma > metastatic carcinoma [Bibbo 1973]. The diagnostic sensitivity increases from about 70% to about 90% when two specimens instead of one are submitted [Ng 1983a,1983b].

T7.3 **Bronchial Cytology**

Advantages	Disadvantages
Can localize lesions, establish spread, and diagnose diffuse disease	Time consuming, unpleasant, some morbidity, not for screening
Accurate diagnosis of malignant tumors	Benign tumors less amenable to diagnosis
Good for both central and peripheral tumors	Very peripheral may not be diagnosable
Smaller tumors can be diagnosed	Limited area sampled

T7.4 **Fine Needle Aspiration Biopsy**

Advantages	Disadvantages
Can diagnose otherwise unreachable areas, eg, pancoast tumor, extrabronchial lesions	Bleeding, pneumothorax, etc
Very peripheral, small tumors amenable to diagnosis	Central tumors not easily reached
Benign tumors, metastases, lymphoma amenable to diagnosis	Diffuse diseases and very large tumors may be less amenable to diagnosis

Bronchoalveolar Lavage

BAL specimens are obtained by wedging a subsegmental bronchus with the bronchoscope and lavaging the area with saline or balanced salt solution. BAL has been particularly useful in diagnosis of opportunistic infections in immunocompromised hosts (eg, patients with AIDS or transplants). It is also used to help diagnose interstitial lung disease, granulomatous disease, including sarcoid, hypersensitivity pneumonia, drug-induced pulmonary toxicity, asbestosis, pulmonary hemorrhage, and cancer (particularly helpful when peripherally located) [Crystal 1976,1981,1984, de Gracia 1993, Fleury-Feith 1987, Haslam 1980, Huang 1989, Hunninghake 1979, Levy 1988, Linder 1987, Pirozynski 1992, Poletti 1995, Ramirez-R 1965, Saltini 1984, Springmeyer 1987, Stoller 1987, Studdy 1984, Taskinen 1992, Weinberger 1978]. BAL can also be useful in evaluation of transplant rejection [Prior 1992, Selvaggi 1992, Walts 1991].

In a BAL specimen, it is important to look for fungus, *Pneumocystis*, virus, hemosiderin-laden macrophages, and atypical or malignant cells [Stover 1984]. A portion of the material should also be submitted for culture.

BAL can help to separate inflammatory processes in which lymphocytes predominate (eg, sarcoid, hypersensitivity pneumonia including drug reaction, berylliosis) from those in which neutrophils or macrophages predominate (eg, idiopathic pulmonary fibrosis, cytotoxic drug reaction, Langerhans' histiocytosis) [Daniele 1985, Huang 1989]. Hemosiderin-laden macrophages are useful in diagnosing occult pulmonary hemorrhage (except during the acute phase), but are also seen in association with infection [Perez-Arellano 1992, Stover 1984]. The sensitivity of BAL in diagnosing lung cancer compares favorably to transbronchial biopsy and Wang needle aspiration, being positive in about two thirds of cases (68.6%) [Linder 1987]. The overall specificity is similar to other types of bronchial specimens, nearly 80% [Linder 1987].

Imprint Cytology

Imprint cytology of forceps tissue biopsies can be performed at the time of flexible fiberoptic bronchoscopy. Imprint cytology of the tissue sample increases the diagnostic sensitivity of the procedure. The sensitivity when all three (brush, biopsy, imprint) methods are used together may be as high as 97%; the specificity approaches 100% [Popp 1991].

Pulmonary Microvascular Cytology

Pulmonary microvascular cytology is the examination of a blood sample drawn through a wedged pulmonary artery catheter to diagnose lymphatic carcinomatosis. The blood must be collected in a heparinized tube. In the laboratory, the specimen is placed on a Ficoll-Hypaque gradient to remove the blood and concentrate diagnostic cells [Abati 1994]. Megakaryocytes, which are present in the capillary bed, are the hallmark of a satisfactory sample and should not be mistaken for tumor cells [Masson 1989].

Cell Blocks

Cytologic detail in cell blocks is inferior to that in smears. Although architectural arrangements may be more obvious in cell blocks than in smears, this seldom aids in the diagnosis [Flint 1993]. Cell blocks generally do not add much to cytologic diagnosis, but do add to the expense, and are time-consuming to prepare [Jay 1980, Johnston 1986]. However, cell blocks are sometimes positive when smears are negative [Flint 1993], and some authors report good results with this method [Böcking 1992]. Preparation of cell blocks is usually not recommended as a routine procedure, although they can be useful for processing coagulated specimens or when the use of a battery of special stains is anticipated.

The Cells

Sputum and bronchial cytology are similar in many ways and different in others. In essence, although the overall morphology is similar, the cells of bronchial cytology appear "fresher" [Hattori 1971]. Cells obtained in bronchial washings and brushings are better preserved, more numerous, more cohesive, and larger than those obtained in sputum cytology, and the lesions can be localized [Zaharopoulos 1982]. In contrast, the cells obtained in sputum cytology are usually less well-preserved, fewer, smaller, and more single, compared with those obtained in bronchial cytology, and lesions cannot be localized [T7.5]. Cells from squamous cell carcinoma in sputum are usually more

T7.5 **Differences Between Sputum Cytology and Bronchial Brushing**

	Sputum	Bronchial Brushing
Background	Dirty	Clean
Cell Arrangement	More single cells	More clusters
Cells	Fewer, smaller, degenerated	More, larger, better preserved
Cytoplasm	Well defined	Poorly defined
Chromatin	Clumped	More open

keratinized (differentiated) than those found in bronchial washing or brushing specimens of the same tumor. All cell types of bronchogenic carcinoma tend to appear less mature in bronchial brushing specimens [Bedrossian 1976]. Papillary groups from adenocarcinoma are more likely to be found in sputum cytology than in bronchial brushing or washing. As a general rule, the presence of single cells is required to diagnose malignancy. However, occasionally single cells may not be apparent in bronchial brushings of malignant tumors.

The sputum and bronchial cytology of the various tissues and lesions will be presented together. Different cytologic appearances, if any, will be discussed in the following presentation.

Squamous Cells

Squamous cells are more common in sputum specimens than in bronchial washings/brushings, in which they should be sparse or absent. Most squamous cells come from the mouth, as contaminants. Patients should at least rinse their mouths (and preferably also brush their teeth) before expectorating. The cytologic appearance of the squamous cells in respiratory cytology is essentially identical to their appearance in the Pap smear. There is usually a predominance of superficial cells. Anucleate squames and intermediate cells may also be found. Benign pearls [1 I7.1] and occasionally spindle squamous cells may be seen. Degenerative changes are common.

Squamous cells originating in the mouth often show mild cytologic atypia. These atypical squamous cells can cause a problem in diagnosis. Although benign, they may suggest dysplasia or even very well-differentiated keratinizing squamous cell carcinoma. Furthermore, it is impossible to determine with certainty, by cytologic criteria alone, whether a cancer originated in the lung, pharynx, or mouth (see also "Squamous Metaplasia," p220).

Glandular Cells

The tracheobronchial tree is lined with a pseudostratified glandular epithelium composed predominantly of ciliated columnar and mucous goblet cells. The purpose of this epithelium is garbage disposal, ie, to clear debris from the airways. Mucous cells secrete a sheet of sticky mucus that, like fly paper, traps particulate matter such as dust. Ciliated cells propel the mucus along the airways, like a conveyer belt, away from the alveoli. Usually there are about 5 to 10 ciliated cells for every mucous goblet cell in the bronchi, with fewer goblet cells in the trachea. The proportion also varies depending on the presence of certain irritants or diseases.

1

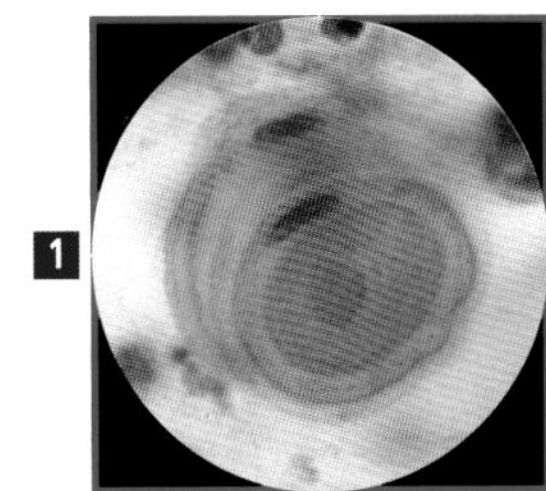

2

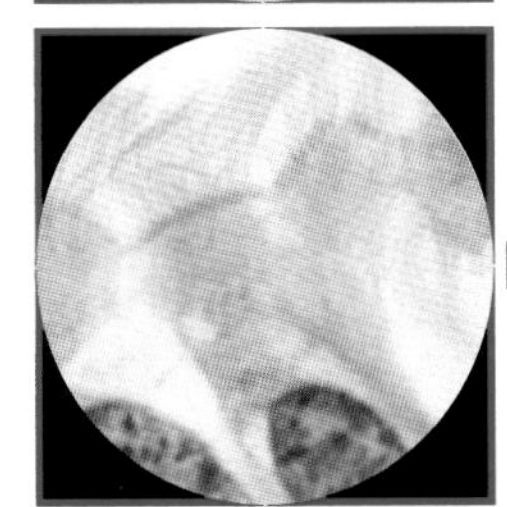

3

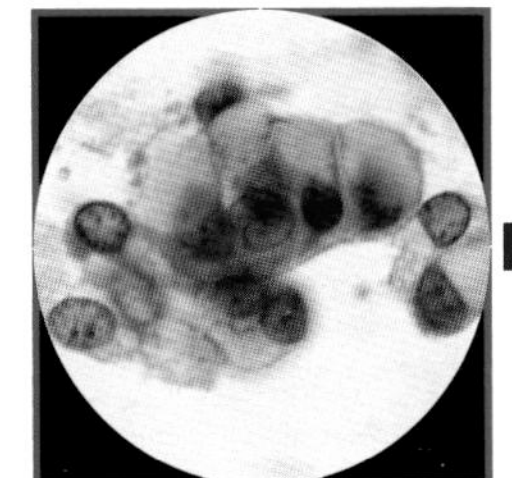

Ciliated Columnar Cells

Except in postbronchoscopy specimens, ciliated columnar cells are few in sputum samples but common in bronchial washing/brushing samples. In bronchial washing/brushing specimens, ciliated cells are frequently found singly and in sheets that may show honeycombing. The most characteristic cytologic feature is, of course, the presence of cilia on the apical surface, anchored into a terminal bar or plate [2 I7.2]. Cilia usually stain bright red, and the terminal bar is seen as a distinct thickening of the apical border of the cell, which may stain red. Tiny red granules, basal bodies, may also be appreciated in the terminal bar. At the basal surface, the ciliated cells often have a slender tail by which they were anchored to the basement membrane.

The cytoplasm is usually basophilic and homogeneous, although pigment granules may be present. The nuclei are round to oval. The relative position of the nucleus in the cell varies during the menstrual cycle in women (nuclei migrate north during the cycle, then return south), but remains constant in men and older women [Chalon 1971]. The chromatin can be fine, but often appears somewhat hyperchromatic and moderately coarse. However, it is regularly distributed and the nuclear membrane is generally smooth. Rarely, intranuclear cytoplasmic invaginations can be seen. Small nucleoli may be present, which increase in prominence when the cells are irritated or reactive.

Cilia are relatively hearty. Loss of cilia indicates bronchial irritation, including thermal injury [Ambiavagar 1974] or dry anesthesia [Chalon 1974b].

Goblet Cells

Goblet cells are not often identified in sputum, in which they degenerate rapidly. However, they are commonly observed in bronchial washing/brushing specimens, often in clusters or sheets, together with ciliated cells, in a ratio of about one goblet cell for every 5 to 10 ciliated cells. In bronchial washing/brushing specimens, goblet cells have a relatively abundant, finely vacuolated, slightly basophilic, delicate cytoplasm filled with mucus [3 I7.3]. Hypersecretory forms may occur. The nuclei are uniform and basally located. Naked nuclei are common, because these cells degenerate readily. Mucous goblet cells are more numerous in asthma, chronic bronchitis, bronchiectasis, and allergies. When mucus cells are abundant, mucinous bronchioloalveolar carcinoma must be excluded.

Clara Cells

Clara cells are nonciliated bronchiolar cells named for an early investigator. They secrete a protein that acts as a clarificant to clear the airways, a function similar to mucus. This protein, possibly related to surfactant, is less sticky than mucus, which is important because some bronchioles collapse on expiration and sticky mucus would interfere with their reinflation [P Smith 1974]. Clara cells become more numerous distally in the bronchi, whereas goblet cells decrease in number. Clara cells are difficult to appreciate without special studies.

Reserve Cells

Reserve cells are small, round, lymphocyte-like cells with central, hyperchromatic nuclei. They can only be specifically identified in clusters. Reserve cells are usually scarce in sputum, but may be seen in reserve cell hyperplasia. In bronchial brushings, reserve cells can also be seen with ulceration associated with acute bronchitis or due to vigorous abrasion of the mucosa with the brush.

Bronchial Irritation Cells

When bronchial cells are irritated due to various infections or toxins, including cigarette smoke, as well as chronic tracheobronchial disease, and recent instrumentation, they can undergo reactive/reparative changes, become atypical or multinucleated [4 I7.4], or lose their cilia (ciliocytophthoria) [5 I7.5] [Chalon 1975, Johnston 1976,1986, Nasiell 1967,1968, Plamenac 1969,1970,1972,1973,1974,1979].

Benign, Reactive Atypia

Benign respiratory cells can undergo reactive changes reminiscent of those seen in endocervical cells in the Pap smear [Kinsella 1959]. Reactive atypia includes enlarged, pleomorphic nuclei, with abnormally coarse, dark chromatin, and prominent nucleoli. Reactive changes are more frequently seen in bronchial washing/brushing specimens than in sputum. In contrast with cancer, benign cells usually have good intercellular cohesion, with fewer single cells. There is a range of atypia in benign conditions, whereas in malignancies, there is usually a discrete population of abnormal cells.

A key diagnostic point is that when a cell is ciliated, it is almost certainly benign, with only very rare exceptions (such as a

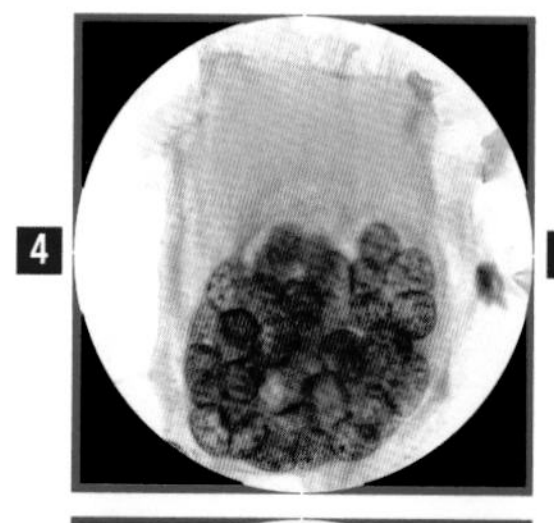
4

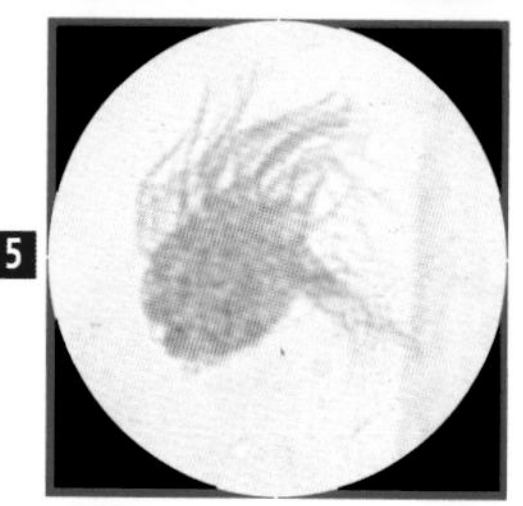
5

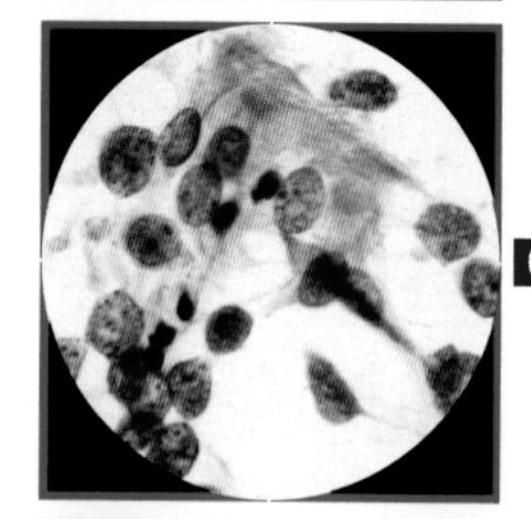
6

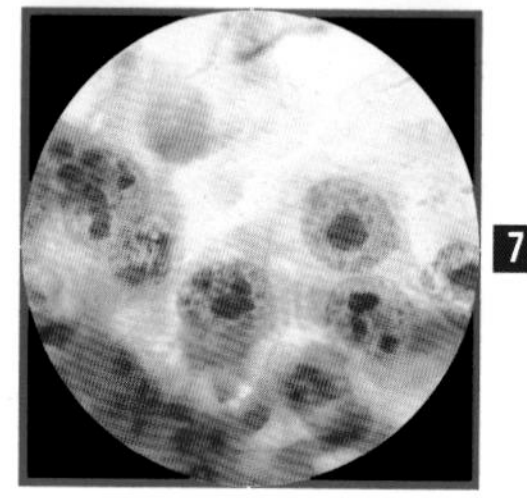
7

rare case of metastatic ovarian carcinoma [P Gupta 1985]). However, cilia can degenerate quickly, leaving only a terminal bar (see also "Ciliocytophthoria"). Although the presence of a terminal bar still suggests a benign process, terminal bar–like apical borders can be seen in certain malignancies (particularly colorectal carcinoma, but also including primary lung cancer, especially bronchioloalveolar carcinoma). With further degeneration, the cells may lose their cytoplasm altogether, leaving only naked nuclei. Never unequivocally diagnose cancer based only on naked nuclei. Another caveat is that cancer can grow underneath a benign epithelium. Therefore, groups of malignant cells may be exfoliated, which are covered on one surface by benign ciliated cells, giving the false impression that the malignant cells are ciliated. Small cell carcinoma is particularly likely to do this [6 I7.68].

Multinucleation

Multinucleation is a very common, nonspecific reaction of bronchial cells to stress (eg, inflammation, infection, toxic gas/fumes, radiation, or chemotherapy). It can occur as a response to instrumentation, air pollution, or other irritants [Shroff 1988]. Multinucleation of bronchial cells has also been described as a "malignancy-associated change," in patients with a wide variety of malignancies not necessarily involving the lung, including colon, breast, female genital tract, and stomach carcinomas [Chalon 1974a,1976,1978].

Multinucleated bronchial cells maintain their basic shape, usually with terminal bars and often cilia [4 I7.4]. The nuclei are more or less basally oriented. The number of nuclei can vary from two to dozens. Highly nucleated cells are probably the result of cell fusion. Although the nuclei may be slightly variable, they maintain their family resemblance, or sibling image (ie, they more or less look alike).

Regenerative/Reparative Bronchial Cells

Regeneration/repair in bronchial cells is similar to that seen in the Pap smear [Saito 1988]. It is a nonspecific response to various noxious stimuli. Cytologic atypia can range from mild to bizarre, and can mimic cancer [7 I7.31]. The entire cell, including both nucleus and cytoplasm, enlarges, so that the nuclear/cytoplasmic (N/C) ratio remains within normal limits. Reparative cells form cohesive, relatively orderly, monolayered sheets, with adequate cytoplasm. Single reparative cells are absent or sparse. Although the nuclei may be remarkably enlarged and pleomorphic, with large, sometimes irregular, nucleoli, they are not crowded, piled up, or disorderly. The chromatin is usually fine, but the nuclei can degenerate and undergo karyopyknosis, karyorrhexis, or karyolysis. Some reparative cells may retain their cilia (almost always benign) or terminal bars (suggestive of a benign process). Transitional forms to ciliated columnar cells may be observed.

Ciliocytophthoria

Ciliocytophthoria refers to small ciliated tufts that appear to be broken-off tops of ciliated bronchial cells [8 I7.5] [Papanicolaou 1956]. Ciliocytophthoria occurs when bronchial cells are insulted or injured. Ciliocytophthoria is a cytopathic effect related to nonspecific injury/insults, including exposure to air pollution [Plamenac 1973], hot or dry air, and viral infections, particularly adenovirus [Kim 1964]. Ciliocytophthoria also occurs in other ciliated epithelia such as the endocervix. Do not mistake ciliocytophthoria for parasites; however, ciliocytophthoria is a warning that there may also be reactive atypia in the bronchial cells.

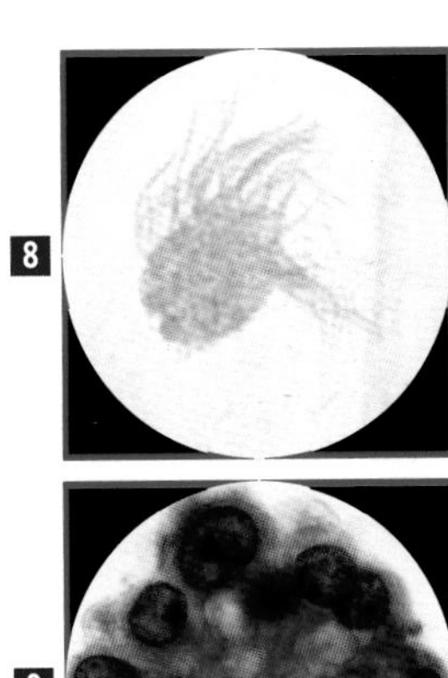
8

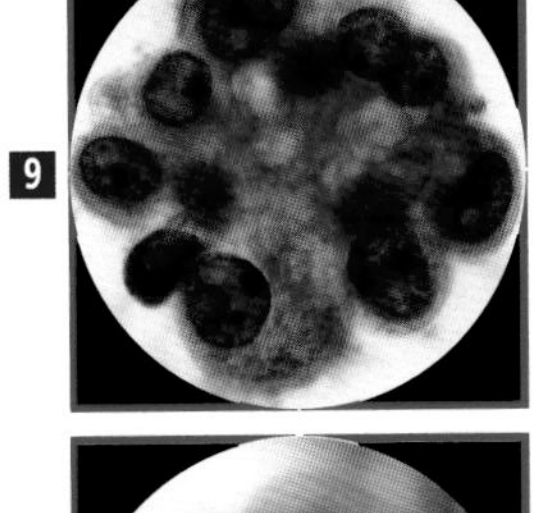
9

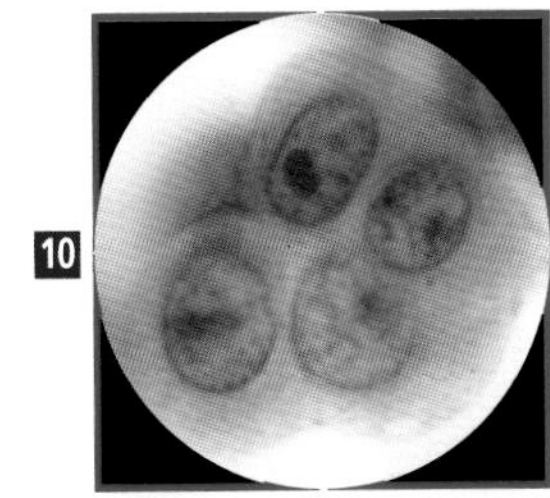
10

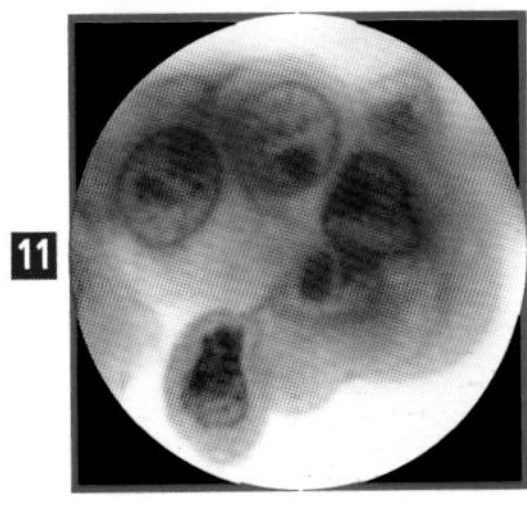
11

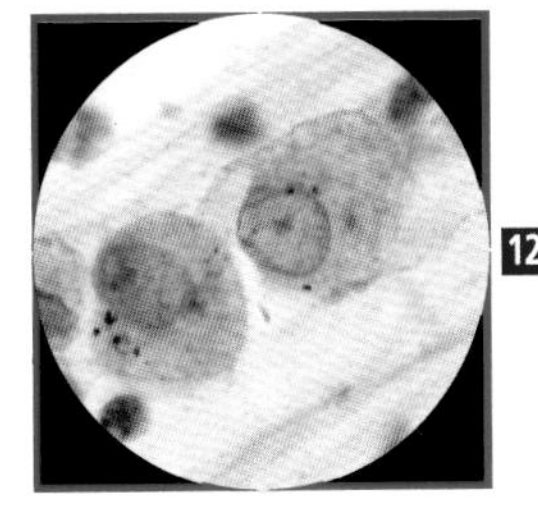
12

Pneumocytes

Type I and II Pneumocytes

Type I pneumocytes are flat (ie, squamous) cells with keratin and long cell processes that line 90% to 95% of the alveolus. Interspersed are type II pneumocytes, also known as granular pneumocytes, that produce surfactant. Ultrastructurally, surfactant granules are lysosomal-sized and laminated. Surfactant is a phospholipid, which acts like a detergent, and lowers surface tension, making it easier to inflate the balloon-like alveolus.

Reactive Pneumocytes

Type I and II pneumocytes are usually not specifically identified in respiratory cytology, unless hyperplastic and in groups [9 I7.6, 10 11 I7.7]. It is primarily the type II granular pneumocytes that proliferate when the lung is injured. Reactive pneumocytes are associated with numerous conditions, particularly pulmonary infarcts and viral infections, but also including other pulmonary injuries, such as pulmonary embolism, organizing pneumonia, pulmonary fibrosis, granulomatous disease including tuberculosis, silicosis, anthracosis, diffuse alveolar damage (also known as "adult respiratory distress syndrome"), congestive heart failure, oxygen toxicity, radiation/chemotherapy, burns, connective tissue diseases, and drug toxicity, such as amiodarone [Cooney 1972, Israel-Biet 1987, Martin 1985, Mermolja 1994, Stein 1987].

Reactive type II pneumocytes can mimic adenocarcinoma [Grotte 1990, Johnston 1992, Kern 1965, Wagner 1989]. They occur singly and in clusters. The cells have cyanophilic cytoplasm that ranges from finely vacuolated to distended by one or more large vacuoles. They show increased N/C ratios, angular or irregular nuclear membranes, chromatin clumping and clearing, and macronucleoli, and can be multinucleated. Pneumocytes usually lack cytoplasmic inclusions and can be associated with ciliated respiratory cells [Johnston 1992].

One of the key differential diagnostic points is that the benign atypical cells are usually sparse [Johnston 1992]. However, these cells can be seen in large numbers in conditions such as infarcts, drug toxicity, and viral infections.

The differential diagnosis primarily includes adenocarcinoma, particularly bronchioloalveolar carcinoma (BAC) [Johnston 1992]. BAC should only be diagnosed in the presence of numerous well-preserved cells. The cells of BAC always lack cilia and tend to form rounded ball-like clusters, with great depth of focus. Favoring a benign process are the following criteria: degenerated and fewer cells, *more* variability among groups than in BAC; lower N/C ratio; scalloped flower petal–like borders of clusters (vs community border); less depth of focus; intercellular windows [Grotte 1990]; and, of course, cilia, if present. Type II pneumocytes share the expression of several antigens with epithelial tumor cells, limiting the usefulness of these immunologic markers in differentiating between reactive and malignant cells [Guzman 1994].

Alveolar Macrophages

Alveolar macrophages, sometimes known as type III alveolar pneumocytes, free alveolar macrophages, or pulmonary alveolar macrophages, are mesenchymal rather than epithelial cells [12 I7.8]. They are bone marrow–derived histiocytes [E Thomas 1976]. Their job is to neutralize foreign material in the alveoli (where the ciliated and mucus-producing bronchial cells are not present). Consequently, a variety of substances can be found ingested by these cells.

Alveolar macrophages are key cells to look for in a sputum specimen. The presence of alveolar macrophages is a necessary, but not sufficient, condition for adequacy of a sputum specimen. Their presence indicates that at least some of the "deep lung" (ie, most peripheral, alveolar part) has been sampled. Ciliated respiratory cells (so-called "bronchial" cells) are insufficient evidence of a deep lung sample, because they could originate from as far away from the deep lung as the nasal passages. If a sputum specimen does not contain alveolar macrophages, it is considered to be only saliva (or spit) rather than sputum. Such a specimen is unsatisfactory for evaluation: it is not a "deep cough". On the other hand, however, the mere presence of alveolar macrophages may not be sufficient evidence for a high-quality specimen since these cells, in lower numbers, are consistently found in sputum specimens with a false-negative cytologic diagnosis [Risse 1987c].

A sputum specimen with the best chance for detecting cancer contains a relatively high proportion of alveolar macrophages. Although no specific minimum number of histiocytes is currently accepted as required for specimen adequacy, as many as 150 macrophages *per slide* in nonsmokers and 300 in smokers have been suggested [Roby 1990b, Schumann 1989]. The presence or absence of alveolar macrophages is not critical in determining the adequacy of bronchial washing/brushing or fine needle aspiration biopsies. However, in BAL specimens, macrophages should not only be present but abundant [Chamberlain 1987]. Alveolar macrophages occasionally also find their way to lymph nodes or effusions through lymphatics.

Alveolar macrophages are essentially identical to other histiocytes [Kern 1970]. Alveolar macrophages vary a great deal in size. They have round to oval or bean-shaped nuclei. They can be uninucleated, binucleated, or multinucleated. Multinucleated alveolar macrophages are found in increased numbers in sarcoid, tuberculosis, and other granulomatous diseases, but are not specific. The chromatin is characteristically "salt-and-pepper," but its texture is variable. One or more nucleoli may be present. The cytoplasm is foamy and stains basophilic to acidophilic to amphophilic. Cell borders may be indistinct or well defined. Occasionally, eosinophilic cytoplasmic processes may be observed [Walker 1971]. Characteristically, the cells are phagocytic and often contain various particles, like carbon (particularly in smokers). These cells are commonly named for the particles found in them.

Carbon Histiocytes

These are carbon-laden alveolar macrophages and are common in smokers and urban dwellers. They are the key cells to identify as one measure of adequacy of a sputum specimen. They are also known as "dust cells" (no mere "dust bunnies" in the corners of the lung) [13 I7.8].

Siderophages

In reaction to bleeding, these macrophages contain the blood pigment hemosiderin (that is, hemosiderin-laden macrophages) [14 I7.9, 15 I7.10]. There is an inverse relationship between the number of siderophages found in the sputum and cardiac index (also known as "heart failure cells" in the appropriate clinical setting) [Friedman-Mor 1978]. However, hemosiderin-laden macrophages are not specific for heart failure; any old hemorrhage will do, including hemorrhagic shock, pulmonary hemorrhage, cardiopulmonary bypass during open heart surgery, idiopathic pulmonary hemosiderosis, and Goodpasture's syndrome [Friedman-Mor 1977].

Lipophages

These are cells with lacy, bubbly cytoplasm due to lipid content. Lipid source can be exogenous (eg, oily nose drops) or endogenous (related to tissue destruction, eg, tuberculosis or cancer) [16 I7.11]. Lipid staining (eg, oil red O) of BAL specimens shows strong positivity in lipid pneumonia, and may be useful in confirming the diagnosis [I7.12] [Pickren 1971, Silverman 1989]. However, lipid-laden macrophages can also be seen in fat embolism due to trauma, acute pancreatitis, use of parenteral lipid emulsions, bone marrow transplant, liposuction, cirrhosis, and fatty liver, and in acutely ill patients with agglutination of lipids by C-reactive protein [Védrinne 1992]. In children, lipid-laden macrophages may be associated with gastroesophageal reflux [Nussbaum 1987]. However, when lipophages are present, particularly in adults, malignancy must be excluded before accepting a benign etiology.

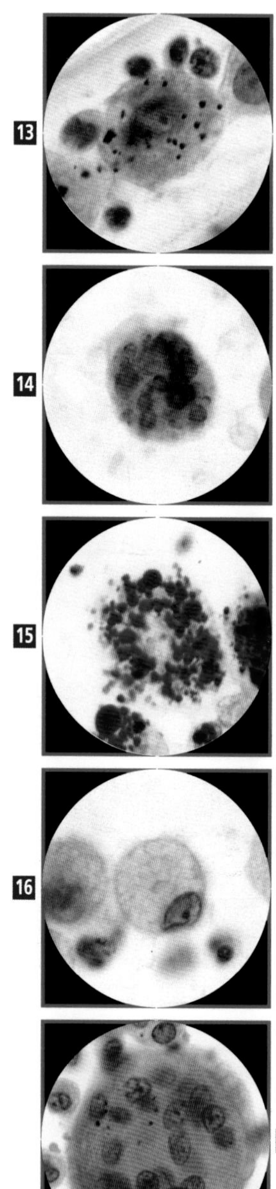

13

14

15

16

17

Muciphages

Muciphages may resemble mucin-producing cells of adenocarcinoma, particularly BAC, but the benign cells are found singly or in loose groups that lack great depth of focus and have bland, histiocytic nuclei.

Multinucleated Giant Cell Histiocytes (Foreign Body, Langhans')

Giant cells can be seen in a wide variety of diseases and even in apparently healthy people [Agusti 1987, Costabel 1985]. However, giant cell histiocytes can be associated with tuberculosis (particularly Langhans' type [Nasiell 1972]), sarcoid, or other granulomatous diseases (eg, fungal infections). The mere presence of giant cells is not diagnostic of a granuloma. Multinucleated histiocytes with dense (epithelioid) cytoplasm are more suspicious for granuloma than multinucleated histiocytes with delicate, bubbly cytoplasm, particularly with carbon particles [17 I7.13].

Giant cells also occur in giant cell interstitial pneumonia [Tabatowski 1988, Valicenti 1979], lipid or aspiration pneumonia, foreign body reactions, silicosis, viral infections, and malignancies [Frable 1977, Harboldt 1994, Mottet 1961, Naib 1968]. Also, pneumothorax, hemorrhage, radiation, cytotoxic drugs, collagen diseases, and bronchoscopy can all be associated with the presence of giant cells [Aisner 1977, Harboldt 1994]. Even specimens from normal lung can have small numbers of giant cell histiocytes [Harboldt 1994].

Bronchial irritation cells may assume multinucleated large to giant forms. Also, megakaryocytes may be found in pulmonary capillaries and sampled with bronchial brushing [Chess 1988, Copeland 1993] or fine needle aspiration biopsy [Chen 1987]. In addition, a number of neoplasms can give rise to giant tumor cells, including not only primary lung cancer, but also numerous metastatic tumors. Some malignancies may be associated with granulomatous inflammation, particularly squamous cell carcinoma [Nasiell 1972].

Atypical Histiocytes

Histiocytes can also become quite atypical, resembling cancer, particularly bronchioloalveolar carcinoma. Atypical histiocytes can have enlarged, pleomorphic, hyperchromatic nuclei and prominent nucleoli. However, the nuclei often appear degenerated, with smudgy rather than distinct chromatin. Further degeneration can also occur, with nuclear pyknosis and cytoplasmic coagulation. This coagulative necrosis can produce orangeophilic cells with pyknotic (ink dot) nuclei that mimic keratinizing squamous cell carcinoma. Phagocytosed particles in the cytoplasm are helpful in the differential diagnosis. Also, histiocytic cytoplasm tends to be foamy to granular, rather than hard and waxy (see also "Pseudokeratosis").

Miscellaneous Cells

Blood

In patients with primary or metastatic cancer in the lung, the presence of blood in the sputum is strongly associated with finding diagnostic malignant cells [Risse 1987a].

Inflammatory Cells

As in the Pap smear, a few inflammatory cells, such as polymorphonuclear leukocytes and lymphocytes, are usually present, even in the absence of infection or inflammation.

A possible exception to the general rule requiring the presence of alveolar macrophages as representatives of "deep lung" may occur in acute pneumonia, in which the alveoli are filled with neutrophils.

Polymorphonuclear Leukocytes

Increased: Associated with necrosis (and smoking)
- Cancer
- Bronchitis
- Abscess
- Pneumonia (including fungal)
- Drug toxicity
- (Smokers)

Absence: Specimen may be unsatisfactory
If satisfactory, cancer unlikely

Lymphocytes: Lymphoid follicles are a normal component of the tracheobronchial tree. Therefore, lymphocytes may be found from a ruptured normal follicle. However, if the lymphocytes are abundant, they are usually associated with chronic inflammation. Lymphocytes may also be indicate lung cancer, lymphomas, and leukemias. Pools of lymphocytes may be seen in malignancy [Tassoni 1963].

Lymphocytes tend to "string out" in mucus strands in sputum, much like cells of small cell carcinoma [18 I7.14]. However, in contrast with small cell carcinoma, lymphocytes show little or no molding, no cohesion, no necrosis, and no malignant features. Immature lymphocytes, which may display mitotic figures, from a ruptured germinal center may suggest malignant lymphoma. However, as with follicular cervicitis in the Pap smear, there is a range of maturation of the lymphoid cells and tingible body macrophages are characteristically present (see Chapters 6, 18, 21).

Increased Lymphocytes

- Chronic bronchitis
- Tuberculosis
- Atelectasis
- Follicular bronchitis
- Hypersensitivity
- Cancer
- (Many others)

18

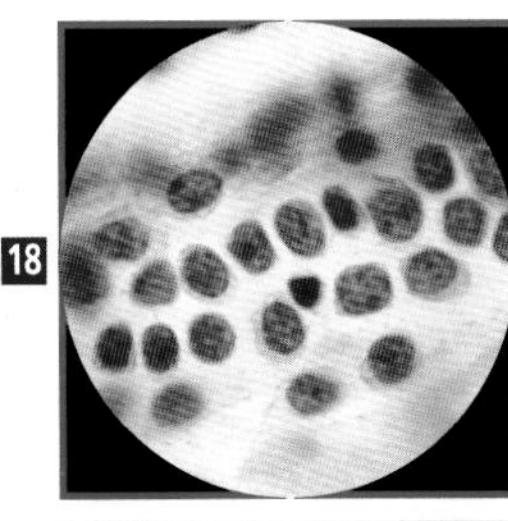

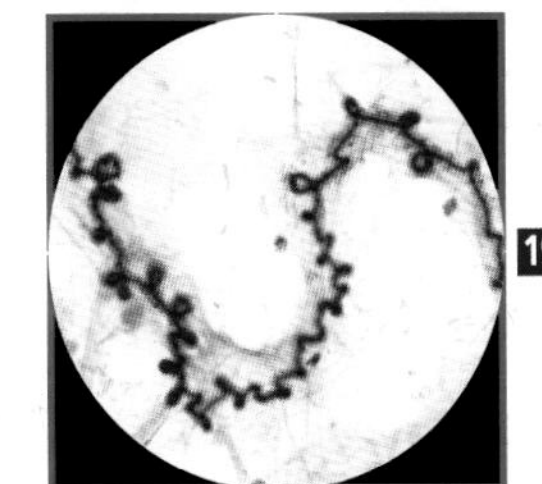

19

Plasma Cells

Plasma cells often originate from the mouth. However, they may indicate chronic pulmonary inflammation, including asthma. They can also be seen in collagen vascular disease, plasma cell interstitial pneumonia (or usual interstitial pneumonia with increased plasma cells), or myeloma [Riazmontazer 1989].

Eosinophils

Eosinophils do not necessarily stain bright red in the Pap stain. Look for relatively large distinct granules and typical bilobed nuclei to distinguish eosinophils from neutrophils, whose individual granules are indistinct with the light microscope and whose nuclei usually have three to five segments. Eosinophils are increased in nasal secretions in allergic conditions [Jean 1988, Rivasi 1988].

Eosinophils

- Allergies
- Asthma
- Eosinophilic (Löffler's) pneumonia
- Wegener's granulomatosis
- Drug toxicity
- Environmental toxins, eg, air pollution, smoking

Smooth Muscle Cells

These cells may be seen in severe tracheobronchial ulceration, including Wegener's granulomatosis [M Takeda 1969]. They have caudate or bizarre shapes, eosinophilic cytoplasm, and pyknotic nuclei that may be mistaken for squamous cell carcinoma.

Acellular Material

Curschmann's Spirals

Curschmann's spirals are usually found in conditions associated with excess mucus production, as in patients with asthma and in smokers [Walker 1970]. Curschmann's spirals usually arise from the deep lung, possibly from bronchial glands [Antonakopoulos 1987]. They are associated with bronchial obstruction, often due to asthma or chronic bronchitis. Although Curschmann's spirals may be inspissated mucus casts of small bronchioles, they can also be found rarely in other sites, such as in cervicovaginal smears [Bornstein 1987, Novak 1984], endometrial washings [Roszel 1985], effusions (often malignant) [Wahl 1986], and gallbladder. Therefore, their formation is probably an intrinsic property of mucus itself, caused by prolonged inspissation in which the components of mucins are altered and a spiral precipitate forms.

Morphologically, Curschmann's spirals have a darkly staining center with a coaxial lighter staining periphery, usually spiraling like a corkscrew [19 I7.15] [Frost 1973]. In patients with asthma, Curschmann's spirals may be associated with eosinophils. They can also be associated with neutrophils, possibly due to air pollution or smoking.

Ferruginous (Asbestos) Bodies

Ferruginous bodies form when iron salts precipitate onto tiny rounded or fibrous inhaled dusts. The fiber is usually asbestos (ergo, "asbestos bodies"), but can be other particles such as fiberglass, carbon, or other minerals. Thus, although ferruginous bodies are likely to contain asbestos, they are not specific for it.

Ferruginous bodies are golden brown, beaded, and have bulbous tips [20 I7.16] Their shape resembles a parade twirler's baton, but may be bent, and range in length up to 200 µm. Ferruginous bodies are often engulfed or surrounded by macrophages [Frost 1973]. The presence of ferruginous bodies correlates with the duration and extent of exposure [Dodson 1983, P Gordon 1976, S Greenberg 1976, P Rosen 1972]. An iron stain can be helpful in detecting ferruginous bodies. Even a rare ferruginous body in a smear suggests that considerably more of the fiber (usually asbestos) is present in the patient [Roggli 1986,1994].

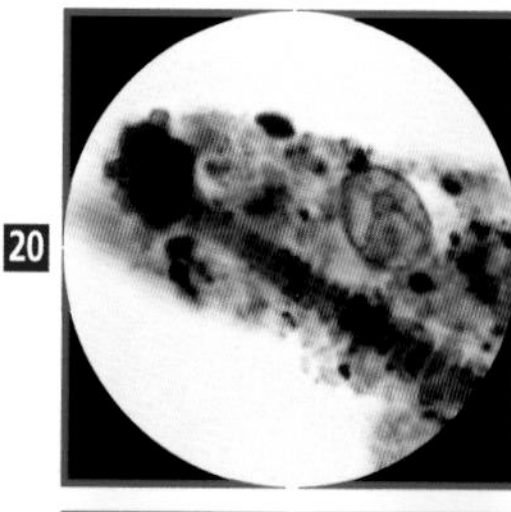
20

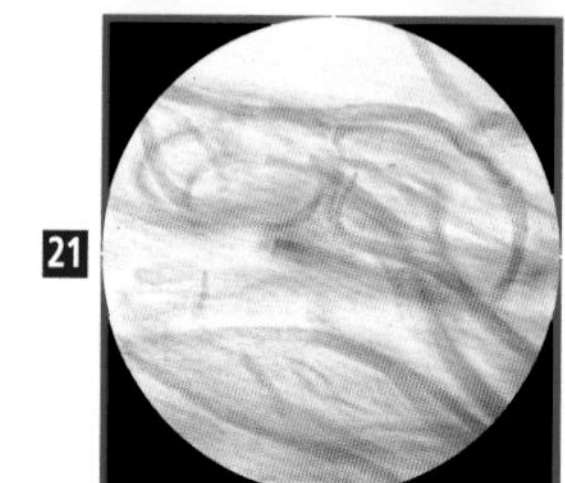
21

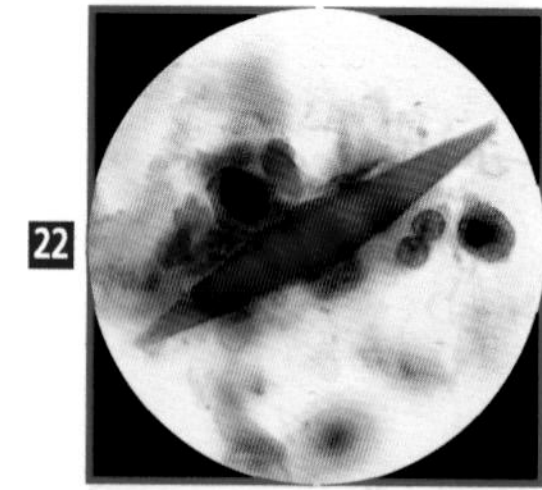
22

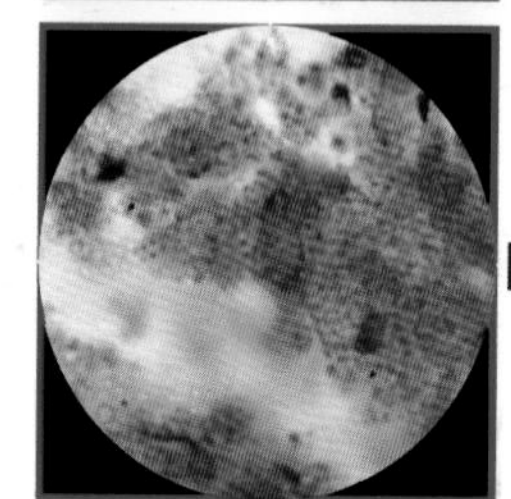
23

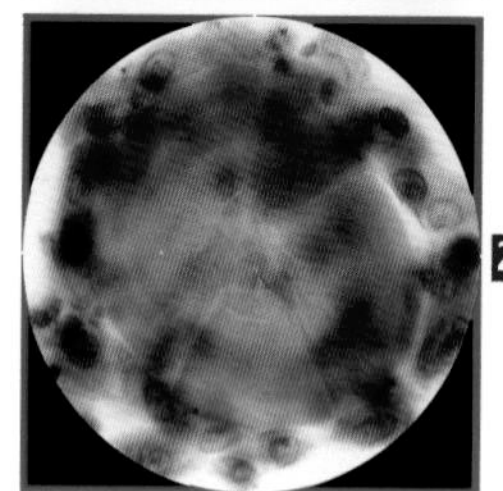
24

Elastin Fibers

The presence of elastin fibers often correlates with tissue destruction (such as seen in acute inflammation, abscess, infarct, bronchiectasis, or cancer), but they may also appear in vigorous brushings or needle aspirations [Shlaes 1983]. Elastin fibers are elongated, curved, often frayed, and though usually poorly stained, appear somewhat refractile [21 I7.17]. They are often seen in bundles and may be associated with necrotic debris. Elastin fibers should not be mistaken for a filamentous fungus (eg, *Aspergillus*), which they somewhat resemble. Elastin fibers lack cell walls, septation, and cytoplasm.

Charcot-Leyden Crystals

Charcot-Leyden crystals are bipyramidal or needle-like red crystals composed of condensed granules derived from eosinophils [22 I7.18], which are usually present near the crystals. The material is predominantly lysophospholipase (phospholipase B), an acidic protein. Its function is to inactivate lysophospholipids, which are found in the cell membrane. This protein is also implicated in prostaglandin metabolism [Sakula 1986]. Charcot-Leyden crystals are particularly associated with asthma, but can also be seen in any condition with excessive turnover of eosinophils (and rarely, basophils [Sakula 1986]), such as allergies, allergic bronchopulmonary aspergillosis [Chen 1993], and healing eosinophilic (Löffler's) pneumonia. Charcot-Leyden crystal formation is probably a degenerative process that occurs in vitro, because they are usually rare or absent in fresh sputum.

Alveolar Proteinosis

Alveolar proteinosis is thought to be due to an enzymatic disorder of macrophages. Macrophages ingest some toxin (such as silica), then die and release more toxins (enzymes, silica), which other macrophages ingest and then they too die, and so on, resulting in a necrotic mess. The alveoli become filled with acidophilic granules of various sizes, consisting of cell debris and phospholipid surfactant material. This intra-alveolar material interferes with gas exchange.

The gross appearance of the fluid is opaque [Mermolja 1994]. The cytology shows a very "dirty" background composed of coarsely granular, eosinophilic "junko" and cell debris [23 I7.19] [Masin 1962]. Staining with PAS, with or without diastase, is positive, but mucicarmine and amyloid stains are negative in alveolar proteinosis [Carlson 1960]. Occasional pink spherules with lipid and cholesterol crystals may be present. The findings are characteristic, but not specific.

Corpora Amylacea

Corpora amylacea are glycoprotein casts of the alveolar space. Their formation is related to previous pulmonary edema. Hence, corpora amylacea are associated with such conditions as congestive heart failure, pulmonary infarcts, and chronic bronchitis.

Corpora amylacea are acidophilic or cyanophilic bodies that are often concentrically laminated, sometimes with a central dot and radial striations, and often crack [24 I7.20]. In contrast with calcospherites and psammoma bodies, corpora amylacea are usually not calcified, but are birefringent [Schmitz 1984]. The differential diagnosis also includes fungus, talc, starch (Maltese cross birefringence), and pollen.

Calcospherites and Psammoma Bodies

Both calcospherites and psammoma bodies are concentrically laminated, calcified, and basophilic in the Pap stain. Psammoma bodies are surrounded by cells; calcospherites are naked of cells. True psammoma bodies are somewhat more likely than mere calcospherites to be associated with cancer (such as bronchioloalveolar carcinoma or metastatic papillary carcinoma). It is important to emphasize that cancer is not necessarily present; these bodies can be seen in benign conditions. Calcospherites can be seen in chronic pulmonary disease, such as tuberculosis, and in rare diseases like pulmonary microlithiasis. Nevertheless, their presence must be viewed with the suspicion of cancer. Calcification differentiates them from corpora amylacea.

Blue Bodies

In addition to psammoma bodies and calcospherites, a variety of other "blue bodies" can be found in respiratory specimens. Some may be related to benign diseases such as chronic obstructive pulmonary disease [Tao 1978a], inflammation, pulmonary fibrosis, emphysema [Schmitz 1984], severe pulmonary hypertension, or oxygen therapy [Mouriquand 1986], but they can also sometimes be seen in malignancy.

Calcium Salt Crystals: Birefringent, laminated, or needle-shaped purplish crystals; may be present in giant cells [Kung 1987, Vigorita 1979].

Microliths: Seen most frequently in cases of chronic obstructive pulmonary disease, but also associated with pulmonary alveolar microlithiasis [Tao 1978a].

Mucus Bodies (Blue Blobs): Occasionally amorphous "blue blobs" possibly representing condensed inspissated mucus can be seen and can mimic naked malignant nuclei. However, they do not have a distinct chromatin pattern or cytoplasm. They can be round or ring shaped [Schmitz 1984]. Mucus bodies may be the nidus for formation of other blue bodies formed by deposition of calcium or oxalate [Schmitz 1984].

Kuhn's Cytoplasmic Hyalin

First described in asbestosis, this accumulation of hyaline material, identical to Mallory's alcoholic hyalin (liver), is now recognized as a nonspecific change [25 I7.21] [Kuhn 1973, Warnock 1980].

Amyloid

Amyloid occurs as multiple, irregular, dense, acellular fragments of eosinophilic material. It may have a waxy, homogeneous appearance, with sharp, often scalloped margins; characteristic apple green birefringence is seen under polarized light with Congo red staining [Chen 1984, Neifer 1985].

Oxalate Crystals

These are sheaf-like (most characteristic), needle, rosette, ellipsoid, biconcave, or dumbbell-shaped crystals, which are strongly birefringent and associated with aspergillosis, particularly *Aspergillus niger* [Farley 1985, Reyes 1979].

Barium Crystals

These are polarizable rhomboid crystals of different sizes [Shahar 1994].

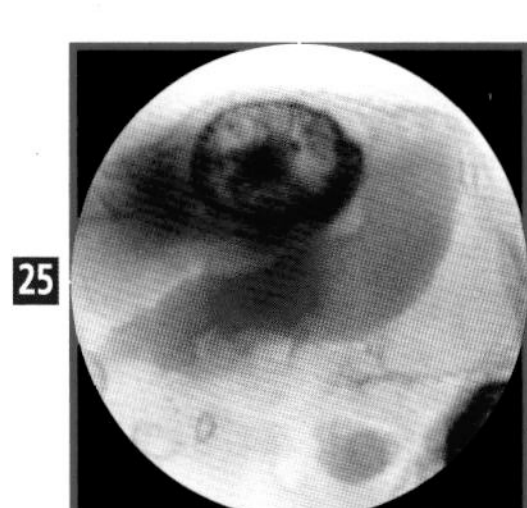
25

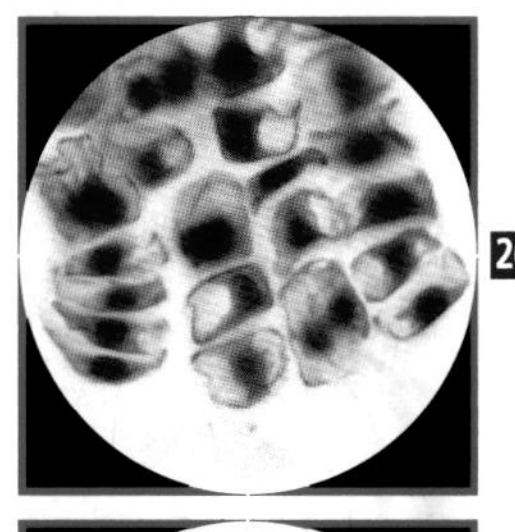
26

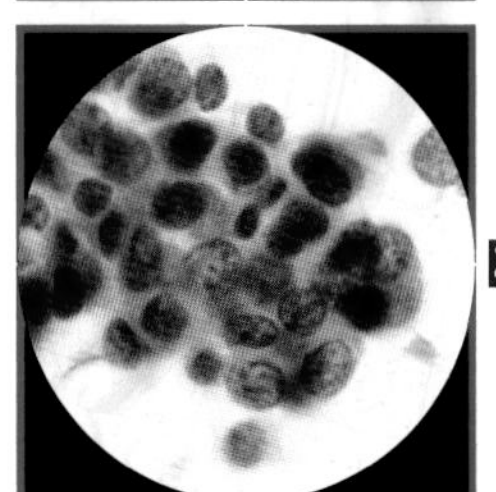
27

Contaminants

Talc/Starch: From glove powder. Talc is no longer used; starch has cracked center and Maltese cross polarization.

Pollen: Colorful bodies with cell walls and spikes.

Plant Cells/Food: Food particles are common in sputum and may be a source of error for the novice [Weaver 1981]. Meat is recognized by cross striations. Plant cells may have very dark nuclei and can resemble adenocarcinoma or squamous cell carcinoma [26 I7.22]. However, plant cells have translucent, refractile cell walls (cellulose), which distinguishes them from members of the animal kingdom.

Benign Proliferation

In response to chronic irritation (including toxins such as cigarette smoke [Nasiell 1968, Saccomanno 1970], air pollution, and inflammation or infections such as asthma, tuberculosis, sarcoid, chronic bronchitis, organizing pneumonia, infarcts, bronchiectasis, mycetomas, especially aspergillosis, as well as radiation and chemotherapy), the bronchial epithelium can undergo a series of transformations, including reserve cell hyperplasia, squamous metaplasia, and bronchial hyperplasia [Iwama de Mattos 1991, Johnston 1976,1986, Kierszenbaum 1965]. Metaplastic changes are similar to those described in the chapter on Pap smear. Squamous epithelium is more mechanically resistant, but less specialized than the respiratory epithelium. As in the uterine cervix, while not considered premalignant, squamous metaplasia is the milieu in which cancer may arise.

Reserve Cell Hyperplasia

Reserve cell hyperplasia (RCH) occurs in response to a variety of stimuli previously mentioned above. RCH is most commonly observed in bronchial brushings. As in the Pap smear, reserve cells resemble lymphocytes or histiocytes, and would probably not be recognizable when occurring singly [27 I7.23]. However, RCH can be recognized as tightly cohesive groups of small, uniform cells, often with small ciliated columnar cells along one surface. Reserve cells have uniform, small, dark round nuclei with a thin rim of basophilic cytoplasm (resulting in a high N/C ratio). The nuclei resemble those of ordinary ciliated cells, but may show some nuclear molding. Nucleoli are usually absent, but may be present when the reserve cells are irritated. RCH is not associated with necrosis or a tumor diathesis.

Perhaps the most important consideration in the differential diagnosis is small cell carcinoma. Compared with RCH, small cell carcinoma displays much more variable nuclei, with more nuclear molding, crush artifact, and a tumor diathesis. The presence of large nucleoli rules out small cell carcinoma, but leaves open the possibility of poorly differentiated non–small cell carcinoma. Lymphocytes, including those deriving from malignant lymphoma, do not form cohesive clusters; therefore, in contrast with RCH, all of the cells are single. Also, lymphoglandular bodies are characteristically present in organized lymphoid tissue, including lymphoma.

Squamous Metaplasia

Squamous metaplasia is extremely common (occurring in 20% to 80% of all patients, with men being affected more commonly than women). Squamous metaplasia peaks in the 50s, and gradually declines in frequency after the age of 60 [Spain 1970]. Squamous metaplasia occurs with various conditions previously discussed, and is also associated with cancer. Squamous metaplasia can vary from focal to extensive to nearly total. It frequently occurs with RCH.

Immature squamous metaplasia in the respiratory system appears similar to that in the cervix, but the respiratory metaplasia cells are often smaller and have more angulated or polygonal outlines than those from the cervix [28 I7.24]. The immature metaplastic cells are about the diameter of a bronchial cell and considerably smaller than mature squamous cells originating in the mouth. As the metaplasia matures, it more closely resembles cervical squamous metaplasia, with larger cells and rounded cell margins.

Metaplastic cells are uniform in size and shape. As in the Pap smear, the cells often appear in loose sheets, in a cobblestone arrangement. The cytoplasm of the metaplastic cells is dense with distinct cell borders. The cytoplasm is usually blue-green, but may stain pink to orange when degenerated. The nuclei are round. The chromatin varies from granular (like normal ciliated cells) to coarse or pyknotic. No nucleoli are present unless the metaplastic cells are irritated (ie, repairish) [29 I7.25, 30 I7.31].

Metaplasia may be difficult to distinguish from small parabasal cells, oral cells, or groups of macrophages [Roby 1990a]. Also, small metaplastic cells with angular outlines, orange cytoplasm, and pyknotic nuclei may be difficult to distinguish from parakeratosis. Atypical squamous metaplasia, often associated with necrotizing pneumonia, is a relatively common source of false-positive diagnoses. The differential diagnosis also includes true squamous dysplasia and metastases (eg, transitional cell carcinoma) [Lachman 1994].

Parakeratosis, Atypical Parakeratosis

Bronchial parakeratosis and atypical parakeratosis are similar to parakeratosis seen in the Pap smear, and are likewise associated with irritation/inflammation or dysplasia/cancer. Parakeratosis [I7.26] and atypical parakeratosis usually arise in the mouth or in the tracheobronchial tree associated with severe irritation, eg, a tracheostomy tube [Cahan 1966, Nunez 1966]. Individual cells from atypical parakeratosis can be very abnormal appearing (pleomorphic, keratinized), and in some cases, may be virtually indistinguishable from keratinizing squamous cell carcinoma, *except* for the small size of the parakeratotic cells [31 I7.27, I7.28]. Look carefully for clear-cut (large) malignant cells to diagnose cancer.

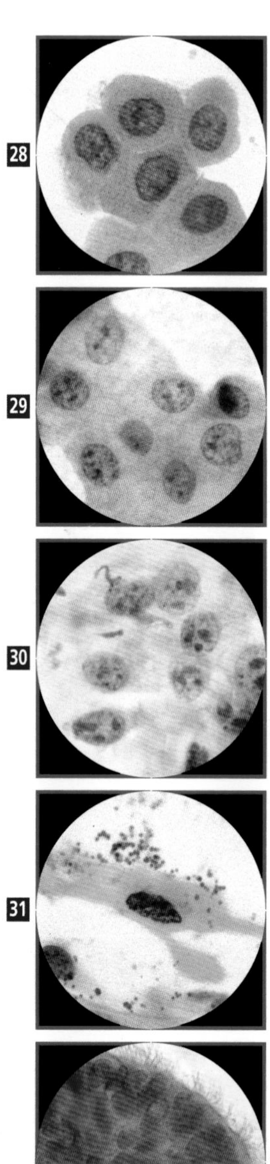
28
29
30
31
32

Bronchial Hyperplasia and Creola Bodies

Bronchial hyperplasia is a response to a variety of acute or chronic pulmonary disorders, including asthma, bronchiectasis, chronic bronchitis, viral pneumonia, Wegener's granulomatosis [Hector 1976], and respiratory distress syndrome. In tissue, the bronchial mucosa is thrown into papillary folds; however, true papillae with fibrovascular cores are not formed. In cytology, compact, pseudopapillary, three-dimensional groups of reactive/atypical bronchial cells, which have been mistaken for cancer, may be exfoliated. These clusters, named for a patient, are also known as "creola bodies" [32 I7.29] [Naylor 1962]. Creola bodies are tightly cohesive, with smooth or knobby outlines. The peripheral cells tend to palisade; smaller, less differentiated cells may be present in the center. Benign, reactive nuclei are fairly uniform in size and shape. They have smooth nuclear membranes, fine to coarse but regularly distributed chromatin, and may have prominent, but regular and uniform, nucleoli. The cytoplasm varies from homogeneous and granular, to finely vacuolated, to highly vacuolated, with cells distended by large vacuoles.

The principal consideration in the differential diagnosis is primary or metastatic adenocarcinoma [Naylor 1964], including papillary adenocarcinoma and bronchioloaveolar carcinoma. Cilia, if present, are the key to the benign nature of creola bodies. They are usually seen along part of the surface but may degenerate, leaving only terminal bars. A mixture of ciliated and goblet cells in a cluster usually indicates a benign process. Large nuclei and nucleoli can be seen in either reactive or malignant conditions; however, in benign conditions the chromatin remains finely granular and the nucleoli are regular and uniform [Johnston 1976,1986]. Large cytoplasmic vacuoles are more common in bronchial hyperplasia or metastatic adenocarcinoma than primary lung cancer [J Smith 1974]. Transitional forms between clearly benign and atypical cells point to a benign process, while a discrete population of abnormal cells suggests malignancy. The time course may also be helpful; creola bodies disappear if the underlying condition resolves, whereas malignant cells remain. (Interestingly, creola body–like fragments have been described in an ovarian teratoma, which showed a typical asthmatic picture, complete with eosinophilic reaction and thickening of the basement membrane [Thomson 1945].)

Miscellaneous

Pap Cells

Pap cells are tiny squamous cells probably deriving from squamous metaplasia or parakeratosis, perhaps originating in the pharynx or upper respiratory tract [Koss 1955]. Pap cells can be seen in patients with pneumonia, tuberculosis, bronchiectasis, or other chronic inflammatory processes.

The cells may appear atypical, but are small. They have regular elliptical or angular outlines, relatively abundant pink to orange cytoplasm, and often occur in dense clusters [33 I7.30]. The ovoid nuclei are hyperchromatic to pyknotic or lysed. (Dr Papanicolaou, for whom the cells are named, first detected these atypical cells in his own sputum; they turned out to be associated with a cold, not cancer.)

Pseudokeratosis

In response to various injuries, glandular cells sometimes undergo coagulative necrosis, resulting in irregularly shaped cells with cytoplasmic orangeophilia (pseudokeratosis), and nuclear pyknosis [DiBonito 1991]. These pleomorphic cells, with deep orange cytoplasm and ink dot nuclei, can resemble keratinizing squamous cell carcinoma. However, such cells usually maintain their nucleocytoplasmic polarity (ie, "basal" nuclei with "apical" cytoplasm), have granular, rather than waxy cytoplasm, and may be associated with better preserved cells still recognizable as glandular. Pseudokeratosis can affect either benign or malignant glandular cells. Similar changes can also occur in histiocytes, as previously described.

33
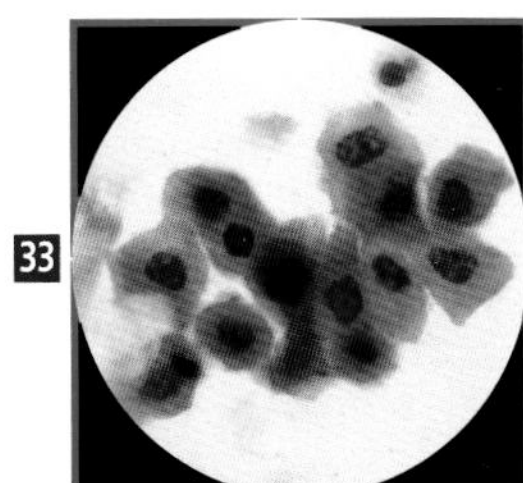

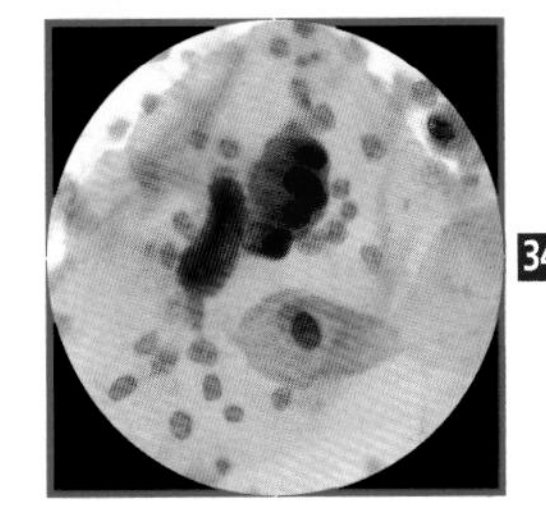
34

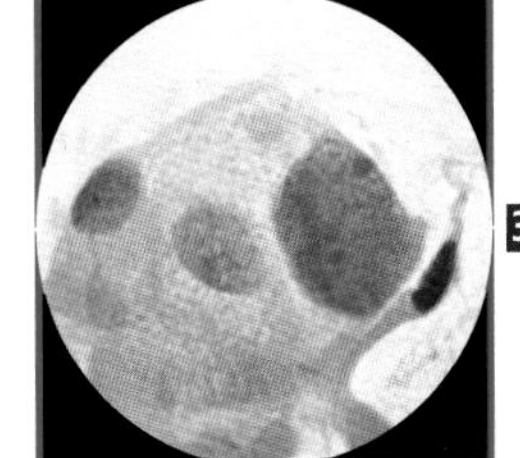
35

Therapeutic Agents

Radiation and chemotherapy can affect virtually any dividing cell, whether benign or malignant. Therapeutic agents can induce severe atypia, which must be distinguished from cancer. Clinical history of radiation or chemotherapy is essential for proper diagnosis. The fact that most of these patients have a history of cancer may make the abnormal cytologic features seem all the more ominous. Smudged and degenerated, rather than crisp and distinct, chromatin is a critical observation in benign atypia associated with therapeutic effect.

Radiation

As in the Pap smear, radiation induces changes that are characterized by the presence of macrocytes, of either squamous or glandular origin. Radiated malignant cells show, in addition to radiation effect, characteristic malignant features. Radiation changes may subside with time or persist for the life of the patient.

Effects on Squamous Cells

Radiation effect on squamous cells causes cytomegaly with enlargement of both cytoplasm and nucleus in concert, so that the N/C ratio remains within normal limits [34 I7.32]. Multinucleation is common. The nuclei may be hyperchromatic, hypochromatic, or sometimes vacuolated. Prominent nucleoli, occasionally macronucleoli, may be seen. The cytoplasm is thick and dense, but frequently vacuolated, and stains polychromatically (two-tone staining). In addition, squamous metaplasia, which may be atypical, can be seen.

Big cells with big nuclei and big nucleoli may be mistaken for malignancy. However, in contrast with cancer cells, the N/C ratio in these benign cells is within normal limits and the chromatin tends to be degenerated or smudgy.

Effects on Glandular Cells

Many of the changes described for bronchial irritation cells, including multinucleation and reactive changes, can be caused by radiation [Albright 1988]. Radiation can also induce squamous metaplasia of the glandular epithelium. As in squamous cells, macrocytic glandular cells, with both nucleomegaly and cytomegaly, can develop due to radiation [35 I7.33]. Occasionally, these benign radiated cells appear quite atypical, giant, or even bizarre, with disorganized groups, large, dark nuclei, coarse (usually smudgy) chromatin, and prominent nucleoli. Such changes may suggest malignancy. However, despite the atypia, benign radiated cells remain relatively well formed (ie, they maintain their columnar shape) and may have remnants of cilia or terminal bars. Radiation can induce coagulative necrosis of the glandular cells, causing pseudokeratosis, which could be mistaken for keratinizing squamous cell carcinoma.

A dirty background may be present in radiation effect, mimicking a tumor diathesis, with necrosis, white blood cells, and degenerated cells.

Chemotherapy

Chemotherapy often causes cytologic changes, particularly affecting glandular cells, similar to those seen with radiation, which can be summed up by the word "macrocyte." The cells are enlarged, pleomorphic, and may have dark chromatin and prominent nucleoli. There may also be an increase in the number of goblet cells and the amount of mucin. Histiocytes and inflammatory cells are typically seen in the background. Although terminal bars may be retained, chemotherapy may cause the atypical cells to lose their cilia, and with them, a valuable clue to benignancy is lost. However, the atypical cells tend to be few, degenerated, and single, and maintain their columnar shape. Clinical history is essential.

Busulfan

Busulfan can have pronounced effects on the lung ("busulfan lung") and also affects other organs (such as the bladder).

Busulfan can cause pulmonary fibrosis resulting in dyspnea, which can be of sudden onset, even months after therapy. It is potentially fatal.

Abnormal cells are seen which may be mistaken for cancer cells [Hankins 1978]. The cells are very large, and have enlarged, hyperchromatic nuclei with slightly irregular membranes and coarse chromatin and an increased N/C ratio. The presence of cilia or terminal bars points to a benign diagnosis. Markedly atypical cells are few.

Other Chemotherapeutic Agents

1,3-bis-(2-chloroethyl)-1-nitrosourea (BCNU): BCNU causes clouding of the lung fields on chest x-ray. The cells are giant and may resemble adenocarcinoma. Mitotic figures can be seen.

Bleomycin: Causes atypia of squamous cells, but may be sparse; columnar cells are not significantly affected [Bedrossian 1978].

Methotrexate: Atypical, but not malignant appearing cells.

Inflammation

In addition to diagnosing an inflammatory process, cytologic examination may be able to identify the specific agent.

Acute Inflammation

Acute inflammation is characterized by neutrophils, histiocytes, debris, and necrosis, including pneumonia, abscess, and purulent bronchitis, resulting in tissue destruction. Look carefully for cancer cells and fungus, which may be obscured by the exudate. Marked acute inflammation is a unique case in which a sputum specimen may be from the deep lung (ie, adequate) without the presence of alveolar macrophages.

Chronic Inflammation

Nonspecific

Nonspecific chronic inflammation is very common.

Follicular Bronchitis

The bronchi normally contain small lymphoid follicles. To diagnose follicular bronchitis, an abundance of immature lymphocytes indicating the presence of large lymphoid follicles must be found. Immature lymphocytes should not be mistaken for malignant lymphoma. The key to this differential diagnosis is the same as for follicular cervicitis in the Pap smear and consists in finding a "range of maturation" of the lymphoid cells and tingible body macrophages. Another tumor to rule out is small cell carcinoma. In contrast to small cell carcinoma, the lymphocytes do not form true groups: lymphocytes are present as single cells with little or no molding.

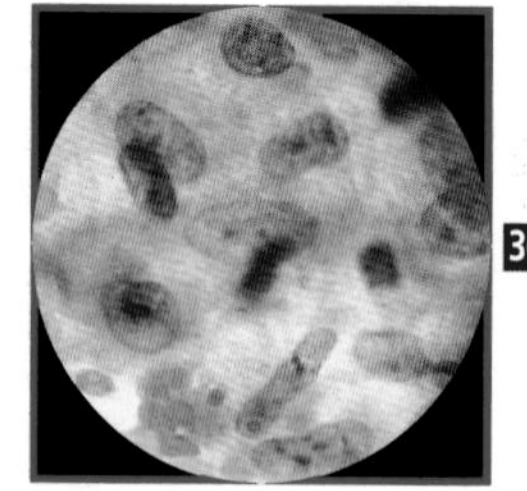

36

Granulomatous Inflammation

Granulomas are nodular collections of epithelioid histiocytes—giant cells are not required to diagnose a granuloma. On cytologic examination, epithelioid histiocytes are usually found in loose clusters with poorly defined cell boundaries [36 I7.34].

In sputum, epithelioid histiocytes are generally about the size of bronchial cells. Epithelioid histiocytes may be shaped like elongated cones that stain pink to orange when degenerated and resemble carrots, hence are termed "carrot cells." Epithelioid histiocytes can also be rounded, in which case they can be difficult to distinguish from ordinary histiocytes. The nucleus is elongated, often with a fold in the nuclear membrane, and has fine, pale chromatin, with a tiny nucleolus. In well-preserved cells, such as in bronchial brushings or aspiration cytology, the cytoplasm is more abundant, eccentrically located around the nucleus, and often has a peculiar fibrillar quality, with poorly defined cell borders. In foreign body granulomas, phagocytosis is prominent. However, in tuberculosis, phagocytosis is absent or minimal.

Tuberculosis

The typical features of tuberculosis are epithelioid histiocytes, giant cells (particularly Langhans' type), lymphocytes, and a necrotic—caseous—background [Tani 1987]. Granulomas per se are not diagnostic of tuberculosis; granulomas can be seen in a wide variety of conditions, including as a reaction to cancer (particularly with squamous differentiation). Moreover, tuberculosis and cancer can coexist.

Although giant cells are seen in sputum in up to half of cases of pulmonary tuberculosis, typical Langhans' giant cells (with peripheral nuclei and relatively dense, epithelioid cytoplasm) are present in only as few as 5% of cases [Roger 1972]. In patients with tuberculosis, epithelioid histiocytes are found in about 25% to 50% of sputum specimens [Roger 1972, Tani 1987]. In sputum specimens in which *either* Langhans' giant cells or epithelioid histiocytes are seen, as many as 60% of the patients have tuberculosis, depending upon the patient population [Nasiell 1972]. The combination of *both* Langhans' giant cells and epithelioid histiocytes is most specific, but not pathognomonic. Identification of beaded acid-fast bacilli or a positive culture clinches the diagnosis of tuberculosis (including typical or atypical forms).

Lymphocytes, plasma cells, granular necrotic (caseous) material as well as neutrophils (particularly early in the course of the disease) can be seen in patients with tuberculosis [Tani 1987]. In addition, reactive bronchial epithelium and squamous metaplasia can occur. Reactive atypia in these cells may be the source of false-positive diagnoses. The differential diagnosis of necrotizing granulomas is long, and includes fungal infections and Wegener's granulomatosis [Granados 1994].

Sarcoid

Sarcoidosis, or simply, sarcoid, is a chronic granulomatous disease of unknown etiology. Epithelioid histiocytes or giant cells may be seen in large numbers, particularly during the interstitial fibrosis and scarring phase of the disease [Aisner 1977], but are not specific. The characteristic cells occur in streaks, either singly or as syncytial collections (ie, granulomas). Giant cells with Schaumann or asteroid bodies are suggestive of sarcoid, but are not specific. Schaumann bodies are concentrically laminated calcifications found in the cytoplasm of the giant cells [37 I7.35]. Asteroid bodies are intracytoplasmic radiate arrays of needle-shaped crystalline material [38 I7.36]. In contrast with tuberculous granulomas, the background in sarcoid is clean (ie, no caseation is seen).

Rheumatoid Granuloma of Lung

Rheumatoid granulomas can exfoliate epithelioid histiocytes with bizarre shapes. These cells may have hyperchromatic, degenerated, smudged nuclei and variously colored cytoplasm, ranging from blue/gray to red/orange. The background shows marked inflammation and necrotic debris. Occasional degenerated multinucleated giant cells may be seen.

Bizarre cells with dark nuclei and pink/orange cytoplasm in a necrotic background can mimic keratinizing squamous cell carcinoma. A clue to the benign diagnosis is that the histiocytic cells tend to be relatively small. Squamous metaplasia, which may show reactive atypia, can further confuse the picture.

Inflammatory Pseudotumor

This is a rare inflammatory lesion of the lung that usually occurs in younger patients, but can be confused with a neoplasm. Cytologic study shows short, spindle-shaped histiocytic cells, with a tendency to be arranged in a storiform pattern, in a background of minimal necrotic debris [Usuda 1990].

Specific Infections

The lung can be affected by a multitude of organisms that may be diagnosed with respiratory cytology. Cytologic methods are increasingly being used to diagnose opportunistic infections, especially in patients with transplants or AIDS. Although many infectious agents can be diagnosed on routine stains, respiratory cytology is least useful for specific identification of bacterial infections (see Chapter 5).

Viral Pneumonia: Viral infections, such as cytomegalovirus, are being seen with increased frequency in immunocompromised patients [Miles 1990]. Viral infection can cause reactive changes in bronchial cells, which in the absence of cilia, may be virtually indistinguishable from bronchioloalveolar carcinoma (BAC) cells. Thus, it may occasionally be difficult or impossible to differentiate viral pneumonia from BAC cytologically, and tissue biopsy may be required for a final diagnosis. However, in infection, atypical cells are generally few; in BAC, many. As a rule, do not diagnose BAC in a patient with an acute illness or fever, unless the evidence is compelling.

Candida, Bacterial Colonies: Suspect oral contamination, overgrowth. *Actinomyces* is commonly a saprophyte in the tonsils.

Miscellaneous Infections: These include fungi, pneumocystis, toxoplasmosis, etc. More commonly diagnosed in immunosuppressed patients, but can also be seen in apparently immunocompetent hosts [S Gordon 1993, Hsu 1993, Wheeler 1994] (see Chapter 5).

37
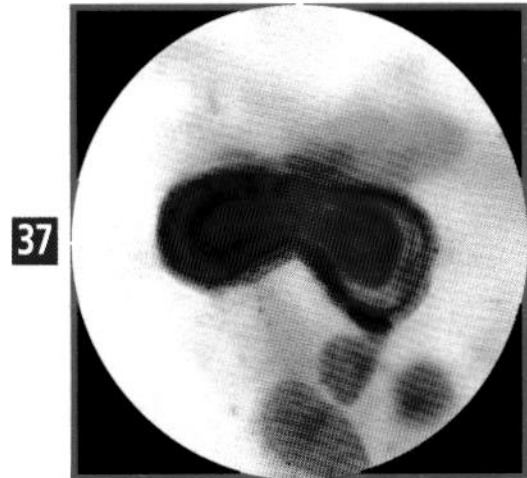

38
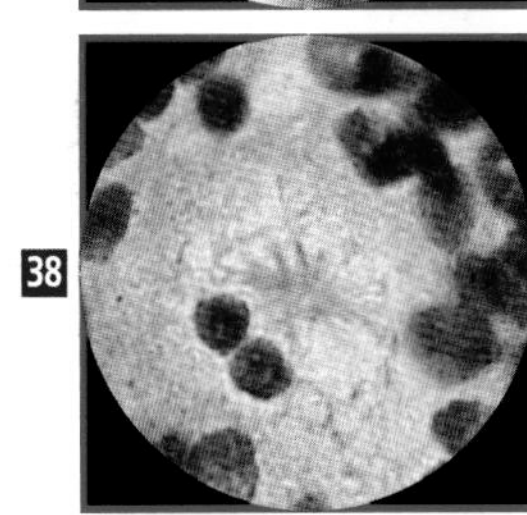

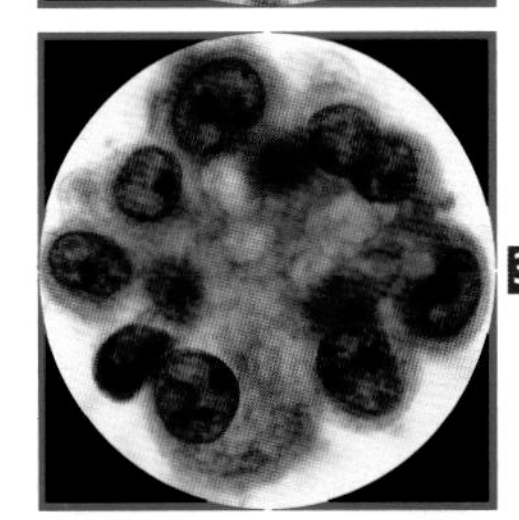
39

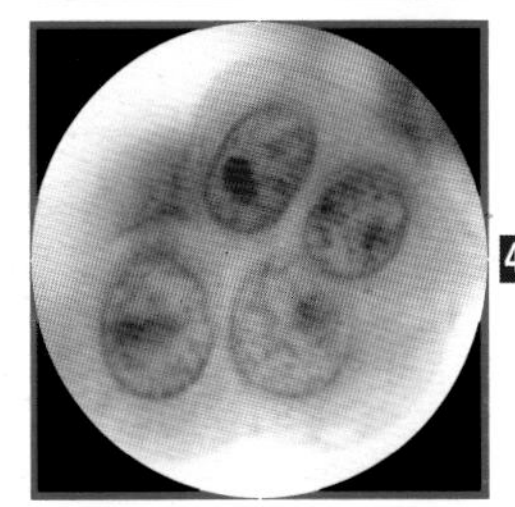
40

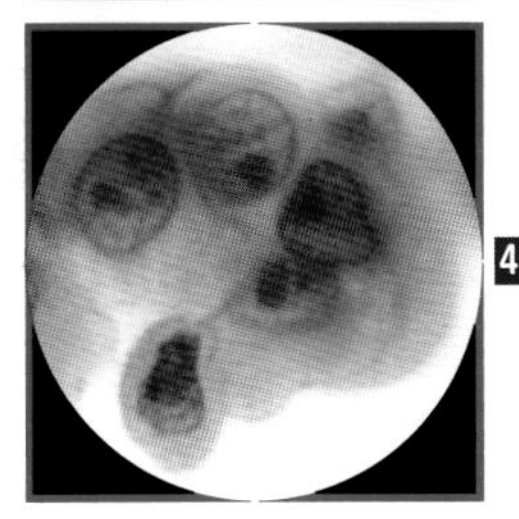
41

Pulmonary Embolism/Infarct

A solitary pulmonary embolism can mimic a peripheral neoplasm clinically. In addition, a few cases exfoliate markedly reactive (atypical) cells that may be confused with malignancy, a pitfall in diagnosis [Kern 1990, Scoggins 1977]. The diagnostic dilemma applies to both sputum and bronchial cytology. The atypical cells may form three-dimensional clusters of reactive bronchioloalveolar glandular epithelium, with pleomorphic, markedly enlarged nuclei, irregular chromatin clearing, and macronucleoli, which can mimic adenocarcinoma [39 I7.6, 40 41 I7.7]. Sheets of cells with orangeophilic cytoplasm and enlarged, hyperchromatic nuclei can mimic squamous cell carcinoma. Atypia is maximal during the second to third postinfarction weeks. In the acute phase, fresh blood, inflammation, and siderophages may be seen in the background. Squamous metaplasia is common. In the chronic phase, the background is nonspecific. Clues to the benign nature of the changes may include sparsity of atypical cells, few or no single atypical cells, variability within groups (ie, typical and atypical cells together), shallow depth of focus, tight cell grouping, presence of cilia, smudgy chromatin, and transience of atypia, with cytologic variability from day to day (as the healing progresses) [Bewtra 1983, Scoggins 1977].

Bronchopulmonary Dysplasia

In response to mechanical ventilation and oxygen toxicity usually associated with respiratory distress syndrome of premature infants (also known as "hyalin membrane disease"), the lung undergoes epithelial hyperplasia, squamous metaplasia, and fibrosis (interstitial, peribronchial). These changes are known as "bronchopulmonary dysplasia" [Northway 1967]. The chronic proliferative and fibrotic stages of the adult respiratory distress syndrome (ARDS) (also known as "diffuse alveolar damage") generally correspond to the changes seen in infants with bronchopulmonary dysplasia.

The tracheobronchial cytology essentially consists of loss of cilia, squamous metaplasia, repair/regeneration, and atypical squamous metaplasia (dysplasia) [D'Ablang 1975, Doshi 1982]. Of note is that all the observed components (bronchial cells, metaplastic cells, macrophages, as well as Curschmann's spirals) are uniformly miniature, about half the size of the adult counterparts [Rothberg 1986].

The changes have been divided into three classes (not to be confused with the Papanicolaou classification system) [Merritt 1981b, Rothberg 1986]. Class I (1–4 days) is characterized by exfoliation of well-preserved, normal-appearing bronchial cells. Class II (4–10 days), the proliferative phase, is characterized by exfoliation of hyperplastic groups of crowded bronchial cells with reactive, enlarged, irregular nuclei, with nucleoli, and loss of cilia. Class III (>10 days), the metaplastic/dysplastic stage, is characterized by squamous metaplasia of the glandular cells (also known as class II/III), and finally, the presence of nuclear features of dysplasia, with hyperchromatic, coarse chromatin (class III).

In the background of class II and III smears are alveolar macrophages, amorphous membranous structures (probably hyaline membranes), Curschmann's spirals, bacteria, blood, and inflammatory cells. Class III smears may allow earlier prediction of the subsequent development of bronchopulmonary dysplasia than radiology alone [Merritt 1981a], although class III smears can also be seen in infants with a normal outcome [Rothberg 1986].

Bronchopulmonary Dysplasia

Class I: Normal
Class II: Hyperplastic
Class II/III: Metaplastic
Class III: Dysplastic

Asthma

Creola bodies are particularly common and conspicuous in asthmatic patients [42 I7.29] [Naylor 1964]. A history of asthma and creola bodies, together with eosinophils, Curschmann's spirals [43 I7.15], and possibly Charcot-Leyden crystals [44 I7.18], aid in the diagnosis [Sanerkin 1965]. Bacteria may be decreased.

Pneumoconioses and Miscellaneous Diseases

Hemosiderosis: Marked increase in hemosiderin-laden macrophages [45 I7.9].

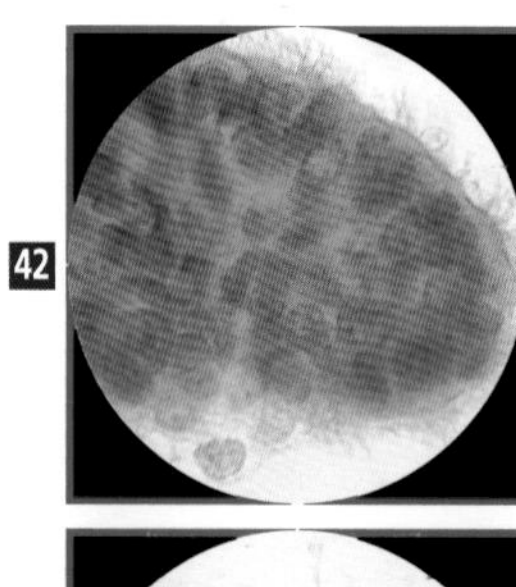

42

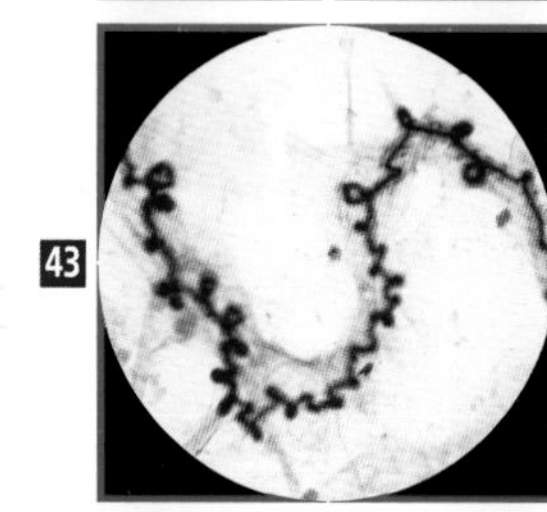

43

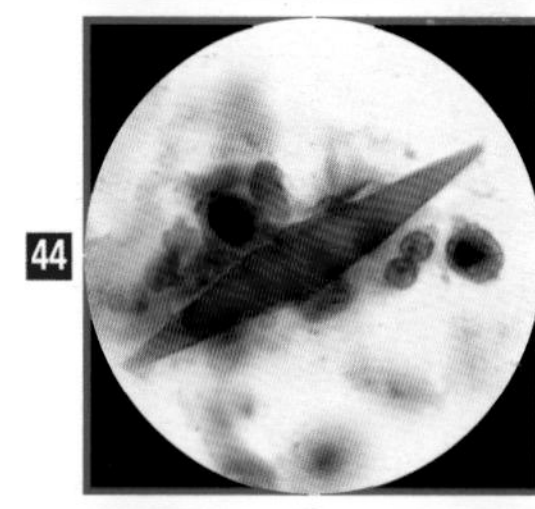

44

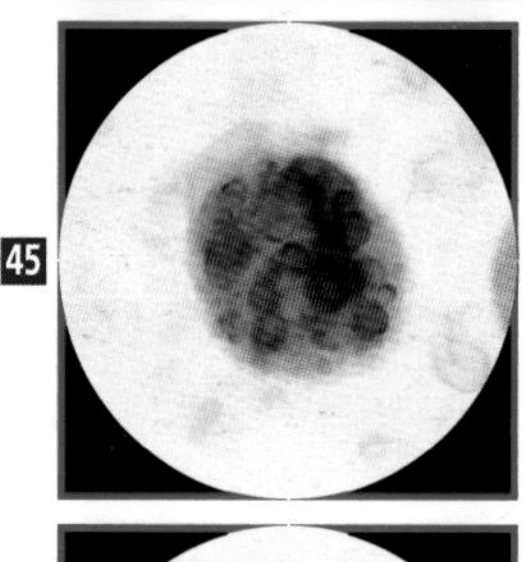

45

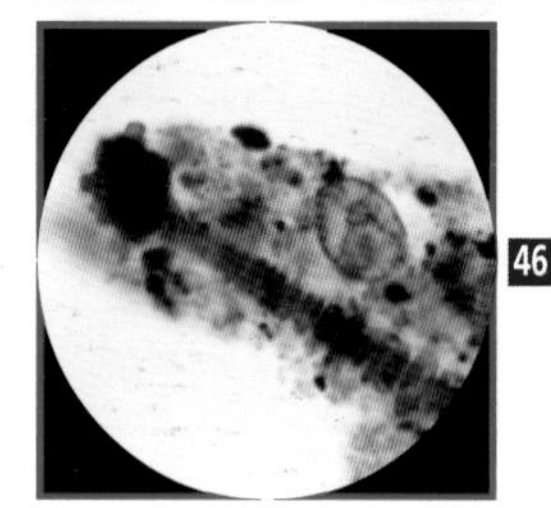

46

Löffler's Pneumonia: Eosinophilic pneumonia.

Silicosis: Weakly birefringent, silvery particles.

Silicate Pneumoconiosis: Brightly birefringent silicates of various sorts may also cause disease.

Asbestosis: Ferruginous bodies suggestive [46 I7.16].

Berylliosis: Causes a disease similar to sarcoid. Beryllium cannot be seen.

Anthracosis: Carbon.

Talc: Strong birefringence, no Maltese cross; may be contaminant with asbestos.

Starch: Maltese cross birefringence. Note that starch has replaced talc as glove powder. Although glove powder is frequently referred to as "talc," it is not.

Byssinosis (Cotton, Flax, Hemp Dust): "Occupational asthma"; cytologic findings similar to chronic bronchitis.

Giant Cell Interstitial Pneumonia: Pneumoconiosis often due to industrial exposure to hard metals [Tabatowski 1988]. Characterized by benign multinucleated giant cell histiocytes which may contain phagocytosed debris or cells [Valicenti 1979].

Storage Diseases: These include Gaucher's disease, a lysosomal storage disease with accumulation of glucocerebroside in phagocytes, and Gaucher's cells, which are characterized by abundant cytoplasm with a "rumpled tissue" appearance [Carson 1994].

Atelectasis: Atypical squamous cells, foreign body macrophages.

Malignant Disease

Although sputum cytology has not been able to prevent lung cancer in the same way that the Pap smear has prevented cervical cancer, the general principle that early diagnosis is the best hope for cure, or at least better survival, still holds true [Melamed 1981]. In essence, the role of respiratory cytology is to detect and classify pulmonary disease, with an emphasis on neoplastic disease, so that proper therapy can be instituted.

Squamous cell carcinoma is the most common type of lung cancer diagnosed by classic exfoliative cytology, although its incidence is decreasing. It is also the most common type diagnosed in men. Adenocarcinoma is increasing in incidence, and is the most commonly diagnosed type of lung cancer in women. Small cell carcinoma is the most aggressive of the common types of lung cancer. Bronchioloalveolar carcinoma is an uncommon form of well-differentiated adenocarcinoma. The diagnostic criteria for large cell carcinoma and adenosquamous carcinoma are variable, and therefore, their incidences are also variable.

General Features of Respiratory Cancer Cytologic Diagnosis

As a general rule, cancer cells are more pleomorphic in size and shape than benign or reactive cells. Malignant cells are typically larger and have higher N/C ratios than their benign counterparts. Abnormal, coarse, dark, and especially irregularly distributed chromatin are key diagnostic features of malignant cells. In exfoliative respiratory cytology, the mere presence of mitotic figures is suspicious for malignancy, and must be adequately explained. On the other hand, ciliated cells are virtually always benign, with only very rare exceptions [P Gupta 1985].

The cytology of the common lung cancers will be discussed in the following sections. The cancers will be presented as if they occurred as pure lesions. However, many (in fact, probably most) lung cancers are mixtures of cell types. Mixtures of adenocarcinoma and squamous cell carcinoma are particularly common. Even a single cell can show evidence of glandular and squamous as well as neuroendocrine differentiation. In practice, a diagnosis of either small cell carcinoma or non–small cell carcinoma in primary lung cancer is usually sufficient to initiate therapy.

Squamous Cell Carcinoma

Patients with squamous cell carcinoma often present with cough and hemoptysis. Squamous cell carcinoma tends to arise centrally and usually can be diagnosed with sputum cytology and bronchial brushing/washing. The tumor can range from well to poorly differentiated or somewhere in between (moderately differentiated). In essence, sputum cytology usually shows more differentiated keratinized cells—with denser cytoplasm, more pyknotic nuclei, and fewer nucleoli compared with bronchial brushing/washing, which tends to select less differentiated, nonkeratinized cells—with more open chromatin and more prominent nucleoli. Bronchial brushing specimens may contain large tissue fragments of malignant cells. The two extremes of differentiation of squamous cell carcinoma will be compared and contrasted [T7.6].

Keratinizing ("Well-Differentiated") Squamous Cell Carcinoma

Keratinizing squamous cell carcinoma is characterized by malignant cells with heavy keratinization. Pearls (squamous eddies, whorls) are pathognomonic of keratinization [47 I7.40, 48 I7.43]. The heavier the keratinization, the more dissociation and single cells that are seen. Cytologic features of keratinization are usually more apparent in sputum than in bronchial washing/brushing specimens.

The tumor is composed of abnormal squamous cells with marked pleomorphism, including bizarre cell shapes (snakes, tadpoles, etc) [49 I7.37] and pumpkin cells (large, round, densely orange cells with abnormal, dark, often ink dot nuclei) [I7.37]. Finding very small cells with high N/C ratios juxtaposed with very large cells with low N/C ratios is characteristic of keratinizing squamous cell carcinoma. (Keratinizing squamous cell carcinoma is an exception to the general rule that malignant cells have high N/C ratios.)

T7.6 **Differences Between Keratinizing and Nonkeratinizing Squamous Cell Carcinoma (SCC)**

Feature	Keratinizing SCC	Nonkeratinizing SCC
Cohesion	More single cells	More groups
Cells	Very pleomorphic to bizarre	More uniform, none bizarre
Stain	Orange, pink	Blue-green
Keratinization	Pearls, rings, ghosts	Occasional dyskeratosis, but no pearls
N/C ratio	Low to high	High
Chromatin	Pyknotic, ink dot	Coarse, but more open
Nucleoli	Less prominent	More prominent

47
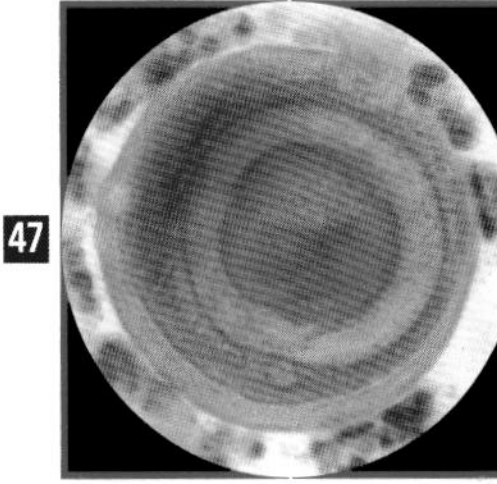

48
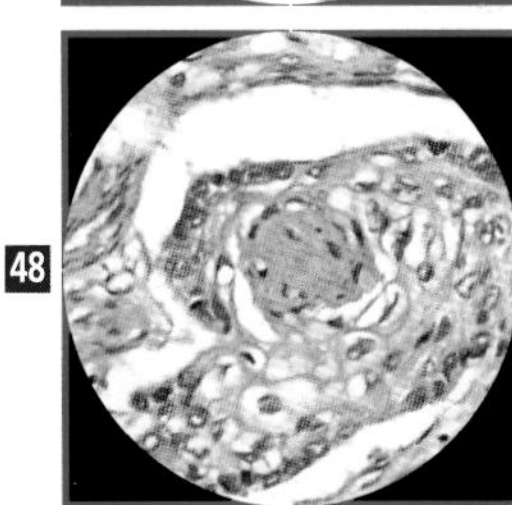

49
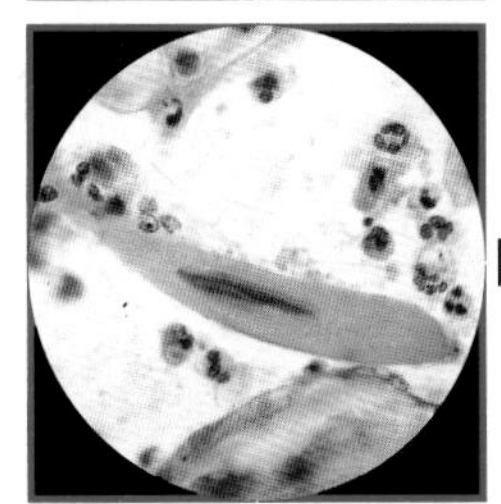

50
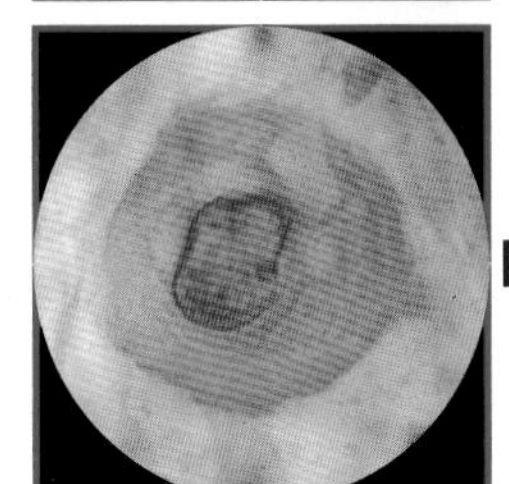

The cytoplasm is dense, waxy, or hard and varies from scant to abundant [I7.41]. The stain can vary from blue to pink to (most characteristically) bright orange. Basophilic tumor cells often predominate in bronchial brushings, and eosinophilic or orangeophilic cells predominate in sputum [49 I7.37, I7.38, 50 I7.39]. Refractile, concentric rings around the nucleus can be seen due to keratinization (best appreciated with the substage condenser diaphragm partially closed) [50 I7.39]. There is frequently a distinct demarcation between the ectoplasm and endoplasm, and the cell borders are sharply defined [Johnston 1986]. Herxheimer's spirals (twisted, ropy aggregates of filaments) are another feature of keratinization [Erozan 1986]. Well-defined intercellular bridges are diagnostically useful. However, they may be difficult to appreciate in routine cytologic specimens, but can be more readily seen in cell blocks.

The nuclei are also pleomorphic, with the chromatin varying from irregular, coarse, and hyperchromatic with clearing and clumping (especially in bronchial brushing/washing specimens) to a pyknotic, ink dot–like appearance (especially in sputum). Further nuclear degeneration (karyorrhexis) is common in keratinizing squamous cell carcinoma, and some cells may lose their nuclei altogether (karyolysis), resulting in pleomorphic, anucleate squames, or "ghosts." Multinucleation occurs and the multiple nuclei often mold one another. Although conspicuous nucleoli can be seen in keratinizing squamous cell carcinoma, particularly in brushing specimens, they are more often inconspicuous to invisible, being concealed by the dense, degenerated chromatin, particularly in sputum specimens. Mitotic figures, including abnormal forms, may occasionally be seen, but are rare.

In respiratory cytology, not as much emphasis is placed upon the presence of a diathesis in the diagnosis of cancer as in the Pap smear, although it is still an important factor to consider. Infiltrating tumors are usually associated with a diathesis. However, inflammation (including tuberculosis or fungus) or infarct can cause a necrotic background that may include atypical (reactive) squamous cells. These findings can mimic squamous cell carcinoma. If inflammation is absent, a necrotic background is more likely to be due to cancer.

Keratinizing squamous cell carcinoma may undergo extensive central necrosis (in part an attempt to recap normal exfoliation), producing a central cavity [51 I7.42]. If the cavity communicates with the bronchus, an abundance of necrotic material, containing markedly pleomorphic, degenerated, keratinized cells (anucleate squames, nuclear pyknosis, etc), and marked inflammation may appear in the specimen [Lavoie 1977]. The differential diagnosis includes fungus cavity (mycetoma) or caseating tuberculoma, which can also be associated with "atypical" (ie, reactive) cells [Weingarten 1981].

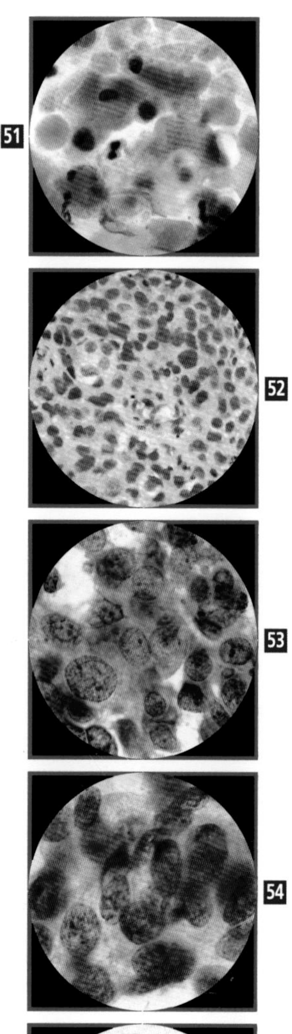

51

52

53

54

55

Differential Diagnosis of Keratinizing Squamous Cell Carcinoma

Various kinds of nonneoplastic, reactive processes (such as pneumonia, fungal infections, tuberculosis, pulmonary infarct, and tracheostomy tubes) can cause inflammatory squamous atypia, regeneration/repair, or atypical parakeratosis that can mimic squamous cell carcinoma [Naryshkin 1993]. These features, as well as bona fide dysplastic changes, are particularly common in necrotizing pneumonias (including fungal infections, especially *Aspergillus*) and pulmonary infarcts. Inflammatory atypia can show some cellular and nuclear pleomorphism, hyperchromatic nuclei and keratinized cytoplasm. Usually, however, the cells and their nuclei remain relatively uniform. The cells form cohesive sheets in mosaic arrangements, with few single cells. Be cautious when diagnosing malignancy in the absence of single cells with malignant features [Koss 1955, Naryshkin 1993]. The nuclei are often poorly preserved and the cytoplasm degenerated in reactive atypia. Single small nucleoli may be seen. Atypical parakeratosis, in particular, can be virtually indistinguishable from keratinizing squamous cell carcinoma, except for one important point—the parakeratotic cells are miniature. Be cautious when diagnosing squamous cell carcinoma in an inflammatory background, but be aware that squamous cell carcinoma can be inflamed too.

Radiation and chemotherapy effect as well as blue blobs and plant cells can mimic cancer, as previously discussed. It is also important to mention that occasionally keratinizing squamous cell carcinoma is so well differentiated that it exfoliates cells which, in the Pap smear, would probably be considered low-grade dysplasia rather than squamous cancer. Such a high degree of differentiation, however, is more likely in metastatic squamous cell carcinoma, particularly from the head and neck area, than in primary lung carcinoma [Matsuda 1988].

Nonkeratinizing "Poorly Differentiated" Squamous Cell Carcinoma

In a sense, nonkeratinizing squamous cell carcinoma is a misnomer [52 I7.46]. The tumor does have cytokeratin, but less than in keratinizing squamous cell carcinoma. In fact, the presence of an occasional heavily keratinized (dyskeratotic) malignant cell can be helpful in determining the nature of a poorly differentiated tumor. However, by definition, no well-formed pearls are present in pure nonkeratinizing squamous cell carcinoma, although an occasional cell-in-cell arrangement or "cannibalism" may be seen.

The malignant cells of nonkeratinizing squamous cell carcinoma are more cohesive than those of keratinizing squamous cell carcinoma, typically forming irregular, disorderly sheets, particularly in brushings [53 I7.44, 54 I7.45]. However, as in most cancers, single cells are also present, particularly in bronchial washing and sputum specimens.

The cells of nonkeratinizing squamous cell carcinoma range from relatively large (which can resemble adenocarcinoma) to small (which can resemble small cell carcinoma). However, in any given tumor, the cells are much more uniform than those of keratinizing squamous cell carcinoma. Bizarre cells, which are so characteristic of keratinizing squamous cell carcinoma, are absent in pure nonkeratinizing squamous cell carcinoma. Enlarged nuclei are accompanied by relatively small amounts of cytoplasm, resulting in increased N/C ratios.

The cytoplasm may be hard and waxy, but is more often cyanophilic (blue-green) than eosinophilic. Heavy keratinization or diffuse orangeophilia is not seen (in well-preserved material), but an occasional orange, dyskeratotic cell is often present. Dense cytoplasm and distinct cell borders are important features of squamous differentiation even in poorly differentiated tumors. There may also be some ectoplasmic/endoplasmic rimming and refractile ringing of the cytoplasm [Johnston 1986].

The nuclei are hyperchromatic. The chromatin is coarse and irregular, and somewhat more open than that of keratinizing squamous cell carcinoma. Pyknotic nuclei are unusual in nonkeratinizing squamous cell carcinoma. One or more prominent nucleoli may be present. Nucleoli are typically more prominent in nonkeratinizing than in keratinizing squamous cell carcinoma, but less so than in adenocarcinoma.

Differential Diagnosis of Nonkeratinizing Squamous Cell Carcinoma

Repair/regeneration with pleomorphic nuclei and prominent nucleoli can mimic nonkeratinizing squamous cell carcinoma, but has benign cytologic features (cohesive, orderly sheets, little nuclear overlap, and fine, even chromatin) 55 I7.25]. Bullous-forming diseases such as pemphigus may be associated with highly abnormal, single squamous cells, with prominent nucleoli and dense cytoplasm, but the benign cells have thick-appearing, smooth nuclear membranes and finely granular, even chromatin [Naryshkin 1993]. Other inflammatory and reactive changes are discussed in the section on keratinizing squamous cell carcinoma.

A common problem is distinguishing poorly differentiated adenocarcinoma [56 I7.49] from poorly differentiated squamous cell carcinoma [57 I7.38, T7.7]. By definition, the less differentiated a tumor, the fewer characteristic features it displays. The problem is compounded (or simplified) in the lung because the tumors are often mixed (eg, glandular and squamous). The presence of dense cytoplasm with distinct cell boundaries is evidence of squamous differentiation, while delicate, vacuolated, often basophilic cytoplasm with nucleocytoplasmic polarity (ie, "basal" nuclei and "apical" cytoplasm) is evidence of glandular differentiation. Mucin secretion and intracytoplasmic lumens are glandular features. Note that vacuolization, per se, is nonspecific. Keratinization is a squamous feature. However, coagulative necrosis of adenocarcinoma cells can mimic keratinization (pseudokeratosis).

An important problem is differentiating poorly differentiated squamous cell carcinoma, composed of small cells, from true small cell carcinoma. Distinct, dense cytoplasm, conspicuous nucleoli, little or no crush artifact, and little nuclear molding are clues to squamous differentiation in this situation. (See also "Small Cell Carcinoma.")

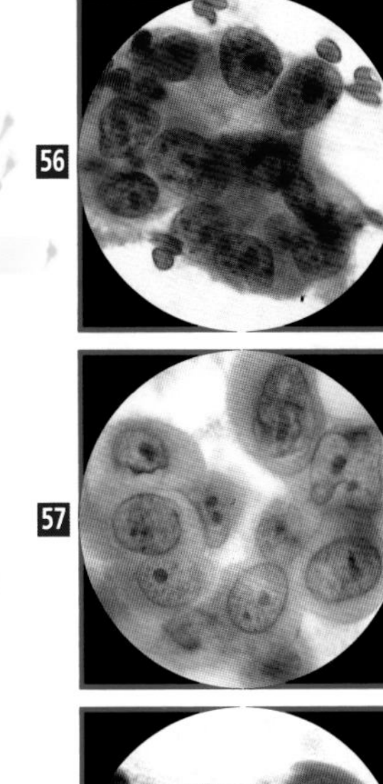
56
57
58

Squamous Dysplasia, Carcinoma In Situ, and Occult Cancers

Squamous cell carcinoma is the only type of lung cancer that is amenable to diagnosis at a preinvasive or an early, radiologically occult stage [Fullmer 1969a,b, Hattori 1964,1965, Matsuda 1990, Melamed 1977,1987, Nasiell 1977, Sassy-Dobray 1970,1975, Woolner 1973]. Localization of the lesion with flexible fiberoptic bronchoscopy is usually possible, but may be tedious [Martini 1980, Sagawa 1994, Sato 1993]. In analogy to the uterine cervix, the respiratory epithelium apparently undergoes premalignant changes over a course of 10 to 20 years before developing invasive cancer [Auerbach 1961, Frost 1973, Saccomanno 1974]. As in the cervix, these changes can be categorized as degrees of dysplasia and carcinoma in situ (or intraepithelial neoplasia or intraepithelial lesion). The abnormal, neoplastic process apparently arises in the milieu of squamous metaplasia [Auerbach 1961, Koprowska 1965, Nasiell 1963,1966, Saccomanno 1965,1974, Schreiber 1975], and therefore is also known as "atypical squamous metaplasia." This designation gives a good clue to its morphology [58 I7.47]. As in the cervix, not all dysplasias progress to cancer. However, even mild dysplasia is associated with a modest increase in risk of subsequently developing lung cancer [Vine 1990].

Low-grade dysplasia resembles metaplasia, but is more pleomorphic in cellular size and nuclear shape [T7.8]. With progressing abnormality, the N/C ratio increases and the chromatin becomes abnormally coarse and dark. The nuclear membrane appears thickened, may be irregular, and small nucleoli may appear.

The cytology of high-grade dysplasia/carcinoma in situ of the lung (or more precisely, the bronchi) is not as well-defined as for the cervix, but the basic features are similar [Papanicolaou 1951, Saccomanno 1982, Tyers 1976]. Carcinoma in situ is composed of small, round to oval, pleomorphic cells, with high N/C ratios. The cells are found singly or in loose clusters; syncytia are not required to diagnose carcinoma in situ in the bronchi. The nuclei are enlarged and hyperchromatic and have irregular membranes. Nucleoli, often basophilic, may be seen. The cytoplasm may be keratinized. There is usually no necrosis, inflammation, or marked pleomorphism. Ordinary squamous metaplastic cells usually outnumber the abnormal cells.

The cytologic distinction of carcinoma in situ from invasive carcinoma is not reliable. However, there are some clues that may suggest invasion. The presence of frankly malignant-appearing cells (ie, bizarre shape, heavy keratinization, irregular chromatin, macronucleoli), high cellularity, and diathesis favor invasive cancer [Erozan 1986, Tao 1982, Woolner 1970]. Because carcinoma in situ typically has a cleaner background than infiltrating carcinoma, the cells of carcinoma in situ may be more readily detected than invasive tumor cells in some cases.

If the lesion exfoliating cancer cells is radiologically visible, it is invasive. Note, however, that a radiologic abnormality does not necessarily correspond to the exfoliating lesion, eg, the patient could also have a granuloma. Many patients (approximately 30%) with positive sputum specimens, but radiologically occult lesions, have primary tumors in the head and neck region [Martini 1980]. However, even advanced primary lung cancer can be radiologically occult, particularly central squamous cell carcinoma (less commonly, peripheral BAC) [Martini 1980]. Multicentric abnormalities and multiple primary cancers are also common [Auerbach 1967, Martini 1980]. Thus, patients with primary lung cancer resected for cure should be monitored cytologically and radiologically on a regular basis [Broghamer 1985].

T7.7 **Differential Diagnosis Between Poorly Differentiated (PD) Squamous Cell Carcinoma (SCC) and PD Adenocarcinoma**

PD SCC	PD Adenocarcinoma
Irregular sheets	Cell balls
Cell-in-cell	Acini
Hard cytoplasm	Delicate cytoplasm
Distinct cell borders	Indistinct cell borders
Central nucleus	Eccentric nucleus
Coarse, dense chromatin	Finer, open chromatin
Smaller nucleoli	Larger nucleoli
Keratin	Mucin
Pitfalls	
Degenerative vacuoles	Pseudokeratosis

Note: Primary lung cancer frequently shows mixed adenosquamous differentiation.

***T7.8* Differential Diagnosis of Metaplasia, Low- and High-Grade Dysplasia, and Cancer**

Feature	Metaplasia	Low-Grade Dysplasia	High-Grade Dysplasia/Carcinoma In Situ	Cancer
No. of cells	As the lesion becomes more advanced, the number of atypical cells that are exfoliated tends to increase			
Groups	Sheets ± single cells	Sheets ± single cells	Single cells predominate + clusters	Fewer clusters
Cell size	Normal	Slightly enlarged	Enlarged up to twice normal	Large
Cellular pleomorphism	Little/none	Mild/moderate	Marked	Bizarre
N/C ratio	Normal	Slight variation	Moderate variation	Marked variation
Nuclei	Uniform	Slight variation	Moderate variation, ± multinucleation	Marked variation, multinucleation
Nuclear membrane	Smooth	Smooth	Lobulated	Irregular
Chromatin	Fine ± chromocenters	Fine ± chromocenters	Coarse, regular	Coarse, irregular
Nucleoli	±	±	Small, basophilic	Large, acidophilic
Cytoplasm	Basophilic	± Acidophilic	Acidophilic predominantly ± cannibalism	Acidophilic or basophilic, more cannibalism
Background	Clean	Clean	Clean	Diathesis; mass → invasion

[Erozan 1986, Papanicolaou 1951, Saccomanno 1974,1982, Tao 1982, Tyers 1976]

Practically speaking, the diagnosis of dysplasia and carcinoma in situ with respiratory cytology, especially sputum study, is tricky. Low-grade dysplasia is difficult to distinguish from reactive atypia, particularly that associated with pneumonia. In fact, low-grade abnormalities are more commonly associated with pneumonia than premalignancy. Severe dysplasia and carcinoma in situ are difficult to reliably distinguish from invasive cancer, and their patients certainly need to be fully investigated clinically. Nearly half the patients with a cytologic diagnosis of severe dysplasia will be found to have invasive cancer [Risse 1988]. Oral contamination of the specimen may result in the presence of atypical parabasal-sized squamous cells resembling metaplastic dysplasia, but deriving from infection, inflammation, or ulceration of the mouth or upper respiratory tract. Other possible sources of diagnostic error include radiation or chemotherapy effect, tracheostomy tubes, bronchiectasis, squamous metaplasia, benign squamous pearls, vegetable cells, as well as degenerated bronchial cells (common in postbronchoscopy specimens).

Adenocarcinoma

Adenocarcinoma usually occurs in the peripheral areas of the lung, but can also be centrally located (which is more typical of squamous cell carcinoma). The number of exfoliated cells is variable, but adenocarcinomas are generally more readily detected with bronchial cytology than sputum cytology, particularly when the tumor is small and peripheral. The incidence of adenocarcinoma is increasing, particularly among women, in whom it has become the most common primary lung cancer [Johnston 1988a]. Adenocarcinoma is associated with smoking, but less strongly than squamous cell carcinoma or small cell carcinoma. The chest x-ray may show a solitary nodule (differential diagnosis includes other "coin" lesions), multiple nodules (differential diagnosis: metastases), or a diffuse infiltrate (differential diagnosis: pneumonia). Adenocarcinoma of the lung can be grossly divided into two types, the usual bronchogenic type [I7.53] and bronchioloalveolar carcinoma [I7.62].

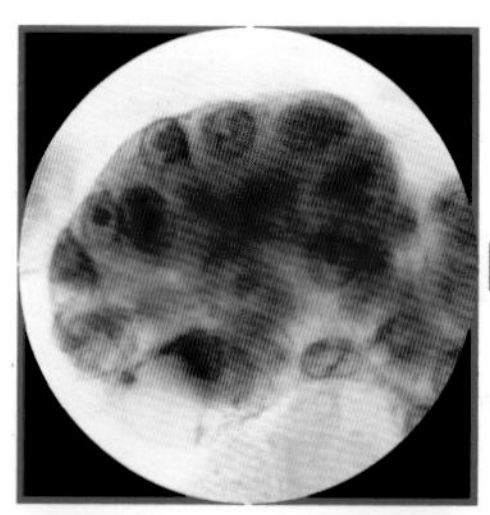
59

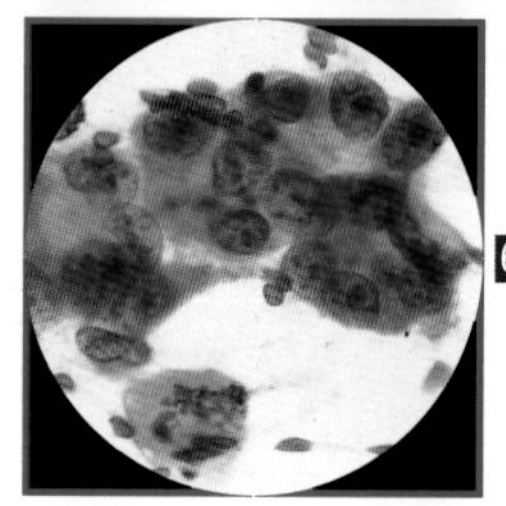
60

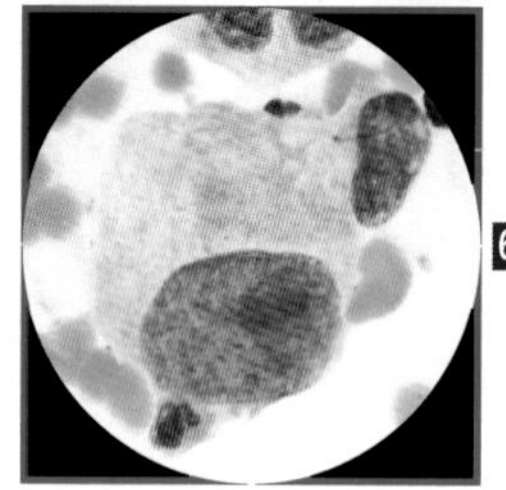
61

Bronchogenic Adenocarcinoma

Cytologically, the cells of ordinary bronchogenic adenocarcinoma may be found singly and in characteristic groups, including acini, tubules, cell balls, and papillae, depending upon the degree of differentiation [59 I7.48, I7.52, I7.53]. Sheets of crowded, irregularly arranged, disorderly cells with poorly defined cell borders can also be seen, particularly in brushings [I7.50]. Poorly differentiated adenocarcinoma grows in syncytial aggregates that may show little evidence of glandular differentiation. However, of interest is that glandular differentiation is often more apparent cytologically than in the corresponding histology. Small microacinar or rosette-like structures, which can be rather obvious cytologically even in poorly differentiated adenocarcinoma, may be inapparent histologically [60 I7.49]. Epithelial malignancies lacking any sign of specific differentiation are classified as undifferentiated carcinomas.

Bronchogenic Adenocarcinoma
- Architecture
  - Crowded Sheets, Cell Balls, Papillae
  - Microacini
- Nuclei
  - Polar orientation
  - Lobulated Border
  - Vesicular Chromatin
  - Prominent Nucleoli
- Cytoplasm
  - Foamy, Granular, or Secretory
  - ± Mucin

The cells of adenocarcinoma are relatively large and vary from cuboidal to columnar. A characteristic feature of adenocarcinoma, even when poorly differentiated, is the presence of nucleocytoplasmic polarity [61 I7.50]. Cell polarity may be also more obvious cytologically than histologically. The cytoplasm varies from homogeneous to foamy or finely vacuolated. However, large vacuoles suggest metastasis or reactive conditions [J Smith 1974]. The cytoplasm usually stains faintly basophilic, but color is not specific. Degenerated cells can stain eosinophilic or even orangeophilic [J Smith 1974]. The cell borders are indistinct and poorly defined compared with those in squamous cell carcinoma. Better-differentiated tumors may contain mucin-positive secretory vacuoles [62 I7.51].

The cells have enlarged nuclei with high N/C ratios. The chromatin is typically more finely granular and the nucleoli more prominent in adenocarcinoma than in squamous cell carcinoma. Classically, a single cherry-red macronucleolus is seen in the center of a relatively pale nucleus [63 I7.52]. However, the chromatin quality and size and number of nucleoli are variable. The nuclear membrane is often irregular or lobulated. Multinucleation is relatively common.

Differential Diagnosis of Adenocarcinoma

Nucleocytoplasmic polarity, three-dimensional clusters, microacini, irregular nuclear membranes, large nucleoli, and cytoplasmic vacuolization are among the most helpful features in the diagnosis of adenocarcinoma. Occasionally, adenocarcinoma undergoes coagulative necrosis—the cells turn pink to orange and the nuclei become pyknotic (dark and ink dot–like), closely resembling keratinizing squamous cell carcinoma ("pseudokeratosis"). On the other hand, squamous cell carcinoma may develop nonspecific, degenerative vacuoles that can mimic secretory vacuoles [Naryshkin 1993]. (For differential diagnosis of adenocarcinoma with reactive changes and BAC, see following section.)

Bronchioloalveolar Carcinoma

BAC is actually a group of tumors that can arise from different cell types, including ciliated terminal bronchiolar cells, Clara cells, and type II alveolar pneumocytes. Mucin production can be abundant, producing copious amounts of sputum (bronchorrhea). BAC begins in the terminal bronchioles or alveoli and grows along the preexisting bronchioloalveolar framework of the lung, *without invasion* (by strict definition) [I7.62]. The pattern of growth can be a single mass, multiple nodules, or massive/diffuse. The classic chest x-ray resembles pneumonia, but does not resolve.

The diagnosis of BAC by exfoliative cytology can be difficult. Among exfoliative cytologic methods, sputum cytology has the highest sensitivity and specificity for diagnosis of BAC [Ng 1983b]. BAL may be helpful in diagnosis [Milman 1992, Poletti 1995]. However, many cases of BAC cannot be recognized as malignant using exfoliative methods (ie, low sensitivity) [Kern 1988, Springmeyer 1983]. Moreover, even when correctly diagnosed as malignant, BAC is commonly misclassified, usually as ordinary bronchogenic adenocarcinoma (ie, low specificity) [Johnston 1981b]. Peripheral, solitary BAC is particularly difficult to diagnose by exfoliative cytology [Tao 1978b]; such tumors are best diagnosed by fine needle aspiration biopsy.

The cytology of BAC is similar to the usual type of adenocarcinoma, although BAC is more often well differentiated.

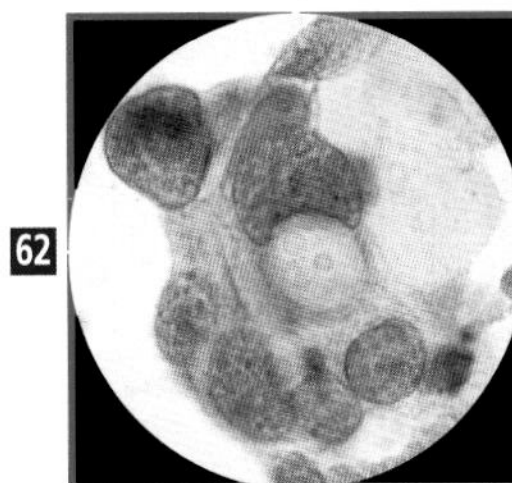

62

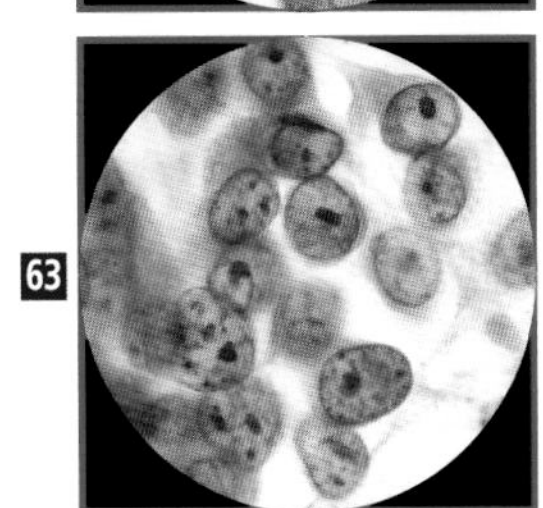

63

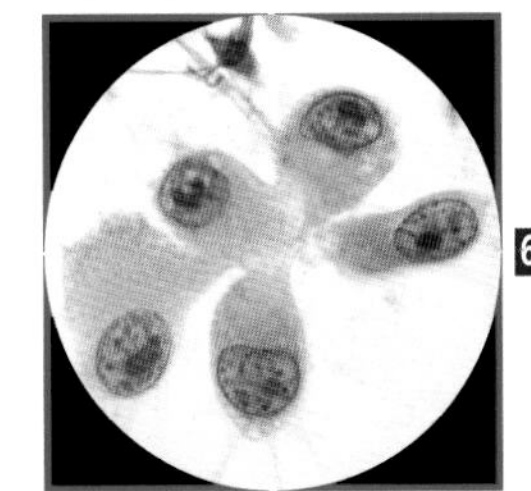

64

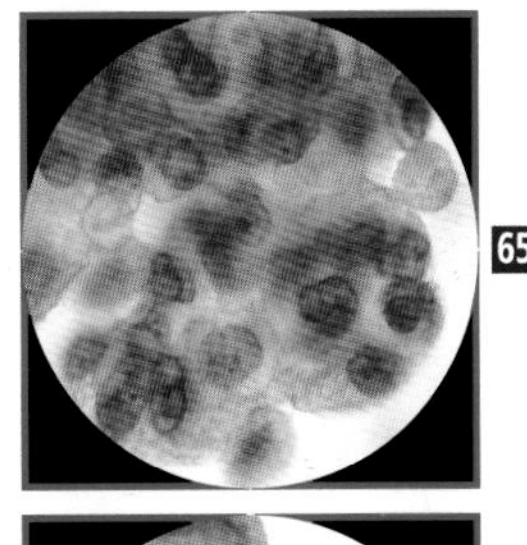

65

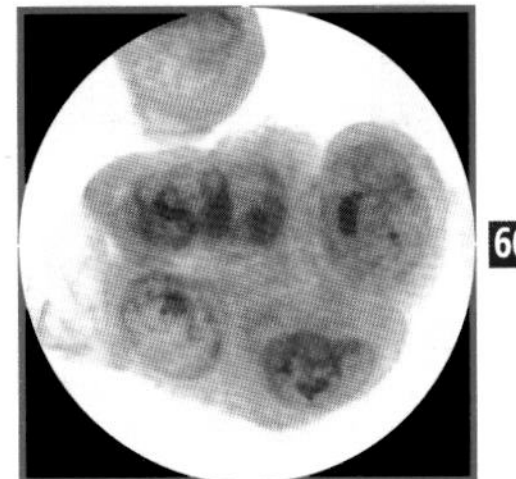

66

Poorly differentiated BACs also exist, but are essentially indistinguishable from ordinary adenocarcinoma. Finding abundant clusters of strikingly uniform cells suggests the diagnosis of BAC [J Smith 1974]. The tumor cells may be present in flat sheets or cell balls with great depth of focus (especially sputum). Cell balls often have flower petal–like or hobnailed outlines and do not mold [64 I7.55]. Papillary growth is a characteristic feature [I7.58-I7.61]. Acinar structures and single cells may also be seen, although single cells may be sparse in sputum [R Gupta 1981, Roger 1976]. Numerous clusters varying in size, texture, and number are a characteristic feature of BAC.

Bronchioloalveolar Carcinoma

Abundant cellularity (but variable)
Three-dimensional groups with great depth of focus
High degree of differentiation
Cells can resemble
- Goblet cells
- Mesothelial cells
- Alveolar macrophages

Two basic types of tumor cells can be recognized cytologically—mucinous and nonmucinous (or serous) [Tao 1978b]. Mucinous tumor cells are large and columnar and resemble goblet cells [65 I7.54], but frequently have prominent nucleoli which provide a clue for the diagnosis. Nonmucinous tumor cells are smaller and cuboidal, and reminiscent of mesothelial cells [64 I7.55]. The tumor cells can also closely resemble reactive alveolar macrophages [66 I7.56]. Benign macrophages may also be present in large numbers [Johnston 1986]. In fact, this mixture of cell types is a clue to the specific diagnosis of BAC. Compared with macrophages, the tumor cells have higher N/C ratios and lack phagocytosed debris [R Gupta 1981].

The cytoplasm varies from scant to abundant and finely granular to clear, depending on cell type. Mucin vacuoles are typical of mucinous tumors. The cells may have microvilli that can mimic cilia or terminal bars, but true cilia are not seen on the tumor cells [Johnston 1986].

The nuclei are round to oval and the chromatin is usually pale and fine, but can be moderately hyperchromatic. Intranuclear cytoplasmic invaginations are common but not specific [I7.57]. Nucleoli, usually one or two, can vary from inconspicuous to prominent, depending upon the cell type and degree of differentiation.

Abundant mucus in the background, when present, is a clue to the diagnosis. Rarely, psammoma bodies are seen [I7.57] [P Gupta 1972].

Differential Diagnosis of BAC (and Adenocarcinoma)

Pulmonary infarcts, bronchiectasis, asthma, viral pneumonia, radiation, or chemotherapy, among many other possibilities, can cause atypical changes closely mimicking adenocarcinoma. In some cases, it may not be possible, on cytologic grounds alone, to differentiate these benign changes from adenocarcinoma, particularly BAC [T7.9]. Be particularly cautious when making a diagnosis of BAC in a patient with an acute pneumonic illness, fever, or other condition known to be

T7.9 **Differential Diagnosis Between Benign Reactive Changes and Adenocarcinoma**

Favors Benign Reactive Changes	Favors Adenocarcinoma
History of acute/chronic respiratory disease	No history of pulmonary disease
Atypia diminishes with time	Atypia increases with time
Cell degeneration	Well preserved cells
Fewer atypical cells	More atypical cells
Transition from benign to atypical	Discrete population of atypical cells
Fewer single cells	More single cells
Orderly groups	Disorderly groups
Mild to moderate nuclear enlargement	Marked nuclear enlargement
N/C ratio within normal limits	High N/C ratio
Smooth nuclear membranes	Irregular nuclear membranes
Regular, micronucleoli	Irregular or macronucleoli
Regular fine to coarse chromatin	Irregular chromatin
Cilia or terminal bar	No cilia

associated with reactive atypia in respiratory cells [I7.58, I7.59, 67 I7.60, 68 I7.61]. The chest x-ray findings should be compatible with the presence of a tumor.

Bronchial hyperplasia (creola bodies), reactive alveolar pneumocytes, and atypical macrophages can mimic adenocarcinoma [Grotte 1990]. In benign conditions, there is usually a relative sparsity of atypical cells and the cells often appear degenerated. In contrast, there tends to be greater numbers of well-preserved cells in patients with adenocarcinoma, including BAC [Johnston 1982]. With serial specimens, reactive atypia should diminish.

Crowded, irregular arrangements of cells are typical of adenocarcinoma, while regularly arranged groups of cells are characteristic of benign reactions. An important clue to a benign process is finding a transition from clearly benign to atypical-appearing cells. In contrast, ordinary adenocarcinoma usually shows a discrete population of atypical cells [Naryshkin 1993]. Unfortunately, this diagnostic clue may be lost in BAC, in which there is frequently a bland component, even in less-differentiated tumors. Although single atypical cells are usually expected in cancer, they may not be apparent in sputum specimens of patients with BAC or bronchial brushing specimens of patients with ordinary adenocarcinoma.

Compared with benign reactive bronchial cells, malignant cells are generally larger, with larger nuclei and higher N/C ratios, abnormal chromatin, and nucleoli, and lack cilia. Benign features include cohesive groups, with peripheral palisading, mixture of cell types (goblet, ciliated), presence of cilia, and few or no atypical single cells. No abnormal nucleoli or macronucleoli should be seen in benign reactions, except in repair/regeneration. Benign muciphages can mimic mucinous BAC; look for typical histiocytic nuclei in the muciphages.

As mentioned, it may be difficult or impossible to distinguish BAC from garden variety bronchogenic adenocarcinoma. In fact, the cytologic differential diagnosis is largely presumptive—well-differentiated tumors, particularly papillary adenocarcinomas, are often presumed to be BAC. Papillae and cells with bland, uniform, round nuclei, and intranuclear cytoplasmic invaginations can be seen in ordinary bronchogenic adenocarcinoma, but are more common in BAC. Evidence of dual adenosquamous differentiation favors ordinary bronchogenic adenocarcinoma. Metastatic adenocarcinoma, especially papillary or clear cell types, may be indistinguishable from BAC. Clinical correlation is required; a diagnosis of BAC in a patient with another known primary adenocarcinoma is difficult to prove.

67

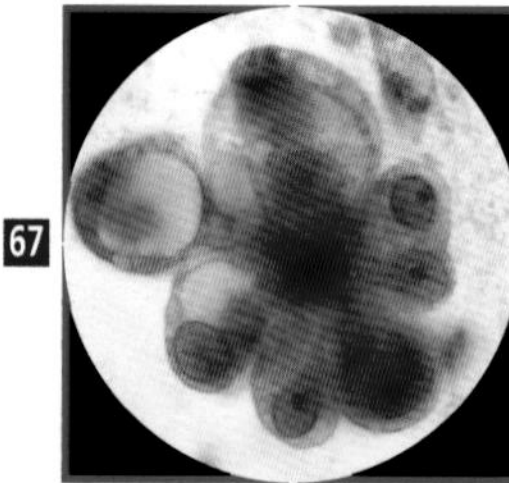

68

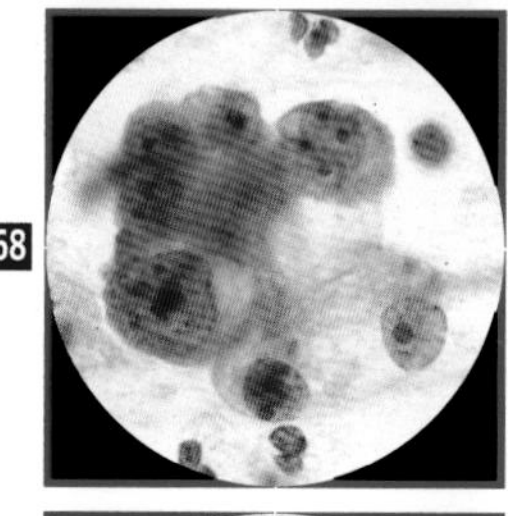

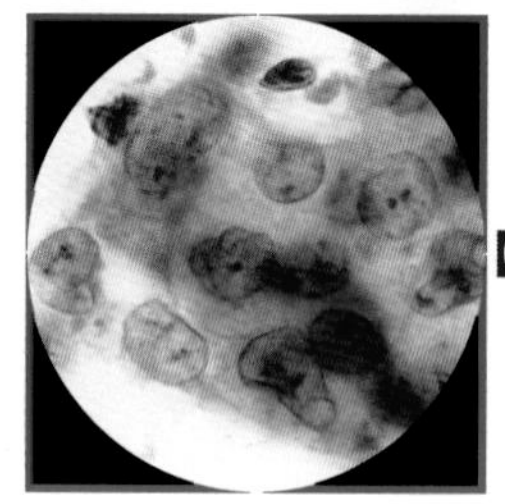

69

Large Cell Undifferentiated Carcinoma

Large cell undifferentiated carcinoma is usually easy to recognize as malignant. However, because it lacks light microscopic features of glandular, squamous, or neuroendocrine differentiation, this category is something of a wastebasket for tumors that are difficult to classify. Rudimentary differentiation is often more apparent cytologically than histologically. Using electron microscopy or immunocytochemistry, most large cell undifferentiated carcinomas are found to have glandular or squamous features, or both [Banner 1985, Hess 1981]. It is likely that large cell undifferentiated carcinoma represents a final common pathway of dedifferentiation of originally more differentiated tumors [Barbazza 1992]. For clinical purposes, tumors are usually classified using light microscopic rather than electron microscopic or immunocytochemical features.

Not surprisingly, the cells of large cell undifferentiated carcinoma are relatively large and undifferentiated [69 I7.71]. They can be fairly uniform in a given case, but are often pleomorphic. Single cells are usually plentiful, although groups are also present. The groups usually form syncytia with irregularly arranged, overlapped nuclei. By definition, neither glandular nor squamous features are seen.

The cytoplasm is relatively abundant and varies from delicate (but not secretory) to dense (but not squamoid) to granular. The staining varies from basophilic to amphophilic to acidophilic. The cell borders can be well or poorly defined. Keratinization and mucin secretion are totally absent.

The nuclei are obviously malignant appearing. They are large, pleomorphic, and round or irregular, with irregular or lobulated nuclear membranes The chromatin can vary from fine to coarse, and is irregularly distributed. Nucleoli can be prominent, multiple, and irregular. A diathesis is usually present in the background.

Differential Diagnosis of Large Cell Undifferentiated Carcinoma

By definition, glands, including acini and cell balls, and papillae are not seen, for this would indicate adenocarcinoma. Also, dense, hard cytoplasm and sharp cell boundaries, which would indicate squamous cell carcinoma, are not present. The relatively abundant cytoplasm, the quality of the nuclear chromatin, and prominent nucleoli exclude small cell carcinoma. However, non–small cell carcinomas may preferentially exfoliate apparently undifferentiated large cells, thus resulting in a misclassification of the tumor as large cell carcinoma.

Occasionally, the tumor cytoplasm has a clear appearance due to lack of organelles, and resembles clear cell carcinoma, such as from the kidney. Large cell undifferentiated carcinoma differs from large cell lymphoma primarily by the formation of at least a few true tissue groups. Germ cell tumors and the syndrome of undifferentiated carcinoma/poorly differentiated adenocarcinoma should also be considered in the differential diagnosis of large cell carcinoma, especially when the tumor occurs in a midline location in a young patient. The diagnosis is important because some patients respond to therapy. (See Chapter 13 and 21, for further discussion.) Sarcoma, melanoma, and metastatic malignancies should also be considered in the differential diagnosis. Radiation and chemotherapy can induce cytomegaly and marked atypia in benign cells, which should not be mistaken for malignancy (see p 221).

Giant Cell Carcinoma

If significant numbers of giant tumor cells are present, the tumor is designated giant cell carcinoma [70 I7.72] [Broderick 1975, Naib 1961, Pfitzer 1968]. This tumor may be extremely aggressive. A spindle cell component may also be present (giant and spindle cell carcinoma). Giant cell change is common after radiation or chemotherapy.

Small Cell Carcinoma

Small cell carcinoma is one of the most aggressive cancers. However, some therapeutic successes have been achieved using aggressive ("big gun") radiation and chemotherapy. Surgery is usually considered contraindicated in primary therapy of small cell carcinoma. Small cell carcinoma is a specific category of tumor thought to arise from or mimic Kulchitsky cells. The tumor often produces polypeptide hormones and therefore may be associated with various paraneoplastic syndromes (see Chapter 21).

The highest level of correlation between cytologic and histologic diagnoses is obtained in small cell carcinoma, which can be better than 95% [Johnston 1981b]. Small cell carcinoma arises in the major bronchi, but rather than forming a large primary tumor, it usually spreads rapidly to the hilar lymph nodes and produces large secondary masses. Thus, patients with small cell carcinoma may have unremarkable bronchoscopic findings or show only extrinsic compression, even in the face of widely disseminated disease [Jay 1980].

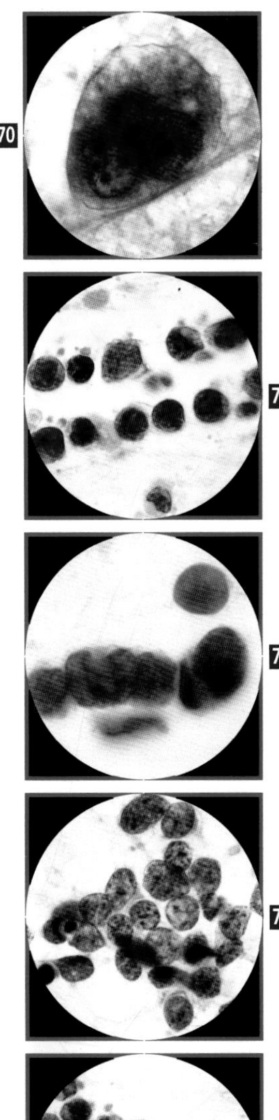

General Features of Small Cell Carcinoma

Small cell carcinoma has been subdivided into different categories: *pure* small cell carcinoma and two variants, *mixed* small/large cell carcinoma and *combined* small cell carcinoma. Pure small cell carcinoma is sometimes divided into oat cell carcinoma (the classic type) and intermediate cell carcinoma.

Small Cell Carcinoma

Cells
- Small, 1–4 times lymphocytes
- Conspicuous molding

Nuclei
- Hyperchromatic to pyknotic
- Inconspicuous nucleoli

Cytoplasm
- Scant, delicate

Diathesis

Tumors composed of both classic oat cells and intermediate cells are common. The variants of small cell carcinoma can have a large cell component (mixed small/large carcinoma) or show adenocarcinoma or squamous cell carcinoma (combined type). Variants are more common after therapy or in metastases. However, mixed and combined types are seldom recognized in exfoliative cytology (see also Chapter 21).

The tumor cells can vary somewhat (two to four times) in size, but marked variation is not a feature of pure small cell carcinoma. In sputum specimens, the tumor cells are often degenerated and nuclear detail may be obscured [71 I7.65]. Nevertheless, the cytologic features may still be sufficiently characteristic to be diagnostic, a rare example in which a definitive diagnosis can sometimes be rendered based on markedly degenerated cells. The characteristic features in sputum are the presence of small, dark cells forming loosely cohesive strings in mucus strands or Indian files with conspicuous nuclear molding and a necrotic background [71 I7.65, 72 I7.66]. In bronchial washing/brushing specimens, more cohesive, markedly molded groups with better preservation are seen [73 I7.68]. Indian file arrangements are also characteristic [74 I7.67].

The pick-and-smear technique may be preferred in sputum cytologic diagnosis of small cell carcinoma to either the Saccomanno or filter methods. The Saccomanno technique disperses the cells, reduces cytologic detail, and decreases nuclear molding, and the characteristic necrotic background (diathesis) may be lost. This can markedly decrease the diagnostic sensitivity [Perlman 1989]. The diagnostic yield may also be decreased with filters due to cellular distortion and decreased depth of focus at high power [Koss 1964].

Small Cell Carcinoma, Oat Cell Type

Oat cell carcinoma is composed of lymphocyte-like tumor cells with high N/C ratios. The cells are arranged in loose clusters reminiscent of cervical carcinoma in situ, or as single cells in variable proportions. In sputum specimens, the small cells are often found in linear arrays ("strings") in mucus strands [71 I7.65]. The cell size ranges from about one to two times the size of a lymphocyte. The tumor cells are smaller and more uniform in sputum, where they are degenerated, but are somewhat larger and more pleomorphic in bronchial washing/

brushing specimens. Fresh, very well-preserved cells may appear unexpectedly large (particularly in brushings and fine needle aspiration biopsy) [75 I7.67].

The cells often exhibit prominent nuclear molding. The nuclei are pleomorphic within their small size range, varying from round to very angular. The nuclear membrane is irregular. The chromatin is intensely hyperchromatic, and varies from finely granular in well-preserved cells (especially in brushing specimens) [75 I7.67] to pyknotic and ink dot–like (especially in sputum) [76 I7.65]. In classic oat cell carcinoma, nucleoli are always invisible or inconspicuous. Prominent nucleoli suggest poorly differentiated squamous cell carcinoma or adenocarcinoma.

The cytoplasm is very scant and delicate, consisting of a thin basophilic wisp. Sparse neurosecretory granules may be present, but their demonstration is not required to make the diagnosis. A diathesis is characteristically present around the tumor cells [Erozan 1986]. Because the tumor cells are very fragile, crush artifact (nuclear DNA streaming) is often present, particularly in brushings [77 I7.69, I7.70].

Small Cell Carcinoma, Intermediate Type

The intermediate type of small cell carcinoma is composed of cells that are generally similar in appearance to those of classic oat cell carcinoma, except that they are somewhat larger, ranging from about two to four times the size of a lymphocyte (or one to two times the size of an oat cell) [I7.67, I7.68]. They are also more pleomorphic (including spindle and polygonal cells), with coarser chromatin, more conspicuous (but not prominent) nucleoli, and more cytoplasm. The chromatin is similar to normal bronchial cells [78 I7.68]. Pyknotic nuclei are less common than in classic oat cell carcinoma. Crush artifact, a characteristic feature, is common, particularly in bronchial brushings.

There are no significant biological or therapeutic differences between classic oat cell carcinoma and intermediate (small) cell carcinoma. Mixtures of cell types are common. Large, prominent nucleoli, or particularly macronucleoli, indicate a diagnosis other than (pure) small cell carcinoma.

Variants of Small Cell Carcinoma

Small cell carcinoma occasionally shows focal glandular (cytoplasmic secretion, microacini) or squamous differentiation (more abundant, dense cytoplasm), which is known as combined small cell carcinoma [Zaharopoulos 1982]. In some cases, small cell carcinoma is mixed with larger, undifferentiated tumor cells, with more abundant cytoplasm and prominent nucleoli. This is known as mixed small/large cell carcinoma [Zaharopoulos 1982]. It may be difficult to distinguish variants of small cell carcinoma from poorly differentiated adenocarcinoma or squamous cell carcinoma. Also, using sputum cytology, which fails to localize lesions, another diagnostic possibility is separate, synchronous primary tumors of different types [Willett 1984]. Benign, reactive glandular or squamous elements in small cell carcinoma should not be mistaken for combined differentiation.

T7.10 **Differences Between Reserve Cell Hyperplasia and Small Cell Carcinoma**

Reserve Cell Hyperplasia	Small Cell Carcinoma
More cohesive	Less cohesive
More uniform	More pleomorphic
Little molding	Prominent molding
Smooth nuclear border	Irregular nuclear border
± Prominent nucleoli	Inconspicuous nucleoli
No diathesis	Diathesis
No crush artifact	Crush artifact (especially with bronchial brushing)
± Cilia	No cilia

75
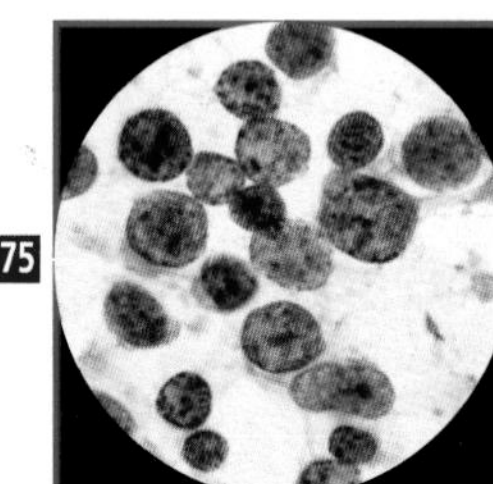

76
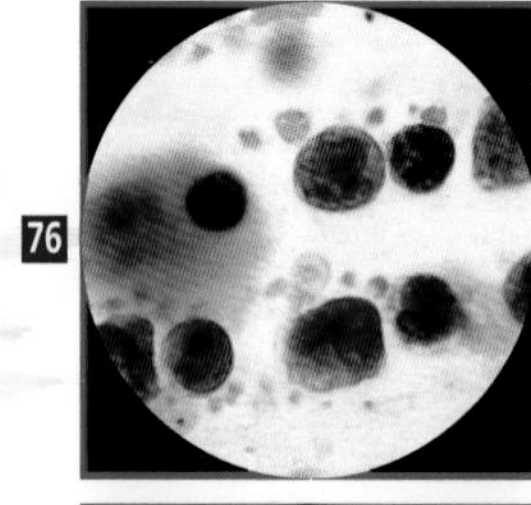

77
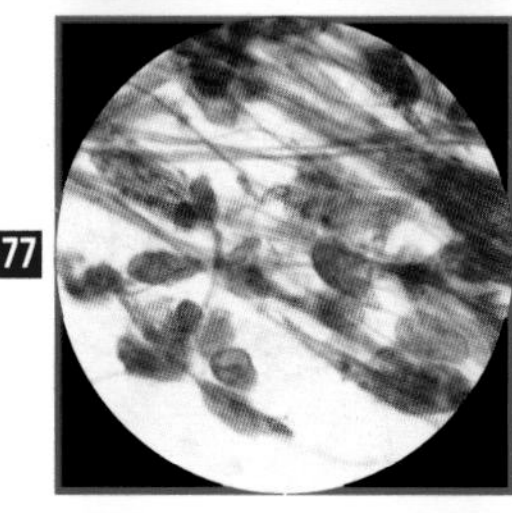

78
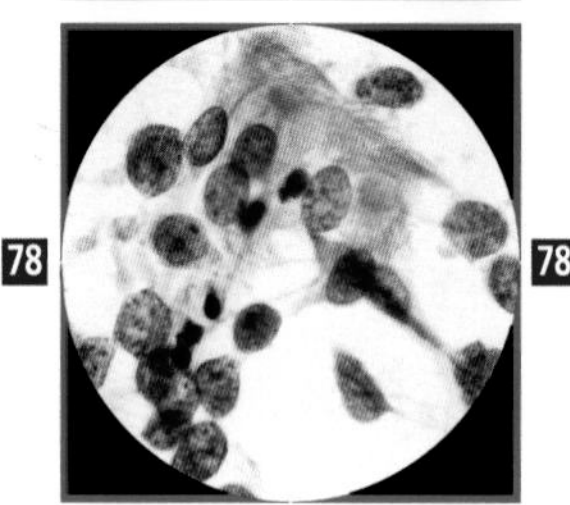
78

Differential Diagnosis

In sputum specimens, schools of lymphocytes in pools of mucus can resemble small cell carcinoma. A characteristic diagnostic feature of both benign and malignant lymphocytes is their failure to form tissue aggregates, while small cell carcinoma is characterized by at least a few cohesive, molded groups of cells. Prominent nucleoli may be seen in large lymphocytes, but not pure small cell carcinoma. Necrosis can be seen in small cell carcinoma, but is not seen in benign lymphocytes and is unusual in lymphoma (except as tingible body macrophages). Lymphoglandular bodies may accompany lymphoid cells.

Reserve cell hyperlpasia (RCH) is composed of small cells with hyperchromatic nuclei and scant cytoplasm, which can exhibit molding, thereby mimicking small cell carcinoma [T7.10]. However, the cells of RCH are more cohesive and uniform, have smooth nuclear borders, and lack a diathesis. At the margins of groups of cells of RCH there may be maturation to columnar cells, sometimes with cilia [Naryshkin 1993]. However, small cell carcinoma can grow underneath a benign epithelium, causing the misleading impression that the tumor cells are ciliated [78 I7.68]. Prominent nucleoli can be seen in reactive conditions, but not pure small cell carcinoma. Diathesis or crush artifact is not seen in benign conditions, but may be seen in small cell carcinoma, particularly in brushings.

Although it is obviously important to distinguish small cell carcinoma from benign conditions, it is also critically important to differentiate small cell carcinoma from all other types of lung cancer (ie, non–small cell carcinoma) because the therapy may be different.

Distinguishing very poorly differentiated squamous cell carcinoma from small cell carcinoma is perhaps the most common differential diagnostic dilemma [T7.11]. In contrast with small cell carcinoma, poorly differentiated squamous cell carcinoma has more prominent nucleoli, more and denser cytoplasm, and little or no crush artifact. Dyskeratotic cells may be seen. The keratin of squamous cell carcinoma, even in so-called nonkeratinizing squamous cell carcinoma, may incite a granulomatous

T7.11 **Differences Between Poorly Differentiated (PD) Squamous Cell Carcinoma and Small Cell Carcinoma**

PD Squamous Cell Carcinoma	Small Cell Carcinoma
Cell-in-cell	Indian file
Less nuclear molding	Prominent nuclear molding
Conspicuous nucleoli	Inconspicuous nucleoli
Slightly more and denser cytoplasm	Very scant, delicate cytoplasm
Little or no crush artifact	Crush artifact (especially with bronchial brushing)
Granulomas may occur	No granulomas

reaction. A confounding problem is that atypical squamous metaplasia, squamous carcinoma in situ, and invasive squamous carcinoma can coexist with small cell carcinoma [Boucher 1995].

Poorly differentiated adenocarcinoma can also be considered in the differential diagnosis. Metastatic adenocarcinoma from the breast is particularly likely to show a small cell pattern. Either adenocarcinoma or small cell carcinoma can grow in Indian files or exhibit molding. Characteristics of adenocarcinoma include the presence of three-dimensional cell balls, eccentric nuclei, and prominent nucleoli. Mucin production is indicative of glandular differentiation. Crush artifact is more often associated with small cell carcinoma than adenocarcinoma.

Carcinoid tumors, particularly atypical carcinoids, can also present a diagnostic problem. In fact, these neoplasms are thought to be in the same family as small cell carcinoma, comprising a spectrum of neuroendocrine tumors. Typical carcinoid cells should not be too difficult to distinguish from the cells of small cell carcinoma because carcinoids are much more uniform, have more cytoplasm, often have typical salt-and-pepper chromatin and variable nucleoli, and may form rosettes. No necrosis is present in typical carcinoid tumors.

The differential diagnosis between small cell carcinoma and atypical carcinoid can be particularly difficult. The cytologic features of atypical carcinoid are intermediate between typical carcinoid and small cell carcinoma. However, in contrast with typical carcinoid, some necrosis may be present, and in contrast with small cell carcinoma, prominent nucleoli may be seen. The more closely atypical carcinoid resembles small cell carcinoma, the worse the prognosis.

Although small cell carcinoma, by far, most commonly arises in the lung, similar or identical tumors are known to arise in a number of other organs. Other types of neuroendocrine tumors, such as paragangliomas/pheochromocytoma, could also be considered in the differential diagnosis [De Jong 1991]. Small cell malignancies of childhood (embryonal rhabdomyosarcoma, neuroblastoma, Wilms' tumor, Ewing's sarcoma) could theoretically be a cytodiagnostic problem, but small cell carcinoma of the lung is exclusively a disease of adults (see Chapter 12).

In summary, the lesions discussed (RCH, lymphocytes, bronchial cells, non–small cell carcinomas, carcinoids, etc) can be associated with conspicuous nucleoli, well-preserved coarse chromatin, distinct cytoplasm, no necrosis, and little or no molding. These five features may help differentiate these entities from small cell carcinoma.

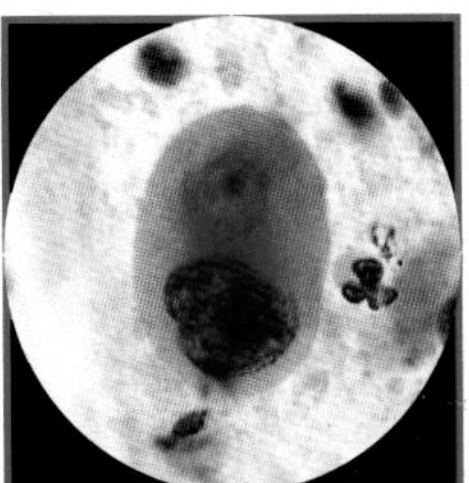

79

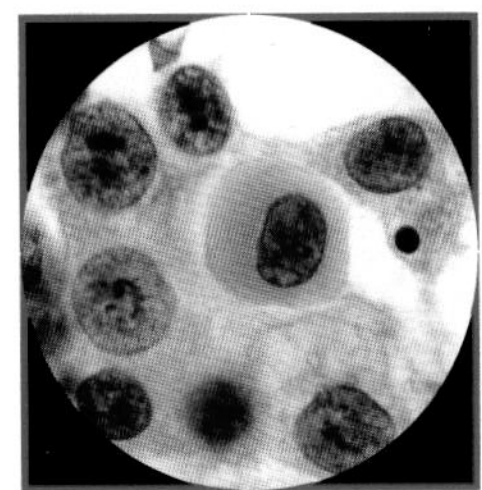

80

Adenosquamous Carcinoma

Cancer of the lung with well-defined adenocarcinomatous and squamous cell carcinomatous components, ie, adenosquamous carcinoma, has been considered relatively rare, particularly histologically. However, cytologically, tumors exhibiting at least minor degrees of dual differentiation are very common [Johnston 1986]. In fact, mixed adenosquamous carcinomas may be the single most common type of lung cancer (see Chapter 21).

A mixed adenosquamous carcinoma is a tumor that shows evidence of both keratin (ie, squamous features such as dense cytoplasm, distinct cell borders, rings, pearls, etc) and secretion (ie, glandular features such as nucleocytoplasmic polarity, acini, mucin). To make the diagnosis, look for cells with nucleocytoplasmic polarity (a grandular feature), but with dense cytoplasm (a squamous feature) [79 I7.64]. Also, look for a sharp contrast between dense squamoid cytoplasm and delicate glandular cytoplasm [80 I7.63]. Double carcinomas, with squamous cell carcinoma in one site and adenocarcinoma in another, could shed into sputum, creating the false impression of dual differentiation [Grunze 1973] (see Chapter 21).

Carcinoids

Carcinoid tumors usually arise in a large bronchus, probably from Kulchitsky cells or their precursors. They are essentially identical to similar neuroendocrine tumors occurring in the gastrointestinal tract, among other sites. Bronchial carcinoids rarely produce the carcinoid syndrome. Because the tumors are usually covered by an intact bronchial mucosa, the tumor cells seldom exfoliate spontaneously. Therefore, this tumor is unlikely to be diagnosed in sputum specimens unless ulcerated or after bronchoscopy, although diagnostic cells may be found in bronchial brushings (or fine needle aspiration biopsies).

The tumor cells are cohesive, forming sheets, ball-like clusters, or rosettes, but are also present singly [W Lozowski 1979]. They are small and monotonous, and round to oval. The appearance of the cells is reminiscent of small histiocytes, lymphocytes, or plasma cells. The cytoplasm is variable in amount (from scant to moderate), delicate, basophilic, and poorly outlined. The nuclei are eccentric, occasionally multiple, usually round, and very uniform. The chromatin classically has a salt-and-pepper appearance, but its texture is variable. Nucleoli are usually small, but may be conspicuous. Occasionally, larger, atypical, or multinucleated cells are present ("endocrine atypia").

The nuclear features are similar to those of normal or reactive bronchial cells, but bronchial cells are columnar and often have cilia [Gephardt 1982]. The small tumor cells should not be mistaken for small cell carcinoma [Kyriakos 1972]. Atypical carcinoids have features intermediate between typical carcinoids and small cell carcinoma, with more pleomorphism, hyperchromasia, mitoses, necrosis, and molding than typical carcinoids but less atypia, more cytoplasm, and more prominent nucleoli than small cell carcinoma [Jordan 1987]. Also, in contrast with both typical carcinoid and small cell carcinoma, atypical carcinoid tends to be peripheral rather than central. Spindle cell carcinoids usually occur in the periphery of the lung. Their nuclear features are similar to those of typical carcinoids, but the cells are elongated or spindle shaped.

Pulmonary tumorlets are minute epithelial growths that have been associated with chronic inflammation and fibrosis, particularly bronchiectasis, but also including tuberculosis [Marchevsky 1982]. Tumorlets are composed of cells resembling spindle cell carcinoids. (See also Chapter 21.)

Granular Cell Tumor

The tumor cells are elongated, spindle, strap-like, or polyhedral cells with abundant, coarsely granular cytoplasm (= lysosomes) present singly or in loose clusters [Chen 1991, Füzesi 1989, Glant 1979, Guillou 1991, Mermolja 1991, Naib 1962, L Thomas 1984]. The granules are PAS positive. The nuclei are usually small and bland, round to spindle, but may be somewhat atypical. The tumors occur endobronchially in the submucosa, and usually do not spontaneously exfoliate cells, but can be diagnosed with bronchial brushing. (See Chapter 14 for illustration.)

Salivary Gland Analog Tumors

A variety of neoplasms analogous to salivary gland tumors occur rarely in the lung (usually trachea or major bronchi). They probably arise from submucous glands. (See also Chapter 16.)

Adenoid-Cystic Carcinoma

This is a rare lung tumor that more commonly arises in the trachea than the bronchi. The tumors may be covered with tracheobronchial epithelium. Thus sputum cytology is usually negative and the tumor is best diagnosed with bronchial brushing (or Wang needle).

The cells are present in cohesive, globular, honeycomb arrangements and may form three-dimensional ball-like clusters, some with cystic spaces containing hyaline, basement membrane material [Buchanan 1988, R Gupta 1992, Hajdu 1969, M Lozowski 1983, Radhika 1993]. The cells are small and uniform, with bland to hyperchromatic nuclei and small nucleoli, but lack conspicuous nuclear molding. The differential diagnosis includes well-differentiated adenocarcinoma, carcinoid, and small cell carcinoma.

Mucoepidermoid Carcinoma

This tumor shows clusters of malignant squamous cells and mucus-secreting glandular cells; a third (intermediate or spindle) cell type may be seen in low-grade malignancies. High-grade mucoepidermoid carcinoma is indistinguishable from ordinary mixed adenosquamous carcinoma [Nguyen 1988].

Oncocytoma

This tumor is characterized by cells with abundant finely granular cytoplasm (due to mitochondria) and round to oval nuclei with somewhat coarse chromatin and occasional nucleoli [Cwierzyk 1985].

Blastoma

This is a biphasic malignant tumor of epithelium (adenocarcinoma) and mesenchyme (stromal cells); the malignant cells tend to be relatively small [Francis 1979, Non 1976, Spahr 1979, Yokoyama 1992]. Only the adenocarcinomatous component may exfoliate in some cases [Meinecke 1976].

Carcinosarcoma

Rarely, these mixed tumors may shed sarcoma cells (eg, rhabdomyoblasts [Ishizuka 1988]) *plus* carcinoma cells [S Takeda 1994]. More commonly, only the carcinomatous component exfoliates cells.

Sarcomas/Rare Tumors

Sarcomas can have spindle, round, or pleomorphic cells, be primary or metastatic, and represent a wide range of possible tumor types [Fleming 1975, Lambird 1970, Sawada 1977]. Germ cell tumors can also be seen in respiratory cytology [Gindhart 1979]. Consider one of these rare neoplasms when diagnosing a tumor that does not fit neatly into one of the more common categories. (See also Chapters 14, 21, and 28.)

Malignant Lymphoma

Primary malignant lymphoma of the lung is rare; large cell non-Hodgkin's lymphoma is the most common type [Schumann

1983], and Hodgkin's disease also occurs. Secondary involvement is more common. The cytologic appearance depends on the specific type of lymphoma. The cells may be reminiscent of oat cell carcinoma, but characteristically do not form groups, and there is no molding [81 I7.73]. Also, the cytoplasm is usually more abundant and the cell outlines are more rounded. The nuclei are usually somewhat uniform and the chromatin is more open. Nuclear protrusions and cleaves may be present. Unlike small cell carcinoma, prominent nucleoli may be seen in some lymphomas. Lymphoglandular bodies are typically present in the background of smears of lymphoma. Reed-Sternberg cells and variants may be seen in Hodgkin's disease [82 I7.74] [Fullmer 1972, Levij 1972, Reale 1983, Stanley 1993, Suprun 1964, Wisecarver 1989]. Atypical cells of mycosis fungoides [Ludwig 1983, S Rosen 1984, Shaheen 1984], hairy cell leukemia [Volpe 1981], or myeloma [Riazmontazer 1989] can also be seen in respiratory material.

Metastases

Metastatic adenocarcinoma is three times more common than primary adenocarcinoma of the lung [83 I7.79]. Virtually any malignant tumor can metastasize to the lung. The most common sites of origin are the gastrointestinal tract, breast, and lymphoma/leukemia [Burke 1968]. Melanoma [84 I7.78] and sarcomas also frequently metastasize to the lung [I7.75-I7.81]

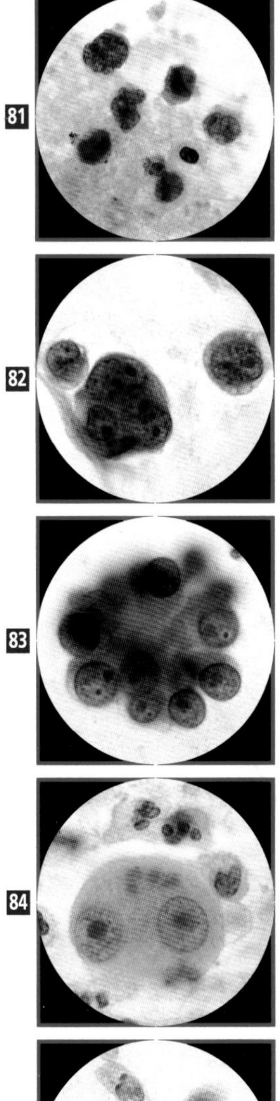

[Khoddami 1993]. Multiple nodules favor metastatic disease. Also to be considered in the differential diagnosis are tumors that have involved the lung by direct extension, such as esophageal carcinoma. Of course, patients with other cancers can also develop primary lung cancer.

Respiratory cytology, particularly the Saccomanno method, may not be quite as good at diagnosing metastatic tumors as primary cancers [Ellis 1950, Kern 1976, Risse 1985]. Small peripheral lesions are more difficult to detect and the differential diagnosis of primary vs metastatic adenocarcinoma can be particularly difficult. A metastatic tumor mass involving a major bronchus is more likely to shed diagnostic cells. The cardinal rule of diagnosis of metastatic malignancy is to review the material from the primary, if available, to see if the new lesion matches or is compatible with the original tumor. Generally, metastases yield cohesive clusters of cells in a clean background (as in the Pap smear). However, some metastases invade locally (approximately 20%), and a diathesis can then be seen. In direct extension, the background may be extremely "dirty."

Consider a metastasis when malignant cells are found that do not resemble ordinary forms of lung cancer. For example, breast carcinoma tends to have tight, thick clusters of cells, molded nuclei with pale chromatin, prominent nucleoli, and intracytoplasmic lumens. Signet ring cells suggest gastric origin [85 I7.75].

Bear in mind that malignant tumor cells deriving from primary lesions in the oral cavity or esophagus, not involving the lung, can also be found in sputum.

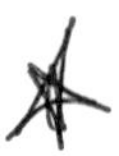

I7.1
Benign squamous pearl. Most squamous cells originate in the mouth, particularly when present in sputum specimens.

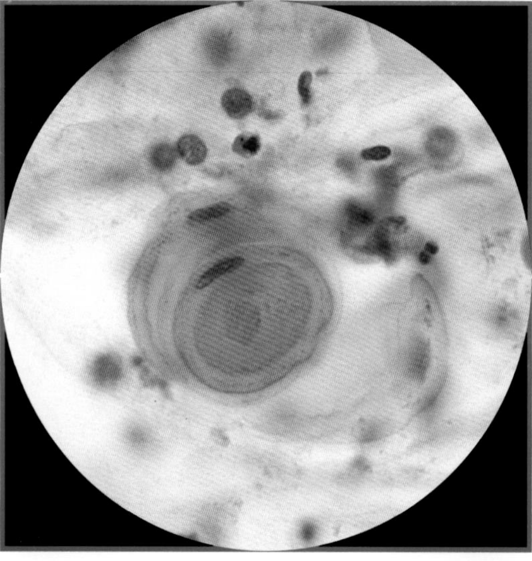

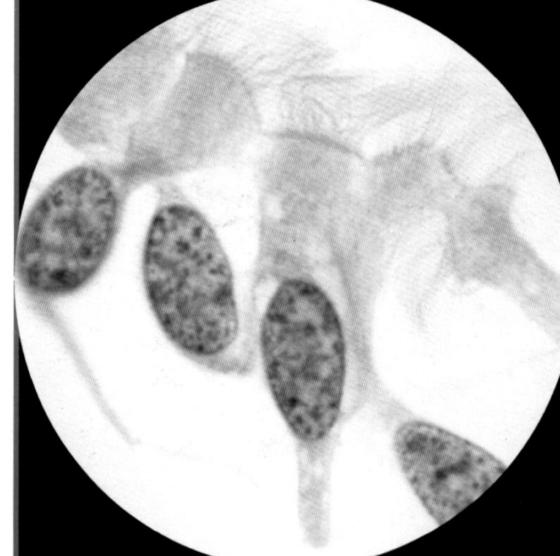

I7.2
Ciliated columnar cells. These so-called "bronchial cells" can actually be found as far away from the lung as the nose. Note the moderately coarse and hyperchromatic chromatin (compare with small cell carcinoma). Also note the little tails where the cells were attached to the basement membrane and, of course, the presence of terminal bars and cilia. (Oil)

I7.3
Goblet cell hyperplasia. Normally, the ciliated cells far outnumber the secretory cells (by at least 5 to 1). However, in asthma, for example, the goblet cells may actually outnumber the ciliated cells. When goblet cells are abundant, exclude bronchioloalveolar carcinoma.

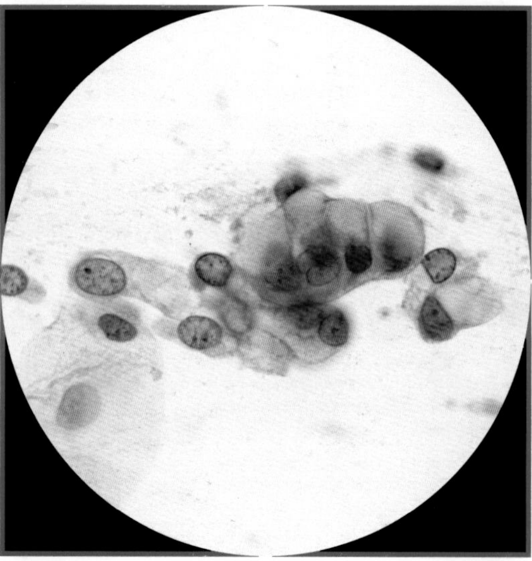

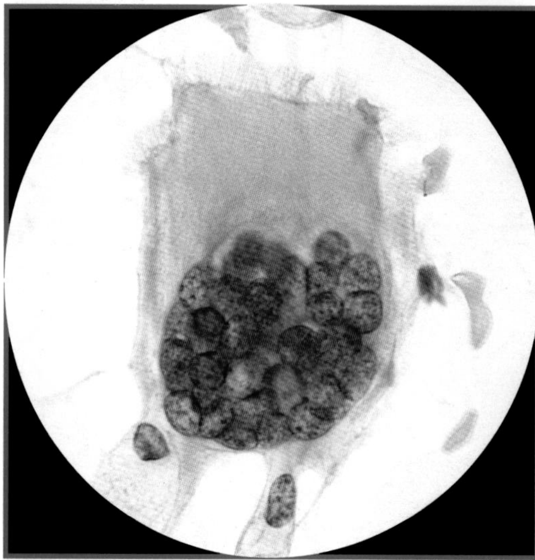

I7.4
Bronchial irritation cell. As a result of injury, bronchial cells commonly undergo various reactive changes, including multinucleation. Occasionally, myriads of nuclei are present. (High dry)

I7.5
Ciliocytophthoria. Detached ciliated tufts are a nonspecific finding related to bronchial cell injury. Do not mistake these for parasites. (Oil)

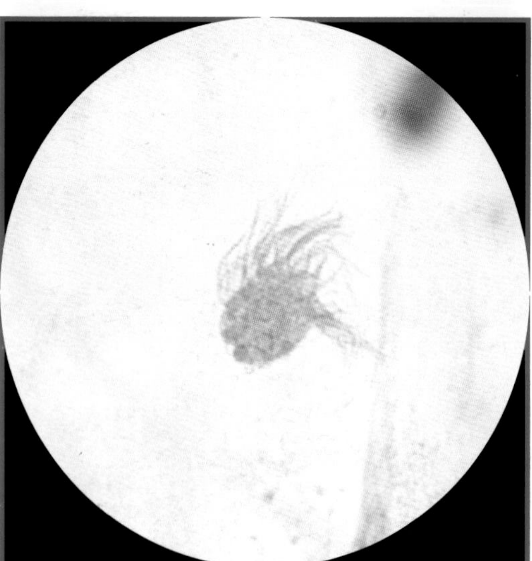

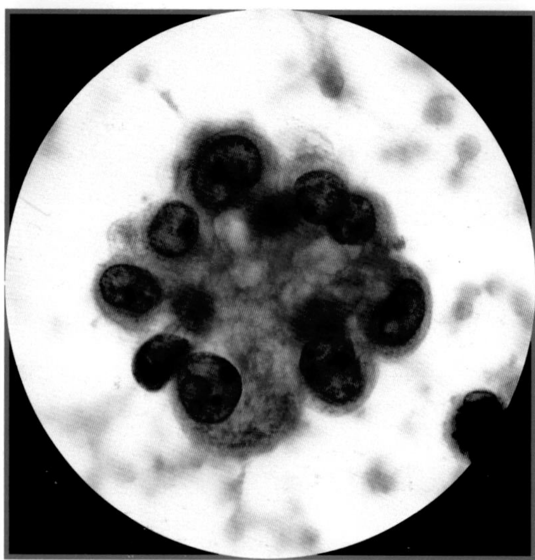

I7.6
Reactive (type II) pneumocytes. In response to severe injury, including infarcts or infections, the type II alveolar pneumocytes proliferate. These cells can show marked atypia, including high N/C ratios, pleomorphism, irregular nuclear membranes, chromatin clumping, and macronucleoli. The reactive cells may be present singly or in glandular clusters that strongly suggest adenocarcinoma.

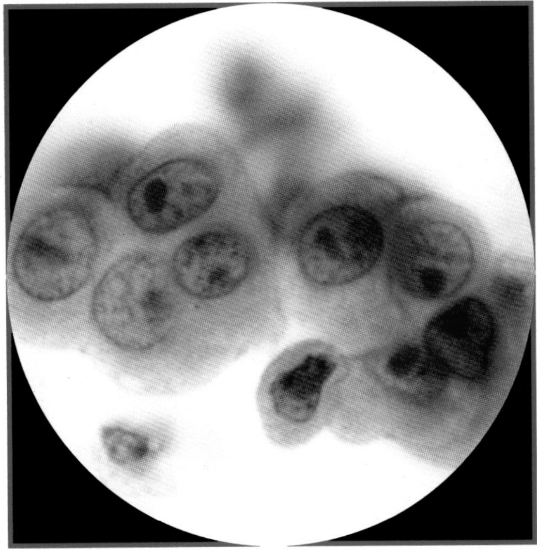

I7.7
Reactive bronchioloalveolar cells. A morphologic expression of the response of pneumocytes to injury that can mimic malignancy. Benign clusters such as these are usually sparse.

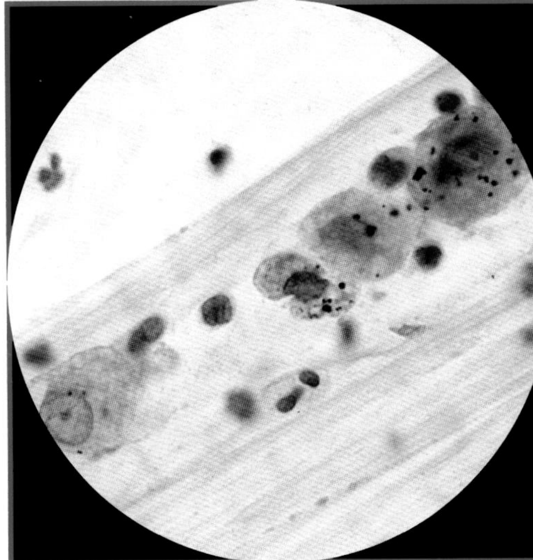

I7.8
Alveolar macrophages (sputum). The presence of alveolar macrophages indicates that the "deep lung" has been sampled. Alveolar macrophages are bone marrow–derived histiocytes that live in the alveoli and phagocytose the various dusts ("dust cells"), including carbon pigment ("carbon histiocytes") and other garbage we breathe.

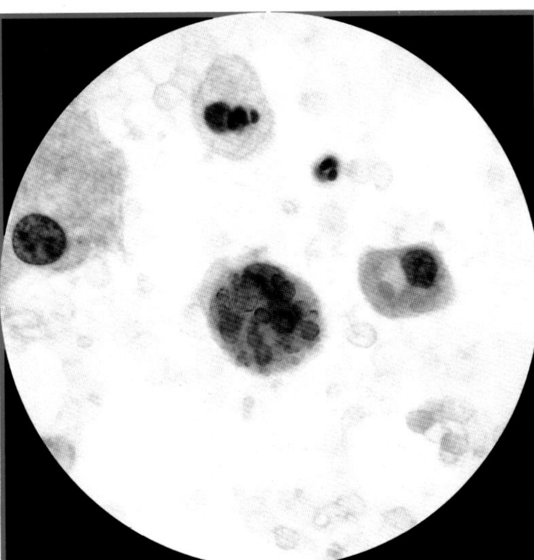

I7.9
Siderophages. Hemosiderin-laden macrophages indicate old bleeding. They are sometimes known as "heart failure cells" but are not specific. Note that hemosiderin is a refractile golden pigment.

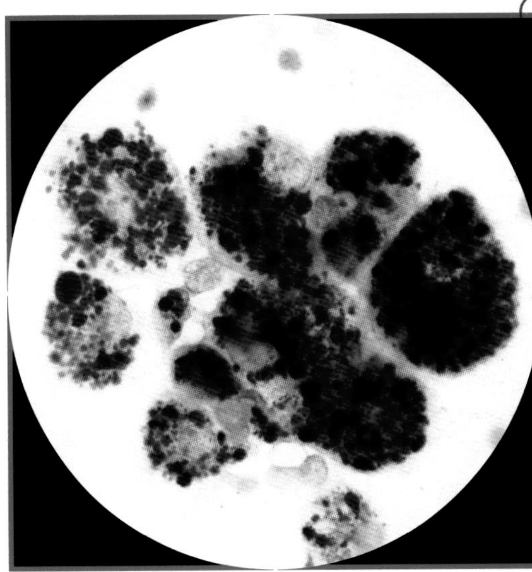

I7.10
Siderophages. Presence of iron confirmed by special stain. (Prussian blue)

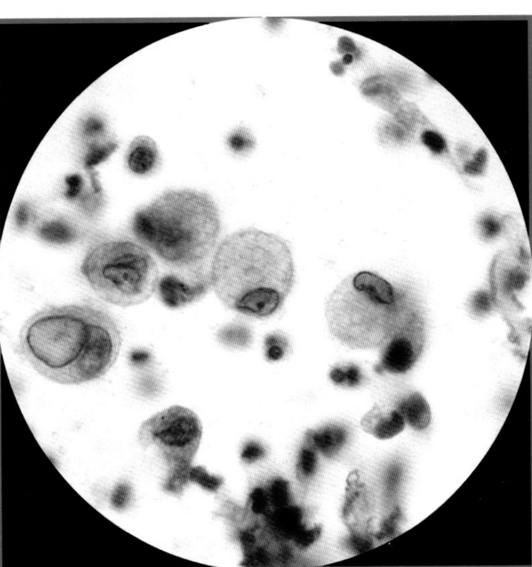

I7.11
Lipophages. Lacy bubbly cytoplasm of macrophage is due to presence of lipid. Lipid source can be exogenous (eg, oily nose drops) or endogenous (related to tissue destruction, including infections and *cancer*).

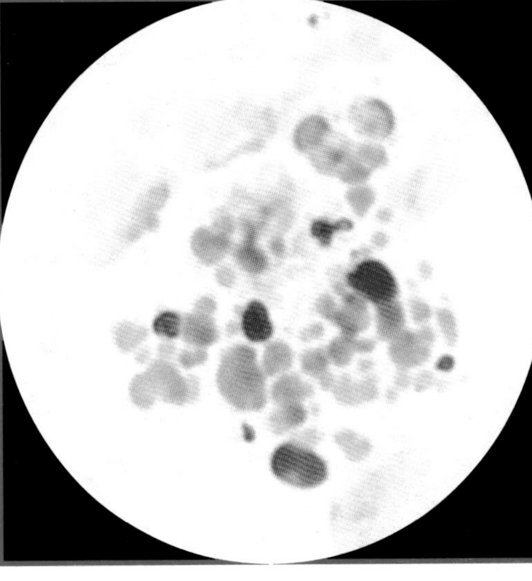

I7.12
Lipophages. Fresh specimen. Lipid stained red. (Oil red stain, oil immersion)

I7.13
Giant cell histiocyte. Giant cell histiocytes can be seen in a wide variety of pulmonary disorders, but can also be seen in apparently healthy people, and therefore do not necessarily indicate the presence of disease.

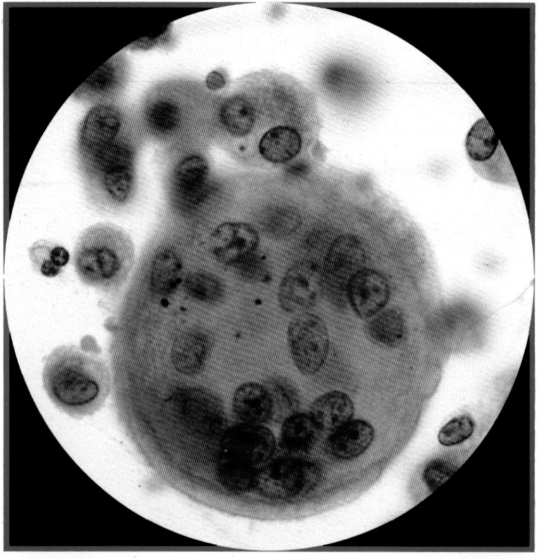

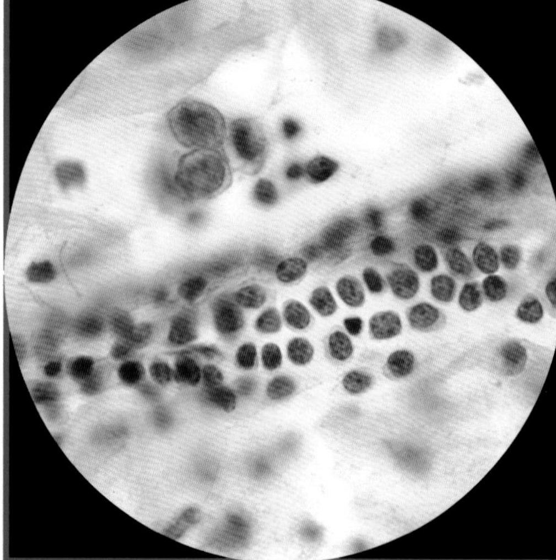

I7.14
Lymphocytes. Lymphocytes are commonly found in strings in mucus in sputum specimens. In contrast with small cell carcinoma (which also may be seen in strings in mucus), lymphocytes are noncohesive and do not mold.

I7.15
Curschmann's spiral. Associated with excess mucus production as seen in asthmatics and smokers. These spiral formations are probably due to an intrinsic property of the mucus itself rather than representing bronchiolar casts. Curschmann's spirals are sometimes associated with neutrophils, which may be related to smoking or air pollution.

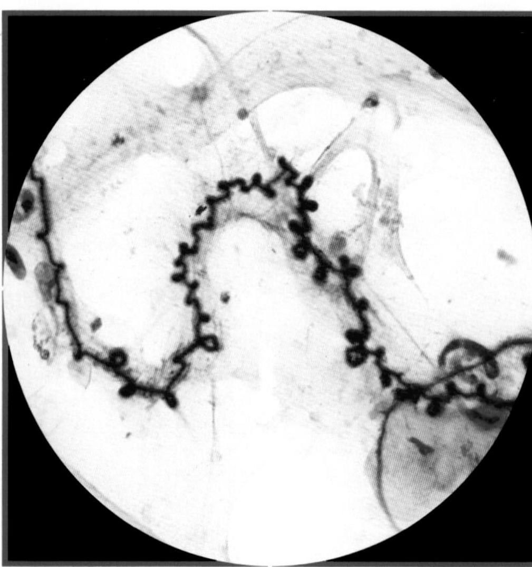

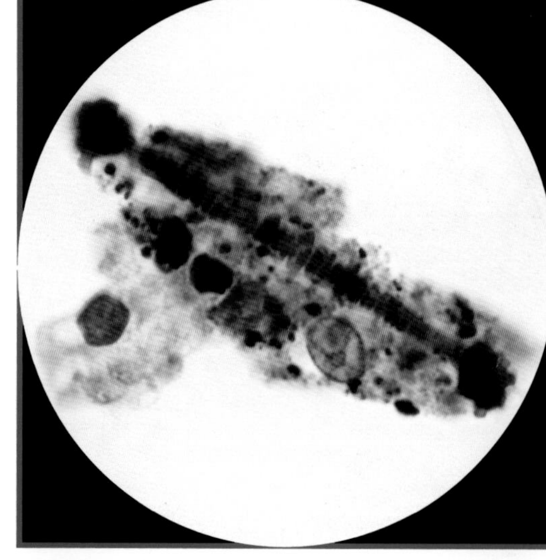

I7.16
Ferruginous bodies. Golden, refractile, iron salts precipitated onto thin fibers, with characteristic beading and baton shape, are usually phagocytosed by histiocytes. They are associated with asbestosis, but are not absolutely specific.

I7.17
Elastin fibers. Glassy, refractile elastin fibers may be associated with tissue destruction, but can also appear in vigorous brushings or needle aspirations. They should not be mistaken for filamentous fungi (lack cell walls, septation, cytoplasm).

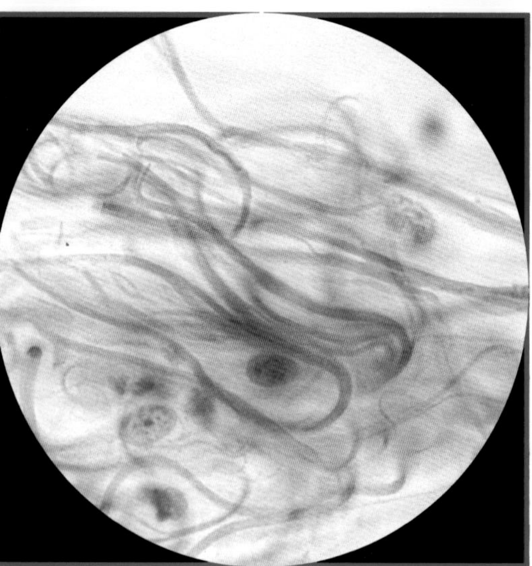

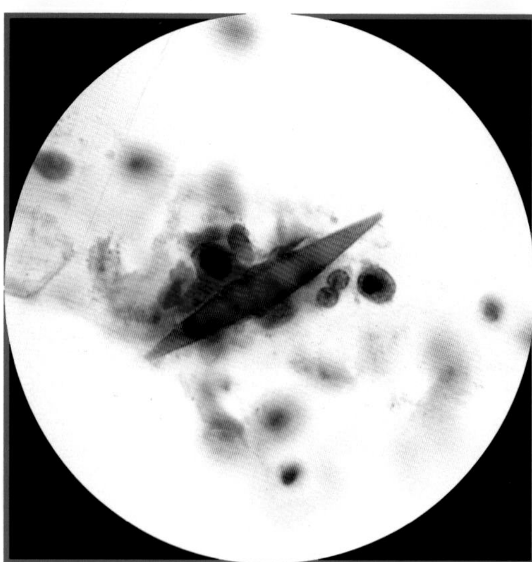

I7.18
Charcot-Leyden crystals. Bipyramidal, needle-shaped crystal of granules derived from eosinophils. They are associated with hypersensitivity, particularly asthma.

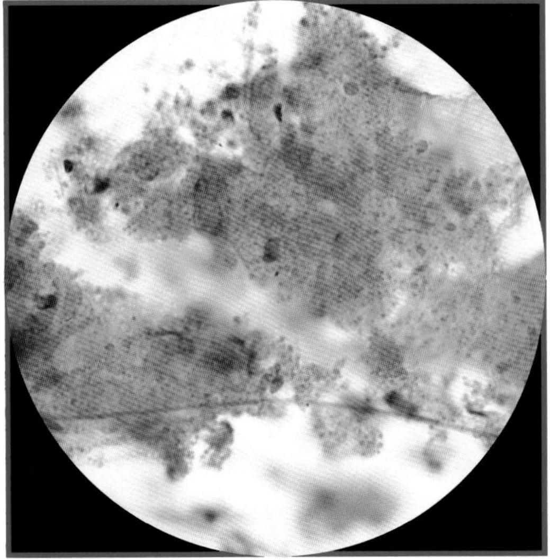

I7.19
Alveolar proteinosis. Granular debris in alveoli, thought to be due to enzymatic disorder of macrophages.

I7.20
Corpora amylacea. Glycoprotein casts of the alveoli are related to previous pulmonary edema. They are acidophilic, concentrically laminated bodies that often crack.

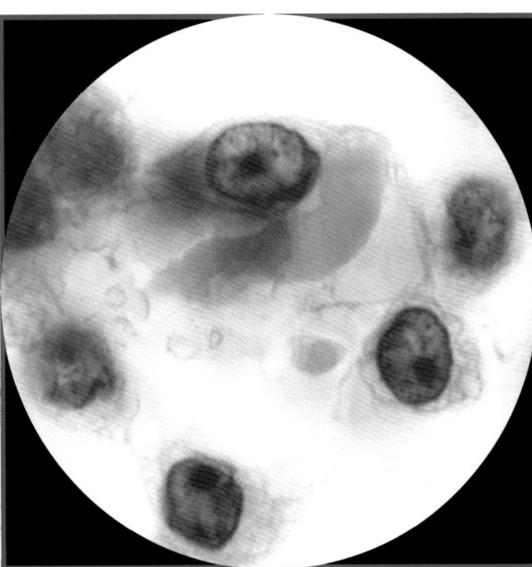

I7.21
Kuhn's cytoplasmic hyalin. Nonspecific accumulation of hyaline material identical to Mallory bodies in the liver.

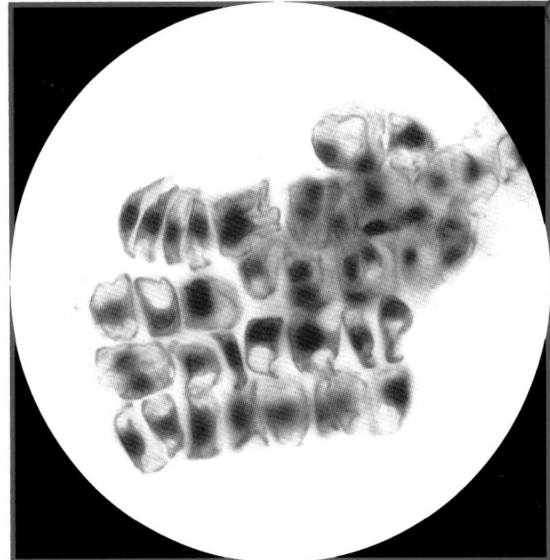

I7.22
Food particles. Illustrated are vegetable cells, a common finding in sputum (note refractile cell walls). The presence of dark nuclei could suggest malignancy.

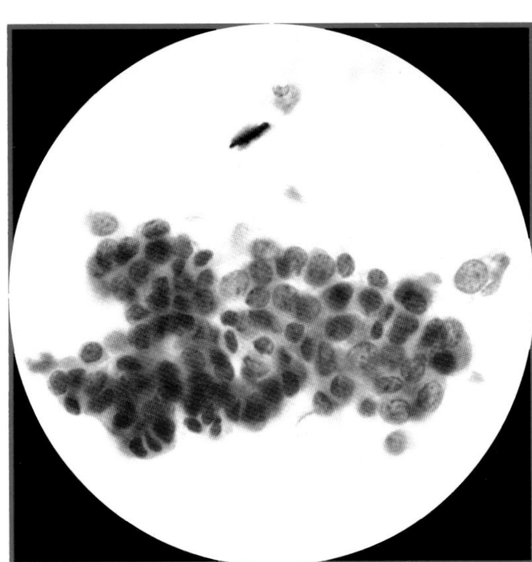

I7.23
Reserve cell hyperplasia. Tightly cohesive groups of small, uniform cells with high N/C ratios. The reserve cells may be associated with ciliated columnar cells or squamous metaplasia. Significant molding, crush artifact, and necrosis are not seen, in contrast with small cell carcinoma.

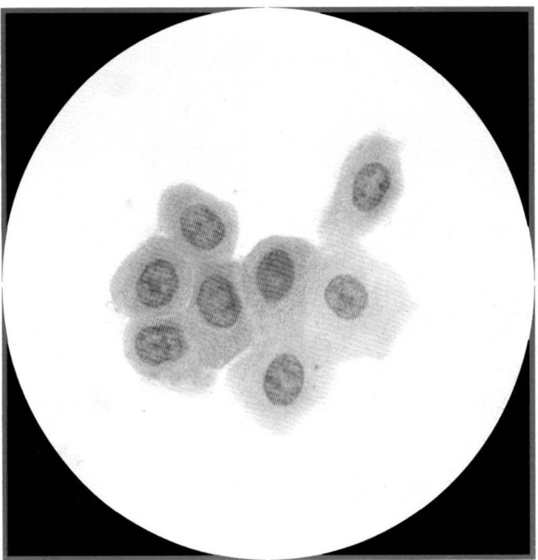

I7.24
Squamous metaplasia. An extremely common process, often manifested by small, angular cells that can stain cyanophilic, eosinophilic, or orangeophilic. As the squamous metaplasia matures, it more closely resembles classic squamous metaplasia as seen in the Pap smear, ie, rounded cells with dense, cyanophilic cytoplasm.

I7.25
Squamous metaplasia, inflamed. As in the Pap smear, inflammatory reactive/ reparative changes such as nuclear enlargement and presence of nucleoli may be observed in exfoliative respiratory cytology.

I7.26
Atypical parakeratosis. Parakeratosis and atypical parakeratosis are associated with severe irritation, such as that seen with a tracheostomy tube (as in this biopsy-proven case of a 28-year-old woman). As in the Pap smear, parakeratosis is similar to miniature superficial cells; atypical parakeratosis mimics keratinizing dysplasia and keratinizing squamous cell carcinoma, *except* that it occurs in small cells.

I7.27
Atypical parakeratosis. Occasional pleomorphic keratinized cell suggests keratinizing squamous cell carcinoma; however, the cell is small. (Same patient as in I7.26.)

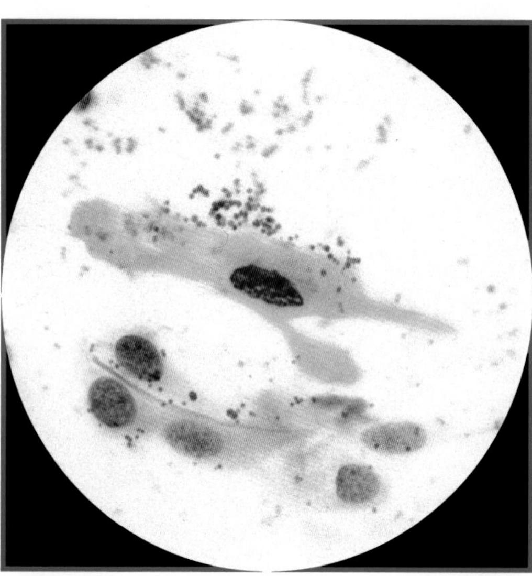

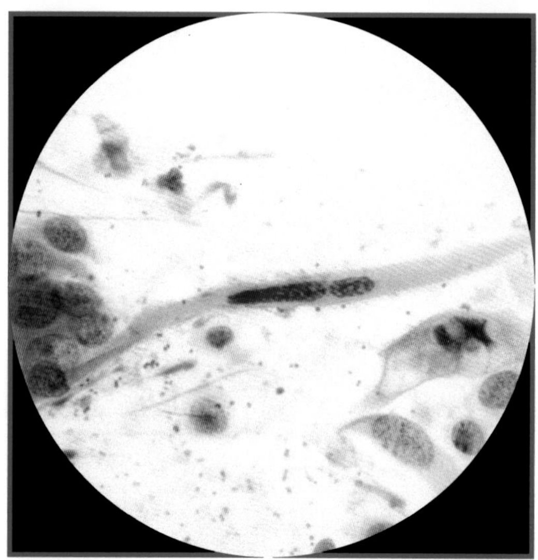

I7.28
Atypical parakeratosis. Spindle or "snake" cell mimicking squamous cell carcinoma. (Same patient as in I7.26 and I7.27.)

I7.29
Bronchial hyperplasia (creola body). Bronchial hyperplasia is a nonspecific response to a variety of pulmonary disorders that result in exfoliation of tightly cohesive, three-dimensional aggregates of reactive glandular cells that may be mistaken for adenocarcinoma. Note presence of cilia, the best clue to a benign diagnosis.

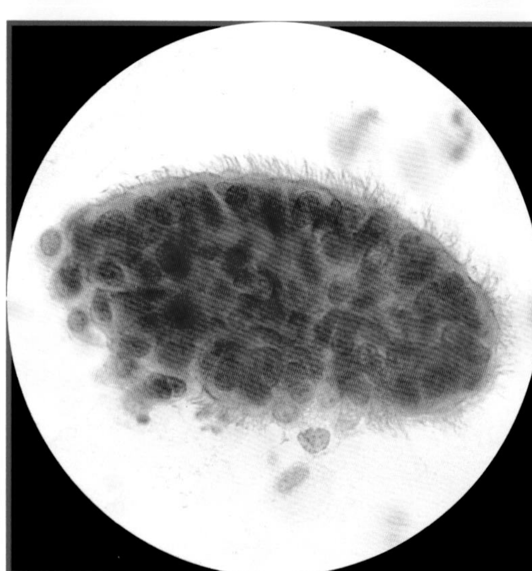

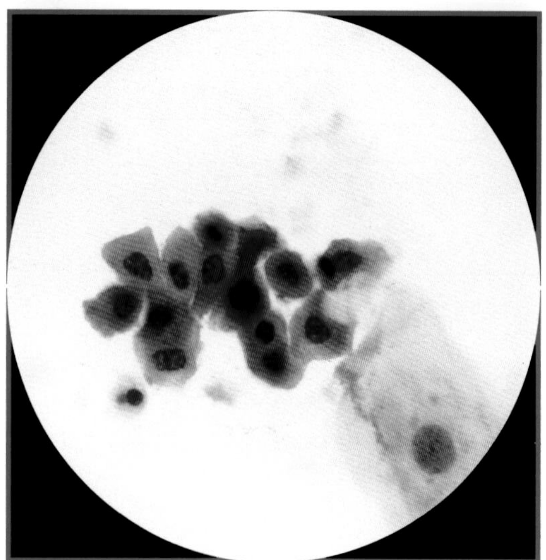

I7.30
Pap cells. Compare cell size with normal intermediate cell. Small angulated cells (squamous metaplasia, parakeratosis) are related to inflammation.

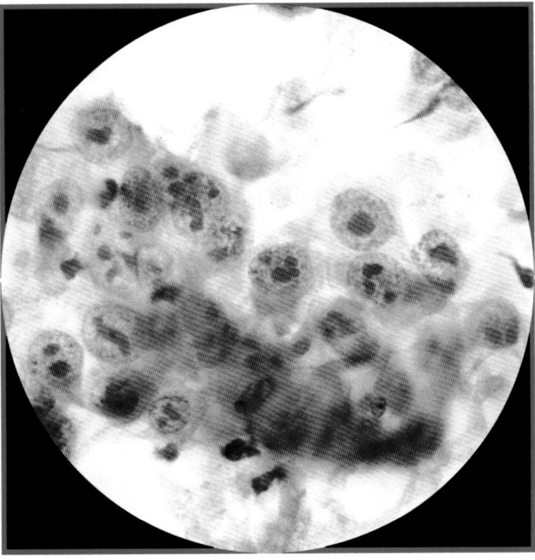

I7.31
Repair in respiratory epithelium. As in the Pap smear, although nuclear atypia can be pronounced (note spectacular nucleoli in this example), the cells remain cohesive and orderly, and the chromatin fine.

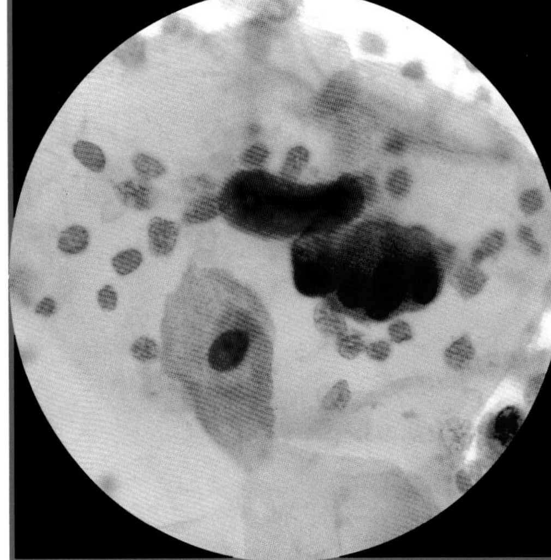

I7.32
Antineoplastic therapy effect. Radiation and radiomimetic drugs can induce cellular changes characterized by the presence of macrocytes of either glandular or squamous origin. Compare the size of the macrocyte, which spills over the edge of the microscopic field, to the normal squamous and bronchial cells. This is an example of the cytologic effect of ARA-C on squamous cells.

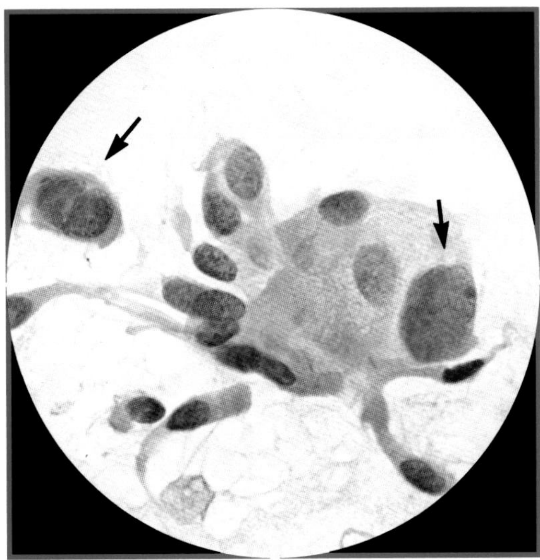

I7.33
Antineoplastic therapy effect. This is an example of the cytologic effect of radiation on glandular cells (arrows). Compare with normal bronchial cells.

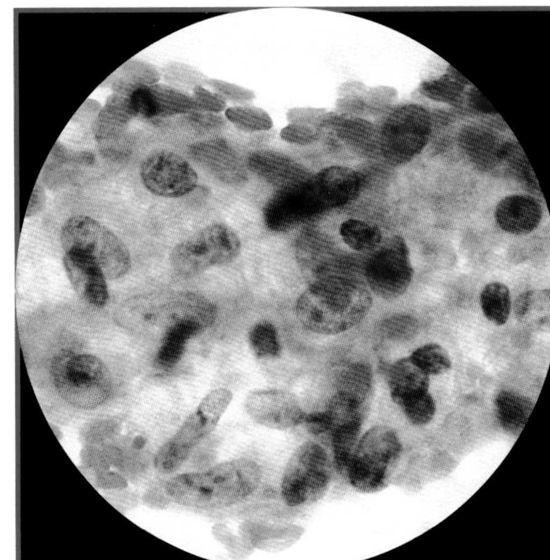

I7.34
Granuloma. Nodular collection of epithelioid histiocytes. Giant cells are not necessary for the diagnosis of a granuloma. Epithelioid histiocytes are characterized by elongated, pale staining nuclei, with tiny nucleoli, and by the fibrillar quality of their cytoplasm.

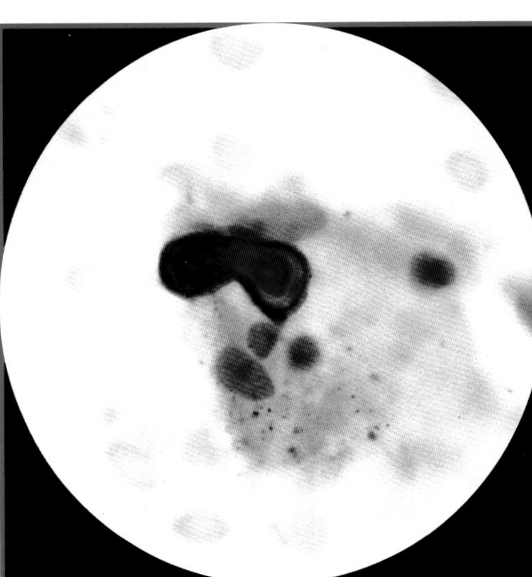

I7.35
Schaumann body. Concentrically laminated calcifications in cytoplasm of giant cell. Like asteroid bodies, these are associated with, but not diagnostic of, sarcoid.

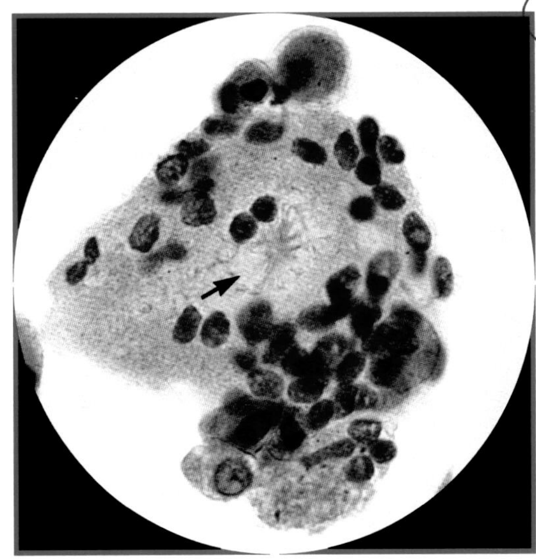

I7.36
Asteroid body. Radiate arrays of needle-shaped crystalline material in cytoplasm of giant cell (arrow); associated with, but not diagnostic of, sarcoid.

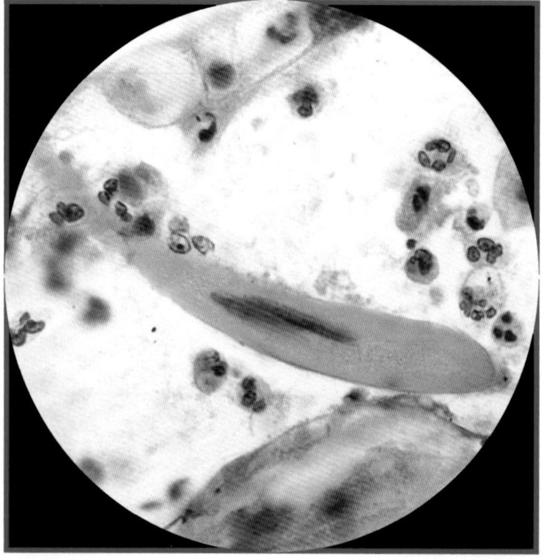

I7.37
Keratinizing squamous cell carcinoma. Bizarre keratinizing cells, often single, are a characteristic feature. Such cells are particularly associated with sputum specimens.

I7.38
Keratinizing squamous cell carcinoma. Basophilic or cyanophilic cells may predominate in bronchial brushing specimens.

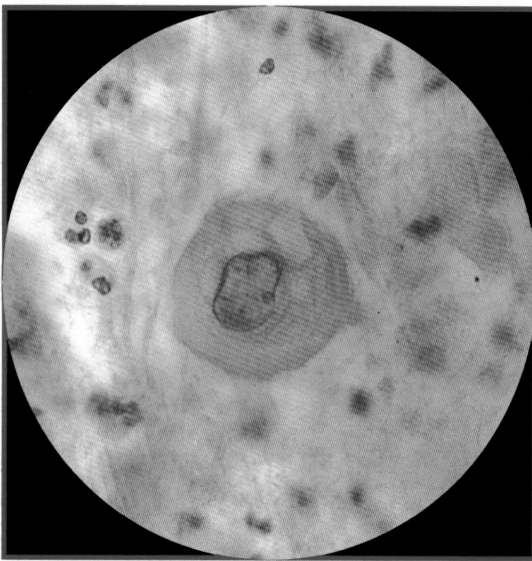

I7.39
Keratinizing squamous cell carcinoma. Eosinophilic cells can also be seen. Note the presence of refractile rings around the nucleus due to cytoplasmic keratinization.

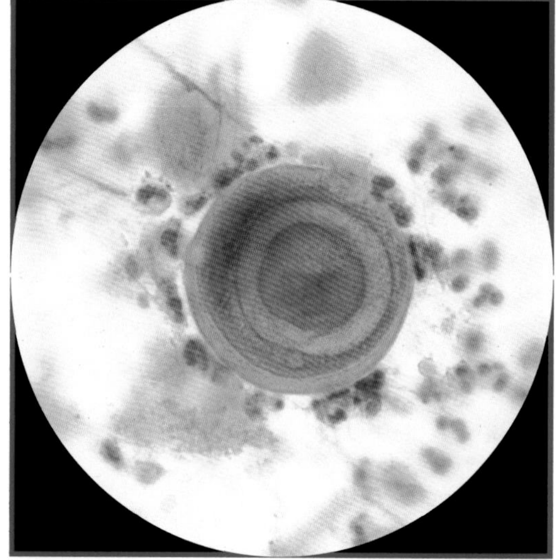

I7.40
Keratinizing squamous cell carcinoma. Pearls are characteristic of keratinizing lesions.

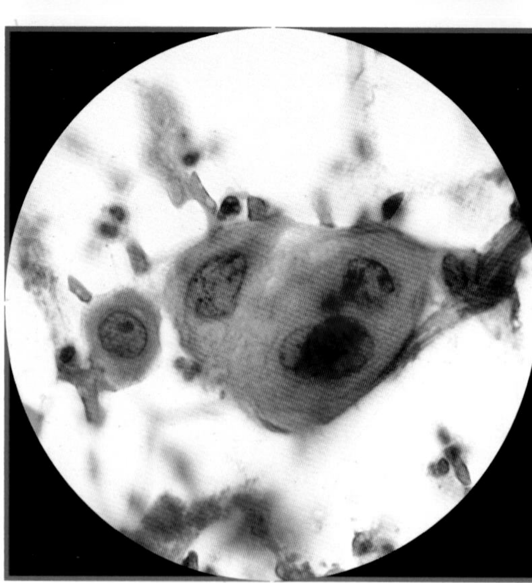

I7.41
Keratinizing squamous cell carcinoma. Nuclear pleomorphism and irregular coarse, hyperchromatic chromatin, with clumping and clearing, are characteristic of the nuclei seen in bronchial washing/brushing specimen (illustrated). Nuclear degeneration and pyknotic ink-dot nuclei are more characteristic of sputum specimens. Note the glassy cytoplasm.

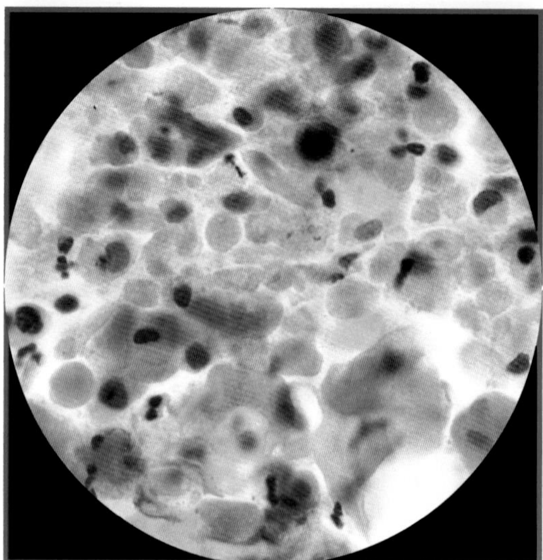

I7.42
Cavitating squamous cell carcinoma. As a result of extensive central degeneration, a cavity containing an abundance of necrotic material may form. Note the presence of keratinized squamous debris.

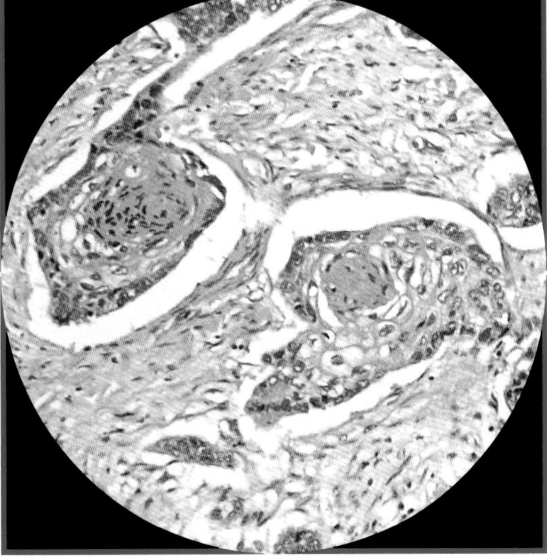

I7.43
Keratinizing squamous cell carcinoma (tissue). Note the presence of squamous eddies, or pearls, which are pathognomonic of keratinization.

I7.44
Nonkeratinizing squamous cell carcinoma. The groups of malignant cells tend to be more cohesive and the cells more uniform than in keratinizing squamous cell carcinoma. Also, basophilia predominates in nonkeratinizing squamous cell carcinoma. Although an occasional dyskeratotic cell can be seen, pearls, extensive keratinization, and bizarre-shaped cells are not present.

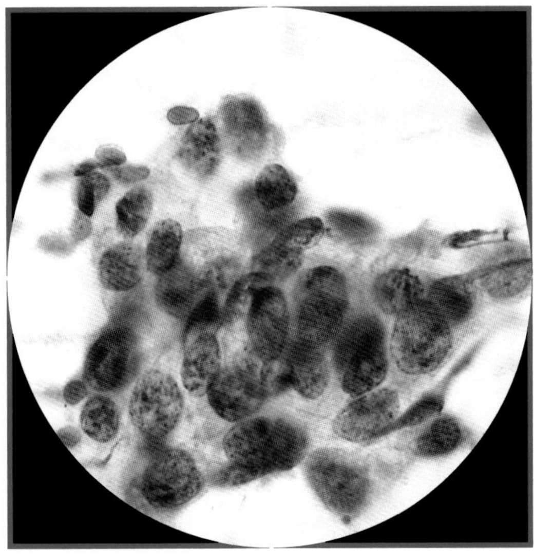

I7.45
Nonkeratinizing squamous cell carcinoma. Syncytial-like aggregate of relatively uniform cells, with high N/C ratios and coarse, dark chromatin. Nucleoli tend to be more prominent in nonkeratinizing squamous cell carcinoma than in the keratinizing counterpart.

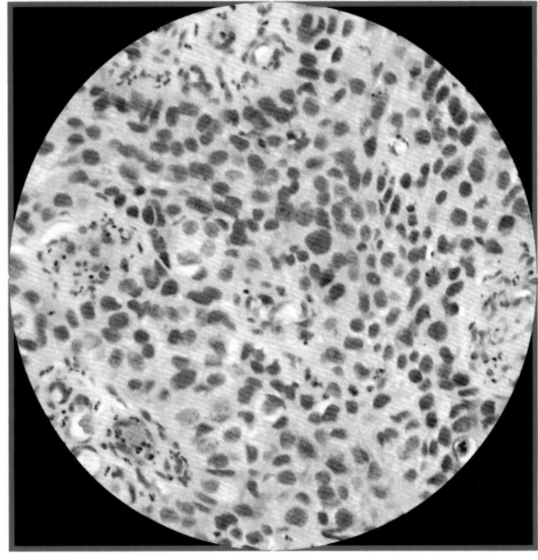

I7.46
Nonkeratinizing squamous cell carcinoma (tissue). Note relative uniformity of cells and absence of bizarre cells and pearls.

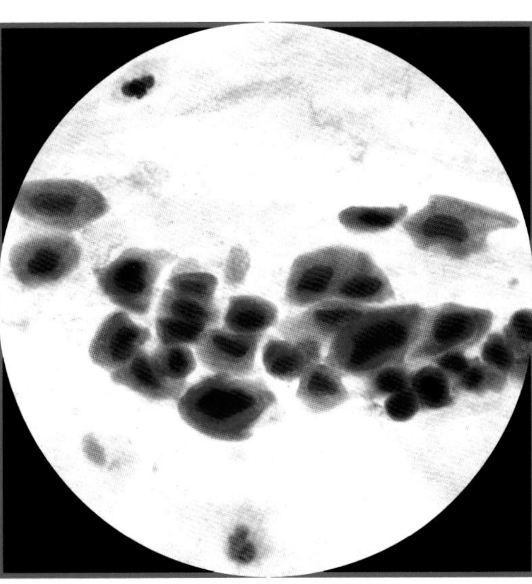

I7.47
Squamous dysplasia (atypical squamous metaplasia). Just as in the uterine cervix, squamous carcinoma of the respiratory tract apparently arises from a precursor lesion, ie, dysplasia and carcinoma in situ. Low-grade respiratory dysplasia resembles squamous metaplasia with nuclear atypia (atypical squamous metaplasia, illustrated). As the abnormality becomes more advanced, distinction from invasive carcinoma may be difficult.

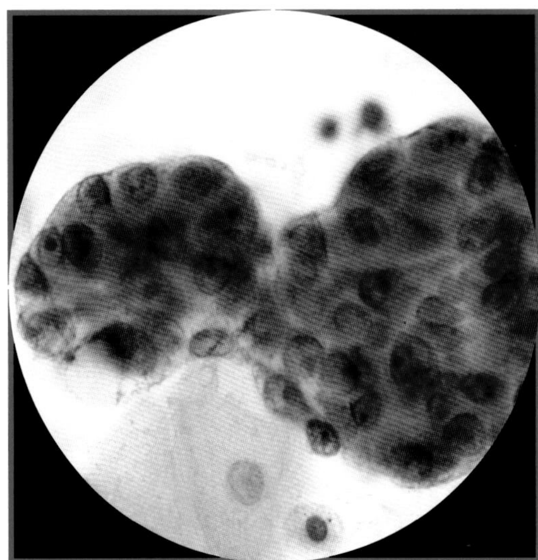

I7.48
Adenocarcinoma. Three-dimensional cell balls or papillary clusters of malignant cells are characteristic architectural features of adenocarcinoma.

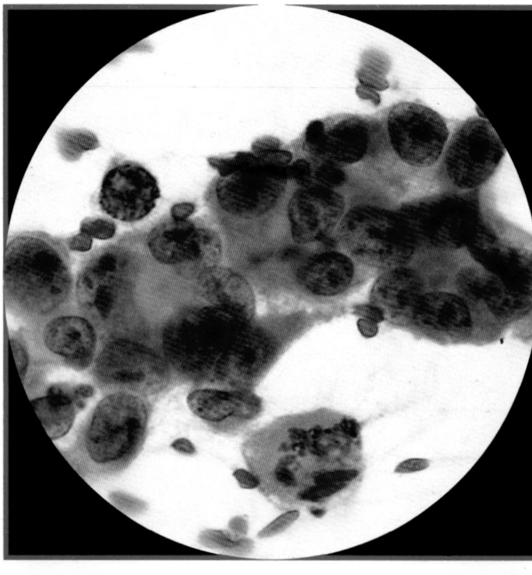

I7.49
Adenocarcinoma. Microacinar or rosette-like structures indicate glandular differentiation. Microacinar complexes (repeated microacinar structures) are a cytologic equivalent of the "gland-in-gland" histologic growth pattern of adenocarcinoma.

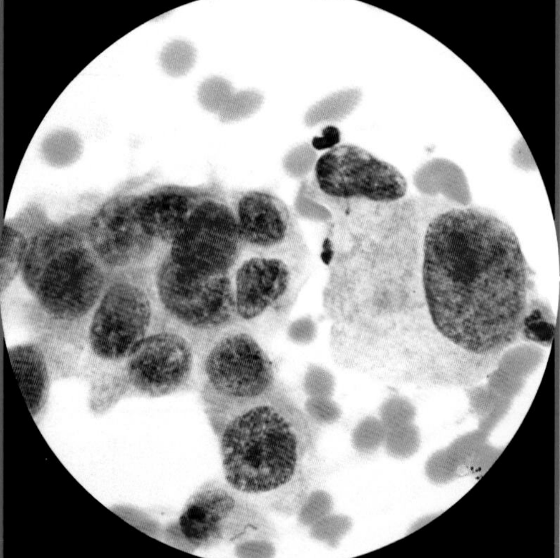

I7.50
Adenocarcinoma. Nuclear-cytoplasmic polarity is a characteristic feature of glandular cells (ie, "basal" nuclei, "apical" cytoplasm).

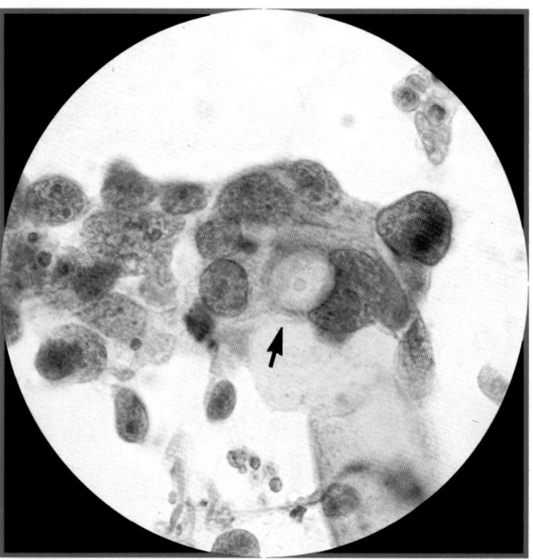

I7.51
Adenocarcinoma. Note intracytoplasmic secretory vacuole containing mucin (arrow).

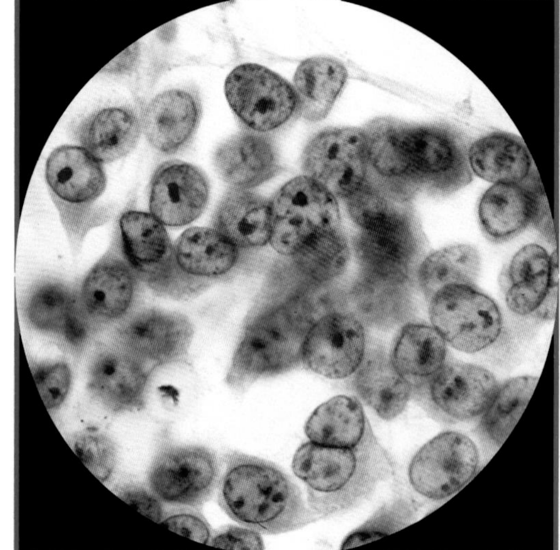

I7.52
Adenocarcinoma. The classic nucleus in adenocarcinoma is open and vesicular and contains a cherry red macronucleolus; however, this feature is not always seen.

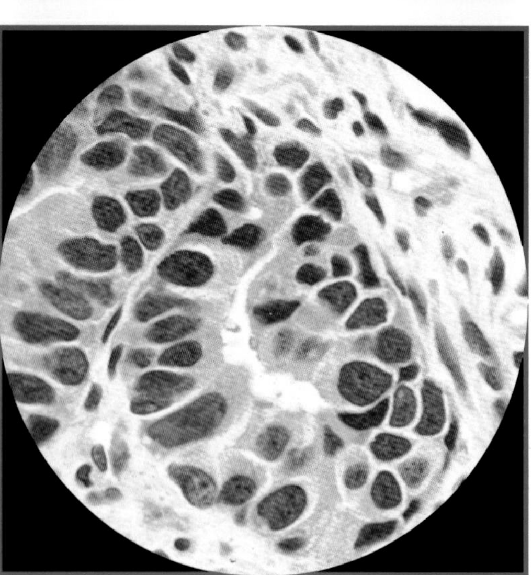

I7.53
Adenocarcinoma (tissue). Malignant gland infiltrating stroma.

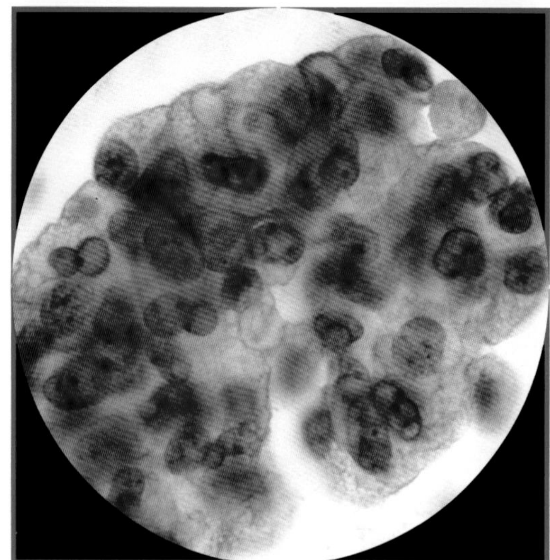

I7.54
Bronchioloalveolar carcinoma. First clue to diagnosis is abundant cellularity, with numerous cell balls or papillae. Individual cells are characteristically very well differentiated and may resemble goblet cells (as here), mesothelial cells, or alveolar macrophages.

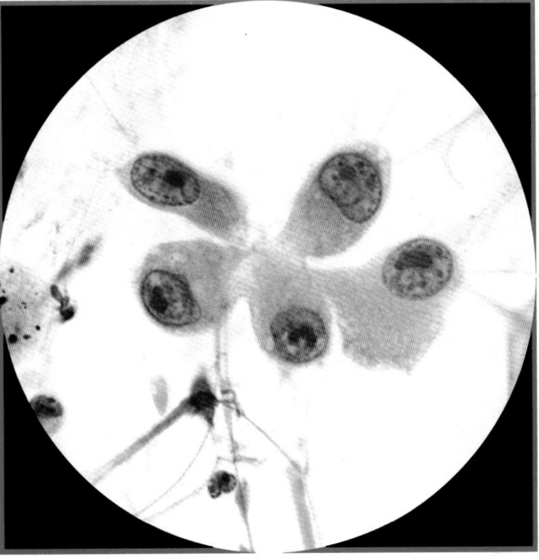

I7.55
Bronchioloalveolar carcinoma. Uniform tumor cells resembling mesothelial cells are shown. Note characteristic "hob nail" arrangement of the malignant cells.

I7.56
Bronchioloalveolar carcinoma. The tumor cells may resemble alveolar macrophages.

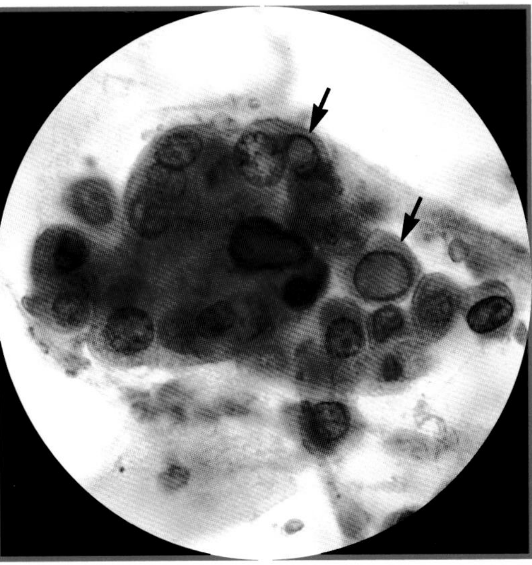

I7.57
Bronchioloalveolar carcinoma. Intranuclear cytoplasmic invaginations can be seen (arrows); nucleoli can be prominent. Although microvilli and terminal bar–like cytoplasmic borders can be seen, cilia are absent. Papillary growth is a characteristic feature in bronchioloalveolar carcinoma; psammoma bodies can be seen, rarely (center of field).

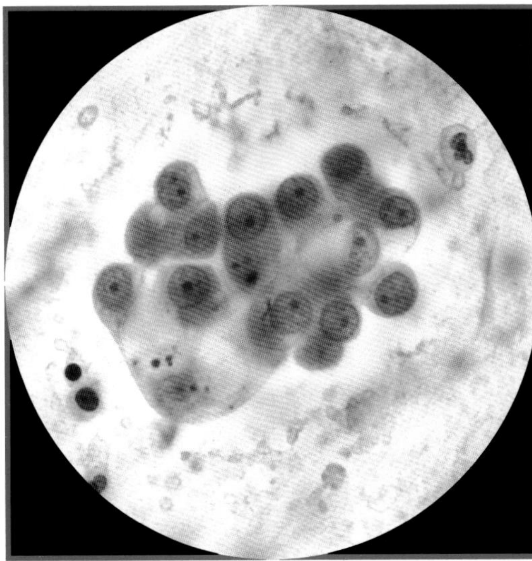

I7.58
Faux bronchioloalveolar carcinoma. These benign, reactive bronchioloalveolar cells were seen in a patient with pneumonia. Individually, these groups of cells may be virtually indistinguishable from bronchoalveolar carcinoma. However, such groups are sparse in benign conditions. As a rule, be cautious when diagnosing bronchioloalveolar carcinoma in a febrile patient.

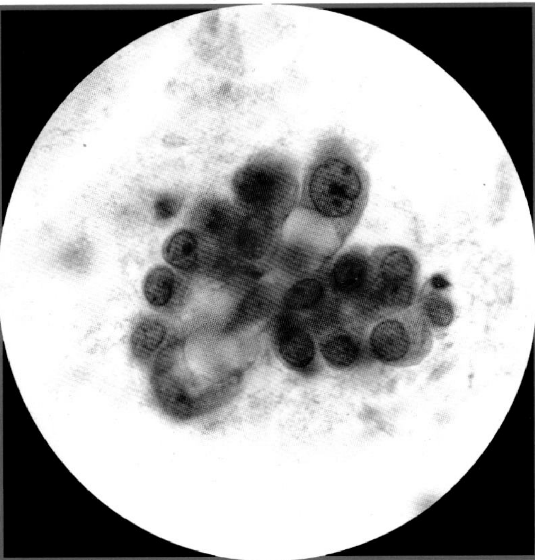

I7.59
Faux bronchioloalveolar carcinoma. Cluster of cells mimicking bronchioloalveolar carcinoma seen in another patient with pneumonia.

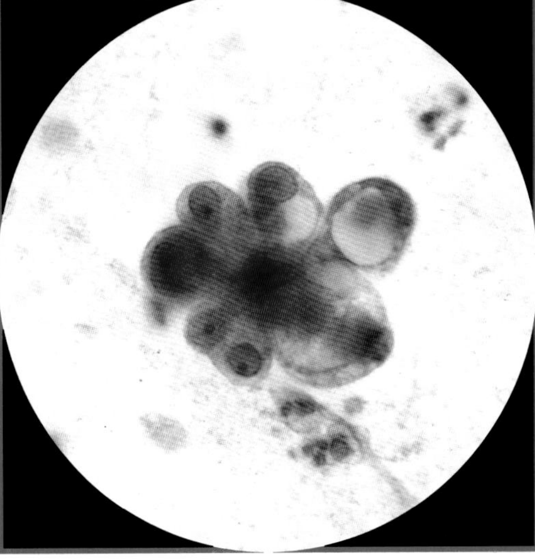

I7.60
Faux bronchioloalveolar carcinoma. Another patient with pneumonia, exfoliating rare clusters of cells mimicking BAC.

I7.61
Faux bronchioloalveolar carcinoma. This cluster is particularly atypical but shows the degree of abnormality that can be seen in benign reactive cells.

I7.62
Bronchioloalveolar carcinoma (tissue). The malignant cells grow along preexisting bronchioloalveolar walls without stromal invasion.

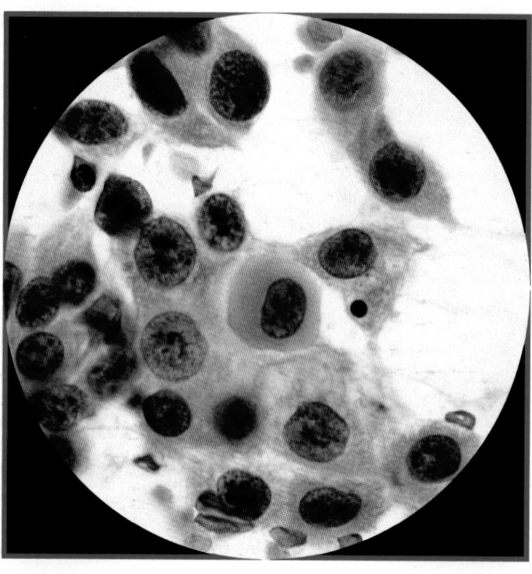

I7.63
Adenosquamous carcinoma. Note sharp contrast between cells with delicate, vacuolated (grandular) cytoplasm and those with dense, squamous cytoplasm. This combination is, perhaps unexpectedly, common in cytologic specimens.

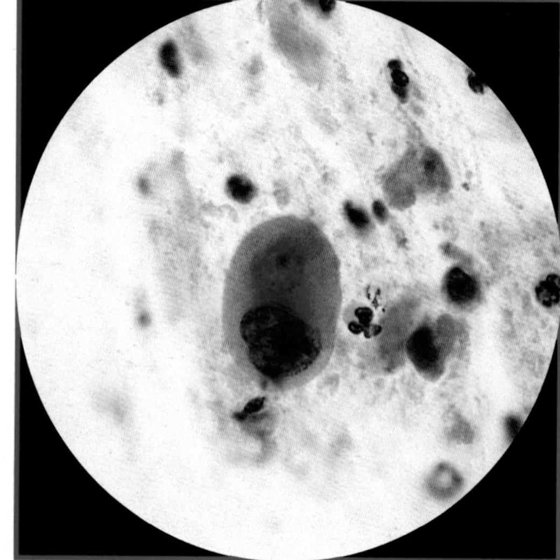

I7.64
Adenosquamous carcinoma. Columnar cell (glandular feature) with dense cytoplasm (squamous feature).

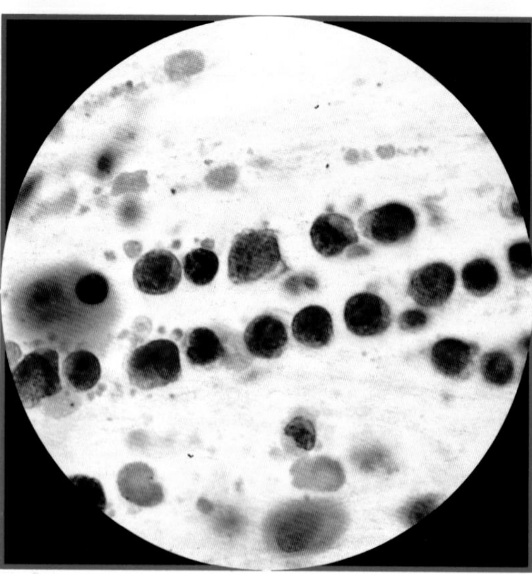

I7.65
Small cell carcinoma (sputum). In sputum specimens prepared with the pick-and-smear technique, the tumor cells characteristically line up in strands of mucus, forming strings of small blue cells that could be mistaken for lymphocytes. The tumor cells are about one to two times the size of a lymphocyte, and are often degenerated (classic oat cells).

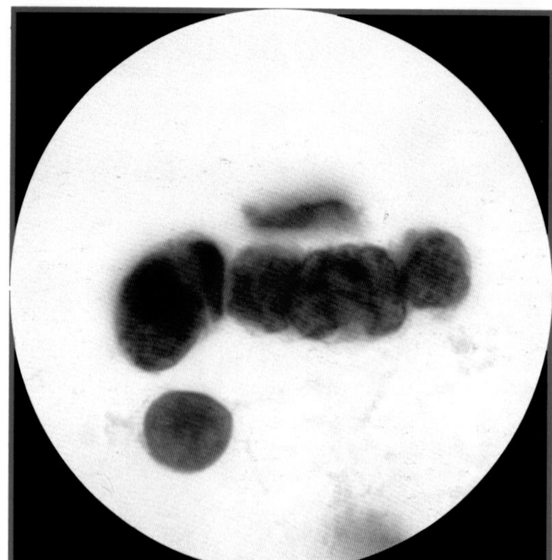

I7.66
Small cell carcinoma (sputum). Cytoplasm is extremely scanty. Marked nuclear molding and Indian files are characteristic features of small cell carcinoma. Nucleoli are inconspicuous or absent. (Oil)

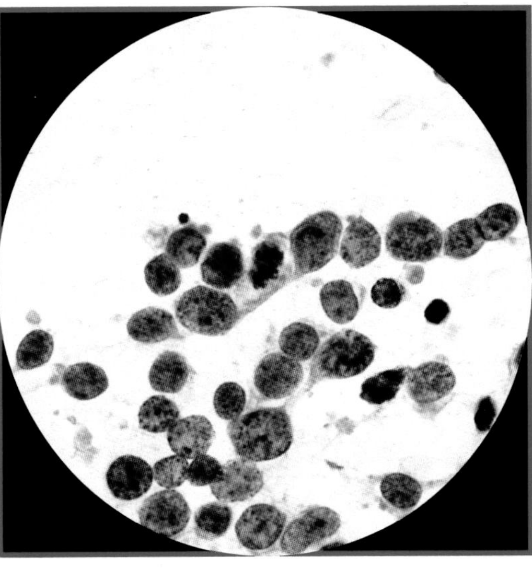

I7.67
Small cell carcinoma (brushing specimen). The cells obtained by direct brushing appear "fresher." In such well-preserved material, the cells appear somewhat larger (intermediate type, two to four times the size of a lymphocyte). A similar fresh appearance is also noted in fine needle aspiration biopsy specimens.

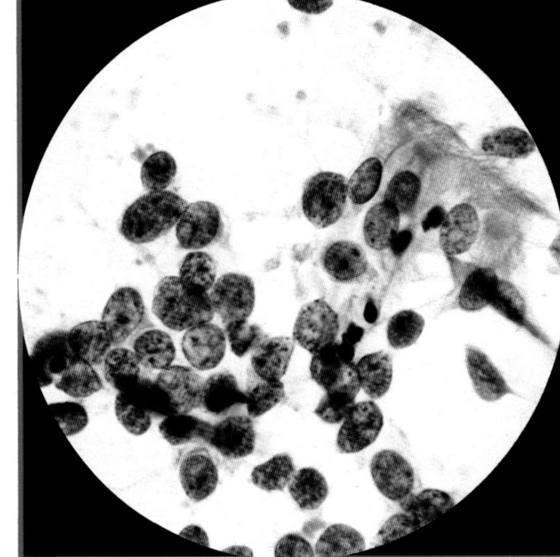

I7.68
Small cell carcinoma (brushing specimen). The tumor cells have very little cytoplasm, relatively fine but very hyperchromatic chromatin, and inconspicuous nucleoli. Note the similarity of bronchial cell nuclear chromatin to that of the tumor cells.

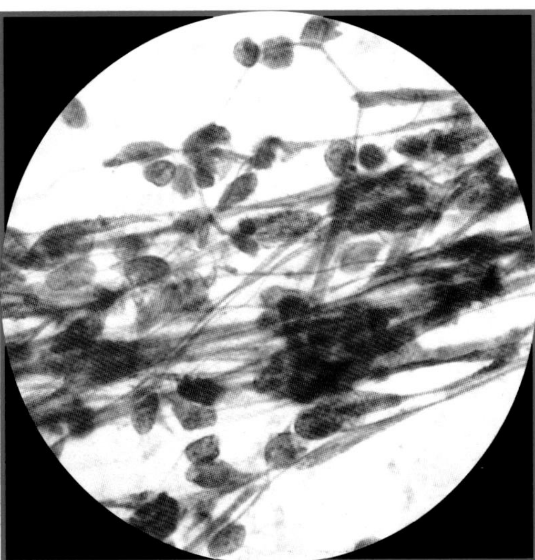

I7.69
Small cell carcinoma (brushing specimen). Crush artifact (nuclear DNA streaming) is usually present, particularly in brushing specimens.

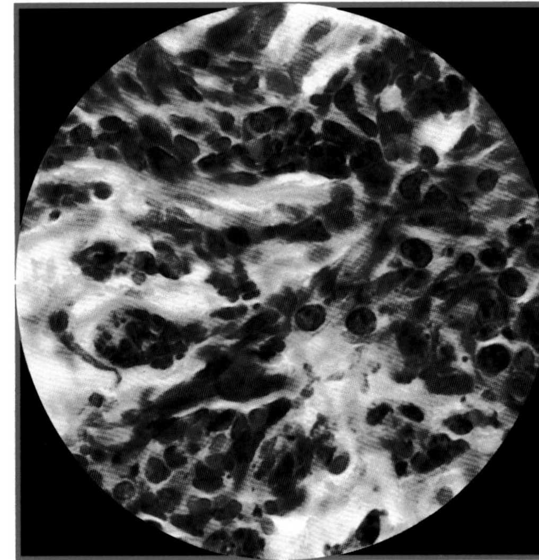

I7.70
Small cell carcinoma (tissue). Because the individual cells can usually be better visualized, it may actually be easier to diagnose small cell carcinoma in cytology than in tissue. Extensive crush artifact is common in small tissue biopsies.

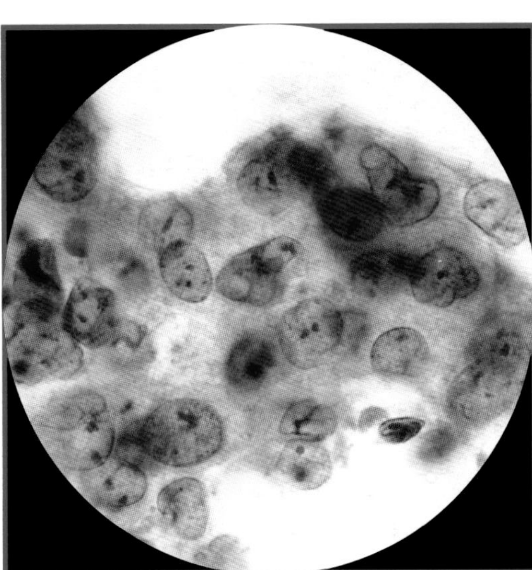

I7.71
Large cell undifferentiated carcinoma. Malignant (non–small cell) epithelial neoplasm without evidence of any special differentiation whatsoever (not glandular, not squamous, not neuroendocrine). In cytology, it is rare to not see any evidence of specific differentiation; in fact, even in this example there is a hint of a glandular acinus.

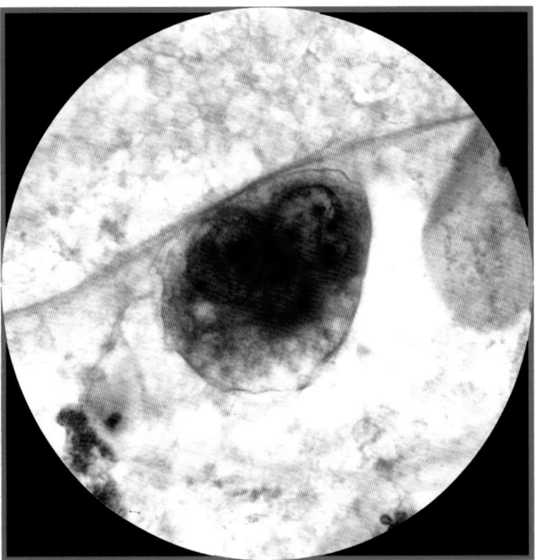

I7.72
Giant cell carcinoma. Highly aggressive malignancy with significant number of giant tumor cells.

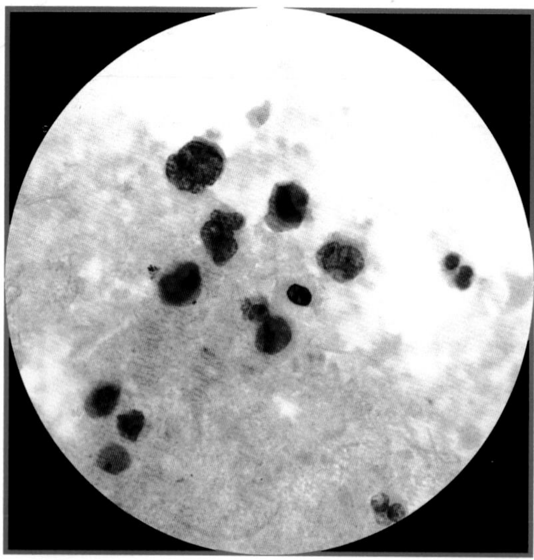

I7.73
Malignant lymphoma. Primary lymphoma occurs, but secondary involvement is more common. The malignant cells characteristically do not form aggregates and do not mold.

I7.74
Hodgkin's disease. Note markedly atypical lymphoid cells that are much larger than even large lymphocytes. Classic Reed-Sternberg cells are rarely observed.

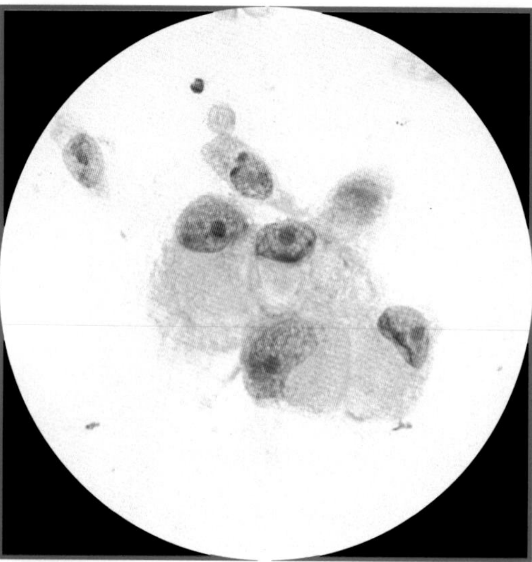

I7.75
Metastatic signet ring carcinoma. Consider metastasis from stomach (first choice) followed by other sites, such as breast.

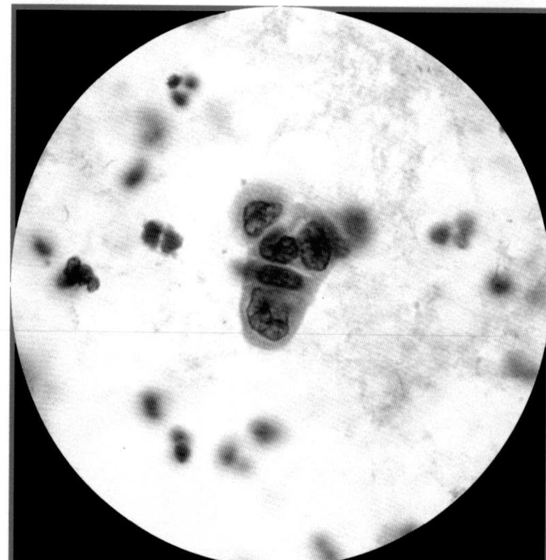

I7.76
Metastatic gastric carcinoma, intestinal pattern (see Chapter 9). As in the Pap smear, metastatic carcinomas usually have a clean background.

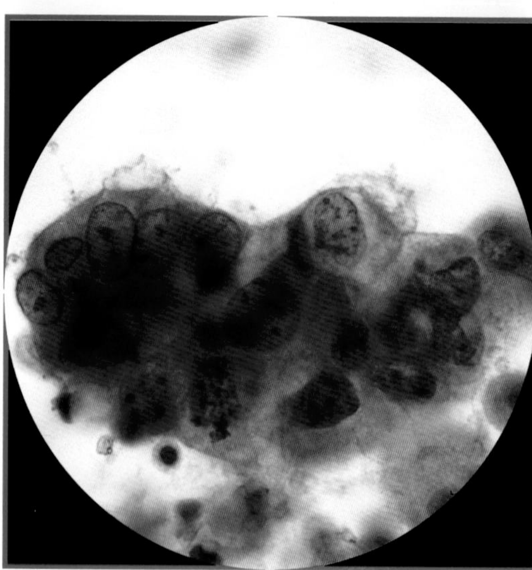

I7.77
Metastatic breast carcinoma. Breast carcinoma tends to exfoliate in tight, thick clusters of malignant cells in a clean background.

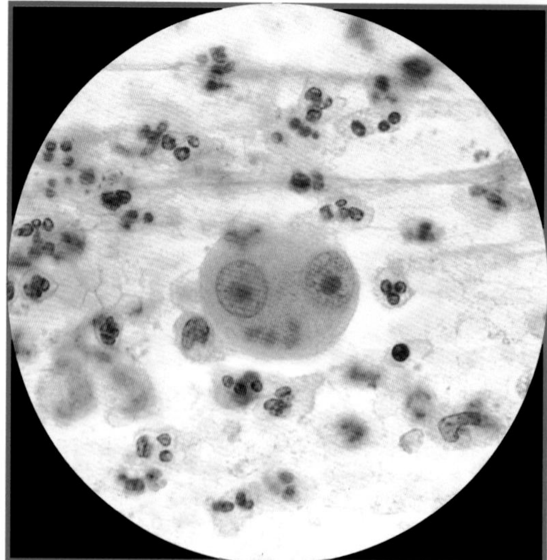

I7.78
Metastatic melanoma. Large, loosely cohesive cells with prominent nucleoli or macronucleoli; frequent binucleation, intranuclear cytoplasmic invaginations, and pigment are the characteristic features.

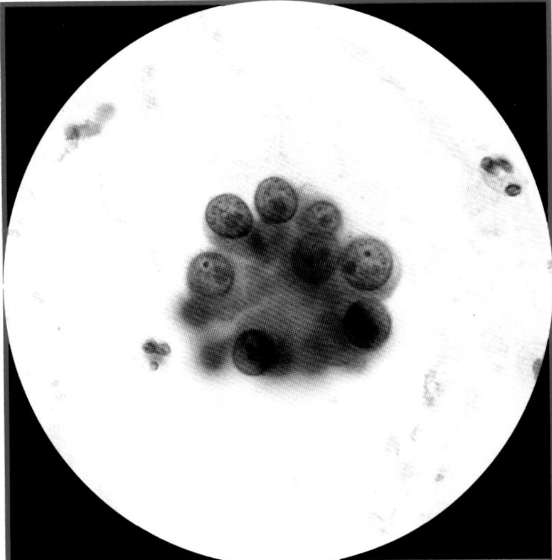

I7.79
Metastatic prostatic carcinoma. Relatively uniform cells with prominent nucleoli and microacinar complex formation.

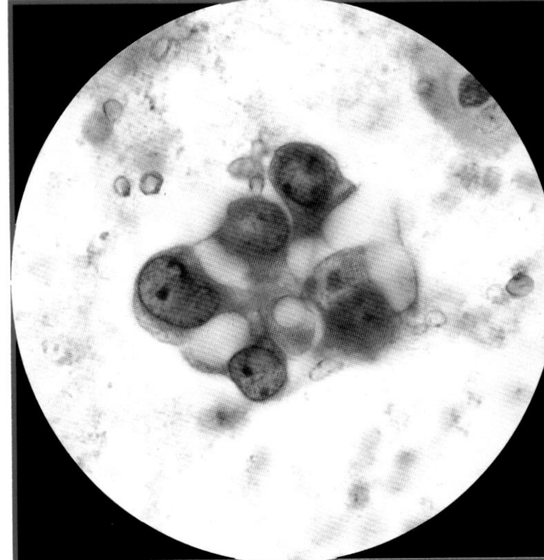

I7.80
Metastatic thyroid carcinoma. The less differentiated the primary, the more likely is lung metastasis.

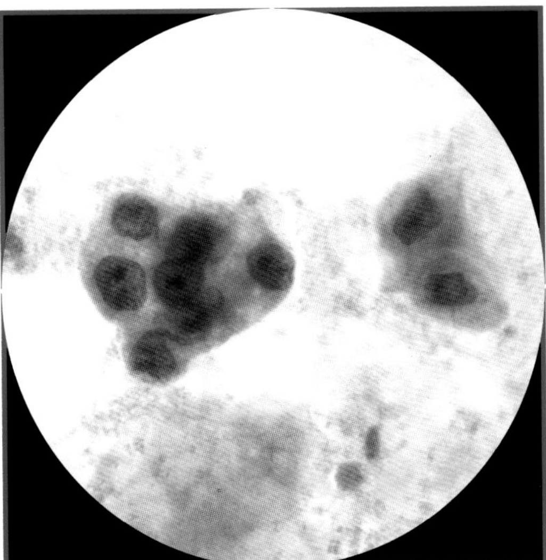

I7.81
Metastatic transitional cell carcinoma. Angular cells with relatively dense cytoplasm. High-grade transitional cell carcinoma may have glandular or squamous components.

References

Abati A, Landucci D, Danner RL, et al: Diagnosis of Pulmonary Microvascular Metastases by Cytologic Evaluation of Pulmonary Artery Catheter-Derived Blood Specimens. *Hum Pathol* 25: 257–262, 1994.

Agusti C, Xaubet A, Arriols R, et al: Multinuclear Giant Cells in Bronchoalveolar Lavage in Interstitial Lung Diseases. *Respiration* 51: 307–311, 1987.

Aisner SC, Gupta PK, Frost JK: Sputum Cytology in Pulmonary Sarcoidosis. *Acta Cytol* 21: 394–398, 1977.

Albright CD, Hafiz MA: Cytomorphologic Changes in Split-Course Radiation-Treated Bronchogenic Carcinomas. *Diagn Cytopathol* 4: 9–13, 1988.

Ambiavagar M, Chalon J, Zargham I: Tracheobronchial Cytologic Changes Following Lower Airway Thermal Injury: A Preliminary Report. *J Trauma* 14: 280–289, 1974.

Antonakopoulos GN, Lambrinaki E, Kyrkou KA: Curschmann's Spirals in Sputum: Histochemical Evidence of Bronchial Gland Ductal Origin. *Diagn Cytopathol* 3: 291–294, 1987.

Athanassiadou PP, Athanissiades PH, Kostopoulos C, et al: Antigen Expression of Alveolar Macrophages in Smokers and Patients With Lung Diseases. *Diagn Cytopathol* 12: 37–41, 1995.

Auerbach O, Stout AP, Hammond EC, et al: Changes in Bronchial Epithelium in Relation to Cigarette Smoking and in Relation to Lung Cancer. *New Engl J Med* 265: 253–267, 1961.

Auerbach O, Stout AP, Hammond EC, et al: Multiple Primary Bronchial Carcinomas. *Cancer* 20: 699–705, 1967.

Banner BF, Gould VE, Radosevich JA, et al: Application of Monoclonal Antibody 44-3A6 in the Cytodiagnosis and Classification of Pulmonary Carcinomas. *Diagn Cytopathol* 1: 300–307, 1985.

Barbazza R, Toniolo L, Pinarello A, et al: Accuracy of Bronchial Aspiration Cytology in Typing Operable (Stage I-II) Pulmonary Carcinomas. *Diagn Cytopathol* 8: 3–7, 1992.

Bedrossian CWM, Rybka DL: Bronchial Brushing During Fiberoptic Bronchoscopy for the Cytodiagnosis of Lung Cancer: Comparison With Sputum and Bronchial Washings. *Acta Cytol* 20: 446–453, 1976.

Bedrossian CWM, Corey BJ: Abnormal Sputum Cytopathology During Chemotherapy With Bleomycin. *Acta Cytol* 22: 202–207, 1978.

Bender BL, Cherock MA, Sotos SN: Effective Use of Bronchoscopy and Sputa in the Diagnosis of Lung Cancer. *Diagn Cytopathol* 1: 183–187, 1985.

Bewtra C, Dewan N, O'Donahue WJ Jr: Exfoliative Sputum Cytology in Pulmonary Embolism. *Acta Cytol* 27: 489–496, 1983.

Bibbo M, Fennessy JJ, Lu C-T, et al: Bronchial Brushing Technique for the Cytologic Diagnosis of Peripheral Lung Lesions: A Review of 693 Cases. *Acta Cytol* 17: 245–251, 1973.

Böcking A, Biesterfeld S, Chatelain R, et al: Diagnosis of Bronchial Carcinoma on Sections of Paraffin-Embedded Sputum: Sensitivity and Specificity of an Alternative to Routine Cytology. *Acta Cytol* 36: 37–47, 1992.

Bornstein J, Stinson-Carter T, Kaufman RH: Curschmann's Spiral in an Endocervical Brushing. *Acta Cytol* 31: 530–531, 1987.

Boucher LD, Yoneda K: Cytologic Characterization of Bronchial Epithelial Changes in Small Cell Carcinoma of the Lung. *Acta Cytol* 39; 69–72, 1995.

Broderick PA, Corvese NL, LaChance T, et al: Giant Cell Carcinoma of Lung: A Cytologic Evaluation. *Acta Cytol* 19: 225–230, 1975.

Broghamer WL Jr, Richards ME, Biscopink RJ: Pulmonary Cytologic Examination in the Identification of the Second Primary Carcinoma of the Lung. *Cancer* 56: 2664–2668, 1985.

Buchanan AJ, Fauck R, Gupta RK: Cytologic Diagnosis of Adenoid Cystic Carcinoma in Tracheal Wash Specimens. *Diagn Cytopathol* 4: 130–132, 1988.

Burke MD, Melamed MR: Exfoliative Cytology in Metastatic Cancer in Lung. *Acta Cytol* 12: 61–74, 1968.

Cahan WG, Melamed MR, Frazell EL: Tracheobronchial Cytology After Laryngectomy for Carcinoma. *Surg Gynecol Obstet* 123: 15–21, 1966.

Carlson DJ, Mason EW: Pulmonary Alveolar Proteinosis: Diagnosis of Probable Case by Examination of Sputum. *Am J Clin Pathol* 33: 48–54, 1960.

Carson KF, Williams CA, Rosenthal DL, et al: Bronchoalveolar Lavage in a Girl With Gaucher's Disease. A Report of a Case. *Acta Cytol* 38: 597–600, 1994.

Caya JG, Wollenberg NJ, Lawrence JC: The Significance of "Positive" Respiratory Cytology Determinations in a Series of 327 Patients. *Am J Clin Pathol* 82: 155–159, 1984.

Caya JG, Wollenberg NJ, Clowry LJ: Respiratory Cytology: Significance of "Suspect" Results in a Series of 435 Patients. *South Med J* 78: 701–703, 1985.

Caya JG, Wollenberg NJ, Clowry LJ, et al: The Diagnosis of Pulmonary Small-Cell Anaplastic Carcinoma by Cytologic Means: A 13-Year Experience. *Diagn Cytopathol* 4: 202–205, 1988.

Caya JG, Gilles L, Tieu TM, et al: Lung Cancer Treated on the Basis of Cytologic Findings: An Analysis of 112 Patients. *Diagn Cytopathol* 6: 313–316, 1990.

Chalon J, Loew DAY, Orking LR: Tracheobronchial Cytologic Changes During the Menstrual Cycle. *JAMA* 218: 1928–1931, 1971.

Chalon J, Katz J, Ramanathan S, et al: Tracheobronchial Epithelial Multinucleation in Malignant Disease. *Science* 183: 525–526, 1974a.

Chalon J: Changes in Tracheobronchial Cytology Noted During Anesthesia. *NY State J Med* 74: 2185–2189, 1974b.

Chalon J, Tayyab MA, Ramanathan S: Cytology of Respiratory Epithelium as a Predictor of Respiratory Complications After Operation. *Chest* 67: 32–35, 1975.

Chalon J, Katz JS, Gorstein F, et al: Malignant Disease and Tracheobronchial Epithelial Multinucleation. *Cancer* 37: 1874–1881, 1976.

Chalon J, Tang C-K, Gorstein F, et al: Diagnostic and Prognostic Significance of Tracheobronchial Epithelial Multinucleation. *Acta Cytol* 22: 316–320, 1978.

Chamberlain DW, Braude AC, Rebuck AS: A Critical Evaluation of Bronchoalveolar Lavage: Criteria for Identifying Unsatisfactory Specimens. *Acta Cytol* 31: 599–605, 1987.

Chaudhary BA, Yoneda K, Burki NK: Fiberoptic Bronchoscopy: Comparison of Procedures Used in the Diagnosis of Lung Cancer. *J Thorac Cardiovasc Surg* 76: 33–37, 1978.

Chen KTK: Cytology of Tracheobronchial Amyloidosis. *Acta Cytol* 28: 133–135, 1984.

Chen KTK: Megakaryocytes in a Fine Needle Aspirate of the Lung. *Acta Cytol* 31: 81–82, 1987.

Chen KTK: Cytology of Bronchial Benign Granular-Cell Tumor. *Acta Cytol* 35: 381–384, 1991.

Chen KTK: Cytology of Allergic Bronchopulmonary Aspergillosis. *Diagn Cytopathol* 9: 82–85, 1993.

Chess Q: Megakaryocytes in Bronchial Brushings. *Acta Cytol* 32: 130–131, 1988.

Chodosh S: Examination of Sputum Cells. *N Engl J Med* 282: 854–857, 1970.

Chopra SK, Genovesi MG, Simmons DH, et al: Fiberoptic Bronchoscopy in the Diagnosis of Lung Cancer: Comparison of Pre- and Post-bronchoscopy Sputa, Washings, Brushings and Biopsies. *Acta Cytol* 21: 524–623, 1977.

Cooney W, Dzuira B, Harper R, et al: The Cytology of Sputum From Thermally Injured Patients. *Acta Cytol* 16: 433–437, 1972.

Copeland AR, O'Tool K, Chadburn A, et al: Megakaryocytes in Bronchial Brush Cytology. A Case Report. *Acta Cytol* 37: 400–402, 1993.

Cortese DA: The Prognostic Value of Sputum Cytology. *Chest* 102: 1315–1316, 1992.

Costabel U, Matthys H, Guzman J, et al: Multinucleated Cells in Bronchoalveolar Lavage. *Acta Cytol* 29: 189–190, 1985.

Crystal RG, Fulmer JD, Roberts WC, et al: Idiopathic Pulmonary Fibrosis: Clinical, Histologic, Radiographic, Physiologic, Scintigraphic, Cytologic, and Biochemical Aspects. *Ann Intern Med* 85: 769–788, 1976.

Crystal RG, Gadek JE, Ferrans VJ, et al: Interstitial Lung Disease: Current Concepts of Pathogenesis, Staging and Therapy. *Am J Med* 70: 342–568, 1981.

Crystal RG, Bitterman PB, Rennard I, et al: Interstitial Lung Diseases of Unknown Cause: Disorders Characterized by Chronic Inflammation of the Lower Respiratory Tract. *New Engl J Med* 310: 154–166, 1984.

Cwierzyk TA, Glasberg SS, Virshup MA, et al: Pulmonary Oncocytoma: Report of a Case with Cytologic, Histologic and Electron Microscopic Study. *Acta Cytol* 29: 620–623, 1985.

D'Ablang G III, Bernard B, Zaharov I, et al: Neonatal Pulmonary Cytology and Bronchopulmonary Dysplasia. *Acta Cytol* 19: 21–27, 1975.

Daniele RP, Elias JA, Epstein PE, et al: Bronchoalveolar Lavage: Role in the Pathogenesis, Diagnosis, and Management of Interstitial Lung Disease. *Ann Intern Med* 102: 93–108, 1985.

DeFine LA, Saleba KP, Gibson BB, et al: Cytologic Evaluation of Bronchoalveolar Lavage Specimens in Immunosuppressed Patients With Suspected Opportunistic Infections. *Acta Cytol* 31: 235–242, 1987.

de Gracia J, Bravo C, Miravitlles M, et al: Diagnostic Value of Bronchoalveolar Lavage in Peripheral Lung Cancer. *Am Rev Resp Dis* 147: 649–652, 1993.

De Jong RS, van den Bergen HA, Boender CA, et al: Extra-Adrenal Pheochromocytoma Presenting as Fulminant Malignant Disease With Tumor Positive Sputum Cytology. *J Intern Med* 230: 355–359, 1991.

DiBonito L, Colautti I, Patriarca S, et al: Cytological Typing of Primary Lung Cancer: Study of 100 Cases with Autopsy Confirmation. *Diagn Cytopathol* 7: 7–10, 1991.

Dodson RF, Williams MG, McLarty JW, et al: Asbestos Bodies and Particulate Matter in Sputum From Former Asbestos Workers: An Ultrastructural Study. *Acta Cytol* 27: 635–640, 1983.

Doshi N, Kanbour A, Fujikura T, et al: Tracheal Aspiration Cytology in Neonates With Respiratory Distress: Histopathologic Correlation. *Acta Cytol* 26: 15–21, 1982.

Druce HM: Diagnosis of Sinusitis in Adults: History, Physical Examination, Nasal Cytology, Echo, and Rhinoscope. *J Allergy Clin Immunol* 90: 436–441, 1992.

Ellis FH Jr, Woolner LB, Schmidt HW: Metastatic Pulmonary Malignancy: A Study of Factors Involved in Exfoliation of Malignant Cells. *J Thorac Surg* 20: 125–135, 1950.

Erozan YS, Frost JK: Cytopathologic Diagnosis of Cancer in Pulmonary Material: A Critical Histopathologic Correlation. *Acta Cytol* 14: 560–565, 1970.

Erozan YS, Frost JK: Cytopathologic Diagnosis of Lung Cancer. *Sem Oncol* 1: 191–198, 1974.

Erozan YS: Cytopathologic Diagnosis of Pulmonary Neoplasms in Sputum and Bronchoscopic Specimens. *Sem Diagn Pathol* 3: 188–195, 1986.

Farley ML, Mabry L, Muñoz LA, et al: Crystals Occurring in Pulmonary Cytology Specimens: Association With *Aspergillus* Infection. *Acta Cytol* 29: 737–744, 1985.

Fennessy JJ, Fry WA, Manalo-Estrella P, et al: The Bronchial Brushing Technique for Obtaining Cytologic Specimens From Peripheral Lung Lesions. *Acta Cytol* 14: 25–30, 1970.

Flehinger BJ, Melamed MR, Zaman MB, et al: Early Lung Cancer Detection: Results of the Initial (Prevalence) Radiologic and Cytologic Screening in the Memorial Sloan-Kettering Study. *Am Rev Respir Dis* 130: 555–560, 1984.

Flehinger BJ, Kimmel M, Polyak T, et al: Screening for Lung Cancer: The Mayo Lung Project Revisited. *Cancer* 72: 1573–1580, 1993.

Fleming WH, Jove DF: Primary Leiomyosarcoma of the Lung With Positive Sputum Cytology. *Acta Cytol* 19: 14–20, 1975.

Fleury-Feith J, Escudier E, Pocholle M-J, et al: The Effects of Cytocentrifugation on Differential Cell Counts in Samples Obtained by Bronchoalveolar Lavage. *Acta Cytol* 31: 606–610, 1987.

Flint A: Detection of Pulmonary Neoplasms by Bronchial Washings: Are Cell Blocks a Diagnostic Aid? *Acta Cytol* 37: 21–23, 1993.

Fontana RS, Sanderson DR, Taylor WF, et al: Early Lung Cancer Detection: Results of Initial (Prevalence) Radiologic and Cytologic Screening in the Mayo Clinic Study. *Am Rev Respir Dis* 130: 561–565, 1984.

Fontana RS, Sanderson DR, Woolner LB, et al: Screening for Lung Cancer: A Critique of the Mayo Lung Project. *Cancer* 67: 1155–1164, 1991.

Foot NC: The Identification of Types of Pulmonary Cancer in Cytologic Smears. *Am J Pathol* 28: 963–983, 1952.

Frable WJ: The Relationship of Pulmonary Cytology to Survival in Lung Cancer. *Acta Cytol* 12: 52–56, 1968.

Frable WJ, Frable MA, Seney FD Jr: Virus Infections of the Respiratory Tract: Cytopathologic and Clinical Analysis. *Acta Cytol* 21: 32–36, 1977.

Francis D, Jacobsen M: Pulmonary Blastoma: Preoperative Cytologic and Histologic Findings. *Acta Cytol* 23: 437–442, 1979.

Friedman-Mor Z, Chalon J, Turndorf H, et al: Tracheobronchial Cytologic Changes and Abnormal Serum Heme Pigments in Hemorrhagic Shock. *J Trauma* 17: 829–834, 1977.

Friedman-Mor Z, Chalon J, Turndorf H, et al: Cardiac Index and Incidence of Heart Failure Cells. *Arch Pathol Lab Med* 102: 418–419, 1978.

Frost JK, Gupta PK, Erozan YS, et al: Pulmonary Cytologic Alterations in Toxic Environmental Inhalation. *Hum Pathol* 4: 521–536, 1973.

Frost JK, Ball WC Jr, Levin ML, et al: Early Lung Cancer Detection: Results of the Initial (Prevalence) Radiologic and Cytologic Screening in The John Hopkins Study. *Am Rev Resp Dis* 130: 549–554, 1984.

Fry WA, Manalo-Estrella P: Bronchial Brushing. *Surg Gynecol Obstet* 130: 67–71, 1970.

Fullmer CD, Parrish CM: Pulmonary Cytology: a Diagnostic Method for Occult Carcinoma. *Acta Cytol* 13: 645–651, 1969a.

Fullmer CD, Short JG, Allen A, et al: Proposed Classification for Bronchial Epithelial Cell Abnormalities in the Category of Dyskaryosis. *Acta Cytol* 13: 459–471, 1969b.

Fullmer CD, Morris RP: Primary Cytodiagnosis of Unsuspected Mediastinal Hodgkin's Disease: (Report of a Case). *Acta Cytol* 16: 77–81, 1972.

Füzesi L, Höer P-W, Schmidt W: Exfoliative Cytology of Multiple Endobronchial Granular Cell Tumor. *Acta Cytol* 33: 516–518, 1989.

Gagneten CB, Geller CE, del Carmen Saenz M: Diagnosis of Bronchogenic Carcinoma Through the Cytologic Examination of Sputum, With Special Reference to Tumor Typing. *Acta Cytol* 20: 530–536, 1976.

Gephardt GN, Belovich DM: Cytology of Pulmonary Carcinoid Tumors. *Acta Cytol* 26: 434–438, 1982.

Gindhart TD, Tsukahara YC: Cytologic Diagnosis of Pineal Germinoma in Cerebrospinal Fluid and Sputum. *Acta Cytol* 23: 341–346, 1979.

Glant MD, Wall RW, Ransburg R: Endobronchial Granular Cell Tumor: Cytology of a New Case and Review of the Literature. *Acta Cytol* 23: 477–482, 1979.

Gordon P, Rosen PP, Savino A: The Ferruginous Body Content of Lungs at Autopsy in Boston 1928–1932. *Acta Cytol* 20: 521–524, 1976.

Gordon SM, Gal AA, Hertzler GL, et al: Diagnosis of Pulmonary Toxoplasmosis by Bronchoalveolar Lavage in Cardiac Transplant Recipients. *Diagn Cytopathol* 9: 650–654, 1993.

Granados R, Constantine NM, Cibas ES: Nasal Scrape Cytology in the Diagnosis of Wegener's Granulomatosis: A Case Report. *Acta Cytol* 38: 463–466, 1994.

Greenberg SD, Hurst GA, Christianson SC, et al: Pulmonary Cytopathology of Former Asbestos Workers: Report of the First Year. *Am J Clin Pathol* 66: 815–822, 1976.

Greenberg SD: Recent Advances in Pulmonary Cytopathology. *Hum Pathol* 14: 901–912, 1983.

Grotte D, Stanley MW, Swanson PE, et al: Reactive Type II Pneumocytes in Bronchoalveolar Lavage Fluid From Adult Respiratory Distress Syndrome Can Be Mistaken for Cells of Adenocarcinoma. *Diagn Cytopathol* 6: 317–322, 1990.

Grunze H: A Critical Review and Evaluation of Cytodiagnosis in Chest Diseases. *Acta Cytol* 4: 175–198, 1960.

Grunze H: Cytologic Diagnosis of Tumors of the Chest. *Acta Cytol* 17: 148–159, 1973.

Guillou L, Gloor E, Anani PA, et al: Bronchial Granular-Cell Tumor: Report of a Case With Preoperative Cytologic Diagnosis on Bronchial Brushings and Immunohistochemical Studies. *Int Acad Cytol* 35: 375–380, 1991.

Gupta PK, Verma K: Calcified (Psammoma) Bodies in Alveolar Cell Carcinoma of the Lung. *Acta Cytol* 16: 59–62, 1972.

Gupta PK, Albritton N, Erozan YS, et al: Occurrence of Cilia in Exfoliated Ovarian Adenocarcinoma Cells. *Diagn Cytopathol* 1: 228–231, 1985.

Gupta RK: Value of Sputum Cytology in the Differential Diagnosis of Alveolar Cell Carcinoma From Bronchogenic Adenocarcinoma. *Acta Cytol* 25: 255–258, 1981.

Gupta RK: Value of Sputum Cytology in the Diagnosis and Typing of Bronchogenic Carcinomas, Excluding Adenocarcinomas. *Acta Cytol* 26: 645–648, 1982.

Gupta RK, McHutchison AGR: Cytologic Findings of Adenoid Cystic Carcinoma in a Tracheal Wash Specimen. *Diagn Cytopathol* 8: 196–197, 1992.

Guzman J, Izumi T, Nagai S, et al: Immunocytochemical Characterization of Isolated Human Type II Pneumocytes. *Acta Cytol* 38: 539–542, 1994.

Hajdu SI, Koss LG: Cytology of Carcinoma of the Trachea. *Acta Cytol* 13: 255–259, 1969.

Hankins DG, Sanders S, MacDonald FM, et al: Pulmonary Toxicity Recurring After a Six Week Course of Busulfan Therapy and After Subsequent Therapy With Uracil Mustard. *Chest* 73: 415–416, 1978.

Harboldt SL, Dugan JM, Tronic BS: Cytologic Diagnosis of Measles Pneumonia in a Bronchoalveolar Lavage. *Acta Cytol* 38: 403–406, 1994.

Haslam PL, Turton CWG, Heard B, et al: Bronchoalveolar Lavage in Pulmonary Fibrosis: Comparison of Cells Obtained With Lung Biopsy and Clinical Features. *Thorax* 35: 9–18, 1980.

Hattori S, Matsuda M, Sugiyama T, et al: Cytologic Diagnosis of Early Lung Cancer: Brushing Method Under X-ray Television Fluoroscopy. *Dis Chest* 45: 129–142, 1964.

Hattori S, Matsuda M, Sugiyama T, et al: Some Limitations of Cytologic Diagnosis of Small Peripheral Lung Cancers. *Acta Cytol* 9: 431–436, 1965.

Hattori S, Matsuda M, Nishihara H, et al: Early Diagnosis of Small Peripheral Lung Cancer–Cytologic Diagnosis of Very Fresh Cancer Cells Obtained by the TV-Brushing Technique. *Acta Cytol* 15: 460–467, 1971.

Hector MF: Sputum Cytology in Two Cases of Wegener's Granulomatosis. *J Clin Pathol* 29: 259–263, 1976.

Herbut PA, Clerf LH: Bronchogenic Carcinoma: Diagnosis by Cytologic Study of Bronchoscopically Removed Secretions. *JAMA* 130: 1006–1012, 1946.

Herf SM, Suratt PM: Complications of Transbronchial Lung Biopsies. *Chest* 73: 759–760, 1978.

Hess FG Jr, McDowell EM, Trump BF: The Respiratory Epithelium: VIII. Interpretation of Cytologic Criteria for Human and Hamster Respiratory Tract Tumors. *Acta Cytol* 25: 111–134, 1981.

Holiday DB, McLarty JW, Farley ML, et al: Sputum Cytology Within and Across Laboratories: A Reliability Study. *Acta Cytol* 39: 195–206, 1995.

Hsu C: Cytologic Diagnosis of Lung Tumors From Bronchial Brushings of Chinese Patients in Hong Kong. *Acta Cytol* 27: 641–646, 1983.

Hsu C-Y: Cytologic Diagnosis of Pulmonary Cryptococcosis in Immunocompetent Hosts. *Acta Cytol* 37: 667–672, 1993.

Huang M-S, Colby TV, Goellner JR, et al: Utility of Bronchoalveolar Lavage in the Diagnosis of Drug-Induced Pulmonary Toxicity. *Acta Cytol* 33: 533–538, 1989.

Hunninghake GW, Gadek JE, Kawanami O, et al: Inflammatory and Immune Processes in the Human Lung in Health and Disease: Evaluation by Bronchoalveolar Lavage. *Am J Pathol* 97: 149–206, 1979.

Ishizuka T, Yoshitake J, Yamada T, et al: Diagnosis of a Case of Pulmonary Carcinosarcoma by Detection of Rhabdomyosarcoma Cells in Sputum. *Acta Cytol* 32: 658–662, 1988.

Israël-Biet D, Venet A, Caubarrére I, et al: Bronchoalveolar Lavage in Amiodarone Pneumonitis: Cellular Abnormalities and Their Relevance to Pathogenesis. *Chest* 91: 214–221, 1987.

Iwama de Mattos MCF, de Oliveira MLS: Pseudoepitheliomatous Proliferation, a Pitfall in Sputum Cytology. *Diagn Cytopathol* 7: 656–657, 1991.

Janower ML, Land RE: Bronchial Brushing and Percutaneous Puncture. *Radiol Clin North Am* 9: 73–83, 1971.

Jay SJ, Wehr K, Nicholson DP, et al: Diagnostic Sensitivity and Specificity of Pulmonary Cytology: Comparison of Techniques Used in Conjunction With Flexible Fiber Optic Bronchoscopy. *Acta Cytol* 24: 304–312, 1980.

Jean R, Lellouch-Tubiana A, Brunet-Langot D, et al: Nasal Eosinophilia in Children: Its Use in the Nasal Allergen Provocation Test. *Diagn Cytopathol* 4: 23–27, 1988.

Johnston WW, Frable WJ: The Cytopathology of the Respiratory Tract: A Review. *Am J Pathol* 84: 372–414, 1976.

Johnston WW, Bossen EH: Ten Years of Respiratory Cytopathology at Duke University Medical Center: I. The Cytopathologic Diagnosis of Lung Cancer During the Years 1970 to 1974, Noting the Significance of Specimen Number and Type. *Acta Cytol* 25: 103–107, 1981a.

Johnston WW, Bossen EH: Ten Years of Respiratory Cytopathology at Duke University Medical Center: II. The Cytopathologic Diagnosis of Lung Cancer During the Years 1970-1974, With a Comparison Between Cytopathology and Histopathology in the Typing of Lung Cancer. *Acta Cytol* 25: 499–505, 1981b.

Johnston WW: Ten Years of Respiratory Cytopathology at Duke University Medical Center: III. The Significance of Inconclusive Cytopathologic Diagnoses During the Years 1970 to 1974. *Acta Cytol* 26: 759–766, 1982.

Johnston WW: Cytologic Diagnosis of Lung Cancer: Principles and Problems. *Pathol Res Pract* 181: 1–36, 1986.

Johnston WW: Histologic and Cytologic Patterns of Lung Cancers in 2,580 Men and Women Over a 15-Year Period. *Acta Cytol* 32: 163–168, 1988a.

Johnston WW: Fine Needle Aspiration Biopsy Versus Sputum and Bronchial Material in the Diagnosis of Lung Cancer: A Comparative Study of 168 Patients. *Acta Cytol* 32: 641–646, 1988b.

Johnston WW: Type II Pneumocytes in Cytologic Specimens: A Diagnostic Dilemma. *Am J Clin Pathol* 97: 608–609, 1992.

Jordan AG, Predmore L, Sullivan MM, et al: The Cytodiagnosis of Well-Differentiated Neuroendocrine Carcinoma: A Distinct Clinicopathologic Entity. *Acta Cytol* 31: 464–470, 1987.

Kern WH: Cytology of Hyperplastic and Neoplastic Lesions of Terminal Bronchioles and Alveoli. *Acta Cytol* 9: 372–379, 1965.

Kern WH, Dermer GB, Tiemann RM: Comparative Morphology of Histiocytes From Various Organ Systems: Quantitative Cytologic and Ultrastructural Studies. *Acta Cytol* 14: 205–215, 1970.

Kern WH, Schweizer CW: Sputum Cytology of Metastatic Carcinoma of the Lung. *Acta Cytol* 20: 514–520, 1976.

Kern WH: The Diagnostic Accuracy of Sputum and Urine Cytology. *Acta Cytol* 32: 651–654, 1988.

Kern WH: The Elusive "False-Positive" Sputum and Urine Cytology. *Acta Cytol* 34: 587–588, 1990.

Khajotia RR, Mohn A, Pokieser L, et al: Induced Sputum and Cytological Diagnosis of Lung Cancer. *Lancet* 338: 976–977, 1991.

Khoddami M: Cytologic Diagnosis of Metastatic Malignant Melanoma of the Lung in Sputum and Bronchial Washings. A Case Report. *Acta Cytol* 37: 403–408, 1993.

Kierszenbaum AL: Bronchial Metaplasia: Observations on its Histology and Cytology. *Acta Cytol* 9: 365–371, 1965.

Kim C-J, Ko I, Bukantz SC: Ciliocytophthoria (CCP) in Asthmatic Children, With References to Viral Respiratory Infection and Exacerbation of Asthma: Preliminary Report. *J Allergy* 35: 159–168, 1964.

Kinsella DL Jr: Bronchial Cell Atypias: A Report of a Preliminary Study Correlating Cytology With Histology. *Cancer* 12: 463–472, 1959.

Koprowska I, An SH, Corsey D, et al: Cytologic Patterns of Developing Bronchogenic Carcinoma. *Acta Cytol* 9: 424–430, 1965.

Korfhage L, Broghamer WL Jr, Richardson ME, et al: Pulmonary Cytology in the Posttherapeutic Monitoring of Patients with Bronchogenic Carcinoma. *Acta Cytol* 30: 351–355, 1986.

Koss LG, Richardson HL: Some Pitfalls of Cytological Diagnosis of Lung Cancer. *Cancer* 8: 937–947, 1955.

Koss LG, Melamed MR, Goodner JT: Pulmonary Cytology: A Brief Survey of Diagnostic Results From July 1st 1952 Until December 31st, 1960. *Acta Cytol* 8: 104–113, 1964.

Kuhn C III, Kuo T-T: Cytoplasmic Hyalin in Asbestosis: A Reaction of Injured Alveolar Epithelium. *Arch Pathol* 95: 190–194, 1973.

Kung ITM, Hsu C, Chan SCW, et al: Frequency of "Blue Bodies" in Pulmonary Cytology Specimens. *Diagn Cytopathol* 3: 284–286, 1987.

Kvale PA, Bode FR, Kini S: Diagnostic Accuracy in Lung Cancer: Comparison of Techniques Used in Association with Flexible Fiberoptic Bronchoscopy. *Chest* 69: 752–757, 1976.

Kyriakos M, Rockoff SD: Brush Biopsy of Bronchial Carcinoid: A Source of Cytologic Error. *Acta Cytol* 16: 261–268, 1972.

Kyriazis AP, Kyriazis AA: Incidence and Distribution of Opportunistic Lung Infections in AIDS Patients Related to Intravenous Drug Use: A Study of Bronchoalveolar Lavage Cytology by the Diff-Quik Stain. *Diagn Cytopathol* 9: 487–491, 1993.

Lachman MF: Morphometric Comparison of a Metastatic Transitional Cell Carcinoma Simulating Squamous Metaplasia in Sputum Cytology: A Case Report. *Acta Cytol* 38: 407–409, 1994.

Lambird PA, Ashton PR: Exfoliative Cytopathology of a Primary Pulmonary Malignant Histiocytoma. *Acta Cytol* 14: 83–86, 1970.

Landa JF: Indications for Bronchoscopy. *Chest* 73: 686–690, 1978.

Lavoie RR, McDonald JR, Kling GA: Cavitation in Squamous Carcinoma of the Lung. *Acta Cytol* 21: 210–214, 1977.

Lee HS, Majima Y, Sakakura Y, et al: Quantitative Cytology of Nasal Secretions Under Various Conditions. *Laryngoscope* 103: 533–537, 1993.

Levij IS: A Case of Primary Cavitary Hodgkin's Disease of the Lungs, Diagnosed Cytologically. *Acta Cytol* 16: 546–549, 1972.

Levy H, Horak DA, Lewis MI: The Value of Bronchial Washings and Bronchoalveolar Lavage in the Diagnosis of Lymphangitic Carcinomatosis. *Chest* 94: 1028–1030, 1988.

Liang XM: Accuracy of Cytologic Diagnosis and Cytotyping of Sputum in Primary Lung Cancer: Analysis of 161 Cases. *J Surg Oncol* 40: 107–111, 1989.

Linder J, Radio SJ, Robbins RA, et al: Bronchoalveolar Lavage in the Cytologic Diagnosis of Carcinoma of the Lung. *Acta Cytol* 31: 796–801, 1987.

Lozowski MS, Mishriki Y, Solitare GB: Cytopathologic Features of Adenoid Cystic Carcinoma: Case Report and Literature Review. *Acta Cytol* 27: 317–322, 1983.

Lozowski W, Hajdu SI, Melamed MR: Cytomorphology of Carcinoid Tumors. *Acta Cytol* 23: 360–365, 1979.

Ludwig RA, Balachandran I: Mycosis Fungoides: The Importance of Pulmonary Cytology in the Diagnosing of a Case with Systemic Involvement. *Acta Cytol* 27: 198–201, 1983.

Lukeman JM: Reliability of Cytologic Diagnosing in Cancer of the Lung. *Cancer Chemother Rep* 4: 79–83, 1973.

Lundgren J, Olofsson J, Hellquist HB, et al: Exfoliative Cytology in Laryngology: Comparison of Cytologic and Histologic Diagnoses in 350 Microlaryngoscopic Examinations—A Prospective Study. *Cancer* 47: 1336–1343, 1981.

MacDougall B, Weinerman B: The Value of Sputum Cytology. *J Gen Intern Med* 7: 11–13, 1992.

Mak VHF, Johnston IDA, Hetzel MR, et al: Value of Washings and Brushings at Fibreoptic Bronchoscopy in the Diagnosis of Lung Cancer. *Thorax* 45: 373–376, 1990.

Marchevsky A, Nieburgs HE, Olenko E: Pulmonary Tumorlets in Cases of "Tuberculoma" of the Lung With Malignant Cells in Brush Biopsy. *Acta Cytol* 26: 491–494, 1982.

Martin WJ II, Osborn MJ, Douglas WW: Amiodarone Pulmonary Toxicity: Assessment by Bronchoalveolar Lavage. *Chest* 88: 630–631, 1985.

Martini N, Melamed MR: Occult Carcinomas of the Lung. *Ann Thorac Surg* 30: 215–223, 1980.

Masin M, Masin F: Pulmonary Alveolar Proteinosis: Cytologic and Cytochemical Observations on Sputum Specimens. *Acta Cytol* 6: 429–438, 1962.

Masson RG, Krikorian J, Lukl P, et al: Pulmonary Microvascular Cytology in the Diagnosis of Lymphangitic Carcinomatosis. *N Engl J Med* 321: 71–76, 1989.

Matsuda M, Nagumo S, Horai T, et al: Cytologic Diagnosis of Laryngeal and Hypopharyngeal Squamous Cell Carcinoma in Sputum. *Acta Cytol* 32: 655–657, 1988.

Matsuda M, Horai T, Doi O, et al: Diagnosis of Squamous-Cell Carcinoma of the Lung by Sputum Cytology: With Special Reference to Correlation of Diagnostic Accuracy With Size and Proximal Extent of Resected Tumor. *Diagn Cytopathol* 6: 248–251, 1990.

Meinecke R, Bauer F, Skouras J, et al: Blastomatous Tumors of the Respiratory Tract. *Cancer* 38: 818–823, 1976.

Melamed MR, Zaman MB, Flehinger BJ, et al: Radiologically Occult In Situ and Incipient Invasive Epidermoid Lung Cancer: Detection by Sputum Cytology in a Survey of Asymptomatic Cigarette Smokers. *Am J Surg Pathol* 1: 5–16, 1977.

Melamed MR, Flehinger BJ, Zaman MB, et al: Detection of True Pathologic Stage I Lung Cancer in a Screening Program and the Effect on Survival. *Cancer* 47: 1182–1187, 1981.

Melamed MR, Flehinger BJ, Zaman MB: Impact of Early Detection on the Clinical Course of Lung Cancer. *Surg Clin North Am* 67: 909–924, 1987.

Mermolja M, Rott T: Cytology of Endobronchial Granular Cell Tumor. *Diagn Cytopathol* 7: 524–526, 1991.

Mermolja M, Rott T, Debeljak A: Cytology of Bronchoalveolar Lavage in Some Rare Pulmonary Disorders: Pulmonary Alveolar Proteinosis and Amiodarone Pulmonary Toxicity. *Cytopathology* 5: 9–16, 1994.

Merritt TA, Puccia JM, Stuard ID: Cytologic Evaluation of Pulmonary Effluent in Neonates With Respiratory Distress Syndrome and Bronchopulmonary Dysplasia. *Acta Cytol* 25: 631–639, 1981a.

Merritt TA, Stuard ID, Puccia J, et al: Newborn Tracheal Aspirate Cytology: Classification During Respiratory Distress Syndrome and Bronchopulmonary Dysplasia. *J Pediatrics* 98: 949–956, 1981b.

Merz B: Is Screening for Early Lung Cancer Worthwhile? *JAMA* 249: 1537–1538, 1983.

Meyer JA, Umiker WO: A Review of Problems Relating to the "Diagnostic Triad" in Lung Cancer: Bronchoscopy, Scalene Lymph Node Biopsy, and Cytopathology of Bronchial Secretions. *Surg Clin North Am* 41: 1233–1244, 1961.

Miles PR, Baughman RP, Linnemann CC Jr: Cytomegalovirus in the Bronchoalveolar Lavage Fluid of Patients With AIDS. *Chest* 97: 1072–1076, 1990.

Milman N, Jacobsen GK: Bronchioloalveolar Lavage in the Diagnosis of Bronchiolo-Alveolar Carcinoma: A Case Report. *Cytopathology* 3: 55–59, 1992.

Miura H, Konaka C, Kawate N, et al: Sputum Cytology–Positive Bronchoscopically Negative Adenocarcinoma of the Lung. *Chest* 192: 1328–1332, 1992.

Mottet NK, Szanton V: Exfoliated Measles Giant Cells in Nasal Secretions. *Arch Pathol* 72: 434–437, 1961.

Mouriquand J, Dumollard J-M: Unidentified Bronchial Objects in Bronchial Secretions. *Acta Cytol* 30: 87–88, 1986.

Mylius EA, Gullvag: Alveolar Macrophage Count as an Indicator of Lung Reaction to Industrial Air Pollution. *Acta Cytol* 30: 157–162, 1986.

Naib ZM: Giant Cell Carcinoma of the Lung: Cytological Study of Exfoliated Cells in Sputa and Bronchial Washings. *Acta Cytol* 5: 69–73, 1961.

Naib ZM, Goldstein HG: Exfoliative Cytology of a Case of Bronchial Granular Cell Myoblastoma. *Dis Chest* 42: 645–647, 1962.

Naib ZM, Stewart JA, Dowdle WR: Cytological Features of Viral Respiratory Tract Infections. *Acta Cytol* 12: 162–171, 1968.

Naryshkin S, Daniels J, Young NA: Diagnostic Correlation of Fiberoptic Bronchoscopic Biopsy and Bronchoscopic Cytology Performed Simultaneously. *Diagn Cytopathol* 8: 119–123, 1992.

Naryshkin S, Young NA: Respiratory Cytology: A Review of Non-Neoplastic Mimics of Malignancy. *Diagn Cytopathol* 9: 89–97, 1993.

Nasiell M: The General Appearance of the Bronchial Epithelium in Bronchial Carcinoma: A Histopathological Study With Some Cytological Viewpoints. *Acta Cytol* 7: 97–106, 1963.

Nasiell M: Metaplasia and Atypical Metaplasia in the Bronchial Epithelium: A Histopathologic and Cytopathologic Study. *Acta Cytol* 10: 421–427, 1966.

Nasiell M: Abnormal Columnar Cell Findings in Bronchial Epithelium: A Cytologic and Histologic Study of Lung Cancer and Non-Cancer Cases. *Acta Cytol* 11: 397–402, 1967.

Nasiell M: Sputum-Cytologic Changes in Smokers and Non-Smokers in Relation to Chronic Inflammatory Lung Diseases. *Acta Path et Microbiol Scand* 74: 205–213, 1968.

Nasiell M, Roger V, Nasiell K, et al: Cytologic Findings Indicating Pulmonary Tuberculosis: I. The Diagnostic Significance of Epithelioid Cells and Langhans' Giant Cells Found in Sputum or Bronchial Secretions. *Acta Cytol* 16: 146–151, 1972.

Nasiell M, Sinner W, Tornvall G, et al: Clinically Occult Lung Cancer with Positive Sputum Cytology and Primarily Negative Radiological Findings. *Scand J Resp Dis* 58: 134–144, 1977.

Naylor B: The Shedding of the Mucosa of the Bronchial Tree in Asthma. *Thorax* 17: 69–72, 1962.

Naylor B, Railey C: A Pitfall in the Cytodiagnosis of Sputum of Asthmatics. *J Clin Pathol* 17: 84–89, 1964.

Neifer RA, Amy RWM: Cytology of Tracheobronchial Amyloidosis. *Acta Cytol* 29: 187–188, 1985.

Ng ABP, Horak GC: Factors Significant in the Diagnostic Accuracy of Lung Cytology in Bronchial Washing and Sputum: I. Bronchial Washings. *Acta Cytol* 27: 391–396, 1983a.

Ng ABP, Horak GC: Factors Significant in the Diagnostic Accuracy of Lung Cytology in Bronchial Washing and Sputum Samples: II: Sputum Samples. *Acta Cytol* 27: 397–402, 1983b.

Nguyen G-K: Cytology of Bronchial Gland Carcinoma. *Acta Cytol* 32: 235–239, 1988.

Non DP Jr, Lang WR, Patchefsky A, et al: Pulmonary Blastoma: Cytopathologic and Histopathologic Findings. *Acta Cytol* 20: 381–386, 1976.

Northway WH Jr, Rosan RC, Proter DY: Pulmonary Disease Following Respirator Therapy of Hyaline-Membrane Disease: Bronchopulmonary Dysplasia. *N Engl J Med* 276: 357–368, 1967.

Novak PM, Kumar NB, Naylor B: Curschmann's Spirals in Cervicovaginal Smears: Prevalence, Morphology, Significance and Origin. *Acta Cytol* 28: 5–8, 1984.

Nunez V, Melamed M, Cahan W: Tracheo-Bronchial Cytology after Laryngectomy for Carcinoma of Larynx: II. Benign Atypias. *Acta Cytol* 10: 38–48, 1966.

Nussbaum E, Maggi JC, Mathis R, et al: Association of Lipid-Laden Alveolar Macrophages and Gastroesophageal Reflux in Children. *J Pediatr* 110: 190–194, 1987.

Oswald NC, Hinson KFW, Canti G, et al: The Diagnosis of Primary Lung Cancer With Special Reference to Sputum Cytology. *Thorax* 26: 623–631, 1971.

Papanicolaou GN, Koprowska I: Carcinoma In Situ of the Right Lower Bronchus: A Case Report. *Cancer* 4: 141–146, 1951.

Papanicolaou GN: Degenerative Changes in Ciliated Cells Exfoliating From the Bronchial Epithelium as a Cytologic Criterion in the Diagnosis of Diseases of the Lung. *New York J State Med* 56: 2647–2650, 1956.

Perez-Arellano JL, Garcia J-EL, Macías MCG, et al: Hemosiderin-Laden Macrophages in Bronchoalveolar Lavage Fluid. *Acta Cytol* 36: 26–30, 1992.

Perlman EJ, Erozan YS, Howdon A: The Role of the Saccomanno Technique in Sputum Cytopathologic Diagnosis of Lung Cancer. *Am J Clin Pathol* 91: 57–60, 1989.

Pfitzer P, Knoblich PG: Giant Carcinoma Cells of Bronchiogenic Origin. *Acta Cytol* 12: 256–261, 1968.

Pickren JW: Identification of Oil-Red-O Stained Granules in Sputum Macrophages. *JAMA* 215: 1985, 1971.

Pilotti S, Rilke F, Gribaudi G, et al: Sputum Cytology for the Diagnosis of Carcinoma of the Lung. *Acta Cytol* 26: 649–654, 1982a.

Pilotti S, Rilke F, Gribaudi G, et al: Cytologic Diagnosis of Pulmonary Carcinoma on Bronchoscopic Brushing Material. *Acta Cytol* 26: 655–660, 1982b.

Pirozynski M: Bronchoalveolar Lavage in the Diagnosis of Peripheral, Primary Lung Cancer. *Chest* 102: 372–374, 1992.

Plamenac P, Nikulin A: Atypia of the Bronchial Epithelium in Wind Instrument Players and in Singers: A Cytopathologic Study. *Acta Cytol* 13: 274–278, 1969.

Plamenac P, Nikulin A, Kahvic M: Cytology of the Respiratory Tract in Advanced Age. *Acta Cytol* 14: 526–530, 1970.

Plamenac P, Nikulin A, Pikula B: Cytology of the Respiratory Tract in Former Smokers. *Acta Cytol* 16: 256–260, 1972.

Plamenac P, Nikulin A, Pikula B: Cytologic Changes of the Respiratory Tract in Young Adults as a Consequence of High Levels of Air Pollution Exposure. *Acta Cytol* 17: 241–244, 1973.

Plamenac P, Nikulin A, Pikula B: Cytologic Changes of the Respiratory Epithelium in Iron Foundry Workers. *Acta Cytol* 18: 34–40, 1974.

Plamenac P, Nikulin A, Pikula B, et al: Cytologic Changes of the Respiratory Tract as a Consequence of Air Pollution and Smoking. *Acta Cytol* 23: 449–453, 1979.

Poletti V, Romagna M, Allen KA, et al: Bronchoalveolar Lavage in the Diagnosis of Disseminated Lung Tumors. *Acta Cytol* 39: 472–477, 1995.

Popp W, Rauscher H, Ritschka L, et al: Diagnostic Sensitivity of Different Techniques in the Diagnosis of Lung Tumors With the Flexible Fiberoptic Bronchoscope: Comparison of Brush Biopsy, Imprint Cytology of Forceps Biopsy, and Histology of Forceps Biopsy. *Cancer* 67: 72–75, 1991.

Popp W, Merkle M, Schreiber B, et al: How Much Brushing Is Enough for the Diagnosis of Lung Tumors? *Cancer* 70: 2278–2280, 1992.

Prior C, Klima G, Gattringer C, et al: Cell Profiles in Serial Bronchoalveolar Lavage After Human Heart-Lung Transplantation. *Acta Cytol* 36: 19–25, 1992.

Radhika S, Dey P, Rajwanshi A, et al: Adenoid Cystic Carcinoma in a Bronchial Washing: A Case Report. *Acta Cytol* 37: 97–99, 1993.

Ramirez-R J, Kieffer RF Jr, Ball WC Jr: Bronchopulmonary Lavage in Man. *Ann Intern Med* 63: 819–828, 1965.

Reale FR, Variakojis D, Compton J, et al: Cytodiagnosis of Hodgkin's Disease in Sputum Specimens. *Acta Cytol* 27: 258–261, 1983.

Reid JD, Carr AH: The Validity and Value of Histological and Cytological Classifications of Lung Cancer. *Cancer* 14: 673–698, 1961.

Reyes CV, Kathuria S, MacGlashan A: Diagnostic Value of Calcium Oxalate Crystals in Respiratory and Pleural Fluid Cytology: A Case Report. *Acta Cytol* 23: 65–68, 1979.

Riazmontazer N, Bedayat G: Cytology of Plasma Cell Myeloma in Bronchial Washing. *Acta Cytol* 33: 519–522, 1989.

Risse EKJ, van't Hof MA, Laurini RN, et al: Sputum Cytology by the Saccomanno Method in Diagnosing Lung Malignancy. *Diagn Cytopathol* 1: 286–290, 1985.

Risse EKJ, van't Hof MA, Vooijs GP: Relationship Between Patient Characteristics and the Sputum Cytologic Diagnosis of Lung Cancer. *Acta Cytol* 31: 159–165, 1987a.

Risse EKJ, Vooijs GP, van't Hof MA: The Quality and Diagnostic Outcome of Postbronchoscopic Sputum. *Acta Cytol* 31: 166–169, 1987b.

Risse EKJ, Vooijs GP, van't Hof MA: Relationship Between the Cellular Composition of Sputum and the Cytologic Diagnosis of Lung Cancer. *Acta Cytol* 31: 170–176, 1987c.

Risse EKJ, Vooijs GP, van't Hof MA: Diagnostic Significance of "Severe Dysplasia" in Sputum Cytology. *Acta Cytol* 32: 629–634, 1988.

Rivasi F, Bergamini G: Nasal Cytology in Allergic Processes and Other Syndromes Caused by Hyperreactivity. *Diagn Cytopathol* 4: 99–105, 1988.

Rizzo T, Schumann GB, Riding JM: Comparison of the Pick-and-Smear and Saccomanno Methods for Sputum Cytologic Analysis. *Acta Cytol* 34: 875–880, 1990.

Roby TJ, Swan GE, Schumann GB, et al: Reliability of a Quantitative Interpretation of Sputum Cytology Slides. *Acta Cytol* 34: 140–146, 1990a.

Roby TJ, Swan GE, Sorensen KW, et al: Discriminant Analysis of Lower Respiratory Tract Components Associated With Cigarette Smoking, Based on Quantitative Sputum Cytology. *Acta Cytol* 34: 147–154, 1990b.

Roby TJ, Hubbard G, Swan GE: Cytomorphologic Features of Sputum Samples From Marijuana Smokers. *Diagn Cytopathol* 7: 229–234, 1991.

Roger V, Nasiell M, Nasiell K, et al: Cytologic Findings Indicating Pulmonary Tuberculosis: II. The Occurrence in Sputum of Epithelioid Cells and Multinucleated Giant Cells in Pulmonary Tuberculosis, Chronic Non-Tuberculous Inflammatory Lung Disease and Bronchogenic Carcinoma. *Acta Cytol* 17: 538–542, 1972.

Roger V, Nasiell M, Linden M, et al: Cytologic Differential Diagnosis of Bronchiolo-Alveolar Carcinoma and Bronchogenic Adenocarcinoma. *Acta Cytol* 20: 303–307, 1976.

Roggli VL, Piantadosi CA, Bell DY: Asbestos Bodies in Bronchoalveolar Lavage Fluid: A Study of 20 Asbestos-Exposed Individuals and Comparison to Patients With Other Chronic Interstitial Lung Diseases. *Acta Cytol* 30: 470–476, 1986.

Roggli VL, Coin PG, MacIntyre NR, et al: Asbestos Content of Bronchoalveolar Lavage Fluid. A Comparison of Light and Scanning Electron Microscopic Analysis. *Acta Cytol* 38: 502–510, 1994.

Rosen P, Melamed M, Savino A: The "Ferruginous Body" Content of Lung Tissue: A Quantitative Study of Eighty-Six Patients. *Acta Cytol* 16: 207–211, 1972.

Rosen SE, Vonderheid EC, Koprowska I: Mycosis Fungoides With Pulmonary Involvement: Cytopathologic Findings. *Acta Cytol* 28: 51–57, 1984.

Roszel JF, Freeman KP, Slusher SH: Curschmann's Spirals in Equine Endometrial Washings. *Acta Cytol* 29: 186, 1985.

Rothberg AD, Miot A, Leiman G: Tracheal Aspirate Cytology and Bronchopulmonary Dysplasia. *Diagn Cytopathol* 2: 212–216, 1986.

Saccomanno G, Saunders RP, Ellis H, et al: Concentration of Carcinoma or Atypical Cells in Sputum. *Acta Cytol* 7: 305–310, 1963.

Saccomanno G, Saunders RP, Arche VE, et al: Cancer of the Lung: The Cytology of Sputum Prior to the Development of Carcinoma. *Acta Cytol* 9: 413–423, 1965.

Saccomanno G, Saunders RP, Klein MG, et al: Cytology of the Lung in Reference to Irritant, Individual Sensitivity and Healing. *Acta Cytol* 14: 377–381, 1970.

Saccomanno G, Archer VE, Auerbach O, et al: Development of Carcinoma of the Lung as Reflected in Exfoliated Cells. *Cancer* 33: 256–270, 1974.

Saccomanno G: Carcinoma In Situ of the Lung: Its Development, Detection, and Treatment. *Sem Resp Med* 4: 156–160, 1982.

Sagawa M, Saito Y, Sato M, et al: Localization of Double, Roentgenographically Occult Lung Cancer: Cytologic Findings From Selective Brushings of All Segmental and Subsegmental Bronchi. *Acta Cytol* 38: 392–397, 1994.

Saito Y, Imai T, Sato M, et al: Cytologic Study of Tissue Repair in Human Bronchial Epithelium. *Acta Cytol* 32: 622–628, 1988.

Sakula A: Charcot-Leyden Crystals and Curschmann Spirals in Asthmatic Sputum. *Thorax* 41: 503–507, 1986.

Saltini C, Hance AJ, Ferrans VJ, et al: Accurate Quantification of Cells Recovered by Bronchoalveolar Lavage. *Am Rev Respir Dis* 130: 650–658, 1984.

Sanerkin NG, Evans DMD: The Sputum in Bronchial Asthma: Pathognomonic Patterns. *J Path Bact* 89: 535–541, 1965.

Sassy-Dobray G: The Evaluation of Cytology in the Early Diagnosis of Pulmonary Carcinoma. *Acta Cytol* 14: 95–103, 1970.

Sassy-Dobray G: Possibilities of Early Diagnosis of Bronchogenic Carcinoma. *Acta Cytol* 19: 351–357, 1975.

Sato M, Saito Y, Nagamoto N, et al: Diagnostic Value of Differential Brushing of All Branches of the Bronchi in Patients With Sputum Positive or Suspected Positive for Lung Cancer. *Acta Cytol* 37: 879–883, 1993.

Sawada K, Fukuma S, Seki Y, et al: Cytologic Features of Primary Leiomyosarcoma of the Lung: Report of a Case Diagnosed by Bronchial Brushing Procedure. *Acta Cytol* 21: 770–773, 1977.

Schmitz B, Pfitzer P: Acellular Bodies in Sputum. *Acta Cytol* 28: 118–125, 1984.

Schreiber H, Schreiber K, Martin DH: Experimental Tumor Induction in a Circumscribed Region of the Hamster Trachea: Correlation of Histology and Exfoliative Cytology. *J Natl Cancer Inst* 54: 187–197, 1975.

Schumann GB, DiFiore K, Johnston JL: Sputum Cytodiagnosis of Disseminated Histiocytic Lymphoma: A Case Report. *Acta Cytol* 27: 262–266, 1983.

Schumann GB, Roby TJ, Swan GE: Quantitative Sputum Cytologic Findings in 109 Nonsmokers. *Am Rev Respir Dis* 139: 601–603, 1989.

Scoggins WG, Smith RH, Frable WJ, et al: False-Positive Cytological Diagnosis of Lung Carcinoma in Patients With Pulmonary Infarcts. *Ann Thorac Surg* 24: 474–480, 1977.

Selvaggi SM: Bronchoalveolar Lavage in Lung Transplant Patients. *Acta Cytol* 36: 674–679, 1992.

Shahar J, Mailman D, Meitzen G: Crystals in Pulmonary Cytologic Preparations in Association With Aspiration of Barium. A Case Report. *Acta Cytol* 38: 415–416, 1994.

Shaheen K, Oertel YC: Mycosis Fungoides Cells in Sputum: A Case Report. *Acta Cytol* 28: 483–486, 1984.

Shlaes DM, Lederman M, Chmielewski R, et al: Elastin Fibers in the Sputum of Patients With Necrotizing Pneumonia. *Chest* 83: 885–889, 1983.

Shroff CP, Khade MV, Srinivasan M: Respiratory Cytopathology in Chlorine Gas Toxicity: A Study in 28 Subjects. *Diagn Cytopathol* 4: 28–32, 1988.

Silverman JF, Turner RC, West RL, et al: Bronchoalveolar Lavage in the Diagnosis of Lipoid Pneumonia. *Diagn Cytopathol* 5: 3–9, 1989.

Skitarelic K, von Haam E: Bronchial Brushings and Washings: A Diagnostically Rewarding Procedure? *Acta Cytol* 18: 321–326, 1974.

Smith JH, Frable WJ: Adenocarcinoma of the Lung: Cytologic Correlation With Histologic Types. *Acta Cytol* 18: 316–320, 1974.

Smith P, Heath D, Moosavi H: The Clara Cell. *Thorax* 29: 147–163, 1974.

Solomon DA, Solliday NH, Gracey DR: Cytology in Fiberoptic Bronchoscopy: Comparison of Bronchial Brushing, Washing and Post-Bronchoscopy Sputum. *Chest* 65: 616–619, 1974.

Spahr J, Draffin RM, Johnston WW: Cytopathologic Findings in Pulmonary Blastoma. *Acta Cytol* 23: 454–459, 1979.

Spain DM, Bradess VA, Tarter R, et al: Metaplasia of Bronchial Epithelium: Effect of Age, Sex, and Smoking. *JAMA* 211: 1331–1334, 1970.

Spjut HJ, Fier DJ, Ackerman LV: Exfoliative Cytology and Pulmonary Cancer: A Histopathologic and Cytologic Correlation. *J Thorac Surg* 30: 90–107, 1955.

Springmeyer SC, Hackman R, Carlson JJ, et al: Bronchiolo-Alveolar Cell Carcinoma Diagnosed by Bronchoalveolar Lavage. *Chest* 83: 278–279, 1983.

Springmeyer SC: The Clinical Use of Bronchoalveolar Lavage. *Chest* 92: 771–772, 1987.

Sproul EE, Huvos A, Britsch C: A Two-Year Follow Up Study of 261 Patients Examined by Use of Superheated Aerosol Induced Sputum. *Acta Cytol* 6: 409–412, 1962.

Stanley C, Wolf P, Haghighi P: Reed-Sternberg Cells in Sputum From a Patient With Hodgkin's Disease: A Case Report. *Acta Cytol* 37: 90–92, 1993.

Stein B, Zaatari GS, Pine JR: Amiodarone Pulmonary Toxicity: Clinical, Cytologic and Ultrastructural Findings. *Acta Cytol* 31: 357–361, 1987.

Stoller JK, Rankin JA, Reynolds HY: The Impact of Bronchoalveolar Lavage Cell Analysis on Clinicians' Diagnostic Reasoning About Interstitial Lung Disease. *Chest* 92: 839–843, 1987.

Stover DE, Zaman MB, Hajdu SI, et al: Bronchoalveolar Lavage in the Diagnosis of Diffuse Pulmonary Infiltrates in the Immunosuppressed Host. *Ann Intern Med* 101: 1–7, 1984.

Strauss GM, Gleason RE, Sugarbaker DJ: Screening for Lung Cancer Re-Examined: A Reinterpretation of the Mayo Lung Project Randomized Trial on Lung Cancer Screening. *Chest* 103: 337S–341S, 1993.

Strigle SM, Gal AA: A Review of Pulmonary Cytopathology in the Acquired Immunodeficiency Syndrome. *Diagn Cytopathol* 5: 44–54, 1989.

Studdy PR, Rudd RM, Gellert AR, et al: Bronchoalveolar Lavage in the Diagnosing of Diffuse Pulmonary Shadowing. *Br J Dis Chest* 78: 46–54, 1984.

Suprun H, Koss LG: The Cytological Study of Sputum and Bronchial Washings in Hodgkin's Disease With Pulmonary Involvement. *Cancer* 17: 674–680, 1964.

Suprun H, Pedio G, Ruttner JR: The Diagnostic Reliability of Cytologic Typing in Primary Lung Cancer With a Review of the Literature. *Acta Cytol* 24: 494–500, 1980.

Swan GE, Schumann GB, Roby TJ, et al: Quantitative Analysis of Sputum Cytologic Differences Between Smokers and Nonsmokers. *Diagn Cytopathol* 7: 569–575, 1991.

Swan GE, Roby TJ, Hodgkin JE, et al: Relationship of Cytomorphology to Spirometric Findings in Cigarette Smokers. *Acta Cytol* 38: 547–553, 1994.

Tabatowski K, Roggli VL, Fulkerson WJ, et al: Giant Cell Interstitial Pneumonia in a Hard-Metal Worker: Cytologic, Histologic and Analytical Electron Microscopic Investigation. *Acta Cytol* 32: 240–246, 1988.

Takeda M, Burechailo FA: Smooth Muscle Cells in Sputum. *Acta Cytol* 13: 696–699, 1969.

Takeda S, Nanjo S, Nakamoto K, et al: Carcinosarcoma of the Lung. Report of a Case and Review of the Literature. *Respiration* 61: 113–116, 1994.

Tanaka T, Yamamoto M, Tamura T, et al: Cytologic and Histologic Correlation in Primary Lung Cancer: A Study of 154 Cases With Resectable Tumors. *Acta Cytol* 29: 49–56, 1985.

Tani EM, Schmitt FCL, Oliveira MLS, et al: Pulmonary Cytology in Tuberculosis. *Acta Cytol* 31: 460–463, 1987.

Tao L-C: Microliths in Sputum Specimens and Their Relationship to Pulmonary Alveolar Microlithiasis. *Am J Clin Pathol* 69: 482–485, 1978a.

Tao LC, Delarue NC, Sanders D, et al: Bronchiolo-Alveolar Carcinoma: A Correlative Clinical and Cytologic Study. *Cancer* 42: 2759–2767, 1978b.

Tao LC, Chamberlain DW, Delarue NC, et al: Cytologic Diagnosis of Radiographically Occult Squamous Cell Carcinoma of the Lung. *Cancer* 50: 1580–1586, 1982.

Taskinen E, Tukiainen P, Renkonen R: Bronchoalveolar Lavage: Influence of Cytologic Methods on the Cellular Picture. *Acta Cytol* 36: 680–686, 1992.

Tassoni EM: Pools of Lymphocytes: Significance in Pulmonary Secretions. *Acta Cytol* 7: 168–173, 1963.

Teir H, Koivuniemi A, Kyllönen KEJ, et al: A Retrospective Study of 2,756 Lung Cytology Specimens. *Ann Chir Urgiae Gynecol Fenniae* 52: 502–512, 1963.

Thomas ED, Ramberg RE, Sale GE: Direct Evidence for a Bone Marrow Origin of the Alveolar Macrophage in Man. *Science* 192: 1016–1018, 1976.

Thomas L, Risbud M, Gabriel J, et al: Cytomorphology of Granular-Cell Tumor of the Bronchus: A Case Report. *Acta Cytol* 28: 129–132, 1984.

Thomson JG: Fatal Bronchial Asthma Showing the Asthmatic Reaction in an Ovarian Teratoma. *J Pathol Bact* 57: 213–219, 1945.

Truong LD, Underwood RD, Greenberg SD, et al: Diagnosis and Typing of Lung Carcinomas by Cytopathologic Methods: A Review of 108 Cases. *Acta Cytol* 29: 379–384, 1985.

Tyers GFO, McGavran MH: Diagnostic and Therapeutic Challenges Following the Cytologic Diagnosing of In Situ Carcinoma of the Lung. *Chest* 69: 33–38, 1976.

Usuda K, Saito Y, Imai T, et al: Inflammatory Pseudotumor of the Lung Diagnosed as Granulomatous Lesion by Preoperative Brushing Cytology: A Case Report. *Acta Cytol* 34: 685–689, 1990.

Valicenti JF Jr, McMaster KR III, Daniell CJ: Sputum Cytology of Giant Cell Interstitial Pneumonia. *Acta Cytol* 23: 217–221, 1979.

Vedrinne JM, Guillaume C, Gagnieu MC, et al: Bronchoalveolar Lavage in Trauma Patients for Diagnosis of Fat Embolism. *Chest* 102: 1323–1327, 1992.

Vigorita VJ, Gupta PK, Bargeron CB, et al: Occurrence and Identification of Intracellular Calcium Crystals in Pulmonary Specimens. *Acta Cytol* 23: 49–52, 1979.

Vine MF, Schoenbach VJ, Hulka BS, et al: Atypical Metaplasia and Incidence of Bronchogenic Carcinoma. *Am J Epidemiol* 131: 781–793, 1990.

Volpe R, Carbone A, Casartelli GL, et al: Positive Sputum Cytology in Hairy Cell Leukemia. *Acta Cytol* 25: 432–434, 1981.

Wahl RW: Curschmann's Spirals in Pleural and Peritoneal Fluids: Report of 12 Cases. *Acta Cytol* 30: 147–151, 1986.

Walker KR, Fullmer CD: Progress Report on Study of Respiratory Spirals. *Acta Cytol* 14: 396–398, 1970.

Walker KR, Fullmer CD: Observations of Eosinophilic Extracytoplasmic Processes in Pulmonary Macrophages Progress Report. *Acta Cytol* 15: 363–364, 1971.

Walts AE, Marchevsky AM, Morgan M: Pulmonary Cytology in Lung Transplant Recipients: Recent Trends in Laboratory Utilization. *Diagn Cytopathol* 7: 353–358, 1991.

Warnock ML, Press M, Churg A: Further Observations on Cytoplasmic Hyaline in the Lung. *Hum Pathol* 11: 59–65, 1980.

Weaver KM, Novak PM, Naylor B: Vegetable Cell Contaminants in Cytologic Specimens: Their Resemblance to Cells Associated With Various Normal and Pathologic States. *Acta Cytol* 25: 210–214, 1981.

Wehle K, Pfitzer P: Nonspecific Esterase Activity of Human Alveolar Macrophages in Routine Cytology. *Acta Cytol* 32: 153–157, 1988.

Weinberger SE, Kelman JA, Elson NA, et al: Bronchoalveolar Lavage in Interstitial Lung Disease. *Ann Intern Med* 89: 459–466, 1978.

Weingarten J: Cytologic and Histologic Findings in a Case of Tracheobronchial Papillomatosis. *Acta Cytol* 25: 167–170, 1981.

Weiss RL, Snow GW, Schumann GB, et al: Diagnosis of Cytomegalovirus Pneumonitis on Bronchoalveolar Lavage Fluid: Comparison of Cytology, Immunofluorescence, and In Situ Hybridization With Viral Isolation. *Diagn Cytopathol* 7: 243–247, 1991.

Wheeler RR, Bardales RH, North PE, et al: Toxoplasma Pneumonia: Cytologic Diagnosis by Bronchoalveolar Lavage. *Diagn Cytopathol* 11: 52–55, 1994.

Willett GD, Schumann GB, Genack L: Primary Cytodiagnosis of Synchronous Small-Cell Cancer and Squamous-Cell Carcinoma of the Respiratory Tract. *Acta Cytol* 28: 610–613, 1984.

Wisecarver J, Ness MJ, Rennard SI, et al: Bronchoalveolar Lavage in the Assessment of Pulmonary Hodgkin's Disease. *Acta Cytol* 33: 527–532, 1989.

Woolner LB, David E, Fontana RS, et al: In Situ and Early Invasive Bronchogenic Carcinoma: Report of 28 Cases With Postoperative Survival Data. *J Thorac Cardiovasc Surg* 60: 275–290, 1970.

Woolner LB, Fontana RS, Bernatz PE: Early Bronchogenic Carcinoma: Problems in Detection, Localization, and Treatment. *Surg Clin North Am* 53: 761–768, 1973.

Woolner LB, Fontana RS, Sanderson DR, et al: Mayo Lung Project: Evaluation of Lung Cancer Screening Through December 1979. *Mayo Clin Proc* 56: 544–555, 1981.

Yokoyama S, Hayashida Y, Nagahama J, et al: Pulmonary Blastoma: A Case Report. *Acta Cytol* 36: 293–298, 1992.

Yoneyama T, Canlas MS: From "Exfoliative" to "Diagnostic" Cytology a Statistical Evaluation of Pulmonary Cytology. *Acta Cytol* 22: 158–161, 1978.

Zaharopoulos P, Wong JY, Stewart GD: Cytomorphology of the Variants of Small-Cell Carcinoma of the Lung. *Acta Cytol* 26: 800–808, 1982.

8

Fluids

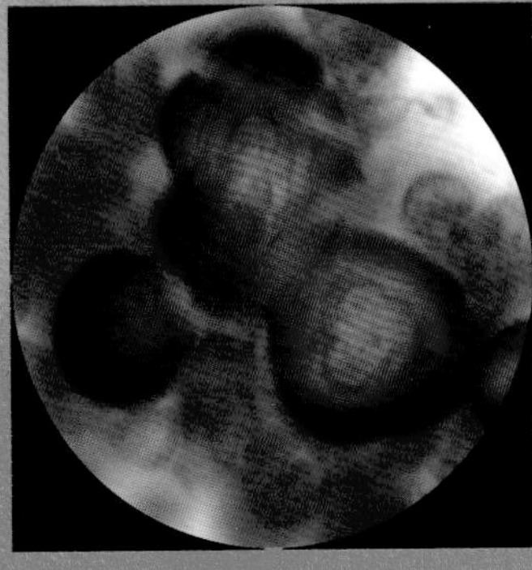

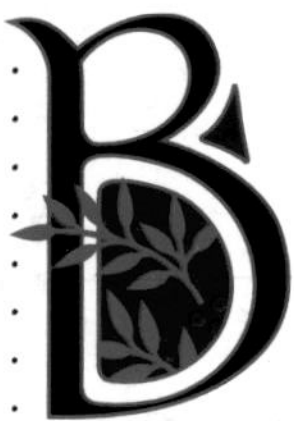

ODY CAVITY FLUIDS

The three major coelomic body cavities are the thorax, the pericardium, and the abdomen. (In men, there is also the tunica vaginalis testis.) The body cavity walls (that is, the parietes) and the surfaces of the organs (or viscera) contained in the body cavities are lined by serous membranes, with parietal and visceral aspects. The pleura covers each lung and lines the hemithorax; the pericardium surrounds and covers the heart; and the peritoneum lines most of the abdomen and covers many of its organs, including the gastrointestinal tract. The pleura, pericardium, and peritoneum share a common embryology, physiology, histology, and cytology. In these respects, the serous membranes are identical and cannot be distinguished with microscopy alone.

Serous membranes consist of a connective tissue support that is rich in capillaries and lymphatics, normally lined by a single layer of flat mesothelial cells which, when irradiated, become cuboidal [1 I8.1]. The serous membranes produce a clear, watery (serum-like or serous) fluid. The visceral and parietal layers are continuous with one another, forming a potential space that is closed (except at the openings of the fallopian tubes in women). The space contains just enough of the serous fluid (a few milliliters) to keep the surfaces moist and act as a lubricant (like a collapsed balloon with a few drops of water in it). This allows the membranes to slide and glide over one another with each breath, heartbeat, or peristaltic contraction. Any excess amount of this fluid—an effusion—is always due to a pathologic process. Thus, the mere presence of an effusion indicates that the patient has a disease.

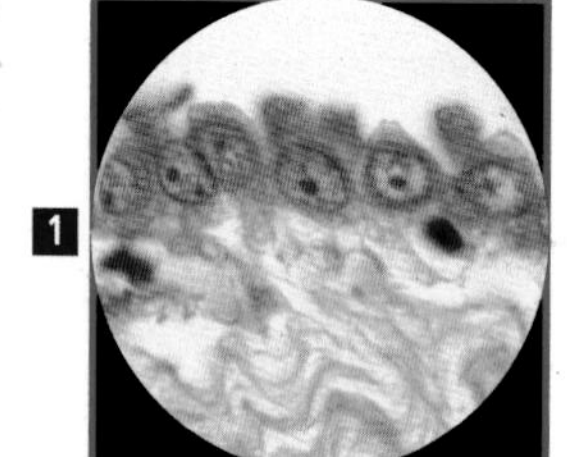

1

Although it usually requires a fairly significant accumulation of fluid before an effusion can be detected clinically—about 300 mL in the pleura and about 500 mL in the peritoneum (ascites)—even as much as 1000 mL of ascites can go clinically undetected. However, smaller effusions can be detected radiologically. More than 1 million effusions occur annually in the United States, about 20% of them due to cancer (lung cancer > breast cancer > lymphoreticular malignancy) [McKenna 1985]. Laboratory investigation of the effusion fluid, including examination of the exfoliated cells, may provide the key to the patient's diagnosis.

Serous fluid is continuously produced by filtration of blood plasma through the semipermeable endothelium of the capillaries of the serous membrane. About 5 to 10 L of fluid are filtered each day. The pH, glucose, and electrolytes approximate that of serum, but the filtrate is normally almost protein-free. The bulk of the fluid (approximately 80% to 90%) is normally resorbed by the venous system and the remaining (10% to 20%) is resorbed by lymphatics.

The amount of fluid in the space depends on the balance between formation and resorption [Black 1972, Broaddus 1987, Hausheer 1985, Olopade 1991]. Formation is influenced by hydrostatic pressure in the capillary (which is affected not only by the heart but also by sodium retention), plasma oncotic pressure (mostly due to albumin), and permeability of the capillary. Resorption is provided by capillaries and venules, which can take up water, electrolytes, and small molecules, and by lymphatics, which in addition can take up proteins and particulate matter.

Physiology of Serous Fluid

- Formation
  - Hydrostatic capillary pressure
  - Plasma oncotic pressure (mostly albumin)
  - Capillary permeability
- Resorption
  - Lymphatics (protein, particulate matter)
  - Capillaries, venules (water, small molecules)
- Effusions can be either:
  - Transudates, caused by mechanical factors
  - Exudates, which imply damage to the serous membrane

Transudate: A transudate is an ultrafiltrate of the plasma, usually through physically intact vessels; the serous membranes, including the capillaries, are normal. The fluid is clear and watery. A transudate is generally due to mechanical factors and associated with systemic disease, resulting in a hydrodynamic imbalance (increased hydrostatic pressure, decreased oncotic pressure). The most common causes of transudates are congestive heart failure (increased hydrostatic pressure) and cirrhosis (decreased plasma oncotic pressure). There are many other causes for the formation of transudates, including nephrotic syndrome, myxedema, peritoneal dialysis, hypoproteinemia, Meig's syndrome, sarcoidosis, and glomerulonephritis [McKenna 1985]. These systemic diseases usually involve all three body cavities and can result in generalized tissue edema or anasarca.

Principal Causes of Transudates

- Increased hydrostatic pressure, often due to congestive heart failure
- Decreased oncotic pressure, eg, cirrhosis, nephrosis, and malnutrition (associated with decreased albumin)

A transudate is typically a clear, pale yellow fluid with low protein content (<3.0 g/dL, some use 2.0 to 2.5 g/dL for ascites) and low specific gravity (<1.015), and does not clot (low protein, including fibrin). If a fluid is a transudate, it is unlikely to contain malignant cells, ie, *a transudate is usually, but not always, benign*.

Microscopically, a transudate usually contains only a few cells, mostly mesothelial. However, the cell count may rise in effusions of long duration. The background of the smear is clean. The mesothelial cells are single or in loose clusters. They are bland appearing and often show various degrees of degeneration. A few histiocytes and chronic inflammatory cells, mostly lymphocytes, will also usually be present.

Exudate: An exudate resembles unfiltered plasma. It is usually due to irritation of the serous membrane and mesothelium. It is associated with damaged vessels resulting in a change in membrane permeability. The membrane disease is frequently due to inflammation or cancer. However, the causes of exudates are legion, and include not only malignant tumors and infections, but also pulmonary infarction, autoimmune diseases (such as rheumatoid arthritis, lupus erythematosus, and Sjögren's syndrome), diseases of the gastrointestinal tract (such as pancreatitis and ruptured or herniated viscus), trauma, drugs (eg, nitrofurantoin, methysergide, methotrexate, bromocriptine), as well as miscellaneous causes such as radiation therapy, postmyocardial infarction syndrome, yellow nail syndrome (associated with malignancy) [DeCoste 1990], sarcoidosis, uremia, and idiopathic causes [McKenna 1985].

Principal Causes of Exudates

Inflammation
- Local or systemic, eg, infection, infarction, hemorrhage, or autoimmune disease

Cancer
- Benign tumors rarely cause an exudate

The specific etiology of an exudate is often more difficult to ascertain than that of a transudate. An exudate is usually cloudy, yellow, or bloody, with high protein content (>3.0 g/dL, or 2.0 to 2.5 g/dL in ascites), high specific gravity (>1.015), and a tendency to clot due to the fibrin content. The lactate dehydrogenase (LDH) level is usually greater than 200 U/L or the ratio of effusion fluid to blood serum LDH is greater than 0.6. LDH correlates with the presence of more cells; it is usually elevated in malignant effusions [Wróblewski 1959]. *Malignant effusions are usually exudates.*

Microscopically, an exudate usually contains many cells, although there is no absolute cut-off number separating a transudate from an exudate. The background is granular and proteinaceous, with cell debris and sometimes microorganisms. There are typically many mesothelial cells present singly and in clusters. The mesothelial cells show reactive changes including variable shape, increased cell size, enlarged nuclei, and prominent nucleoli. There is usually an increase in the number of macrophages (which may contain debris) and white blood cells, both fresh and old.

Some of the major differences between a transudate and an exudate are shown [T8.1]. However, a clear-cut distinction cannot always be made. For example, lymphatic blockage could lead to an increased protein level with a normal serous membrane; or diuresis could result in a high protein level due to its concentration as a result of fluid loss. Therefore, as always, clinical correlation with the laboratory results is required. When the cause of an effusion is cured, the fluid is resorbed and debris is removed by macrophages. The effects and possible causes of effusions are summarized [T8.2].

Specimen Adequacy: It is recommended that at least 30 to 50 mL of fluid be sent for cytologic analysis [Walshe 1992]. The optimum number of specimens to diagnose malignancy is three [Salyer 1975, Venrick1993].

T8.1 **Differences Between a Transudate and an Exudate**

Feature	Transudate	Exudate
Gross appearance	Watery, clear	Variable, cloudy
Specific gravity	<1.015	>1.015
Protein	<3 (<2 in ascites)	>3 (or 2 in ascites)
Clots	No	Maybe
Lactate dehydrogenase	<200 U/L (or <0.6)	>200 U/L (or >0.6)
Cells	Few; usually benign	Many; can be malignant

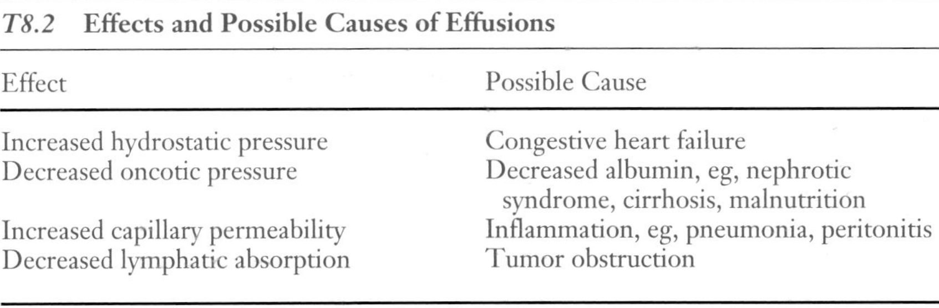

T8.2 **Effects and Possible Causes of Effusions**

Effect	Possible Cause
Increased hydrostatic pressure	Congestive heart failure
Decreased oncotic pressure	Decreased albumin, eg, nephrotic syndrome, cirrhosis, malnutrition
Increased capillary permeability	Inflammation, eg, pneumonia, peritonitis
Decreased lymphatic absorption	Tumor obstruction

Some tests for effusions are as follows:

Glucose: Low in tuberculosis, rheumatoid disease, bacterial infections, postpneumonic syndrome, occasionally cancer.

Amylase: High in pancreatitis, esophageal perforation, occasionally cancer.

pH: Low (<7.3) in rheumatoid disease, tuberculosis, hemothorax, systemic acidosis, esophageal perforation; parapneumonic effusion. Low pH in malignancy, suggests positive cytology, poor prognosis.

Ammonia: Intestinal necrosis, perforation. Presence can help differentiate effusion (-) from urine (+).

Creatinine: Effusion (negative) vs urine (positive).

Alkaline Phosphatase: Small intestinal necrosis, perforation.

Bile: Included in the differential diagnosis of a green appearance of effusion.

Hyaluronic acid: High values (>8 mg/dL) are suggestive of mesothelioma (specific but insensitive) [Rasmussen 1967]. Atypical mesothelial cells plus elevated hyaluronic acid level is consistent with mesothelioma [Castor 1967]. Adding 50% glacial acetic acid causes a heavy, milky turbidity.

Carcinoembryonic Antigen: Associated with adenocarcinoma, rather than mesothelioma, but can also be somewhat elevated in benign conditions, eg, empyema, tuberculosis, cirrhosis, and pancreatitis [Pinto 1987].

Culture: Key diagnostic procedure in certain infections.

Cell Block: Cell blocks usually do not contribute to the information obtained from the cytologic smears alone, except by virtue of examining more material [Saphir 1949, Starr 1991]. However cell blocks can be useful for clotted specimens, electron microscopy, and special staining procedures, including immunocytochemistry [Dekker 1978, Sears 1987]. Pericellular lacunae are associated with adenocarcinoma, but are not specific for malignancy [McNeely 1993, Price 1992].

Electron Microscopy: Can be helpful in distinguishing between mesothelial cells and adenocarcinoma as well as demonstrating specific subcellular diagnostic features [Beals 1992, Domagala 1975, Duane 1985, Gondos 1978, Hanna 1985, Murad 1973a, Nance 1992, Posalaky 1983, Woyke 1977a,b].

Immunocytochemistry: Can be helpful in determining if cells are malignant as well as in determining the type of tumor [Al-Nafussi 1990, Athanassiadou 1994, Cajulis 1993, Daste 1991, Diaz-Arias 1993, Ferrandez-Izquierdo 1994, Flynn 1993, Gioanni 1991, Guzman 1988a,b, 1990, Johnston 1987, Linari 1989, Mason 1987, Nance 1991a,1992, Permanetter 1987, Tickman 1990].

Flow Cytometry: Can make a contribution to diagnosis, particularly when applied to hematopoietic malignancies [Banks 1994, Croonen 1988, El-Naggar 1991, Frierson 1988, M Jones 1991, Leslie 1990, Nance 1992, Rijken 1991].

Morphometry: Aid to diagnosis of epithelial and mesothelial malignancies in effusions [Banks 1994, Marchevsky 1987].

Cytogenetics: Helpful in patient with negative cytologic/biopsy findings, but in whom a malignancy is still suspected. May be helpful in diagnosis of mesothelioma [Granados 1994]. Also useful in assessing prognosis [Cajulis 1992, Dewald 1976, Miles 1973, Watts 1983].

The gross appearance of the effusion can be important in the differential diagnosis [T8.3].

Pleural Effusions

Pleural effusions can arise in the thorax (primary) or can be secondary to ascites [Leuallen 1955]. The abdominal lymphatic drainage is via the diaphragm, especially on the right side. Therefore, any disease causing ascites can occasionally cause a pleural effusion, especially right sided. Right-sided pleural effusions resulting from abdominal disease are commonly due to cirrhosis; also subdiaphragmatic abscess, hepatic abscess, and Meig's syndrome (pleural effusion and ovarian fibroma). Pancreatitis is noteworthy for more often being associated with a left-sided pleural effusion. Anywhere from approximately 40% to 80% of pleural exudates are malignant, depending upon the patient population. Exudates can also be caused by pneumonia, infarcts, abscess, pleuritis, or a secondarily infected transudate. Most patients with malignant effusions are symptomatic (dyspnea, cough, chest pain) [Hausheer 1985] and such symptoms are often the presenting problem. However, about a quarter of patients with malignant effusions are asymptomatic. The most common sources of malignant pleural effusions are: lung > breast > lymphoreticular system > gastrointestinal tract [DiBonito 1992, Järvi 1972, Olopade 1991, Sears 1987]. Many cases have primaries of unknown origin. Massive pleural effusions are often malignant (approximately two of three) and are most commonly associated with the lung followed by breast cancer [Maher 1972].

Pleural Effusions

- Pleural transudates
  - *Cirrhosis*
  - *Nephrosis*
  - *Congestive heart failure*
  - *Malnutrition*
- Pleural exudates
  - *Pneumonia (bacterial, tubercular, fungal, viral, parasitic)*
  - *Abscess*
  - *Infarct, pulmonary embolism, trauma*
  - *Pleuritis*
  - *Autoimmune disease (eg, rheumatoid disease, systemic lupus erythematosus)*
  - *Secondary infection of transudate*
  - *Malignancy (especially lung, breast, ovary, gastrointestinal tract)*
- Massive pleural effusion (ie, entire hemithorax)
  - *Often malignant (~2/3), especially lung, then breast*
  - *Also, cirrhosis, congestive heart failure, infections*

T8.3 Gross Examination of Effusion Fluid

Characteristic	Due to	Associated With
Watery, clear, pale yellow	Transudate	CHF, cirrhosis, nephrosis, malnutrition
Cloudy, turbid, yellow-white	Increased WBC count	Infection, pancreatitis, malignancy
Milky white or green, chylous (chylous effusion)	Chyle or increased fat	Thoracic duct obstruction due to trauma, malignancy (especially lymphoma/leukemia)
Milky green, silky sheen, "gold paint" (pseudochylous effusion)	Cholesterol crystals	Tuberculosis, rheumatoid disease, long-standing effusion or cyst (years), usually not cancer
Watery, brown	Transudate	Bilirubin
Bloody or dark chocolate brown	Hemorrhage (also, melanin)	Trauma, malignancy, pancreatitis, infarction, infection, occasionally CHF (also melanoma)
Green	Bile	Biliary tract disease, ruptured bowel
Viscid, gelatinous	Hyaluronic acid Epithelial mucin	Mesothelioma Pseudomyxoma peritonei
Anchovy paste	"Chopped liver"	Amoebic abscess with rupture

CHF = congestive heart failure.

Ascites

Ascites can result from portal venous hypertension, hypoproteinemia, excess secretion of aldosterone (resulting in salt retention and volume expansion), neoplasia, or a combination of factors. Malignant ascites occurs commonly with cancers of the ovary, breast, stomach, pancreas, liver, colon, and lymphoreticular system, as well as with mesothelioma [Ceelen 1964, Olopade 1991, Sears 1987]. In malignant ascites of unknown origin, consider the ovary, endometrium, and cervix in women, and colorectal and stomach cancers in men [Ringenberg 1989]. Unfortunately, the median survival in patients with malignant ascites and occult primaries may be measured in days [Ringenberg 1989].

Ascites

- Transudates
  - *see pleural transudates*
- Exudates
  - *Visceral injury*
  - *Tuberculosis, other peritonitides (bacterial)*
  - *Inflammation of female genital tract (pelvic inflammatory disease), bowel, pancreas*
  - *Malignancy (gastrointestinal tract, ovary, others)*

Pericardial Effusions

Most pericardial effusions result from damage to the pericardial membrane, with increased capillary permeability, and are therefore exudates. Congestive heart failure is the most common cause of a pericardial transudate [Wiener 1991]. Although the cytologic features are more or less similar to effusions from other body cavities [Ramsey 1970], pericardial effusions may contain *extremely* reactive mesothelial cells, perhaps because of the beating they take from the heart. Since these benign, reactive cells can closely mimic cancer, extra caution is advised when interpreting a pericardial effusion.

Many diseases can cause pericardial effusions, including radiation, drugs (eg, hydralazine, procainamide), hypothyroidism, uremia, congestive heart failure, fluid overload, hypoproteinemia, autoimmune disease, infection, cancer, and AIDS [Zakowski 1993]. Some cases are idiopathic. Infectious etiologies are more common in immunosuppressed patients (see also section on pericarditis). The majority of pericardial effusions in patients with cancer are due to metastases [Wiener 1991]. Lung carcinoma, breast carcinoma, lymphoma, sarcoma, and melanoma are among the possible causes [Olopade 1991, Wiener 1991, Yazdi 1980]. Rarely, primary cardiac lymphomas arise, which can be diagnosed by exfoliative cytology [Castelli 1989, Pozniak 1986].

Pericardial Effusions

- Transudates
  - Congestive heart failure
  - Fluid overload
  - Hypoproteinemia
- Exudates
  - Cancer
  - Drugs
  - Rheumatoid disease
  - Radiation
  - Tuberculosis
  - Uremia
  - Bacterial, viral, other infections
  - Autoimmune disease

Special Types of Effusions

Chylous Effusion

A chylous effusion is due to leakage of the thoracic duct or its blockage, which causes rupture of lacteals. The thoracic duct is the main lymph duct, has its origin in the cisterna chyli of the abdomen, and receives lymph from most of the body (except the right side of the head and neck and right shoulder, thorax, and arm). A chylous effusion is classically milky white, but is also frequently milky yellow, green, or bloody. True chylous effusions are rare, but likely causes include cancer, trauma, and tuberculosis [Fife 1992]. The most common cause of a chylous effusion is lymphoreticular malignancy, and this may be the presenting sign. Other possible causes include mediastinal fibrosis, congenital abnormality, adhesions, parasitic infection, and lymphangiomyomatosis.

Turbid effusions (due to tumor or white blood cells) and pseudochylous effusions must be distinguished from true chylous effusions. Chylous effusions, unlike the others, contain neutral lipid.

Pseudochylous Effusions

Pseudochylous effusions are cloudy and milky greenish appearing. They classically have a shimmering metallic sheen, like gold paint. Pseudochylous effusions are caused by a breakdown of cellular lipids. Their characteristic metallic appearance is caused by cholesterol crystals, lecithin-globulin complexes, and cell debris. The lipids are dissolved when the specimen is processed, and therefore are not seen in Pap-stained material. Pseudochylous effusions are rare, although they may be associated with any chronic, long-standing effusion, usually tuberculosis, rheumatoid lung, or myxedema. Cyst fluids can also take on a pseudochylous appearance. In contrast with true chylous effusions, pseudochylous effusions do not contain neutral lipid.

Empyema

Empyema means pus in a body cavity. It is usually secondary to infection in a contiguous structure, especially in the lungs. It can also occur when the effusion itself becomes infected.

Bile-Stained Effusions

Bile-stained effusions result in greenish fluid and are associated with cholecystitis, acute pancreatitis, and gastrointestinal perforation (duodenal ulcer, intestine, gall bladder). A spot test for bile can be used to confirm the nature of the effusion.

Bloody or Dark Brown ("Chocolate") Effusions

Bloody fluids can be due to a traumatic tap, a hemorrhagic effusion, or actual hemorrhage. A traumatic tap tends to clear as the fluid is withdrawn. A hemorrhagic effusion has a low hematocrit, while true hemorrhage has a high hematocrit. Many benign effusions are bloody. Among malignant effusions, about half are bloody [Broghamer 1984]. Thus, blood in an effusion is neither sensitive nor specific for the presence of cancer. A dark brown effusion can also be caused by melanin pigment produced by metastatic melanoma.

Bloody Effusions

- Hemorrhagic Effusion
  - Neoplasm
  - Organ infarct
  - Infection
  - Pancreatitis
  - Uremia
  - Others, eg, autoimmune disease, congestive heart failure, cirrhosis, endometriosis
- Hemorrhage
  - Trauma (especially, spleen, liver)
  - Perforated vessel, atrium
  - Leaking aneurysm

Air and Fluid

Air can be introduced into a body cavity from penetrating wounds, including surgery as well as radiologic, diagnostic, or therapeutic procedures (resulting in development of pneumothorax, pneumopericardium, or pneumoperitoneum). Bronchopulmonary fistulae due to tuberculosis, bacterial pneumonia, lung abscess, or tumor are other possible causes. Microscopically, the fluid frequently contains numerous eosinophils.

Mucinous Effusions

Mucinous effusions ("jelly belly") can be due to pseudomyxoma peritonei caused by mucinous cysts (eg, ovary or appendix) [Costa 1990, R Gupta 1993, Rammou-Kinia 1986] or colloid carcinomas (eg, stomach, breast, colon, or ovary) producing neutral epithelial mucins. Cytologic findings include clusters and single cells. The cells are relatively bland, with fine chromatin and inconspicuous nucleoli, and resemble reactive mesothelial cells or histiocytes [2 I8.47]. Mesotheliomas can produce mesenchymal mucins rich in hyaluronic acid.

Effusions of Unknown or Occult Etiology

When the origin of an effusion is unknown, suspect cirrhosis, carcinomatosis, or tuberculosis. Most perplexing exudates will be due to cancer, including hepatocellular carcinoma, or to connective tissue disease, rather than infections [McKenna 1985]. Other occult causes to consider include constrictive pericarditis, hepatic vein obstruction (Budd–Chiari syndrome), myxedema, and Meig's syndrome (benign ovarian fibroma with pleural effusion). In about a third of cases, no cause can be found [Gunnels 1978].

The Cells

Mesothelial Cells

Mesothelial cells are mesodermally derived epithelial cells. Under normal circumstances, they form a single layer of cells that are flat, ie, squamous in the traditional histologic sense. In addition, ultrastructurally, mesothelial cells do indeed show some squamous features, including desmosomes and tonofibrils [Wang 1985]. However, the most characteristic ultrastructural feature is the presence of numerous long, slender microvilli extending from the cell surface. The most important function of the microvilli is to trap mesenchymal mucin (rich in hyaluronic acid), which acts as a lubricant to reduce friction [Spriggs 1961, Wang 1985]. The microvilli also increase the surface area for absorption of fluid. It is possible that mesothelial cells can differentiate into macrophages for phagocytosis or fibroblasts that can produce collagenous scars [McKenna 1985, Spriggs 1983].

When mesothelial cells are injured or irritated they proliferate (benign mesothelial proliferation). The mesothelium may stratify, and can even become papillary (known as papillary hyperplasia). The cells become plump and cuboidal, about the size of parabasal squamous cells, and the nuclei become active. These "reactive mesothelial cells" can be confused with cancer cells, and therein lies the essence of the diagnostic dilemma in fluid cytology—distinguishing reactive mesothelial cells from malignant tumor.

2
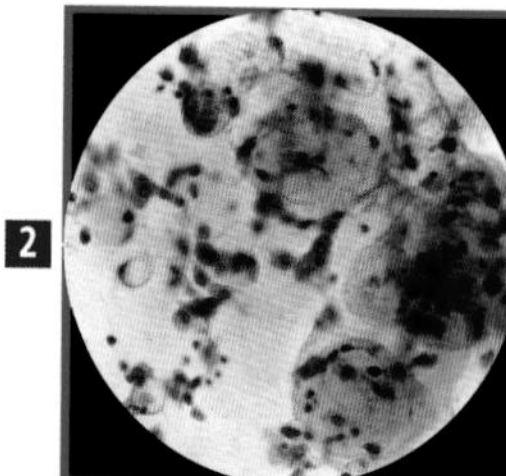

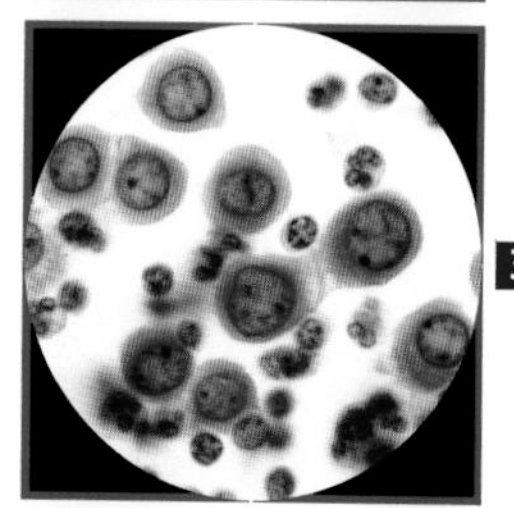
3

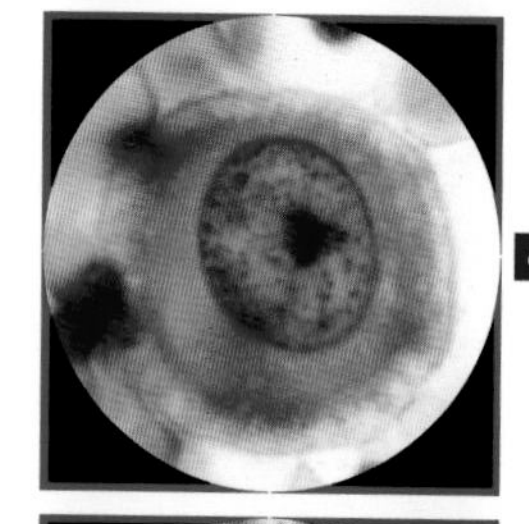
4

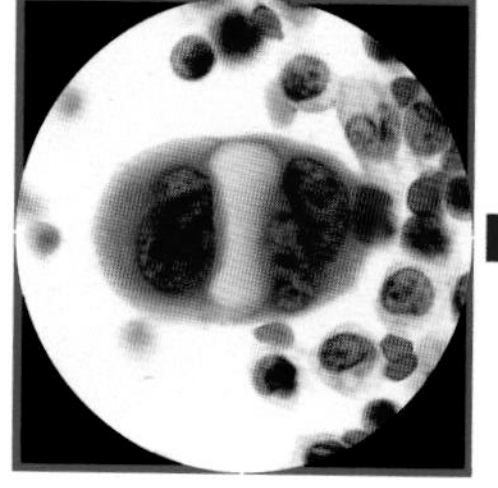
5

Effusion fluid accumulates for protection, but it is also a good culture medium, with nutrients, oxygen, and carbon dioxide, as well as body temperature and pH. Cells exfoliated into this environment can not only survive but may in fact divide and proliferate. Tumor cells can even differentiate (and therefore, can appear somewhat different from the primary neoplasm). Mitotic figures can be seen. Cells that divide after exfoliation tend to form three-dimensional, morula-like cell balls. Furthermore, due to surface tension effects, all cells tend to round up in fluids.

Many of the exfoliated mesothelial cells in fluid are present singly [3 I8.2]. (See "Body Cavity Washings," p 286.) However, groups of mesothelial cells are also seen. These groups can take a variety of forms that can mimic formations of tumor cells [T8.4]. Clusters, balls, pseudopapillae, cell-in-cell, and "Indian files" can be seen in benign mesothelial cells.

Mesothelial cells can vary from small to large; even giant multinucleated forms can be seen in reactive conditions [Luse 1954a]. Mesothelial cells often appear to have a lacy "skirt" around them, due at least in part to the presence of long surface microvilli [4 I8.3]. Although the microvilli are usually not seen in the Pap-stained material, occasionally metachromatic red "whiskers" or fringes, which are prominent microvilli, can be seen with the Diff-Quik® stain [I8.4]. Mesothelial cells can also have blunt cytoplasmic processes or blebs, which are degenerative in nature.

The cell borders of mesothelial cells are fairly distinct, but not dense and sharply demarcated. A characteristic feature of mesothelial cells in groups is the presence of a clear space or "window" between adjacent cells [5 I8.6]. This is also due to the presence of long microvilli on the surface of the cells, stiff arming adjacent cells, forcing them to keep their distance. In contrast, cancer cells seldom have windows between them.

Mesothelial cells frequently exhibit molding between adjacent cells. Orderly mosaic-like sheets of cells, occasional cell-in-cell patterns, and hugging (in which two cytoplasmic arms reach out and embrace an adjacent cell) are also characteristic of mesothelial cells [I8.7]. In contrast with histiocytes, mesothelial cells are usually not phagocytic, but occasionally they can become macrophages. Histiocytes do not mold one another to any significant degree.

T8.4 **Benign Mesothelial Cells That Mimic Cancer Cells**

Benign Formation	Mimics
Two-dimensional rosettes	Adenocarcinoma
Three-dimensional cell balls	Adenocarcinoma
Papillae	Papillary adenocarcinoma
Indian files	Breast, small cell carcinoma
Cell-in-cell	Squamous cell carcinoma
Signet rings	Signet ring carcinoma
Single cells	Carcinoma, lymphoma

A characteristic feature of mesothelial cells in fluids is that the cytoplasm is dense in the central area or endoplasm (due to perinuclear accumulation of filaments [Herrera 1985]), and has a paler ectoplasmic rim [6 I8.3]. Sometimes, a differential staining of the endoplasm (eosinophilic to orangeophilic) and the ectoplasm (basophilic to cyanophilic) is seen with the Pap stain. The cytoplasm is otherwise relatively homogeneous and granular, with a ground-glass appearance [Luse 1954a]. However, a variety of vacuoles can be seen in mesothelial cells. For example, with degeneration, which is common, degenerative vacuoles appear in the cytoplasm, which can vary from minute to large. Degenerative vacuoles are often multiple, but when a single, large vacuole forms, pushing the nucleus to the side, the cells resemble signet rings, and must be differentiated from cancer cells [7 I8.8, I8.13] [Foot 1937]. Degenerative vacuoles are crystal clear and glassy. Such vacuoles can be seen in either benign or malignant cells. Secretory vacuoles, on the other hand, have some substance to them, because they contain the secretory product, usually epithelial mucin, which is a glycoprotein and stains lightly. The presence of secretory (epithelial mucin) vacuoles in cells in an effusion is indicative of malignancy. Also, mesothelial cells may contain central fat or peripheral glycogen vacuoles. Thus, mesothelial cells may be periodic acid–Schiff (PAS)–positive due to glycogen content, but usually stain negative with PAS following diastase digestion (DPAS) and with mucicarmine. (See also section on mesothelioma.)

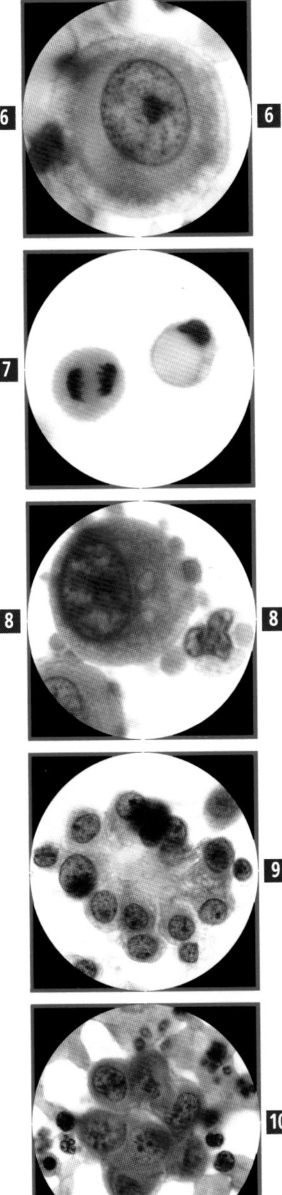

The nuclei of mesothelial cells vary from one to many, and are not necessarily of the same size, even in a single cell. The cells can be small with a high N/C ratio, large with a low N/C ratio, or rarely, giant and multinucleated [I8.9]. The nuclei are usually round to oval, but occasionally can be bean-shaped, like a histiocyte nucleus. The nuclei are usually central or paracentral, but can be eccentric, especially if there is vacuolar degeneration. The nuclear membrane appears prominent and well defined. It is usually smooth, but can also be folded or convoluted. Intranuclear cytoplasmic invaginations are rare—but have been identified—in benign mesothelial cells. Normally the chromatin is fine, although commonly a few chromocenters are present. With reactive changes, the chromatin becomes coarser. Nucleoli range from small to prominent. Mitoses are uncommon in the absence of cancer, but their presence is not indicative of malignancy [7 I8.8]. Although slightly abnormal mitoses have been reported in benign mesothelial cells [Bottles 1991, Melamed 1963], extreme caution is urged in issuing a benign diagnosis when abnormal mitotic figures are seen.

Reactive Changes in Mesothelial Cells

Reactive changes are commonly seen in mesothelial cells in effusions as a result of mitosis and proliferation (benign mesothelial hyperplasia). Reactive mesothelial cells with cytologic atypia can present a diagnostic problem [6 I8.3, 8 I8.5] [Hansen 1984].

Reactive hyperplasia is characterized by an abundant, but uniform, population of mesothelial cells. Usually, the mesothelial cells form flat sheets or small groups, often with windows. However, papillae and pseudoacini as well as psammoma bodies can sometimes be seen in benign proliferations [9 I8.11, I8.12] [Becker 1976, Kern 1969, Luse 1954a,b, Zakowski 1993]. Clusters of cells with lobulated, flower-like "knobby" borders, favor a mesothelial origin [10 I8.10,I8.11] compared with adenocarcinoma, which more often has smooth, "community" borders.

Some Possible Causes of Atypical Mesothelial Cells

- Effusions of long standing
- Asbestos
- Chronic renal failure, uremia
- Peritoneal dialysis
- Thromboembolism with organ infarct
- Radiation or chemotherapy
- Active liver disease (cirrhosis, hepatitis)
- Pericardial effusions
- Acute serositis, including pancreatitis
- Neoplasm

The nuclei of reactive cells enlarge, but remain central or paracentral, unless displaced by degenerative vacuoles [6 I8.3, 8 I8.5]. Binucleation or multinucleation can be seen in reactive cells, but multinucleation with atypia favors malignancy. Marked nuclear pleomorphism or markedly irregular membranes also indicate malignancy [Stevens 1992]. Reactive chromatin can become somewhat coarse, but remains evenly distributed; chromocenters and nucleoli may become prominent. However, multiple or macronucleoli suggest malignancy. Intranuclear cytoplasmic invaginations have been reported, but are rare, in benign effusions [Baddoura 1990, Stevens 1992].

The cytoplasm of reactive mesothelial cells is characteristically dense, with accentuation of the endoectoplasmic demarcation. Blebs and skirts may be seen in benign or malignant mesothelial cells [6 I8.3, 8 I8.5] [Stevens 1992]. Cell borders are usually definite, but not sharp or crisp. Inclusions may be seen in the cytoplasm (eg, debris, pigments, blood, glycogen, lipid—in wet preparation, but not epithelial mucin).

Because reactive cells may be pleomorphic and atypical, with enlarged nuclei, hyperchromasia, prominent nucleoli, and mitotic figures, caution is urged in diagnosis. Reactive mesothelial cells can mimic mesothelioma or adenocarcinoma [P Gupta 1981]. Malignant effusions are usually exudates, while reactive mesothelial cells can be seen in either transudates or exudates. Marked inflammation—common in benign effusions with reactive mesothelial cells—is unusual in malignant effusions. Inflammation can also cause marked reactive atypia in mesothelial cells. Therefore, diagnose cancer cautiously in the presence of marked inflammation. Also be cautious when diagnosing malignancy based on degenerated cells. A second tap may help resolve diagnostic difficulties. Look for clear-cut cancer cells to make a malignant diagnosis. As always, clinical history may be crucial in diagnosis.

Numerous cell-in-cell arrangements; irregular, three-dimensional cell aggregates; and obvious nuclear atypia, including macronucleoli in mesothelial cells, favor a diagnosis of mesothelioma. On the other hand, less complex aggregates and monolayered sheets of less atypical mesothelial cells with fine, even chromatin favor a benign diagnosis [Stevens 1992]. Even highly atypical mesothelial cells, when present in flat, squamoid sheets, are likely to be benign [Whitaker 1984]. (See "Mesothelioma," p 278.)

In distinguishing reactive mesothelial cells from metastatic carcinoma, the key to correct diagnosis is a uniform vs foreign population of cells. Even the most atypical, reactive mesothelial cells maintain a strong family resemblance (or sibling image) to clearly benign mesothelial cells, whereas metastatic carcinoma typically forms a discrete, foreign population of tumor cells. Well-formed glands or papillae are suspicious for malignancy, while windows favor a mesothelial origin. Characteristically, mesothelial cytoplasm is dense; therefore, the nucleus and cytoplasm stain with about equal intensity. In contrast, in adenocarcinoma, the nucleus is often much darker than the delicate, pale-staining cytoplasm. Intracellular mucin positivity (ie, epithelial mucin) is diagnostic of malignancy in a fluid. If the atypical cells are attached to clearly benign mesothelial cells, it is a good indication that the cells are benign [T8.5]. (See also section on adenocarcinoma.)

Histiocytes

Histiocytes are usually present in effusions [11 I8.14]. They may be particularly prominent in cancer, tuberculosis, and embolism. It can be difficult to distinguish histiocytes from mesothelial cells [T8.6]. Fortunately, both are benign so the distinction is rarely critical. Morphologically transitional forms are frequently seen, which might suggest that mesothelial cells give rise to the histiocytes [Efrati 1976]. However, histiocytes have been demonstrated to originate from blood monocytes, and thus ultimately from bone marrow [Radzun 1982]. Mesothelial cells can sometimes become phagocytic (macrophages).

Histiocytes can range from small to large, although giant forms are rarely seen in effusions (except in rheumatoid effusions). Most are of medium size or about the size of mesothelial cells. Histiocytes occur singly or in loose sheets, without molding, hugging, windows, tight groups, or papillae. With scanning electron microscopy, histiocytes are seen to have sail-like protrusions or ridges, in contrast with mesothelial cells, which have microvilli or blebs [Domagala 1979].

Histiocytes have indistinct cell borders, in contrast with mesothelial cells, which have better defined borders. The cytoplasm can be granular, but is often vacuolated. As in mesothelial cells, degenerative vacuoles may be seen. Phagocytosis is a characteristic feature of histiocytes. Therefore, particles may be seen in their cytoplasm, eg, RBCs [12 I8.16], hemosiderin [13 I8.15], or debris. When lipid is present (ie, lipophages), which is best appreciated in wet preparations, it implies that tissue destruction has occurred, and cancer must be excluded (although other causes, like pancreatitis, are also possible). RBCs (erythrophagocytosis) or hemosiderin (siderophages) imply recent or old bleeding, respectively. Melanin may be found in histiocytes in patients with metastatic melanoma (melanophages).

11

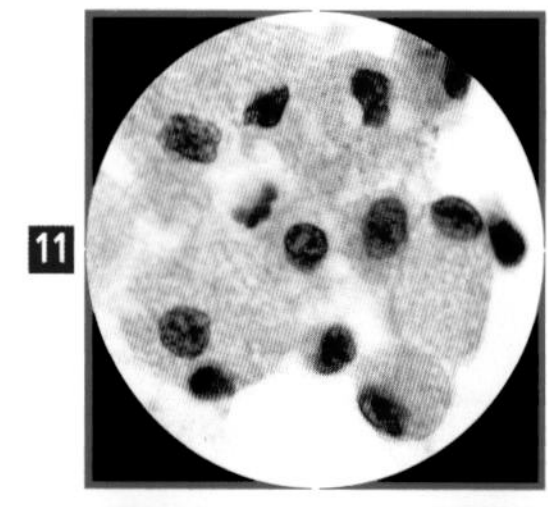

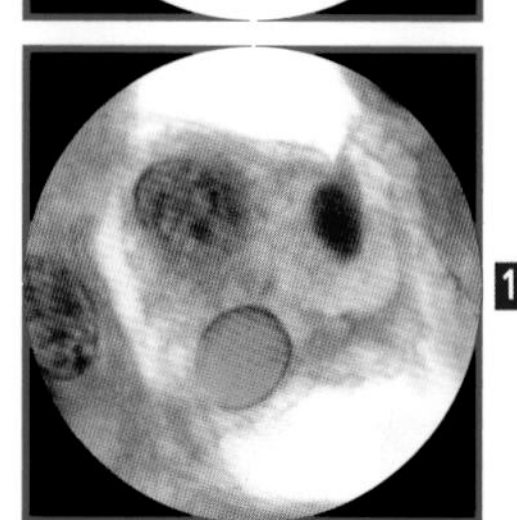

12

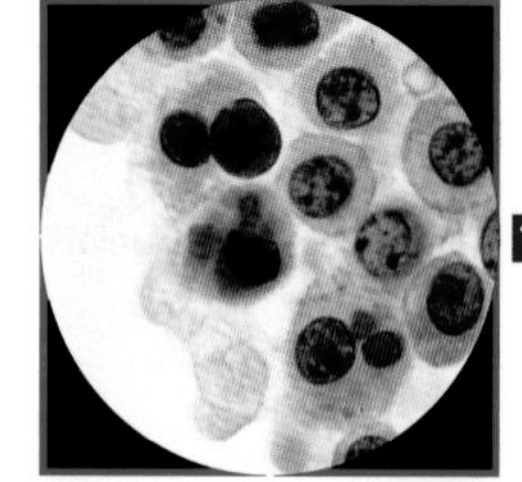

13

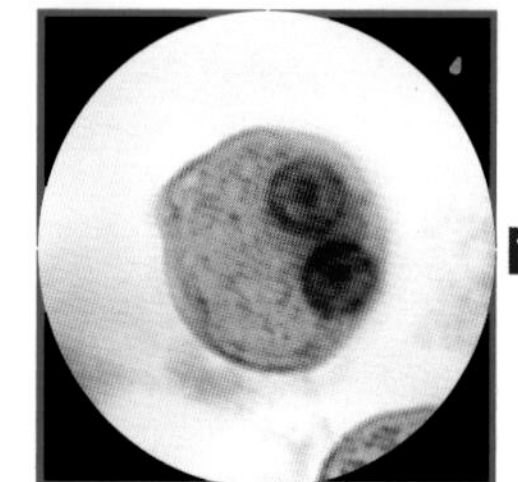

14

T8.5 Notes on Differential Diagnosis With Cancer
Do not diagnose cancer based on degenerated cells.
Cancer cells should show cancer atypia. Clinical history can be critical in diagnosis. Cancer unlikely in transudate (but not impossible). Marked inflammation is unusual with cancer. In equivocal cases, suggest second tap if fluid reaccumulates. Cells Definite acini or papillae: Must rule out malignancy. Nuclear and cytoplasmic stain. About equal intensity: Mesothelial cells. Nucleus much darker: Metastatic cancer. Epithelial mucin positive: Diagnostic of adenocarcinoma.

The nuclei of histiocytes are variably sized and classically bean shaped, but can also be round or oval. Binucleation or multinucleation are common. The nuclei are usually eccentrically located. The chromatin texture varies from fine to "salt and pepper" to coarse. It has a very characteristic "raked sand" appearance in air-dried material. Nucleoli are often small and indistinct. However, reactive histiocytes may have large, red nucleoli. Mitotic figures can be seen.

A characteristic feature of histiocytes not associated with mesothelial cells is their ability to actively take up supravital stains such as neutral red or Janis green. Histiocytes are acid phosphatase–positive (a measure of lysosomal content) and PAS-negative.

Other Blood Cells

Lymphocytes: At least a few lymphocytes are usually present in an effusion. Their presence is nonspecific and can be seen in a wide range of conditions [Yam 1967]. Lymphocytes are particularly prominent in effusions of long duration (such as those associated with congestive heart failure). When numerous, but benign, a range of maturation may be seen, including lymphocytes with more open chromatin and prominent nucleoli. Occasionally, plasmacytoid lymphocytes and plasma cells are seen.

Smears dominated by an abundance of immature, monotonous lymphocytes suggest lymphoma or leukemia. However, there are some potential pitfalls in diagnosis. For example, malignant lymphoma is often associated with a nondiagnostic lymphocytosis. Also, benign lymphocytes may have more prominent nucleoli and more irregular nuclear membranes in fluids than in peripheral blood. Of particular note, benign, mature small lymphocytes in an effusion often develop irregular nuclear membranes (probably a form of crenation) when they "hit glass." This artifact should not be misinterpreted as small cleaved (poorly differentiated lymphocytic) lymphoma.

Eosinophils: Effusion eosinophilia is associated with a wide variety of conditions [14 I8.18] [Contino 1966, Curran 1963, MacMurray 1950]. It is not itself

Lymphocytes

Congestive heart failure
Idiopathic pleuritis
Cirrhosis
Constrictive pericarditis
Nephrosis
Rheumatoid disease
Cancer/lymphoma
Systemic lupus erythematosus
Tuberculosis
Sarcoid
Viral
Nonspecific: Many other causes

T8.6 **Differences Between Histiocytes and Mesothelial Cells**

Histiocytes	Mesothelial Cells
Cytoplasm	Cytoplasm
Homogeneous, foamy, pale	Dense center, pale periphery
Frequently contains inclusions	Usually no inclusions
No molding	Frequent molding
Vacuoles common	Vacuoles uncommon (except degenerative)
Indistinct cell borders	More distinct cell borders
No windows	"Windows" between cells
Nucleus	Nucleus
Somewhat darker chromatin	Somewhat paler chromatin
Eccentric	Central
Bean shaped	Round to oval
Indistinct nucleoli	Distinct nucleoli
Special Stains	Special Stains
Acid phosphatase–positive	PAS-positive periphery
Takes cytologic supravital stain	

a disease—only a laboratory finding [Bower 1967]. Eosinophilia is usually defined as an eosinophil count of at least 10% of the white blood cell count of the effusion [Adelman 1984, Bower 1967, Kokkola 1974, Sahn 1987a, Veress 1979]. Eosinophilic effusions occur most commonly in the pleural cavity, are rare in the peritoneum, and rarer still in the pericardium. Eosinophilic pleural effusions are always exudates, account for about 5% to 8% of pleural exudates [Adelman 1984], are almost always unilateral, and can occur at any age, in either sex.

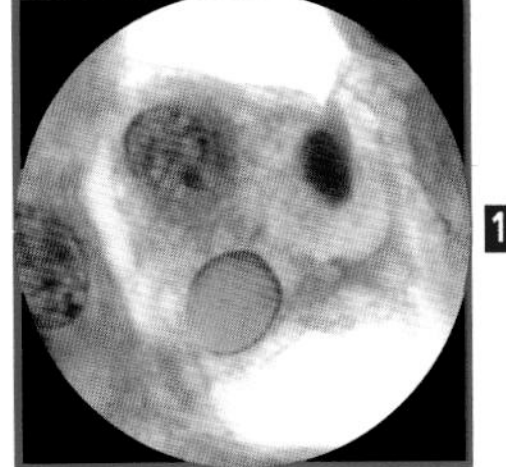

15

Eosinophilic effusions are nonspecific, but often associated with infections, hypersensitivity reactions, and trauma, including pneumothorax, asbestos, and cancer. The single most common category (about one third of cases) is idiopathic, in which a cause is never identified. In fact, the cause of an eosinophilic effusion is three times more likely to never be identified than that of an ordinary pleural effusion [Adelman 1984]. More important, however, is that an eosinophilic effusion considerably reduces the chance of finding cancer (by more than half) or tuberculosis (by ten-fold), while increasing the likelihood of an underlying benign disorder [Adelman 1984]. Nevertheless, about 5% of malignant effusions are eosinophilic; therefore, finding eosinophils does not completely exclude malignancy [Campbell 1964, Martensson 1985]. Hodgkin's disease is often mentioned as a possible cause of eosinophilic pleural effusion. However, Hodgkin's disease is itself rather rare and it is rarer still for it to produce an eosinophilic effusion.

About a third to a half of the cases of pleural eosinophilic effusions are associated with a simultaneous peripheral blood eosinophilia. In eosinophilic effusions *with* peripheral eosinophilia, consider hydatid disease, Loeffler's syndrome, polyarteritis nodosa, dialysis, and Hodgkin's disease (rarely, trauma) [Kuma 1975]. In the presence of an eosinophilic effusion *without* peripheral blood eosinophilia, consider pulmonary infarct, pneumonia, or trauma.

Many cases of eosinophilic effusion are apparently caused by the introduction of air into a cavity (usually pleural). Pleural eosinophilia is apparently the normal reaction of the pleura to air, perhaps as an allergic reaction to dust particles of animal or vegetable origin [Spriggs 1979a]. In fact, the incidence of eosinophilic effusion is directly related to the number of times the effusion is "tapped": the more taps, the more likely that air is introduced, and the higher the incidence of eosinophilic effusions. This fact makes it difficult to evaluate the true incidence of primary eosinophilic effusions reported in the literature, since it is often not stated whether the eosinophils were present from the beginning or appeared only after numerous taps.

Charcot-Leyden crystals may form [S Krishnan 1983]. This seems particularly likely if processing is delayed and the specimen sits in a refrigerator [Naylor 1985].

In summary, although many eosinophilic effusions have a prolonged course, they are usually self limiting, resolve spontaneously, and usually have a good prognosis. The risk of cancer is significantly reduced, but not eliminated.

Eosinophilic Effusions (mostly Pleural)

- Idiopathic (single most common)
- Trauma, especially with air introduction
  - Pneumothorax
- Pulmonary infection
  - Bacterial, viral, fungal, parasite, tuberculosis*
- Pulmonary infarction
- Hypersensitivity
  - Asthma, rheumatoid arthritis, allergies, drug reaction, peritoneal dialysis
- Asbestos
- Pleural tumor
- Malignancy*
- Others: Congenital heart failure, eosinophilic gastroenteritis, sarcoid, hydatid disease, Loeffler's syndrome, allergic vasculitis, tropical eosinophilia, hypereosinophilic syndrome

* Reduced risk, but possible cause.

Neutrophils: A few neutrophils are usually present in effusions; however, a neutrophil count of more than 25% is considered abnormal. Purulent effusions are usually found in the pleural cavity. In noninfectious pleural effusions the neutrophils are usually well preserved, while in infectious effusions, the neutrophils are often degenerated. It should be kept in mind that early tuberculosis can be a cause of a neutrophilic pleural effusion. Numerous neutrophils are nonspecific and can be present for many reasons.

There are usually relatively few neutrophils present in a malignant effusion unless there is secondary infection. Therefore, the presence of numerous neutrophils suggests that the effusion is benign. Furthermore, in the presence of acute inflammation, reactive mesothelial atypia is expected, so exercise caution in the diagnosis of cancer.

Neutrophils

- Infection, abscess, empyema
- Infarction (eg, due to embolism)
- Gastrointestinal disease, including rupture
- Foreign body
- Tuberculosis (early)
- Malignancy*

* Usually sparse, unless secondary infection.

Plasma Cells: Plasma cells may be present in rheumatoid effusions, tuberculosis, cancer, Hodgkin's disease, multiple myeloma, and effusions with lymphocytosis.

Red Blood Cells: If there are few red blood cells, they are likely insignificant, probably the result of traumatic tap. If there are many, especially if associated with erythrophagocytosis [15 I8.16], consider hematoma due to infarct, trauma, or neoplasm, or dialysis. Sickled cells can be seen in sickle cell anemia [I8.17] [Dekker 1975]. Rouleaux (wet preparation) or massive clumping may be seen in Waldenström's macroglobulinemia (See also "Hemorrhagic Effusions.")

Miscellaneous Findings

Lung, Liver, Muscle, Cartilage, Skin and Appendages, Fat, or Gut: These cells can all be seen from time to time in fluid specimens. Usually, they represent "pick ups" from the needle [I8.19]. Rarely, they may represent a fistula, which is more likely if vegetable matter, bacteria, etc, are also present.

Squamous Metaplasia: This is rare, but has been reported [Schatz 1991].

Ciliated Cells: These include bronchial cells, ovarian cystadenoma, teratoma, and endosalpingiosis. Proliferation of microvilli can mimic cilia in the light microscope [Palaoro 1992]. Ciliated cells are benign until proven otherwise.

Ciliocytophthoria: This is represented by detached ciliated tufts of fallopian tube origin; it is relatively common in peritoneal specimens from females, and usually found in the second half of the menstrual cycle (indicating cyclic shedding) [16 I8.20] [Papanicolaou 1956a, Poropatich 1986, Sidawy 1987a]. Ciliocytophthoria should not be mistaken for a protozoan or parasite [Ashfaq-Drewett 1990, D Coleman 1986, Mahoney 1993].

Microorganisms: A careful search may be needed in some cases to identify microorganisms. Virtually every organism ever described has been reported in effusions, such as parasites, fungi, and viruses, including but not limited to *Echinococcus, Paragonimus, Strongyloides, Trichomonas, Giardia, Balantidium, Schistosoma*, ameba, Filaria, *Pneumocystis carinii*, and cytomegalovirus [Delfs-Jegge 1994, Mathews 1992].

Megakaryocytes: These are large cells with multilobated nuclei and granular platelet-forming cytoplasm [17 I8.21]. They are rare in effusions or washes, but can be seen in any condition associated with extramedullary hematopoiesis, such as myeloid metaplasia, myeloproliferative disorder, and metastatic carcinoma [Calle 1968, Kumar 1980, Pedio 1985, Silverman 1985]. They are also associated with anticoagulant therapy [Bartziota 1986]. Factor VIII positivity is a potential aid in differentiating megakaryocytes from cancer cells [Yazdi 1986].

Malignant Giant Cells: The presence of these suggests origin in the lung (pleura) or pancreas (peritoneum), or a sarcoma. However, benign giant cells are more common. Multinucleated tumor giant cells are unusual in an untreated malignant effusion.

LE (Lupus Erythematosus) Cells: These are polymorphonuclear leukocytes with relatively large cytoplasmic inclusions of antinuclear antibody–coated, degenerated nuclear material, the hematoxylin body, which is chemotactic [18 I8.22]). Presence of these cells is suggestive of systemic lupus erythematosus (hence, the term "LE cell"), but these cells can also be associated with rheumatoid arthritis and drugs (such as procainamide, hydralazine) [Kelley 1971, Naylor 1992]. LE cells can also be seen in multiple myeloma and Hodgkin's disease.

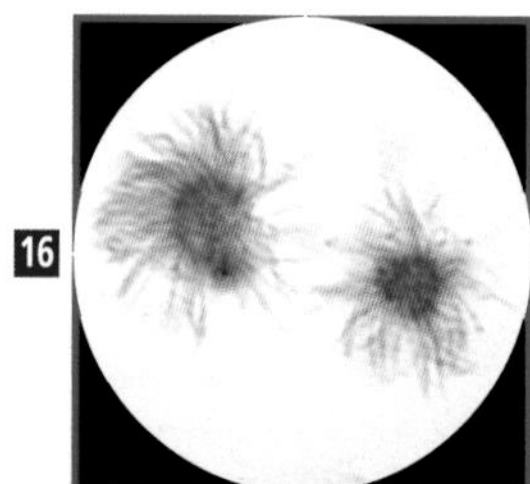
16

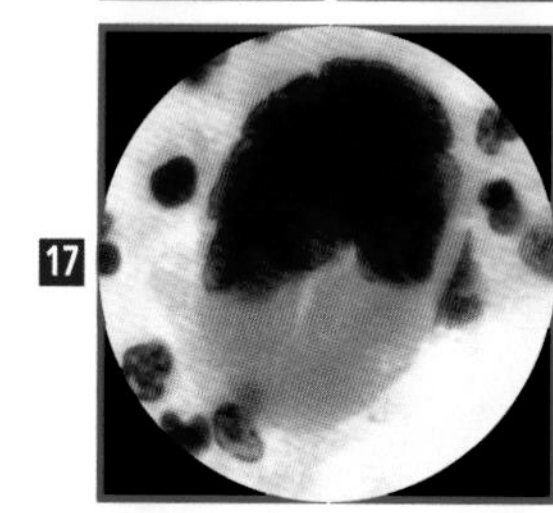
17

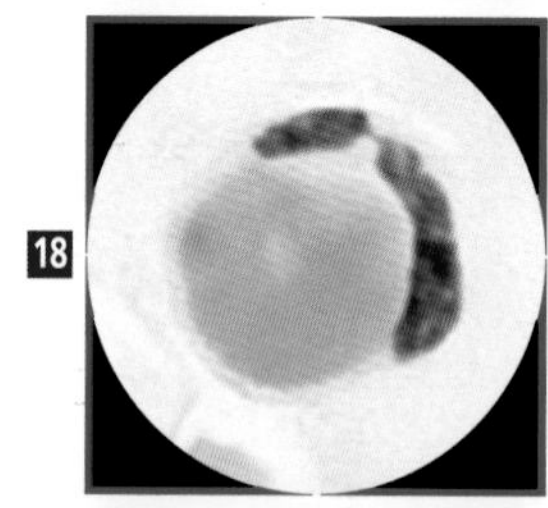
18

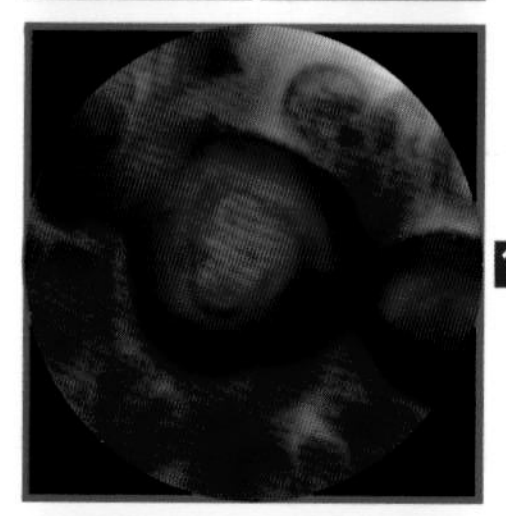
19

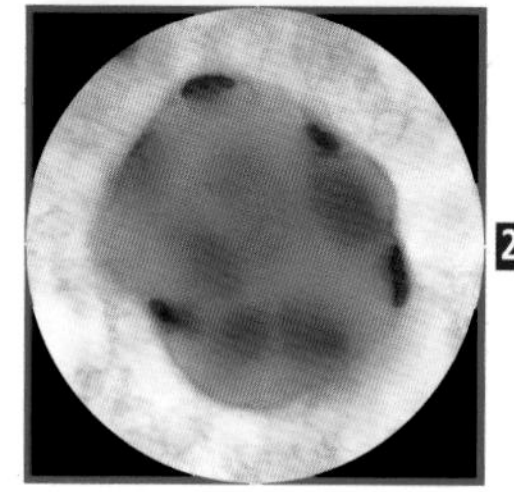
20

Tart Cells: Tart cells are similar to LE cells, but chromatin structure can be detected in the hematoxylin body. They are more common, but less diagnostic, than LE cells.

Curschmann's Spirals: These have been described in effusions with and without an obvious source of mucin (eg, adenocarcinoma) [I8.23] [Naylor 1990a, Wahl 1986].

Charcot-Leyden Crystals: They are more likely to form with delayed processing of an eosinophilic effusion [Naylor 1985]. (See Chapter 7.)

Other Crystals: These include hemoglobin [Zaharopoulos 1987], oxalate [Reyes 1979], cholesterol, cryoglobulin [A Martin 1987]

Psammoma Bodies: These are not diagnostic of malignancy; in fact, in fluids, they are more commonly found in benign conditions, eg, mesothelial hyperplasia and endosalpingiosis. The most common malignant effusion associated with psammoma bodies is ovarian cancer. Psammoma bodies are also seen with other cancers, such as cancers of the breast, lung, pancreas, and colon, mesothelioma, and others [19 I8.24] [Spieler 1985]. (See Chapter 13.)

Psammoma Bodies

Benign
- Mesothelial hyperplasia
- Endosalpingiosis
- Many others

Malignant
- Ovarian cancer
- Many others

Ferruginous Bodies: Presence of these is evidence of asbestosis, most commonly in pleural effusion. They are not pathognomonic.

Collagen Balls: Cell balls with collagen cores can be seen in benign mesothelial proliferations and mesothelioma, but are rarely observed in adenocarcinoma [Becker 1976, Delahaye 1990, Y Kobayashi 1978, Leong 1992, Spriggs 1979b, Stevens 1992, Triol 1984, Whitaker 1977, Wojcik 1992]. They are more or less spheroidal hyaline bodies that have smooth or lobulated outlines and are usually covered with mesothelium [20 I8.25] [Wojcik 1992].

Benign Effusions

Some conditions that produce effusions deserve special mention because they can cause benign atypia mimicking malignancy.

Active Liver Disease

Active liver disease (active cirrhosis or hepatitis) is a notorious cause of markedly reactive mesothelial cells that can closely mimic cancer [I8.26] [Saphir 1949]. The reactive cells may be present singly or in papillary clusters, acini, or rosettes. There may be marked nuclear atypia, including nuclear enlargement, hyperchromasia, and prominent nucleoli. Although the atypia can be severe, it affects the cells more or less uniformly, resulting in the "sibling image" characteristic of benign cells without a foreign population. Multinucleated giant mesothelial cells may be seen.

Macrophages with irregular chromatin can also mimic cancer. Rarely, atypical mitoses or abnormal karyotypes have been described in benign effusions from patients with active liver disease [To 1981]; however, in general, an atypical mitosis is highly suggestive of malignancy. Be cautious when diagnosing malignancy in an effusion, especially ascites, in a patient with acute or chronic active liver disease [21 I8.26].

Uremia

Uremia can cause many very atypical, reactive mesothelial cells with prominent nucleoli to appear in a fluid [22 I8.27]. These cells can be even more atypical than those associated with active liver disease. The reactive cells can have irregular nuclei, multinucleation, and multiple, prominent nucleoli, which can have irregular shapes. Again, be cautious when diagnosing malignancy in an effusion from a uremic patient.

Long-Term Dialysis

Dialysis can result in pleural, peritoneal, or pericardial effusions [Carlon 1983, Gotloib 1976, Rodriguez 1974]. Pleural effusions are usually unilateral. Paradoxically, ascites may develop after renal transplantation [Marcel 1977]. Lymphocytes are usually predominant. Erthythrophagocytosis and effusion eosinophilia, occasionally with peripheral blood eosinophilia, can also be seen [Lee 1967]. Severe atypia, including large nuclei, increased N/C ratios, irregular nuclear membranes, granular hyperchromatic chromatin, and prominent nucleoli, as well as pseudoacinar and papillary clusters, may be seen in the mesothelial cells [Carlon 1983, Fok 1988,1989, Selvaggi 1990].

Acute Pancreatitis

Acute pancreatitis can be associated with left-sided pleural effusion or can be bilateral. The cells are predominantly polymorphonuclear leukocytes. The fluid characteristically has a high amylase level. Occasionally, very atypical mesothelial cells are present that must be differentiated from malignancy [23 I8.32] [Kutty 1981]. They have abnormal chromatin, prominent nucleoli, and may form gland-like clusters. The nuclei can also be irregular or multiple. Fatty change can occur in the cytoplasm.

Pericarditis

Pericarditis can be bacterial or viral (especially coxsackie) in origin. Postmyocardial infection is another common cause. When bacterial, the cells are predominantly polymorphonuclear leukocytes. Beware of markedly reactive mesothelial cells mimicking cancer in a pericardial effusion.

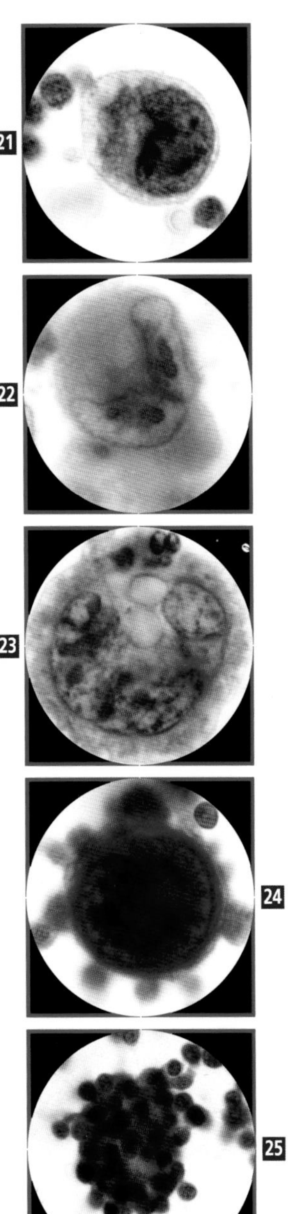

Radiation/Chemotherapy

As a result of radiation or chemotherapy, effusions often decrease in size, but increase in cellularity (mesothelial cells, histiocytes, inflammatory cells) and become hemorrhagic [24 I8.28]. The concentration of protein increases.

The mesothelial cells may show classic radiation (or chemotherapy) effect, consisting of cellular enlargement, more variation in shape, multinucleation, hyperchromasia, and cytoplasmic vacuolization [de Torres 1981]. Nuclear vacuolization is common [McGowan 1976], but intranuclear cytoplasmic invaginations are not. Bizarre cells may be seen after radiation therapy [Wojno 1994]. Benign mesothelial cell balls with "community borders" (a feature associated with metastatic adenocarcinoma) can also be seen [de Torres 1981]. These features could result in a false-positive diagnosis, particularly since the patients are likely to have a history of cancer. Thus, caution is warranted in diagnosis.

Tuberculosis

The gross appearance of a tuberculous effusion is typically turbid and yellow or may have a silky green, metallic sheen (pseudochylous effusion). Microscopically, early in the course of the disease, the inflammatory exudate is composed of neutrophils and mesothelial cells. Later, lymphocytes predominate, and mesothelial cells become sparse or absent, especially in a pleural effusion. The absence of mesothelial cells is very characteristic of a tuberculous pleural effusion [25 I8.29] [Spriggs 1960]. A mesothelial cell count of >5% in a pleural effusion virtually excludes the diagnosis of tuberculous pleurisy [Sahn 1987a]. Sparsity of mesothelial cells is a result of fibrin exudation, which traps mesothelial cells and inhibits their exfoliation. Thus their absence is a nonspecific reaction to inflammation and is not diagnostic of tuberculosis. Also, mesothelial cells can be seen in peritoneal specimens of patients with tuberculosis. Note that macrophages can be present in tuberculous fluids and should be differentiated from mesothelial cells [Light 1973, Sahn 1987a]. However, giant cell histiocytes, especially Langhans' type, are seldom seen.

In most cases, a tuberculous effusion is rich in lymphocytes [Spieler 1979]. Pleural fluid lymphocytosis, particularly a count of 85% to 90% of total cells, is highly suggestive of tuberculous pleurisy; however, other diagnoses such as lymphoma and sarcoid must also be considered [Sahn 1987a]. There is typically an abundance of small, mature lymphocytes. However, in fluids, the mature lymphocytes may be slightly larger than normal and possess some nuclear clefts and small nucleoli. These features (many cells, some atypia) may suggest a small cell type of malignant lymphoma.

The fibrin exudation characteristic of infectious processes may trap lymphocytes, causing them to form aggregates [25 I8.29]. Lymphomas are not usually associated with fibrin exudation; therefore, the neoplastic lymphocytes are single. (Of course, clinical history can be critical in the differential diagnosis.)

Most (approximately 80%) of the benign lymphocytes of tuberculosis are T cells immunologically. In contrast, most lymphomas (approximately 80%), particularly of the small cell type, are of B-cell origin [Katz 1987]. Thus, most of the lymphocytes in lymphomatous effusions are likely to be B cells [Domagala 1981]. Sarcoid has a mixture of B and T cells. Flow cytometry can be considered for cases in which the nature of the lymphocytes is in doubt.

Lymphoid Effusions

Tuberculosis: Most lymphocytes are T cells
Lymphoma: Often B cells
Sarcoid: Mixed B and T cells

Parapneumonic Effusion

A parapneumonic effusion is usually associated with pneumonia (often bacterial), lung abscess, or sometimes cancer. It is exudative in about half of the cases. Small parapneumonic effusions can also be seen with viral or mycoplasmal pneumonia. Empyema occurs with virulent, purulent infections.

Pulmonary Embolism, Infarct

Effusions occur in about half the cases of pulmonary embolism or infarct; however, the effusions are nonspecific. Unfortunately, highly atypical cells may be seen, which could lead to a mistaken diagnosis of cancer. In addition, siderophages, eosinophils, neutrophils, or lymphocytes may be found.

Rheumatoid Effusion

Although rheumatoid arthritis is much more common in women than men, rheumatoid effusions are slightly more common in men than women [Naylor 1990b]. A rheumatoid effusion is usually associated with active arthritis, but its occurrence is independent of severity or duration of disease [Naylor 1990b], and rarely may precede the onset of arthritic symptoms [Boddington 1971]. The effusion may be present for months or even years, producing effusion-related symptoms in about half of the cases. The effusions are almost always pleural and unilateral. Pericardial and peritoneal rheumatoid effusions are rare.

On gross examination, the effusion appears yellow to green, turbid, or pseudochylous (metallic sheen). The glucose level is characteristically very low. Cholesterol crystals may be identified in wet preparations.

The pathognomonic microscopic picture of a rheumatoid effusion reflects the histology of a rheumatoid nodule, ie, a necrotizing granuloma with central necrotic debris surrounded by palisaded epithelioid histiocytes and multinucleated giant cell histiocytes [26 I8.30, 27 I8.31] [Geisinger 1985, Naylor 1990b, Zufferey 1993] Necrotic debris in a fluid is almost sufficient by itself to make the diagnosis. The debris consists of granular, amorphous, necrotic material from the center of the nodule. It stains blue to pink to orange and has a "fluffy" appearance. The palisaded epithelioid histiocytes from tissue are seen in fluids as slender spindle, elongated, or carrot-shaped cells that resemble fibroblasts or "snake cells" of squamous cell carcinoma [27 I8.31]. The spindle cells show various degrees of degeneration and the nuclei are frequently pyknotic. The cytoplasm is dense and stains blue to pink or even orange. It often has a dense, granular quality in contrast with the glassy appearance of keratinized squamous cancer cells (squamous cell carcinoma is rare in fluids). Multinucleated giant cell histiocytes, which are also often elongated, represent large, multinucleated versions of the spindle epithelioid histiocytes [26 I8.30]. Transitional forms of histiocytes are also encountered.

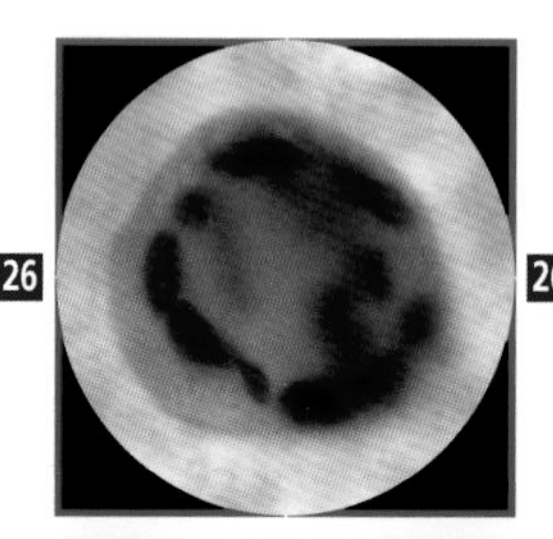

26

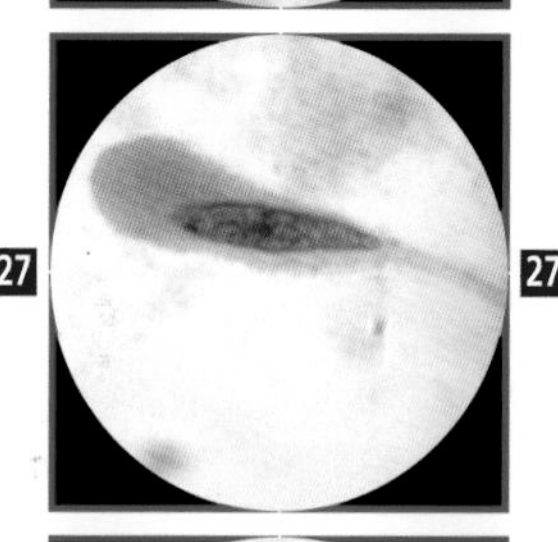

27

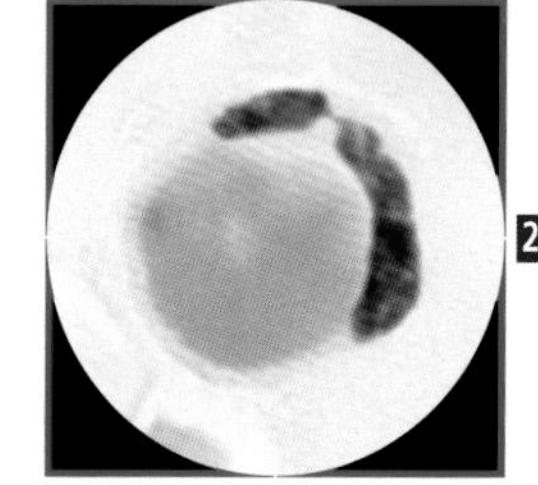

28

In addition, polymorphonuclear leukocytes, lymphocytes, and small mononuclear histiocytes may be seen, but mesothelial cells are rare or absent. A rheumatoid effusion is one of the few benign entities in which cells with peculiar shapes can be seen in a fluid. Otherwise, bizarrely shaped cells are usually malignant.

Rheumatoid Effusion

Debris
Spindle cells
Multinucleated giant cells
Few/no mesothelial cells
Note: Peculiar cell shapes, yet benign.

Systemic Lupus Erythematosus

Patients with systemic lupus erythematosus commonly develop pleural effusions (and to a lesser degree, pericardial effusions). Effusions are usually a late manifestation of the disease, but can occur early in the course, before the diagnosis is well established. Effusions in systemic lupus erythematosus are usually exudates. The glucose level is usually normal, in contrast with rheumatoid effusion (low).

Microscopically, polymorphonuclear leukocytes or lymphocytes predominate. Plasmacytoid lymphocytes may be seen. Infection must be ruled out. A characteristic feature is the LE cell (a polymorphonuclear leukocyte or less commonly, a macrophage, which contains a homogeneous hematoxylin body [28 I8.22] [Naylor 1992, Reda 1980]). The number of LE cells can vary from rare to numerous; they are more commonly observed if the specimen stands at room temperature before processing. LE cells are not specific for systemic lupus erythematosus and may be seen in drug-induced lupus erythematosus–like syndromes (eg, procainamide [Kaplan 1978]). In a woman of childbearing age with an unexplained pleural effusion, suspect and look for LE cells.

Tart cell
cytoplasmic inclusions? Not homogeneous as compared to LE cells and can be found in any serous effusions

Asbestos Effusions

Asbestos may be a cause of unexplained pleural effusion [Becklake 1976, P Gupta 1981, Lancet 1982, Pisani 1988]. Pleural effusions are one of the most common manifestation of asbestosis in the first 20 years after exposure [Epler 1982]. Occasionally, peritoneal or pericardial effusion can also occur [P Gupta 1981]. Many benign asbestos effusions are eosinophilic.

Talc

Talc is a silicate that is closely related to asbestos chemically. It produces a chronic granulomatous reaction in the lung when inhaled. Instillation of talc into the pleural space (talc poudrage), sometimes used to treat intractable pleural effusion, causes intense pleuritis and subsequent obliteration of the space [Leff 1978]. Also, there is a syndrome of fever and ascites without infection, due to surgical glove talc. Talc is no longer used for glove powder, having been replaced with starch.

Endometriosis

Endometriosis can be associated with body cavity effusions [Yu 1991]. The fluid is bloody to chocolate brown [Gaulier 1983, Zaatari 1982]. The triad of endometrial glands (small columnar cells similar in appearance to mesothelial cells), endometrial stroma (similar in appearance to histiocytes or lymphocytes), and evidence of old bleeding, eg, hemosiderin-laden macrophages, is diagnostic, but rarely are all elements seen. Similarity of endometrial cells to mesothelial cells and histiocytes makes endometriosis even more difficult to specifically diagnose; clinical history (and cell block) may help. Rarely, neoplastic transformation of the epithelial component, or very rarely, the stromal component, can occur [Labay 1971].

Hydrocele

Although any chronic, long-standing effusion can result in cytologic abnormalities, hydroceles are particularly associated with mesothelial hyperplasia, including marked proliferation of mesothelial cells and cytologic atypia.

Fistula

Suspect a fistula if vegetable matter, squamous cells, benign glandular cells, bacteria, or debris are present in an effusion.

Malignant Effusions

Malignancy is second only to congestive heart failure as a cause of effusions. Cancer can produce effusions directly or indirectly. When direct seeding and irritation of the serous membranes cause an effusion, tumor cells are usually plentiful in the fluid. With indirect causes, tumor cells may be sparse or absent. Indirect causes of malignant effusions include bronchial obstruction with postobstructive pneumonia, resulting in a parapneumonic effusion; lymphatic obstruction, resulting in decreased reabsorption of fluid; hypercoagulable state, with pulmonary embolism and infarction; and reaction to radiation or chemotherapy [Sahn 1987b]. Also note that although most effu-

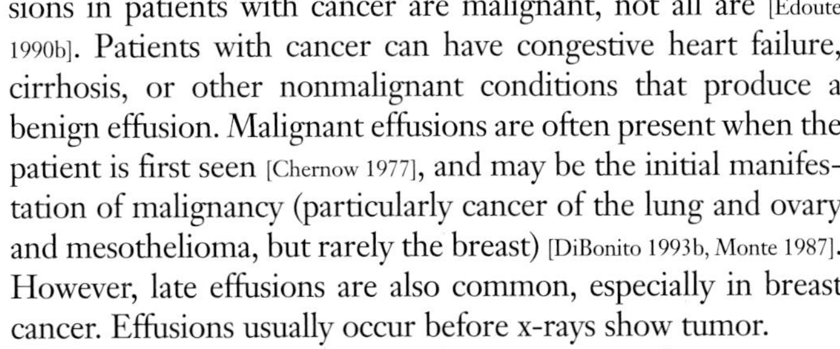

sions in patients with cancer are malignant, not all are [Edoute 1990b]. Patients with cancer can have congestive heart failure, cirrhosis, or other nonmalignant conditions that produce a benign effusion. Malignant effusions are often present when the patient is first seen [Chernow 1977], and may be the initial manifestation of malignancy (particularly cancer of the lung and ovary and mesothelioma, but rarely the breast) [DiBonito 1993b, Monte 1987]. However, late effusions are also common, especially in breast cancer. Effusions usually occur before x-rays show tumor.

Lung, breast, ovarian, and gastrointestinal cancers are particularly likely to cause malignant effusions. Carcinoma and malignant lymphoma are the most common causes of bilateral pleural effusions in the absence of congestive heart failure. Mesothelioma and other rare tumors such as sarcomas can also cause malignant effusions. In fact, virtually any cancer could result in an effusion. Up to 90% of pleural effusions from lung, breast, and ovarian malignancies are ipsilateral to the primary tumor [Canto-Armengod 1990, Chernow 1977]. Most of the rest are bilateral.

The site of the primary determines the cavity of spread. Abdominal tumors usually cause ascites before causing a pleural effusion. Pleural metastases from primaries below the diaphragm or from the breast usually indicate the presence of liver metastases. Bilateral pleural effusions in lung cancer also usually imply the presence of liver metastasis.

The development of an effusion is a poor prognostic sign in patients with cancer [Edoute 1990a, Sahn 1987b, Van de Molengraft 1989]. The mean survival time for a patient with a malignant pleural effusion is on the order of a few months [DiBonito 1992]. Malignant ascites is even more ominous, with survival measured in days or weeks [Garrison 1986, Ringenberg 1989]. Not all effusions in patients with cancer are malignant, and some may be treatable [Edoute 1990a]. However, few cancers are resectable when an effusion develops, even when the fluid is "negative" for malignant cells [Decker 1978]. A "positive" fluid sample is a poor prognostic sign that correlates with disseminated disease, and is independent of the number of malignant cells found [Towers 1979]. Of important note, however, is that certain subsets of patients, eg, women with peritoneal carcinomatosis, patients with lymphomas, and children with small blue cell tumors, may be amenable to treatment.

Since a positive fluid sample could result in either withholding or intensifying therapy, diagnostic conservatism is warranted, particularly since fluid cytology can be diagnostically difficult and the cells are often degenerated. Requesting the clinician to submit more material if the fluid reaccumulates can be extremely useful. First of all, if the fluid does not reaccumulate, the effusion was probably not malignant (assuming no intervening therapy was administered). In a first tap, the cells may have been degenerating for a long time at body temperature. Be cautious when making a malignant diagnosis on degenerated cells. With a second tap, the cells are often better preserved. If the atypia was due to inflammation or therapy, it should resolve with time. On the other hand, atypia due to cancer, if anything, increases with time (resulting in more cells with more atypical features).

At least two thirds of malignant effusions can be diagnosed cytologically. The optimum number of specimens is three; after that, few additional cases are picked up [Salyer 1975, Venrick 1993]. Up to 90% of cases can be diagnosed on the first specimen [Hausheer 1985, Hsu 1987, Johnston 1985]. Alcohol-fixed, Papanicolaou-stained material is most commonly used in diagnosis, but adding the Diff-Quik stain increases diagnostic sensitivity [Venrick 1993]. Cytologic examination is generally superior to histologic examination (eg, pleural biopsy) in diagnosing malignant effusions and is cost-effective [DiBonito 1993b, Frist 1979, Nance 1991b, Prakash 1985, Storey 1976, Winkelmann 1981]. Adding histology increases sensitivity and may be particularly helpful in diagnosis of mesothelioma [Edmondstone 1990]. Although generally safe, fatal hemothorax has occurred as a result of pleural biopsy [Nance 1991b].

General Features of a Malignant Effusion

Most malignant effusions are exudates; however, a significant number, up to 20%, are transudates [Chernow 1977, Dines 1975, Light 1972]. The number of malignant cells is extremely variable [Leff 1978]. *The key to diagnosis of malignancy in fluids is foreign cells with foreign features* [29 I8.33], ie, finding a discrete or extra population of cells with malignant features, particularly malignant chromatin, but also including such features as mucus, melanin, or heavy keratinization. In general, both small and large cell cancers are easier to diagnose than cancers with medium-sized cells, because mesothelial cells are also medium sized. Thus cells at the size extremes more clearly stand out as a foreign population. Mesothelioma is an exception to the general diagnostic rule, because the cells are native, rather than "foreign." Also, rarely, metastatic carcinoma, particularly of the ovary or breast, produces an effusion that is composed of an essentially pure population of tumor cells or of cells that closely mimic mesothelial cells; thus an extra population of cells may not be apparent [Ehya 1986].

Malignant Cells

None: Secondary effusion, eg, parapneumonic
Few: eg, blocked lymphatics
Moderate: Tumor implants, direct extension
Many: Carcinomatosis, free growing cells in fluid

Tumor Diagnosis: Unfortunately, no single feature is diagnostic of malignancy. However, several features regarding cell clusters, the cells per se, and the background are helpful in cytodiagnosis.

Cell Groups: Tumor cells, particularly from adenocarcinoma, are frequently present in large clumps, cell balls, papillae, or gland-like groups. These clusters may be easily—even best—seen at low power [I8.34, 30 I8.36, I8.37]. Benign mesothelial cells usually do not form very large aggregates, although they can. When large aggregates are present, metastases and mesothelioma must be considered. On the other hand, some tumors, particularly lymphomas [31 I8.35], but also melanomas, sarcomas, and some carcinomas, shed single cells exclusively.

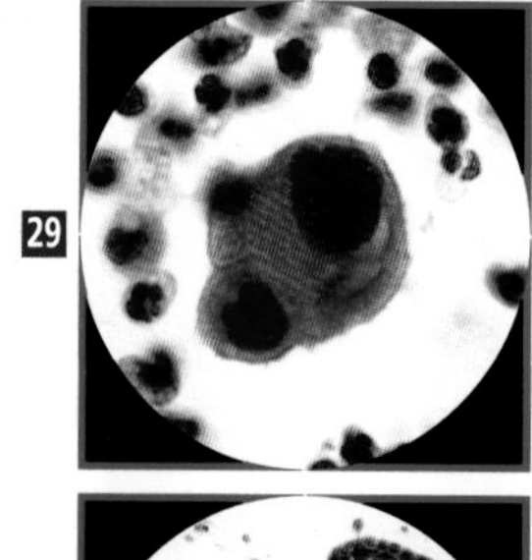
29

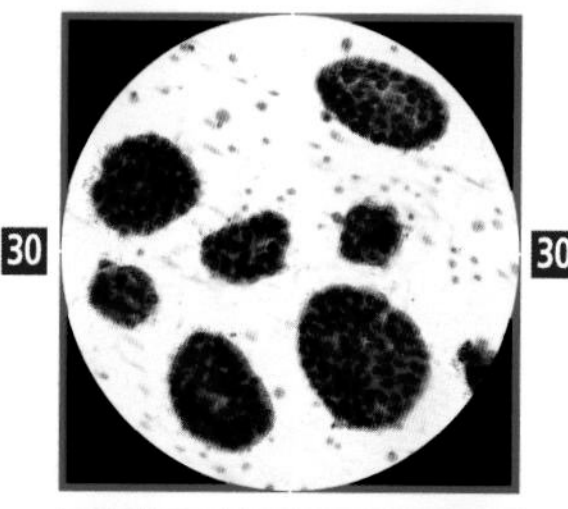
30

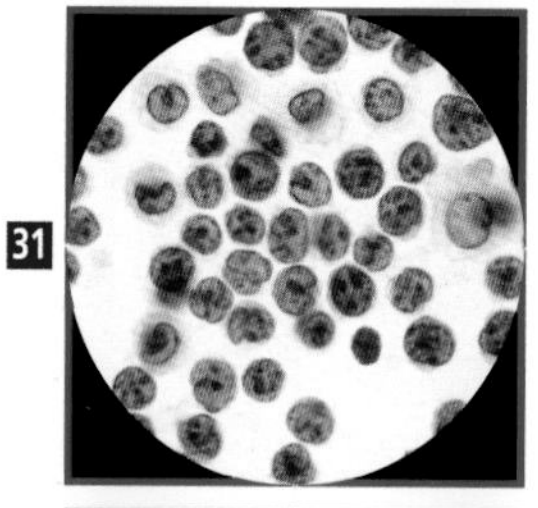
31

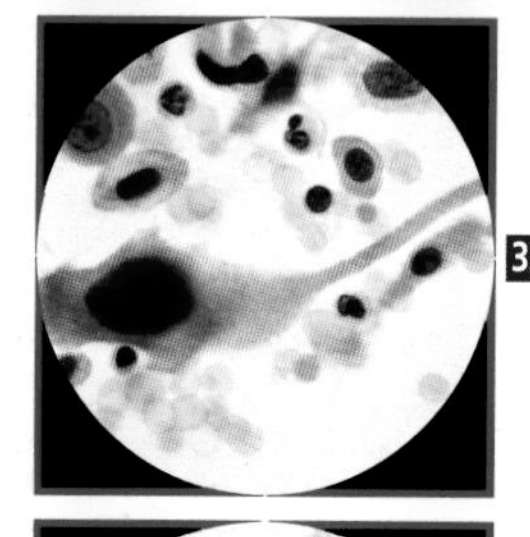
32

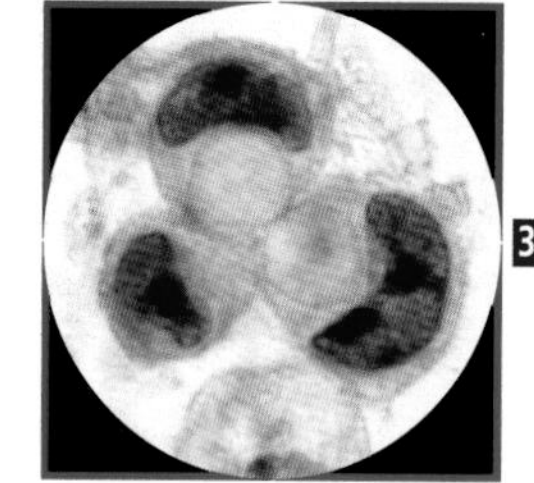
33

Cluster formation in adenocarcinoma is a form of differentiation. Tumors forming large clusters may have a somewhat more favorable prognosis than those with a predominance of single cells [Dieterich 1994, Wiley 1990, Yamada 1983].

Group Contours: The contours of cellular aggregates of metastatic tumors also tend to be different from those of mesothelial cells. Adenocarcinoma usually forms aggregates with smooth outlines (community border)[30 I8.36], while benign (or malignant) mesothelial cell aggregates usually have knobby, flower-like outlines [I8.10]. Unfortunately, although helpful, these outlines are not specific (ie, mesothelial cells can form aggregates with smooth outlines, carcinoma can have irregular outlines).

Cell Shape: Tumor cells usually appear distinctly different from benign cells. Malignant cells can vary from monomorphic to pleomorphic. However, all cells tend to round up in fluid. This factor lends a certain degree of uniformity to various cell types. However, when a cell has an unusual, abnormal, or bizarre shape in a fluid, this feature alone is highly suggestive of malignancy (rheumatoid effusion is an exception) [I8.39, 32 I8.41] [Foot 1937]. Tumor cells may grow and even differentiate in the culture medium–like effusion fluid. Therefore, metastases do not necessarily exactly resemble the primary tumor.

Cell Surface: The cell borders of individual malignant cells are often very well defined, in contrast with mesothelial cells, or particularly, histiocytes. Ciliated malignant cells are so rare as to be reportable [P Gupta 1985, T Kobayashi 1988]. However, long microvilli, which can resemble cilia, may be seen in malignancy, especially ovarian cancer, and can also be seen on benign mesothelial cells.

Cytoplasm: The cytoplasm is often basophilic, but may contain secretory vacuoles. However, the mere presence of cytoplasmic vacuoles is nonspecific and often degenerative in nature. Degenerative vacuoles are usually crystal clear. The presence of (epithelial) mucin in a cell in fluid is virtually diagnostic of adenocarcinoma [I8.46]. Intracytoplasmic lumens commonly observed in breast cancer, with well-defined borders and an inspissated dot of mucin, as well as secretory signet ring cells (not due to degeneration) are essentially diagnostic of adenocarcinoma in fluids [33 I8.44] [Spriggs 1975]. Other cytoplasmic products, including melanin, heavy keratinization, and cross-striations are equally important.

Nuclei: Malignant nuclei are usually enlarged, and the cells often have high N/C ratios [I8.42]. Nuclei also tend to round up in fluids, but are of variable size. Irregular nuclear membranes may be a clue to malignancy. Intranuclear cytoplasmic invaginations are rare in benign, nonneoplastic mesothelial cells. Therefore, malignancy must be excluded when these nuclear inclusions are present (eg, melanoma). Tongue-like nuclear protrusions (or nuclear knobs) are another abnormal feature and suggest malignant lymphoma (if the cells are single). Malignant-appearing, coarse, irregular chromatin is usually the single most important diagnostic feature of a cancer cell. Hyperchromasia is not always as prominent as expected, however, since the cells can proliferate in fluids. Massive karyorrhexis suggests malignant lymphoma. The presence of extra Barr bodies, except in rare genetic diseases, is virtually diagnostic of cancer, and suggests an origin in the breast. Large, and especially abnormal-shaped, nucleoli are also important diagnostic clues. Mitotic figures per se are just about meaningless in a fluid specimen unless they are abnormal. However, prophase nuclei (very coarse, dark chromatin, dissolved nuclear membrane) may be diagnostically important.

Background: The background of a fluid specimen is usually nonspecific. Acute inflammation is unusual in cancer, unless it is secondarily infected. True chylous effusions are associated with malignant lymphomas. A bloody background is common in cancer but nonspecific, and is usually only a microscopic finding. However, in the absence of trauma, a massive bloody effusion is frequently due to cancer. Some other features, such as lymphocytosis or histiocytosis, are associated with malignant effusions, but again are nonspecific.

Typical Malignant Background

Blood (usually microscopic)
Lymphocytosis
Histiocytosis, especially lipophages
(Polymorphonuclear leukocytes usually not prominent)

When these features are present, look carefully for malignant cells. Lipophages, in particular, imply tissue destruction, and should serve as a warning to the possible presence of cancer.

In malignancy, psammoma bodies are most commonly found in metastatic ovarian carcinoma, but are not specific, and can also be associated with benign processes, such as papillary hyperplasia of the mesothelium with psammoma bodies [Zakowski 1993]. Fibrin can trap cells, giving the false impression of cell aggregation and clumping. Many problems in diagnosis are due to cell degeneration (submit more specimens). Be cautious when diagnosing malignancy in degenerated cells. Reactive mesothelial cells and histiocytes can mimic cancer. These benign cells can therefore result in a false-positive diagnosis, but they can also result in a false-negative diagnosis by camouflaging malignant cells. Causes of malignant effusions are shown [T8.7]. Clinical information is the single most useful feature in determining the primary site of a tumor. Unknown primaries most commonly arise in the ovary followed by the lung and then the lymphoreticular system. Bilateral pleural effusions in lung cancer usually indicate the presence of liver metastasis. Pleural metastases from primaries below the diaphragm or from the breast also indicate the presence of liver metastasis.

Causes of Malignant Effusions

Frequent
- Lung
- Breast
- Ovary
- Lymphoma
- Kidney

Occasional
- Pancreaticobiliary
- Prostate
- Bladder
- Liver
- Mesothelioma
- Germ cell
- Many others

Malignant Effusions

Groups: large clusters
Contours: community vs knobby borders
Cell shape: bizarre or unusual shapes
All cells tend to round up in fluids
Cell surface: well defined vs fuzzy
Ciliated cells are benign until proven otherwise
Cytoplasm: secretory vs degenerative vacuoles
Nuclei: Irregular membranes, abnormal chromatin
Background: Nonspecific blood, chronic—not acute—inflammation

T8.7 **Malignant Effusions***

	Men	Women	Children
	Pleural		
Ratio	2	3	
Sources	Lung Lymphoreticular Mesothelioma Gastrointestinal tract Pancreas Liver Others	Breast Lung Lymphoreticular Ovary Gastrointestinal tract Uterus Others	Lymphoreticular Wilms' tumor Neuroblastoma Others
	Ascites		
Ratio	1	3	
Sources	Gastrointestinal tract Pancreas Prostate Lymphoreticular Others	Ovary Breast Uterus Gastrointestinal tract Lymphoreticular; others	Lymphoreticular Neuroblastoma Rhabdomyosarcoma Wilms' tumor Others

* Note: Unknown primaries are common.

Adenocarcinoma

Adenocarcinoma is, by far, the most common cause of a malignant effusion. Among the most useful features in the diagnosis of adenocarcinoma are increased N/C ratio, irregular nuclear membranes, large nucleoli, secretory vacuoles, and three-dimensional aggregates [Bottles 1991].

Nuclear enlargement, pleomorphism, and hyperchromasia can also be seen. However, many of these features can also be seen in benign effusions. True glandular acini or papillae may be formed. Epithelial mucin, if present in cells, is virtually diagnostic of adenocarcinoma. However, vacuolization per se is virtually meaningless. Degenerative vacuoles can be very large. Ciliated cells are benign until proven otherwise.

Adenocarcinoma

Increased N/C ratio
Irregular nuclear membranes
Large nucleoli
Secretory vacuoles
Three-dimensional aggregates

General Patterns of Adenocarcinoma

The general patterns of adenocarcinomas in fluids include cell balls (morulas), papillary or acinar groups, signet ring cells, other vacuolated cells, single cells, chains of cells (Indian files), and bizarre or giant cells.

Cell balls (morulas) [34 I8.36] are multiple, round (ie, spherical) aggregates with smooth, community borders. Very large cell balls with community borders are known as "cannonballs" (also, proliferation spheres [Foot 1955]). Cannonballs are diagnostic of malignancy and suggest origin in the breast, particularly if the cells are uniform and not prominently vacuolated. Other common sources of cannonballs include carcinoma of the ovary (in which the cells are more pleomorphic and contain prominent vacuoles) and non–small cell carcinoma of the lung. Mesothelial cells, benign or malignant, and other cancers, including those of gastrointestinal origin, are among other possible sources of cannonballs.

Acini are three-dimensional cell balls with hollow cores, corresponding to gland lumens. They are characteristic of adenocarcinomas in general. Papillae are three-dimensional clusters that are longer in one dimension than in the other two [35 I8.37]. In effusions, they are particularly characteristic of carcinomas of gastric and colorectal origin. In pleural effusions, papillae are commonly associated with carcinomas of the lung and breast. In ascitic fluids, papillae are commonly seen in ovarian and uterine cancers (endometrial > endocervical carcinomas). When papillae are encountered in fluids, also consider mesothelioma and papillary mesothelial hyperplasia. Note that papillary carcinoma of the thyroid rarely produces a malignant effusion.

Signet ring cells are cells with large cytoplasmic vacuoles that compress the nucleus to the periphery of the cell [36 I8.54]. Large signet ring cells are characteristic of carcinoma of the stomach, in particular, as well as other gastrointestinal cancers. Small signet ring cells are more commonly associated with breast cancer. Intracytoplasmic lumens are similar to signet rings, except that the vacuoles are small and sharply defined, and usually do not indent the nucleus [I8.44]. Intracytoplasmic lumens are particularly characteristic of breast cancer, but can be seen in any tumor associated with signet rings. Extreme vacuolization of malignant cells is most characteristic of ovarian carcinoma, but is nonspecific, and can also be seen in lung and pancreatic carcinomas, among others. The differential diagnosis of these large vacuoles, which are degenerative in nature, includes benign cells with nonspecific degenerative vacuoles. Evidence of secretion (epithelial mucin) in the vacuoles indicates a malignant process.

A predominance of single malignant cells suggests carcinoma of the breast (particularly lobular type; look for intracytoplasmic lumens) [I8.45]. Gastric cancer can also present as single cells (often signet ring cells). Cuboidal to columnar shape of the single cells suggests carcinoma. Other tumors that characteristically shed isolated tumor cells include lymphoma (classic presentation), melanoma, sarcomas, and occasionally, mesothelioma.

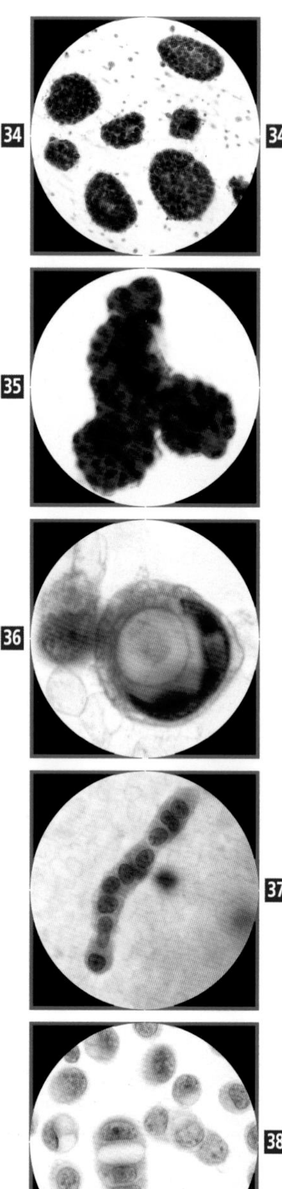

Chains of tumor cells, also known as "Indian files" [37 I8.38, I8.82], suggest origin in the breast (particularly when the chains are very long). "Indian files" can also be seen with pancreatic carcinoma [DiBonito 1991, 1993b], gastric cancer, small cell carcinoma [I8.49], mesothelioma [I8.82], and carcinoid tumors [Lozowski 1979].

Bizarre cells or giant cells [I8.39, I8.62, I8.71] are particularly associated with carcinomas of the lung, pancreas, or thyroid. They can also be seen in squamous cell carcinoma[I8.62], sarcomas [I8.71], and melanomas, among others. Rheumatoid effusion is one of the few benign explanations for bizarre or giant cells in an effusion.

Clear cells are associated with carcinomas of the kidney and ovary [Zirkin 1984], as well as with germ cell tumors [I8.40]. Clear cells in fluids may have an unexpectedly dense cytoplasm.

"Specific" Patterns of Adenocarcinoma

Breast Cancer: About half the patients with breast cancer eventually develop effusions. Effusions may be an early or late manifestation of the disease. Breast cancer is the most common source of malignant effusions in women. 80% are ipsilateral to the primary lesion and 10% are bilateral; contralateral effusions are unusual.

The cells are usually uniform, with fine chromatin and dense cytoplasm [Danner 1975, Spieler 1985]. Multiple Barr bodies may be seen in the nucleus. Intracytoplasmic lumens are a common and characteristic feature [I8.44]. The tumor cells also frequently contain neutral lipid in the cytoplasm. Most breast cancers are of ductal origin. Lobular carcinoma is suggested by the presence of isolated, small, bland tumor cells with intracytoplasmic lumens, occasionally forming Indian files.

Several patterns of breast carcinoma in effusions have been described [Danner 1975].

Cannonballs (blastulas, proliferation spheres) [34 I8.36] are cohesive, tightly packed large balls of cells with smooth community borders. The cells have homogeneous cytoplasm. Very large cannonballs are particularly characteristic of breast cancer (favors ductal carcinoma) [Ashton 1975] and are more favorable prognostically [Dieterich 1994].

Indian files [37 I8.38] are commonly seen in breast cancer; very long chains are considered virtually diagnostic of breast origin. If the component cells are small, this favors lobular carcinoma; medium to large cells favor ductal carcinoma.

Signet ring cells, when small, are characteristic of breast cancer (particularly lobular carcinoma).

The "mesothelial pattern" of breast cancer consists of medium-sized, bland cells that are very difficult to distinguish from benign, reactive mesothelial cells [38 I8.45]. This is potentially one of the most difficult cytologic diagnoses of all, especially when the cells are present predominantly as single cells. Unfortunately, this is a relatively common pattern. Diagnostic clues include irregular or thick nuclear membrane; extra Barr bodies; prominent nucleoli; and particularly, secretory vacuoles or intracytoplasmic lumens. Mucin stain (eg, mucicarmine) can be extremely helpful [I8.46].

A predominance of single tumor cells in a breast cancer effusion is associated with lobular carcinoma [I8.48]. The differential diagnosis includes macrophages and mesothelial cells.

Lung Cancer: Lung cancer is the single most common cause of malignant effusions. Adenocarcinomas tend to arise peripherally; therefore, they are likely to cause pleural effusions. In essence, the common forms of lung cancer can be divided into small cell [**39** I8.49] and non–small cell types [I8.50, **40** I8.51]. The non–small cell pattern shows large, pleomorphic cells, with or without evidence of mucus formation; multinucleation may be prominent [Spieler 1985]. Many lung cancers show combined glandular and squamous differentiation; therefore, adenocarcinoma of the lung frequently has cells with relatively dense, squamoid cytoplasm, which provides a clue to their origin [**40** I8.51]. (See also "Small Cell Carcinoma" and "Squamous Cell Carcinoma.") The cells may be present as papillary or acinar groups, or as isolated columnar cells. They can range from very well differentiated (characteristic of bronchioloalveolar carcinoma) to giant and anaplastic. Highly vacuolated cells may be seen, similar to those associated with ovarian carcinoma. Similar cells can also be seen in pancreatic carcinoma (including adenocarcinoma cells with squamoid cytoplasm, highly vacuolated cells, and giant tumor cells).

Kidney Cancer: The tumor cells can exfoliate in papillary or acinar groups. The cytoplasm can be clear or granular. Note that "clear" cytoplasm may appear unexpectedly dense in effusions. A characteristic finding in renal cell carcinoma is tumor cells with a granular center and a clear periphery [**41** I8.52]. The cells characteristically contain glycogen and lipid, but not mucin.

Stomach Cancer: The tumor cells are frequently isolated, but can also form papillae or acini [I8.53]. The tumor cells are either large columnar cells or most characteristically, signet ring cells [I8.54], depending on whether the primary tumor is intestinal or gastric type, respectively. The nuclei, particularly of the intestinal type, may have bizarre shapes, with very coarse, hyperchromatic chromatin [Spieler 1985]. Most gastric cancers are mucin positive. The differential diagnosis of the signet ring type of gastric cancer includes degenerative changes in mesothelial cells (look for malignant criteria in the nuclei) and breast cancer (the tumor cells are usually smaller than those of gastric cancer).

Colorectal Cancer: Colorectal carcinomas characteristically exfoliate cells in papillary or acinar aggregates. The component cells are usually large, and have a tall, columnar configuration. Nuclear palisading and deep nuclear membrane irregularities together with apical cytoplasmic densities suggesting terminal bars are characteristic cytologic features of colorectal carcinomas [Posalaky 1983] [**42** I8.55]. Signet ring cells, as well as pleomorphic spindle to columnar shaped cells, can also be seen [Spieler 1985]. Most cases are mucin positive.

39

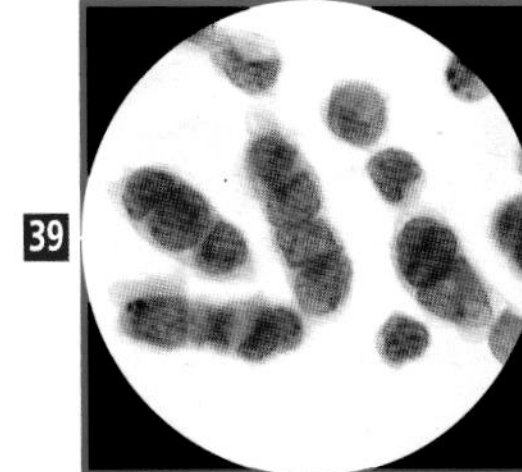

40

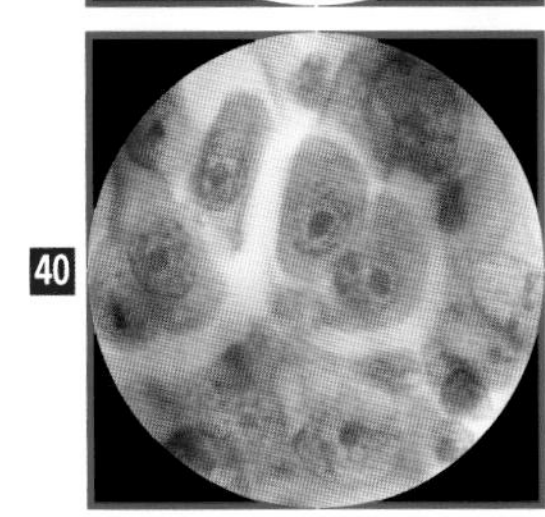

41

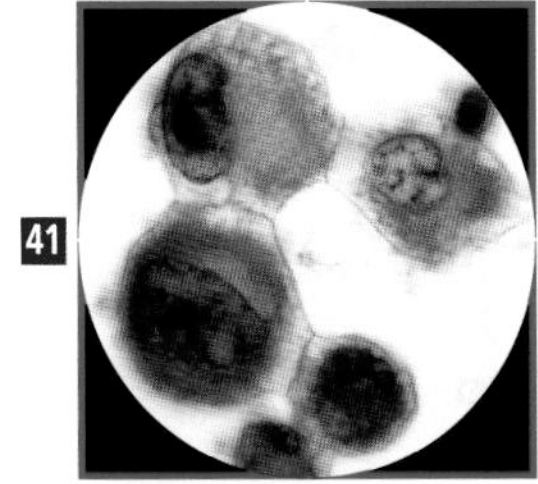

42

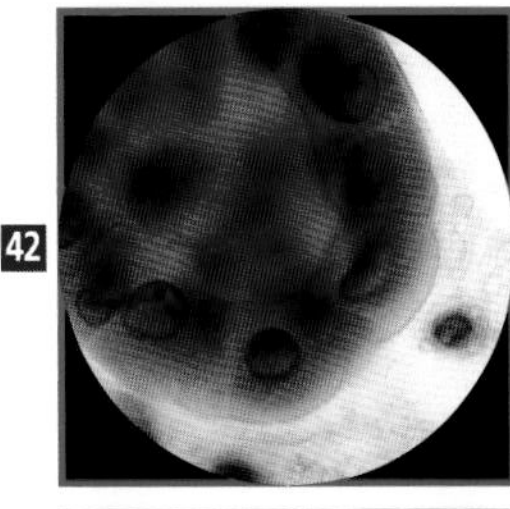

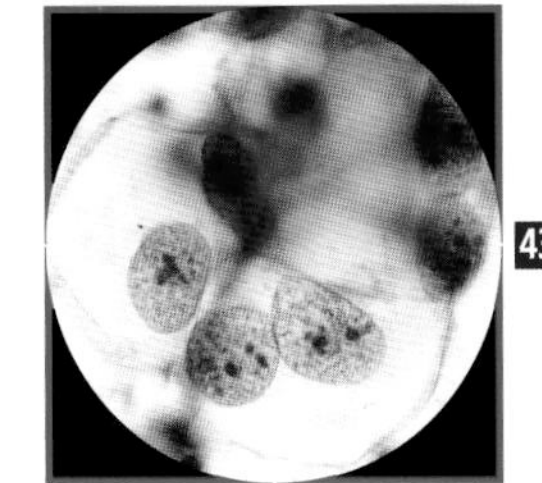

43

Pancreaticobiliary Cancer: Carcinomas of the pancreas and bile ducts are morphologically indistinguishable, although those of the bile duct tend to be better differentiated. The cells may form Indian files with nuclear molding or rounded clusters [DiBonito 1991]. The cells may be similar to those of lung cancer, with adenosquamous features [I8.56], or to those of ovarian carcinoma, with large cytoplasmic vacuoles [I8.58]. These tumors can be mucinous, with mucus-producing cells [I8.57] or serous, with eosinophilic cytoplasm and indistinct cell borders. Mixed cell patterns also occur, composed of small columnar cells in clusters with palisaded edges and large single cells with large cytoplasmic vacuoles [Spieler 1985]. A characteristic feature of pancreaticobiliary carcinoma is that there is often a very well-differentiated component, even in otherwise poorly differentiated tumors.

Ovarian Cancer: Ovarian carcinoma is usually characterized by the presence of large, irregular, transparent clusters of large, pleomorphic tumor cells, distended with large, degenerative vacuoles [**43** I8.43, I8.59] [Spieler 1985]. The nuclei often have large nucleoli. In some cases, dense apical, terminal bar-like cell borders may be seen. Very rarely, the tumor cells are ciliated. Psammoma bodies, if present with tumor cells, suggests ovarian origin. Note that in ovarian cancer, pleural effusions are rarely seen without ascites. The differential diagnosis includes non–small cell lung cancer, mesothelioma, and thyroid cancer, all of which can have similar cells, including the possibility of Psammoma bodies.

There are three common types of neoplasms of the ovary: mucinous (cells generally resemble endocervical cells or cells of gastrointestinal malignancies, including pseudomyxoma peritonei); serous (cells generally resemble fallopian tube cells, and can also be virtually indistinguishable from reactive mesothelial cells or mesothelioma [I8.60]); and endometrioid (identical to endometrial carcinoma [Nagai 1983]). Most mucinous or serous ovarian carcinomas contain a mixture of serous and mucinous cells; therefore, even in so-called serous tumors, an occasional cell may be mucin positive. Other rare tumors, including small cell carcinoma [Selvaggi 1994] and germ cell tumors, can also arise in the ovary.

Pseudomyxoma Peritonei: Pseudomyxoma peritonei is a low-grade neoplasm characterized by slow but relentless growth in the peritoneal cavity. Treatment is difficult. The sources of the tumor cells include the ovary (mucinous cystadenoma, cystadenocarcinoma), appendix (mucocele), and other gastrointestinal or pancreatic cancers. Endocervical carcinoma and colloid carcinomas, such as occur in the breast, are other possible sources. The effusion fluid is characteristically composed of thick mucus (mucinous ascites) which is difficult to smear [Green 1975]. The tumor cells tend to be sparse and present in cohesive sheets [Rona 1969]. They are well differentiated, bland, and tall columnar cells, with large mucin vacuoles. Few or no mesothelial cells, histiocytes, or leukocytes are present in the background. The essence of the diagnosis is the presence of endocervical-like cells in mucous lakes.

Liver Cancer: Hepatocellular carcinoma is frequently associated with ascites because the tumor usually arises in the setting of cirrhosis. However, it is unusual to find tumor cells in the fluid [Runyon 1988], leading to the paradox of malignant disease, but benign effusion. If tumor cells were present, they would have malignant nuclear features, granular cytoplasm, and possibly, evidence of bile production.

Thyroid Cancer: Papillae, intranuclear cytoplasmic invaginations, and psammoma bodies may suggest thyroid cancer, but this is a rare cause of effusions, particularly as an unknown primary.

Prostate Cancer: Prostate cancer is associated with microacinar complexes, uniform tumor cells, and prominent nucleoli [I8.61].

Squamous Cell Carcinoma

Squamous cell carcinoma is a common cancer, frequently originating in the skin, lung, esophagus, genital tract, or head and neck area, which also commonly metastasizes [Hoda 1992, Sears 1987]. However, squamous cell carcinoma rarely sheds diagnostic cells into an effusion [Spriggs 1954]. Less than 1% of all effusions contain cells of squamous carcinoma [Smith-Purslow 1989]. Only about one in 20 malignant pleural effusions [Johnston 1985, Sears 1987], even fewer malignant ascites (about 1% to 2%) [Sears 1987], and still fewer malignant pericardial effusions will demonstrate malignant squamous cells.

Squamous cell carcinoma of the lung tends to arise centrally, in large bronchi, and can cause bronchial obstruction, with atelectasis or postobstructive pneumonia, producing a parapneumonic effusion without diagnostic cells. If squamous carcinoma of the lung exfoliates cells, the less differentiated (nonkeratinized) invading front will be more likely to shed into a pleural effusion, compared with more differentiated (keratinized), maturing surface cells found in sputum. Thus, there may be a discrepancy between the cells found in fluid and those in the sputum. Moreover, the nonkeratinized squamous cancer cells in fluid are frequently vacuolated and can be mistaken for adenocarcinoma or reactive mesothelial cells. Some cases, particularly when arising in the lung, occur as a component of adenosquamous carcinoma.

Diagnostic Features of Squamous Cell Carcinoma

Keratinization
- Cytoplasmic rings
- Pearls

Abnormal cell shapes
- Tadpoles, bizarre

Differential diagnosis includes vacuolated, nonkeratinized squamous cells that resemble adenocarcinoma or reactive mesothelial cells.

When squamous cell carcinoma sheds diagnostic cells into a fluid specimen, the diagnosis is usually apparent. Malignant squamous cells can be present singly or in clusters. Characteristically, they have thick, dense cytoplasm with very distinct cell borders. Rings of heavy keratinization (seen best with the substage condenser diaphragm partially closed) and pearls are diagnostic of keratinization. All cells tend to round up in fluids, but if abnormally shaped cells (like snakes, tadpoles, etc) are present, it not only suggests malignancy, but also squamous origin (differential diagnosis includes sarcomas and rheumatoid effusion).

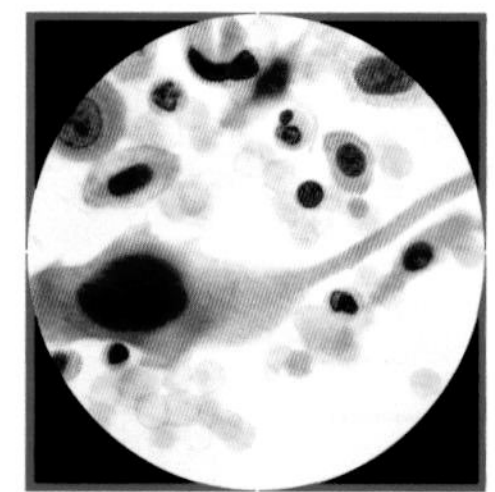
44

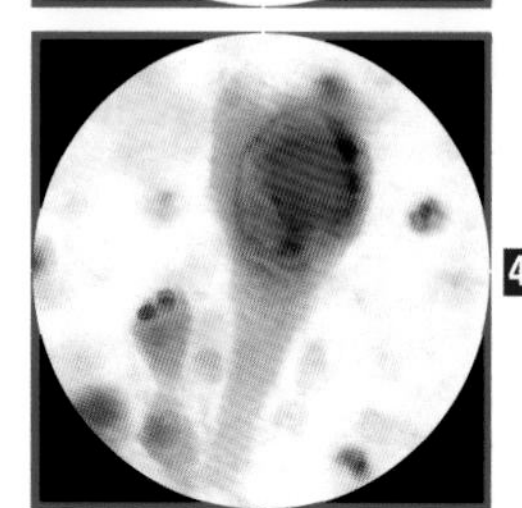
45

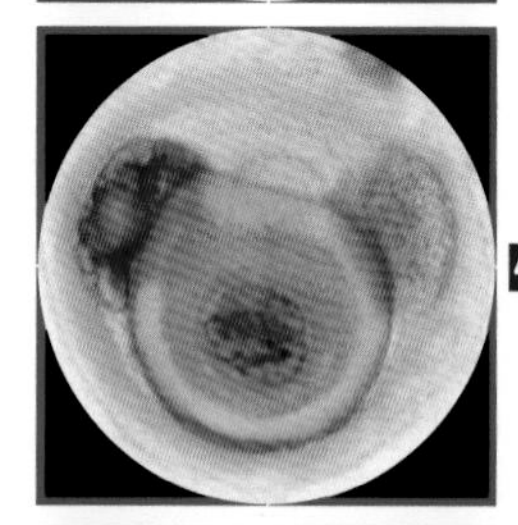
46

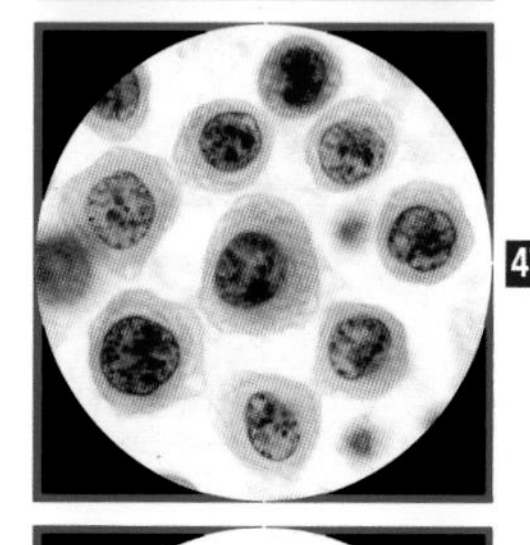
47

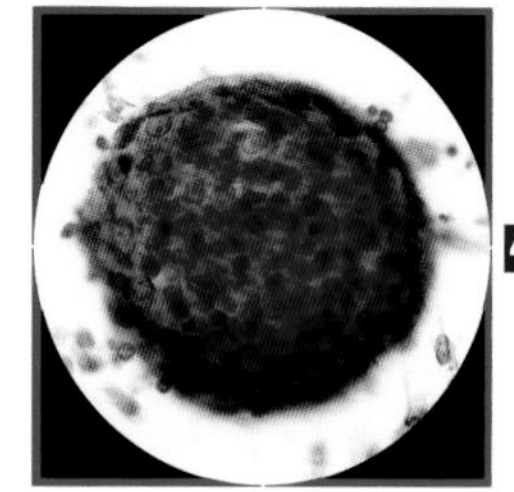
48

Keratinizing squamous cell carcinoma is particularly rare in fluid specimens. Only about 10% of cases of squamous cell carcinoma in fluids show evidence of heavy keratinization [Johnston 1985]. However, when heavily keratinized cells, particularly with abnormal shapes, or pearls are present, the diagnosis is usually easy, even though there may be little nuclear atypia in highly differentiated squamous cell carcinomas [44 I8.41, 45 I8.62, 46 I8.63]. The nuclei are characteristically opaque and pyknotic. The cytoplasm is characteristically orange or eosinophilic. The differential diagnosis may include benign squamous cells that can be seen in ruptured dermoid cysts [Cobb 1985], fistulae, "pick ups," contamination, and possibly, squamous metaplasia [Schatz 1991].

Nonkeratinizing squamous cell carcinoma is relatively more common in fluid specimens than keratinizing squamous cell carcinoma. Unfortunately, it can also be more of a diagnostic problem. Nonkeratinizing squamous cell carcinoma can mimic adenocarcinoma, which is much more common in fluids. Nonkeratinized cytoplasm often stains basophilic, and the cells may form balls like adenocarcinoma [47 I8.64, 48 I8.65]. Reactive mesothelial cells can mimic nonkeratinizing squamous cell carcinoma, including the presence of thin rings of keratinization. Reactive mesothelial cells are far more common than nonkeratinizing squamous cell carcinoma in fluids; therefore, exercise caution in making a diagnosis of nonkeratinizing squamous cell carcinoma. A positive mucin stain or definite evidence of keratinization are helpful diagnostic features of malignancy. As previously emphasized, the key to diagnosis of metastatic carcinoma is the presence of a distinctly different, or discrete, population of cells that have malignant nuclear features.

Small Cell Carcinoma

The individual cells of small cell carcinoma resemble large, immature lymphocytes. However, small cell carcinoma is composed of cells that are more variable in size and shape than benign lymphocytes. Most cells are rounded or angular, but some may be elongated to spindle shaped. The chromatin appears somewhat coarser in fluids than bronchial brushes. Nucleoli are usually indistinct, but may be slightly more conspicuous in fluid specimens. Also, the malignant cells may be larger than expected (approximately the size of mesothelial cells). Cytoplasm is scant [I8.49].

In contrast with benign lymphocytes or lymphoma, small cell carcinoma usually forms definite tissue aggregates, often forming Indian files or branching columns of cells [49 I8.49]. Distinct, even marked, nuclear molding is characteristic of small cell carcinoma [Spriggs 1976]. Cell-in-cell arrangement can also be seen. However, in some cases the malignant cells may be sparse or single [Spriggs 1954].

Small Cell Carcinoma

Small- to medium-sized cells
Scant cytoplasm, inconspicuous nucleoli
Prominent molding and Indian files

Prominent molding and Indian files together give a highly characteristic pattern of small cell carcinoma, variously referred to as "stacks of dishes," "piles of coins," or "vertebral columns" [Salhadin 1976]. The presence of small cells and Indian file groups may suggest breast cancer. However, the cells of small cell carcinoma have distinctly less cytoplasm, with very high N/C ratios, and molding is more prominent than in breast cancer. Mucin may be positive in breast cancer, but is negative in small cell carcinoma (a possible exception is the rare variant of combined small cell carcinoma/adenocarcinoma). Also, breast cancer is rare in men, in contrast with small cell carcinoma. Small cell carcinoma is a disease of older adults; consider other "small blue cell tumors" (eg, neuroblastoma, rhabdomyosarcoma, Ewing's sarcoma, or Wilms' tumors) in children or young adults.

Small Cell Effusions

Small cell carcinoma
Breast
Gastrointestinal
(Pediatric tumors)

Lymphoma/Leukemia

Malignant lymphomas, including Hodgkin's disease and non-Hodgkin's lymphomas, as well as various leukemias involving serosal surfaces can be diagnosed with exfoliative cytology [Billingham 1975]. Patients with lymphoma or leukemia seldom present with effusions without a known history of malignancy [S Graham 1990]. Because effective therapy may be available, effusions due to lymphoreticular malignancy can be exceptions to the generally dismal prognosis of malignant effusions. In contrast with carcinoma, direct serous membrane involvement is uncommonly the major factor in fluid formation. Rather, effusions in lymphoreticular malignancy are usually due to lymphatic blockage caused by enlarged lymph nodes [Weick 1973]. The majority of chylous effusions are due to lymphoma/leukemia [Hansen 1983, Weick 1973].

The most characteristic feature of this whole class of diseases is that no tissue aggregates are formed; all the cells are single [50 I8.35, 51 I8.66, 52 I8.67] [Melamed 1963]. If true tissue aggregates of cells are present (not just trapped in fibrin, etc), lymphoma/leukemia can be excluded. In general, the larger the cell type, the more easily is it recognized as malignant. Occasionally, the cells are so bizarre it is not possible to recognize them as lymphoid in origin [Yam 1967]. Small cell and mixed lymphomas may be difficult to distinguish from reactive lymphocytosis, such as is seen in tuberculosis.

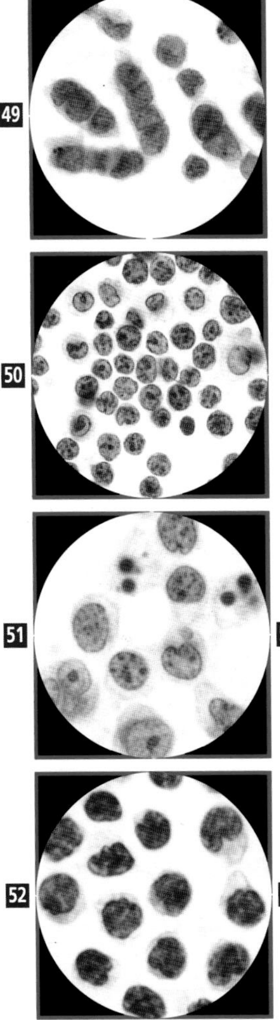

The cells often have scant, delicate cytoplasm, with relatively high N/C ratios; however, some large cell lymphomas may have more abundant cytoplasm. Nuclear abnormalities are often present, including prominent nucleoli and irregular nuclear membranes (cleaves, nuclear knobs, etc) [51 I8.66, 52 I8.67]. Massive karyorrhexis (nuclear fragmentation pattern) also suggests malignant lymphoma, and is particularly common with high-grade lymphomas or after therapy [51 I8.66] [Melamed 1963]. Air-dried, Diff-Quik–stained slides may be useful in precise classification of lymphoma/leukemia, since the cytoplasmic features, including various granules, are better seen with the Diff-Quik stain than with the Papanicolaou stain.

Cell blocks are usually not too helpful in diagnosing lymphoma/leukemia, except when performing special staining procedures. Immunocytochemistry and flow cytometry can be helpful in diagnosis and classification of these tumors [Guzman 1991, I Peterson 1991]. However, in most cases, the type of lymphoreticular malignancy will have been previously determined. Most lymphoma/ leukemia in effusions will be of the B-cell type [Katz 1987], a helpful feature in differential diagnosis with tuberculous effusions (mostly T cell, as previously discussed). Of course, T-cell lymphomas such as mycosis fungoides/Sézary syndrome can also be found in fluids [Vernon 1979].

Marked chronic inflammation, such as that seen in tuberculosis, may be difficult to distinguish from malignant lymphoma. A possible diagnostic clue to the differential diagnosis is the presence of groups of lymphocytes trapped in fibrin exudate, which suggests an inflammatory condition. A mixed pattern of chronic inflammatory cells, in which small lymphocytes predominate and plasma cells may be present, also favors a reactive process. Eosinophils may be observed, rarely, in Hodgkin's disease.

Lymphoid Leukemia, Non-Hodgkin's Lymphoma

Compared with chronic inflammation, there may be more marked size variation in lymphoma/leukemia. Large malignant cells often have prominent nucleoli, malignant chromatin, and irregular nuclear membranes. However, benign lymphocytes may show more membrane irregularity and nucleolar prominence in fluids than in peripheral blood or lymph node.

Small Lymphocytic Lymphoma/ Chronic Lymphocytic Leukemia

This neoplasm is composed of small, well-differentiated lymphocytes. In some cases, however, the cells may be slightly larger than usually expected for small lymphocytes and the chromatin may clump ("cellulées grumeles"). The differential diagnosis includes marked chronic inflammation, as may be seen in tuberculosis. A diagnostic clue is that in inflammation, the lymphocytes may be trapped in fibrin exudation, causing the lymphocytes to form loose aggregates or clumps. In neoplasia, clumps of lymphocytes are usually not seen because the lesion is noninflammatory. Special studies can be performed to determine whether the cells are monoclonal (neoplastic) or polyclonal (inflammatory), as well as whether they are of T or B cell origin. Clinical history, as usual, may be crucial in diagnosis.

Small Cleaved (Poorly Differentiated) Lymphoma

This is the most common type of lymphoma in effusions [53 I8.67]. The malignant cells are small, cleaved lymphocytes, ie, small round to oval lymphoid cells with irregular (cleaved) nuclear membranes, small but conspicuous nucleoli, and scant cytoplasm. The tumor may show conspicuous size variation, including the presence of large lymphoid cells (up to 25% of the malignant cells). Do not "overread" irregular, crenated lymphocytic nuclei as cleaved nuclei.

Large Cell Lymphoma

Large cell lymphoma is characterized by malignant lymphocytes whose nuclei are larger than histiocytic nuclei [54 I8.66]. The cells may be relatively uniform, or show considerable variation in size and shape. The nuclear membranes can be smooth (noncleaved) or irregular (cleaved). Nuclear protrusions ("knobs") are common and suggest the diagnosis of lymphoma. Abnormal nucleoli (more, larger, irregular) may be seen. The cytoplasm ranges from sparse to abundant, and appears delicate in the Papanicolaou stain. B-cell immunoblastic lymphoma is characterized by large, plasmacytoid lymphocytes (best appreciated in Diff-Quik) with eccentric nuclei, large prominent single nucleoli, and relatively abundant blue cytoplasm, which may have a perinuclear clearing.

Lymphoblastic Lymphoma

Lymphoblastic lymphoma is composed of small to medium-sized lymphoid cells with smooth or irregularly convoluted nuclear membranes, fine powdery chromatin, inconspicuous nucleoli, and scant cytoplasm. The pleural effusion is usually either left sided or bilateral [Das 1987].

Burkitt's Lymphoma

The malignant cells are small to medium-sized lymphocytes, with noncleaved nuclei; prominent, multiple nucleoli; and scant to moderate cytoplasm. Cytoplasmic or nuclear vacuoles may be present (best appreciated in Diff-Quik) [Haddad 1995].

53

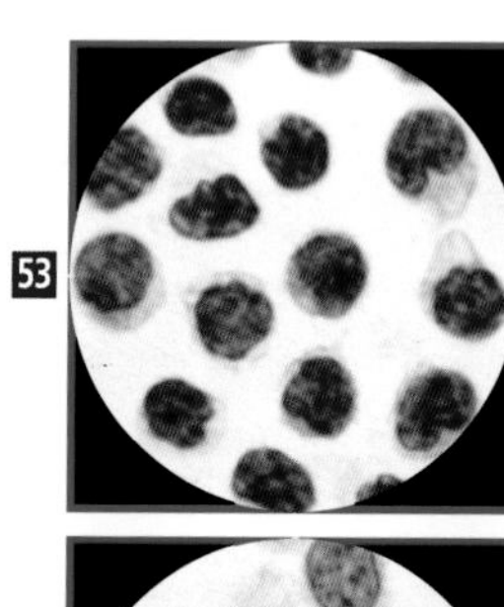

54

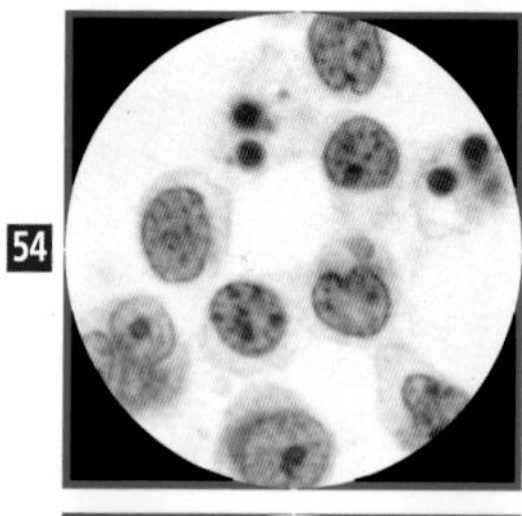

55

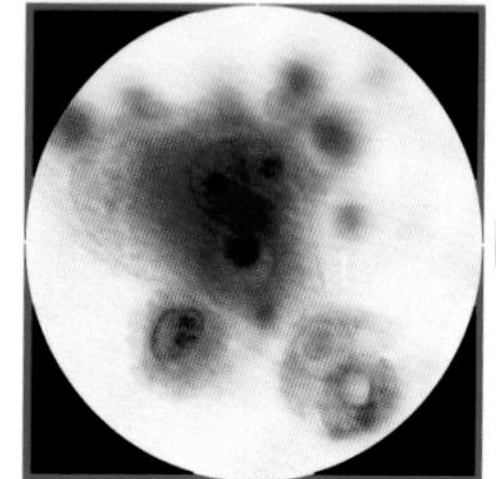

Hodgkin's Disease

Hodgkin's disease is relatively commonly associated with pleural effusions; however, it is rare to find diagnostic Reed-Sternberg cells in a fluid specimen. Hodgkin's cells are more commonly observed, but may also be sparse or absent. The tumor cells are large and very pleomorphic [55 I8.68]. The nuclei are irregular in shape and eccentrically located. The chromatin is fine and nucleoli are large and irregular. The cytoplasm may be relatively abundant.

Markedly reactive mesothelial cells and a nonspecific, reactive inflammatory pattern with lymphocytes, plasma cells, and neutrophils are usually present, but eosinophils may be sparse. It may be difficult to distinguish the Hodgkin's cells from large cells of non-Hodgkin's lymphomas. Also, any of these atypical cells could be mistaken for carcinoma or melanoma.

Leukemias

Leukemias are cytologically similar to lymphomas in fluid specimens, ie, they are composed of malignant hematopoietic cells in a dispersed, single cell pattern. Cytoplasmic features can be helpful in classification (best appreciated in Diff-Quik). For example, myelogenous leukemias may have cytoplasmic granules or Auer rods as evidence of granulocytic differentiation. The differential diagnosis of acute myelogenous leukemia includes large cell lymphoma, and the differential diagnosis of chronic myelogenous leukemia includes marked acute inflammation. Hairy cell leukemia is characterized by singly dispersed malignant cells with "hairy" cytoplasmic projections [Okabe 1991].

Multiple Myeloma, Plasmacytoma

This class of disease rarely causes an effusion; however, in some cases, an effusion is the presenting sign [Badrinas 1974, Gabriel 1965, Karp 1987, Kleinholz 1973, Koeffler 1977]. An effusion is a grave prognostic finding, with survival measured in weeks [Geisinger 1986]. When an effusion occurs, numerous malignant plasma cells may be present, allowing diagnosis in about half the cases [Geisinger 1986]. While large numbers of plasma cells suggest the diagnosis, a small number is nondiagnostic and can be observed in a wide variety of diseases, ranging from congestive heart failure to malignancy [Sahn 1987a].

The malignant plasma cells are present singly and lack cohesive aggregates [Khoddami 1992]. Diff-Quik stain is superior to the Papanicolaou stain in identifying plasmacytoid differentiation [Kapadia 1977]. The most characteristic feature is the presence of mature, and particularly immature, plasma cells [L-M Chen 1991, Favis 1960, Safa 1973, Sasser 1990, Scullin 1979]. However, malignant plasma cells in fluid may be more mature than the corresponding cells in tissue. The malignant plasma cells are frequently binucleated or multinucleated and many of the cells may have prominent nucleoli. The classic cartwheel chromatin pattern is only infrequently observed in malignant plasma cells in effusions [Geisinger 1986]. Perinuclear clear areas (hof) may be scanty. Mitotic figures may be seen [Khoddami 1992]. Russell or Dutcher bodies may be seen to aid in identification.

Melanoma

The effusion fluid in melanoma may appear dark brown or black due to either old bleeding or melanin pigment. The cells are mostly single [Hajdu 1973, Walts 1986]. They are relatively large, with large eccentrically located nuclei [56 I8.69]. Binucleation is common. The nuclei usually have large, prominent nucleoli and frequently have intranuclear cytoplasmic invaginations. The presence of melanin pigment in malignant cells is diagnostic. Melanoma is known for late recurrences, but effusions can also be the presenting sign in patients with melanoma. In either case, the diagnosis may not be suspected clinically. Melanoma is notorious for its protean manifestations, including its ability to mimic a wide variety of other neoplasms. Also, the chromatin may be bland, and cytoplasmic pigment, if present, could be mistaken for hemosiderin, leading to a false-negative diagnosis [Walts 1986].

Carcinoid Tumors

Carcinoid tumors can shed diagnostic cells into fluids. The most characteristic pattern shows monotonously uniform, small, round tumor cells arranged in loose clusters or singly. In fluids, the cells tend to round up and may form small Indian files with cellular molding. The nuclei are single and may have typical "salt and pepper" chromatin. The cytoplasm is scant and neurosecretory granules may be demonstrable with special stains [Lozowski 1979]. The differential diagnosis includes small cell carcinoma and small cell adenocarcinoma. The presence of mitotic figures is strong evidence against a diagnosis of typical carcinoid tumor [Lozowski 1979].

Transitional Cell Carcinoma

Transitional cell carcinoma is rarely associated with malignant effusions containing diagnostic malignant cells [Spieler 1985]. When present, the cells have variable, nonspecific cytologic features, including dark chromatin and dense cytoplasm with perinuclear clearing. There may also be evidence of glandular or squamous differentiation.

56

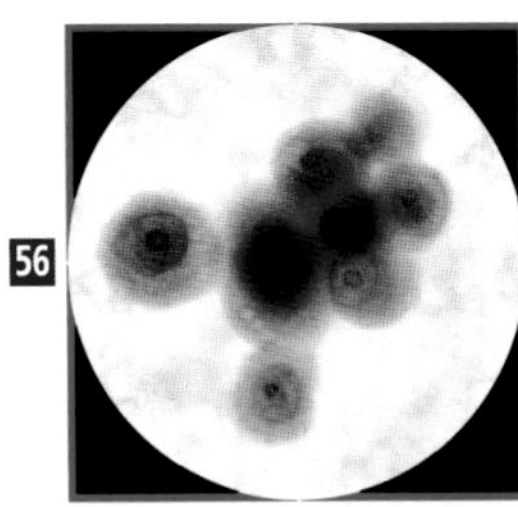

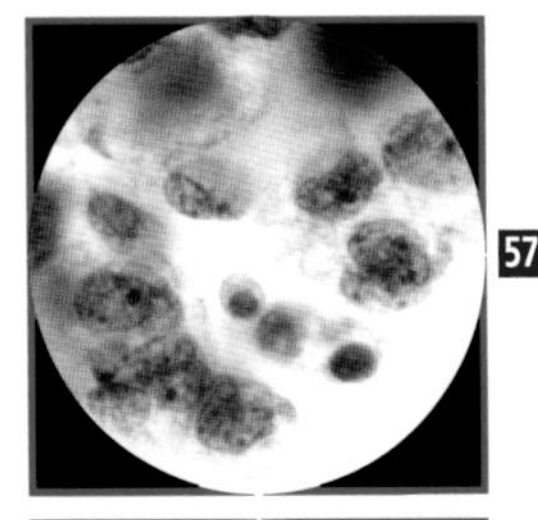

57

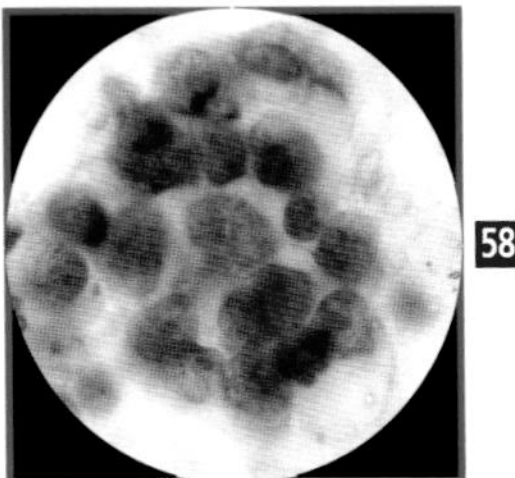

58

Germ Cell Tumors

Germ cell tumors may shed diagnostic cells into fluids [Hajdu 1975, Kapila 1983]. The morphology depends on the type of tumor.

Germinoma

Germinoma (dysgerminoma in women and seminoma in men) is the most common germ cell tumor producing an effusion. The cells are present in flat sheets, small clusters, and singly. They are large and polyhedral with pale to clear or foamy cytoplasm, which is PAS-positive due to glycogen content [57 I8.40]. The nuclei are large and vesicular and have prominant nucleoli [Kashimura 1986, Valente 1992]. Lymphocytes associated with clusters of tumor cells are diagnostically important, but lymphocytes in the background is essentially meaningless. Multinucleated giant cells (syncytiotrophoblasts) may be present. It is important to diagnose germinoma correctly, because cure is possible with proper therapy.

Embryonal Carcinoma

Patients with embryonal carcinoma often have effusions. The cytologic findings resemble those seen in papillary adenocarcinoma, but occur in young patients. Papillary clusters and single cells are typically present [58 I8.70]. The cells are medium sized and contain prominent vacuoles. The nuclei are obviously malignant appearing—pleomorphic and hyperchromatic, with macronucleoli. Alpha-fetoprotein may be helpful in diagnosis.

Endodermal Sinus (Yolk Sac) Tumor

Endodermal sinus (yolk sac) tumor is characterized by clusters of plump, round cells, with large, hyperchromatic nuclei, fine chromatin, multiple, prominent nucleoli, and vacuolated cytoplasm. In contrast with most other germ cell tumors, the cells may contain mucin, thereby suggesting adenocarcinoma [Cho 1991, Kashimura 1986, Kimura 1984, Roncalli 1988]. PAS-positive hyaline globules and Schiller-Duval (glomeruloid) bodies may be seen [Valente 1992].

Mature Teratoma

Large sheets of squamous cells and squames in all stages of degeneration and debris are seen [Grunz 1964].

Immature Teratoma

The most diagnostic features of immature teratoma are immature neuroglial cells (ie, neuroblasts) and benign squamous cells. Neuroblasts may form rosettes with central lumens.

Choriocarcinoma

Hemorrhagic effusion with malignant giant cells (syncytiotrophoblasts) and smaller, more uniform cells (cytotrophoblasts) may be seen.

Sertoli-Leydig Cell Tumor

This is a sex cord stromal tumor composed of tightly packed clusters of molded cells with high N/C ratios. The cells are rounded, with clear cytoplasm, oval nuclei, occasional nuclear grooves, and delicate chromatin. Heterologous elements may be seen [Valente 1992].

Sarcomas

Patients with sarcomas may develop effusions, but sarcomas almost never present in effusions with an unknown primary. Thus, the two questions to be answered are: (1) Are malignant cells present? (2) Are they morphologically compatible with the primary? It can be quite helpful to compare the cells with the primary lesion. Special studies, including electron microscopy and immunocytochemistry, can be used, if necessary, to help classify the tumors.

The cells can vary from large and bizarre (pleomorphic sarcoma [59 I8.71]), to relatively small and uniform (round cell sarcoma [60 I8.72, I8.73]), to spindle shaped (spindle cell sarcoma [61 I8.74]). Spindle-shaped sarcoma cells are particularly uncommon in effusions, since cells tend to round up in effusions. Because there may be no obvious special differentiation, the differential diagnosis of sarcomas may include practically all malignant tumors [T8.8] [Berry 1991].

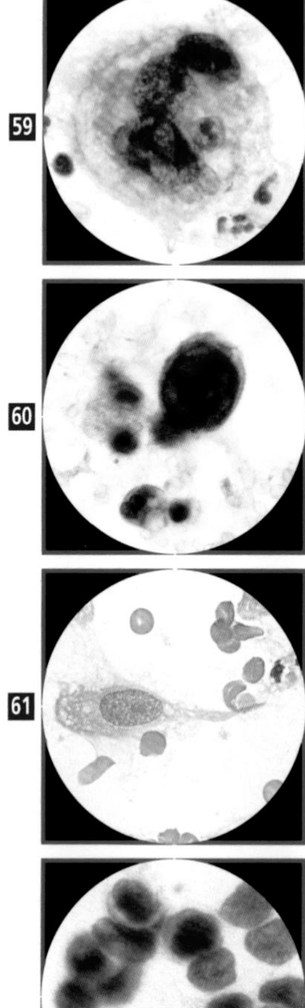

Malignant Effusions in Children

Almost all pediatric effusions are benign [Hallman 1994]. Most malignant effusions are of the small cell type, chiefly lymphomas. Nonlymphoreticular neoplasms, neuroblastomas, germ cell tumors, and bone sarcomas are also common diagnoses in malignant effusions in children [Geisinger 1984]. Distinguishing small cell malignancies from benign mononuclear inflammatory cells can be difficult.

Small cell malignancies in children are as follows:

Lymphoma/Leukemia: These tumors are characterized by exclusively single cells (as previously discussed).

Neuroblastoma: The tumor is composed of small cells that mold one another, a picture similar to the appearance of small cell carcinoma of the lung; however, the patient's age is different. Rosettes may be seen, rarely [62 I8.75]. The cells are usually PAS-negative [Farr 1972, Geisinger 1984].

Wilms' Tumor: This tumor is characterized by small malignant cells, reminiscent of those of small cell carcinoma of the lung [I8.76]. The cells are typically present in clusters and cell balls and have coarse chromatin and prominent nucleoli. A spindle cell component may be present [Geisinger 1984, Hajdu 1971].

Ewing's Sarcoma: The tumor is composed of relatively monomorphic, lymphoma-like cells, but which form small, loose or molded clusters [I8.77]. The cells are typically PAS-positive [Geisinger 1984].

Rhabdomyosarcoma, Embryonal Type: Although the tumor cells are relatively small, they are characteristically pleomorphic and include elongated, spindle, and strap shaped cells [I8.78]. The cells are PAS-positive. Cross striations in the cytoplasm are diagnostic, but rarely observed [Geisinger 1984, Hajdu 1969].

***T8.8* Differential Diagnosis of Sarcomas**

Pleomorphic sarcoma 59	Osteosarcoma, liposarcoma*, malignant fibrous histiocytoma, etc
Round cell sarcoma 60	Rhabdomyosarcoma†, neuroblastoma, Wilms' tumor, Ewing's sarcoma, synovial sarcoma, desmoplastic round cell tumor‡, etc
Spindle cell sarcoma (Note: cells may round up in effusion) 61	Fibrosarcoma, malignant nerve sheath tumor, leiomyosarcoma§, mesothelioma, etc (differential diagnosis includes rheumatoid effusion, squamous cell carcinoma)

* Geisinger 1980
† Daste 1993, Hajdu 1969
‡ Bian 1993
§ Hajdu 1969

Mesothelioma

Mesotheliomas can be either benign or malignant. However, usually only the malignant varieties are associated with effusions. Malignant mesothelioma (or simply, mesothelioma) can grow in either an epithelial (carcinomatous) or fibrous (sarcomatous) pattern or as a mixture of the two (biphasic or mixed). Half the cases are carcinomatous, 20% sarcomatous, and 30% mixed [Roggli 1987]. The carcinomatous and mixed types are most likely to result in an effusion containing diagnostic cells. Sarcomatous mesotheliomas seldom cause an effusion (about 20%) and when they do, rarely exfoliate diagnostic cells [Tao 1979]. Therefore, the following discussion will pertain primarily to carcinomatous mesothelioma. (See also section on fine needle aspiration biopsy of the pleura, Chapter 20.)

Mesothelioma is a rare tumor. Although its incidence is apparently on the rise, heightened awareness of its association with asbestos exposure may be responsible for its overdiagnosis [Wright 1984]. The primary consideration in the differential diagnosis is adenocarcinoma, particularly of the lung. Whether mesothelioma or adenocarcinoma, any malignant tumor with extensive pleural spread is essentially incurable. However, the diagnosis of mesothelioma may be crucial from a medicolegal point of view because of the potential for lucrative litigation based on personal injuries (pulmonary fibrosis, cancer) related to asbestos.

Asbestos is a white, flaky mineral that has been known since antiquity. In modern times, asbestos has been used for its fire-retardant properties. From the 1940s to the 1960s, asbestos found increased use in various industries. Although its use and manufacture have now declined, injuries are only beginning to become apparent. By the year 2000, approximately 200,000 asbestos-related deaths are expected in the United States alone. Asbestos is still found in a wide variety of products, from brake linings to small appliances, as well as roof, ceiling, and floor tiles. In the past, many (still existing) buildings were insulated with asbestos, including hospitals and schools.

Asbestos is the commercial name for a family of hydrated fibrous silicate minerals [Craighead 1982]. The carcinogenic effects of asbestos seem to be related to the physical properties of the fiber rather than its chemical makeup. Amphibole fibers (including amosite [brown asbestos], crocidolite [blue asbestos]), which are long (>8 µm) and thin (<0.25 µm), are more carcinogenic than curled, serpentine chrysotile fibers [Stanton 1981]. Amphiboles are carried to the periphery of the lung by laminar air flow, where they tend to remain intact and accumulate. Chrysotile fibers are deposited more centrally, tend to disintegrate, and are removed by the body's defense mechanisms. Chrysotile accounts for over 90% of the total asbestos marketed in the United States [Craighead 1982].

In patients who develop mesothelioma, the exposure to asbestos is often heavy (eg, shipyard or insulation workers, asbestos miners), but need not be. Workers at high risk include brake mechanics, railroad workers, and construction workers [Huncharek 1992]. However, the lifetime risk of developing mesothelioma is less than 10%, even with prolonged, heavy exposure [Antman 1980a,b, Craighead 1982, Ribak 1988, Selikoff 1979]. On the other hand, 50% of male patients with mesothelioma and as many as 95% of female patients have no history of asbestos exposure [Antman 1980a, Churg 1986, Roggli 1987]. Thus, mesothelioma occurs in many patients who have no significant history of exposure to asbestos [Huncharek 1992]. However, asbestos is ubiquitous in the urban environment and exposure is, in fact, virtually universal. These facts suggest that factors other than, or in addition to, asbestos are important in many cases of mesothelioma [J Peterson 1984]. But because industrial exposure to asbestos can apparently cause mesothelioma, and the carcinogenic threshold is unknown, asbestos-related disease, particularly mesothelioma, has become the subject of intense litigation [Craighead 1982].

Contrary to the impression given in the popular press, asbestos is associated with more cases of ordinary lung cancer than mesothelioma by a factor of 2.75 times. In addition, many other types of cancer, including gastrointestinal and kidney carcinomas, occur with increased frequency in exposed individuals [Becklake 1976, Craighead 1982, Selikoff 1980]. Perhaps surprisingly, asbestos-exposed cigarette smokers seem to have little or no increased risk of developing mesothelioma, compared with asbestos-exposed nonsmokers [Ribak 1988]. However, smoking potentiates the development of lung cancer in asbestos-exposed patients, with an 80- to 90-fold greater predisposition to carcinoma of the lung [Craighead 1982]. (In fact, ironically, smoking may actually lower the risk of mesothelioma by increasing the chance of dying of lung cancer [Tagnon 1980].) It is also worth noting that smokers in the general population are at a substantially higher risk of developing lung cancer than asbestos workers who do not smoke [Craighead 1982].

There is a long latency period (approximately two to four decades) between exposure and the onset of disease [Selikoff 1980]. More than 90% of inhaled fibers are removed from the lung, but are then swallowed, thereby gaining entrance to the gastrointestinal tract. Thus, prolonged, heavy exposure favors development of peritoneal mesotheliomas over the otherwise more common pleural mesotheliomas [Ribak 1988]. Of the remaining fibers in the lung, about a fifth are coated with iron (ferruginous or "asbestos" bodies) and may be phagocytosed by macrophages [Churg 1981,1982, Greenberg 1982]. Coated fibers are apparently harmless, but the uncoated fibers may cause asbestosis or cancer [Becklake 1976, Greenberg 1982]. "Asbestos bodies" are actually more commonly seen in lung cancer than in mesothelioma, and are therefore not useful in determining that a lesion is a mesothelioma.

Although still a rare tumor, the incidence of mesothelioma is rapidly increasing [Huncharek 1992, Pisani 1988, Spirtas 1986, K Wolf 1987]. Mesothelioma can arise in the pleura, peritoneum, or pericardium, in a ratio of approximately 6:2:1, respectively [Antman 1981], as well as in rarer sites, such as the tunica vaginalis testis (examine hydrocele fluid cytologically) [Ehya 1985, Japko 1982]. Pleural mesotheliomas are 1.5 to 2 times more common on the right side than the left [Antman 1981, Sridhar 1992], perhaps for the same reason aspiration pneumonia is more common on the right side (ie, it is an anatomical "straight shot" for foreign material to enter the right lung through the bronchi). About 75% to 80% of cases occur in men [Antman 1981, Sridhar 1992]. Two thirds of cases occur between the ages of 50 and 70 years, but many other cases occur before age 50 years [Antman 1980a,1981, Ribak 1988]. Rarely, mesothelioma can even occur in children [Grundy 1972].

Patients with pleural mesotheliomas usually present with the insidious onset of aching, nonpleuritic chest pain or shortness of breath. In the early stages, a large majority (75% to 95%) have a pleural effusion, although it may be asymptomatic for quite some time [Chahinian 1982, Hasan 1977, Oels 1971, Whitaker 1984, 1986a,1991, Wright 1984]. Approximately 1 in 500 malignant pleural effusions are due to mesothelioma [McKenna 1985]. The clinical triad of unilateral chest pain, weight loss, and bloody pleural effusion suggests the diagnosis [Greenberg 1983]. However, other malignancies metastatic to the pleura may produce similar symptoms. Late in course, the effusion may subside or disappear as the pleural space becomes obliterated by tumor growth. About 15% of patients have lymphadenopathy and 10% have hepatomegaly at presentation [Pisani 1988]. Clubbing of the fingers is seen in less than 10% of patients [Pisani 1988]. Elevated erythrocyte sedimentation rate and thrombocytosis (>400,000 platelets/mm^3) are usual [Pisani 1988].

Peritoneal mesotheliomas may produce abdominal cramps, bowel obstruction, and ascites [Roggli 1987]. Unusually, peritoneal mesothelioma presents as a hernia [Ribak 1988]. Pericardial mesotheliomas can cause cardiac failure, arrhythmias, and pericardial effusions [Roggli 1987].

In the past, the presence of metastases had been considered evidence against a diagnosis of mesothelioma. However, it is now well documented that mesothelioma can metastasize [Adams 1984, Edge 1978, McCaughey 1965, G Roberts 1976]. Metastases occur with about the same frequency as non–small cell lung cancer, particularly to regional lymph nodes and lung (See chapter on "Fine Needle Aspiration Biopsy"). Uncommonly, lymphadenopathy can be the initial manifestation of mesothelioma [Sussman 1988]. Distant metastases to kidney, the adrenal glands, liver, and bone are also relatively common, although in contrast with lung cancer, brain metastases are rare [Roberts 1976]. Sputum cytology is only rarely positive (findings include papillary aggregates of epithelial-like cells, which may be indistinguishable from adenocarcinoma) [M Nakajima 1992, Whitaker 1986b].

One of the most characteristic features of mesothelioma is growth by encasement, forming a thick rind of tissue that superficially invades the underlying viscera. Because there is no cleavage plane, the tumor does not strip easily at surgery. Pleural mesotheliomas also tend to grow into interlobular fissures. However, a significant number (approximately 10%) of pleural mesotheliomas form a solitary lesion or dominant mass like lung cancer [Adams 1986]. Conversely, lung cancer can sometimes grow by encasement [Braganza 1978, Broghamer 1978, Harwood 1976].

Because lung cancer can so closely mimic the clinical, gross, and microscopic features of mesothelioma (pseudomesotheliomatous carcinoma [Braganza 1978, Broghamer 1978, Harwood 1976]), it has been suggested that thoracotomy or even full autopsy may be required to establish the diagnosis [Adams 1986, Antman 1981b, Butchart 1981, Greenberg 1983, Hasan 1977, Prakash 1985, Whitaker 1991]. Unfortunately, thoracotomy can be hazardous. The tumor tends to spread, including invasion of surgical incisions, which may cause intractable pain [Pisani 1988]. However, a definitive diagnosis of mesothelioma can usually be made based on the triad of compatible clinical history, diagnostic imaging, and morphological findings. Metastatic carcinoma, particularly from the lung, pancreas, or ovary, must be excluded. Be cautious when diagnosing mesothelioma in patients with a known history of malignancy.

Diagnostic imaging techniques are useful in determining the pattern of growth, and thus aid in the differential diagnosis. The characteristic findings in pleural mesothelioma are diffuse, nodular pleural thickening, especially at the basal and posterior surfaces, often with irregular, thick interlobular fissures and encasement of the lung, resulting in decreased lung volume. In contrast, adenocarcinoma is more likely to cause hilar adenopathy, pulmonary nodules, and bilateral, discrete, pleural masses [T8.9] [Adams 1986]. Unfortunately, the radiologic findings may be indeterminate.

T8.9 **Radiologic Findings in Mesothelioma and Adenocarcinoma**

Favors Mesothelioma	Favors Adenocarcinoma
Diffuse, nodular pleural thickening	Discrete, nodular pleural masses
Often unilateral	Often bilateral
Nodular thickening of fissures	Intraparenchymal lung nodules
Encasement, invasion of bone, lung, decreased lung volume	Encasement unusual but can occur
Can metastasize	Often associated with hilar adenopathy

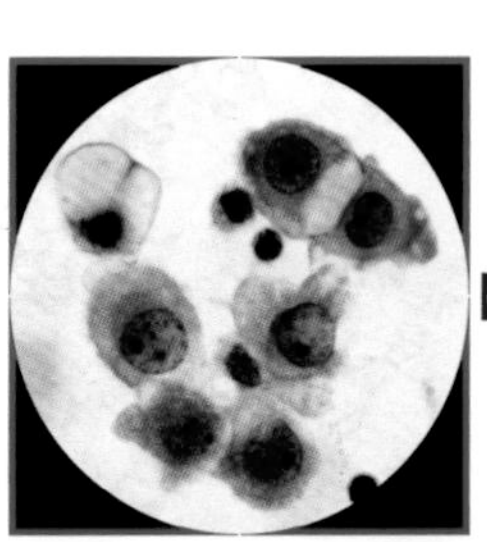

63

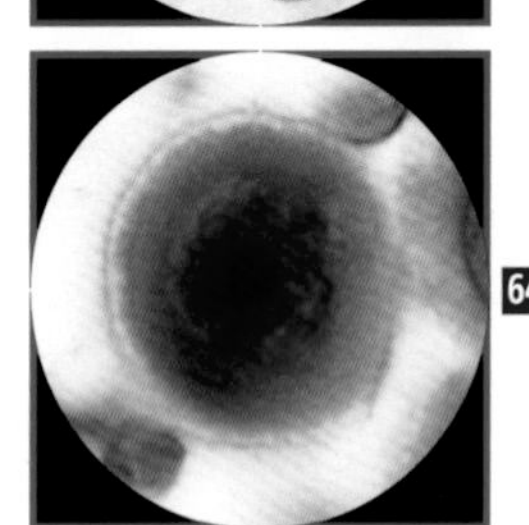

64

Cytologic Findings

The classic clinical history of pleural mesothelioma is one of asbestos exposure, persistent pleural effusions, chest pain, and evidence of pleural thickening. The diagnosis should be suspected in a middle-aged man who complains of shortness of breath, has persistent effusions, and in whom sputum cytologic and bronchoscopic findings are negative for malignancy. Because gross and radiologic features of lung cancer and mesothelioma overlap, microscopy is the key to proper diagnosis, and because patients with mesotheliomas frequently present with effusions, fluid cytology is frequently the first diagnostic study.

The fluid is usually yellowish in color, but many cases are bloody or hemorrhagic [Antman 1981, Pisani 1988, Ribak 1988]. Most are exudates [Pisani 1988]. The fluid is characteristically viscous to gelatinous (like synovial fluid), which is primarily due to hyaluronic acid (an acid mucopolysaccharide, mesenchymal mucin). Hyaluronic acid can be elevated in both benign disease and nonmesotheliomatous cancers, but very high levels of hyaluronic acid (>8 mg/dL) are more specific for mesothelioma [Rasmussen 1967]. An elevated hyaluronic acid concentration plus atypical mesothelial cells is consistent with mesothelioma [Castor 1967].

General Cytodiagnostic Features

The essence of the diagnosis of mesothelioma is that the malignant cells look like mesothelial cells [63 I8.79, 64 I8.80]. There is no "foreign," extra, or discrete population of tumor cells, in contrast with metastatic malignancy. Rather, there is a morphologic kinship of the malignant cells with native mesothelial cells forming a continuum from apparently benign to atypical to malignant appearing [Ehya 1986, Klempman 1962, Naylor 1963, G Roberts 1972, Sherman 1990, Triol 1984, Whitaker 1978,1984].

Unfortunately, the "kinship" that is characteristic of mesothelioma is a double-edged sword. This same morphologic feature that makes the diagnosis possible can also make the diagnosis impossible in some cases. Some mesotheliomas have only subtle cytologic abnormalities [Ehya 1986, Naylor 1963]. Thus, in some cases, malignant mesothelial cells are indistinguishable from benign, reactive mesothelial cells. Some cases shed exclusively benign-appearing cells that resemble benign macrophages [Guffanti 1985, Spriggs 1983]. It is the rare case that has numerous highly abnormal cells [Triol 1984].

An important clue to the diagnosis of mesothelioma—a low-power observation—is the presence of "more and bigger cells in more and bigger clusters" [65 I8.81]. Extreme mesothelial cellularity suggests the diagnosis of mesothelioma [DiBonito 1993a, Leong 1992, Naylor 1963, G Roberts 1972]. Similarly, finding numerous, large clusters of cells suggests a diagnosis of malignancy, particularly in pleural effusions [Whitaker 1991]. Aggregates containing 30 to 200 or more cells are characteristic of mesothelioma [Berge 1965, Whitaker 1984]. However, single cells are also usually present and may predominate in a significant number of cases [Sherman 1990, Triol 1984].

Cell Groups

The cell aggregates take various forms. Thick clusters of cells with highly irregular or knobby, flower-like outlines are characteristic of mesothelioma [65 I8.81] [DiBonito 1993a, G Roberts 1972]. In contrast, cell clusters in benign effusions are fewer, smaller, and less complex [Leong 1992, Whitaker 1984]. Benign aggregates are usually flatter and rarely form large three-dimensional clusters [Whitaker 1984]. Even highly atypical cells in flat, monolayered sheets are likely to be benign [Whitaker 1984]. Cell clusters in adenocarcinoma tend to have smooth community borders. Unfortunately, exceptions to these general rules occur [Ehya 1986].

Papillary clusters are seen more commonly in mesothelioma than in adenocarcinoma or benign effusions, reflecting the growth pattern of mesothelioma (often seen in tissue) [DiBonito 1993a, Stevens 1992]. True acinar formation is indicative of adenocarcinoma, but intercellular spaces in mesothelial cells can mimic acini [Ehya 1986, Leong 1992, G Roberts 1972]. Numerous "cell-in-cell" patterns (also known as "cell-embracing," "pincer-like grip," "cell engulfment," and "cannibalism") [66 I8.83] and long chains of cells (Indian files) [67 I8.82] are common in mesothelioma and rare in benign effusions [DiBonito 1993a, Ehya 1986, Stevens 1992, Whitaker 1978]. Collagen cores may be seen in the center of cell aggregates of benign or malignant mesothelial cells[I8.25], but are rarely observed in adenocarcinoma [Becker 1976, Delahaye 1990, Y Kobayashi 1978, Leong 1992, Spriggs 1979b, Stevens 1992, Triol 1984, Whitaker 1977,1978,1984,1991, Wojcik 1992].

Cells

The individual malignant mesothelial cells are usually larger and more variable than benign mesothelial cells [T8.10] [Ehya 1986, Kwee 1982]. Giant mesothelial cells, including multinucleated forms, are relatively common in mesothelioma [I8.85], in contrast with both benign effusions and metastatic carcinomas, in which giant cells are rare [Ehya 1986, Klempman 1962, Sherman 1990]. Malignant giant mesothelial cells maintain morphologic features suggestive of mesothelial origin (kinship). Although the cells of mesothelioma can be quite variable in size, the nucleus

T8.10 Malignant Mesothelioma

(Key = Morphologic kinship with mesothelial cells)
"More and bigger cells, in more and bigger clusters"

Groups
- Irregular papillae and knobby three-dimensional clusters
- Cell-in-cell arrangements
- Long chains (Indian files)

Nuclei
- Increased bi/multinucleation
- Nuclear enlargement and pleomorphism
- Macronucleoli

Cytoplasm
- Windows, skirts, blebs
- Dense, may show two-tone staining
- Fine vacuoles (lipid, glycogen, not epithelial mucin)

Background
- Hyaluronic acid
- Fluffy to bubbly in Papanicolaou stain
- Metachromatic precipitate in Diff-Quik® stain
- May show chronic inflammation, otherwise clean

65
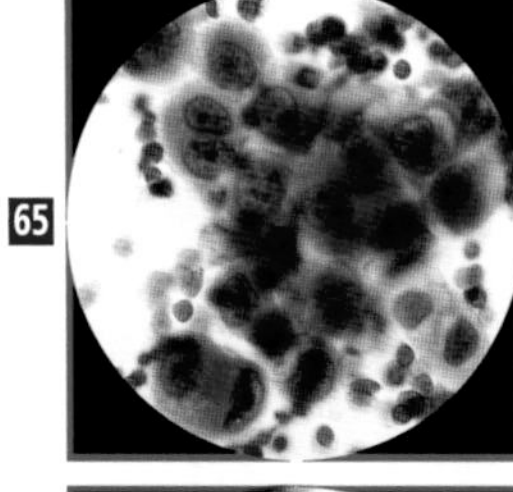

66
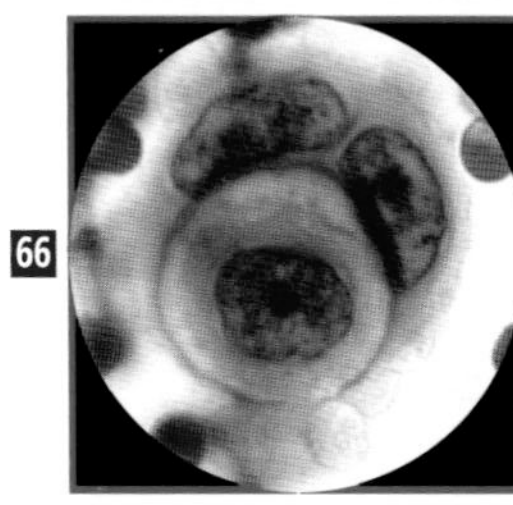

67
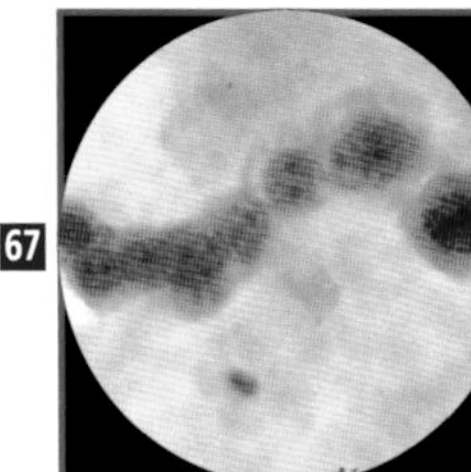

and cytoplasm tend to vary in proportion to one another, thereby maintaining a relatively constant N/C ratio. This imparts a certain degree of uniformity to the malignant mesothelial cells, which is usually not seen in adenocarcinoma [Adams 1984]. Frankly bizarre-appearing cells favor carcinoma.

Cytoplasm

Mesothelial cytoplasm is characteristically dense, particularly in the central, perinuclear area (the endoplasm), but often fades to a delicate, lacy appearance toward the edges (the ectoplasm) [I8.80] [Naylor 1963]. Occasionally, the endoplasm stains pink to orange and the ectoplasm blue to green (two-tone staining) [Whitaker 1991]. Thin rings of keratinization may be observed in the endoplasm, which is highlighted when the substage condenser diaphragm is partially closed. Sometimes, dense, coagulated mummified cells (analogous to Councilman bodies in the liver) are seen in mesothelioma [Whitaker 1991]. Cytoplasmic density is a fairly consistent finding in mesothelioma, and is often helpful in distinguishing it from adenocarcinoma, which usually has diffusely delicate, pale to foamy cytoplasm [Whitaker 1991].

Cell Borders

"Windows" (well-defined gaps or clefts between adjacent cells) are a characteristic feature of benign or malignant mesothelial cells, but are less commonly observed between cells of adenocarcinoma [I8.84]. Peripheral cytoplasmic blebs (prominent cytoplasmic outpouchings) and lacy skirts (microvilli), are often accentuated in malignant mesothelial cells, compared with benign ones, and are uncommonly seen on cells of adenocarcinoma [Stevens 1992].

Cytoplasmic Vacuoles

Cytoplasmic vacuoles can be helpful in diagnosis [T8.11] [Boon 1984, Sherman 1990, Stevens 1992]. Vacuoles are best appreciated with the Diff-Quik stain. Two kinds of vacuoles can be seen in mesothelioma, one containing lipid, the other glycogen. Lipid vacuoles are small and uniform and usually found in a perinuclear location, in the center of the cytoplasm [Boon 1984]. Glycogen can form a peripheral ring of small, somewhat more variable, PAS-positive vacuoles, particularly prominent in cytoplasmic blebs. Occasionally large, crescent-shaped glycogen lakes are present; glycogen stains golden yellow with the Papanicolaou stain (as in navicular cells in the Pap smear) [Whitaker 1991].

(Note: Adenocarcinoma also has lipid or glycogen in approximately 10% of cases. Mesothelioma may produce mesenchymal mucins, particularly hyaluronic acid, but not epithelial mucin. These vacuoles are more prominent in malignant than benign mesothelial cells. Ultimately, vacuolization is nonspecific, since any cell type can undergo vacuolar degeneration.)

Adenocarcinoma more often has large, irregular, eccentric vacuoles containing epithelial mucin, sometimes forming signet rings or coarse, balloon vacuoles. However, vacuolization, per se, is nonspecific. Degenerative vacuoles, which can be seen in any cell type, can produce a signet ring or balloon appearance. Large vacuoles containing hyaluronic acid can also be seen in mesothelioma [Whitaker 1991]. Rarely, secretory signet ring mesothelioma has been reported [Boon 1981,G Roberts 1972, Spriggs 1983, Whitaker 1984].

Nucleus

Central or paracentral location of the nucleus in the cytoplasm favors mesothelial cell origin [68 I8.80], while an eccentric location is more characteristic of adenocarcinoma [Klempman 1962, Sherman 1990]. Although binucleation and multinucleation are common in both benign and malignant mesothelial cells, the presence of numerous large, multinucleated mesothelial cells, particularly with nuclear atypia, favors mesothelioma [Stevens 1992, Tao 1979].

The usual nuclear criteria of malignancy, ie, pleomorphic and enlarged nuclei that are irregular in size and shape, apply in diagnosis of mesothelioma [69 I8.84] [Whitaker 1991]. Unfortunately, diagnostic features of malignancy can be subtle in some cases [Triol 1984]. Nevertheless, on careful search, at least a few cells with clear-cut evidence of malignancy can usually be found. Prominent nuclear membrane irregularity is indicative of malignancy. Intranuclear cytoplasmic invaginations are rare in benign mesothelial cells [Baddoura 1990], but may be seen more commonly in either mesothelioma or adenocarcinoma [Herrera 1985, Sherman 1990]. The chromatin stains variably dark and may be irregularly distributed. Nucleoli are usually present and may be enlarged, multiple, or irregular in outline [P Gupta 1981]. Macronucleoli are associated with malignancy and may be the sole criterion of malignancy in some cases of mesothelioma [Whitaker 1991]. Macronucleoli (red blood cell sized) are rare in benign effusions. Mitotic figures are not helpful in diagnosis unless they are atypical, but atypical mitoses are rarely seen.

68

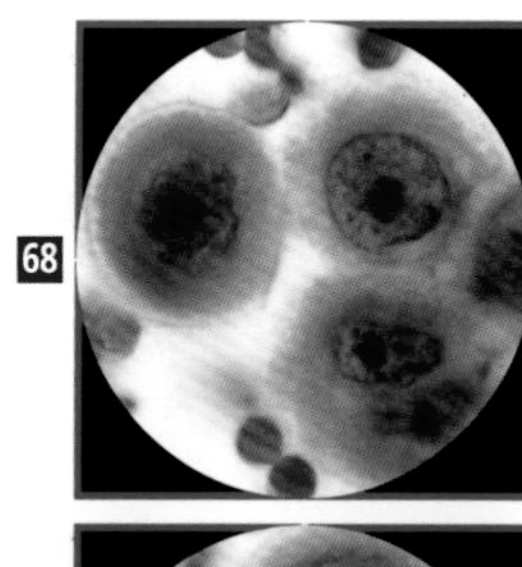

69

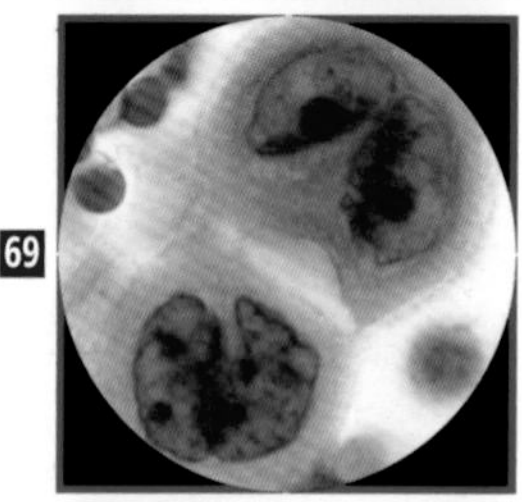

70

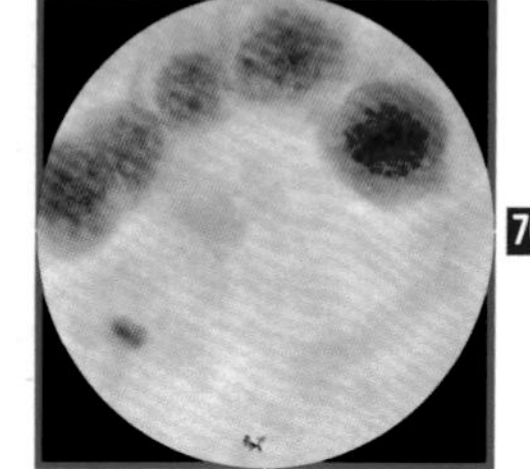

T8.11 **Cytoplasmic Vacuole Differences in Mesothelioma and Adenocarcinoma**

	Size/Shape	Location	Content
Mesothelioma	Small, uniform	Perinuclear	Lipid
	Small, slight variation	Peripheral	Glycogen
Adenocarcinoma	Large, marked variation	Eccentric	Mucin

Background

Although spindle cells are rarely identified in effusions, the combination of epithelial and spindle cells in a fluid specimen suggests a diagnosis of mesothelioma [Klempman 1962, Sherman 1990]. Although psammoma bodies can be seen rarely [Japko 1982, Sherman 1990], they are more commonly observed in metastatic carcinoma, eg, ovary, and in benign effusions than in mesothelioma [Stevens 1992]. Thus, psammoma bodies are not diagnostic of mesothelioma or even of malignancy. Significant lymphocytic infiltration can be observed in mesothelioma, which may suggest an inflammatory process [Klempman 1962, Leong 1992]. Necrosis and debris are usually not present [Sherman 1990]. However, an unusual flocculent material corresponding to hyaluronic acid may be seen in some cases [Naylor 1963]. In the Pap stain, it ranges from fluffy to bubbly in appearance [70 I8.82] [Whitaker 1986a]. With the Diff-Quik stain, it appears as a stippled, metachromatic precipitate [Spriggs 1983].

Diagnostic Problems

With adequate specimens, cytologic analysis can make a diagnosis of malignant mesothelioma in about two of three cases [Sherman 1990, Whitaker 1984,1991]. Pleural biopsy alone can diagnose about 40% to 60% of cases [Whitaker 1984]. The two techniques are complementary, however, and a diagnosis can be made in up to 80% of cases using a combination of cytologic and histologic examination and history [Whitaker 1984]. Diagnostic accuracy improves with experience and interest [Whitaker 1987,1991].

False-negative diagnoses are well known in mesothelioma; even when the cells are recognized as malignant, they may be misclassified as adenocarcinoma [Adams 1986, Antman 1980b, Brenner 1982, Jara 1977, Law 1984, Lewis 1981, Martensson 1984, Nauta 1982, Oels 1971, Pisani 1988, Ribak 1988, Scamurra 1991, Shearin 1976, Sridhar 1992, Strankinga 1987]. Most false-negative diagnoses occur in specimens that contain few or no mesothelial cells (unsatisfactory specimens) [Whitaker 1991]. Excess blood can dilute the diagnostic cells. Occasionally, a fibrinous pleuritis develops, which prevents exfoliation of tumor cells [Sherman 1990, Tao 1979]. This can result in an effusion with numerous lymphocytes but few mesothelial cells, a situation similar to tuberculous pleural effusions [Sherman 1990, Whitaker 1984]. Also, it is rare to be able to diagnose the pure sarcomatous variety of mesothelioma in exfoliative cytology, since few or no diagnostic cells are exfoliated [Kobayashi 1988, Tao 1979]. However, the presence of atypical spindle cells in an effusion suggests the diagnosis.

Benign mesothelial proliferations with reactive or atypical mesothelial cells can be difficult to distinguish from mesotheliomas (see below) [P Gupta 1981]. Conversely, bland mesotheliomas, sometimes composed of cells resembling histiocytes, are difficult to recognize as malignant [Boon 1981, Guffanti 1985, Spriggs 1983]. A possible cytologic clue in such cases is the presence of multinucleated giant cell histiocytes, a rare finding in benign effusions other than those associated with rheumatoid disease. A clinical clue to the diagnosis of a bland mesothelioma is that the malignant effusion does not resolve like most benign effusions. Peritoneal mesotheliomas can be particularly bland [Boon 1981,1982]. Squamous metaplasia has been reported in peritoneal mesotheliomas [Matsuo 1993]. At the other extreme, sometimes the malignant cells are very large and pleomorphic, with clearly malignant features. In such cases, the diagnosis of malignancy may be obvious, but the cell origin may not be evident [Whitaker 1984,1987]. The differential diagnosis of mesothelioma with papillary serous carcinoma of the ovary can be particularly difficult or impossible [Berge 1965, Bollinger 1989, Ehya 1986, Klempman 1962].

False-positive diagnoses of mesothelioma are rare [Whitaker 1991]. Although large clusters of benign mesothelial cells can occasionally be seen, particularly in pericardial effusions or ascites, they are rare in benign pleural effusions [Becker 1976, Rosai 1975, Selvaggi 1990, Spriggs 1979b, Whitaker 1991]. Diagnosis of mesothelioma based on complex aggregates of atypical mesothelial cells is reliable, but diagnosis based on single atypical mesothelial cells is more difficult [Whitaker 1991].

Mesothelioma vs Reactive Mesothelial Cells: Benign effusions show fewer mesothelial cells compared with effusions associated with mesothelioma, which may show extreme cellularity. Reactive mesothelial cells typically form smaller, less complex groups than those of mesothelioma, which show larger, more complex aggregates. Reactive mesothelial cells form flat sheets or knobby, flower-like clusters. Mesotheliomas form irregular, more three-dimensional aggregates. Papillary formations and numerous cell-in-cell arrangements are more common in mesothelioma. Benign mesothelial cells frequently have reactive nuclear changes, but mesothelioma characteristically shows malignant nuclear features. Benign nuclei are more monomorphic, malignant nuclei more pleomorphic. Nucleoli can be prominent in either reactive mesothelial cells or mesothelioma, but multiple or macronucleoli suggest mesothelioma.

Nonkeratinizing Squamous Cell Carcinoma vs Mesothelioma: Nonkeratinizing squamous cell carcinoma, like other metastatic malignancies, is characterized by a discrete population of malignant cells. Mesothelioma, on the other hand, characteristically shows a continuum of cells (morphologic kinship). The cytoplasm of squamous cells is denser and more homogeneous than that of mesothelial cells and the cell borders are more sharply defined. Mesothelial cells tend to have ectoplasmic rims, skirts, and less distinct cell borders. Pearls and bizarre cells are characteristic of squamous carcinoma, while papillae, knobby "flower-like" aggregates, and "windows" are more characteristic of mesothelial cells. Either cell type can show cell-in-cell patterns. Heavy keratinization with thick cytoplasmic rings is a feature of squamous cells, but mesothelial cells may have thin rings of keratinization. Peripheral PAS positive cytoplasmic staining is characteristic of mesothelial cells.

Adenocarcinoma vs Mesothelioma: Unfortunately, in a number of cases, the cells of adenocarcinoma closely resemble mesothelial cells; thus, the fact that they are "foreign" may not be obvious [Stevens 1992]. Papillary adenocarcinomas, particularly bronchioloalveolar carcinoma of the lung and papillary carcinoma of the thyroid, may shed clusters of cells mimicking mesothelioma [Lozowski 1987]. Any of these tumors may have psammoma bodies and intranuclear cytoplasmic invaginations. Either adenocarcinoma or mesothelioma can have vacuolated tumor cells [DiBonito 1993a]. Many differential diagnostic features of adenocarcinoma were considered in the above description. Among the most useful features separating mesothelioma from adenocarcinoma are true papillary aggregates, multinucleation with atypia, and windows (which favor mesothelioma), vs acinar structures and secretory vacuoles (which favor adenocarcinoma) [T8.12] [Stevens 1992]. Note that neoplasms, including lung cancer, can cause atypical mesothelial hyperplasia [Yokoi 1991].

Special Studies in Diagnosis of Mesothelioma

Distinguishing adenocarcinoma from mesothelioma can be particularly problematic. Here, various special studies can be helpful in diagnosis.

Special Stains: Due to different embryologic origins, mesotheliomas and adenocarcinomas may have different secretory products that can be demonstrated using special stains. Mesotheliomas are mesodermally derived and in some cases secrete the acid (mesenchymal) mucin, hyaluronic acid. Adenocarcinomas are derived from either endoderm (eg, lung, gastrointestinal tract) or ectoderm (eg, breast) and may secrete neutral (epithelial) mucins. Adenocarcinomas can also produce a variety of acid mucins other than hyaluronic acid.

Most adenocarcinomas of the lung produce stainable intracellular neutral (epithelial) mucin, which reacts with the mucicarmine or DPAS stain. Mesotheliomas very rarely take up neutral mucin stains. Although mucin-positive mesotheliomas have been reported [MacDougall 1992], definite intracytoplasmic epithelial (mucicarmine, DPAS positive) mucin is strong evidence against a diagnosis of mesothelioma. However, a negative reaction is not helpful. Also, extracellular mucin-posi-

T8.12 **Cytologic Differences Between Adenocarcinoma and Mesothelioma**

	Adenocarcinoma	Mesothelioma
Key	Foreign cells	Continuum
Groupings	Less complex Community borders Collagen cores rare Windows unusual	More complex Irregular knobby outlines Collagen cores common Windows common
Cells	Columnar shape	Blebs, skirts
Nucleus	Usually eccentric	Usually central or paracentral
	Often pleomorphic, occasionally bizarre	Often less pleomorphic, not bizarre
	Less hyperchromatic	More hyperchromatic
Cytoplasm	Delicate, homogeneous	Dense center, with lacy edges
	Uniform stain	Two-tone staining
Vacuoles	Secretory Random, irregular size	Degenerative Perinuclear, small, regular
Multinucleated giant cells	Rare (at first)	Common
Mucin (epithelial)	May be present	Not present
PAS stain	May be positive (droplet, diffuse)	Positive (peripheral)

tive material or mucin in histiocytes should not be misinterpreted as evidence of adenocarcinoma.

PAS Stain: Mesothelioma produces intracytoplasmic glycogen much more commonly than does adenocarcinoma. However, mesothelioma does not secrete neutral mucin, while many adenocarcinomas do. Both neutral mucin and glycogen are PAS-positive. But glycogen staining can be removed by prior digestion with diastase (DPAS). Therefore, DPAS positivity correlates with mucin production. Unfortunately, mucin is not the only DPAS-positive material; some proteins or lipoproteins are also DPAS-positive [Whitaker 1984].

With PAS, mesotheliomas most characteristically show an abundant, usually peripheral, finely granular stain, while adenocarcinomas characteristically display intracellular droplets of positivity, although the staining can be diffuse. Intracellular DPAS positivity, particularly when present as hard-edged or target-shaped inclusions, virtually excludes mesothelioma [Roggli 1987, Whitaker 1991].

Mucicarmine: In theory, mucicarmine stains only neutral (epithelial) mucin. Thus, mucicarmine positivity in cells in an effusion would not only exclude mesothelioma, but would in and of itself be diagnostic of adenocarcinoma. Unfortunately, in practice, mucicarmine also stains hyaluronic acid in a few cases (5% to 10%), leading to unexpected positive reactions [Churg 1986, Triol 1984]. This staining can be abolished with hyaluronidase.

Alcian Blue/Colloidal Iron With and Without Hyaluronidase: Acid mucopolysaccharides (AMPS) react with the alcian blue or colloidal iron stains. The degree of staining removed by hyaluronidase digestion is (theoretically) due to hyaluronic acid. Therefore, the combination of these acid mucin stains, with and without predigestion with hyaluronidase, can be used to assess the presence of hyaluronic acid. However, there are several caveats and the FDA has declared it a carcinogen.

Some adenocarcinomas produce a mucin that will react with the alcian blue stain [T8.13]; however, this staining is usually not sensitive to hyaluronidase. In addition, abundant hyaluronic acid can be present in either mesothelioma or in the stroma of carcinoma. Thus, the mere presence of hyaluronic acid means little or nothing: it must be demonstrated intracellularly to be diagnostically useful. AMPS tend to wash out in processing; thus the apparent absence of hyaluronic acid can be misleading. The type of hyaluronidase used in digestion is also important. *Streptomyces* hyaluronidase is specific for hyaluronic acid, but the more commonly used testicular hyaluronidase also removes chondroitin sulfate [Kawai 1985, MacDougall 1992]. Hyaluronic acid is neither the sole, nor even the predominant, mucin in most mesotheliomas [Chiu 1984, Kawai 1985, Roggli 1987]. Only slightly more than half (56%) of epithelial mesotheliomas have demonstrable hyaluronic acid at all, and only about 30% have the classic feature of alcian blue positivity removed by hyaluronidase [Roggli 1987]. Digestion-resistant alcian blue positivity is seen in approximately 60% of adenocarcinomas.

Oil Red O: Most mesotheliomas, but only about 10% of adenocarcinomas, contain oil red O (neutral lipid)–positive cytoplasmic vacuoles indicating the presence of neutral lipid [Boon 1984]. In mesothelioma, the vacuoles are fine and centrally located. In adenocarcinoma, the vacuoles are large and eccentrically located.

Other Special Studies

Because of atypical or peculiar staining reactions, there has been considerable interest in electron microscopy and immunostaining in helping to make a diagnosis of mesothelioma.

Electron Microscopy: Mesothelioma is characterized, ultrastructurally, by the presence of abundant intermediate filaments, often distributed perinuclearly and frequently condensed into tonofibrils; long, slender, bushy microvilli,

T8.13 **Special Stains in Differential Diagnosis of Mesothelioma and Adenocarcinoma**

Stain	Mesothelioma	Adenocarcinoma
Mucicarmine, DPAS	Usually (–)	Often (+)
Alcian blue	Usually (+)	Often (+)
After hyaluronidase digestion	Digested (–)	Remains (+)

which tend to branch; and, frequently, prominent accumulations of glycogen [71 I8.86] [Barsotti 1989, Coleman 1989, Kobzik 1985, Leong 1992, Suzuki 1980]. Although the microvilli have cores in both types of tumors, rootlets and terminal webs identify adenocarcinoma [Leong 1992]. There are no true intercellular gland lumens in mesothelioma (although apparent intracellular lumens can be seen). In contrast, adenocarcinoma has relatively few intermediate filaments and microvilli that tend to be short, stubby, and blunt [T8.14]. True glands, mucin droplets, or other secretory granules such as lamellar bodies may be seen in adenocarcinoma but not in mesothelioma [Dewar 1987].

Unfortunately, there is some degree of overlap of these features, making a clear-cut distinction impossible in some cases, particularly with poorly differentiated tumors [Burns 1985, Coleman 1989, Dewar 1987]. Electron microscopy cannot resolve the dilemma of benign vs malignant mesothelial cells [Kobzik 1985].

Immunocytochemistry: More recently, immunostains for various cellular antigens have come into vogue to aid in the differential diagnosis [Esteban 1990, Motoyama 1995]. Because many of these stains lack specificity, caution must be exercised in their interpretation [DiBonito 1993a]

Cytokeratins are found in both mesothelioma and adenocarcinomas [Duggan 1987]. Although high-molecular-weight keratins are more characteristic of epithelial mesothelioma [72 I8.88], keratin positivity, per se, is not helpful in making the distinction. Sarcomatous mesotheliomas may be negative for high-molecular-weight keratin [Leong 1992]. However, cytokeratin-positive spindle cells suggest mesothelioma in the proper setting [Walz 1990].

The pattern of keratin staining may be somewhat specific [Kahn 1982]. Mesotheliomas show a peripheral ring of keratin in air-dried specimens and perinuclear keratin in alcohol-fixed material. Adenocarcinomas have an arborizing, web-like network of keratin.

Vimentin is theoretically limited to mesenchymal cells. It was hoped that the combination of cytokeratin plus vimentin positivity would point at least to a diagnosis of mesothelial origin [Blobel 1985] (which would still leave open the question of benign vs malignant). However, this combination has now been found in a variety of cancers, including metastatic carcinomas in effusions [Kuhlmann 1991, Leong 1992, Ramaekers 1983, Upton 1986].

T8.14 **Electron Microscopic Differences Between Mesothelioma and Adenocarcinoma**

Finding	Mesothelioma	Adenocarcinoma
True glands	No	Yes
Intermediate filaments	Abundant	Sparse
Microvilli	Long, slender branching	Short, stubby rootlets and terminal web
Glycogen	Common	Unusual
Mucin (epithelial)	No	Common

T8.15 **Typical Immunostaining Patterns**

Tumor	CEA	Keratin*	Vimentin	EMA	Leu-M1	Secretory Component
Mesothelioma	(–)	(+)	(+)	(+)†	(–)	(–)
Lung adenocarcinoma	(+)	(+)	(–)	(+)	(+)	(+)

CEA = carcinoembryonic antigen; EMA = epithelial membrane antigen.
* High-molecular-weight keratin is characteristic of mesothelioma.
† Thick cell membranes.

71

72

73

Carcinoembryonic antigen (CEA) is abundant in tumors of endodermal origin, including lung and gastrointestinal cancers, and theoretically absent in mesothelioma [73 I8.87] [Wang 1979]. CEA staining is useful diagnostically—a positive reaction (intense staining of the glycocalyx) is strong evidence against mesothelioma [Duggan 1987, Mezger 1990, Motoyama 1995, Whitaker 1982]. However, many adenocarcinomas are CEA-negative and some mesotheliomas are CEA-positive, but the staining is usually weak and focal [Adams 1984, Battifora 1985, DiBonito 1993a, Otis 1987, Walz 1990, Whitaker 1984]. Also, caution must be exercised in interpretation of CEA positivity, particularly in single cells, because macrophages and other inflammatory cells may stain [Whitaker 1991].

It has been suggested that the ratio of CEA to keratin staining may be useful in differentiating mesothelioma from adenocarcinoma [Corson 1982, Roggli 1987]. Keratin staining stronger than CEA favors mesothelioma; CEA stronger than keratin favors adenocarcinoma. Sarcomatous mesotheliomas may be negative for both CEA and keratin [Roggli 1987].

Both mesothelioma and adenocarcinoma express epithelial membrane antigen, but mesothelioma shows a characteristic "thick cell membrane" staining reaction [Leong 1990]. Strong staining of cell clusters is not seen in benign conditions, although occasional cells may partially stain [Whitaker 1991].

Leu-M1 (CD 15) and secretory component may be positive in adenocarcinoma, but are typically negative in mesothelioma [Sheibani 1992]. A variety of more specific monoclonal antibodies are being developed and tested [Abati 1995, Donna 1992, Maguire 1994, Motoyama 1995, Spagnolo 1991].

A summary of typical immunostaining patterns and special studies is given [T8.15, T8.16].

Cytogenetics: Cytogenetic analysis has identified clonal abnormalities in most malignant pleural fluids, including some from malignant mesotheliomas. Cytogenetic aberrations, including del (1p), del (3p), and del (22q), have been associated with malignant mesothelioma [Granados 1994].

Culdocentesis

Culdocentesis (cul-de-sac aspiration) is a simple, safe, and inexpensive procedure, that can be performed in the office, to

T8.16 **Summary of Special Studies**		
Feature	Mesothelioma	Adenocarcinoma
Glycogen	More common	Less common
Mucins	HA	Neutral, AMPS (other than HA)
EM		
Microvilli	Long, slender, more	Short, stubby, fewer
Filaments	Abundant, ± tonofibrils	Scanty
Keratin	Both high and low molecular weight	Low molecular weight
CEA/Keratin	Keratin > CEA	CEA > Keratin
Vimentin	Usually (+)	Usually (–)

AMPS = acid mucopolysaccharide; HA = hyaluronic acid; EM = electron microscopy; CEA = carcinoembryonic antigen.

obtain cytologic specimens from the pelvic cavity [McGowan 1972]. It enjoyed a brief popularity as a possible means of early detection of ovarian cancer [Funkhouser 1975, J Graham 1964, R Graham 1962]. Unfortunately, a review of more than 3000 reported cul-de-sac aspirations found 35% of the specimens to be inadequate, with very few positive results (1.2%). Moreover, among the positive results, at least a quarter (10/37) were false positive, and not a single case of unsuspected ovarian carcinoma was detected [Keettel 1974]. Because the procedure is time consuming and painful and has no proven efficacy in early cancer detection, it has been abandoned for use as a screening test for ovarian cancer. However, culdocentesis provides a means of detection of recurrent ovarian cancer [VillaSanta 1980], although there is still a significant rate of false negative and inadequate specimens [I Jones 1981].

Culdocentesis can also be used as a diagnostic aid in other kinds of pelvic disease [T8.17] [Beacham 1958]. However, newer techniques such as ultrasonography are usually employed instead.

74

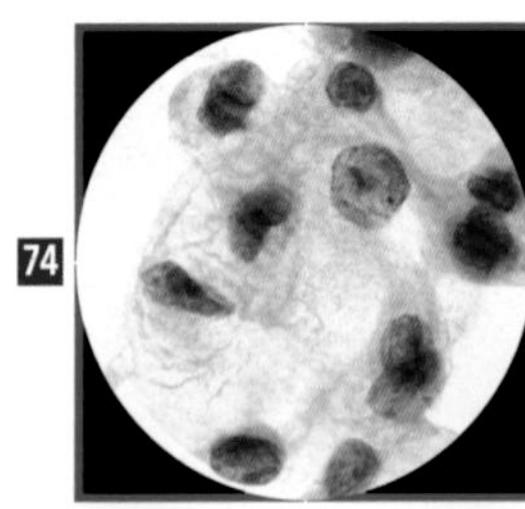

75

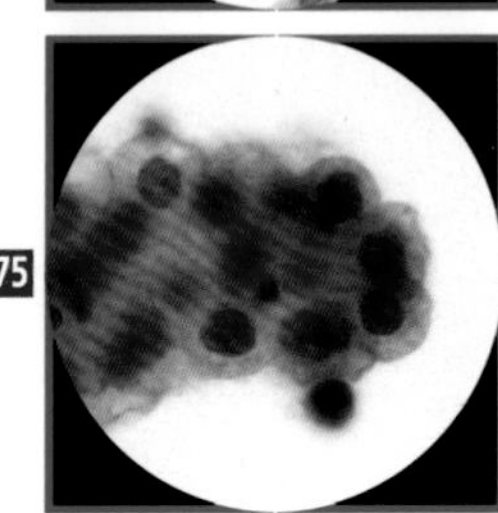

Body Cavity Washings

Finding malignant cells in peritoneal fluid is an accepted, important prognostic factor in assessing some gynecologic cancers. Body cavity washings may also be important in predicting prognosis of other malignancies such as cancers of the lung, gastrointestinal tract, and pancreas [74 I8.102] and possibly others such as kidney [75 I8.103] [Buhr 1990, Kondo 1993, J Martin 1986, T Nakajima 1978, Okumura 1991, Quan 1966, Warshaw 1991].

Peritoneal Wash Cytology

Using cytologic examination of peritoneal washings, subclinical disease such as early ovarian cancer can be detected, although in some cases, even patients with grossly apparent disease can have negative findings on cytologic examination [Creasman 1971]. Patients with negative cytologic findings generally have a better prognosis than patients with positive cytologic findings, who generally have a poor prognosis. However, patients with positive cytologic findings are more likely also to also have other poor prognostic factors (such as lymph node metastases or extrauterine spread) [Abu-Ghazaleh 1984, Creasman 1971,1981, Imachi 1987, Jacques 1991, Kilgore 1984, W Roberts 1986], and do poorly regardless of cytologic status. On the other hand, favorable prognostic indicators are neutralized by positive cytology. Therefore, cytologic findings are particularly important in patients with good prognostic factors [Creasman 1981].

Peritoneal Wash Cytology
Staging gynecologic or other cancers
Detecting occult carcinoma
Document persistent/recurrent cancers

Peritoneal wash cytology is most useful in documenting persistent or recurrent cancer, and can sometimes detect occult carcinoma during surgery for benign disease. The value of peritoneal wash cytology is well established in evaluation of ovarian cancer, in which cytologic status is an independent variable in assessing prognosis [Creasman 1971, Kudo 1990]. The value of peritoneal cytology in endometrial cancer is less well substantiated [Grimshaw 1990, Hirai 1989, Konski 1988, Yazigi 1983], but seems also to be important in prognosis [Creasman 1981, Harouny 1988, Heath 1988, Imachi 1988, Kadar 1994, , Mazurka 1988, McLellan 1989, Morrow 1991, Sutton 1989, Szpak 1981, Turner 1989]. Although positive peritoneal cytology correlates with poor prognosis in cervical cancer, it is not an independent prognostic variable [Abu-Ghazaleh 1984, Imachi 1987, Kilgore 1984, Morris 1992, W Roberts 1986, Trelford 1995]. Cytologic status is incorporated in International Federation of Gynecology and Obstetrics staging protocols for both ovarian and endometrial carcinoma.

Samples for cytologic examination should be taken when the peritoneal cavity is first opened during surgery. If ascitic fluid is present, a sample should be collected, and there is no

T8.17 **Culdocentesis**	
Gross Appearance	Possible Diagnosis
Clear, slightly cloudy	Usually peritoneal, occasionally adnexal cyst
Pink, blood tinged	Salpingo-oophoritis, torsion of the ovary
Blood	
Does not clot	Hemoperitoneum
Clots	Bloody tap
Old blood	Ectopic pregnancy
Pus	Abscess, peritonitis (recommend culture)
Chocolate	Endometrioma
Sebaceous	Dermoid cyst

need to obtain a washing specimen [Spriggs 1987, Yoshimura 1984]. The mere presence of ascitic fluid in a patient with cancer is a poor prognostic sign and usually correlates with positive cytologic findings [Pretorius 1986, Spriggs 1987]. If no ascitic fluid is present, washes from the cul-de-sac, left and right paracolic gutters, and diaphragm are usually collected, although the value of multiple specimens has been questioned [Jacques 1991].

What constitutes an adequate body cavity wash specimen is not well defined in the literature. Among more than 3,000 reported specimens, not a single one was reported as unsatisfactory for evaluation [Abu-Ghazaleh 1984, Coffin 1985, Covell 1985, Creasman 1971,1981, Geszler 1986, Kanbour 1989, Kilgore 1984, Marcus 1962, Pretorius 1986, Ravinsky 1986, Yazigi 1983, Ziselman 1984, Zuna 1988,1989]. In the few studies that did report unsatisfactory specimens, the rates were remarkably high, ranging from 15% to nearly 58% [Jacques 1991, Keettel 1956,1958, Luesley 1990]. The implication is that many of the cases reported as "negative for malignant cells" may actually have been negative for cells altogether. An analysis of false-negative peritoneal wash cytologic specimens showed that a significant number of false negatives are due to scant cellularity [Zuna 1989], which may be a result of specimen collection technique, sampling error (including adhesions), or meager exfoliation of malignant cells [Pretorius 1986, Sneige 1992].

False negatives are a serious problem with rates ranging as high as 66% in patients with gross residual disease and up to 86% for patients with only microscopic disease [Copeland 1985, Jacques 1991, E Rubin 1988]. In some cases, the surgeon fails to obtain a cytologic specimen at all [McGowan 1985]. Unfortunately, the rate of false-positive diagnoses is also significant (up to 9%) [Creasman 1971, Keettel 1974, McLellan 1989]. False positives are often due to misinterpretation of reactive mesothelial cells, endometriosis, endosalpingiosis, psammoma bodies, and miscellaneous causes such as ectopic pancreas [McLellan 1989, Ravinsky 1986, Sams 1990, Sneige 1992].

It is possible that the practice of reporting a negative diagnosis on what was in fact inadequate material has at least contributed to ironic findings, such as negative cytologic findings in the face of grossly evident disease, or more ominously, observing recurrence in patients with negative cytologic findings [Kudo 1990]. It is important to resist making a diagnosis on inadequate material. At a minimum, at least a few mesothelial cells must be present for specimen adequacy [McGowan 1989].

Cytology of Body Cavity Washings

The body cavity washing specimen consists of traumatically exfoliated sheets of mesothelial cells, white blood cells, macrophages, blood, fibrin, and debris, often including glove powder [Bercovici 1978, McGowan 1967,1968,1974,1975]. Other cells such as endometrial (including endometriosis) or fallopian tube (including endosalpingiosis) as well as psammoma bodies may be seen in benign disease [K Chen 1983]. Excess blood or debris may obscure the specimen and result in an unsatisfactory specimen.

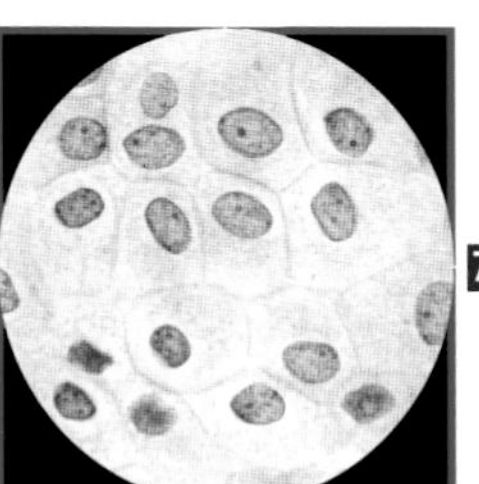

76

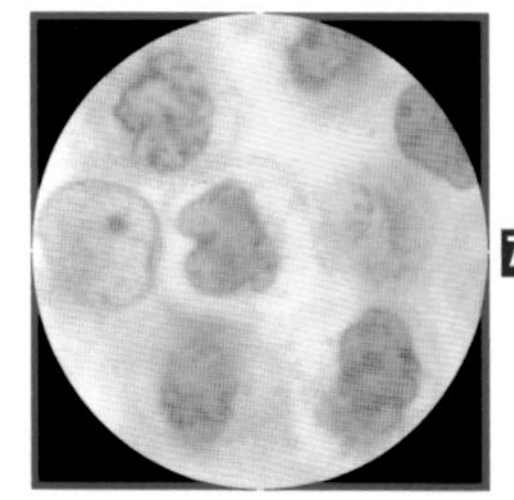

77

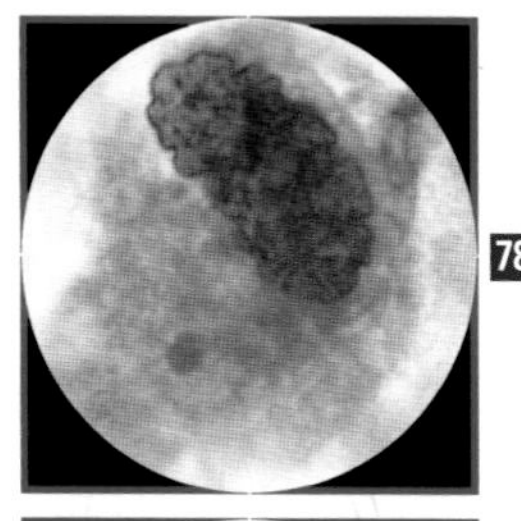

78

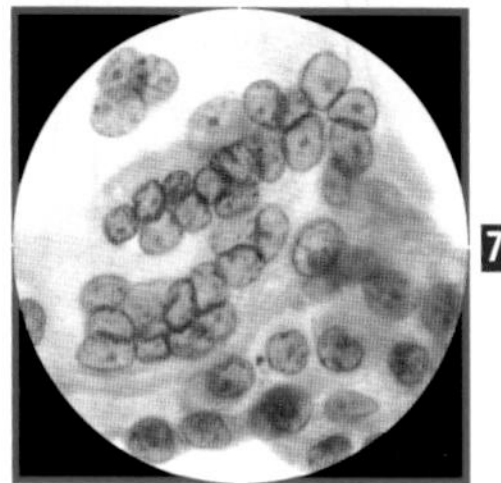

79

Mesothelial Cells

Nonreactive Mesothelial Cells

In contrast with serous effusions, in which the mesothelial cells always show at least minimal reactive changes, in washes, normal, nonreactive mesothelial cells are frequently obtained. Nonreactive mesothelial cells form flat sheets of polygonal cells [76 I8.89]. The cytoplasm is moderate in amount, delicate, and lightly basophilic. Despite the delicate cytoplasm, the cells usually have well-defined borders. They can form large, orderly sheets or mosaics of cells reminiscent of the honeycomb arrangement characteristic of benign glandular cells. The nuclei are single, tend to be paracentrically located, and are generally round to oval, with smooth membranes, fine chromatin, and small nucleoli. The nuclei can vary slightly in size and shape. Occasionally, the nuclei have lobulated outlines, like a flower in bloom (daisy cells) [77 I8.90]. This peculiar but benign change is apparently related to estrogen, and is seen most commonly in women at midcycle [McGowan 1970].

Reactive Mesothelial Cells

In response to a variety of conditions (such as pelvic inflammatory disease, endometriosis, hemorrhage, pelvic mass, radiation or chemotherapy, previous surgery, ectopic pregnancy, tubo-ovarian abscess—as well as any of the causes of reactive change discussed for effusions, such as cirrhosis, uremia, pancreatitis) the mesothelial cells may undergo reactive changes essentially identical to those previously described for reactive mesothelial cells in an effusion [78 I8.92]. The reactive cells can be seen in large clusters or flat sheets or singly. Balls of cells and papillary structures, as well as psammoma bodies, can also be seen in benign conditions [K Chen 1983, Kern 1969]. However, complex, branching clusters or papillae usually indicate neoplasia. Benign reactive cells are plump and cuboidal instead of thin and flat, and vary more in size and shape. The cytoplasm becomes dense and distinct. However, in contrast with effusions, degenerative vacuoles in mesothelial cells are less common in body cavity washes [Marcus 1962]. The reactive nuclei enlarge and the N/C ratio may increase somewhat. Multinucleation may be observed [79 I8.91]. The chromatin of reactive nuclei can vary from bland to hyperchromatic to somewhat coarse, but is not frankly malignant appearing. Nucleoli can range from small to prominent.

The diagnosis of malignancy in body cavity washes generally requires abnormal cells present both singly and in groups; a known history of the cancer being diagnosed; and that the tumor cells be distinct from reactive mesothelial cells [Ziselman 1984]. It is important to compare the cytologic findings with the history and histologic findings [Ravinsky 1986, Sneige 1992, Ziselman 1984]. As in effusion cytology, reactive mesothelial cells usually show a morphologic continuum with clearly benign mesothelial cells, while cancer usually shows a foreign population of cells.

(Certain ovarian lesions are an exception to this general rule, however.) Large flat sheets of orderly cells usually exclude cancer. Also, special studies, such as mucin staining or immunocytochemistry, may help to resolve diagnostic difficulties [Crosby 1992, Sneige 1992]. Certain benign conditions can also be diagnosed.

Gynecologic Peritoneal Wash Cytology

There is a morphologic spectrum from reactive mesothelial cells to endosalpingiosis to borderline serous tumors to low-grade serous adenocarcinoma. The cells of any of these conditions can appear quite similar to one another, with only subtle differences. In general, reactive mesothelial cells are characterized by orderly, flat sheets of cells with smooth nuclear membranes and bland chromatin. In contrast, low-grade serous adenocarcinoma shows disorderly, three-dimensional clusters of cells with irregular nuclear membranes and coarser chromatin. Note that irregular nuclear membranes can also be seen in benign cells due to osmotic or degenerative effects (crenation).

Diagnosis of Tumors and Other Conditions

Endosalpingiosis (Müllerian Glandular Inclusions): Endosalpingiosis is ectopically located benign epithelium composed of cells morphologically identical to those lining the fallopian tube (the endosalpinx). Endosalpingiosis probably derives from metaplasia of coelomic epithelium. The most common locations are the pelvic peritoneum, pelvic lymph nodes, and the omentum [Sneige 1992].

Cytologically, the most characteristic feature is tightly cohesive aggregates and simple nonbranching papillae of small cells [80 I8.93], which may form a single layer surrounding psammoma bodies [Carlson 1986, Sidawy 1987b, Sneige 1986,1992]. Few single epithelial cells are present. The cells are orderly and uniform, with scant basophilic cytoplasm and high N/C ratios. The nuclei are eccentrically located, round to oval, and uniform, with smooth membranes. The chromatin is fine and even. Nucleoli are inconspicuous and mitoses are absent or rare.

Groups of epithelial cells with psammoma bodies should not be misinterpreted as evidence of malignancy. A helpful feature is that ciliated cells can usually be identified, pointing to tubal-type epithelium. The presence of cilia usually excludes a diagnosis of malignancy. On the other hand, more than mild atypia or complex, branching papillae usually exclude a diagnosis of endosalpingiosis [Sneige 1992]. However, pregnancy-related changes, including numerous papillary structures, single cells, and more marked cytologic atypia with hyperchromatic nuclei, prominent nucleoli, and mitotic figures may be a pitfall in the diagnosis [Sneige 1992].

Serous Cystadenoma and Cystadenofibroma: Papillary clusters of epithelial cells that resemble fallopian tube epithelium and therefore endosalpingiosis, are characteristic of serous cystadenoma or adenofibroma. Although the papillary groups may have lobulated borders or bulges here and there, they have smooth surfaces. There may also be slight variation in size and shape of the cells [Zuna 1988]. The cells are tall columnar and may have cilia. The nuclei have smooth membranes, fine chromatin, and one or two small nucleoli [Ravinsky 1986]. Psammoma bodies may be seen.

80

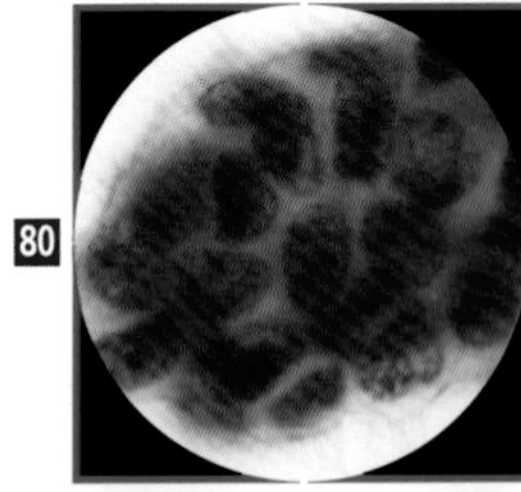

81

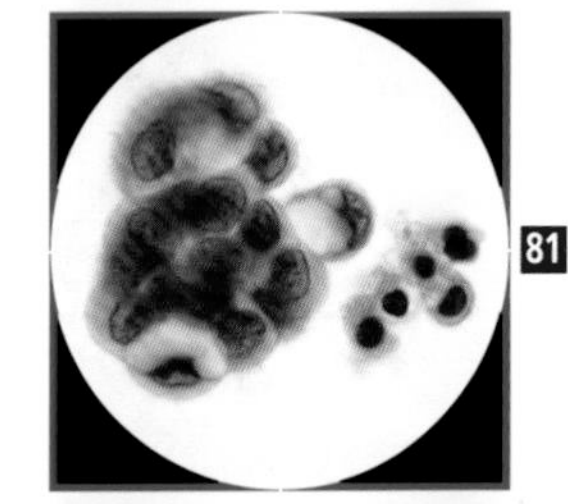

82

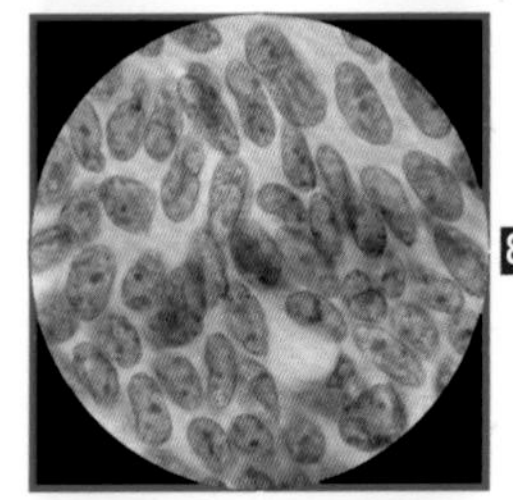

83

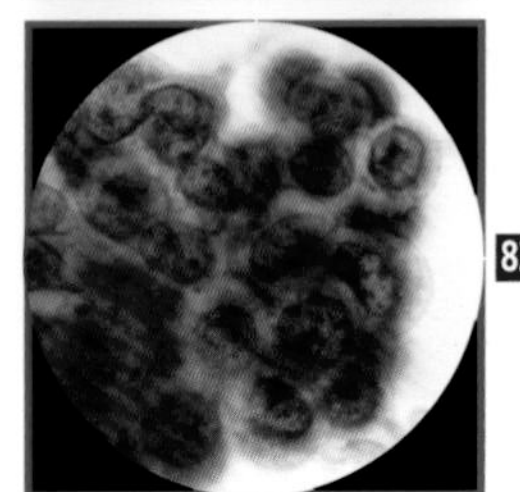

Borderline (Low Malignant Potential) Serous Ovarian Tumors: Ovarian tumors of low malignant potential, or so-called borderline tumors, are noninvasive histologically. Clinically, borderline tumors have a significantly better prognosis and different therapy than does outspoken cancer.

Cytologically, these tumors are characterized by the presence of cohesive, often branching, papillary structures [81 I8.94, 82 I8.95] [Johnson 1988]. The papillae are of variable but often large size and usually have smooth borders. The cells are overlapping, with variable degrees of atypia. Single tumor cells may be seen [Sneige 1992].

The cells are mostly small, but less uniform, and have well-defined cell borders and high N/C ratios. Occasionally, ciliated cells are seen. The cytoplasm is scant, basophilic, and contains few vacuoles. The nuclei are usually monomorphic, with smooth or slightly irregular nuclear membranes, and inconspicuous or invisible nucleoli. Although slight to moderate atypia consisting of more variation in size, irregular nuclear membranes, coarse chromatin, and occasional prominent nucleoli may be seen, mitoses are rare or absent [Covell 1985, Sneige 1992]. Psammoma bodies may be present.

Ovarian Adenocarcinoma: Both the architecture of the papillae as well as the cellular morphology aid in differentiating borderline tumors from frank adenocarcinoma [Gurley 1994, Johnson 1988, Kashimura 1986]. Unfortunately, there is no sharp cytologic cutoff but rather a morphologic continuum of change between the two entities [T8.18].

Compared with borderline tumors, adenocarcinoma is characterized by a predominance of smaller, less cohesive clusters and papillae, with more irregular outlines, and an increase in single cells [I8.96, 83 I8.97]. The cells are larger, more pleomorphic, and appear syncytial with indistinct cell borders. The cytoplasm is more abundant and usually vacuolated. The nuclei vary in size and shape, have irregular membranes, coarser chromatin, and usually have prominent nucleoli. Mitoses may be frequent. Psammoma bodies can be seen. Serous psammocarcinoma of the ovary and peritoneum is a rare form of low-grade

T8.18 **Differences Between Endosalpingiosis, Borderline Tumor, and Adenocarcinoma**

Feature	Endosalpingiosis	Borderline Tumor	Adenocarcinoma
Papillae	Simple, nonbranching	Branching, large	Irregular, smaller
Cells	Cohesive, orderly	Crowded + single	Increased single
Atypia	Little or none	Mild to moderate	Obvious

T8.19 **Differential Diagnosis Between Borderline Tumors and Adenocarcinoma***

Feature	Borderline	Adenocarcinoma
Papillae		
Size	Variable, often large, branching	Predominantly small
Borders	Smoother	More irregular
Pleomorphism, atypia	Slight to moderate	Moderate to marked
Cytoplasmic vacuoles	Usually absent	Usually present
Cilia	Occasionally present	Extremely rare
Nuclear borders	Less irregular	More irregular
Chromatin	Less dense	More dense
Nucleoli	Usually inconspicuous	Usually prominent
Mitoses	None	Often present
Psammoma bodies	No significant difference	No significant difference

* Johnson 1988, Sneige 1992

serous carcinoma characterized by extensive psammoma body formation and bland cytologic features [K Chen 1994].

Well-differentiated ovarian adenocarcinoma can be very difficult to distinguish from borderline tumors [T8.19]. However, on careful search, at least a few clearly malignant cells may be found in adenocarcinoma [Covell 1985]. Aneuploidy is rare in borderline tumors, but common in ovarian adenocarcinomas [Gurley 1994]. Poorly differentiated adenocarcinomas, including clear cell carcinoma, are obviously malignant appearing [Ravinsky 1986]. Ciliated malignant cells are rare, but have been reported in ovarian adenocarcinoma [P Gupta 1985, Kobayashi 1988]. Also, the differential diagnosis of papillary serous adenocarcinoma with peritoneal mesothelioma can be very difficult [Bollinger 1989].

Endometriosis: If the triad of endometrial glandular cells, endometrial stromal cells, and hemosiderin-laden macrophages can be identified in the body cavity wash, endometriosis can be safely diagnosed. However, it is unusual to find all three components in such specimens. More likely is the finding of numerous mesothelial cells with varying degrees of reactive atypia (due to irritation) and siderophages. These findings are nonspecific, but consistent with the diagnosis of endometriosis [Zuna 1988].

Endometrial Adenocarcinoma: Papillary clusters or single atypical cells may be identified in patients with endometrial adenocarcinoma [84 I8.98]. High-grade cancers are obviously malignant. Low-grade endometrial adenocarcinoma may resemble reactive mesothelial cells, forming loose, three-dimensional clusters of cells with delicate cytoplasm, which ranges from scant to abundant. The nuclei have coarse chromatin and prominent or macronucleoli. Peritoneal washings can be positive in stage I endometrial carcinoma [Creasman 1981, Szpak 1981, Yazigi 1983, Zuna 1989], but it is not entirely clear why. Positive cytology portends a worse prognosis.

Endolymphatic Stromal Myosis (Low-Grade Stromal Sarcoma): Endolymphatic stromal myosis is characterized by tight clusters of small cells with scant cytoplasm. The nuclei have irregular membranes and coarse, dark chromatin [Ravinsky 1986].

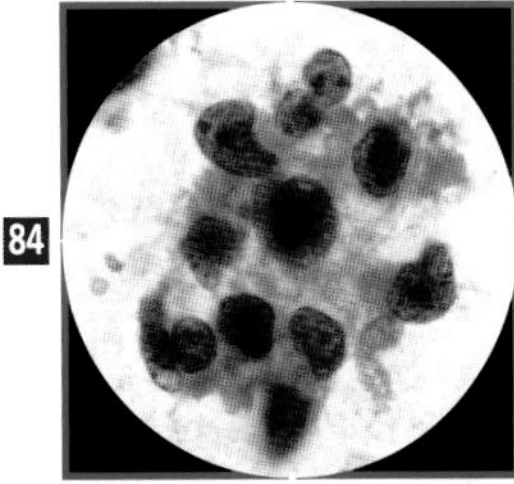
84

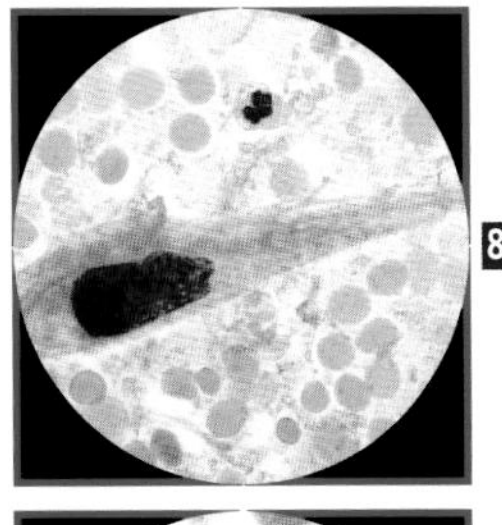
85

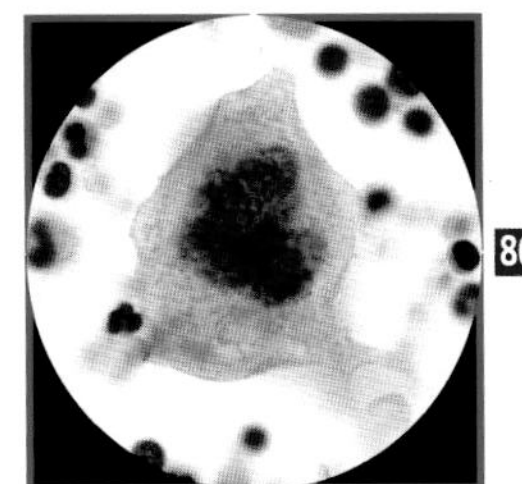
86

Malignant Mixed Mesodermal (Müllerian) Tumor (MMMT): The majority of MMMTs exfoliate only adenocarcinomatous cells or both adenocarcinoma and sarcomatous cells. The minority shed only sarcomatous cells [Kanbour 1989, Valente 1992]. Adenocarcinoma may form papillary or acinar clusters of cells with enlarged, irregular, pleomorphic nuclei with abnormal chromatin and prominent nucleoli, as well as cytoplasmic vacuolization [I8.99]. Sarcomatous features include the presence of isolated or loose aggregates of cells with elongated or caudate shapes and cyanophilic cytoplasm [85 I8.100]. Stromal sarcoma cells are small and round to spindle with scant, wispy, cyanophilic cytoplasm (comet cells [Kanbour 1989]). A positive washing specimen is prognostically important in low-stage tumors [Geszler 1986].

Squamous Cell Carcinoma: Squamous cell carcinoma is rarely identified in peritoneal washings, just as it is rarely found in effusions [86 I8.101] [Abu-Ghazaleh 1984, Kilgore 1984]. However, the small cell (poorly differentiated) type is more apt to exfoliate diagnostic cells [Abu-Ghazaleh 1984].

Germ Cell Tumors and other rare neoplasms can also be detected in peritoneal washings (see section on body cavity effusions).

"Ovarian" Tumors Arising in the Peritoneum: The peritoneum, the lymph node sinusoidal mesoderm, the ovarian capsule (germinal epithelium), and the serous cavities of the genital canal share a common embryologic origin in the coelomic epithelium [F8.1]. The peritoneal mesothelium and ovarian surface cells are structurally similar [Blaustein 1984]. These facts help explain why the peritoneum can give rise to all manner of ovarian and other genital tract–like tumors and tumor-like conditions as well as why the ovary can give rise to mesotheliomas, etc [Bollinger 1989, Dalrymple 1989, Genadry 1981, Mills 1988, Shen 1983, Truong 1990, Wick 1989]. In particular, the differential diagnosis of reactive mesothelial cell vs serous adenocarcinoma can be extremely difficult because the cells are so similar, both morphologically and embryologically.

Ovarian-like tumors arising by müllerian metaplasia of peritoneum are: endometriosis (mimics endometrium), endometrioid carcinoma (mimics endometrium), endosalpingiosis (mimics fallopian tube), serous cystadenoma/carcinoma (mimics fallopian tube), mucinous cystadenoma/carcinoma (mimics endocervix), decidualization.

The different types of müllerian structures are produced by the multipotential coelomic epithelium which forms müllerian ducts during embryogenesis [Lauchlan 1968,1984]. Also, tumors are not necessarily composed of a single cell type. For example, both serous and mucinous, even decidual, type cells are often present in the same tumor or lesion. Tubal metaplasia of the endometrium and endocervix also occurs. Endosalpingiosis, which is ectopic location of all three cell types of fallopian tube epithelium (ciliated, nonciliated, and intercalated), also arises from coelomic metaplasia. Ovarian mesotheliomas are another example.

F8.1 **Diagnostic Map**

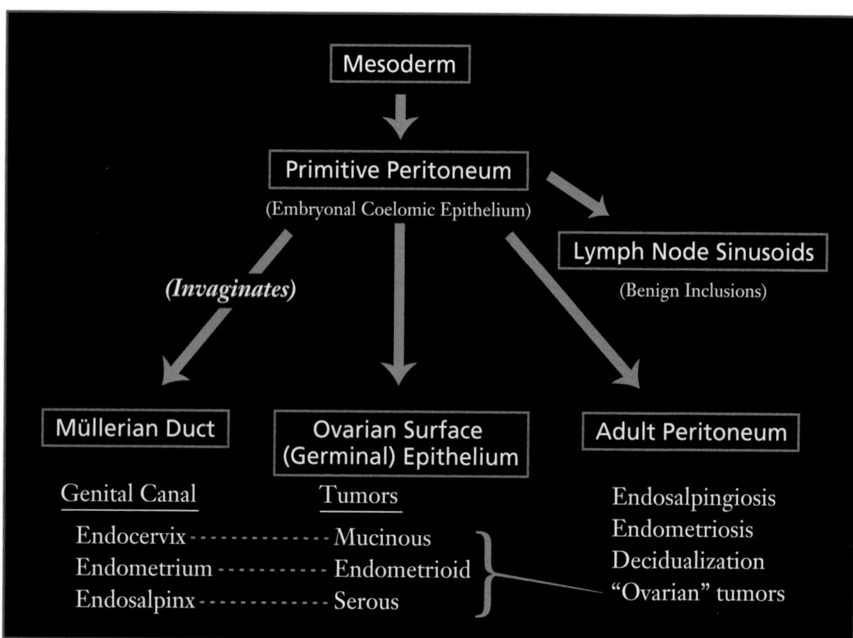

This map explains the origin of peritoneal "ovarian" tumors; endometriosis, endosalpingiosis, and decidualization of the peritoneum; benign peritoneal implants (whatever induces the ovarian tumor might also affect the peritoneum); benign lymph node inclusions; morphologic similarity of mesothelial cells and serous ovarian cells.

In diagnosing metastatic ovarian tumors, the question arises: "What is an implant (or inclusion) and what is borderline or fully malignant?"

Little nuclear atypia: Some nuclear pleomorphism, and nuclear membrane irregularity, but no significant abnormality (associated with inclusion or implant).

Moderate nuclear atypia: Prominent nucleoli, nuclear membrane infolding (associated with borderline tumor).

Marked nuclear atypia: Malignant criteria (associated with adenocarcinoma).

Positive cytology correlates with decreased survival in ovarian (and other) cancer.

Summary

The Rule: If a foreign population of cells can be identified in the fluid, it is malignant until proven otherwise.

The Corollary: If no foreign population of cells is present in the fluid, the fluid is benign until proven otherwise.

The Exceptions:

1. Mesothelioma. Continuum from benign appearing to malignant appearing cells. No foreign cell population.
2. Breast cancer (occasionally others). Mesothelial pattern of medium-sized bland cells.
3. Serous tumors (usually ovary). Tumor cells may closely resemble reactive mesothelial cells.
4. Lymphoma/leukemia. Mononuclear leukocytes usually present, thus not foreign population.
5. Virtually every cell malignant. Thus, no obviously foreign population.
6. Benign needle pickups. Liver, lung, muscle, fat, etc. (Foreign—but benign—population of cells.)

The Cheater:

Mucin (ie, epithelial mucin) positive cells in a fluid specimen are malignant.

Other Body Fluids

Synovial Fluid

The body cavities and joint space share similar features. Synovial fluid is formed by ultrafiltration of the plasma, to which synovial cells add the mesenchymal mucin, hyaluronic acid. Synovial fluid acts as a lubricant for joints and also provides nutrients to the articular cartilage. Normally, there is little fluid in the joint; increased fluid, or an effusion, indicates a pathologic process. Normal synovial fluid is transparent, straw colored, and highly viscous [Naib 1973]. The fluid must be heparinized for cytologic examination to prevent clotting. Examination of synovial fluid can lead to rapid definitive diagnosis of infections, crystals, and tumors as well as strongly suggesting diagnoses such as lupus erthythematosus [Broderick 1976, Currey 1976, Eisenberg 1984, Schumacher 1977, Villanueva 1987, A Wolf 1978].

Viscosity Test: Take a small amount of synovial fluid between fingers, pull apart. Normal synovial fluid will form a strand at least an inch long before breaking.

Mucin Clot Test: On addition of 5% acetic acid, normal synovial fluid forms a thick clot.

The Cells, etc

Synovial Cells: Synovial cells are usually present, but sparse [87 I8.104]. They resemble reactive mesothelial cells, with round to oval nuclei, fine chromatin, and abundant cytoplasm.

Inflammatory Cells: Inflammatory cells are normally scant, consisting mostly of monocytes and histiocytes [Naib 1973]. Mature lymphocytes and a few neutrophils may also be seen normally. The histiocytes have round to oval or bean-shaped nuclei, which are usually single, containing vesicular chromatin and often enlarged nucleoli. The cytoplasm is foamy and may contain azurophilic granules (Diff-Quik). Increased numbers of histiocytes are seen in such conditions as pigmented villonodular synovitis, hemarthrosis (due to trauma or hemophilia), rheumatoid arthritis, Reiter's syndrome, osteoarthritis, psoriatic arthritis, systemic lupus erythematosus, viral infections (especially parvovirus), tuberculosis, and glycoprotein storage disease [B Krishnan 1994]. Abundant neutrophils are characteristic of septic arthritis [88 I8.106], as well as in tuberculous arthritis, crystal-induced arthritis, Reiter's syndrome, and psoriatic arthritis. Lymphocytosis can be seen in rheumatoid arthritis, collagen vascular disease, and chronic infections. Monocytosis can be seen in crystal-induced and viral arthritis. A few eosinophils can occasionally be seen in hemorrhagic fluids and in the presence of systemic diseases such as rheumatoid arthritis, rheumatic fever, hypereosinophilic syndrome, parasitic disease, and many others. Numerous eosinophils, a rare finding, can be seen in parasitic infections, malignant effusions, postarthrography (in which air or contrast material was injected), or idiopathically [Brown 1986]. Mast cells are also commonly present in synovial fluid of diseased joints [Malone 1986].

Mott Cells: Mott cells are plasma cells with large numbers of Russell bodies [89 I8.107].

Cartilage Cells (Chondrocytes): Cartilage cells have a thick capsule-like structure surrounding granular or homogeneous cytoplasm [90 I8.105]. The nuclei are central, round, and often multiple, with granular chromatin and prominent nucleoli [Naib 1973]. The capsule is intensely metachromatic in Diff-Quik. These cells are not normally present, but can be seen following injury.

Crystals: Starch crystals and lipid droplets can be seen in polarized light as Maltese crosses [Reginato 1985, Ugai 1988]. (See also sections on gout and pseudogout for discussions on urate and calcium pyrophosphate.) Crystals are not normally present in synovial fluid.

Lipid-Laden Macrophages: Lipid-laden macrophages have been described in a variety of conditions, including traumatic arthritis, rheumatoid arthritis, chylous joint effusions, systemic fat necrosis, after transplantation, and in certain familial disorders of lipid metabolism, among others [Baer 1987].

LE Cells: LE cells are phagocytic neutrophils or monocytoid mononuclear cells containing relatively large pink or blue (Papanicolaou) homogeneous cytoplasmic inclusions that distend the cytoplasm and compress the nuclei [Freemont 1991]. They consist of degenerated nuclear material (with no recognizable chromatin pattern).

Tart Cells: Tart cells are similar in appearance to LE cells, but the inclusion has recognizable chromatin [Freemont 1991].

Ragocytes: Ragocytes are monolobulated or multilobulated neutrophils containing up to a dozen or so dark blue (Papanicolaou), coarse cytoplasmic inclusions, possibly abnormal immunoglobulin or DNA, ranging in size from 0.5 to 1.5 µm [Malinin 1967]. In unstained specimens, the inclusions are green [Freemont 1991]. Ragocytes are suggestive of, but not diagnostic of rheumatoid arthritis; they become more specific as their numbers increase.

Rieder Cells: Rieder cells are cells with N/C ratios greater than 70% and multilobed nuclei, with lobes showing symmetry around a pale central region [Freemont 1991].

88

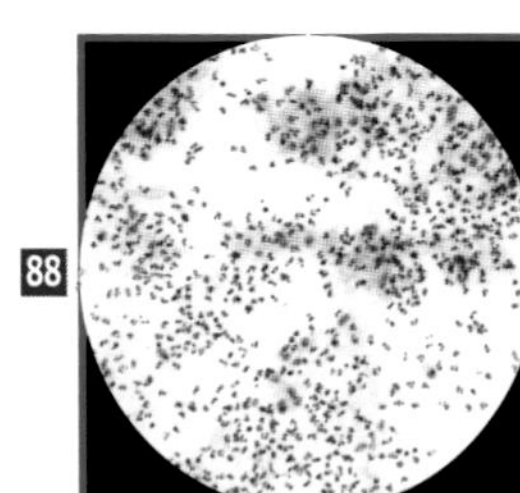

89

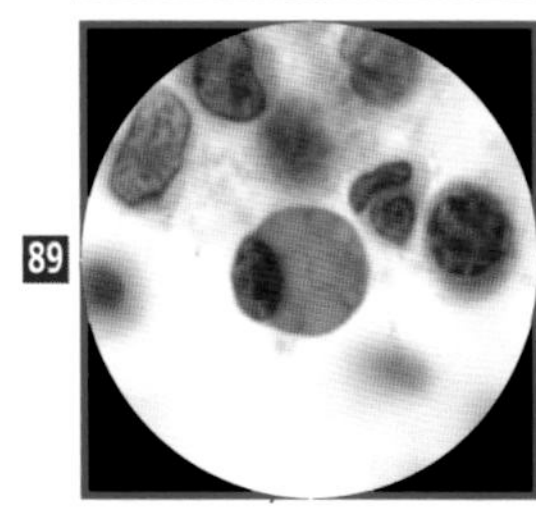

90

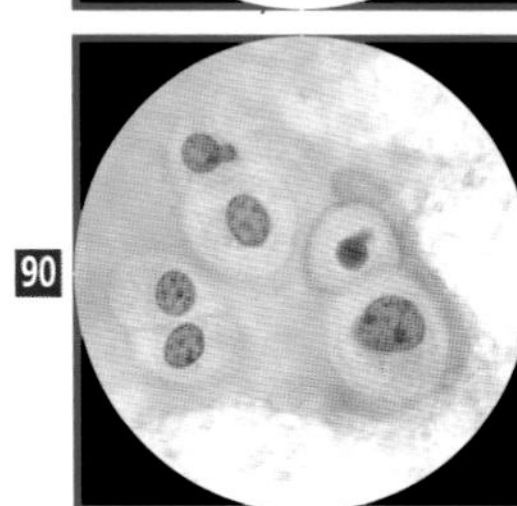

Diseases of Synovium and Joints

Rheumatoid Arthritis

In rheumatoid arthritis, the synovial fluid varies from clear to cloudy to yellow green. The viscosity is decreased and the mucin clot test produces a small, friable, irregular clot [Naib 1973]. However, the specimen rapidly clots without anticoagulant. In the acute phase, a moderate number of inflammatory cells (mostly neutrophils) are present [Bjelle 1982]. Later, marked chronic inflammation, including immature lymphocytes (lymphoblasts, immunoblasts), may be present [Eghtedari 1980, Traycoff 1976]. The diagnosis of rheumatoid arthritis is based on the presence of significant numbers of rheumatoid arthritis cells or ragocytes. The synovial cells are scattered and single. In the background, cholesterol crystals, cellular debris, and protein precipitate are present.

Rheumatic Arthritis

During the early, acute phase, the synovial fluid is scant, yellow, and cloudy. The viscosity test is negative, but the mucin clot test is about normal [Naib 1973]. Numerous inflammatory cells are present, mostly neutrophils and lymphocytes. Many of the cells are ragocytes. Papillary clusters of synovial cells may be seen, particularly late in the infection. Occasionally, histiocytes or giant cells are present, but Aschoff's bodies are not seen cytologically [Naib 1973]. No cartilage cells or crystals are present. The background contains debris and fibrin.

Degenerative Arthritis (Osteoarthritis)

The synovial fluid is usually scant, clear to yellow, and may contain occasional white cartilaginous particles [Naib 1973]. The viscosity and mucin clot tests are positive, as in normal fluid, but the fluid will not spontaneously coagulate. Inflammatory cells are few, mostly mature lymphocytes. Normal or reactive synovial cells may be present singly or in small sheets. The most characteristic feature is the presence of multinucleated cartilage cells, often in sheets or clusters rather than singly. The background is particularly clean. No ragocytes, crystals, or debris are present.

Systemic Lupus Erythematosus

Joint involvement occurs in about 90% of patients with systemic lupus erythematosus at some time during the course of their disease, but is usually mild [Labowitz 1971]. The amount of fluid is variable, but usually scant. The synovial fluid is yellow, transparent to slightly cloudy, and the viscosity and mucin clot test results are strongly positive [Naib 1973]. A variable (but not abundant) number of inflammatory cells, mostly neutrophils, are present. The synovial cells are few and single. No cartilage cells or crystals are present. The most characteristic feature is LE cells, which are usually present and easy to find [Naib 1973].

Infectious Arthritis

Septic arthritis can be due to different kinds of microbiologic agents such as virus, fungus, or bacteria, including mycobacteria [Clarris 1975, Cunningham 1979, Fraser 1981, George 1985]. (See "Reiter's Syndrome," below.)

In septic arthritis, the synovial fluid is usually abundant, gray or purulent, with decreased viscosity and negative mucin clotting test. The cytologic findings include abundant neutrophils (>100,000/µL) [91 I8.106]. Synovial cells are few, but occur in sheets rather than singly, and show advanced degenerative changes [Naib 1973]. Crystals are absent. Organisms are frequently identifiable, either free or in the cytoplasm of inflammatory cells.

Tuberculous arthritis can show either milky or purulent synovial fluid. Inflammatory cells are less abundant, and contain proportionately more lymphocytes [Naib 1973]. Cartilage cells are usually not seen. It may be difficult to identify acid-fast bacilli. Culture is preferable for diagnosis.

Reiter's Syndrome

Reiter's syndrome is chlamydial polyarthritis. The patients have a triad of nongonococcal urethritis, arthritis, and conjunctivitis [Spriggs 1978]. Mucocutaneous lesions are also frequent [Pekin 1967]. The synovial fluid is creamy and contains gray-yellow fibrin flakes [Naib 1973]. The viscosity and mucin clot test results are decreased. Numerous inflammatory cells are usually present, mostly monocytes, lymphocytes, and macrophages, early. Paradoxically, neutrophils appear later. The synovial cells are reactive and pleomorphic. Typical chlamydial cytoplasmic inclusions are found in many of the synovial cells, best appreciated using the Diff-Quik stain using a green filter [Naib 1973]. The background contains debris, fibrin, and protein, but no cartilage cells or crystals. Prompt therapy with appropriate antibiotics prevents irreversible joint injury.

91

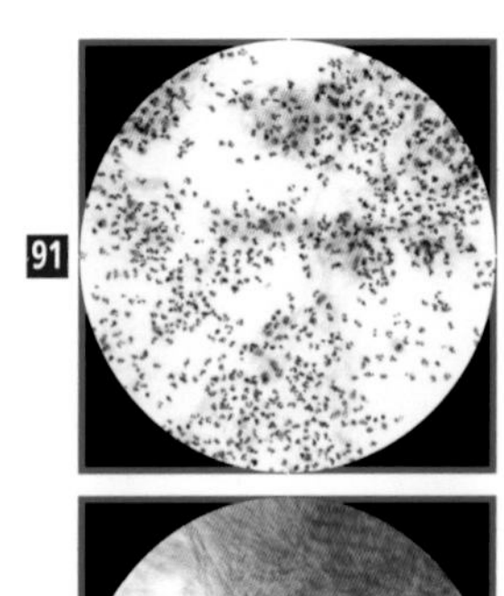

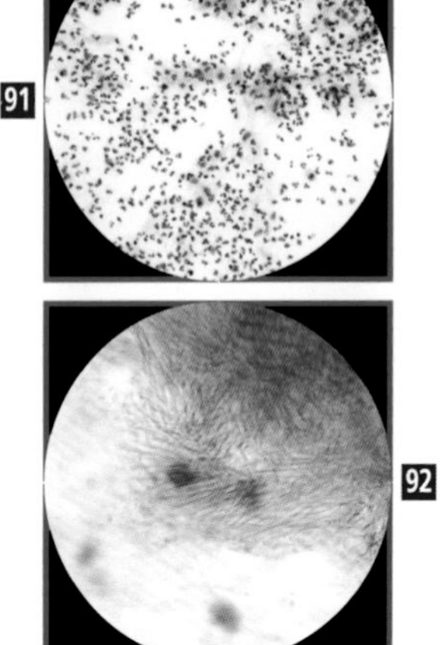

92

Traumatic Arthritis

Traumatic arthritis is one of the most common causes of a hemorrhagic synovial effusion. The fluid may be grossly bloody or xanthochromic. The viscosity and mucin clotting test findings are strongly positive [Naib 1973]. The findings are similar to septic arthritis, except that hemosiderin-laden macrophages as well as tissue fragments, including cartilage cells, muscle, or ligament, may be seen [Naib 1973]. Lipid-laden macrophages may also be present [Baer 1987]. The background contains debris and protein.

Villonodular Synovitis

Villonodular synovitis is inflammation of unknown etiology of the synovial membrane, usually involving the knee of young adult males. The fluid is pink or brown due to bleeding, with variable findings on viscosity and mucin-clotting tests, depending on the duration of the inflammation [Naib 1973]. Hemosiderin-laden histiocytes, synovial cells, and giant cells are seen. The most characteristic feature is the presence of multinucleated giant cells containing hemosiderin. However, giant cells also occur in other forms of synovitis as well as giant cell tumors. Papillary clusters of synovial cells may be seen. Birefringent (Maltese cross) lipid microspherules and foam cells may also be seen [Ugai 1988]. No other inclusions or crystals are present. The background contains RBCs and protein debris.

Gout

Gout is an autosomal dominant, inherited defect in purine metabolism. Gout is characterized by hyperuricemia and deposition of monosodium urate crystals in and about the joints. The effusion is relatively large. The synovial fluid is dense, yellow, and cloudy, with low viscosity. The mucin clot test produces an abnormal, fragile, small clot [Naib 1973]. During an acute attack, a modest number of inflammatory cells are present, mostly degenerated neutrophils. No cytoplasmic inclusions are present. Synovial cells are few, and usually markedly degenerated. Occasional poorly preserved cartilage cells may be seen in advanced, chronic disease. The diagnostic feature, however, is the presence of birefringent, needle-shaped urate crystals with pointed ends, which may be free or phagocytosed by neutrophils [92 I8.108] [Suprun 1973]. Platelike crystals and spherulites have also been reported [Sen 1993]. Using compensated polarization, the crystals show strong negative birefringence [Currey 1968, Zaharopoulos 1980]. The crystals are about 5 to 10 µm long, but may be broken into dust-like fragments [Naib 1973].

Pseudo-Gout/Chondrocalcinosis

Pseudogout is an autosomal recessive, inherited abnormality of inorganic pyrophosphate metabolism, resulting in deposition of calcium pyrophosphate dihydrate crystals in the matrix of fibrocartilaginous structures of major joints. The volume of the effusion is variable. The synovial fluid is yellow, cloudy, and has an abnormally low viscosity. The mucin clot test result is positive. A variable (but not abundant) number of inflammatory cells is present, depending on the stage of the lesion. Ragocytes are seen in many cases, but are fewer than in rheumatoid arthritis. Scattered, single, often degenerated synovial cells are present. Occasional cartilage cells may be seen, particularly in long-standing cases. The diagnostic feature is the presence of calcium pyrophosphate crystals, which are birefringent, rhomboid or rod shaped crystals with square ends. Using compensated polarization, the crystals show weak positive birefringence [Currey 1968, Zaharopoulos 1980]. They are about 5 µm long and are seldom fragmented [Naib 1973].

Reactive Arthritis

Reactive arthritis refers to development of oligoarthropathy in association with gastrointestinal or urinary tract infection, but without demonstrable organisms in the joint [Freemont 1991].

Tumors

A variable amount of hemorrhagic effusion may accumulate in joints involved by primary or secondary tumors. Suspect this diagnosis in effusions that reaccumulate rapidly after aspiration [Naib 1973]. Results of viscosity and mucin clot tests are variable. Usually few inflammatory cells are present. Occasional single synovial cells or degenerated cartilage cells may be seen. No crystals are present. The key diagnostic feature is the presence of tumor cells, singly or in clusters, the morphology of which depends on the particular type of tumor. The most common tumor types are squamous cell carcinoma, adenocarcinoma, and lymphoma/leukemia [Li 1991, Meisels 1961, Moutsopoulos 1975, Newton 1984, Weinberger 1981]. The lung is the most common source of metastatic carcinoma [Fam 1980, Newton 1984]. Primary neoplasms, including osteosarcoma and giant cell tumor, also occur. Note, however, that synovial sarcoma rarely arises in the joints. Recognizing tumor cells is usually straightforward, since they are foreign to the joint space.

Nipple Discharge

There are both physiologic and pathologic nipple discharges [Kline 1964, Saphir 1950]. Physiologic nipple discharge is usually bilateral, arises from multiple ducts, is nonspontaneous, and is usually produced by suction or manual expression. True pathologic nipple discharges are usually unilateral and arise from a single duct (but can be bilateral or involve multiple ducts), are spontaneous, persistent (but may be intermittent), and caused by pathologic lesions of the intraductal epithelium [Urban 1978]. Areolar gland discharge should be differentiated from nipple discharge.

Abnormal nipple discharge is an important clinical finding, ranking second only to the presence of a breast mass as the presenting complaint of patients undergoing breast surgery [Leis 1988]. In women with dominant breast masses, about 10% to 15% of benign lesions and about 2.5% to 3% of malignant lesions are associated with a nipple discharge [Barnes 1966, Leis 1988,1989a,b, Urban 1978]. Thus, the large majority of abnormal nipple discharges are associated with benign conditions [Devitt 1985, Holleb 1966, Johnson 1991, Leis 1988,1989a,b, Murad 1982, Rimsten 1976, Tyler 1982], most commonly fibrocystic disease, physiologic disturbances, and papillomas. A wide range of other benign conditions can be associated with an abnormal nipple discharge. Milk secretion under appropriate conditions is normal (lactation); however, milk secretion can be abnormal (galactorrhea). Brain lesions or encephalitis as well as pituitary or other endocrine abnormalities, including hypothyroidism, can cause galactorrhea [Groll 1975, Leis 1988,1989a,b, Newman 1983]. Drugs such as oral contraceptives (particularly when used irregularly), phenothiazines, antihypertensives, tranquilizers, and psychotropics are other possible causes [Lancet 1983, Tetirick 1980]. Stimulation of the nipple, coitus, and stress can also cause a milky discharge [Lancet 1983, Newman 1983, Rohn 1984, Tetirick 1980]. Milky discharges can be seen in newborns ("witches' milk"); bloody nipple discharges have also been reported in infants [Berkowitz 1983, Fenster 1984, Miller 1990, Sigalas 1985, Stringel 1986]. In many cases, the cause remains undetermined [Johnson 1991].

Abnormal nipple discharges should be examined cytologically, because cases of cancer can be picked up with this simple diagnostic technique [Papanicolaou 1956b,1958, Rangwala 1989]. Malignant nipple discharges are usually unilateral, bloody, and occur in older patients [Funderburk 1969, Johnson 1991, Seltzer 1970]. Although bloody nipple discharges are suspicious, they are more often caused by benign lesions, such as papilloma, duct ectasia, fibrocystic disease/fibroadenoma, or lactation, than by cancer [Chaudary 1982, Devitt 1985, Funderburk 1969, Lafreniere 1990, McDermott 1987, Rimsten 1976]. Most patients with a nipple discharge and breast cancer will also have an abnormal mammogram and a palpable breast mass, but a few patients have no other abnormality [Fischermann 1969, Johnson 1991, Leis 1988, Takeda 1990, Tetirick 1980].

Patients with an abnormal nipple discharge from a single duct may be considered for duct excision, particularly when the cytologic findings are abnormal [Fung 1990, Locker 1988]. Galactography (injection of contrast medium into lactiferous ducts followed by mammography) or injection of dye can help select the area for surgery [Choudhury 1989, Detraux 1985, Grillo 1990, Philip 1984, S Rubin 1988, Tabár 1983]. However, these procedures are not only cumbersome but provide little diagnostic information (only localizes the lesion) [Devitt 1985, Inaji 1987]. Biochemical tests, such as LDH or carcinoembryonic antigen determination, may be used as adjuncts in diagnosis of nipple discharges [Inaji 1987, Scanlon 1981].

Nipple discharges are rare in men, but are always abnormal. Gynecomastia is the most common cause. Although male breast cancer is rare, given a nipple discharge, particularly a bloody discharge, a man's relative risk of cancer is greater than a woman's [Holleb 1966, Johnson 1991, Leis 1988,1989a,b]. The cytology of breast cancer in men is similar to that in women [Fujii 1986].

Although nipple discharge cytology is highly specific, a malignant diagnosis should be confirmed with other appropriate techniques (fine needle aspiration or tissue biopsy) before proceeding with definitive therapy such as mastectomy. False positives occur, eg, due to atypical hyperplasia in fibrocystic disease [Knight 1986]. Unfortunately, nipple discharge cytology is not sensitive to the presence of malignancy [Ciatto 1986]. False negatives are common; moreover, most breast cancers are not associated with a nipple discharge. However, when special sampling devices (eg, breast pumps) are employed, early cancer may be detected [Abe 1985, Buehring 1979, Leif 1980, Sartorius 1977]. *Any patient with a suspicious breast mass or abnormal mammogram must be appropriately investigated* regardless of the presence or absence of a nipple discharge or its cytologic findings.

The Cells

Duct Cells: Normal duct cells are small epithelial cells that can be seen singly or in small, compact clusters [King 1975a, Papanicolaou 1958]. They are round to oval when single, but may be somewhat molded in clusters. The nucleus has smooth nuclear membranes and is hyperchromatic with granular chromatin; nucleoli are rarely prominent [Papanicolaou 1958, Vilaplana 1975]. The cytoplasm is scant and homogeneous. Good intercellular cohesion and uniformity of the cells are clues to a benign process.

Large or papillary clusters and, of course, cytologic atypia are suspicious findings. Hyperplasia and atypical hyperplasia show progressive increase in the number of cells, with increasing pleomorphism, N/C ratios, chromatin abnormalities, and nucleoli [King 1983, Sartorius 1977]. The degree of atypia directly correlates with the risk of breast cancer [Wrensch 1992].

Apocrine Metaplastic Cells: Apocrine cells are medium sized [93 I8.110]. Apocrine change is recognized by the presence of more abundant, finely granular cytoplasm that usually stains orange or occasionally blue with the Papanicolaou stain [Vilaplana 1975]. The nuclei are regular, hyperchromatic, and may have prominent nucleoli [King 1975a].

Foam Cells: Foam cells are the most commonly observed cells in nipple discharges. Foam cells are always benign, but their presence does not exclude malignancy. Foam cells are large, with abundant, vacuolated—or foamy—cytoplasm due to lipid content [94 I8.109]. They usually appear singly, but can form loose clusters. The nuclei are small and eccentric, with low N/C ratios. The nuclei frequently exhibit various signs of degeneration, particularly pyknosis [Papanicolaou 1958]. Nucleoli may be prominent in some cases [King 1975a]. Foam cells can vary considerably in size and may exhibit binucleation or multinucleation [Papanicolaou 1956b,1958]. The origin of these cells (epithelial vs histiocytic) has been controversial, but they are apparently derived from bone marrow monocytes [Dabbs 1993].

Miscellaneous Cells: Squamous cells and anucleate squames from the nipple may be seen. Also, inflammatory cells, including neutrophils, lymphocytes, and histiocytes, as well as giant cells and necrotic cells can occur in various diseases. Microcalcifications can also be seen [King 1975b, Zimmerman 1977].

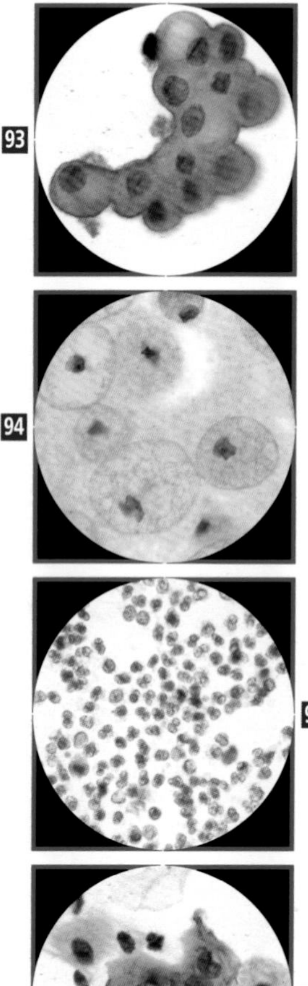

Cytology of Abnormal Nipple Discharge

Nipple secretions can range from watery to thick, and can be colorless, milky, serous, green, brown, black, purulent, or bloody [Johnson 1991, Leis 1988,1989a,b]. Any of these appearances can be associated with malignancy [Johnson 1991], although a bloody discharge is most suspicious [Leis 1988, Rimsten 1976, Takeda 1982,1990]. Milky discharges are most common, but diagnostic attention should be focused on the brain and endocrine system, rather than the breast [Tetirick 1980].

Most nipple discharge specimens have a variably stained proteinaceous background [Johnson 1991]. In many cases, the smear is acellular [Johnson 1991]. Foam cells or a few uniform duct cells are benign findings, but do not exclude malignancy. Neutrophils correlate with clinical mastitis. RBCs correlate with discharges described clinically as bloody.

Suspicious Findings

Bloody discharge
Papillary aggregates
Cytologic atypia

Ductal cells with atypia are suspicious for malignancy. Papillary aggregates are also suspicious, particularly if there is cytologic atypia [Takeda 1982,1990]. These findings require further investigation. However, even the presence of frankly malignant-appearing cells should be confirmed before definitive therapy. Conversely, absence of any of the features does not exclude malignancy.

Galactorrhea: Galactorrhea is abnormal secretion of milky fluid from the nipple. It can be caused by a variety of conditions, including pituitary adenoma. The cytology shows foam cells in a heavy lipoproteinaceous background [Murad 1973b]. Blood is usually absent.

Duct Ectasia: Duct ectasia refers to duct obstruction and dilatation, with accumulation of secretions [O'Brien 1982]. The discharge tends to be bilateral and to exit from multiple ducts [Lorenzen 1986]. The secretion varies from bloody to green, brown, gray, black, or sometimes clear, and may have an odor. Multicolored, sticky secretion is most characteristic; often each duct discharges material of a different color [Devitt 1985, Leis 1988]. The smear may be very cellular, showing numerous foam cells, including large, multinucleated forms, and small clusters of duct cells in a proteinaceous background [Insabato 1992].

Infection/Inflammation

A variety of infectious agents can be identified in nipple discharge specimens, including virus [Kobayashi 1993], fungus [Bertini 1975, Masukawa 1972], microfilaria [Lahiri 1975], and mites [Fidler 1978]. Bacterial infections are associated with acute inflammation [95 I8.111]

Tuberculosis of the breast can mimic breast cancer clinically, including displaying the presence of a breast mass, peau d'orange, and a bloody nipple discharge [Barnes 1966]. The cytology may show epithelioid histiocytes and giant cells; in addition, neutrophils, foam cells, necrotic material, and sometimes acid-fast bacilli may be identified [Nayar 1984].

Lactating sinus granuloma also is associated with squames and a giant cell reaction [96 I8.112].

Intraductal Papilloma

Intraductal papilloma is a relatively common benign disease that may be associated with a bloody nipple discharge. A bloody discharge limited to a single duct is particularly characteristic of this lesion [Lorenzen 1986, Tetirick 1980]. Duct excision can be curative without disfiguring the breast. The cytology shows cohesive papillary clusters of ductal cells, which may show slight nuclear pleomorphism [97 I8.113, 98 I8.114]. In addition, foam and apocrine cells may be present, which suggests a benign diagnosis. Red blood cells are frequently seen in the background [Insabato 1992, Papanicolaou 1956b]. The differential diagnosis with papillary carcinoma may be difficult or impossible in exfoliative cytology [Kjellgren 1964, Papanicolaou 1956b]. Benign papillomas may shed atypical cells, while papillary carcinoma may exfoliate bland uniform cells [99 I8.115, 100 I8.116]. Therefore, the mere presence of papillary clusters is a suspicious finding [Fleming 1955]. A possible diagnosis would be "papillary clusters, neoplasm not excluded."

Breast Cancer

Carcinoma of the breast, whether in situ or invasive, can shed cells into the ductal system. Therefore, malignant cells are sometimes observed in nipple discharge.

Cytologic examination shows abnormal cells singly or in crowded clusters. The malignant cells are typically enlarged, with pleomorphic, hyperchromatic nuclei, irregular nuclear membranes, coarse chromatin, and prominent or macronucleoli [101 I8.117, I8.118] [Murad 1973b, Papanicolaou 1956b]. Papillary or spherical cell clusters, often with smooth outlines (community borders), are an abnormal finding suggestive of malignancy [99 I8.115] [Uei 1980]. Loss of cohesion also suggests malignancy [Murad 1973b]. The background may be clean, hemorrhagic, or necrotic (tumor diathesis). Benign foam cells may be present. Calcification, and rarely, psammoma bodies, can also be seen [Masukawa 1972, Uei 1980].

Benign papillomas can show similar clusters of cells, including nuclear atypia; therefore, caution is warranted in diagnosis of malignancy. Definitive therapy should not be based on exfoliative nipple cytology. However, positive cytologic findings may convince the patient of the need for further investigation [Fleming 1955]. Negative cytology does not exclude cancer.

97

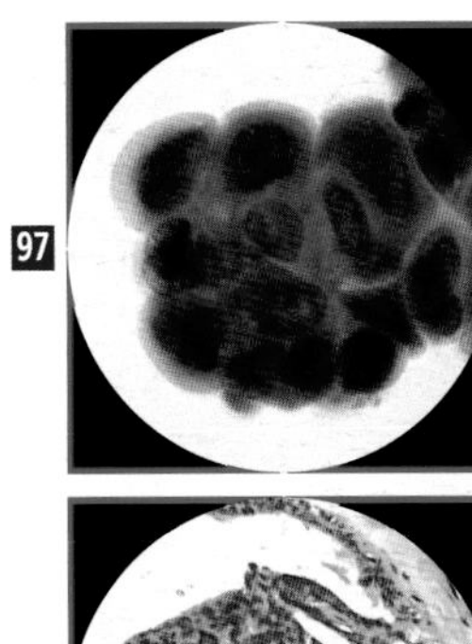

98

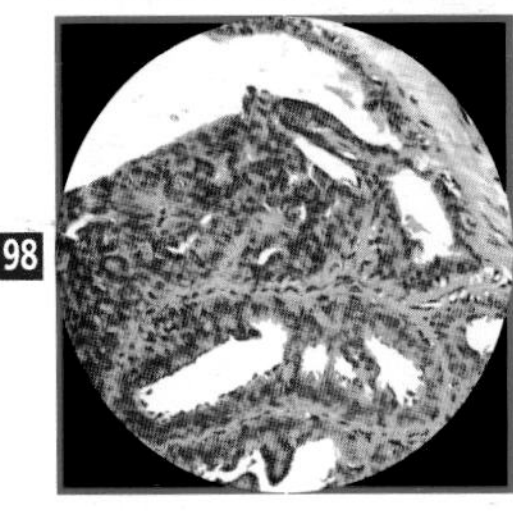

99

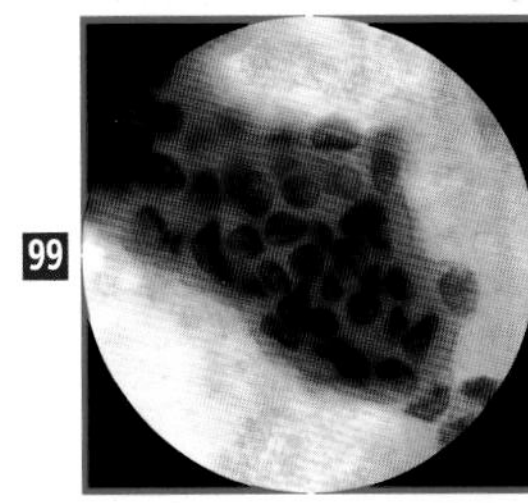

100

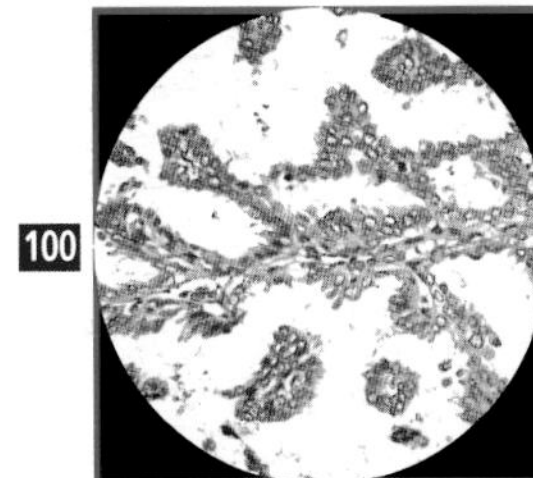

101

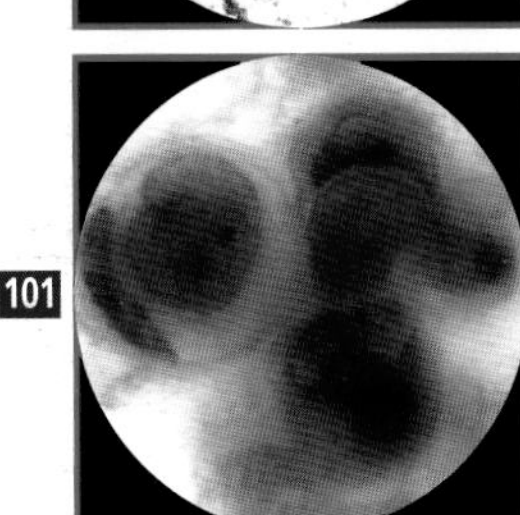

Paget's Disease

Paget's disease is involvement of the nipple ducts by an underlying breast cancer, which can be either in situ or invasive. Clinically, Paget's disease may present as an eczematous, crusting, or ulcerating lesion. There may be a nipple discharge, or the lesion can be directly sampled by scraping the nipple. The cytology shows Paget cells, which are large carcinoma cells with abnormal nuclei, prominent nucleoli, and abundant dense or vacuolated cytoplasm that may contain mucin [Masukawa 1975, Samarasinghe 1993]. Cell balls, papillae, or acinar arrangement may be seen. A characteristic feature is the presence of cell-in-cell patterns, which may suggest squamous differentiation. A background of keratinous debris and reactive squamous cells may add to the impression of a squamous lesion [Samarasinghe 1993]. Rarely, primary (pure) squamous cell carcinoma arises in the breast and can present with a nipple discharge containing malignant squamous cells [Uzoaru 1994]. Melanoma is also frequently mentioned in the differential diagnosis of Paget's disease. However, melanoma of the nipple is exceedingly rare, and mucin positivity, if present, rules out this diagnosis.

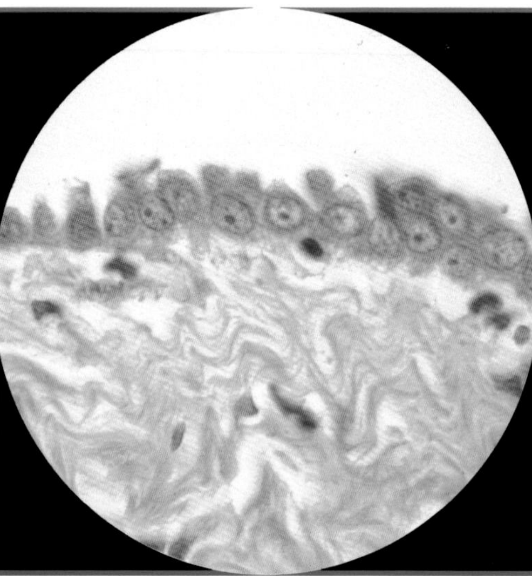

I8.1
Serous membrane. Connective tissue support is lined by single layer of mesothelial cells. Normally the mesothelial cells are flat (squamous in the traditional histologic sense), but when irritated the mesothelial cells become plump and cuboidal, with reactive changes in the nuclei (eg, prominent nucleoli), and may stratify or even form papillae (papillary hyperplasia) complete with psammoma bodies.

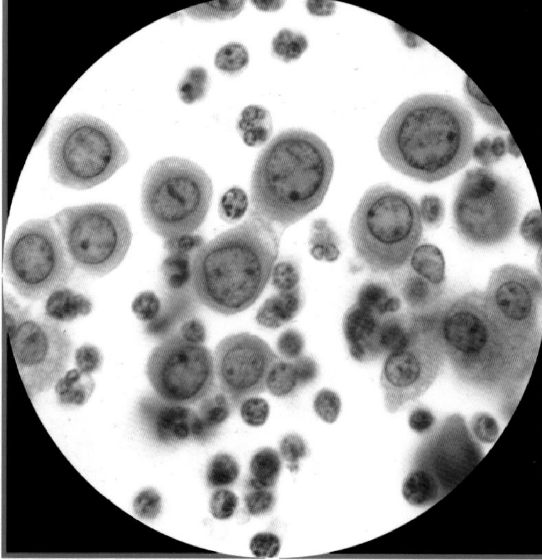

I8.2
Mesothelial cells. An effusion is always a pathologic condition, and mesothelial cells in an effusion always show reactive changes of various degrees. Note nuclear enlargement and a prominent nucleolus but fine chromatin and a smooth nuclear membrane.

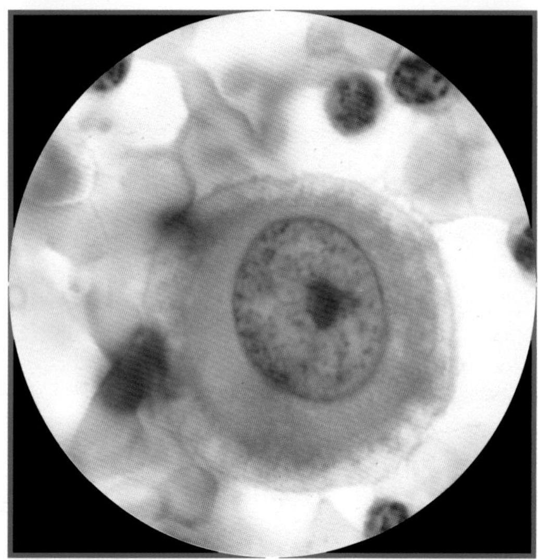

I8.3
Mesothelial cells. The cytoplasm of the reactive cells is frequently rather dense, particularly in the central portion of the cell. There is often a lacy skirt around the cell, a characteristic feature of reactive mesothelial cells. (Oil)

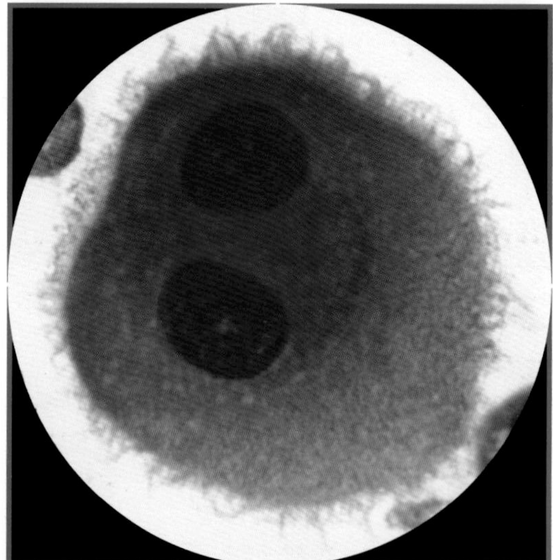

I8.4
Mesothelial cell. Occasionally metachromatic red "whiskers" or fringes, which are prominent microvilli, can be seen in Diff-Quik. (Oil)

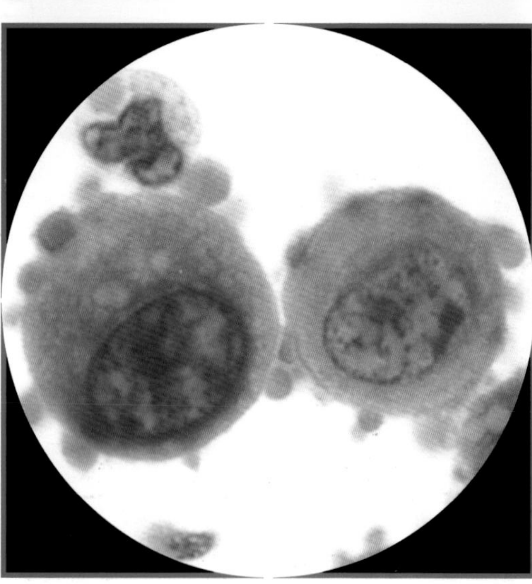

I8.5
Mesothelial cells. Reactive nuclear changes (enlargement, pleomorphism, and prominent nucleoli as well as chromatin degeneration) may suggest malignancy. In contrast with malignancy, marked pleomorphism, irregular nuclear membranes, and multiple or macronucleoli are not present. A key benign feature is that all of the (noninflammatory) cells look like mesothelial cells, ie, there is no foreign population of cells. (Oil)

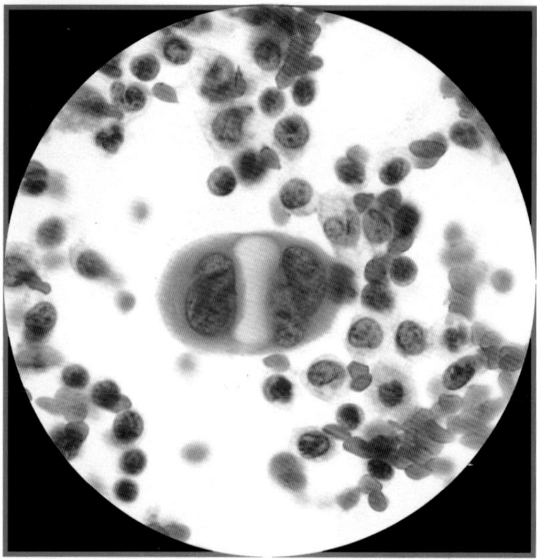

I8.6
Mesothelial cells. Characteristic window can be seen between adjacent cells. Windows are seldom found between malignant glandular cells.

I8.7
Mesothelial cells. An example of characteristic mesothelial cell "hugging" is seen at the center of the field.

I8.8
Mesothelial cells. Mitotic figures can be seen in benign mesothelial cells; their presence is not diagnostic of malignancy unless definitely abnormal.

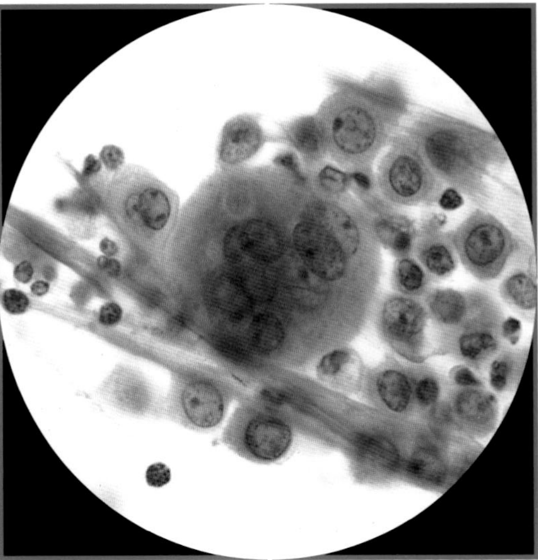

I8.9
Mesothelial cells. Occasional, multinucleated giant mesothelial cells can be seen in reactive conditions.

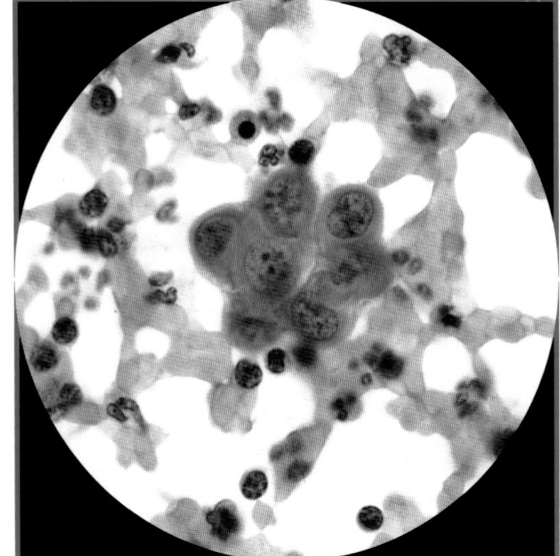

I8.10
Mesothelial cells. Clusters of mesothelial cells usually have knobby or flower-like outlines; in contrast, metastatic carcinoma usually has smooth, community borders.

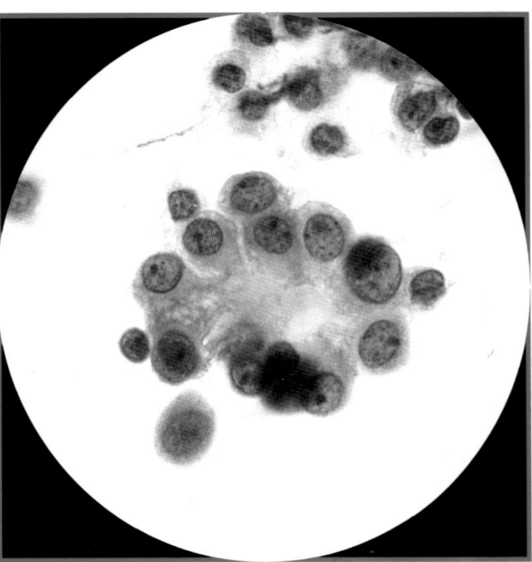

I8.11
Mesothelial cells. Gland-like cluster of benign mesothelial cells mimicking adenocarcinoma. Note that the component cells are identical to the other reactive mesothelial cells, and do not constitute a foreign population.

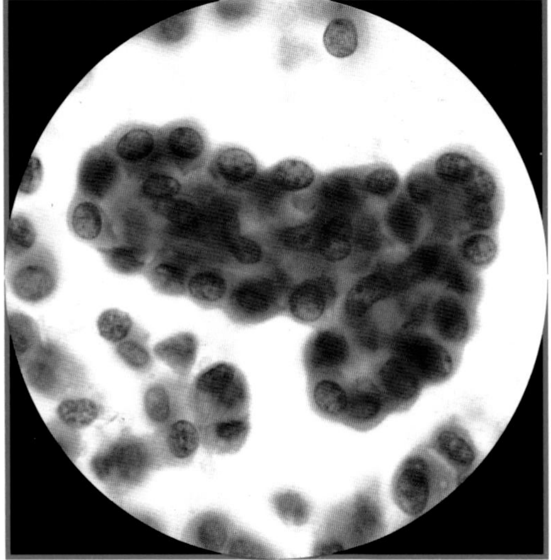

I8.12
Mesothelial cells. Papillary clusters suggestive of papillary carcinoma can be seen in papillary hyperplasia of the mesothelium.

I8.13
Mesothelial cells. Degenerative vacuoles (crystal clear because they only contain water and electrolytes—no secretory products) are common in mesothelial cells and sometimes give the cells a signet ring appearance (not to be mistaken for signet ring cell carcinoma). A mucicarmine stain, if performed, would be negative in benign mesothelial cells.

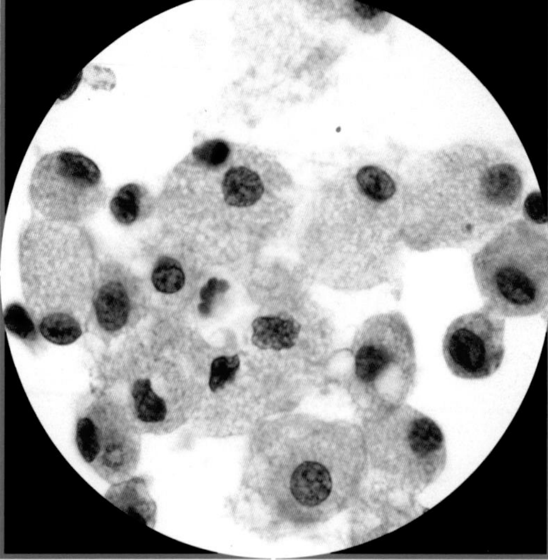

I8.14
Histiocytes. Usually present in fluids, particularly prominent in cancer, tuberculosis, and embolism. Histiocytes vary from small to large to even giant (rare). They do not form molded groups and no windows are seen between cells (in contrast with mesothelial cells). The cytoplasm varies from foamy to granular, and may contain inclusions. Nuclei are eccentrically located and classically bean-shaped, but vary from round to oval, and typically have salt-and-pepper chromatin.

I8.15
Hemosiderin-laden histiocyte. Hemosiderin is a refractile golden brown pigment. The presence of hemosiderin indicates old bleeding.

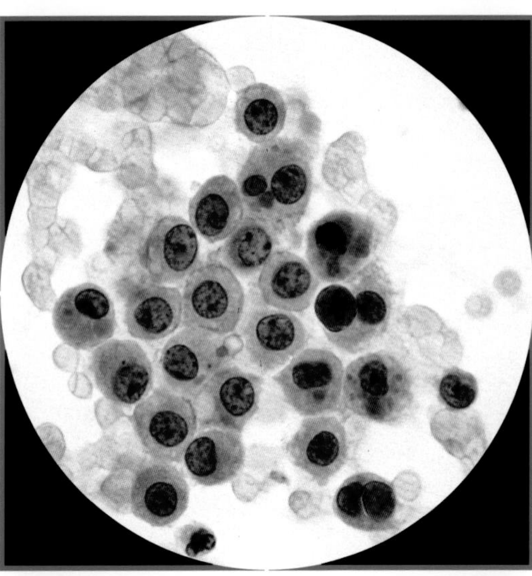

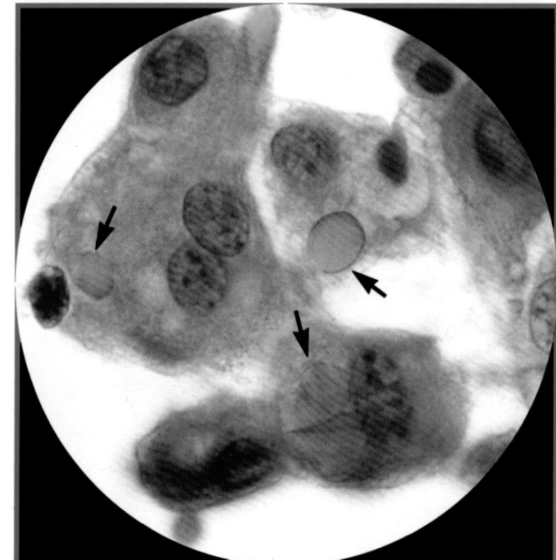

I8.16
Erythrophagocytosis. Hematoma due to infarct, trauma, or neoplasm is suggested. Erythrophagocytosis can also be seen in association with dialysis therapy. Note phagocytosed red blood cells (arrows).

I8.17
Sickled cells. Crescent or shallow S-shaped red blood cells are associated with sickle cell anemia. (Oil)

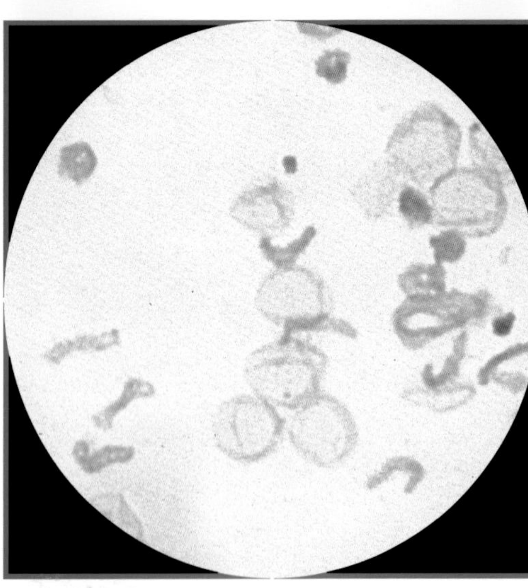

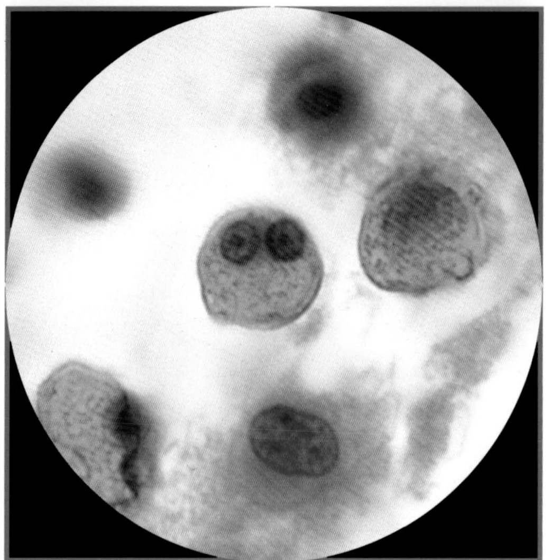

I8.18
Eosinophilic effusion. Most cases are thought to be related to repeated taps, with introduction of air into a body cavity. This case was a drug-related hypersensitivity reaction (Tegretol®).

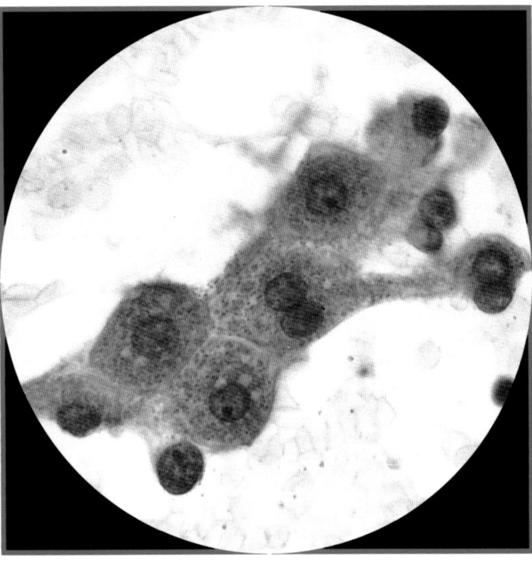

I8.19
Hepatocytes. A variety of unexpected cell types may be encountered as incidental "pickups" by the needle used to obtain the specimen. This is an example of hepatocytes that may be obtained at the time of paracentesis or, less commonly, thoracentesis. Although they represent a "foreign" population of cells, they are benign.

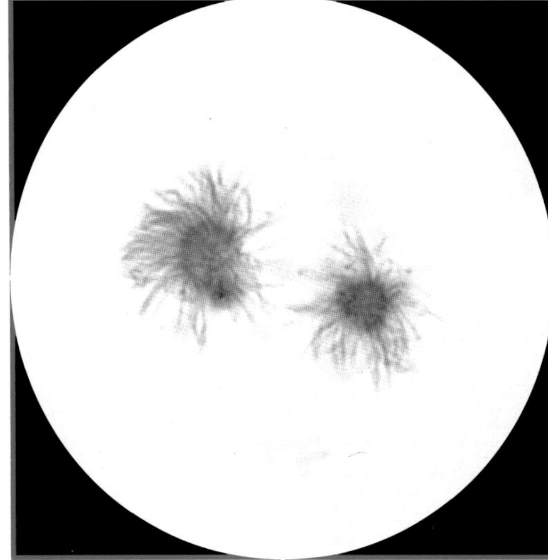

I8.20
Ciliocytophthoria. Detached ciliated tufts, usually of fallopian tube origin, are relatively common in peritoneal specimens from women. Cilia usually stain reddish. Do not mistake them for an organism.

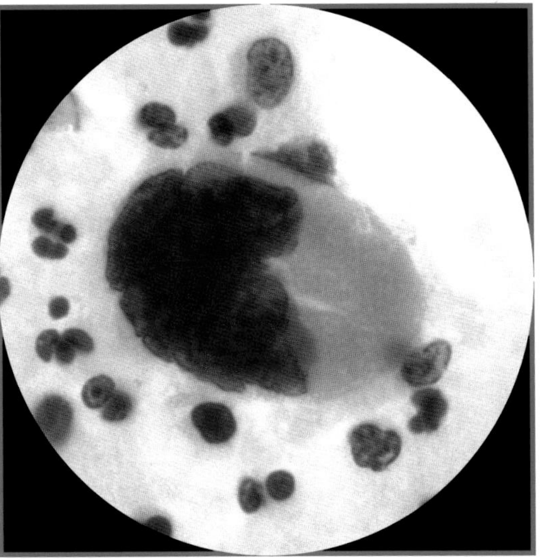

I8.21
Megakaryocyte. Giant cell with multilobated nucleus and granular cytoplasm. Although a rare finding, megakaryocytes are usually associated with conditions causing extramedullary hematopoiesis.

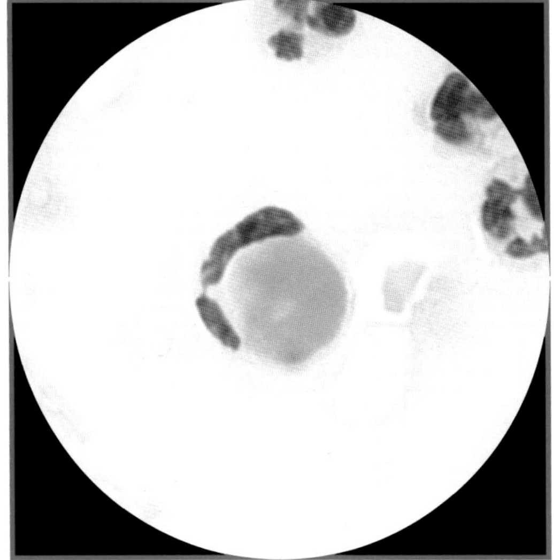

I8.22
LE cell. Neutrophil containing a homogeneous hematoxylin body. LE cells are associated with systemic lupus erythematosus, but can also be seen in drug-induced lupus erythematosus–like syndromes (eg, procainamide). (Oil)

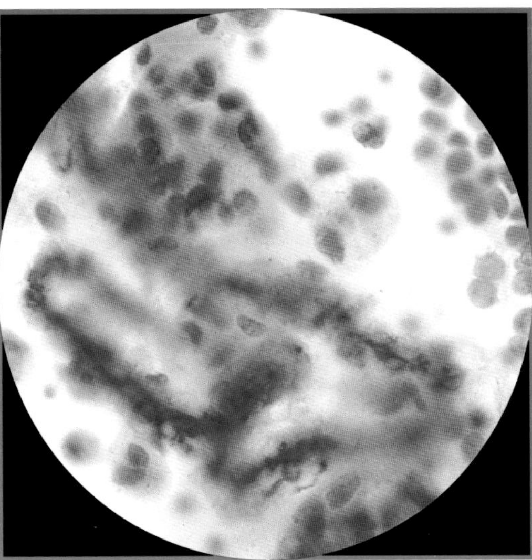

I8.23
Curschmann's spiral. Source of mucin may not be obvious, but in this case, the spiral was associated with malignancy (mixed müllerian tumor).

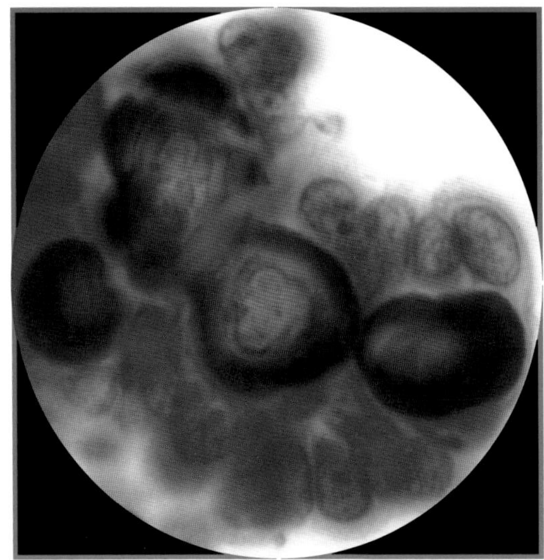

I8.24
Psammoma body. Not necessarily associated with malignancy, can also be seen in benign mesothelial hyperplasia, endosalpingiosis, etc. Ovarian cancer is illustrated.

I8.25
Collagen ball. Hyaline balls of collagen surrounded by mesothelial cells can be seen in benign or malignant mesothelial proliferations; not to be mistaken for adenocarcinoma.

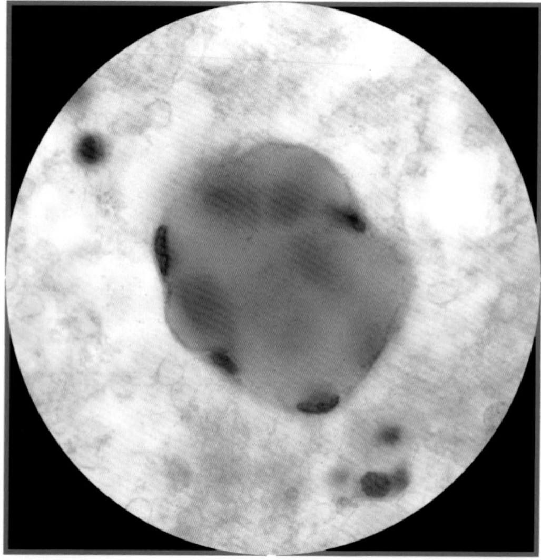

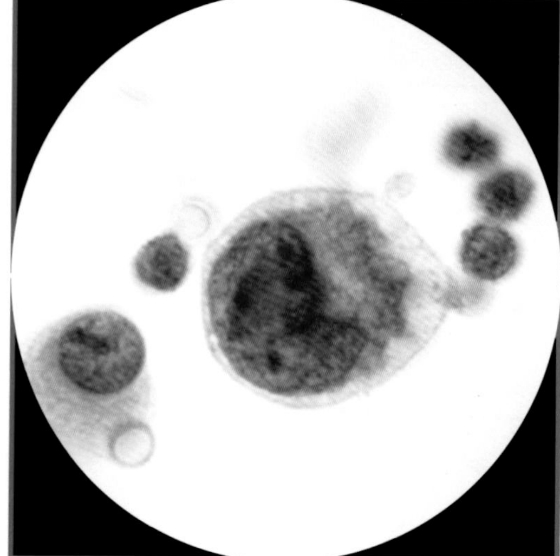

I8.26
Active hepatitis. Marked reactive atypia of mesothelial cells can be seen in active liver disease (hepatitis, active cirrhosis). When the entire slide is observed, there is a spectrum of abnormality, without a foreign population of cells. Be cautious when diagnosing malignancy in an effusion from a patient with active liver disease. (Oil)

I8.27
Uremia. Patients with uremia can have even more atypical mesothelial cells than those associated with hepatitis; atypical features include irregular, multiple nuclei and prominent nucleoli. Caution is warranted when diagnosing malignancy in an effusion from a uremic patient. (Oil)

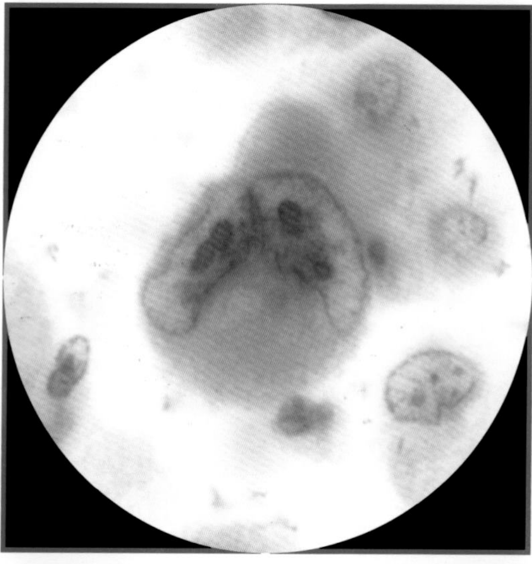

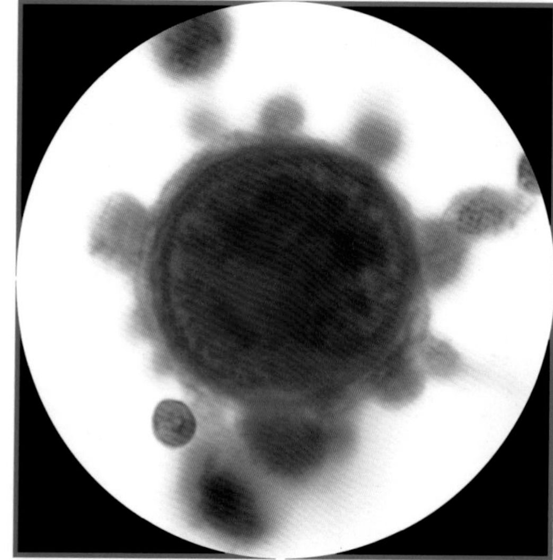

I8.28
Radiation/chemotherapy. Antineoplastic therapy can cause reactive changes in benign mesothelial cells, mimicking malignancy. The differential diagnosis may be particularly difficult because the patients usually have a history of cancer. An important clue is the absence of an extra or foreign population of tumor cells. (Oil)

I8.29
Tuberculous effusion. Abundance of lymphocytes and virtual absence of mesothelial cells are characteristic of tuberculous pleural effusions. In contrast with malignant lymphoma, the reactive lymphoid cells have a tendency to form aggregates, probably because they are trapped in fibrin associated with the inflammatory reaction. Although histiocytes may be seen, giant cells are unusual in a tuberculous effusion.

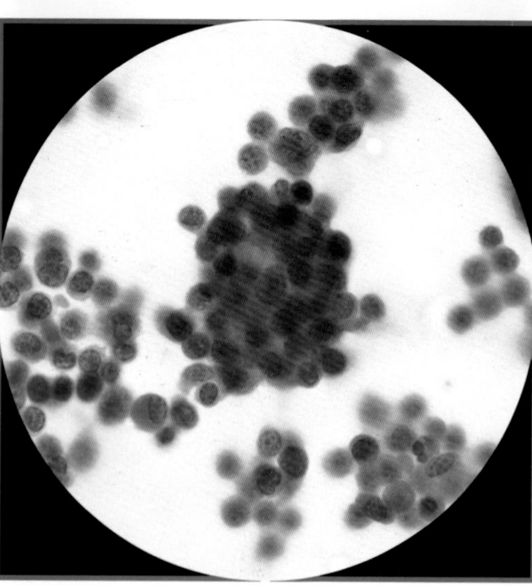

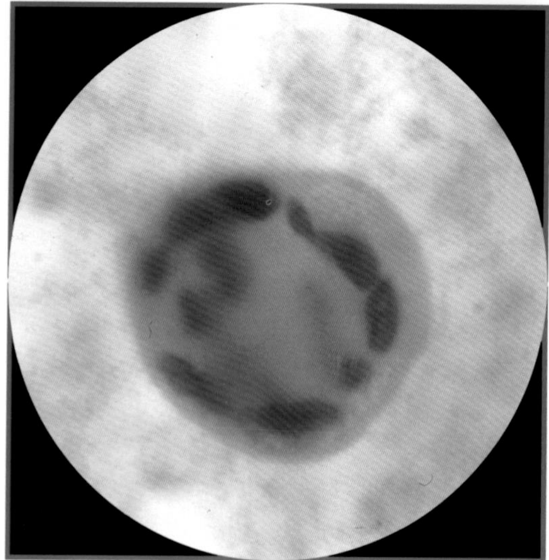

I8.30
Rheumatoid effusion. Rheumatoid effusions are characterized by a triad of giant cells (illustrated), epithelioid histiocytes, and necrotic debris. Mesothelial cells are sparse.

I8.31
Rheumatoid effusion. Epithelioid histiocytes frequently take on elongated carrot, spindle, or bizarre cell shapes, which may suggest keratinizing squamous cell carcinoma.

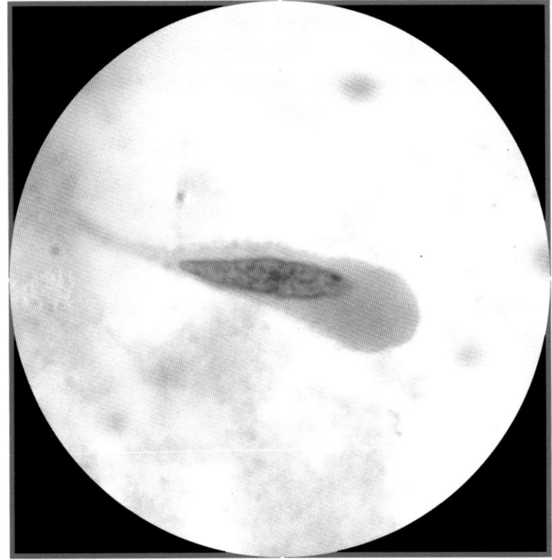

I8.32
Acute pancreatitis. Classically associated with a left-sided pleural effusion (but can be bilateral). Pancreatitis can also cause marked reactive atypia of the mesothelial cells. (Oil)

I8.33
Malignant effusion. A foreign population of cells in an effusion is malignant until proven otherwise. On the other hand, some tumors are composed of bland cells that mimic mesothelial cells, making the diagnosis difficult. Malignant effusions are a poor prognostic sign, but not all effusions in patients with cancer are due to their tumors, eg, the patient may have congestive heart failure.

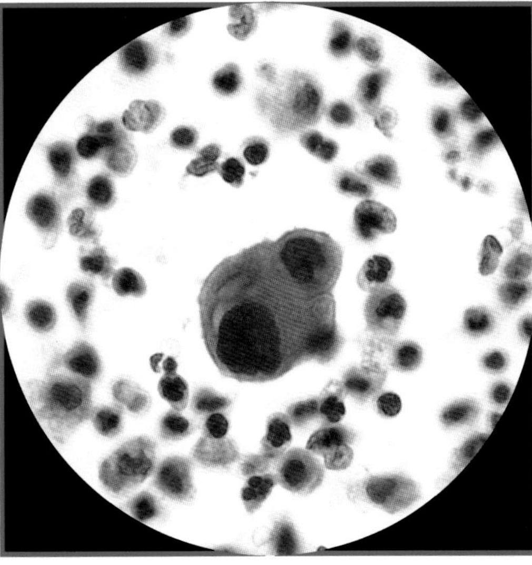

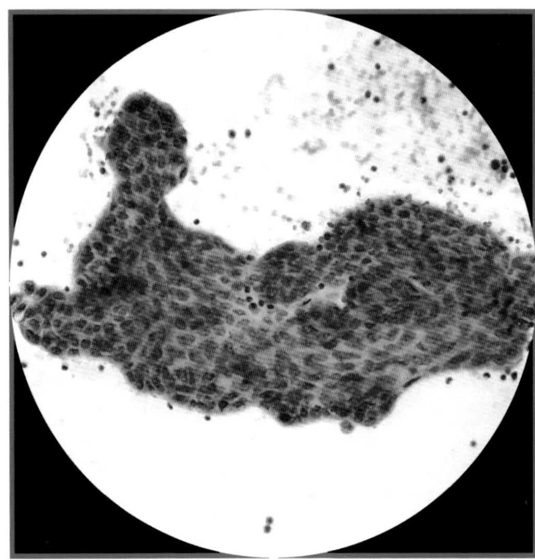

I8.34
Large cell groups. The presence of very large groups of cells strongly suggests malignancy. Benign mesothelial cells rarely exfoliate in very large groups. This is a very low power view of metastatic pancreatic cancer. (4×)

I8.35
Single cell pattern. Certain tumors, classically lymphomas (illustrated), but also melanomas, sarcomas, and some carcinomas (eg, lobular carcinoma), shed exclusively single cells.

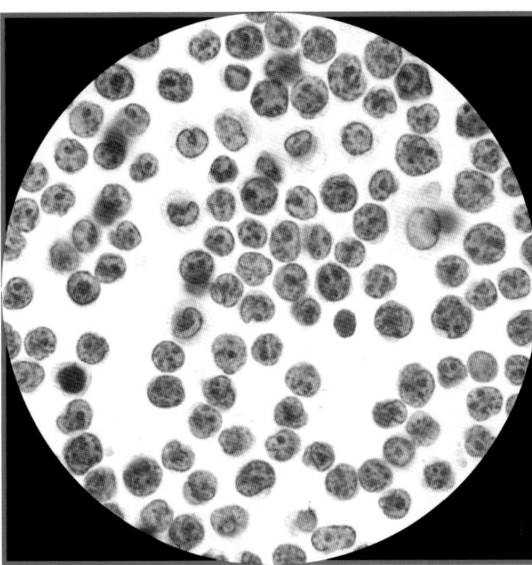

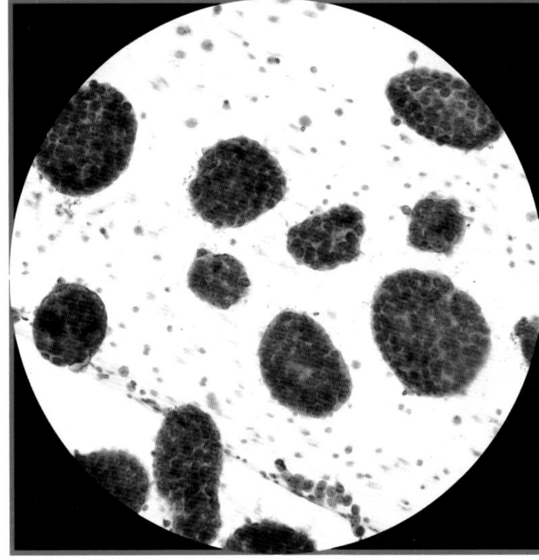

I8.36
Cell balls. Cell balls or morulas with smooth, community borders are a characteristic feature of metastatic adenocarcinoma. In contrast, irregular, knobby, flower-like outlines are more characteristic of groups of mesothelial cells, but neither finding is specific. Large proliferation spheres (also known as "cannonballs") are particularly characteristic of breast cancer (favors ductal type).

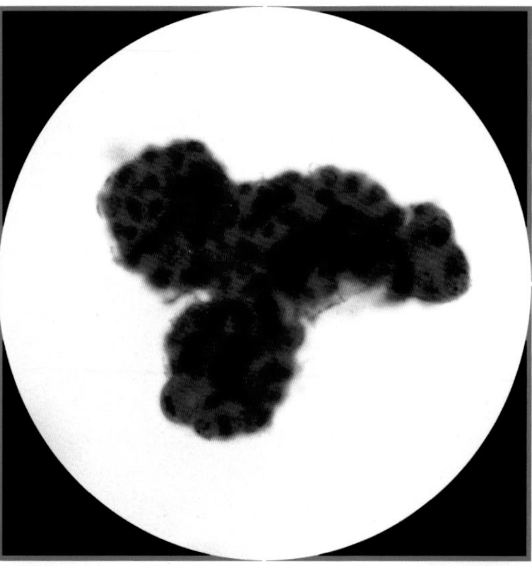

I8.37
Papillary groups. Papillary groups are elongated, three-dimensional aggregates. Psammoma bodies may be present. Adenocarcinomas of the lung (illustrated here), breast, and female genital tract are common sources; papillary thyroid carcinoma rarely produces effusions. Malignant mesothelioma and benign papillary mesothelial hyperplasia are among numerous other possibilities.

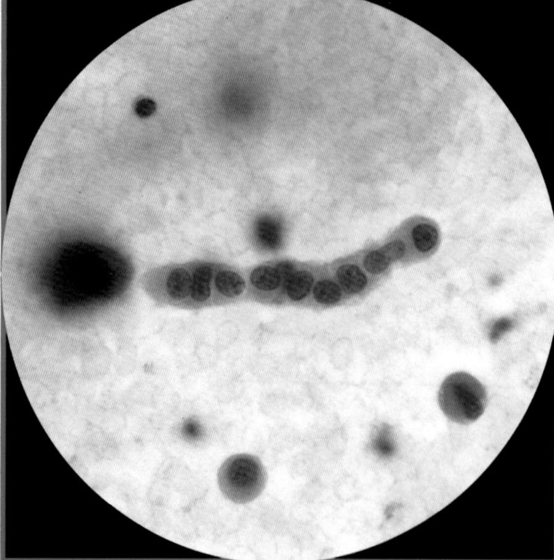

I8.38
Indian files. Chains of cells, particularly when long, suggest breast cancer (illustrated). However, other possibilities, such as pancreas or lung cancers as well as mesothelioma, must also be considered.

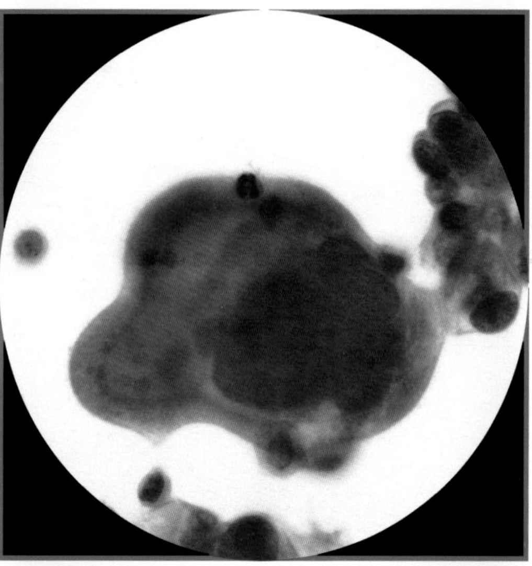

I8.39
Bizarre giant tumor cells. There are many diagnostic possibilities for sources of giant tumor cells, including sarcomas and melanoma. Among adenocarcinomas, lung and pancreas would be the first two choices for primary lesions. However, the example illustrated derived from carcinoma of the ovary.

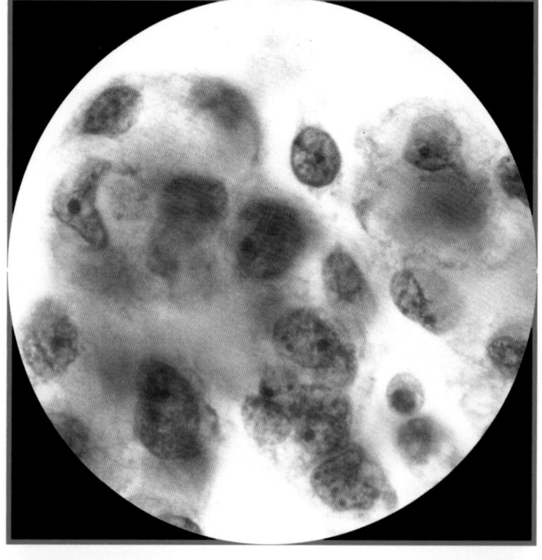

I8.40
Clear cells. Clear cells cytologically have abundant finely vacuolated cytoplasm and therefore are not actually optically clear, and in fluid specimens, the cytoplasm may appear unexpectedly dense. The presence of clear tumor cells suggests carcinoma of the ovary or kidney, as well as germ cell tumors (seminoma is illustrated).

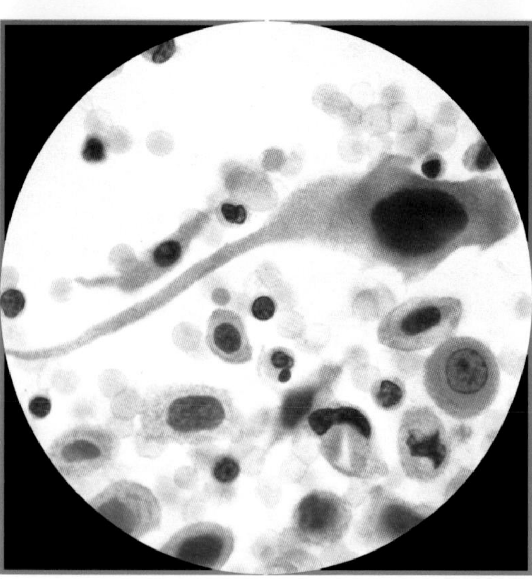

I8.41
Irregularly shaped cells. Due to surface tension effects, all cells tend to round up in fluids, which results in a certain degree of uniformity, even in malignant effusions. Irregularly shaped cells are abnormal and suggest malignancy, such as keratinizing squamous cell carcinoma (illustrated), but can also be seen in rheumatoid effusions.

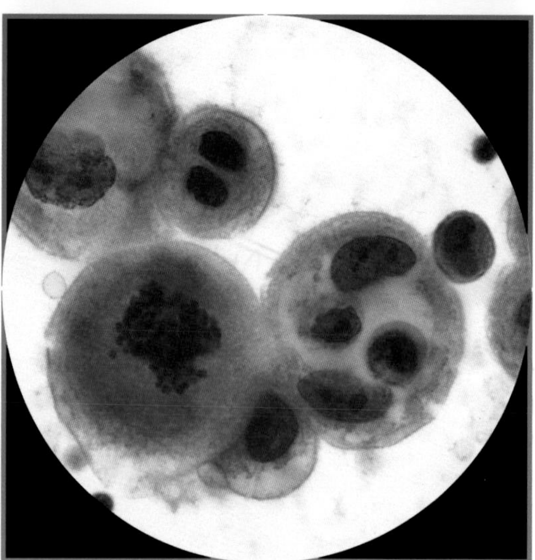

I8.42
Nuclear abnormalities. Nuclear enlargement, pleomorphism, irregular nuclear membranes, and abnormal nucleoli—the usual features of malignancy—are important diagnostically. However, since malignant cells can proliferate in fluids, the nuclei are not necessarily prominently hyperchromatic. Normal mitotic figures are common in benign and malignant fluid specimens, and therefore not particularly useful in diagnosis. However, clearly abnormal mitotic figures indicate malignancy.

I8.43
Extreme cytoplasmic vacuolization. Enormous crystal clear degenerative vacuoles (containing water and electrolytes) are a characteristic feature of ovarian cancer (illustrated), but are also common in lung and pancreatic cancer (among various other possibilities).

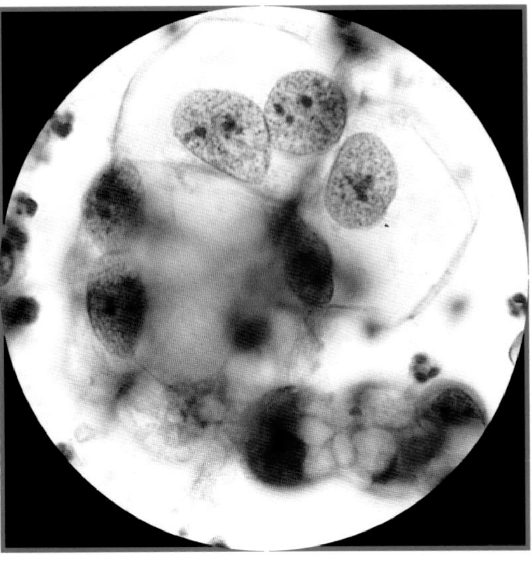

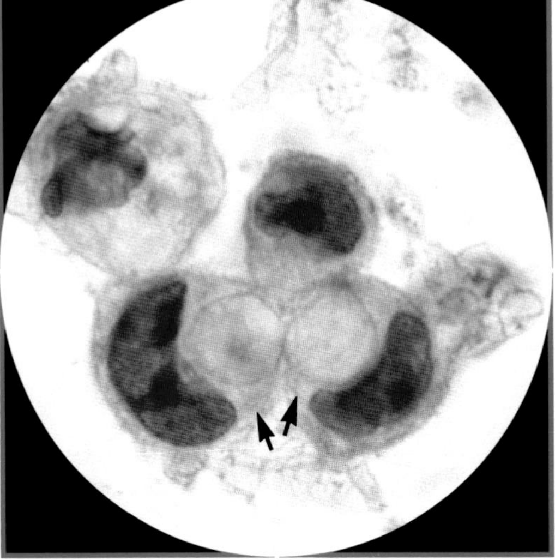

I8.44
Intracytoplasmic lumens. The presence of intracytoplasmic lumens (sharply demarcated secretory vacuoles containing mucin, arrows) is a characteristic feature of metastatic breast cancer, but can be seen in other adenocarcinomas, such as gastric carcinoma. Although commonly associated with the lobular type of breast carcinoma, the case illustrated here represents ductal carcinoma of the breast. Compare the staining of these secretory vacuoles to degenerative vacuoles, which are crystal clear.

I8.45
Bland mesothelial pattern (breast cancer). Virtually every cell in this field is malignant—a potential pitfall in diagnosis since an extra foreign population of cells may not be apparent. Note the strong similarity of the malignant cells to reactive mesothelial cells, complete with a "window" between two of the malignant cells. On careful examination, however, many of the cells have intracytoplasmic lumens.

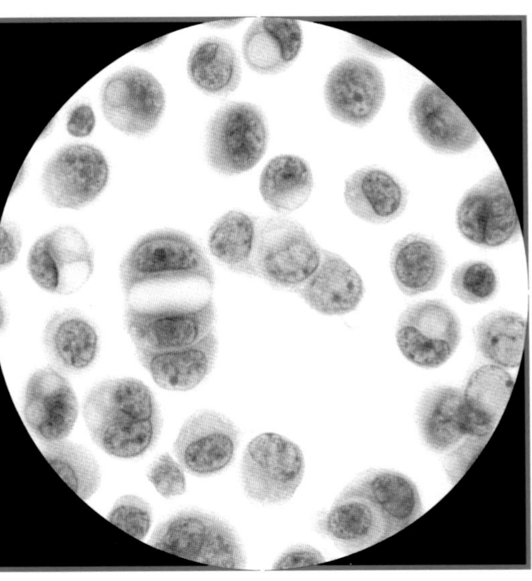

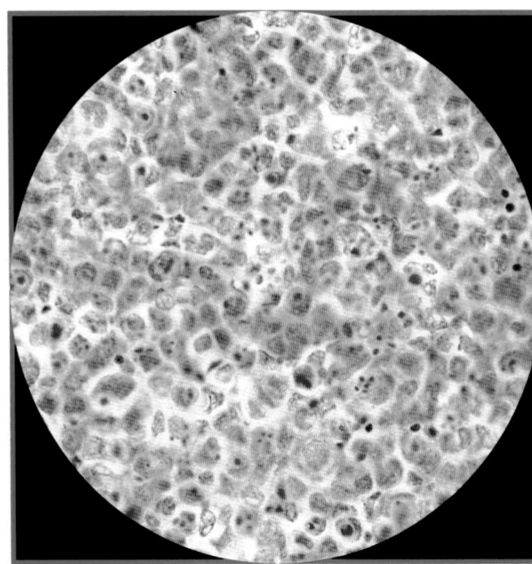

I8.46
Mucicarmine stain. A mucicarmine stain can be one of the most useful special stains in all of cytology: a positive result in a body cavity fluid indicates adenocarcinoma. Note that most of the cells have red dots (positive staining) indicating malignancy. This is the same case illustrated in I8.45.

I8.47
Mucinous effusion. Mucinous effusions can be due to pseudomyxoma peritonei, colloid carcinomas (gastrointestinal tract, ovary, breast cancers), or mesothelioma (mesenchymal mucin).

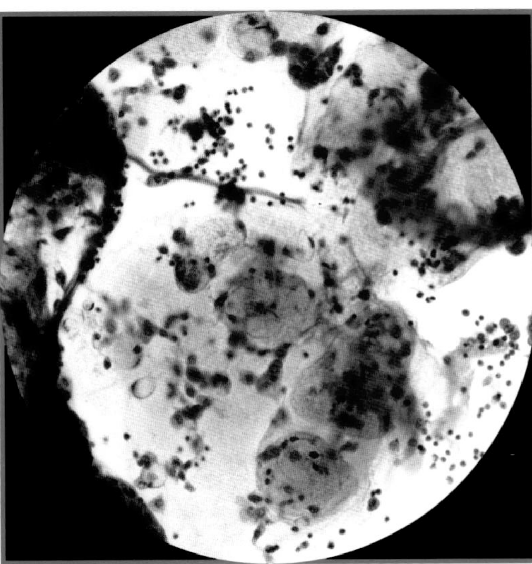

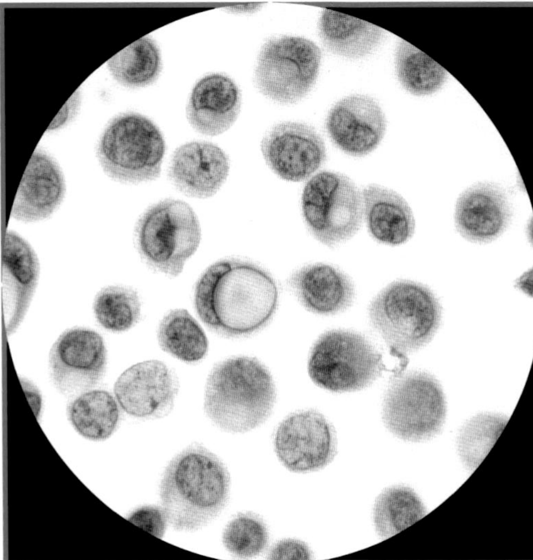

I8.48
Breast carcinoma. This is the most common cause of a malignant pleural effusion in women; most are ductal type. Breast cancer probably has more patterns than any other type of cancer. Several examples have already been illustrated. In general, the cells are relatively uniform, with fine chromatin and dense cytoplasm in which intracytoplasmic lumens may be seen. The single cell pattern is illustrated. Note intracytoplasmic lumen.

I8.49
Lung carcinoma. Lung carcinoma is, overall, the single most common cause of malignant effusions. In essence, there are two major types: small cell and non–small cell. Small cell (neuroendocrine) carcinoma, illustrated here, is characterized by small to medium-sized cells with scant cytoplasm, inconspicuous nucleoli, and prominent molding. Indian file arrangements (also known as "stacks of coins," "vertebral bodies") are also common.

I8.50
Lung carcinoma. Non–small cell carcinoma can be glandular or squamous in origin, but squamous cell carcinoma rarely sheds diagnostic cells in an effusion. Adenocarcinoma of the lung is illustrated.

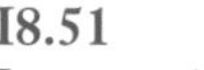

I8.51
Lung carcinoma. Very commonly in non–small cell lung carcinoma, the tumors show evidence of dual differentiation (note the dense cytoplasm and distinct cell boundaries in this cluster otherwise consistent with adenocarcinoma).

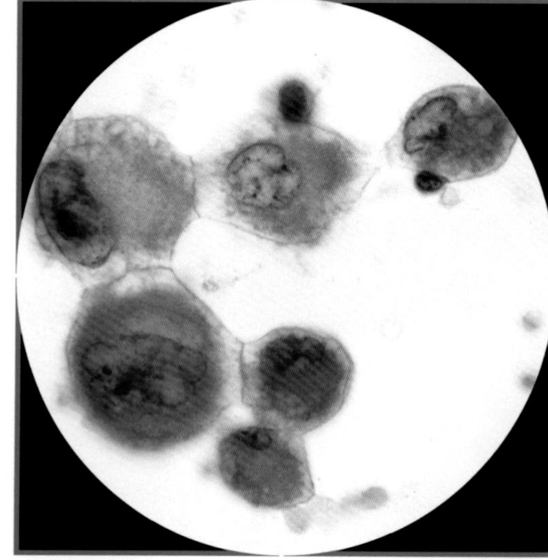

I8.52
Kidney carcinoma. Renal cell carcinoma can have either clear or granular cytoplasm. A characteristic feature is cells with a granular center and clear periphery, as illustrated here. Also note that clear cytoplasm usually appears denser in fluids.

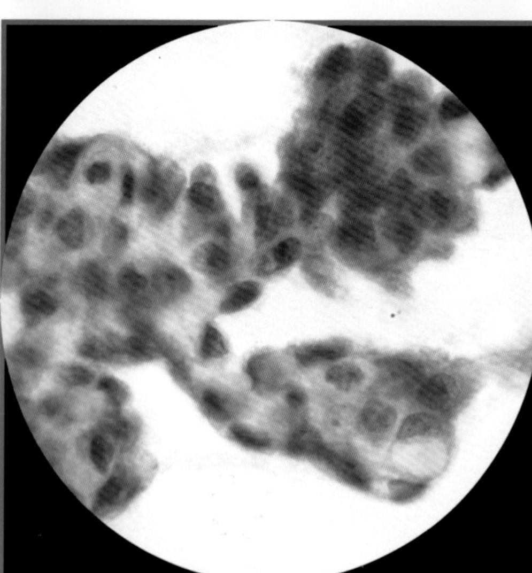

I8.53
Gastric carcinoma. Two common patterns can be seen: papillary/acinar clusters of large columnar cells (illustrated), which sometimes have bizarre nuclei, and isolated signet ring cells.

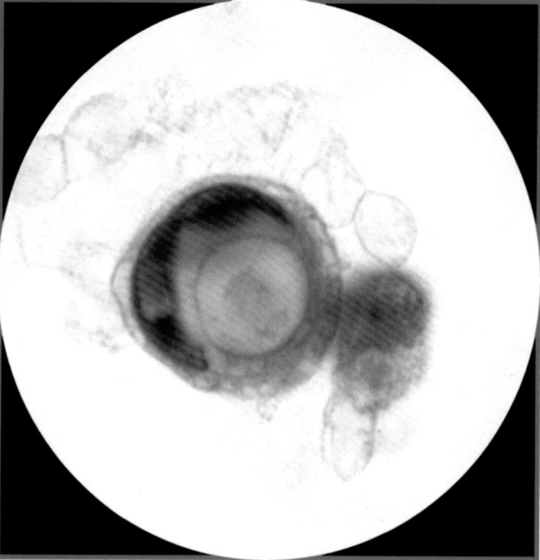

I8.54
Gastric carcinoma. Signet ring cell pattern. This tumor metastasized to the ovary, the classic Krukenberg tumor. (Oil)

I8.55
Colorectal carcinoma. Typically large columnar cells are seen with nuclear palisading and apical cytoplasmic densities suggesting a terminal bar (arrows).

I8.56
Pancreatic carcinoma. May shed cells similar to either non–small cell lung cancer (with mixed adenosquamous features, as illustrated here—note dense cytoplasm in which there is faint keratin ringing) or ovarian cancer (with mucus or serous-like cells or large degenerative cytoplasmic vacuoles). (Oil)

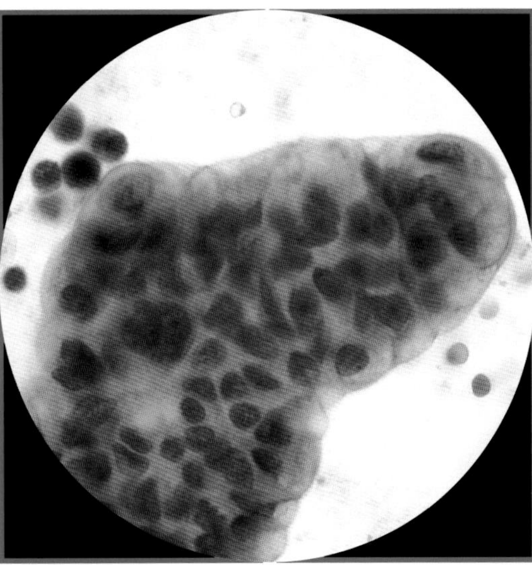

I8.57
Pancreatic carcinoma. Papillary group of relatively well-differentiated mucus cells.

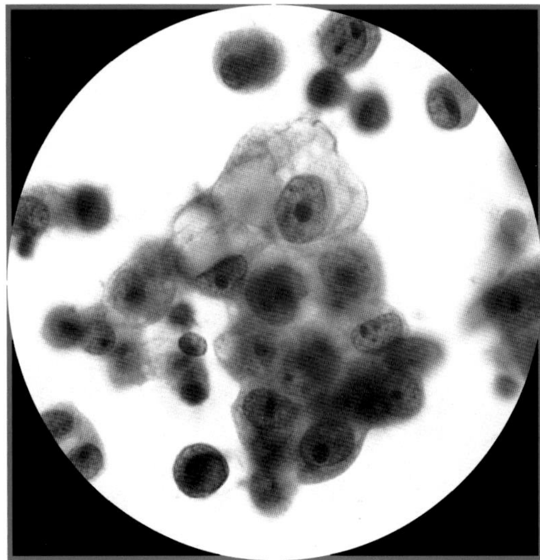

I8.58
Pancreatic carcinoma. Large degenerative vacuoles; also commonly seen in ovarian carcinoma.

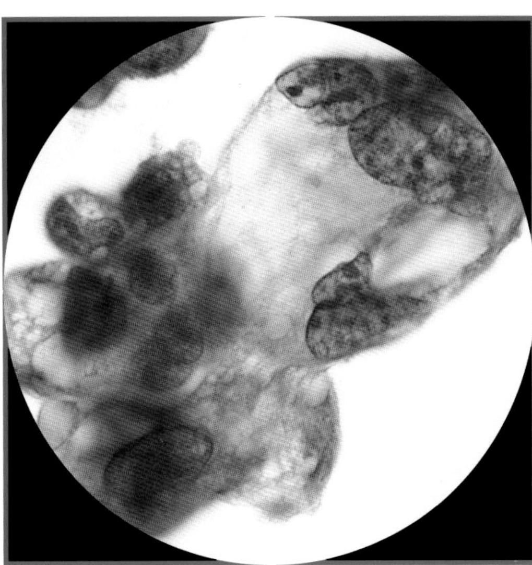

I8.59
Ovarian carcinoma. Probably the most common pattern is very irregular clusters of cells distended with large, clear, degenerative vacuoles. The presence of psammoma bodies (previously illustrated) in a malignant effusion from a woman suggests ovarian carcinoma. Note that patients with ovarian carcinoma rarely have a malignant pleural effusion in the absence of ascites.

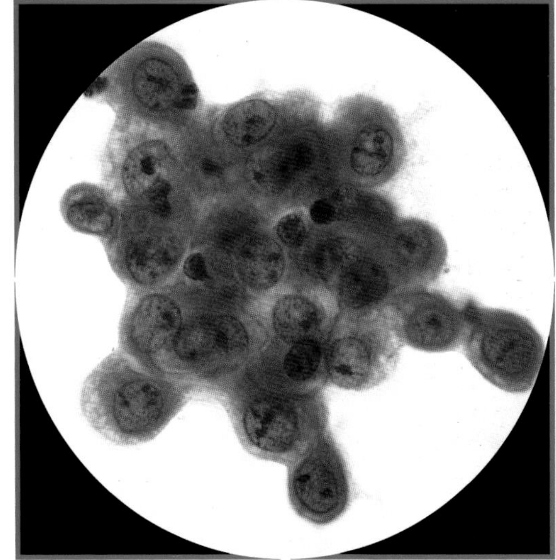

I8.60
Ovarian carcinoma. The differential diagnosis of serous tumors of the ovary is reactive mesothelial cells and mesothelioma (they share a common embryonic origin).

I8.61
Prostate. Microacinar complexes, uniform cells, and prominent nucleoli are characteristic.

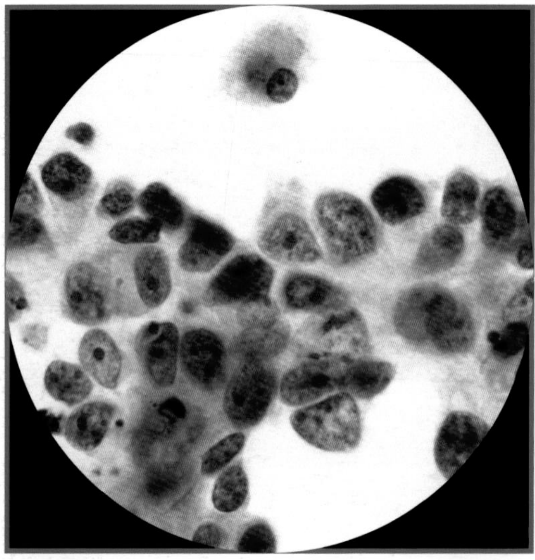

I8.62
Squamous cell carcinoma. Although squamous cell carcinoma is a common malignancy, it rarely sheds diagnostic cells into an effusion. The two key diagnostic features are evidence of keratinization (eg, cytoplasmic rings, pearls) and abnormal cell shapes (tadpoles, etc, as illustrated).

I8.63
Squamous cell carcinoma. Malignant pearls are characteristic of keratinizing squamous cell carcinoma.

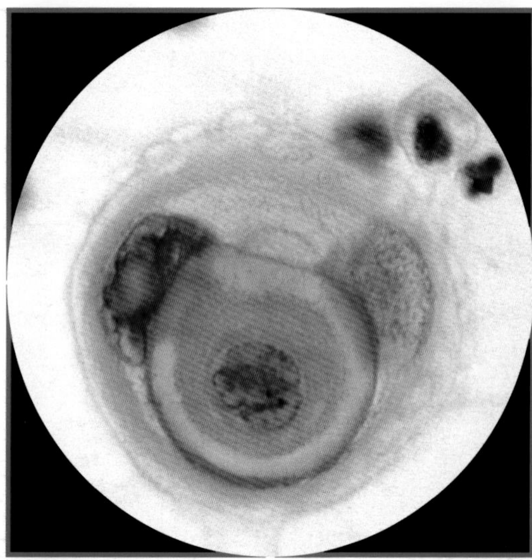

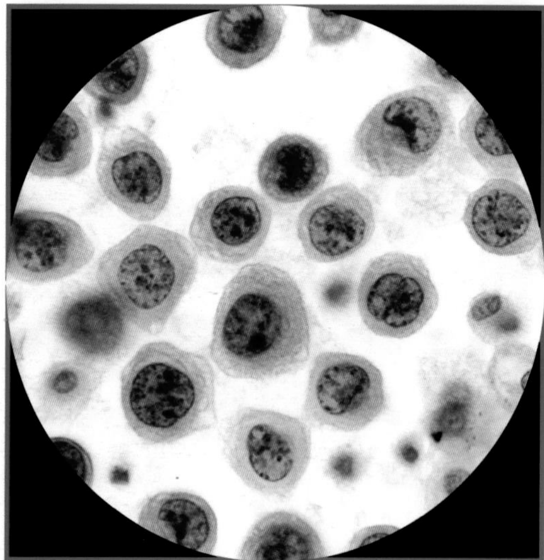

I8.64
Squamous cell carcinoma. Nonkeratinizing squamous cell carcinoma can mimic reactive or neoplastic mesothelial cells.

I8.65
Squamous cell carcinoma. Nonkeratinized squamous cell carcinoma may grow in cohesive balls of tightly wrapped cells with basophilic cytoplasm mimicking adenocarcinoma. The individual cells are reminiscent of reactive mesothelial cells (which are far more common).

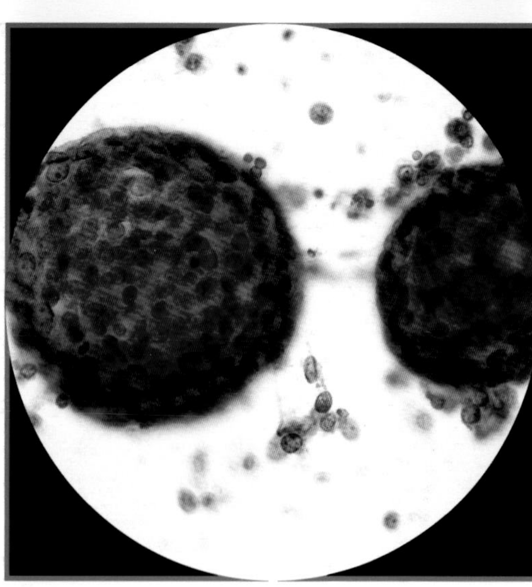

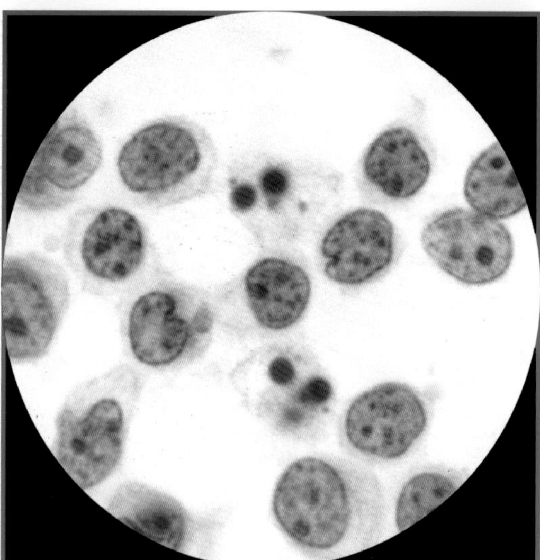

I8.66
Non-Hodgkin's lymphoma, large cell type. The most characteristic feature of lymphoma/leukemia is that all of the cells are single, without formation of true tissue aggregates. Note karyorrhexis; massive karyorrhexis suggests the diagnosis of lymphoma. (Oil)

I8.67
Non-Hodgkin's lymphoma, small cleaved cell type. Dispersed, atypical, small lymphoid cells show nuclear membrane irregularities (cleaves). (Oil)

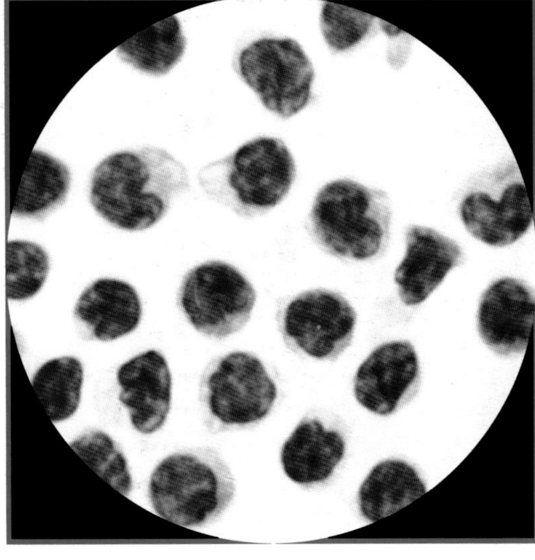

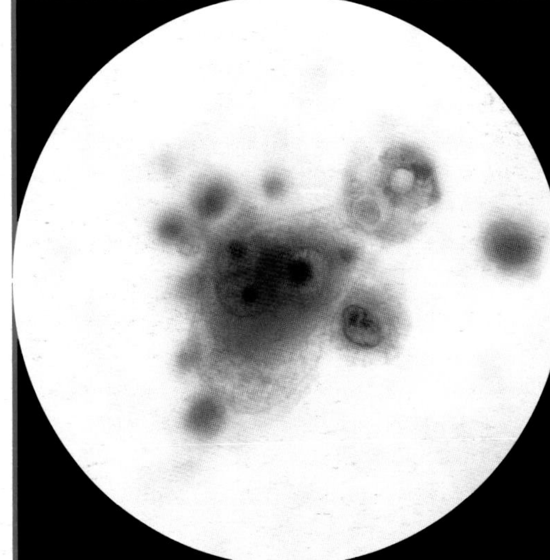

I8.68
Hodgkin's disease. Large, pleomorphic single tumor cells with macronucleoli are characteristic; however, diagnostic Reed-Sternberg cells are rarely found. (Filter preparation)

I8.69
Melanoma. Single cells or loose aggregates, large nuclei with macronucleoli, intranuclear cytoplasmic invaginations, and cytoplasmic pigment are the characteristic features. However, melanoma does not necessarily follow the rules; in particular, cytoplasmic pigment is often sparse or absent, especially in metastases.

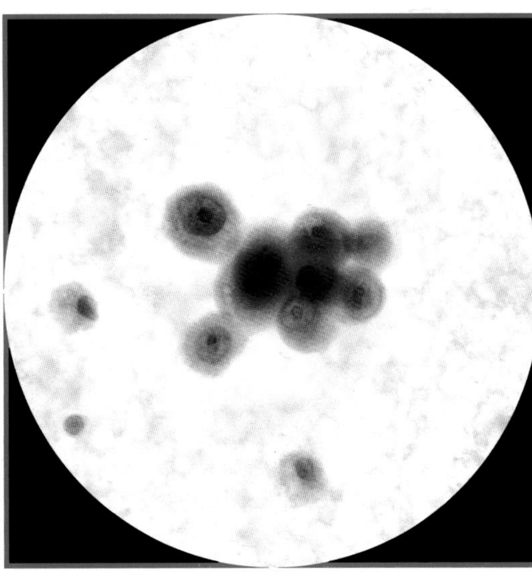

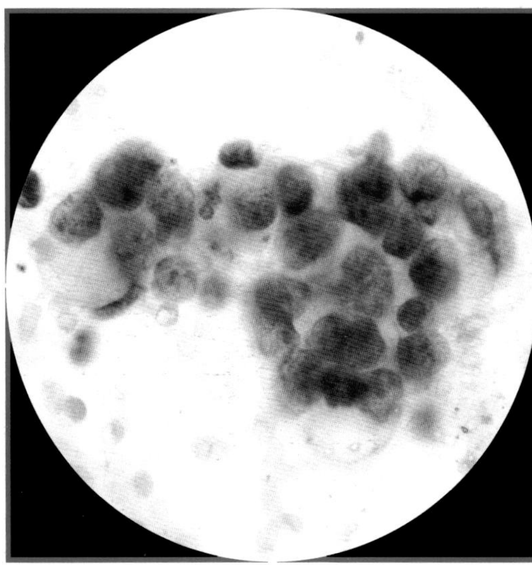

I8.70
Germ cell tumors. Germinomas (dysgerminoma in women and seminoma in men) shed large cells with foamy (clear) PAS-positive cytoplasm (due to glycogen). A case was illustrated previously (see I8.40). Embryonal carcinoma, illustrated here, sheds papillary clusters of obviously malignant cells with prominent nucleoli and mimics adenocarcinoma.

I8.71
Sarcoma. Like lymphoma and melanoma, sarcomas tend to shed singly dispersed cells. For purposes of simplifying the differential diagnosis, sarcomas can be divided into pleomorphic, round, and spindle cell types. Illustrated here is a cell from a pleomorphic sarcoma. The differential diagnosis includes osteosarcoma, liposarcoma, and malignant fibrous histiocytoma.

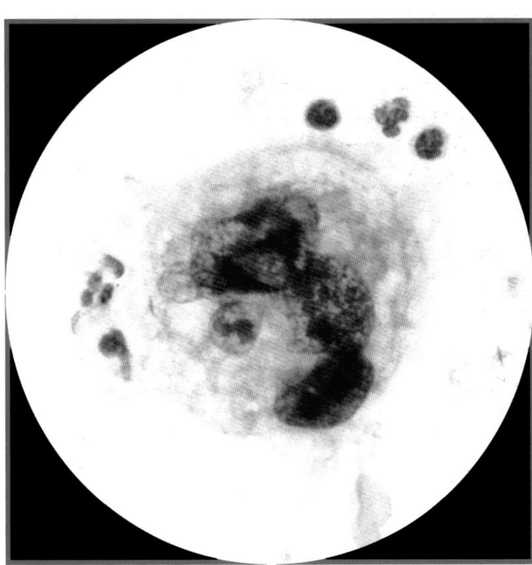

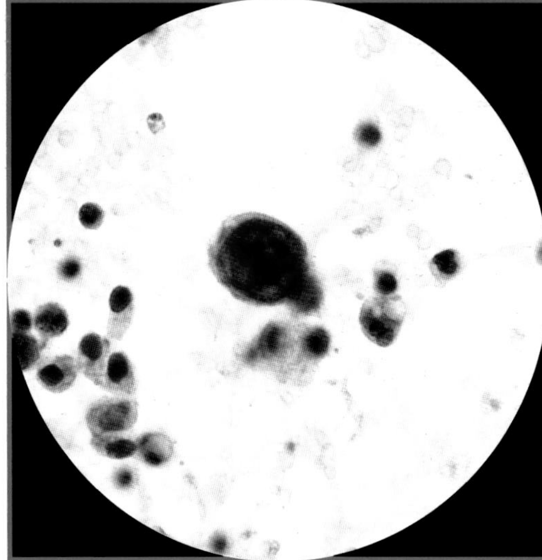

I8.72
Sarcoma. Round cell sarcomas include the "small, blue cell tumors" of childhood such as rhabdomyosarcoma, neuroblastoma, Wilms' tumor, and Ewing's sarcoma. Other possible sources of round cell sarcomas include angiosarcoma, synovial sarcoma, leiomyoblastoma, osteosarcoma or chondrosarcoma, and round cell liposarcoma (illustrated here).

I8.73
Sarcoma. The biphasic sarcoma, synovial sarcoma (illustrated) may exfoliate only as a round cell sarcoma, since spindle cells tend to round up in fluids. Also, spindle cell sarcomas can be considered in the differential diagnosis of round cell sarcomas in an effusion.

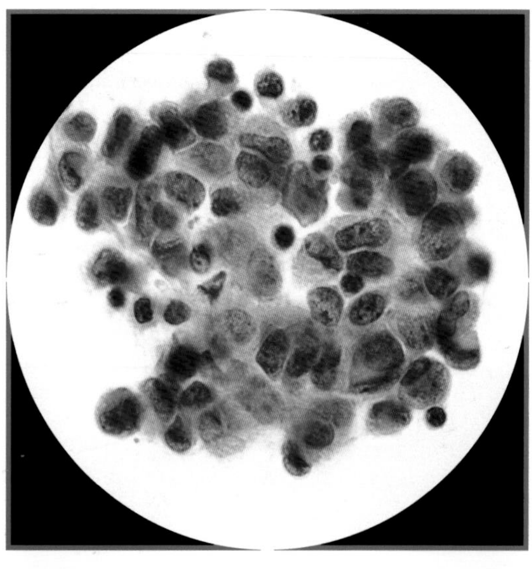

I8.74
Sarcoma. Spindle cell sarcomas include fibrosarcoma (illustrated), leiomyosarcoma, malignant schwannoma, and monophasic synovial sarcoma. The differential diagnosis of spindle cells in an effusion includes not only sarcomas but also squamous cell carcinoma, mesothelioma, and rheumatoid effusions.

I8.75
Neuroblastoma. "Small, blue cell tumor" with monomorphic cells forming small clusters or rosette-like structures (illustrated). The cells are typically PAS negative.

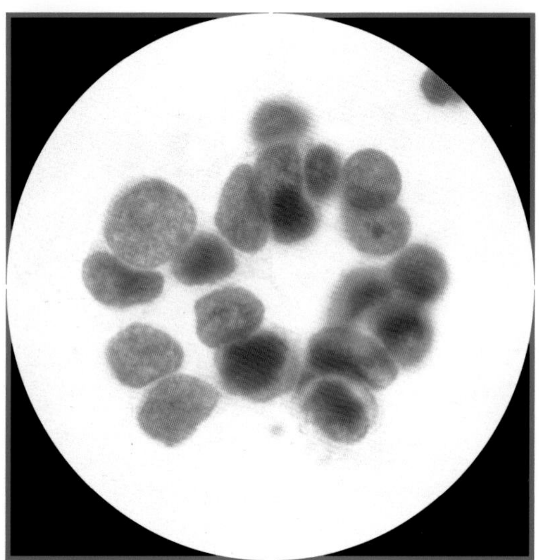

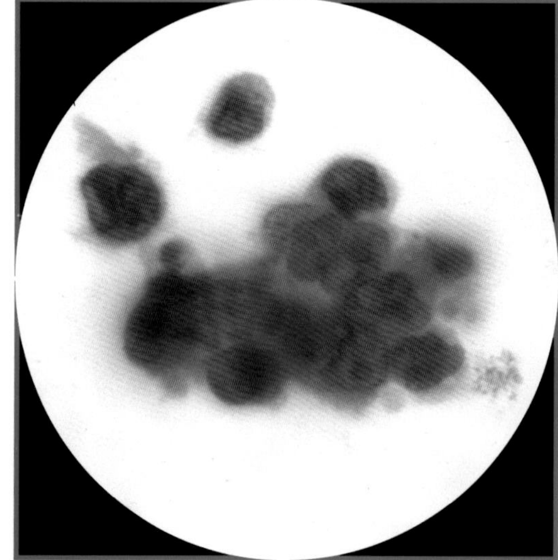

I8.76
Wilms' tumor. "Small blue cells" with coarse chromatin, prominent nucleoli, and sometimes spindle cells.

I8.77
Ewing's sarcoma. "Small blue cell tumor" forms small, loose or molded clusters. Nucleoli may be more prominent than expected in fluid specimens. The cells are typically PAS positive.

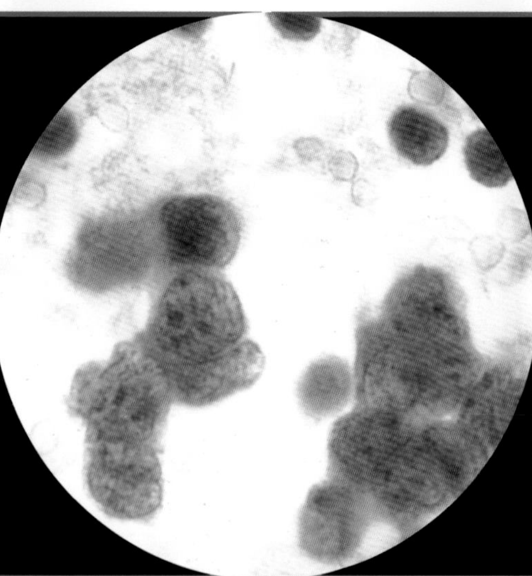

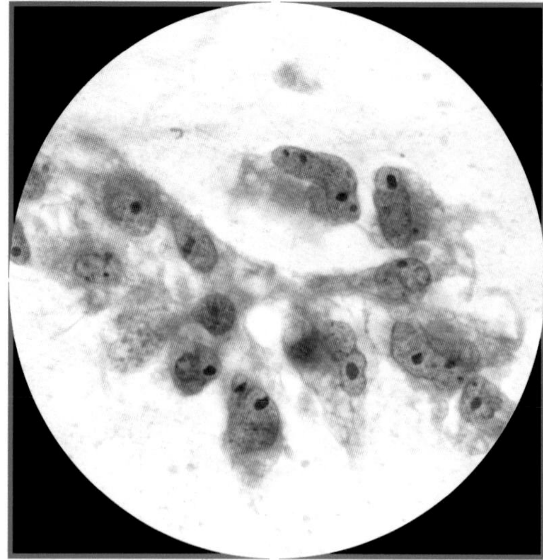

I8.78
Rhabdomyosarcoma. More pleomorphic small cells, including spindle and strap forms. Cross striations are diagnostic but rarely observed. The cells are typically PAS positive.

I8.79
Mesothelioma. The key diagnostic feature is the "morphologic kinship" of the malignant cells with mesothelial cells, ie, the malignant cells look mesothelial (including dense central cytoplasm that fades to delicate and lacy toward the edges, as well as skirts, blebs, and windows, etc).

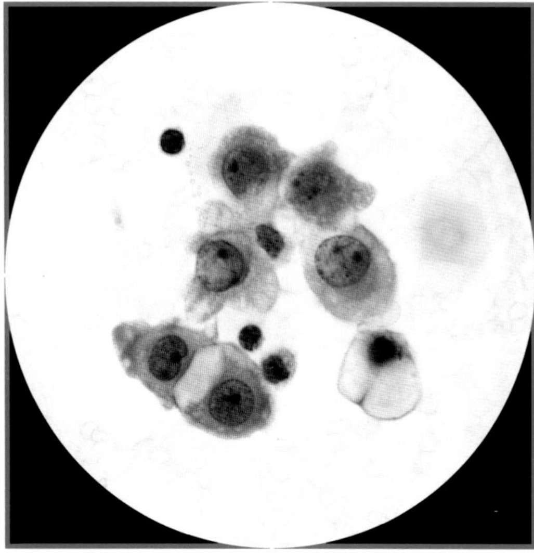

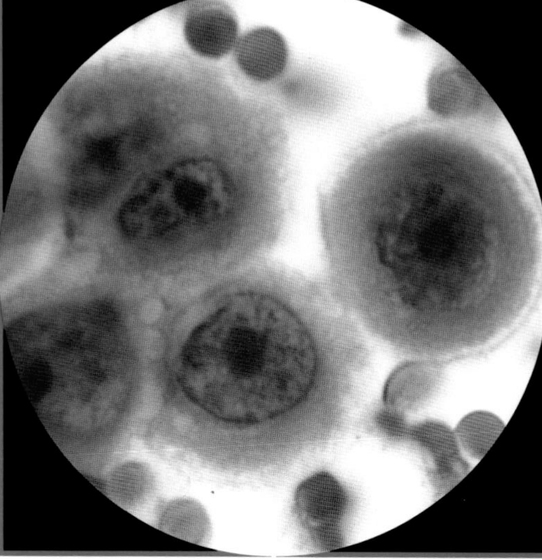

I8.80
Mesothelioma. The diagnosis can be difficult for two reasons. In contrast with most malignant effusions, there is no foreign population—the malignant cells are mesothelial. Without clear malignant features, the cells may be indistinguishable from benign/reactive mesothelial cells. Note the thin rings in the cytoplasm; cytoplasmic density is usually apparent and helps distinguish this tumor from adenocarcinoma. Also note skirts, a characteristic feature of mesothelial cells. (Oil)

I8.81
Mesothelioma. A clue to the diagnosis is "more and bigger cells, in more and bigger clusters." The groups often have very irregular outlines.

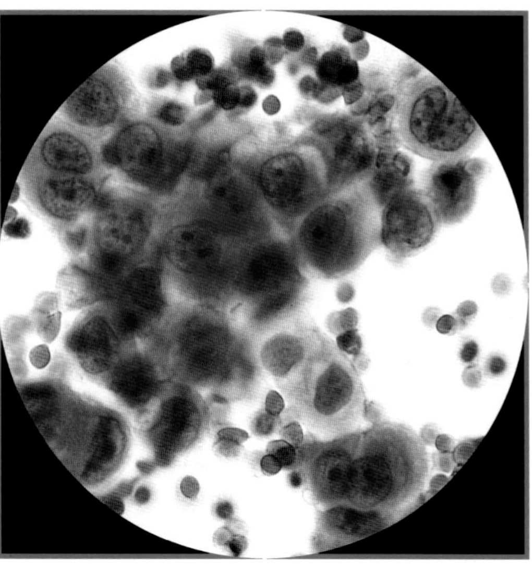

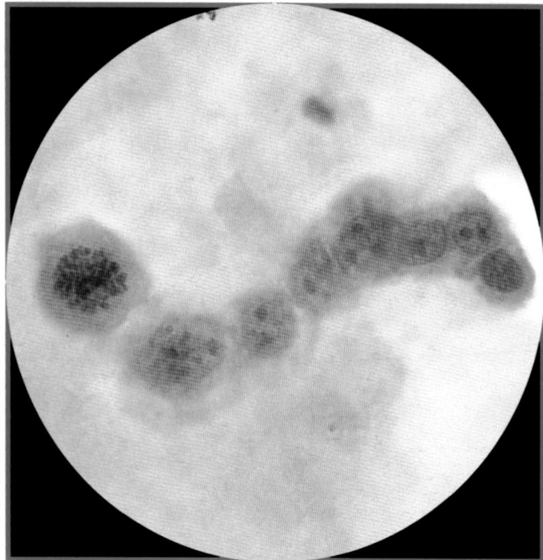

I8.82
Mesothelioma. Long chains of cells (Indian files) may be seen. A fluffy, hyaluronic, and rich background is characteristic and may interfere with staining. This material forms a metachromatic precipitate in Diff-Quik.

I8.83
Mesothelioma. Cell-in-cell arrangements are often numerous. Note malignant nuclear features (enlargement, irregular nuclear membranes, and prominent nucleoli). (Oil)

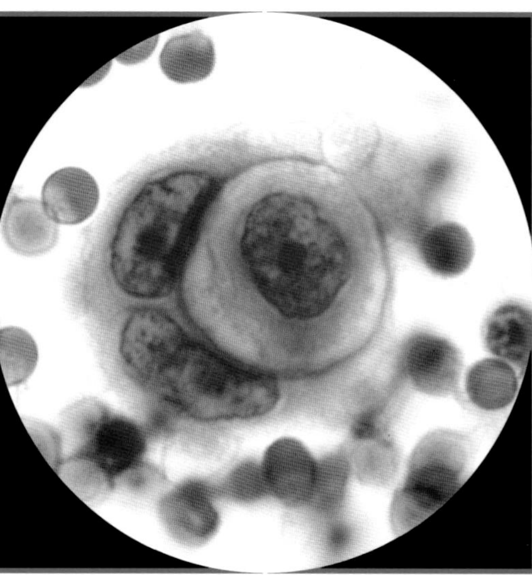

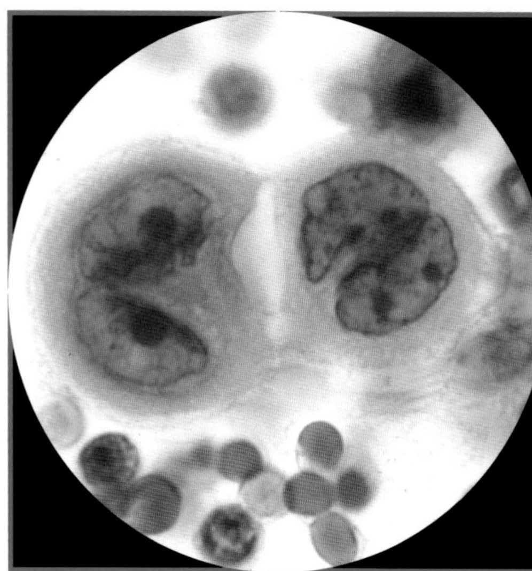

I8.84
Mesothelioma. Cytoplasmic features and windows indicate mesothelial origin; nuclear features indicate malignancy. Nuclear abnormalities may be subtle in some cases. Nucleoli are usually present and may be enlarged, multiple, or irregular. Macronucleoli (some as large as red blood cells) strongly suggest malignancy. (Oil)

I8.85
Mesothelioma. An increased number of cells are binucleated or multinucleated; multinucleated giant tumor cells may be seen in mesothelioma (illustrated).

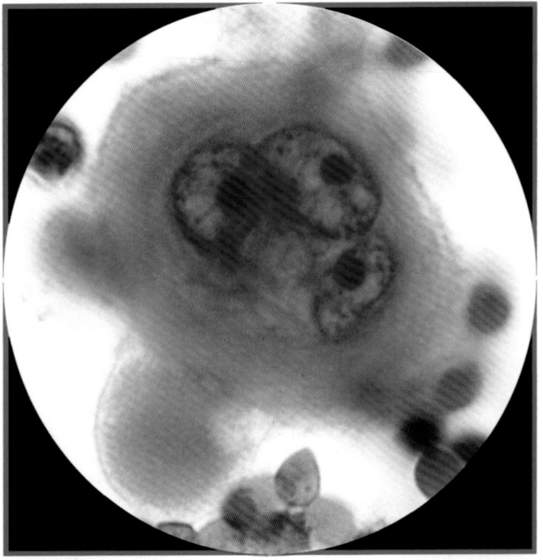

I8.86
Mesothelioma (electron micrograph). Note characteristic long, thin microvilli. In contrast, adenocarcinoma is characterized by short, stubby microvilli.

I8.87
Mesothelioma (carcinoembryonic antigen immunocytochemistry). In contrast with many adenocarcinomas, mesothelioma is usually carcinoembryonic antigen–negative (illustrated) and high-molecular-weight keratin–positive.

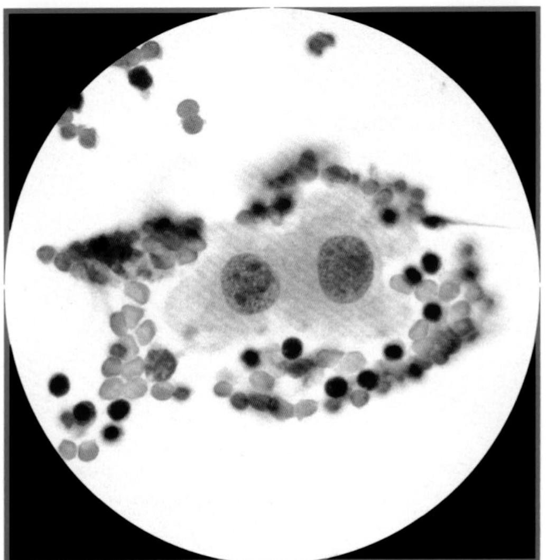

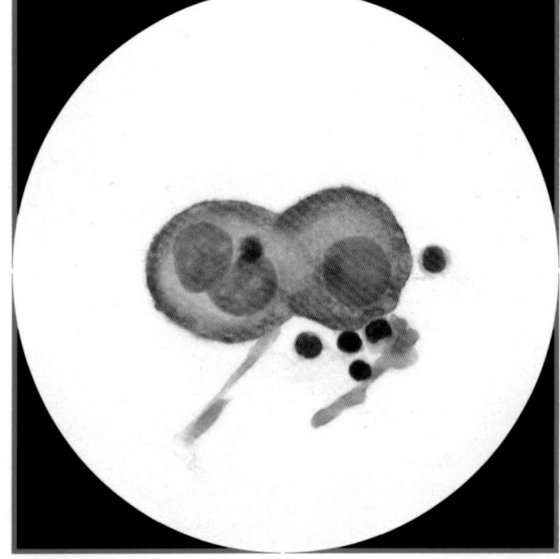

I8.88
Mesothelioma (high-molecular-weight keratin immunocytochemistry). Although both adenocarcinoma and mesothelioma have keratin, high-molecular-weight keratin positivity (illustrated) is more characteristic of mesothelioma. Adenocarcinomas usually express low-molecular-weight keratins.

I8.89
Mesothelial cells. In contrast with body cavity effusions, in which the mesothelial cells are always reactive, directly obtained mesothelial cells do not necessarily show reactive changes. Nonreactive mesothelial cells have very delicate cytoplasm, yet may have well-defined cell borders. The nuclei are round to oval, with fine, even chromatin, and tiny, inconspicuous nucleoli.

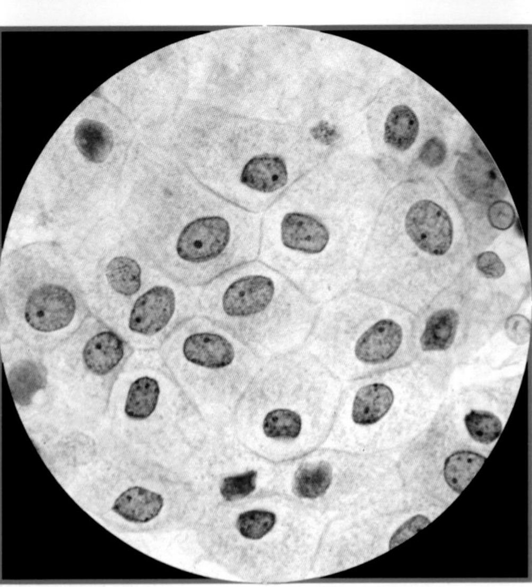

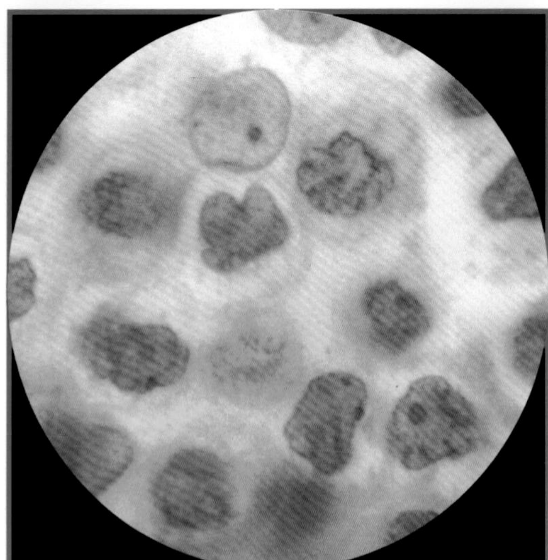

I8.90
Mesothelial cells. Occasionally, the nuclei have very irregular contours, sometimes like a flower ("daisy cells"), a finding more common at midcycle in women. (Oil)

I8.91
Mesothelial cells. Multinucleation may be seen.

I8.92
Mesothelial cells. Reactive, degenerative, and giant forms can be seen after chemotherapy. (Oil)

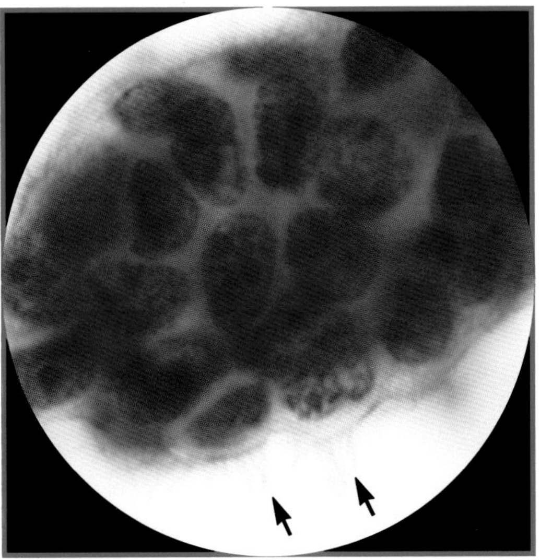

I8.93
Endosalpingiosis (müllerian glandular inclusions). In essence, endosalpingiosis is ectopic fallopian tube epithelium. The cells are seen as tightly cohesive groups of small uniform cells with little or no atypia. Cilia are usually present (arrows); psammoma bodies can be seen. (Oil)

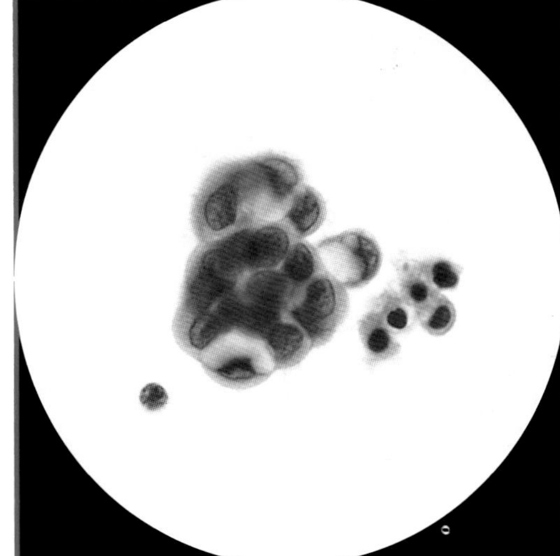

I8.94
Borderline serous ovarian tumor. Borderline tumors, also known as "low malignant potential tumors," are characterized by the presence of cohesive papillary structures that may branch. A few single cells may also be seen. The cells are small, with high N/C ratios, and resemble reactive mesothelial cells. The nuclei are fairly uniform, with smooth nuclear membranes and inconspicuous nucleoli.

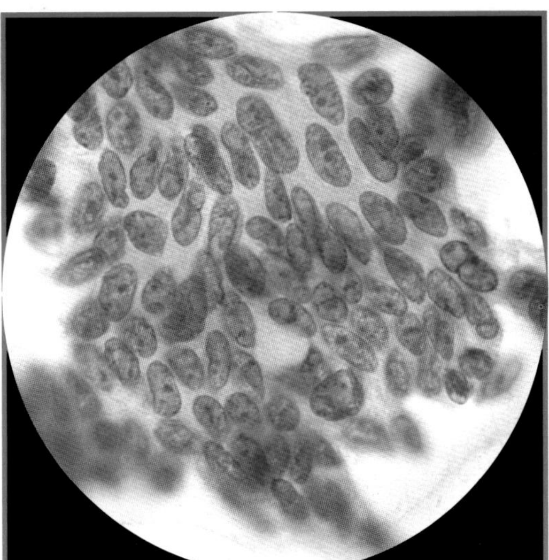

I8.95
Borderline serous ovarian tumor. In some cases, the cells show mild to moderate atypia, including some pleomorphism, irregular nuclear membranes, and occasional prominent nucleoli. Psammoma bodies as well as cilia can also be present.

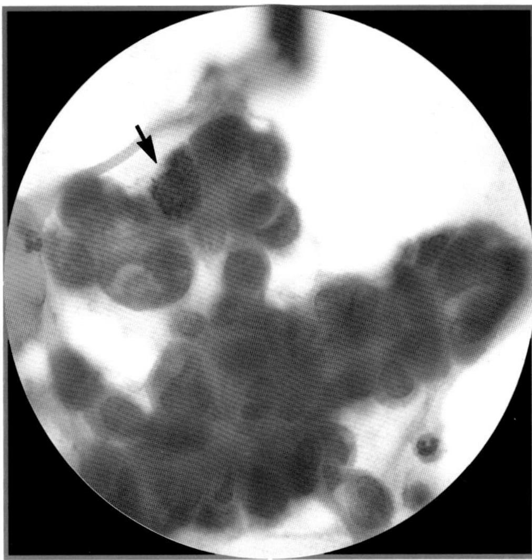

I8.96
Papillary serous carcinoma. Compared with borderline tumors, the papillae are smaller but more irregular in outline. Note mitotic figure (arrow).

I8.97
Papillary serous carcinoma. Moderate to marked nuclear pleomorphism; very irregular nuclear membranes; coarse, dark chromatin, and prominent nucleoli are characteristic findings.

I8.98
Endometrial adenocarcinoma. Clusters and single malignant appearing cells. Positive cytologic findings are an important prognostic sign in stage I endometrial carcinoma.

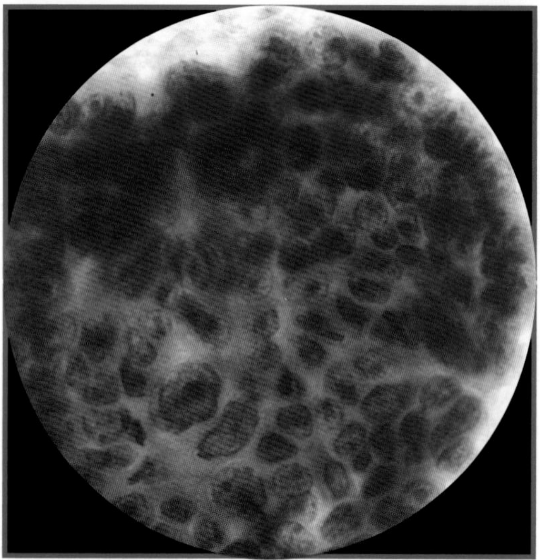

I8.99
Malignant mixed mesodermal tumor. Although the tumor is a carcinosarcoma, usually only the adenocarcinomatous component exfoliates. It is rare for only the sarcomatous elements to be seen.

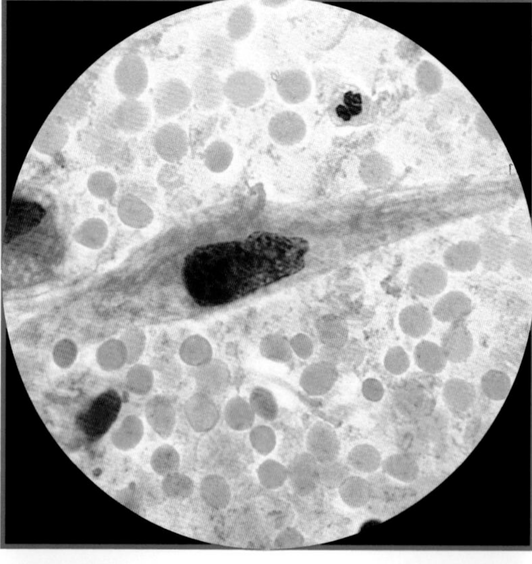

I8.100
Sarcoma. This uterine sarcoma exfoliated malignant appearing spindle cells.

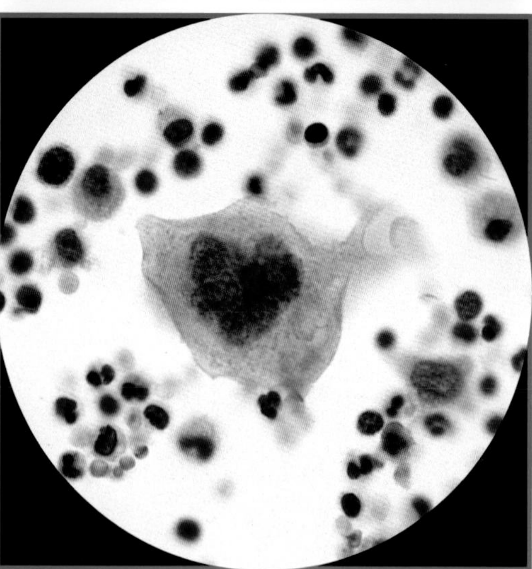

I8.101
Squamous cell carcinoma. This tumor was detected in a patient with squamous cell carcinoma of the cervix. Note irregular cell outline and cytoplasmic density. Peritoneal cytology is not an independent prognostic factor in cervical cancer.

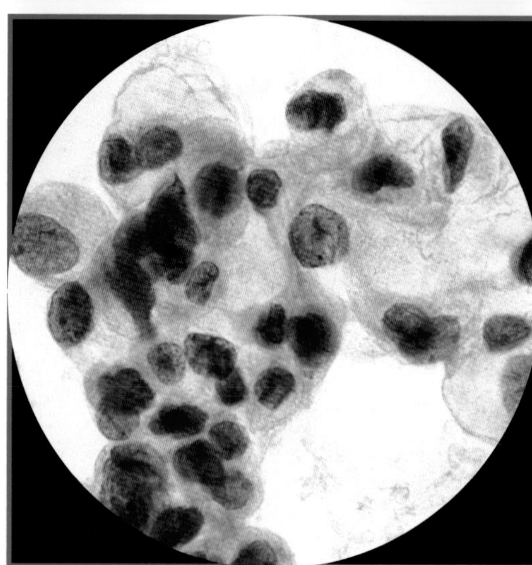

I8.102
Pancreatic carcinoma. The cytology may be very similar to that seen in ovarian carcinoma.

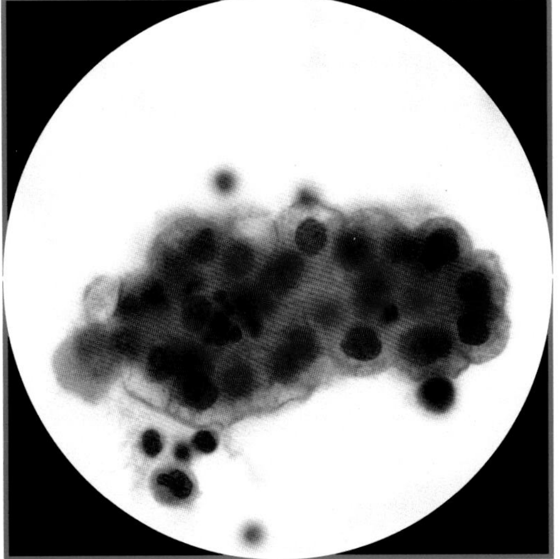

I8.103
Renal cell carcinoma. Papillary aggregate of clear tumor cells.

I8.104
Synoviocytes. They resemble reactive mesothelial cells with round to oval nuclei, fine chromatin, and relatively abundant cytoplasm. Note fluffy hyaluronic acid–rich background.

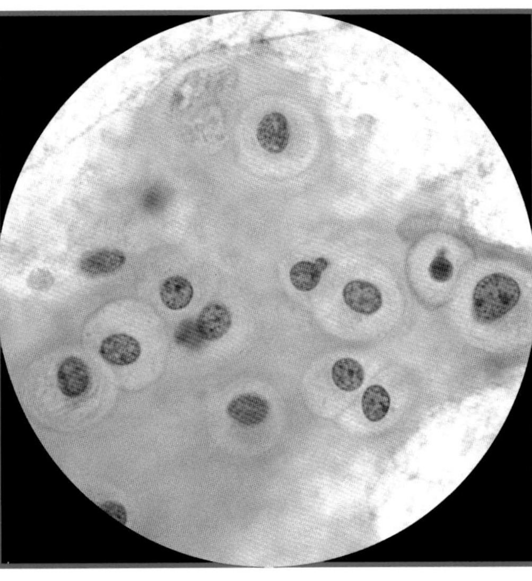

I8.105
Chondrocytes. The cells are not normally present, but can be seen following injury. Chondrocytes are characterized by a thick capsule-like structure surrounding pale staining cytoplasm. The nuclei are central, round, with smooth outlines, granular chromatin, and prominent nucleoli. Binucleation is common. In degenerative arthritis, normal/reactive synoviocytes, little inflammation, and cartilage fragments are seen.

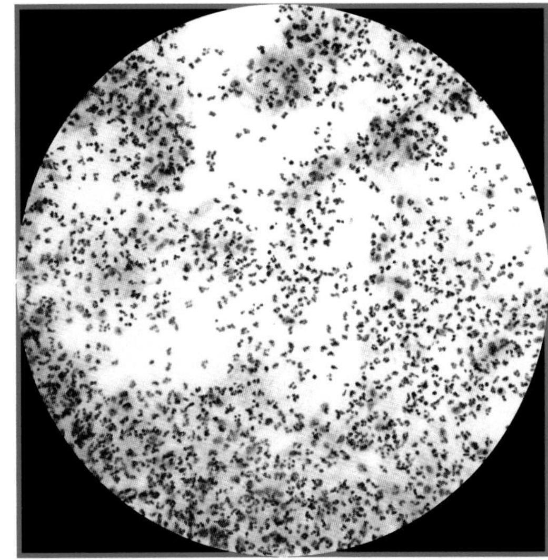

I8.106
Acute (septic) arthritis. Abundant acute inflammation is characteristic. Bacteria are frequently identifiable.

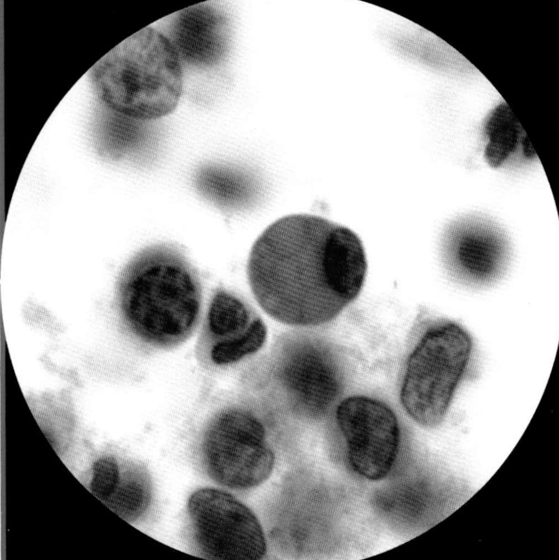

I8.107
Mott cell. Plasma cells with numerous Russell bodies containing immunoglobulin. This cell is associated with chronic inflammation.

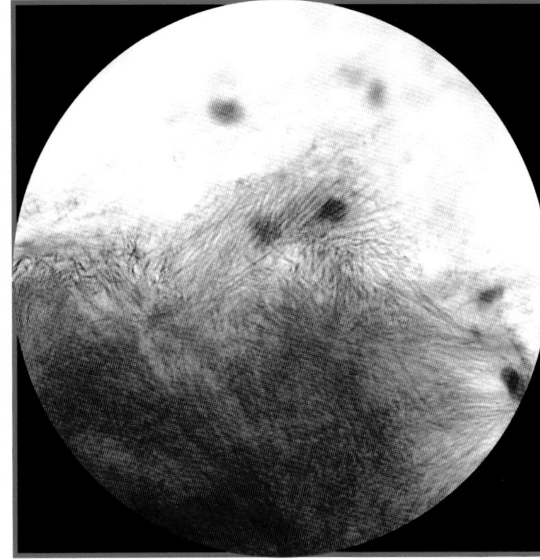

I8.108
Gout. Clusters of needle-shaped urate crystals with pointed ends can be seen. Crystals are not normally present in synovial fluid. Both urate and calcium pyrophosphate crystals are birefringent, but differences can be noted using compensated polarization. Calcium pyrophosphate crystals (pseudogout) are rhomboid or rod shaped with square ends.

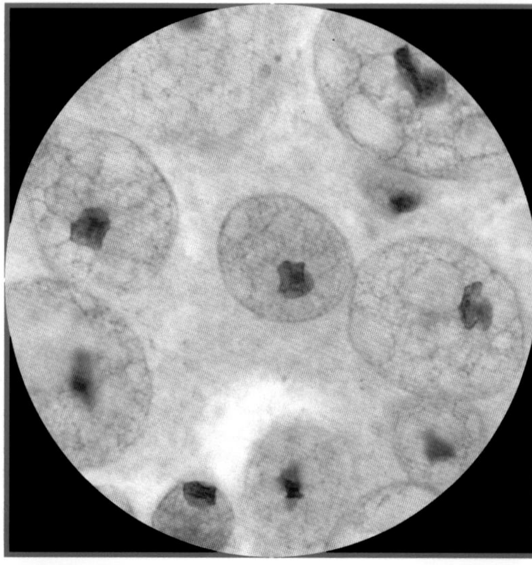

I8.109
Foam cells. These are the most common cell type observed in abnormal nipple discharges; probably bone marrow–derived histiocytes. They have abundant, foamy cytoplasm and low N/C ratios, although they may be binucleated or multinucleated and have prominent nucleoli. Although these cells are benign, their presence does not exclude malignancy.

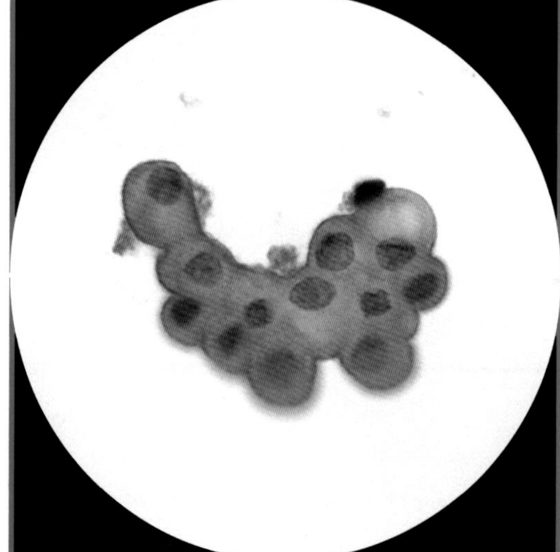

I8.110
Apocrine metaplasia. Medium-sized cells are primarily characterized by finely granular cytoplasm. The cells may have prominent nucleoli but are associated with fibrocystic change and benignancy.

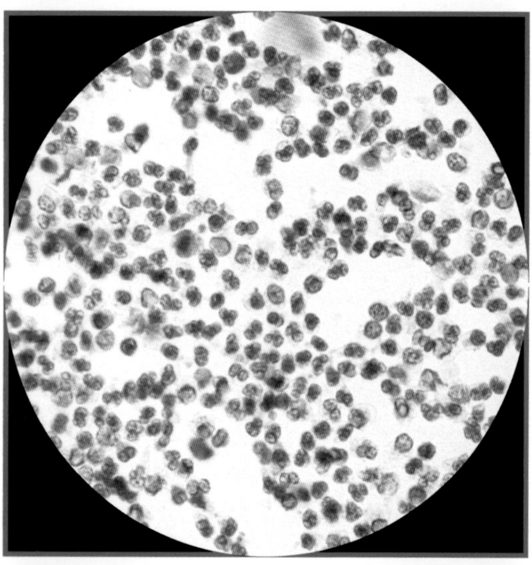

I8.111
Acute inflammation. A variety of infectious agents can cause an abnormal nipple discharge, including bacterial infections associated with acute inflammation.

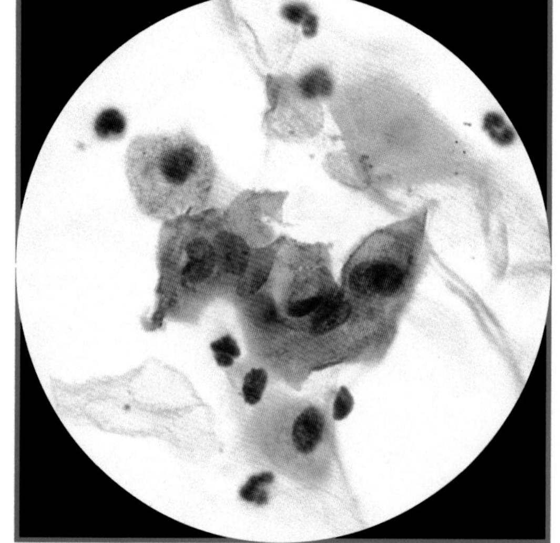

I8.112
Lactating sinus granuloma. Rupture of keratin plug of lactiferous sinus causes acute inflammation and histiocytic/granulomatous response. Giant cells may be seen.

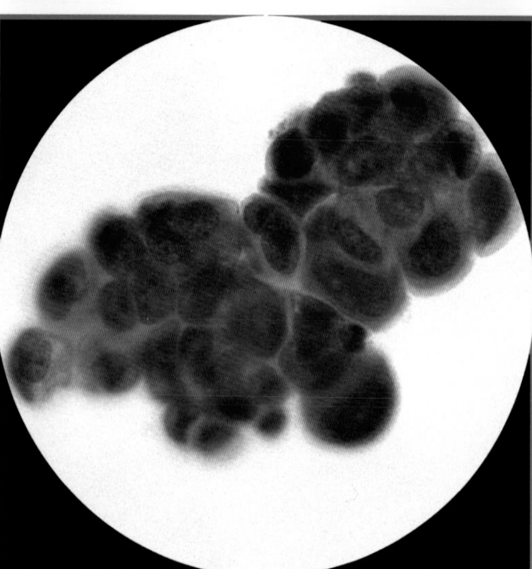

I8.113
Papilloma. This may be indistinguishable from papillary carcinoma on nipple discharge cytology. Diagnosis of papillary clusters, neoplasm not excluded, can be made.

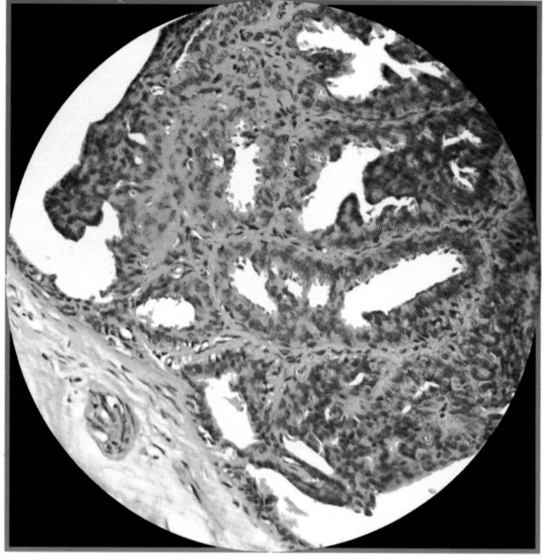

I8.114
Intraductal papilloma. Corresponding tissue.

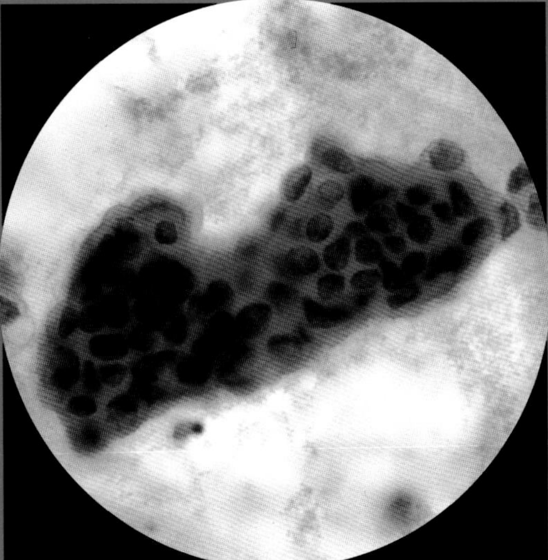

I8.115
Papillary carcinoma. Compare with benign papilloma. Any differences are subtle, at best.

I8.116
Papillary carcinoma. Corresponding tissue.

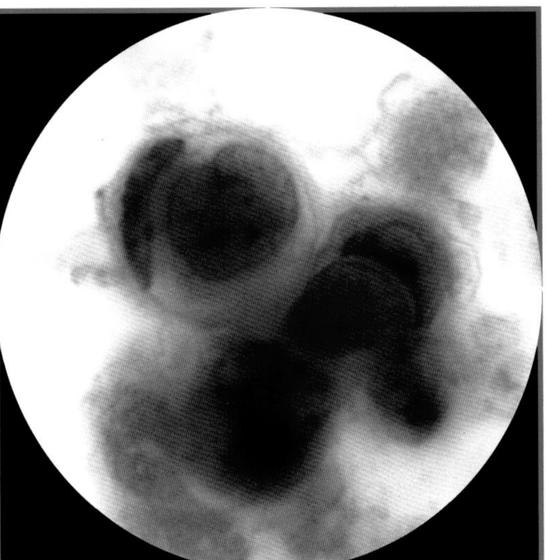

I8.117
Carcinoma of the breast. Abnormal cells with nuclear enlargement, hyperchromasia, and irregular membranes, present singly or in crowded clusters.

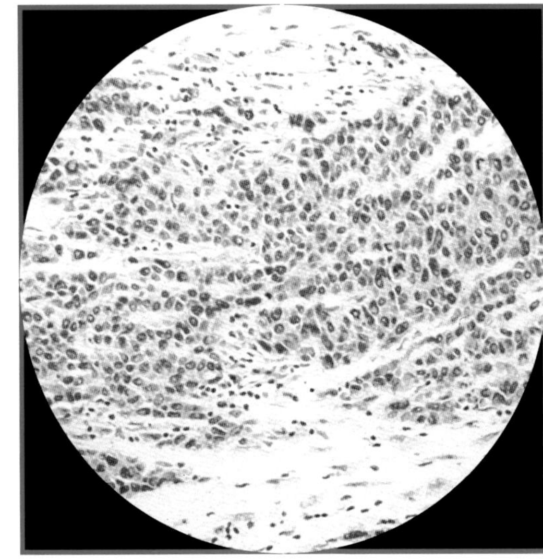

I8.118
Infiltrating ductal carcinoma. Corresponding tissue.

References

Abati A, Fetsch PA: OV632 as a Possible Marker for Malignant Mesothelioma: High Expectations; Low Specificity. *Diagn Cytopathol* 12: 81–82, 1995.

Abe R, Kimura M, Sato T, et al: Trial of Early Detection of Breast Cancer by Mass Screening. *Cancer* 56: 1479–1483, 1985.

Abu-Ghazaleh S, Johnston W, Creasman WT: The Significance of Peritoneal Cytology in Patients With Carcinoma of the Cervix. *Gynecol Oncol* 17: 139–148, 1984.

Adams VI, Unni KK: Diffuse Malignant Mesothelioma of Pleura: Diagnostic Criteria Based on an Autopsy Study. *Am J Clin Pathol* 82: 15–23, 1984.

Adams VI, Unni KK, Muhm JR, et al: Diffuse Malignant Mesothelioma of Pleura: Diagnosis and Survival in 92 Cases. *Cancer* 58: 1540–1551, 1986.

Adelman M, Albelda SM, Gottlieb J, et al: Diagnostic Utility of Pleural Fluid Eosinophilia. *Am J Med* 77: 915–202, 1984.

Al-Nafussi A, Carder PJ: Monoclonal Antibodies in the Cytodiagnosis of Serous Effusions. *Cytopathology* 1: 119–128, 1990.

Antman KH: Malignant Mesothelioma. *N Engl J Med* 303: 200–202, 1980a.

Antman KH, Blum RH, Greenberger JS, et al: Multimodality Therapy for Malignant Mesothelioma Based on a Study of Natural History. *Am J Med* 68: 356–362, 1980b.

Antman KH: Clinical Presentation and Natural History of Benign and Malignant Mesothelioma. *Semin Oncol* 8: 313–319, 1981.

Ashfaq-Drewett R, Allen C, Harrison RL: Detached Ciliary Tufts: Comparison With Intestinal Protozoa and a Review of the Literature. *Am J Clin Pathol* 93: 541–545, 1990.

Ashton PR, Hollingsworth AS Jr, Johnston WW: The Cytopathology of Metastatic Breast Cancer. *Acta Cytol* 19: 1–6, 1975.

Athanassiadou P, Athanassiades P, Lazaris D, et al: Immunocytochemical Differentiation of Reactive Mesothelial Cells and Adenocarcinoma Cells in Serous Effusions With the Use of Carcinoembryonic Antigen and Fibronectin. *Acta Cytol* 38: 718–722, 1994.

Baddoura FK, Varma VA: Cytologic Findings in Multicystic Peritoneal Mesothelioma. *Acta Cytol* 34: 524–528, 1990.

Badrinas F, Rodriguez-Roisin R, Rives A, et al: Multiple Myeloma With Pleural Involvement. *Am Rev Resp Dis* 110: 82–87, 1974.

Baer AN, Wright EP: Lipid Laden Macrophages in Synovial Fluid: A Late Finding in Traumatic Arthritis. *J Rheumatol* 14: 848–851, 1987.

Banks ER, Jennings CD, Jacobs S, et al: Comparative Assessment of DNA Analysis in Effusions by Image Analysis and Flow Cytometry. *Diagn Cytopathol* 10: 62–67, 1994.

Barnes AB: Diagnosis and Treatment of Abnormal Breast Secretions. *N Engl J Med* 275: 1184–1187, 1966.

Barsotti P, Muda AO, Ascoli V, et al: Ultrastructural Histochemistry of Mesotheliomas and Adenocarcinomas in Malignant Effusions. *Diagn Cytopathol* 5: 154–161, 1989.

Bartziota EV, Naylor B: Megakaryocytes in a Hemorrhagic Pleural Effusion Caused by Anticoagulant Overdose. *Acta Cytol* 30: 163–165, 1986.

Battifora H, Kopinski MI: Distinction of Mesothelioma From Adenocarcinoma: An Immunohistochemical Approach. *Cancer* 55: 1679–1685, 1985.

Beacham WD, Beacham DW: Culdocentesis. *Clin Obstet Gynecol* 1: 607–609, 1958.

Beals TF: Scanning Electron Microscopy of Body Fluids. *Diagn Cytopathol* 8: 266–271, 1992.

Becker SN, Pepin DW, Rosenthal DL: Mesothelial Papilloma: A Case of Mistaken Identity in a Pericardial Effusion. *Acta Cytol* 20: 266–268, 1976.

Becklake MR: Asbestos-Related Diseases of the Lung and Other Organs: Their Epidemiology and Implications for Clinical Practice. *Am Rev Respir Dis* 114: 187–227, 1976.

Bercovici B, Gallily R: The Cytology of the Human Peritoneal Fluid. *Acta Cytol* 22: 194–127, 1978.

Berge T, Gröntoft O: Cytologic Diagnosis of Malignant Pleural Mesothelioma. *Acta Cytol* 9: 207–212, 1965.

Berkowitz CD, Inkelis SH: Bloody Nipple Discharge in Infancy. *J Pediatr* 103: 755–756, 1983.

Berry GJ, Anderson CJ, Pitts WC, et al: Cytology of Angiosarcoma in Effusions. *Acta Cytol* 35: 538–542, 1991.

Bertini B, Kuttin ES, Beemer AM: Cytopathology of Nipple Discharge Due to *Pityrosporum orbiculare* and Cocci in an Elderly Woman. *Acta Cytol* 19: 38–42, 1975.

Bian Y, Jordan AG, Rupp M, et al: Effusion Cytology of Desmoplastic Small Round Cell Tumor of the Pleura: A Case Report. *Acta Cytol* 37: 77–82, 1993.

Billingham ME, Rawlinson DG, Berry PF, et al: The Cytodiagnosis of Malignant Lymphomas and Hodgkin's Disease in Cerebrospinal, Pleural and Ascitic Fluids. *Acta Cytol* 19: 547–556, 1975.

Bjelle A, Norberg B, Sjögren G: The Cytology of Joint Exudates in Rheumatoid Arthritis. *Scand J Rheum* 11: 124–128, 1982.

Black LF: The Pleural Spacer and Pleural Fluid. *Mayo Clin Proc* 47: 493–506, 1972.

Blaustein A: Peritoneal Mesothelium and Ovarian Surface Cells–Shared Characteristics. *Int J Gynecol Pathol* 3: 361–375, 1984.

Blobel DA, Moll R, Franke WW, et al: The Intermediate Filament Cytoskeleton of Malignant Mesotheliomas and Its Diagnostic Significance. *Am J Pathol* 121: 235–247, 1985.

Boddington MM, Spriggs AI, Morton JA, et al: Cytodiagnosis of Rheumatoid Pleural Effusions. *J Clin Pathol* 24: 95–106, 1971.

Bollinger DJ, Wick MR, Dehner LP, et al: Peritoneal Malignant Mesothelioma Versus Serous Papillary Adenocarcinoma: A Histochemical and Immunohistochemical Comparison. *Am J Surg Pathol* 13: 659–670, 1989.

Boon ME, Posthuma HS, Ruiter DJ, et al: Secreting Peritoneal Mesothelioma: Report of a Case With Cytological, Ultrastructural, Morphometric and Histologic Studies. *Virchows Arch Pathol Anat* 392: 33–44, 1981.

Boon ME, Kwee HS, Alons CL, et al: Discrimination Between Primary Pleural and Primary Peritoneal Mesotheliomas by Morphometry and Analysis of the Vacuolization Pattern of the Exfoliated Mesothelial Cells. *Acta Cytol* 26: 103–108, 1982.

Boon ME, Veldhuizen RW, Ruinaard C, et al: Qualitative Distinctive Differences Between the Vacuoles of Mesothelioma Cells and of Cells From Metastatic Carcinoma Exfoliated in Pleural Fluid. *Acta Cytol* 28: 443–449, 1984.

Bottles K, Reznicek MJ, Holly EA, et al: Cytologic Criteria Used to Diagnose Adenocarcinoma in Pleural Effusions. *Mod Pathol* 4: 677–681, 1991.

Bower G: Eosinophilic Pleural Effusion: A Condition With Multiple Causes. *Am Rev Respir Dis* 95: 746–751, 1967.

Braganza JM, Butler EB, Fox H, et al: Ectopic Production of Salivary Type Amylase by a Pseudomesotheliomatous Carcinoma of the Lung. *Cancer* 41: 1522–1525, 1978.

Brenner J, Sordillo PP, Magill GB, et al: Malignant Mesothelioma of the Pleura: Review of 123 Patients. *Cancer* 49: 2431–2435, 1982.

Broaddus C, Staub NC: Pleural Liquid and Protein Turnover in Health and Disease. *Semin Respir Med* 9: 7–12, 1987.

Broderick PA, Corvese N, Pierik MG, et al: Exfoliative Cytology Interpretation of Synovial Fluid in Joint Disease. *J Bone Joint Surg* 58-A: 396–399, 1976.

Broghamer WL Jr, Collins WM, Mojsejenko IK: The Cytohistopathology of a Pseudomesotheliomatous Carcinoma of the Lung. *Acta Cytol* 22: 239–242, 1978.

Broghamer WL Jr, Richardson ME, Faurest SE: Malignancy-Associated Serosanguinous Pleural Effusions. *Acta Cytol* 28: 46–50, 1984.

Brown JP, Rola-Pleszczynski M, Menard H-A: Eosinophilic Synovitis: Clinical Observations on a Newly Recognized Subset of Patients With Dermatographism. *Arthritis Rheum* 29: 1147–1151, 1986.

Buehring GC: Screening for Breast Atypias using Exfoliative Cytology. *Cancer* 43: 1788–1799, 1979.

Buhr J, Berghauser K-H, Morr H, et al: Tumor Cells in Intraoperative Pleural Lavage: An Indicator for the Poor Prognosis of Bronchogenic Carcinoma. *Cancer* 65: 1801–1804, 1990.

Burns TR, Greenberg SD, Mace ML, et al: Ultrastructural Diagnosis of Epithelial Malignant Mesothelioma. *Cancer* 56: 2036–2040, 1985.

Butchart EG, Ashcroft T, Barnsley WC, et al: The Role of Surgery in Diffuse Malignant Mesothelioma of the Pleura. *Semin Oncol* 8: 321–328, 1981.

Cajulis RS, Frias-Hidvegi D: Detection of Numerical Chromosomal Abnormalities in Malignant Cells on Body Fluids by Fluorescence In Situ Hybridization of Interphase Cell Nuclei With Chromosome-Specific Probes. *Diagn Cytopathol* 8: 627–631, 662, 1992.

Cajulis RS, Szumel R, Frias-Hidvegi D, et al: Monoclonal Antibody 44-3A6 as an Adjunct in Cytodiagnosis of Adenocarcinomas in Body Fluids. *Diagn Cytopathol* 9: 179–183, 1993.

Calle S: Megakaryocytes in an Abdominal Fluid. *Acta Cytol* 12: 78–80, 1968.

Campbell GD, Webb WR: Eosinophilic Pleural Effusion: A Review With the Presentation of Seven New Cases. *Am Rev Respir Dis* 90: 194–201, 1964.

Canto-Armengod A: Macroscopic Characteristic of Pleural Metastases Arising From the Breast and Observed by Diagnostic Thoracoscopy. *Am Rev Respir Dis* 142: 616–618, 1990.

Carlon G, Della Giustina D: Atypical Mesothelial Cells in Peritoneal Dialysis Fluid. *Acta Cytol* 27: 706–708, 1983.

Carlson GJ, Samuelson JJ, Dehner LP: Cytologic Diagnosis of Florid Peritoneal Endosalpingiosis: A Case Report. *Acta Cytol* 30: 494–496, 1986.

Castelli MJ, Mihalov ML, Posniak HV, et al: Primary Cardiac Lymphoma Initially Diagnosed by Routine Cytology: Case Report and Literature Review. *Acta Cytol* 33: 355–358, 1989.

Castor CW, Naylor B: Acid Mucopolysaccharide Composition of Serous Effusions: Study of 100 Patients With Neoplastic and Non-neoplastic Conditions. *Cancer* 20: 462–466, 1967.

Ceelen GH: The Cytologic Diagnosis of Ascitic Fluid. *Acta Cytol* 8: 175–185, 1964.

Chahinian AP, Pajak TF, Holland JF, et al: Diffuse Malignant Mesothelioma: Prospective Evaluation of 69 Patients. *Ann Intern Med* 96(Part I): 746–755, 1982.

Chaudary MA, Millis RR, Davies GC, et al: Nipple Discharge: The Diagnostic Value of Testing for Occult Blood. *Ann Surg* 196: 651–655, 1982.

Chen KTK: Psammoma Bodies in Pelvic Washings. *Acta Cytol* 27: 377–379, 1983.

Chen KTK: Psammocarcinoma of the Peritoneum. *Diagn Cytopathol* 10: 224–228, 1994.

Chen L-M, Hwang W-S: Myeloma With Pleural Involvement. *Acta Cytol* 35: 372–373, 1991.

Chernow B, Sahn SA: Carcinomatous Involvement of the Pleura: An Analysis of 96 Patients. *Am J Med* 63: 695–702, 1977.

Chiu B, Churg A, Tengblad A, et al: Analysis of Hyaluronic Acid in the Diagnosis of Malignant Mesothelioma. *Cancer* 54: 2195–2199, 1984.

Cho K-J, Myong N-H, Jang J-J: Effusion Cytology of Endodermal Sinus Tumor of the Colon: Report of a Case. *Acta Cytol* 35: 207–209, 1991.

Choudhury A, Wengert PA Jr, Smith JS Jr: A New Surgical Localization Technique for Biopsy in Patients With Nipple Discharge. *Arch Surg* 124: 874–875, 1989.

Churg AM, Warnock ML: Asbestos and Other Ferruginous Bodies: Their Formation and Clinical Significance. *Am J Pathol* 102: 447–456, 1981.

Churg A: Fiber Counting and Analysis in the Diagnosis of Asbestos-Related Disease. *Hum Pathol* 13: 381–392, 1982.

Churg A: Malignant Mesothelioma. *Chest* 89: 367S–368S, 1986.

Ciatto S, Bravetti P, Cariaggi P: Significance of Nipple Discharge Clinical Patterns in the Selection of Cases for Cytologic Examination. *Acta Cytol* 30: 17–20, 1986.

Clarris BJ, Doherty RL, Fraser JRE, et al: Epidemic Polyarthritis: A Cytological, Virological and Immunochemical Study. *Aust N Z J Med* 5: 450–457, 1975.

Cobb CJ, Wynn J, Cobb SR, et al: Cytologic Findings in an Effusion Caused by Rupture of a Benign Cystic Teratoma of the Mediastinum Into a Serous Cavity. *Acta Cytol* 29: 1015–1020, 1985.

Coffin CM, Adcock LL, Dehner LP: The Second-Look Operation for Ovarian Neoplasms: A Study of 85 Cases Emphasizing Cytologic and Histologic Problems. *Int J Gynecol Pathol* 4: 97–109, 1985.

Coleman DV: Ciliated Organisms in Dialysis Fluid. *Lancet* (i): 1030, 1986.

Coleman M, Henderson DW, Mukherjee TM: The Ultrastructural Pathology of Malignant Pleural Mesothelioma. *Pathol Annu* 241: 305–353, 1989.

Contino CA, Vance JW: Eosinophilic Pleural Effusion. *NY State J Med* 66: 2044–2048, 1966.

Copeland LJ, Gershenson DM, Wharton JT, et al: Microscopic Disease at Second-Look Laparotomy in Advanced Ovarian Cancer. *Cancer* 55: 472–478, 1985.

Corson JM, Pinkus GS: Mesothelioma: Profile of Keratin Proteins and Carcinoembryonic Antigen: An Immunoperoxidase Study of 20 Cases and Comparison With Pulmonary Adenocarcinomas. *Am J Pathol* 108: 80–87, 1982.

Costa M, Oertel YC: Cytology of Pseudomyxoma Peritonei: Report of Two Cases Arising From Appendiceal Cystadenomas. *Diagn Cytopathol* 6: 201–203, 1990.

Covell JL, Carry JB, Feldman PS: Peritoneal Washings in Ovarian Tumors: Potential Sources of Error in Cytologic Diagnosis. *Acta Cytol* 29: 310–316, 1985.

Craighead JE, Mossman BT: The Pathogenesis of Asbestos-Associated Diseases. *N Engl J Med* 306: 1446–1455, 1982.

Creasman WT, Rutledge F: The Prognostic Value of Peritoneal Cytology in Gynecologic Malignant Disease. *Am J Obstet Gynecol* 110: 773–781, 1971.

Creasman WT, Disaia PJ, Blessing J, et al: Prognostic Significance of Peritoneal Cytology in Patients With Endometrial Cancer and Preliminary Data Concerning Therapy With Intraperitoneal Radiopharmaceuticals. *Am J Obstet Gynecol* 141: 921–929, 1981.

Croonen AM, Van Der Valk P, Herman CJ, et al: Cytology, Immunopathology and Flow Cytometry in the Diagnosis of Pleural and Peritoneal Effusions. *Lab Invest* 58: 725–732, 1988.

Crosby JH, Allsbrook WC Jr, Pantazis CG, et al: Cytology and DNA Flow Cytometry of Peritoneal Washings in Gynecologic Patients. *Mod Pathol* 5: 153–157, 1992.

Cunningham AL, Fraser JRE, Hobbs JB: A Study of Synovial Fluid and Cytology in Arthritis Associated With Herpes Zoster. *Aust N Z J Med* 9: 440–443, 1979.

Curran WS, Williams AW: Eosinophilic Pleural Effusion: A Clue in Differential Diagnosis. *Arch Intern Med* 111: 809–813, 1963.

Currey HLF: Investigation of Joint Fluids. *Proc R Soc Med* 61: 969–971, 1968.

Currey HLF, Vernon-Roberts B: Examination of Synovial Fluid. *Clin Rheum Dis* 2(1): 149–177, 1976.

Dabbs DJ: Mammary Ductal Foam Cells: Macrophage Immunophenotype. *Hum Pathol* 24: 977–981, 1993.

Dalrymple JC, Bannatyne P, Russell P, et al: Extraovarian Peritoneal Serous Papillary Carcinoma: A Clinicopathologic Study of 31 Cases. *Cancer* 64: 110–115, 1989.

Danner DE, Gmelich JT: A Comparative Study of Tumor Cells From Metastatic Carcinoma of the Breast in Effusions. *Acta Cytol* 19: 509–518, 1975.

Das DK, Gupta SK, Ayyagari S, et al: Pleural Effusions in Non-Hodgkin's Lymphoma: A Cytomorphologic, Cytochemical and Immunologic Study. *Acta Cytol* 31: 119–121, 1987.

Daste G, Serre G, Mauduyt MA, et al: Immunophenotyping of Mesothelial Cells and Carcinoma Cells With Monoclonal Antibodies to Cytokeratins, Vimentin, CEA and EMA Improves the Cytodiagnosis of Serous Effusions. *Cytopathology* 2: 19–28, 1991.

Daste G, Voigt JJ, Rubie H, et al: Cytodiagnosis of Rhabdomyosarcoma in Serous Effusions: Cytological and Immunocytochemical Findings of Two Unusual Cases. *Cytopathology* 4: 315–320, 1993.

Decker DA, Dines DE, Payne WS, et al: The Significance of a Cytologically Negative Pleural Effusion in Bronchogenic Carcinoma. *Chest* 74: 640–642, 1978.

DeCoste SD, Imber MJ, Baden HP: Yellow Nail Syndrome. *Acad Dermatol* 22: 608–611, 1990.

Dekker A, Graham T, Bupp PA: The Occurrence of Sickle Cells in Pleural Fluid: Report of a Patient With Sickle Cell Disease. *Acta Cytol* 19: 251–254, 1975.

Dekker A, Bupp PA: Cytology of Serous Effusions: An Investigation into the Usefulness of Cell Blocks Versus Smears. *Am J Clin Pathol* 70: 855–860, 1978.

Delahaye M, de Jong AA, Versnel MA, et al: Cytopathology of Malignant Mesothelioma. Reappraisal of the Diagnostic Value of Collagen Cores. *Cytopathology* 1: 137–145, 1990.

Delfs-Jegge S, Dalquen P, Hurwitz N: Cytomegalovirus-Infected Cells in a Pleural Effusion From an Acquired Immunodeficiency Syndrome Patient. A Case Report. *Acta Cytol* 38: 70–72, 1994.

de Torres EF, Guevara EC: Pleuritis by Radiation: Report of Two Cases. *Acta Cytol* 25: 427–429, 1981.

Detraux P, Benmussa M, Tristant H, et al: Breast Disease in the Male: Galactographic Evaluation. *Radiology* 154: 605–606, 1985.

Devitt JE: Management of Nipple Discharge by Clinical Findings. *Am J Surg* 149: 789–792, 1985.

Dewald G, Dines DE, Weiland LH, et al: Usefulness of Chromosome Examination in the Diagnosis of Malignant Pleural Effusions. *N Engl J Med* 295: 1494–1500, 1976.

Dewar A, Valente M, Ring NP, et al: Pleural Mesothelioma of Epithelial Type and Pulmonary Adenocarcinoma: An Ultrastructural and Cytochemical Comparison. *J Pathol* 152: 309–316, 1987.

Diaz-Arias AA, Loy TS, Bickel JT, et al: Utility of BER-EP4 in the Diagnosis of Adenocarcinoma in Effusions: An Immunocytochemical Study of 232 Cases. *Diagn Cytopathol* 9: 516–521, 1993.

DiBonito L, Dudine S, Falconieri G: Cytopathology of Exocrine Pancreatic Carcinoma in Effusions. *Acta Cytol* 35: 311–314, 1991.

DiBonito L, Falconieri G, Colautti I, et al: The Positive Pleural Effusion: A Retrospective Study of Cytopathologic Diagnoses With Autopsy Confirmation. *Acta Cytol* 36: 329–332, 1992.

DiBonito L, Falconieri G, Colautti I, et al: Cytopathology of Malignant Mesothelioma: A Study of Its Patterns and Histological Bases. *Diagn Cytopathol* 9: 25–31, 1993a.

DiBonito L, Falconieri G, Colautti I, et al: The Positive Peritoneal Effusion: A Retrospective Study of Cytopathologic Diagnoses With Autopsy Confirmation. *Acta Cytol* 37: 483–488, 1993b.

Dieterich M, Goodman SN, Rojas-Corona RR, et al: Multivariate Analysis of Prognostic Features in Malignant Pleural Effusions From Breast Cancer Patients. *Acta Cytol* 38: 945–952, 1994.

Dines DE, Pierre RV, Franzen S: The Value of Cells in the Pleural Fluid in the Differential Diagnosis. *Mayo Clin Proc* 50: 571–572, 1975.

Domagala W, Woyke S: Transmission and Scanning Electron Microscopic Studies of Cells in Effusions. *Acta Cytol* 19: 214–224, 1975.

Domagala W, Koss LG: Surface Configuration of Mesothelial Cells in Effusion: A Comparative Light Microscopic and Scanning Electron Microscopic Study. *Virchows Arch B Cell Pathol* 30: 231–243, 1979.

Domagala W, Emeson EE, Koss LG: T and B Lymphocyte Enumeration in the Diagnosis of Lymphocyte-Rich Pleural Fluids. *Acta Cytol* 25: 108–110, 1981.

Donna A, Betta P-G, Bellingeri D, et al: Cytologic Diagnosis of Malignant Mesothelioma in Serous Effusions Using an Antimesothelial-Cell Antibody. *Diagn Cytopathol* 8: 361–365, 1992.

Duane GB, Kanter MH: Light and Electron Microscopic Characteristics of Signet-Ring Adenocarcinoma Cells in Serous Effusions and Their Distinction From Mesothelial Cells. *Acta Cytol* 29: 211–218, 1985.

Duggan MA, Masters CB, Alexander F: Immunohistochemical Differentiation of Malignant Mesothelioma, Mesothelial Hyperplasia and Metastatic Adenocarcinoma in Serous Effusions, Utilizing Staining for Carcinoembryonic Antigen, Keratin and Vimentin. *Acta Cytol* 31: 807–814, 1987.

Edge JR, Choudhury SL: Malignant Mesothelioma of the Pleura in Barrow-in-Furness. *Thorax* 33: 26–30, 1978.

Edmondstone WM: Investigation of Pleural Effusion: Comparison Between Fiberoptic Thoracoscopy, Needle Biopsy and Cytology. *Respir Med* 84: 23–26, 1990.

Edoute Y, Malberger E, Kuten A, et al: Symptomatic Pericardial Effusion in Lung Cancer Patients: The Role of Fluid Cytology. *J Surg Oncol* 45: 121–123, 1990a.

Edoute Y, Kuten A, Ben-Haim SA, et al: Symptomatic Pericardial Effusion in Breast Cancer Patients: The Role of Fluid Cytology. *J Surg Oncol* 45: 265–269, 1990b.

Efrati P, Nir E: Morphological and Cytochemical Investigation of Human Mesothelial Cells From Pleural and Peritoneal Effusions: A Light and Electron Microscopy Study. *Isr J Med Sci* 12: 662–673, 1976.

Eghtedari AA, Bacon PA, Collins A: Immunoblasts in Synovial Fluid and Blood in the Rheumatic Diseases. *Ann Rheum Dis* 39: 318–322, 1980.

Ehya H: Cytology of Mesothelioma of the Tunica Vaginalis Metastatic to the Lung. *Acta Cytol* 29: 79–84, 1985.

Ehya H: The Cytologic Diagnosis of Mesothelioma. *Semin Diagn Pathol* 3: 196–203, 1986.

Eisenberg JM, Schumacher HR, Davidson PK, et al: Usefulness of Synovial Fluid Analysis in the Evaluation of Joint Effusions: Use of Threshold Analysis and Likelihood Ratios to Assess a Diagnostic Test. *Arch Intern Med* 144: 715–719, 1984.

El-Naggar AK, Ordonez NG, Garnsey L, et al: Epithelioid Pleural Mesotheliomas and Pulmonary Adenocarcinomas: A Comparative DNA Flow Cytometric Study. *Hum Pathol* 22: 972–978, 1991.

Epler GR, McLoud TC, Gaensler EA: Prevalence and Incidence of Benign Asbestos Pleural Effusion in a Working Population. *JAMA* 247: 617–622, 1982.

Esteban JM, Yokota S, Husain S, et al: Immunocytochemical Profile of Benign and Carcinomatous Effusions. *Am J Clin Pathol* 94: 698–705, 1990.

Fam AAG, Kolin A, Lewis AJ: Metastatic Carcinomatous Arthritis and Carcinoma of the Lung: A Report of Two Cases Diagnosed by Synovial Fluid Cytology. *J Rheumatol* 7: 98–104, 1980.

Farr GH, Hajdu SI: Exfoliative Cytology of Metastatic Neuroblastoma. *Acta Cytol* 16: 203–206, 1972.

Favis EA, Kerman HD, Schildecker W: Multiple Myeloma Manifested as a Problem in the Diagnosis of Pulmonary Disease. *Am J Med* 33: 323–327, 1960.

Fenster DL: Bloody Nipple Discharge. *J Pediatr* 104: 640, 1984.

Ferrandez-Izquierdo A, Navarro-Fos S, Gonzalez-Devesa M, et al: Immunocytochemical Typification of Mesothelial Cells in Effusions: In Vivo and In Vitro Models. *Diagn Cytopathol* 10: 256–262, 1994.

Fidler WJ: Demodex Folliculorum in a Nipple Imprint. *Acta Cytol* 22: 168–169, 1978.

Fife KM, Talbot DC, Mortimer P, et al: Chylous Ascites in Kaposi's Sarcoma: A Case Report. *Br J Dermatol* 126: 378–379, 1992.

Fischermann K, Bech I, Foged P, et al: Nipple Discharge: Diagnosis and Treatment. *Acta Chir Scand* 135: 403–406, 1969.

Fleming RM: Cytological Studies in Lesions of the Breast: Findings in Nipple Secretions and Aspirates From Tumors. *South Med J* 48: 74–78, 1955.

Flynn MK, Johnston W, Bigner S: Carcinoma of Ovarian and Other Origins in Effusions. Immunocytochemical Study With a Panel of Monoclonal Antibodies. *Acta Cytol* 37: 439–447, 1993.

Fok F, Bewtra C, Hammeke M: The Study of Peritoneal Fluid Cytology in Renal Dialysis Patients. *Acta Cytol* 32: 767, 1988.

Fok FK, Bewtra C, Hammeke MD: Cytology of Peritoneal Fluid From Patients on Continuous Ambulatory Dialysis. *Acta Cytol* 33: 595–598, 1989.

Foot NC: The Identification of Tumor Cells in Sediments of Serous Effusions. *Am J Pathol* 13: 1–11, 1937.

Foot NC: Identification of Cells in Exudates and Effusates. *Ann NY Acad Sci* 63: 1324–1330, 1955.

Fraser JRE, Cunningham AL, Clarris BJ, et al: Cytology of Synovial Effusions in Epidemic Polyarthritis. *Aust N Z J Med* 11: 168–173, 1981.

Freemont AJ, Denton J, Chuck A, et al: Diagnostic Value of Synovial Fluid Microscopy: A Reassessment and Rationalisation. *Ann Rheum Dis* 50: 101–107, 1991.

Frierson HF Jr, Mills SE, Legier JF: Flow Cytometric Analysis of Ploidy in Immunohistochemically Confirmed Examples of Malignant Epithelial Mesothelioma. *Am J Clin Pathol* 90: 240–243, 1988.

Frist B, Kahan AV, Koss LG: Comparison of the Diagnostic Values of Biopsies of the Pleura and Cytologic Evaluation of Pleural Fluids. *Am J Clin Pathol* 72: 48–51, 1979.

Fujii M, Ishii Y, Wakabayashi T, et al: Cytologic Diagnosis of Male Breast Cancer With Nipple Discharge: A Case Report. *Acta Cytol* 30: 21–24, 1986.

Funderburk WW, Syphax B: Evaluation of Nipple Discharge in Benign and Malignant Diseases. *Cancer* 24: 1290–1296, 1969.

Fung A, Rayter Z, Fisher C, et al: Preoperative Cytology and Mammography in Patients With Single-Duct Nipple Discharge Treated by Surgery. *Br J Surg* 77: 1211–1212, 1990.

Funkhouser JW, Hunter KK, Thompson NJ: The Diagnostic Value of Cul-de-Sac Aspiration in the Detection of Ovarian Carcinoma. *Acta Cytol* 19: 538–541, 1975.

Gabriel S: Multiple Myeloma Presenting as Pulmonary Infiltration: Report of a Case. *Dis Chest* 47: 123–126, 1965.

Garrison RN, Kaelin LD, Heuser LS, et al: Malignant Ascites: Clinical and Experimental Observations. *Ann Surg* 203: 644–651, 1986.

Gaulier A, Jouret-Mourin A, Marsan C: Peritoneal Endometriosis: Report of a Case With Cytologic, Cytochemical and Histopathologic Study. *Acta Cytol* 27: 446–449, 1983.

Geisinger KR, Naylor B, Beals TF, et al: Cytopathology, Including Transmission and Scanning Electron Microscopy, of Pleomorphic Liposarcomas in Pleural Fluids. *Acta Cytol* 24: 435–441, 1980.

Geisinger KR, Hajdu SI, Helson L: Exfoliative Cytology of Nonlymphoreticular Neoplasms in Children. *Acta Cytol* 28: 16–28, 1984.

Geisinger KR, Vance RP, Prater T, et al: Rheumatoid Pleural Effusion. A Transmission and Scanning Electron Microscopic Evaluation. *Acta Cytol* 29: 239–247, 1985.

Geisinger KR, Buss DH, Kawamoto EH, et al: Multiple Myeloma: The Diagnostic Role and Prognostic Significance of Exfoliative Cytology. *Acta Cytol* 30: 334–340, 1986.

Genadry R, Poliakoff S, Rotmensch J, et al: Primary, Papillary Peritoneal Neoplasia. *Obstet Gynecol* 58: 730–734, 1981.

George AL Jr, Hays JT, Graham BS: Blastomycosis Presenting as Monarticular Arthritis: The Role of Synovial Fluid Cytology. *Arthritis Rheum* 28: 516–521, 1985.

Geszler G, Szpak CA, Harris RE, et al: Prognostic Value of Peritoneal Washings in Patients With Malignant Mixed Müllerian Tumors of the Uterus. *Am J Obstet Gynecol* 155: 83–89, 1986.

Gioanni J, Caldani C, Zanghellini E, et al: A New Epithelial Membrane Antigen (Calam 27) as a Marker of Carcinoma in Serous Effusions. *Acta Cytol* 35: 315–319, 1991.

Gondos B, McIntosh KM, Renston RH, King EB: Application of Electron Microscopy in the Definitive Diagnosis of Effusions. *Acta Cytol* 22: 297–304, 1978.

Gotloib L, Servadio C: Ascites in Patients Undergoing Maintenance Hemodialysis: Report of Six Cases and Physiopathologic Approach. *Am J Med* 61: 465–470, 1976.

Graham JB, Graham RM, Schueller EF: Preclinical Detection of Ovarian Cancer. *Cancer* 17: 1414–1432, 1964.

Graham RM, Bartels JD, Graham JB: Screening for Ovarian Cancer by Cul-de-Sac Aspiration. *Acta Cytol* 6: 492–495, 1962.

Graham SJ, Duval-Arnould B, Mercado TC, et al: Burkitt's Lymphoma: A Pericardial Presentation. *Cytopathology* 1: 239–242, 1990.

Granados R, Cibas ES, Fletcher JA: Cytogenetic Analysis of Effusions From Malignant Mesothelioma. A Diagnostic Adjunct to Cytology. *Acta Cytol* 38: 711–717, 1994.

Green N, Gancedo H, Smith R, et al: Pseudomyxoma Peritonei–Nonoperative Management and Biochemical Findings: A Case Report. *Cancer* 36: 1834–1837, 1975.

Greenberg SD: Asbestos Lung Disease. *Semin Respir Med* 4: 130–137, 1982.

Greenberg SD: Recent Advances in Pulmonary Cytopathology. *Hum Pathol* 14: 901–912, 1983.

Grillo M, Lehmann-Willenbrock E, Gent H-J: Chromogalactography Preceding Ductal-Lobular Unit Excision for Nipple Discharge With Special Reference to Diagnostic Galactography and Histology. *Ann Chir Gynaecol* 79: 6–9, 1990.

Grimshaw RN, Tupper WC, Fraser RC, et al: Prognostic Value of Peritoneal Cytology in Endometrial Carcinoma. *Gynecol Oncol* 36: 97–100, 1990.

Groll M, Takeda M, Rakoff A: Breast and Vaginal Hormonal Cytology in Patients With Breast Secretions. *Acta Cytol* 19: 429–430, 1975.

Grundy GW, Miller RW: Malignant Mesothelioma in Childhood: Report of 13 Cases. *Cancer* 30: 1216–1218, 1972.

Grunz H: The Comparative Diagnostic Accuracy, Efficiency and Specificity of Cytologic Technics Used in the Diagnosis of Malignant Neoplasm in Serous Effusions of the Pleural and Pericardial Cavities. *Acta Cytol* 8: 150–163, 1964.

Guffanti MC, Faleri ML: Benign-Appearing Mesothelioma Cells in a Serous Effusion. *Acta Cytol* 29: 90–92, 1985.

Gunnels JJ: Perplexing Pleural Effusion. *Chest* 74: 390–393, 1978.

Gupta PK, Frost JK: Cytologic Changes Associated With Asbestos Exposure. *Semin Oncol* 8: 283–289, 1981.

Gupta PK, Albritton N, Erozan YS, et al: Occurrence of Cilia in Exfoliated Ovarian Adenocarcinoma Cells. *Diagn Cytopathol* 1: 228–231, 1985.

Gupta RK, Naran S: Cytodiagnosis of Pseudomyxoma Peritonei in Cases Suspected of Ovarian Tumours. *Diagn Cytopathol* 9: 682–684, 1993.

Gurley AM, Hidvegi DF, Cajulis RS, et al: Morphologic and Morphometric Features of Low Grade Serous Tumours of the Ovary. *Diagn Cytopathol* 11: 220–225, 1994.

Guzman J, Costabel U, Bross KJ, et al: The Value of the Immunoperoxidase Slide Assay in the Diagnosis of Malignant Pleural Effusions in Breast Cancer. *Acta Cytol* 32: 188–192, 1988a.

Guzman J, Hilgarth M, Bross KJ, et al: Lymphocyte Subpopulations in Malignant Ascites of Serous Papillary Ovarian Adenocarcinoma: An Immunocytochemical Study. *Acta Cytol* 32: 811–815, 1988b.

Guzman J, Bross KJ, Costabel U: Malignant Pleural Effusions Due to Small Cell Carcinoma of the Lung: An Immunocytochemical Cell-Surface Analysis of Lymphocytes and Tumor Cells. *Acta Cytol* 34: 497–501, 1990.

Guzman J, Bross KJ, Costabel U: Malignant Lymphoma in Pleural Effusions: An Immunocytochemical Cell Surface Analysis. *Diagn Cytopathol* 7: 113–118, 1991.

Haddad MG, Silverman JF, Joshi VV, et al: Effusion Cytology in Burkitt's Lymphoma. *Diagn Cytopathol* 12: 3–7, 1995.

Hajdu SI, Koss LG: Cytologic Diagnosis of Metastatic Myosarcomas. *Acta Cytol* 13: 545–551, 1969.

Hajdu SI: Exfoliative Cytology of Primary and Metastatic Wilms' Tumors. *Acta Cytol* 15: 339–342, 1971.

Hajdu SI, Savino A: Cytologic Diagnosis of Malignant Melanoma. *Acta Cytol* 17: 320–327, 1973.

Hajdu SI, Nolan MA: Exfoliative Cytology of Malignant Germ Cell Tumors. *Acta Cytol* 19: 255–260, 1975.

Hallman JR, Geisinger KR: Cytology of Fluids From Pleural, Peritoneal and Pericardial Cavities in Children: A Comprehensive Survey. *Acta Cytol* 38: 209–217, 1994.

Hanna W, Kahn HJ: The Ultrastructure of Metastatic Adenocarcinoma in Serous Fluids: An Aid in Identification of the Primary Site of the Neoplasm. *Acta Cytol* 29: 202–210, 1985.

Hansen RM, Komaki R, Hanson GA, et al: Indolent Diffuse Histiocytic Lymphoma With Sclerosis and Chylous Effusions. *Cancer* 51: 2144–2146, 1983.

Hansen RM, Caya JG, Clowry LJ Jr, et al: Benign Mesothelial Proliferation With Effusion: Clinicopathologic Entity That May Mimic Malignancy. *Am J Med* 77: 887–892, 1984.

Harouny VR, Sutton GP, Clark SA, et al: The Importance of Peritoneal Cytology in Endometrial Carcinoma. *Obstet Gynecol* 72: 394–398, 1988.

Harwood TR, Gracey DR, Yokoo H: Pseudomesotheliomatous Carcinoma of the Lung: A Variant of Peripheral Lung Cancer. *Am J Clin Pathol* 65: 159–167, 1976.

Hasan FM, Nash G, Kazemi H: The Significance of Asbestos Exposure in the Diagnosis of Mesothelioma: A 28-Year Experience From a Major Urban Hospital. *Am Rev Respir Dis* 115: 761–768, 1977.

Hausheer FH, Yarbro JW: Diagnosis and Treatment of Malignant Pleural Effusion. *Semin Oncol* 12: 54–75, 1985.

Heath R, Rosenman J, Varia M, et al: Peritoneal Fluid Cytology in Endometrial Cancer: Its Significance and the Role of Chromic Phosphate (^{32}P) Therapy. *Int J Radiat Oncol Biol Phys* 15: 815–822, 1988.

Herrera GA, Wilkerson JA: Ultrastructural Studies of Malignant Cells in Fluids. *Diagn Cytopathol* 1: 272–275, 1985.

Heyman RB, Rauh JL: Areola Gland Discharge in Adolescent Females. *J Adolesc Health Care* 4: 285–286, 1983.

Hirai Y, Fujimoto I, Yamauchi K, et al: Peritoneal Fluid Cytology and Prognosis in Patients With Endometrial Carcinoma. *Obstet Gynecol* 73: 335–338, 1989.

Hoda SA, Rosen PP: Cytologic Diagnosis of Metastatic Penile Carcinoma in Pleural Effusion. *Arch Pathol Lab Med* 116: 198–199, 1992.

Holleb AI, Farrow JH: Nipple Discharge. *CA Cancer J Clin* 16: 182–185, 1966.

Hsu C: Cytologic Detection of Malignancy in Pleural Effusion: Review of 5, 255 Samples From 3, 811 Patients. *Diagn Cytopathol* 3: 8–12, 1987.

Huncharek M: Changing Risk Groups for Malignant Mesothelioma. *Cancer* 69: 2704–2711, 1992.

Imachi M, Tsukamoto N, Matsuyama T, et al: Peritoneal Cytology in Patients With Carcinoma of the Uterine Cervix. *Gynecol Oncol* 26: 202–207, 1987.

Imachi M, Tsukamoto N, Matsuyama T, et al: Peritoneal Cytology in Patients With Endometrial Carcinoma. *Gynecol Oncol* 30: 76–81, 1988.

Inaji H, Yayoi E, Maeura Y, et al: Carcinoembryonic Antigen Estimation in Nipple Discharge as an Adjunctive Tool in the Diagnosis of Early Breast Cancer. *Cancer* 60: 3008–3013, 1987.

Insabato L: Nipple Secretions in Breast Diseases. *Diagn Cytopathol* 8: 200–201, 1992.

Jacques SM, Selvaggi SM: Multiple Peritoneal Cytologies Collected During Laparotomy for Gynecologic Malignancy. *Diagn Cytopathol* 7: 482–486, 1991.

Japko L, Horta AA, Schreiber K, et al: Malignant Mesothelioma of the Tunica Vaginalis Testis: Report of First Case With Preoperative Diagnosis. *Cancer* 49: 119–127, 1982.

Jara F, Takita H, Rao UNM: Malignant Mesothelioma of Pleura: Clinicopathologic Observation. *NY State J Med* 77: 1885–1888, 1977.

Järvi OH, Kunnas RJ, Laitio MT, et al: The Accuracy and Significance of Cytologic Cancer Diagnosis of Pleural Effusions (A Followup Study of 338 Patients). *Acta Cytol* 16: 152–158, 1972.

Johnson TL, Kumar NB, Hopkins N, et al: Cytologic Features of Ovarian Tumors of Low Malignant Potential in Peritoneal Fluids. *Acta Cytol* 32: 513–518, 1988.

Johnson TL, Kini SR: Cytologic and Clinicopathologic Features of Abnormal Nipple Secretions: 225 Cases. *Diagn Cytopathol* 7: 17–22, 1991.

Johnston WW: The Malignant Pleural Effusion: A Review of Cytopathologic Diagnoses of 584 Specimens From 472 Consecutive Patients. *Cancer* 56: 905–909, 1985.

Johnston WW: Applications of Monoclonal Antibodies in Clinical Cytology as Exemplified by Studies With Monoclonal Antibody B72.3: The George N. Papanicolaou Award Lecture. *Acta Cytol* 31: 537–556, 1987.

Jones ISC, Khoo SK, Whitaker SV, et al: The Assessment of Residual Ovarian Cancer by Cytological Examination of Peritoneal Washings Obtained by Culdocentesis. *Gynecol Oncol* 11: 131–135, 1981.

Jones MA, Hitchcox S, D'Ascanio P, et al: Flow Cytometric DNA Analysis versus Cytology in the Evaluation of Peritoneal Fluids. *Gynecol Oncol* 43: 226–232, 1991.

Kadar N, Homesley HD, Malfetano JH: Prognostic Factors in Surgical Stage III and IV Carcinoma of the Endometrium. *Obstet Gynecol* 84: 983–986, 1994.

Kahn HJ, Hanna W, Yeger H, et al: Immunohistochemical Localization of Prekeratin Filaments in Benign and Malignant Cells in Effusions: Comparison With Intermediate Filament Distribution by Electron Microscopy. *Am J Pathol* 109: 206–214, 1982.

Kanbour AI, Buchsbaum HJ, Hall A, et al: Peritoneal Cytology in Malignant Mixed Müllerian Tumors of the Uterus. *Gynecol Oncol* 33: 91–95, 1989.

Kapadia SB: Cytological Diagnosis of Malignant Pleural Effusion in Myeloma. *Arch Pathol Lab Med* 101: 534–535, 1977.

Kapila K, Hajdu SI, Whitmore WF Jr, et al: Cytologic Diagnosis of Metastatic Germ-Cell Tumors. *Acta Cytol* 27: 245–251, 1983.

Kaplan AI, Zakher F, Sabin S: Drug-Induced Lupus Erythematosus With In Vivo Lupus Erythematosus Cells in Pleural Fluid. *Chest* 73: 875–876, 1978.

Karp SJ, Shareef D: Ascites as a Presenting Feature of Multiple Myeloma. *J R Soc Med* 80: 182–184, 1987.

Kashimura M, Matsukuma K, Kamura T, et al: Cytologic Findings in Peritoneal Fluids From Patients With Ovarian Serous Carcinoma. *Diagn Cytopathol* 2: 13–16, 1986.

Katz RL, Raval P, Manning JT, et al: A Morphologic, Immunologic, and Cytometric Approach to the Classification of Non-Hodgkin's Lymphoma in Effusions. *Diagn Cytopathol* 3: 91–101, 1987.

Kawai T, Suzuki M, Shinmei M, et al: Glycosaminoglycans in Malignant Diffuse Mesothelioma. *Cancer* 56: 567–574, 1985.

Keettel WC, Elkins HB: Experience With Radioactive Colloidal Gold in the Treatment of Ovarian Carcinoma. *Am J Obstet Gynecol* 71: 553–568, 1956.

Keettel WC, Pixley E: Diagnostic Value of Peritoneal Washings. *Clin Obstet Gynec* 1: 592–606, 1958.

Keettel WC, Pixley EE, Buchsbaum HJ: Experience With Peritoneal Cytology in the Management of Gynecologic Malignancies. *Am J Obstet Gynecol* 120: 174–182, 1974.

Kelley S, McGarry P, Hutson Y: Atypical Cells in Pleural Fluid Characteristic of Systemic Lupus Erythematosus. *Acta Cytol* 15: 357–362, 1971.

Kern WH: Benign Papillary Structures With Psammoma Bodies in Culdocentesis Fluid. *Acta Cytol* 13: 178–180, 1969.

Khoddami M, Esphehani FN, Aslani FS: Ascites as a Presenting Feature of Relapsed Multiple Myeloma: Report of a Case Diagnosed by Aspiration Cytology. *Acta Cytol* 36: 325–328, 1992.

Kilgore LC, Orr JW Jr, Hatch KD, et al: Peritoneal Cytology in Patients With Squamous Cell Carcinoma of the Cervix. *Gynecol Oncol* 19: 24–29, 1984.

Kimura N, Namiki T, Wada T, et al: Peritoneal Implantation of Endodermal Sinus Tumor of the Pineal Region Via a Ventriculoperitoneal Shunt: Cytodiagnosis With Immunocytochemical Demonstration of Alpha-Fetoprotein. *Acta Cytol* 28: 143–147, 1984.

King EB, Barrett D, King M-C, et al: Cellular Composition of the Nipple Aspirate Specimen of Breast Fluid, I: The Benign Cells. *Am J Clin Pathol* 64: 728–738, 1975a.

King EB, Barrett D, Petrakis NL: Cellular Composition of the Nipple Aspirate Specimen of Breast Fluid, II: Abnormal Findings. *Am J Clin Pathol* 64: 739–748, 1975b.

King EB, Chew KL, Petrakis NL, et al: Nipple Aspirate Cytology for the Study of Breast Cancer Precursors. *J Natl Cancer Inst* 71: 1115–1121, 1983.

Kjellgren O: The Cytologic Diagnosis of Cancer of the Breast. *Acta Cytol* 8: 216–223, 1964.

Kleinholz EJ Jr, Tennebaum MJ: Pleural Plasmacytoma Presenting as Pleural Effusion. *Va Med Monthly* 100: 1035–1040, 1973.

Klempman S: The Exfoliative Cytology of Diffuse Pleural Mesothelioma. *Cancer* 15: 691–704, 1962.

Kline TS, Lash SR: The Bleeding Nipple of Pregnancy and Postpartum Period: A Cytologic and Histologic Study. *Acta Cytol* 8: 336–340, 1964.

Knight DC, Lowell DM, Heimann A, et al: Aspiration of the Breast and Nipple Discharge Cytology. *Surg Gynecol Obstet* 163: 415–420, 1986.

Kobayashi TK, Teraoka S, Tsujioka T, et al: Ciliated Ovarian Adenocarcinoma Cells in Ascitic Fluid Cytology: Report of a Case With Immunocytochemical Features. *Diagn Cytopathol* 4: 234–238, 1988.

Kobayashi TK, Okamoto H, Yakushiji M: Cytologic Detection of Herpes Simplex Virus DNA in Nipple Discharge by In Situ Hybridization: Report of Two Cases. *Diagn Cytopathol* 9: 296–299, 1993.

Kobayashi Y, Takeda S, Yamamoto T, et al: Cytologic Detection of Malignant Mesothelioma of the Pericardium. *Acta Cytol* 22: 344–349, 1978.

Kobzik L, Antman KH, Warhol MJ: The Distinction of Mesothelioma From Adenocarcinoma in Malignant Effusions by Electron Microscopy. *Acta Cytol* 29: 219–225, 1985.

Koeffler HP, Cline MJ: Multiple Myeloma Presenting as Ascites. *West J Med* 127: 248–250, 1977.

Kokkola K, Valta R: Aetiology and Findings in Eosinophilic Pleural Effusion. *Scand J Respir Dis Suppl* 89: 159–165, 1974.

Kondo H, Asamura H, Suemasu K, et al: Prognostic Significance of Pleural Lavage Cytology Immediately After Thoracotomy in Patients With Lung Cancer. *J Thorac Cardiovasc Surg* 106: 1092–1097, 1993.

Konski A, Poulter C, Keys H, et al: Absence of Prognostic Significance, Peritoneal Dissemination and Treatment Advantage in Endometrial Cancer Patients With Positive Peritoneal Cytology. *Int J Radiation Oncol Biol Phys* 4: 49–55, 1988.

Krishnan B, Mody DR, Ramzy I: Alpha-Mannosidosis. Report of a Case With Morphologic, Cytologic and Immunohistochemical Considerations. *Acta Cytol* 38: 441–445, 1994.

Krishnan S, Statsinger AL, Kleinman M, et al: Eosinophilic Pleural Effusion With Charcot-Leyden Crystals. *Acta Cytol* 27: 529–532, 1983.

Kudo R, Takashina T, Ito E, et al: Peritoneal Washing Cytology at Second-Look Laparotomy in Cisplatin-Treated Ovarian Cancer Patients. *Acta Cytol* 34: 545–548, 1990.

Kuhlmann L, Berghäuser K-H, Schäffer R: Distinction of Mesothelioma From Carcinoma in Pleural Effusions: An Immunocytochemical Study on Routinely Processed Cytoblock Preparations. *Pathol Res Pract* 187: 467–471, 1991.

Kuma UN, Varkey B, Mathai G: Posttraumatic Pleural-Fluid and Blood Eosinophilia. *JAMA* 234: 625–626, 1975.

Kumar NB, Naylor B: Megakaryocytes in Pleural and Peritoneal Fluids: Prevalence, Significance, Morphology, and Cytohistological Correlation. *J Clin Pathol* 33: 1153–1159, 1980.

Kutty CPK, Remeniuk E, Varkey B: Malignant-Appearing Cells in Pleural Effusion Due to Pancreatitis: Case Report and Literature Review. *Acta Cytol* 25: 412–416, 1981.

Kwee W-S, Veldhuizen RW, Alons CA, et al: Quantitative and Qualitative Differences Between Benign and Malignant Mesothelial Cells in Pleural Fluid. *Acta Cytol* 26: 401–406, 1982.

Labay GR, Feiner F: Malignant Pleural Endometriosis. *Am J Obstet Gynecol* 110: 478–480, 1971.

Labowitz R, Schumacher HR: Articular Manifestations of Systemic Lupus Erythematosus. *Ann Intern Med* 74: 911–921, 1971.

Lafreniere R: Bloody Nipple Discharge During Pregnancy: A Rationale for Conservative Treatment. *J Surg Oncol* 43: 228–230, 1990.

Lahiri VL: Microfilariae in Nipple Secretion. *Acta Cytol* 19: 154, 1975.

Lancet: Mysterious Pleural Effusions. *Lancet* (i): 1226, 1982.

Lancet: Discharge From the Nipple. *Lancet* (i): 1405, 1983.

Lauchlan SC: Conceptual Unity of the Müllerian Tumor Group: Histologic Study. *Cancer* 22: 601–610, 1968.

Lauchlan SC: Metaplasias and Neoplasias of Müllerian Epithelium. *Histopathology* 8: 543–557, 1984.

Law MR, Hodson ME, Turner-Warwick M: Malignant Mesothelioma of the Pleura: Clinical Aspects and Symptomatic Treatment. *Eur J Respir Dis* 65: 162–168, 1984.

Lee S, Schoen I: Eosinophilia of Peritoneal Fluid and Peripheral Blood Associated With Chronic Peritoneal Dialysis. *Am J Clin Pathol* 47: 638–640, 1967.

Leff A, Hopewell PC, Costello J: Pleural Effusion From Malignancy. *Ann Intern Med* 88: 532–537, 1978.

Leif RC, Bobbit D, Railey C, et al: Centrifugal Cytology of Nipple Aspirate Cells. *Acta Cytol* 24: 255–261, 1980.

Leis HP, Greene FL, Cammarata A, et al: Nipple Discharge: Surgical Significance. *South Med J* 81: 20–26, 1988.

Leis HP Jr: Management of Nipple Discharge. *Br J Clin Pract* 68(suppl): 58–65, 1989a.

Leis HP Jr: Management of Nipple Discharge. *World J Surg* 13: 736–742, 1989b.

Leong AS-Y, Parkinson R, Milios J: "Thick" Cell Membranes Revealed by Immunocytochemical Staining: A Clue to the Diagnosis of Mesothelioma. *Diagn Cytopathol* 6: 9–13, 1990.

Leong AS-Y, Stevens MW, Mukherjee TM: Malignant Mesothelioma: Cytologic Diagnosis With Histologic, Immunohistochemical, and Ultrastructural Correlation. *Semin Diagn Pathol* 9: 141–150, 1992.

Leslie DS, Johnston WW, Daly L, et al: Detection of Breast Carcinoma Cells in Human Bone Marrow Using Fluorescence-Activated Cell Sorting and Conventional Cytology. *Am J Clin Pathol* 94: 8–13, 1990.

Leuallen EC, Carr DT: Pleural Effusion: A Statistical Study of 436 Patients. *N Engl J Med* 252: 79–83, 1955.

Lewis RJ, Sisler GE, Mackenzie JW: Diffuse, Mixed Malignant Pleural Mesothelioma. *Ann Thorac Surg* 31: 53–60, 1981.

Li C-Y, Yam LT: Blast Transformation in Chronic Myeloid Leukemia With Synovial Involvement. *Acta Cytol* 35: 543–545, 1991.

Light RW, MacGregor MI, Luchsinger PC, et al: Pleural Effusions: The Diagnostic Separation of Transudates and Exudates. *Ann Intern Med* 77: 507–513, 1972.

Light RW, Erozan YS, Ball WC Jr: Cells in Pleural Fluid: Their Value in Differential Diagnosis. *Arch Intern Med* 132: 854–860, 1973.

Linari A, Bussolati G: Evaluation of Impact of Immunocytochemical Techniques in Cytological Diagnosis of Neoplastic Effusions. *J Clin Pathol* 42: 1184–1189, 1989.

Locker AP, Galea MH, Ellis IO, et al: Microdochectomy for Single-Duct Discharge From the Nipple. *Br J Surg* 75: 700–701, 1988.

Lorenzen JR, Gravdal JA: Bloody Nipple Discharge. *Am Fam Physician* 34(1): 151–154, 1986.

Lozowski W, Hajdu SI, Melamed MR: Cytomorphology of Carcinoid Tumors. *Acta Cytol* 23: 360–365, 1979.

Lozowski W, Hajdu SI: Cytology and Immunocytochemistry of Bronchioloalveolar Carcinoma. *Acta Cytol* 31: 717–725, 1987.

Luesley DM, Williams DR, Ward K, et al: Prospective Comparative Cytologic Study of Direct Peritoneal Smears and Lavage Fluids in Patients With Epithelial Ovarian Cancer and Benign Gynecologic Disease. *Acta Cytol* 34: 539–544, 1990.

Luse SA, Reagan JW: A Histocytological Study of Effusions: I. Effusions Not Associated With Malignant Tumors. *Cancer* 7: 1155–1166, 1954a.

Luse SA, Reagan JW: A Histocytological Study of Effusions: II. Effusions Associated With Malignant Tumors. *Cancer* 7: 1167–1181, 1954b.

MacDougall DB, Wang SE, Zidar BL: Mucin-Positive Epithelial Mesothelioma. *Arch Pathol Lab Med* 116: 874–880, 1992.

MacMurray FG, Katz S, Zimmerman HJ: Pleural-Fluid Eosinophilia. *N Engl J Med* 243: 330–334, 1950.

Maguire B, Whitaker D, Carrello S, et al: Monoclonal Antibody Ber-EP4: Its Use in the Differential Diagnosis of Malignant Mesothelioma and Carcinoma in Cell Blocks of Malignant Effusions and FNA Specimens. *Diagn Cytopathol* 10: 130–134, 1994.

Maher GG, Berger HW: Massive Pleural Effusion: Malignant and Nonmalignant Causes in 46 Patients. *Am Rev Resp Dis* 105: 458–460, 1972.

Mahoney CA, Sherwood N, Yap EH, et al: Ciliated Cell Remnants in Peritoneal Dialysis Fluid. *Arch Pathol Lab Med* 117: 211–213, 1993.

Malinin TI, Pekin TJ, Zvaifler NJ: Cytology of Synovial Fluid in Rheumatoid Arthritis. *Am J Clin Pathol* 47: 203–208, 1967.

Malone DG, Irani A-M, Schwartz LB, et al: Mast Cell Numbers and Histamine Levels in Synovial Fluids From Patients With Diverse Arthritides. *Arthritis Rheum* 29: 956–963, 1986.

Marchevsky AM, Hauptman E, Gill J, et al: Computerized Interactive Morphometry as an Aid in the Diagnosis of Pleural Effusions. *Acta Cytol* 31: 131–136, 1987.

Marcel BR, Koff RS, Cho SI: Ascites Following Renal Transplantation. *Digest Dis* 22: 137–139, 1977.

Marcus CC: Cytology of the Pelvic Peritoneal Cavity in Benign and Malignant Disease. *Obstet Gynecol* 20: 701–712, 1962.

Martensson G, Hagmar B, Zettergren L: Diagnosis and Prognosis in Malignant Pleural Mesothelioma: A Prospective Study. *Eur J Respir Dis* 65: 169–178, 1984.

Martensson G, Pettersson K, Thringer G: Differentiation Between Malignant and Non-Malignant Pleural Effusion. *Eur J Respir Dis* 67: 326–334, 1985.

Martin AW, Carstens PHB, Yam LT: Crystalline Deposits in Ascites in a Case of Cryoglobulinemia. *Acta Cytol* 31: 631–636, 1987.

Martin JK, Goellner JR: Abdominal Fluid Cytology in Patients With Gastrointestinal Malignant Lesions. *Mayo Clin Proc* 61: 467–471, 1986.

Mason MR, Bedrossian CWM, Fahey CA: Value of Immunocytochemistry in the Study of Malignant Effusions. *Diagn Cytopathol* 3: 215–221, 1987.

Masukawa T: Discovery of Psammoma Bodies and Fungus Organism in the Nipple Secretion With Improved Breast Cytology Technique. *Acta Cytol* 16: 408–415, 1972.

Masukawa T, Kuzma JF, Straumfjord JV: Cytologic Detection of Early Paget's Disease of Breast With Improved Cellular Collection Method. *Acta Cytol* 19: 274–278, 1975.

Mathews WC, Bozzette SA, Harrity S, et al: *Pneumocystis carinii* Peritonitis: Antemortem Confirmation of Disseminated Pneumocystosis by Cytologic Examination of Body Fluids. *Arch Intern Med* 152: 867–869, 1992.

Matsuo T, Ito H, Anami M, et al: Malignant Peritoneal Mesothelioma With Squamous Metaplasia. *Cytopathology* 4: 373–378, 1993.

Mazurka JL, Krepart GV, Lotocki RJ: Prognostic Significance of Positive Peritoneal Cytology in Endometrial Carcinoma. *Am J Obstet Gynecol* 158: 303–309, 1988.

McCaughey WTE: Criteria for Diagnosis of Diffuse Mesothelial Tumors. *Ann NY Acad Sci* 132: 603–613, 1965.

McDermott E, Boyle T, Murray M, et al: Nipple Discharge: Clinical and Histological Diagnosis. *Ir Med J* 80: 324–325, 1987.

McGowan L, Davis RH, Stein DB, et al: Cytologic Differential of Pelvic Cavity Aspiration Specimens in Normal Women. *Obstet Gynecol* 30: 821–829, 1967.

McGowan L, Davis RH, Stein DB, et al: The Cytology of the Pelvic Peritoneal Cavity in Normal Women. *Am J Clin Pathol* 49: 506–511, 1968.

McGowan L, Davis RH: Peritoneal Fluid Cellular Patterns in Obstetrics and Gynecology. *Am J Obstet Gynecol* 106: 979–995, 1970.

McGowan L, Bunnag B, Arias LB: Peritoneal Fluid Cytology Associated With Benign Neoplastic Ovarian Tumors in Women. *Am J Obstet Gynecol* 113: 961–966, 1972.

McGowan L, Bunnag B: Morphology of Mesothelial Cells in Peritoneal Fluid From Normal Women. *Acta Cytol* 18: 203–209, 1974.

McGowan L: Peritoneal Fluid Profiles. *Natl Cancer Inst Monogr* 42: 75–79, 1975.

McGowan L, Bunnag B: The Evaluation of Therapy for Ovarian Cancer. *Gynecol Oncol* 4: 375–383, 1976.

McGowan L, Lesher LP, Norris HJ, et al: Misstaging of Ovarian Cancer. *Obstet Gynecol* 65: 568–572, 1985.

McGowan L: Peritoneal Fluid Washings. *Acta Cytol* 33: 414–415, 1989.

McKenna RJ Jr, Ali MK, Ewer MS, et al: Pleural and Pericardial Effusions in Cancer Patients. *Curr Probl Cancer* 9: 1–44, 1985.

McLellan R, Dillon MB, Currie JL, et al: Peritoneal Cytology in Endometrial Cancer: A Review. *Obstet Gynecol Surv* 44: 711–719, 1989.

McNeely TBD: Pericellular Lacunae in Effusions. *Diagn Cytopathol* 9: 503–507, 1993.

Meisels A, Berebichez M: Exfoliative Cytology in Orthopedics. *Can M A J* 84: 957–959, 1961.

Melamed MR: The Cytological Presentation of Malignant Lymphomas and Related Diseases in Effusions. *Cancer* 16: 413–431, 1963.

Mezger J, Lamerz R, Permanetter W: Diagnostic Significance of Carcinoembryonic Antigen in the Differential Diagnosis of Malignant Mesothelioma. *J Thorac Cardiovasc Surg* 100: 860–866, 1990.

Miles CP, Wolinsk W: A Comparative Analysis of Chromosomes and Diagnostic Cytology in Effusions From 58 Cancer Patients. *Cancer* 32: 1458–1469, 1973.

Miller JD, Brownell MD, Shaw A: Bilateral Breast Masses and Bloody Nipple Discharge in a 4-year-old boy. *J Pediatr* 116: 744–747, 1990.

Mills SE, Andersen WA, Fechner RE, et al: Serous Surface Papillary Carcinoma: A Clinicopathologic Study of 10 Cases and Comparison With Stage III-IV Ovarian Serous Carcinoma. *Am J Surg Pathol* 12: 827–834, 1988.

Monte SA, Ehya H, Lang WR: Positive Effusion Cytology as the Initial Presentation of Malignancy. *Acta Cytol* 31: 448–452, 1987.

Morris PC, Haugen J, Anderson B, et al: The Significance of Peritoneal Cytology in Stage 1B Cervical Cancer. *Obstet Gynecol* 80: 196–198, 1992.

Morrow CP, Bundy BN, Kurman RJ, et al: Relationship Between Surgical–Pathological Risk Factors and Outcome in Clinical Stage I and II Carcinoma of the Endometrium: A Gynecologic Oncology Group Study. *Gynecol Oncol* 40: 55–65, 1991.

Motoyama T, Watanabe T, Okazaki E, et al: Immunohistochemical Properties of Malignant Mesothelioma Cell in Histologic and Cytologic Specimens. *Acta Cytol* 39: 164–170, 1995.

Moutsopoulos HM, Fye KH, Pugay PI, et al: Monarthric Arthritis Caused by Metastatic Breast Carcinoma: Value of Cytologic Study of Synovial Fluid. *JAMA* 234: 75–76, 1975.

Murad TM: Electron Microscopic Studies of Cells in Pleural and Peritoneal Effusions. *Acta Cytol* 17: 401–409, 1973a.

Murad, TM, Snyder ME: The Diagnosis of Breast Lesions From Cytologic Material. *Acta Cytol* 17: 418–422, 1973b.

Murad T, Contesso G, Mouriesse H: Nipple Discharge From the Breast. *Ann Surg* 195: 259–264, 1982.

Nagai S, Nozawa S, Kurihara S, et al: Cytologic and Biologic Studies of Endometrioid Carcinoma of the Ovary. *Acta Cytol* 27: 676–682, 1983.

Naib ZM: Cytology of Synovial Fluids. *Acta Cytol* 17: 299–309, 1973.

Nakajima M, Manabe T, Yagi S: Appearance of Mesothelioma Cells in Sputum: A Case Report. *Acta Cytol* 36: 731–736, 1992.

Nakajima T, Harashima S, Hirata M, et al: Prognostic and Therapeutic Values of Peritoneal Cytology in Gastric Cancer. *Acta Cytol* 22: 225–229, 1978.

Nance KV, Silverman JF: Immunocytochemical Panel for the Identification of Malignant Cells in Serous Effusions. *Am J Clin Pathol* 95: 867–874, 1991a.

Nance KV, Shermer R, Askin FB: Diagnostic Efficacy of Pleural Biopsy as Compared With That of Pleural Fluid Examination. *Mod Pathol* 4: 320–324, 1991b.

Nance KV, Silverman JF: The Utility of Ancillary Techniques in Effusion Cytology. *Diagn Cytopathol* 8: 185–189, 1992.

Nauta RJ, Osteen RT, Antman KH, et al: Clinical Staging and the Tendency of Malignant Pleural Mesotheliomas to Remain Localized. *Ann Thorac Surg* 34: 66–70, 1982.

Nayar M, Saxena HMK: Tuberculosis of the Breast: A Cytomorphologic Study of Needle Aspirates and Nipple Discharges. *Acta Cytol* 28: 325–328, 1984.

Naylor B: The Exfoliative Cytology of Diffuse Malignant Mesothelioma. *J Pathol Bact* 86: 293–298, 1963.

Naylor B, Novak MP: Charcot-Leyden Crystals in Pleural Fluids. *Acta Cytol* 29: 781–784, 1985.

Naylor B: Curschmann's Spirals in Pleural and Peritoneal Effusions. *Acta Cytol* 34: 474–478, 1990a.

Naylor B: The Pathognomonic Cytologic Picture of Rheumatoid Pleuritis: The 1989 Maurice Goldblatt Cytology Award Lecture. *Acta Cytol* 34: 465–473, 1990b.

Naylor B: Cytological Aspects of Pleural, Peritoneal and Pericardial Fluids From Patients With Systemic Lupus Erythematosus. *Cytopathology* 3: 1–8, 1992.

Newman HF, Klein M, Northrup JD, et al: Nipple Discharge: Frequency and Pathogenesis in an Ambulatory Population. *NY State J Med* 83: 928–933, 1983.

Newton P, Freemont AT, Noble J, et al: Secondary Malignant Synovitis: Report of Three Cases and Review of the Literature. *Q J Med* 53: 135–143, 1984.

O'Brien PH, Kreutner A Jr: Another Cause of Nipple Discharge: Mammary Duct Ectasia With Periductal Mastitis. *Am Surg* 48: 577–578, 1982.

Oels HC, Harrison EG Jr, Carr DT, et al: Diffuse Malignant Mesothelioma of the Pleura: A Review of 37 Cases. *Chest* 60: 564–570, 1971.

Okabe H, Yoshida T, Yoshimura M, et al: Cytologic Detection of Malignant Lymphoma Cells With a Hairy Appearance in Ascitic Fluid: Report of a Case With Immunofluorocytometric Analysis. *Acta Cytol* 35: 529–532, 1991.

Okumura M, Ohshima S, Kotake Y, et al: Intraoperative Pleural Lavage Cytology in Lung Cancer Patients. *Ann Thorac Surg* 51: 599–604, 1991.

Olopade OI, Ultmann JE: Malignant Effusions. *CA Cancer J Clin* 41: 166–179, 1991.

Otis CN, Carter D, Cole S, Battifora H: Immunohistochemical Evaluation of Pleural Mesothelioma and Pulmonary Adenocarcinoma: A Bi-institutional Study of 47 Cases. *Am J Surg Pathol* 11: 445–456, 1987.

Palaoro L, Rofrano J, Di Roma D, et al: 'Ciliated' Tumour Cells in Ascitic Fluid From Two Cases of Cystadenocarcinoma of the Ovary. *Cytopathology* 3: 183–190, 1992.

Papanicolaou GN: Degenerative Changes in Ciliated Cells Exfoliating From the Bronchial Epithelium as a Cytologic Criterion in the Diagnosis of Diseases of the Lung. *NY State J Med* 56: 2647–2650, 1956a.

Papanicolaou GN, Bader GM, Holmquist DG, et al: Cytologic Evaluation of Breast Secretions. *Ann NY Acad Sci* 63: 1409–1421, 1956b.

Papanicolaou GN, Holmquist DG, Bader GM, et al: Exfoliative Cytology of the Human Mammary Gland and Its Value in the Diagnosis of Cancer and Other Diseases of the Breast. *Cancer* 11: 377–409, 1958.

Pedio G, Krause M, Jansova I: Megakaryocytes in Ascitic Fluid in a Case of Agnogenic Myeloid Metaplasia. *Acta Cytol* 29: 89–90, 1985.

Pekin TJ, Malinin TI, Zvaifler NJ: Unusual Synovial Fluid Findings in Reiter's Syndrome. *Ann Intern Med* 66: 677–684, 1967.

Permanetter W, Wiesinger H: Immunohistochemical Study of Lysozyme, Alpha$_1$-Anti-chymotrypsin, Tissue Polypeptide Antigen, Keratin and Carcinoembryonic Antigen in Effusion Sediments. *Acta Cytol* 31: 104–112, 1987.

Peterson IM, Raible M: Malignant Pleural Effusion in Hodgkin's Lymphoma: Report of a Case With Immunoperoxidase Studies. *Acta Cytol* 35a: 300–305, 1991.

Peterson JT Jr, Greenberg SD, Buffler PA: Non-Asbestos-Related Malignant Mesothelioma: A Review. *Cancer* 54: 951–960, 1984.

Philip J, Harris WG: The Role of Ductography in the Management of Patients With Nipple Discharge. *Br J Clin Pract* 38: 293–297, 1984.

Pinto MM, Bernstein LH, Brogan DA, et al: Carcinoembryonic Antigen in Effusions: A Diagnostic Adjunct to Cytology. *Acta Cytol* 31: 113–118, 1987.

Pisani RJ, Colby TV, Williams DE: Malignant Mesothelioma of the Pleura. *Mayo Clin Proc* 63: 1234–1244, 1988.

Piver MS, Barlow JJ, Lele SB: Incidence of Subclinical Metastasis in Stage I and II Ovarian Carcinoma. *Obstet Gynecol* 52: 100–104, 1978.

Poropatich C, Ehya H: Detached Ciliary Tufts in Pouch of Douglas Fluid. *Acta Cytol* 30: 442–444, 1986.

Posalaky Z, McGinley D, Posalaky IP: Electron Microscopic Identification of the Colorectal Origins of Tumor Cells in Pleural Fluid. *Acta Cytol* 27: 45–48, 1983.

Pozniak AL, Thomas RD, Hobbs CB, et al: Primary Malignant Lymphoma of the Heart: Antemortem Cytologic Diagnosis. *Acta Cytol* 30: 662–664, 1986.

Prakash LBS, Reiman HM: Comparison of Needle Biopsy With Cytologic Analysis for the Evaluation of Pleural Effusion: Analysis of 414 Cases. *Mayo Clin Proc* 60: 158–164, 1985.

Pretorius RG, Lee KR, Papillo J, et al: False-Negative Peritoneal Cytology in Metastatic Ovarian Carcinoma. *Obstet Gynecol* 68: 619–623, 1986.

Price BA, Ehya H, Lee JH: Significance of Pericellular Lacunae in Cell Blocks of Effusions. *Acta Cytol* 36: 333–337, 1992.

Quan SHQ: Cul-de-sac Smears; A Follow-up Study. *Surgery* 60: 1170–1174, 1966.

Radzun HJ, Dommes M, Henselmans M, et al: Resident Human Peritoneal Macrophages: A Monocytic Cell Line. *Acta Cytol* 26: 363–366, 1982.

Ramaekers FCS, Haag D, Kant A, et al: Coexpression of Keratin-and-Vimentin-Type Intermediate Filaments in Human Metastatic Carcinoma Cells. *Proc Natl Acad Sci* 80: 2618–2622, 1983.

Rammou-Kinia R, Sirmakechian-Karra T: Pseudomyxoma Peritonei and Malignant Mucocele of the Appendix: A Case Report. *Acta Cytol* 30: 169–172, 1986.

Ramsey SJ, Tweeddale DN, Bryant LR, et al: Cytologic Features of Pericardial Mesothelium. *Acta Cytol* 14: 283–290, 1970.

Rangwala AF, Perez-Blanco M, Reilly J: Cytological Diagnosis of Breast Cancer. *NJ Med* 86: 8459–865, 1989.

Rasmussen KN, Faber V: Hyaluronic Acid in 247 Pleural Fluids. *Scand J Respir Dis* 48: 366–371, 1967.

Ravinsky E: Cytology of Peritoneal Washings in Gynecologic Patients: Diagnostic Criteria and Pitfalls. *Acta Cytol* 30: 8–16, 1986.

Reda M, Baigelman W: Pleural Effusion in Systemic Lupus Erythematosus. *Acta Cytol* 24: 553–557, 1980.

Reginato AJ, Schumacher HR, Allan DA, et al: Acute Monarthritis Associated With Lipid Liquid Crystals. *Ann Rheum Dis* 44: 537–543, 1985.

Reyes CV, Kathuria S, MacGlashan A: Diagnostic Value of Calcium Oxalate Crystals in Respiratory and Pleural Fluid Cytology: A Case Report. *Acta Cytol* 23: 65–68, 1979.

Ribak J, Lilis R, Suzuki Y, et al: Malignant Mesothelioma in a Cohort of Asbestos Insulation Workers: Clinical Presentation, Diagnosis, and Causes of Death. *Br J Industr Med* 45: 182–187, 1988.

Rijken A, Dekker A, Taylor S, et al: Diagnostic Value of DNA Analysis in Effusions by Flow Cytometry and Image Analysis: A Prospective Study of 102 Patients as Compared With Cytologic Examination. *Am J Clin Pathol* 95: 6–12, 1991.

Rimsten A, Skoog V, Stenkvist B: On the Significance of Nipple Discharge in the Diagnosis of Breast Disease. *Acta Chir Scand* 142: 513–518, 1976.

Ringenberg QS, Doll DC, Loy TS, et al: Malignant Ascites of Unknown Origin. *Cancer* 64: 753–755, 1989.

Roberts GH, Campbell GM: Exfoliative Cytology of Diffuse Mesothelioma. *J Clin Pathol* 25: 577–582, 1972.

Roberts GH: Distant Visceral Metastases in Pleural Mesothelioma. *Br J Dis Chest* 70: 246–250, 1976.

Roberts WS, Bryson SCP, Cavanagh D, et al: Peritoneal Cytology and Invasive Carcinoma of the Cervix. *Gynecol Oncol* 24: 331–336, 1986.

Rodriguez HJ, Walls J, Slatopolsky E, et al: Recurrent Ascites Following Peritoneal Dialysis: A New Syndrome? *Arch Intern Med* 134: 283–287, 1974.

Roggli VL, Kolbeck J, Sanfilippo F, et al: Pathology of Human Mesothelioma: Etiologic and Diagnostic Considerations. *Pathol Annu* 22(2): 91–131, 1987.

Rohn RD: Benign Galactorrhea/Breast Discharge in Adolescent Males Probably Due to Breast Self-Manipulation. *J Adolesc Health Care* 5: 210–212, 1984.

Rona A, Marshall K, Raymont E: The Cytologic Diagnosis of an Ovarian Mucinous Cystoma From a Virtually Acellular Specimen of Abdominal Fluid. *Acta Cytol* 13: 672–674, 1969.

Roncalli M, Gribaudi G, Simoncelli D, et al: Cytology of Yolk-Sac Tumor of the Ovary in Ascitic Fluid: Report of a Case. *Acta Cytol* 32: 113–116, 1988.

Rosai J, Dehner LP: Nodular Mesothelial Hyperplasia in Hernia Sacs: A Benign Reactive Condition Simulating a Neoplastic Process. *Cancer* 35: 165–175, 1975.

Rubin E: Galactography in the Investigation of Nipple Discharge. *Ala J Med Sci* 25: 280–282, 1988.

Rubin SC, Dulaney ED, Markman M, et al: Peritoneal Cytology as an Indicator of Disease in Patients With Residual Ovarian Carcinoma. *Obstet Gynecol* 71: 851–853, 1988.

Runyon BA, Hoefs JC, Morgan TR: Ascitic Fluid Analysis in Malignancy-Related Ascites. *Hepatology* 8: 1104–1109, 1988.

Safa AM, Van Ordstrand HS: Pleural Effusion Due to Multiple Myeloma. *Chest* 64: 246–248, 1973.

Sahn SA: Pleural Fluids Analysis: Narrowing the Differential Diagnosis. *Semin Respir Med* 9: 22–29, 1987a.

Sahn SA: Malignant Pleural Effusions. *Semin Respir Med* 9: 43–53, 1987b.

Salhadin A, Nasiell M, Nasiell K, et al: The Unique Cytologic Picture of Oat Cell Carcinoma in Effusions. *Acta Cytol* 20: 298–302, 1976.

Salyer WR, Eggleston JC, Erozan YS: Efficacy of Pleural Needle Biopsy and Pleural Fluid Cytopathology in the Diagnosis of Malignant Neoplasm Involving the Pleura. *Chest* 67: 536–539, 1975.

Samarasinghe D, Frost F, Sterrett G, et al: Cytological Diagnosis of Paget's Disease of the Nipple by Scrape Smears: A Report of Five Cases. *Diagn Cytopathol* 9: 291–295, 1993.

Sams VR, Benjamin E, Ward RHT: Ectopic Pancreas: A Cause of False-Positive Peritoneal Cytology. *Acta Cytol* 34: 641–644, 1990.

Saphir O: Cytologic Diagnosis of Cancer From Pleural and Peritoneal Fluids. *Am J Clin Pathol* 19: 309–314, 1949.

Saphir O: Cytologic Examination of Breast Secretions. *Am J Clin Pathol* 20: 1001–1010, 1950.

Sartorius OW, Smith HS, Morris P, et al: Cytologic Evaluation of Breast Fluid in the Detection of Breast Disease. *J Natl Cancer Inst* 59: 1073–1080, 1977.

Sasser RL, Yam LT, Li C-Y: Myeloma With Involvement of the Serous Cavities: Cytologic and Immunochemical Diagnosis and Literature Review. *Acta Cytol* 34: 479–485, 1990.

Scamurra D: Effusion Cytology in the Diagnosis of Malignant Epithelioid and Biphasic Pleura Mesothelioma. *Arch Pathol Lab Med* 115: 210, 1991.

Scanlon EF: The Early Diagnosis of Breast Cancer. *Cancer* 48: 523–526, 1981.

Schatz JE, Colgan TJ: Squamous Metaplasia of the Peritoneum. *Arch Pathol Lab Med* 115: 397–398, 1991.

Schumacher HR: Analyzing Synovial Fluid: A Useful Diagnostic Aid for Practitioners. *Mod Med* pp 58–63, January 1, 1977.

Scullin DC Jr, Cohen HJ: Myelomatous Pleural Effusion: Clinical Course and Immunologic Characterization of the Pleural Fluid Cells. *Am J Hematol* 6: 267–273, 1979.

Sears D, Hajdu SI: The Cytologic Diagnosis of Malignant Neoplasms in Pleural and Peritoneal Effusions. *Acta Cytol* 31: 85–97, 1987.

Selikoff IJ: Mortality Experience of Insulation Workers in the United States and Canada, 1943-1976. *Ann NY Acad Sci* 130: 91–116, 1979.

Selikoff IJ, Hammond EC, Seidman H: Latency of Asbestos Disease Among Insulation Workers in the United States and Canada. *Cancer* 46: 2736–2740, 1980.

Seltzer MH, Perloff LJ, Kelley RI, et al: The Significance of Age in Patients With Nipple Discharge. *Surg Gynecol Obstet* 131: 519–522, 1970.

Selvaggi SM, Migdal S: Cytologic Features of Atypical Mesothelial Cells in Peritoneal Dialysis Fluid. *Diagn Cytopathol* 6: 22–26, 1990.

Selvaggi SM: Small-Cell Carcinoma of the Ovary in Peritoneal Fluid. *Diagn Cytopathol* 11: 266–270, 1994.

Sen B, Arora VK, Gupta K, et al: Platelike Urate Crystals in Gouty Tophi. *Acta Cytol* 37: 640–641, 1993.

Shearin JC Jr, Jackson D: Malignant Pleural Mesothelioma: Report of 19 Cases. *J Thorac Cardiovasc Surg* 71: 621–627, 1976.

Sheibani K, Esteban JM, Bailey A, et al: Immunopathologic and Molecular Studies as an Aid to the Diagnosis of Malignant Mesothelioma. *Hum Pathol* 23: 107–116, 1992.

Shen SC, Bansal M, Purrazzella R, et al: Benign Glandular Inclusions in Lymph Nodes, Endosalpingiosis, and Salpingitis Isthmica Nodosa in a Young Girl With Clear Cell Adenocarcinoma of the Cervix. *Am J Surg Pathol* 7: 293–300, 1983.

Sherman ME, Mark EJ: Effusion Cytology in the Diagnosis of Malignant Epithelioid and Biphasic Pleural Mesothelioma. *Arch Pathol Lab Med* 114: 845–851, 1990.

Shield PW, Callan JJ, Devine PL: Markers for Metastatic Adenocarcinoma in Serous Effusion Specimens. *Diagn Cytopathol* 11: 237–245, 1994.

Sidawy MK, Chandra P, Oertel YC: Detached Ciliary Tufts in Female Peritoneal Washings: A Common Finding. *Acta Cytol* 31: 841–844, 1987a.

Sidawy MK, Silverberg SG: Endosalpingiosis in Female Peritoneal Washings: A Diagnostic Pitfall. *Int J Gynecol Pathol* 6: 340–346, 1987b.

Sigalas J, Roilides E, Tsanakas J, et al: Bloody Nipple Discharge in Infants. *J Pediatr* 107: 484, 1985.

Silverman JF: Extramedullary Hematopoietic Ascitic Fluid Cytology in Myelofibrosis. *Am J Clin Pathol* 84: 125–128, 1985.

Smith-Purslow MJ, Kini SR, Naylor B: Cells of Squamous Cell Carcinoma in Pleural, Peritoneal and Pericardial Fluids: Origin and Morphology. *Acta Cytol* 33: 245–253, 1989.

Sneige N, Fernandez T, Copeland LJ, et al: Müllerian Inclusions in Peritoneal Washings: Potential Source of Error in Cytologic Diagnosis. *Acta Cytol* 30: 271–276, 1986.

Sneige N, Fanning CV: Peritoneal Washing Cytology in Women: Diagnostic Pitfalls and Clues for Correct Diagnosis. *Diagn Cytopathol* 8: 632–642, 1992.

Spagnolo DV, Whitaker D, Carrello S, et al: The Use of Monoclonal Antibody 44-3A6 in Cell Blocks in the Diagnosis of Lung Carcinoma, Carcinomas Metastatic to Lung and Pleura, and Pleural Malignant Mesothelioma. *Am J Clin Pathol* 95: 322–329, 1991.

Spieler P: The Cytologic Diagnosis of Tuberculosis in Pleural Effusions. *Acta Cytol* 23: 374–379, 1979.

Spieler P, Gloor F: Identification of Types and Primary Sites of Malignant Tumors by Examination of Exfoliated Tumor Cells in Serous Fluids: Comparison With the Diagnostic Accuracy on Small Histologic Biopsies. *Acta Cytol* 29: 753–767, 1985.

Spirtas R, Beebe GW, Connelly RR, et al: Recent Trends in Mesothelioma Incidence in the United States. *Am J Industr Med* 9: 397–407, 1986.

Spriggs AI: Malignant Cells in Serous Effusions Complicating Bronchial Carcinoma. *Thorax* 9: 26–34, 1954.

Spriggs AI, Boddington MM: Absence of Mesothelial Cells From Tuberculous Pleural Effusions. *Thorax* 15: 169–171, 1960.

Spriggs AI, Meek GA: Surface Specialisations of Free Tumour Cells in Effusions. *J Pathol Bact* 82: 151–159, 1961.

Spriggs AI, Jerrome DW: Intracellular Mucous Inclusions: A Feature of Malignant Cells in Effusions in the Serous Cavities, Particularly Due to Carcinoma of the Breast. *J Clin Pathol* 28: 929–926, 1975.

Spriggs AI, Boddington MM: Oat-Cell Bronchial Carcinoma Identification of Cells in Pleural Fluid. *Acta Cytol* 20: 525–529, 1976.

Spriggs AI, Boddington MM, Mowat AG: Joint Fluid Cytology in Reiter's Syndrome. *Ann Rheum Dis* 37: 557–560, 1978.

Spriggs AI: Pleural Eosinophilia Due to Pneumothorax. *Acta Cytol* 23: 425, 1979a.

Spriggs AI, Jerrome DW: Benign Mesothelial Proliferation With Collagen Formation in Pericardial Fluid. *Acta Cytol* 23: 428–430, 1979b.

Spriggs AI, Grunze H: An Unusual Cytologic Presentation of Mesothelioma in Serous Effusions. *Acta Cytol* 27: 288–292, 1983.

Spriggs AI: Cytology of Peritoneal Aspirates and Washings. *Br J Obstet Gynaecol* 94: 1–3, 1987.

Sridhar KS, Doria R, Raub WA Jr, et al: New Strategies Are Needed in Diffuse Malignant Mesothelioma. *Cancer* 70: 2969–2979, 1992.

Stanton MF, Layard M, Tegeris A, et al: Relation of Particle Dimension to Carcinogenicity in Amphibole Asbestoses and Other Fibrous Minerals. *J Natl Cancer Inst* 67: 965–975, 1981.

Starr RL, Sherman ME: The Value of Multiple Preparations in the Diagnosis of Malignant Pleural Effusions: A Cost-Benefit Analysis. *Acta Cytol* 35: 533–537, 1991.

Stevens MW, Leong AS-Y, Fazzalari NL, et al: Cytopathology of Malignant Mesothelioma: A Stepwise Logistic Regression Analysis. *Diagn Cytopathol* 8: 333–341, 1992.

Storey DD, Dines DE, Coles DT: Pleural Effusion: A Diagnostic Dilemma. *JAMA* 236: 2183–2186, 1976.

Strankinga WFM, Sperber M, Kaiser MC, et al: Accuracy of Diagnostic Procedures in the Initial Evaluation and Follow-up of Mesothelioma Patients. *Respiration* 51: 179–187, 1987.

Stringel G, Perelman A, Jimenez C: Infantile Mammary Duct Ectasia: A Cause of Bloody Nipple Discharge. *J Pediatr Surg* 21: 671–674, 1986.

Suprun H, Mansoor I: An Aspiration Cytodiagnostic Test for Gouty Arthritis. *Acta Cytol* 17: 198–199, 1973.

Sussman J, Rosai J: Lymphadenopathy as the Initial Manifestation of Malignant Mesothelioma. *Lab Invest* 58: 90A, 1988.

Sutton GP, Geisler HE, Stehman FB, et al: Features Associated With Survival and Disease-Free Survival in Early Endometrial Cancer. *Am J Obstet Gynecol* 160: 1385–1393, 1989.

Suzuki Y: Pathology of Human Malignant Mesothelioma. *Semin Oncol* 8: 268–282, 1980.

Szpak CA, Creasman WT, Vollmer RT, et al: Prognostic Value of Cytologic Examination of Peritoneal Washings in Patients With Endometrial Carcinoma. *Acta Cytol* 25: 640–646, 1981.

Tabár L, Dean PB, Péntek Z: Galactography: The Diagnostic Procedure of Choice for Nipple Discharge. *Radiology* 149: 31–38, 1983.

Tagnon I, Blot WJ, Stroube RB, et al: Mesothelioma Associated With the Shipbuilding Industry in Coastal Virginia. *Cancer Res* 40: 3875–3879, 1980.

Takeda T, Suzuki M, Sato Y, et al: Cytologic Studies of Nipple Discharges. *Acta Cytol* 26: 35–36, 1982.

Takeda T, Matsui A, Sato Y, et al: Nipple Discharge Cytology in Mass Screening for Breast Cancer. *Acta Cytol* 34: 161–164, 1990.

Tao L-C: The Cytopathology of Mesothelioma. *Acta Cytol* 23: 209–213, 1979.

Tetirick JE: Nipple Discharge. *AFP* 22: 101–103, 1980.

Tickman RJ, Cohen C, Varma VA, et al: Distinction Between Carcinoma Cells and Mesothelial Cells in Serous Effusions: Usefulness of Immunohistochemistry. *Acta Cytol* 34: 491–496, 1990.

Tiniakos DG, Healicon RM, Hair T, et al. p53 Immunostaining as a Marker of Malignancy in Cytologic Preparations of Body Fluids. *Acta Cytol* 39: 171–176, 1995.

To A, Boyo-Ekwueme HT, Posnansky MC, et al: Chromosomal Abnormalities in Ascitic Fluid From Patients With Alcoholic Cirrhosis. *Br Med J* 282: 1659–1660, 1981.

Towers KJ, Melamed MR: Absence of Prognostic Features in the Cytology of Effusions Due to Mammary Cancer. *Acta Cytol* 23: 30–34, 1979.

Traycoff RB, Pascual E, Schumacher HR Jr: Mononuclear Cells in Human Synovial Fluid: Identification of Lymphoblasts in Rheumatoid Arthritis. *Arthritis Rheum* 19: 743–748, 1976.

Trelford JD, Kinney W, Vogt P: Positive Peritoneal Cytology in Stage I Carcinoma of the Cervix. *Acta Cytol* 39: 177–179, 1995.

Triol JH, Conston AS, Chandler SV: Malignant Mesothelioma: Cytopathology of 75 Cases Seen in a New Jersey Community Hospital. *Acta Cytol* 28: 37–45, 1984.

Truong LD, Maccato ML, Awalt H, et al: Serous Surface Carcinoma of the Peritoneum: A Clinicopathologic Study of 22 Cases. *Hum Pathol* 21: 99–110, 1990.

Turner DA, Gershenson DM, Atkinson N, et al: The Prognostic Significance of Peritoneal Cytology for Stage I Endometrial Cancer. *Obstet Gynecol* 74: 775–780, 1989.

Tyler JR, Baird L, Jones T, et al: Cytology: A Useful Adjunct in the Management of Nipple Discharge. *Aust N Z J Surg* 52: 610–612, 1982.

Uei Y, Watanabe Y, Hirota T, et al: Cytologic Diagnosis of Breast Carcinoma With Nipple Discharge: Special Significance of the Spherical Cell Cluster. *Acta Cytol* 24: 522–528, 1980.

Ugai K, Kurosaka M, Hirohata K: Lipid Microspherules in Synovial Fluid of Patients With Pigmented Villonodular Synovitis. *Arthritis Rheum* 31: 1442–1446, 1988.

Upton MP, Hirohashi S, Tome Y, et al: Expression of Vimentin in Surgically Resected Adenocarcinomas and Large Cell Carcinomas of Lung. *Am J Surg Pathol* 10: 560–567, 1986.

Urban JA, Egeli RA: Non-Lactational Nipple Discharge. *CA Cancer J Clin* 28: 130–140, 1978.

Uzoaru I, Adeyanju M, Ray V, et al: Primary Squamous Cell Carcinoma of the Breast Presenting as a Nipple Discharge. *Acta Cytol* 38: 112–114, 1994.

Valente PT, Schantz HD, Edmonds PR, et al: Peritoneal Cytology of Uncommon Ovarian Tumors. *Diagn Cytopathol* 8: 98–106, 1992.

Van de Molengraft FJJM, Vooijs GP: Survival of Patients With Malignancy-Associated Effusions. *Acta Cytol* 33: 911–916, 1989.

Venrick MG, Sidaway MK: Cytologic Evaluation of Serous Effusions: Processing Techniques and Optimal Number of Smears for Routine Preparation. *Am J Clin Pathol* 99: 182–186, 1993.

Veress JF, Koss LG, Schreiber K: Eosinophilic Pleural Effusions. *Acta Cytol* 23: 40–44, 1979.

Vernon SE, Rosenthal DL: Sézary Cells in Ascitic Fluid. *Acta Cytol* 23: 408–411, 1979.

Vilaplana EV, Jiménez-Ayala M: The Cytologic Diagnosis of Breast Lesions. *Acta Cytol* 19: 519–526, 1975.

Villanueva TG, Schumacher HR: Cytologic Examination of Synovial Fluid. *Diagn Cytopathol* 3: 141–147, 1987.

VillaSanta U, Jovanovski D: Follow-up Study of Ovarian Carcinoma by Cytology of Cul-de-Sac Aspirates. *Gynecol Oncol* 10: 58–62, 1980.

Wahl RW: Curschmann's Spirals in Pleural and Peritoneal Fluids: Report of 12 Cases. *Acta Cytol* 30: 147–151, 1986.

Walshe ADP, Douglas JG, Kerr KM, et al: An Audit of the Clinical Investigation of Pleural Effusions. *Thorax* 47: 734–737, 1992.

Walts AE: Malignant Melanoma in Effusions: A Source of False-Negative Cytodiagnoses. *Diagn Cytopathol* 2: 150–153, 1986.

Walz R, Koch HK: Malignant Pleural Mesothelioma: Some Aspects of Epidemiology, Differential Diagnosis and Prognosis: Histological and Immunohistochemical Evaluation and Follow-up of Mesotheliomas Diagnosed From 1964 to January 1985. *Pathol Res Pract* 186: 124–134, 1990.

Wang N-S, Huang S-N, Gold P: Absence of Carcinoembryonic Antigen-like Material in Mesothelioma: An Immunohistochemical Differentiation From Other Lung Cancers. *Cancer* 44: 937–943, 1979.

Wang N-S: Anatomy and Physiology of the Pleural Space. *Clin Chest Med* 6: 3–16, 1985.

Warshaw AL: Implications of Peritoneal Cytology for Staging of Early Pancreatic Cancer. *Am J Surg* 161: 26–30, 1991.

Watts KC, Boyo-Ekwueme H, To A, et al: Chromosome Studies on Cells Cultured From Serous Effusions: Use in Routine Cytologic Practice. *Acta Cytol* 27: 38–44, 1983.

Weick JK, Kiely JM, Harrison EG Jr, et al: Pleural Effusion in Lymphoma. *Cancer* 31: 848–853, 1973.

Weinberger A, Schumacher HR, Schimmer BM, et al: Arthritis in Acute Leukemia: Clinical and Histopathological Observations. *Arch Intern Med* 141: 1183–1187, 1981.

Whitaker D: Cell Aggregates in Malignant Mesothelioma. *Acta Cytol* 21: 236–239, 1977.

Whitaker D, Shilkin KB: The Cytology of Malignant Mesothelioma in Western Australia. *Acta Cytol* 22: 67–70, 1978.

Whitaker D, Sterrett GF, Shilkin KB: Detection of Tissue CEA-Like Substance as an Aid in the Differential Diagnosis of Malignant Mesothelioma. *Pathology* 14: 255–258, 1982.

Whitaker D, Shilkin KB: Diagnosis of Pleural Malignant Mesothelioma in Life—A Practical Approach. *J Pathol* 143: 147–175, 1984.

Whitaker D: Hyaluronic Acid in Serous Effusions Smears. *Acta Cytol* 30: 90–91, 1986a.

Whitaker D, Sterrett G, Shilkin K, et al: Malignant Mesothelioma Cells in Sputum. *Diagn Cytopathol* 2: 21–24, 1986b.

Whitaker D: The Validity of a Cytological Diagnosis of Mesothelioma. *Aust NZ J Med* 17(S2): 519, 1987. Abstract.

Whitaker D, Shilkin KB, Sterrett GF: Cytological Appearances of Malignant Mesothelioma. In: Henderson DW, Shilkin KB, Langlois SLP, et al, eds. *Malignant Mesothelioma*. New York: Hemisphere Publishing Corp; 167-182, 1991.

Wick MR, Mills SE, Dehner LP, et al: Serous Papillary Carcinomas Arising From the Peritoneum and Ovaries: A Clinicopathologic and Immunohistochemical Comparison. *Int J Gynecol Pathol* 8: 179–188, 1989.

Wiener HG, Kristensen IB, Haubek A, et al: The Diagnostic Value of Pericardial Cytology: An Analysis of 95 Cases. *Acta Cytol* 35: 149–153, 1991.

Wiley EL, Von Roenn J: Metastatic Breast Carcinoma in Pleural Fluid: Correlation of Morphology With Estrogen Receptor Activity and Morphology of the Primary Carcinoma. *Acta Cytol* 34: 169–174, 1990.

Winkelmann M, Pfitzer P: Blind Pleural Biopsy in Combination With Cytology of Pleural Effusions. *Acta Cytol* 25: 373–376, 1981.

Wojcik EM, Naylor B: "Collagen Balls" in Peritoneal Washings: Prevalence, Morphology, Origin and Significance. *Acta Cytol* 36: 466–470, 1992.

Wojno KJ, Olson JL, Sherman ME: Cytopathology of Pleural Effusions After Radiotherapy. *Acta Cytol* 38: 1–8, 1994.

Wolf AW, Benson DR, Shoji H, et al: Current Concepts in Synovial Fluid Analysis. *Clin Orthop Rel Res* 134: 261–265, 1978.

Wolf KM, Pitrowski ZH, Engel JD, et al: Malignant Mesothelioma With Occupational and Environmental Asbestos Exposure in an Illinois Community Hospital. *Arch Intern Med* 147: 2145–2149, 1987.

Woyke S, Czerniak B: The Surface Coat of the Human Effusion Cells. *Acta Cytol* 21: 447–454, 1977a.

Woyke S, Czerniak B: The Morphology of Cells in Effusions Settled on Glass. *Acta Cytol* 21: 508–513, 1977b.

Wrensch MR, Petrakis NL, King EB, et al: Breast Cancer Incidence in Women With Abnormal Cytology in Nipple Aspirates of Breast Fluid. *Am J Epidemiol* 135: 130–141, 1992.

Wright WE, Sherwin RP, Dickson EA, et al: Malignant Mesothelioma: Incidence, Asbestos Exposure, and Reclassification of Histopathology. *Br J Industr Med* 41: 39–45, 1984.

Wróblewski F: The Significance of Alterations in Lactic Dehydrogenase Activity of Body Fluids in the Diagnosis of Malignant Tumors. *Cancer* 12: 27–39, 1959.

Yam LT: Diagnostic Significance of Lymphocytes in Pleural Effusions. *Ann Intern Med* 66: 972–982, 1967.

Yamada S, Takeda T, Matsumoto K: Prognostic Analysis of Malignant Pleural and Peritoneal Effusions. *Cancer* 51: 136–140, 1983.

Yazdi HM, Hajdu SI, Melamed MR: Cytopathology of Pericardial Effusions. *Acta Cytol* 24: 401–412, 1980.

Yazdi HM: Cytopathology of Extramedullary Hemopoiesis in Effusions and Peritoneal Washings: A Report of Three Cases With Immunohistochemical Study. *Diagn Cytopathol* 2: 326–329, 1986.

Yazigi R, Piver MS, Blumenson L: Malignant Peritoneal Cytology as Prognostic Indicator in Stage I Endometrial Cancer. *Obstet Gynecol* 62: 359–362, 1983.

Yokoi T, Mark EJ: Atypical Mesothelial Hyperplasia Associated With Bronchogenic Carcinoma. *Hum Pathol* 22: 695–699, 1991.

Yoshimura S, Scully RE, Taft PD, et al: Peritoneal Fluid Cytology in Patients With Ovarian Cancer. *Gynecol Oncol* 17: 161–167, 1984.

Yu J, Grimes DA: Ascites and Pleural Effusions Associated With Endometriosis. *Obstet Gynecol* 78: 533–534, 1991.

Zakowski MF, Ianuale-Shanerman A: Cytology of Pericardial Effusions in AIDS Patients. *Diagn Cytopathol* 9: 266–269, 1993.

Zaatari GS, Gupta PK, Bhagavan BS, et al: Cytopathology of Pleural Endometriosis. *Acta Cytol* 26: 227–232, 1982.

Zaharopoulos P, Wong JY: Identification of Crystals in Joint Fluids. *Acta Cytol* 24: 197–202, 1980.

Zaharopoulos P, Wong JY: Hemoglobin Crystals in Fluid Specimens From Confined Body Spaces. *Acta Cytol* 31: 777–782, 1987.

Zimmerman AL, King EB, Barrett DL, et al: The Incidence and Significance of Intracytoplasmic Calcifications in Nipple Aspirate Specimens. *Acta Cytol* 21: 685–692, 1977.

Zirkin HJ: Cytology of Clear-Cell Carcinoma of the Ovary in Ascitic Fluid. *Acta Cytol* 28: 777–778, 1984.

Ziselman EM, Harkavy SE, Hogan M, et al: Peritoneal Washing Cytology: Uses and Diagnostic Criteria in Gynecologic Neoplasms. *Acta Cytol* 28: 105–110, 1984.

Zufferey P, Ruzicka J, Gerster JC: Pleural Fluid Cytology as an Indicator of an Effusion of Rheumatoid Origin. *J Rheumatol* 20: 1449–1451, 1993.

Zuna RE, Mitchell ML: Cytologic Findings in Peritoneal Washings Associated With Benign Gynecologic Disease. *Acta Cytol* 32: 139–147, 1988.

Zuna RE, Mitchell ML, Mulick KA, et al: Cytohistologic Correlation of Peritoneal Washing Cytology in Gynecologic Disease. *Acta Cytol* 33: 327–336, 1989.

9

The Gastrointestinal Tract

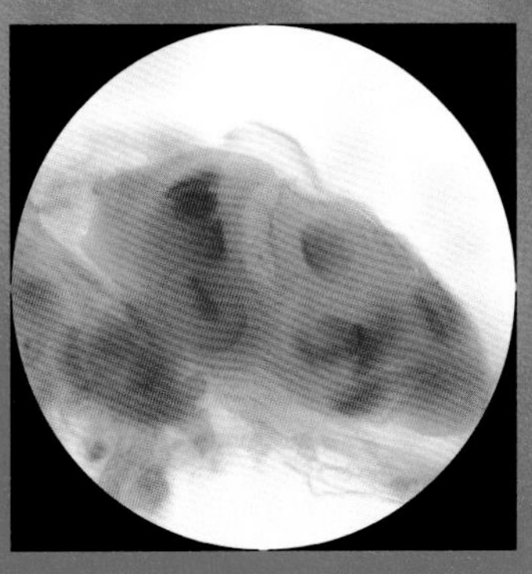

Oropharyngoesophagogastroduodenojejunoileocecocolorectoanal, or gastrointestinal, tract, also known as the GI tract, is topologically an exterior body surface, much like the inside of the hole of a donut. Therefore, the things that pass through it (mostly food) are not actually part of the body until absorbed through the wall of the gut. Only part of the GI tract is normally sterile (the small intestine); the remainder contains a variety of organisms that are normally not pathogenic. Cancer of the GI tract is common; lung and breast cancers are the only more common visceral malignancies. Oral cancer, including cancer of the lips, tongue, mouth, and pharynx, accounts for more than 28,000 new cases of cancer per year and over 8,000 deaths per year in the United States alone [Wingo 1995]. Cancer of other parts of the GI tract accounts for nearly a quarter of a million new cases of cancer annually in the United States and more than 120,000 deaths [Boring 1994, Wingo 1995]. Thus, malignancy of the GI tract is responsible for about one of every four cancer deaths in the United States. The majority of the cancers are squamous cell carcinomas, especially oral, esophageal, and anal, or adenocarcinomas, especially stomach, duodenum, and colorectal. A variety of other malignant tumors also occur, eg, lymphomas, sarcomas, and neuroendocrine tumors.

Direct sampling, using a wooden spatula, tongue blade, or brush, as well as suction cytology, can be performed on accessible lesions [Camp 1992, Main 1990, Ogden 1992, Sandler 1964]. However, except for oral and anal lesions, today most GI cytology is obtained by means of an endoscope [Dawson 1970, Fukuda 1967, Kasugai 1968,1974, Prolla 1971b, Winawer 1976a,b]. Blind lavages, washes, or enemas are obsolete for cytologic purposes [Bardawil 1990]. The most useful cytologic technique is usually direct brushings of visible lesions. The patient can also swallow abrasive balloons or brush capsules to collect cells from lesions of the upper GI tract [D Chapman 1953, Cooper 1953, Jaskiewicz 1987]. Endoscopically directed lavage is technically more difficult to perform, prepare, and interpret than brush cytology and seldom adds to diagnostic yield [Winawer 1978]. Unfortunately, because of the relative difficulty of obtaining samples from most of the GI tract, cytologic examination is not useful as a mass-screening technique [Wuerker 1993]. For this reason, gastrointestinal cytology is used primarily in diagnosing symptomatic or high-risk patients and is generally more useful for screening lesions than screening patients.

Although cytology may be diagnostically more sensitive than histology [Behmard 1978, Kasugai 1978, Moreno-Otero 1983, Prolla 1977, Shroff 1988], cytology and histology are complementary, and the highest diagnostic yields usually occur when both techniques are used together [Behmard 1978, I Cook 1988, Cussó 1993, Geisinger 1992, Kobayashi 1978, Lan 1990, Prolla 1977, Qizilbash 1980, Wang 1991b, Witzel 1976]. Multiple biopsies yield a correct diagnosis in about 80% to 85% of cases of gastrointestinal cancer. When cytology is added, the correct diagnosis can be made in over 90% of cases

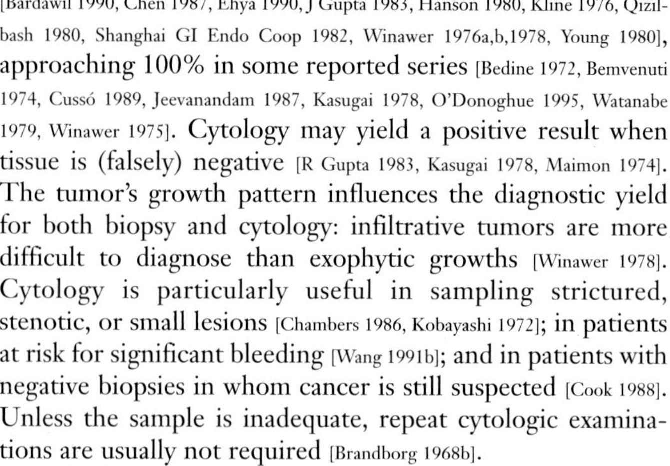

[Bardawil 1990, Chen 1987, Ehya 1990, J Gupta 1983, Hanson 1980, Kline 1976, Qizilbash 1980, Shanghai GI Endo Coop 1982, Winawer 1976a,b,1978, Young 1980], approaching 100% in some reported series [Bedine 1972, Bemvenuti 1974, Cussó 1989, Jeevanandam 1987, Kasugai 1978, O'Donoghue 1995, Watanabe 1979, Winawer 1975]. Cytology may yield a positive result when tissue is (falsely) negative [R Gupta 1983, Kasugai 1978, Maimon 1974]. The tumor's growth pattern influences the diagnostic yield for both biopsy and cytology: infiltrative tumors are more difficult to diagnose than exophytic growths [Winawer 1978]. Cytology is particularly useful in sampling strictured, stenotic, or small lesions [Chambers 1986, Kobayashi 1972]; in patients at risk for significant bleeding [Wang 1991b]; and in patients with negative biopsies in whom cancer is still suspected [Cook 1988]. Unless the sample is inadequate, repeat cytologic examinations are usually not required [Brandborg 1968b].

The best results are obtained when cytology is performed before biopsy, with vigorous and repeated brushing [Zargar 1991a]. Brushing does not interfere with interpretation of the tissue biopsy [H Thompson 1977, Zargar 1991a]. To prepare slides, brushes should be rapidly rolled, rather than rubbed or scrubbed, over an area about the size of a quarter on untreated plain glass slides [Ogden 1991a]. The slides should be immediately fixed in 95% ethanol for Papanicolaou staining or air dried for Diff-Quik® staining. Do not prepare an excessive number of slides, because that makes it more likely that the cells will be poorly preserved and increases the difficulty of screening. Cell blocks do not improve accuracy [Brandborg 1968a, Richardson 1949] and are only recommended for clotted specimens, tissue fragments, or when the use of numerous special stains is anticipated.

Rinsing the brush or needle with balanced salt solution and recovering the cells with filters or cytocentrifugation may decrease the number of unsatisfactory specimens and increase diagnostic sensitivity (yield) [Batra 1982, M Smith 1980]. Various other modifications, eg, washing the channel through which the biopsy forceps or cytology brush have been withdrawn (salvage cytology [Caos 1986, D Graham 1979, Green 1990]) or suctioning the lesion (suction cytology [Bhasin 1988]), have also been applied. Imprints or crush preparations of histologic biopsy material are rapid, require little tissue, and may increase diagnostic yield [Kochhar 1990a, Tamura 1977, Vallilengua 1995, Yoshi 1970], but one must be careful not to crush the tissue to be submitted for histologic examination.

A basic principle of exfoliative cytology is that it is primarily useful in diagnosing lesions that involve a tissue surface. Unfortunately, many tumors of the GI tract (eg, lymphoma or leiomyosarcoma) are found in the deeper tissue layers of the gut. For example, they could be submucosal, subserosal, or in the wall. Unless these tumors are ulcerated, exfoliative cytology may be unable to obtain diagnostic cells [Kobayashi 1970b]. Fine needle aspiration biopsy, which can be endoscopically directed, has been successfully used to diagnose some of these deep, infiltrative, ulcerative, or exophytic lesions and has also been applied to the oral/pharyngeal region [Benya 1993, Castelli 1993, Das 1993,1994, Graham 1989, Iishi 1986, Kochhar 1987,1990b,1991, Layfield 1992, Scher 1988, Singh

1994, Wiersema 1992,1994, Zargar 1991b]. Endoscopic fine needle aspiration may be positive when brush cytology and tissue biopsy are negative [Ingoldby 1987], thus increasing diagnostic sensitivity (yield) [Kochhar 1988].

Alimentary tract cytopathology has assumed renewed importance in diagnosis of diseases associated with AIDS, including infections, lymphomas, and sarcomas [Strigle 1990]. This chapter primarily concerns exfoliative GI cytology. Each division of the GI tract will be discussed separately. Topics in fine needle aspiration biopsy, eg, of the head and neck, pancreas, liver, and soft tissue, are covered in separate chapters.

Oral Cavity

Oral cancer occurs principally in patients with well-defined risk factors, such as alcohol and tobacco use, including the use of smokeless tobacco [Connolly 1986, Winn 1981, Wynder 1957]. Men are twice as likely as women to develop oral cancer, and almost all patients (>95%) are at least 40 years old.

Risk Factors for Oral Cancer

Tobacco*
Alcohol abuse
Male gender (2: 1)
Age ≥40 (>95% of patients)

* Including smokeless tobacco.

The carcinogenic effects of alcohol and tobacco are synergistic and seem to be related to field change rather than to a clonal abnormality [Ogden 1991b]. Although smoking has been emphasized as a major factor in the development of oral cancer, the data suggest that heavy drinking, particularly of beer or wine, is a greater risk factor than previously suspected [Mashberg 1981]. Oral cancer is rare in people who neither smoke nor drink, or do so only minimally [Mashberg 1981]. Other risk factors include sunlight (lip cancer), syphilis, and Plummer-Vinson syndrome (sideropenic dysphagia, also associated with increased risk of esophageal cancer). Trauma and dental irritation are apparently not risk factors [Wynder 1957]. Patients with a history of aerodigestive cancer have a high risk of developing a new primary cancer [Day 1992, Shedd 1971]. The question of whether human papilloma virus is involved in oral carcinogenesis has not been answered conclusively, but as yet there is little evidence that the virus is critical in the development of oral cancer [Koss 1993].

In the United States, nearly all early oral cancers (>95%) occur in one of three sites: the floor of the mouth, the soft palate complex, or the ventrolateral tongue, in a ratio of about 3:2:1, respectively [Mashberg 1976]. These areas are designated the "high-risk" areas. Buccal cancers occur more commonly in cigar and pipe smokers [Mashberg 1984]. Unfortunately, most oral cancers are advanced by the time they are discovered, so the mortality is relatively high, with less than 50% of patients cured [S Silverman 1988]. Early detection (ie, cancers <3 cm, no metastases) can increase the cure rate to about 80% and improve the patient's quality of life by reducing the need for radical surgery [S Silverman 1988]. It has been said that "no lethal disease is easier to cure than oral cancer less than 1 cm in diameter" [Mashberg 1984].

Detection of early oral cancer can be challenging. Because early cancers are usually asymptomatic, the patient may not seek medical attention until symptoms develop—a relatively late occurrence that often indicates advanced disease. The absence of pain does not guarantee the absence of invasive cancer [Shedd 1971]. Also, the clinical diagnosis of early oral cancer may be difficult. Any unhealing sore, irritation, or induration must be considered suspicious for malignancy. However, significant, visible oral lesions, including red or white patches, ulcers, and bumps, are extremely common [Allegra 1973, King 1965]. Most of these are benign, but they can mimic carcinoma. On the other hand, some carcinomas may be mistaken for benign lesions. Thus, even an experienced clinician may not be able to differentiate reliably between the numerous benign and the few malignant oral lesions [Folsom 1972, S Silverman 1988].

Leukoplakia ("white plaque") is statistically associated with the development of carcinoma and has been considered a premalignant condition. However, the malignant potential of leukoplakia has probably been overemphasized [Einhorn 1967]. Although many oral cancers (60%–75%) have a leukoplakic (ie, white) component, only a minority (3%–18%) are entirely white [Mashberg 1977, S Silverman 1984]. Conversely, only a small percentage (~2%–5%) of primarily white lesions are cancer, either in situ or invasive [Mashberg 1977, S Silverman 1984, Waldron 1975]. However, nonsmokers with leukoplakia have a much greater risk (~8 times greater) of malignancy than smokers, which suggests that a more potent carcinogen causes the white lesion in nonsmokers [Einhorn 1967, S Silverman 1984,1988].

Erythroplasia of Queyrat, a red, velvety lesion, is the most common sign of early, asymptomatic oral cancer [Mashberg 1977,1984]. About 80% to 95% of early oral cancers are primarily red, with or without a white component [Koss 1993, Mashberg 1973,1977, S Silverman 1984]. The red appearance is due to an inflammatory immune reaction to the tumor and mimics benign inflammation. There is no color difference between in situ and invasive carcinoma, although the presence of induration implies invasion. However, even when invasive, early oral cancers are usually not indurated, ulcerated, or palpable, nor are they associated with lymphadenopathy. When detected at this early, asymptomatic stage, 84% are no more than 2 cm in diameter (stage T1) and half of those (42%) are no larger than 1 cm [Mashberg 1977]. Unfortunately, minimal size does not rule out the possibility of invasion. More than two thirds (70.6%) of lesions less than 2 cm are invasive [Mashberg 1976]. Nevertheless, treatment results for early oral cancer are usually excellent, with minimal soft tissue or bone loss [Mashberg 1977].

Oral cytology is an accurate diagnostic adjunct that can be of significant value in early cancer detection [JAMA 1968]. Since the vast majority of oral cancers are squamous cell carcinomas arising from the mucosal surface, they lend themselves to early detection via exfoliative cytology. Cytology is not a substitute for biopsy, but it is impractical to surgically biopsy every oral lesion. For this reason, all visible oral lesions should be sampled cytologically [Folsom 1972]. Cytologic preparations have the advantage of being easily, painlessly, and directly obtained, much like a Pap smear, without having to maneuver an endoscope. Patients readily consent to repeat cytologic examinations, but repeated histologic biopsies may cause the patient to fail to return for follow-up. Using cytologic techniques, dentists could screen for oral cancer, and oral surgeons or otolaryngologists could monitor patients with a history of oropharyngeal cancer. Yet even though many oral cancers (up to 50%) may be clinically unsuspected prior to cytologic screening [King 1971, Tiecke 1966], oral cytology is seldom employed. The diagnostic accuracy of oral cytology can be excellent [JAMA 1968, von Haam 1965], but screening is hampered by false-negative diagnoses [Hayes 1969, Reddy 1975, Rovin 1967,1971, Sandler 1966, Shapiro 1964, Shklar 1970, S Silverman 1977]. False negatives are related to necrosis, crusting, or leukoplakia of the lesion, as well as screening the wrong population (ie, a low-risk population), sampling the wrong area, and unsatisfactory diagnostic techniques. False negatives can also be due to the difficulty of assessing malignant criteria in very well-differentiated tumor cells [S Silverman 1977]. However, it is unlikely that a completely normal cytologic specimen will be obtained from a cancerous lesion [Sandler 1964].

Factors That Contribute to a False-Negative Diagnosis

Well-differentiated tumor
Surface keratosis eschar
Extensive necrosis, inflammation
Cell sample not representative of site
Poor quality specimen

Like the Pap smear, exfoliative oral cytology can detect early cancer, complementing but not replacing tissue biopsy. Any clinically suspected or obvious malignancy should be biopsied. A malignant diagnosis made by oral cytology should be confirmed histologically prior to definitive therapy. Although a negative result does not exclude cancer, positive cytology is a safeguard against accepting a false-negative tissue biopsy [Sandler 1966].

Oral cytology is also useful for clinical follow-up, selecting the site for biopsy, detecting multiple lesions, or when the patient refuses biopsy or biopsy is contraindicated. Any ulcer, swelling, or red or white lesion for which there is no clinical explanation (eg, trauma, infection) should be considered suspicious for malignancy [Rovin 1967,1971]. Lesions persisting more than two weeks with therapy should be biopsied. No patient should be discharged from care until the lesion has been adequately diagnosed or has healed. Patients with head and neck cancer who continue to smoke are at high risk (~33%) of developing a new head and neck primary cancer.

Toluidine blue staining can be used to help select an area for biopsy [Mashberg 1980]. Dark-blue staining is a positive result. False positives are common, particularly with inflammatory lesions, but toluidine blue staining is a screening tool and should lead only to close follow-up or biopsy, not definitive therapy. Some patients may present with a lump in the neck that could be due to metastatic disease or inflammation.

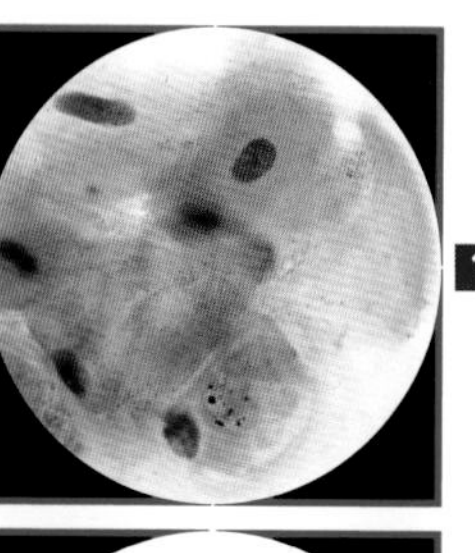
1

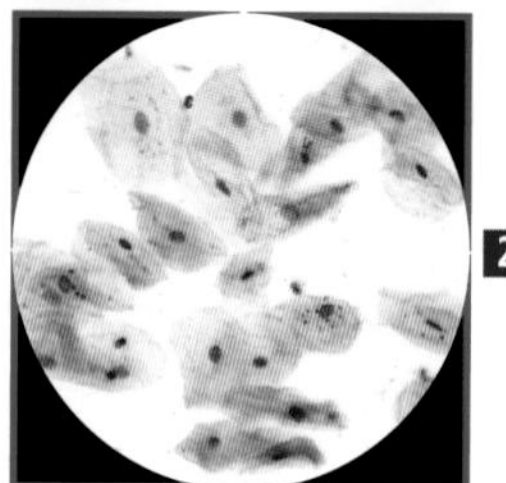
2

The Cells

The lips, hard palate, gingiva, and dorsal surface of the tongue are covered with a keratinized squamous mucosa [Koss 1993, Miller 1951, Montgomery 1951]. Most of the rest of the oral cavity, including the buccal mucosa, is lined by a nonkeratinizing, stratified, squamous epithelium similar to that of the uterine cervix [Miller 1951, Montgomery 1951, S Silverman 1965]. However, the oral mucosa shows little or no cyclic hormonal variation in maturation [Dokumov 1970, S Silverman 1965], though it may show atrophy that will respond to estrogen therapy [Anderson 1969]. Smokers of all ages have a higher maturation index of the oral mucosa than do nonsmokers [Brown 1970]. The oral mucosa renews itself about every five days [G Gillespie 1969].

Cytologically, the appearance of the cells depends on the site sampled. The keratinizing mucosa shows anucleate squames and superficial squamous cells. Keratinized surfaces, particularly the lips and gingiva, and leukoplakia may not be amenable to exfoliative cytologic diagnosis [1 I9.2] [Folsom 1972]. A smear of the nonkeratinized mucosa is composed predominantly of intermediate squamous cells, with few superficial cells and usually no parabasal cells [2 I9.1]. The presence of parabasal cells suggests an ulcer or an excessively vigorous scrape. Barr bodies are best studied from oral (ie, buccal) cytologic preparations. The number of visible Barr bodies is quite variable [Hagy 1972, Platt 1969], but they are typically demonstrated in about 20% to 80% of cells from normal females [Douglass 1969, S Silverman 1965]. Respiratory glandular cells, deriving from the nasopharynx or the ducts of the salivary glands, are occasionally obtained [Koss 1993]. Some inflammatory cells are usually present; an increased number suggests an inflammatory process or infection.

Benign nuclear enlargement can be seen in apparently normal cells, as well as in response to certain drugs, radiation, chemotherapy, mucosal irritations (eg, canker sores or recurrent aphthous ulcers), infections (eg, herpes), and mineral and vitamin deficiencies (iron, folate, B_{12}) [Boddington 1959a,b, S Silverman 1965, Staats 1969].

Benign Nuclear Enlargement

Apparently normal people
Anemia: Fe, B_{12}, Folate
Radiation/chemotherapy
Viral infections, eg, herpes
Mucosal irritations

Longitudinal condensation of the nuclear chromatin, forming a bar similar to that of Anitschkow myocytes seen in rheumatic heart disease, has been described in smears from the labial fold of the lower lip, more commonly in patients with a history of aphthous ulcers [Wood 1975].

Benign Lesions

Hyperkeratosis, Parakeratosis, and Atypical Parakeratosis

Chronic irritation, which is common in the mouth (eg, from dentures, cigarette smoking, or poor dentition), can result in hyperkeratosis (anucleate squames), parakeratosis (miniature superficial cells), or atypical parakeratosis (pleomorphic small cells, as in the cervix). About 80% or more of clinical leukoplakia ("white plaque") is due to various combinations of hyperkeratosis and parakeratosis [3 I9.2]. Benign white lesions must be differentiated from squamous cell carcinoma, which can have a similar clinical appearance. Less than 10% of cases of leukoplakia represent high-grade dysplasia or invasive cancer [Waldron 1975].

Although benign keratoses far outnumber dysplastic or malignant white lesions, cytologic techniques are not a reliable means of detecting epithelial atypia associated with leukoplakia [Dabelsteen 1971, Shklar 1968]. Most false negatives are associated with marked keratosis. As a surface reaction, keratosis may mask an underlying malignancy [Shklar 1968]. Leukoplakic lesions should be scraped with a relatively sharp, nonabsorbent instrument, such as an amalgam spatula [Allegra 1973].

Inflammatory Atypia and Repair/Regeneration

In response to ulceration or various inflammations, the oral mucosa may undergo reactive or reparative changes similar to those seen in the Pap smear [4 I9.3]. The nuclei may be enlarged, with high nuclear/cytoplasmic (N/C) ratios and prominent chromocenters in parabasal-sized cells. Prominent or multiple nucleoli and multinucleation may be seen. The type and amount of inflammatory component is variable. The presence of these deep cells with high N/C ratios may suggest a significant epithelial abnormality [Koss 1993]. In inflammatory atypia (inflammatory "change" in the Bethesda System), the nuclei are relatively uniform, with evenly distributed chromatin. However, the cytoplasm may be poorly preserved. Specific infectious agents (described below) include herpes, *Candida*, *Actinomyces*, and Epstein-Barr virus, but specific infectious agents are rarely identified in individual cases. (For further description of repair/regeneration, see Chapter 6; for further description of microbiologic agents, see Chapter 5.)

Herpes: Usual diagnostic features: multinucleation, molding, and margination (the 3 Ms), as well as possible intranuclear inclusions.

Candida: Often found as a commensal; causes thrush.

Actinomyces: Usually only a saprophyte occurring in the tonsil but can cause invasive disease, rarely.

Other oral flora, including saprophytic fungi, bacteria, and *Entamoeba gingivalis*, can be seen in the absence of infection, particularly in patients with poor oral hygiene [Koss 1993]. *Entamoeba gingivalis* is a multinucleated organism that is larger than *E histolytica* and does not phagocytose red blood cells.

Hairy Leukoplakia: One of the most common oral manifestations of human immunodeficiency virus (but can affect HIV-negative patients as well). It is an Epstein-Barr virus infection with no malignant potential. Characteristic findings include intranuclear Cowdry type-A inclusions, intranuclear inclusions with the appearance of ground glass, and clumping and margination of the chromatin. Bacterial colonies or *Candida* are also often present [Fraga-Fernandez 1992].

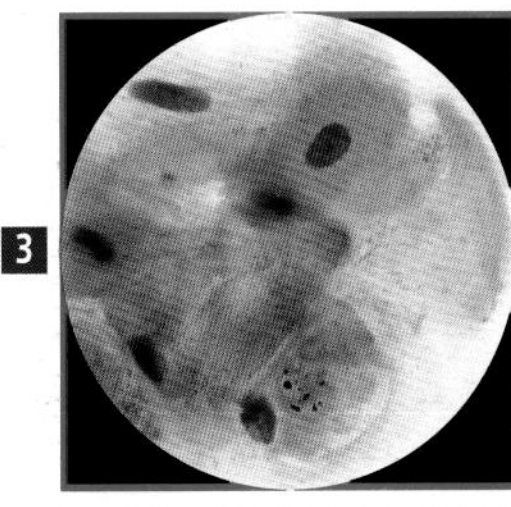
3

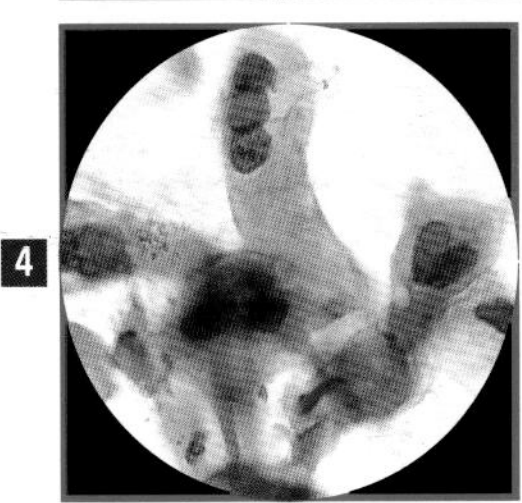
4

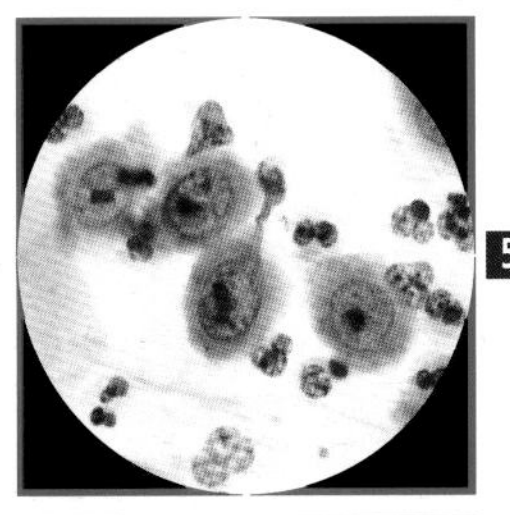
5

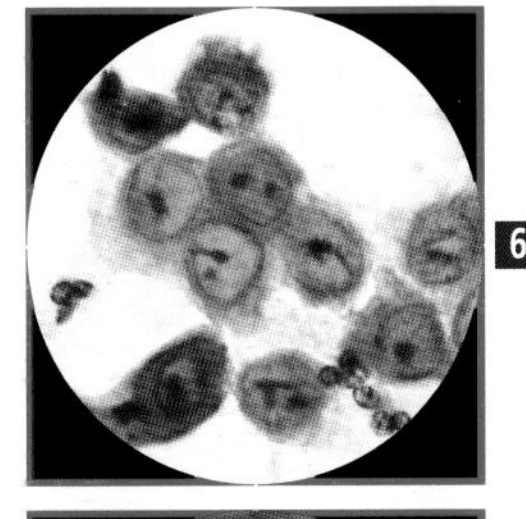
6

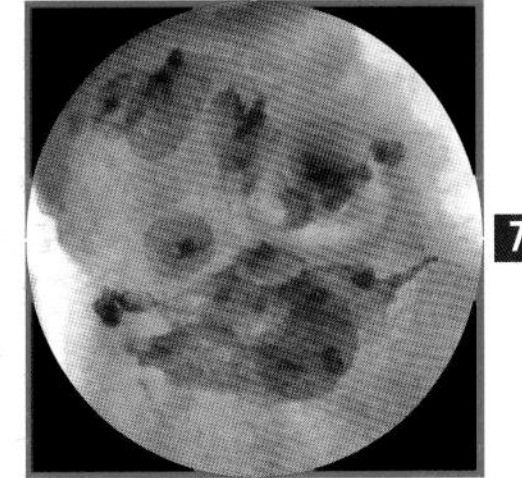
7

Pemphigus Vulgaris

Pemphigus vulgaris is an autoimmune disease that attacks the intercellular junctions (desmosomes) and causes a suprabasilar bleb or blister, acantholysis, and intercellular IgG deposition in skin and mucous membranes [Faravelli 1984]. The mouth, particularly the vermilion border with the skin, is frequently affected and is often the initial site of involvement. Other sites of involvement, including the esophagus [F Kaneko 1985, Raque 1970] and cervix (see Chapter 6), have been described. When seen clinically, the blisters usually have broken, leaving a painful ulcer that is covered with exudate and bleeds easily.

Scrapings from the vesicles obtain very atypical, immature parabasal squamous cells known as acantholytic or Tzanck cells [5 I9.4] [Koss 1993]. Many single cells and loosely cohesive sheets of cells are usually present in the smears [Coscia-Porrazzi 1985]. The cytologic appearance of the individual cells is very much like the cytologic appearance of repair, except that there are many single cells because of autoimmune destruction of intercellular junctions. The combination of cytologic atypia plus numerous single cells may strongly suggest cancer. Cytology can be used to distinguish pemphigus vulgaris from other bullous diseases (eg, pemphigoid, lichen planus, erythema multiforme, aphthous ulcers, herpes, and systemic lupus erythematosus [Coscia-Porrazzi 1985, Medak 1970]) as well as provide a specific diagnosis.

Differential Diagnosis: Bullous Diseases

- Lichen planus
- Erythema multiforme
- Bullous pemphigoid
- Herpes
- Darier's disease
- Pemphigus foliaceous
- (Also, cicatricial pemphigoid, aphthous stomatitis, Behçet's disease, systemic lupus erythematosus)

Numerous acantholytic cells are usually present [5 I9.4]. The characteristic cells are round to polygonal, uniform, parabasal-sized cells that are poorly cohesive or single. The cytoplasm is dense and stains variably blue to red. Perinuclear acidophilic staining of the cytoplasm is common [6 I9.5] [Coscia-Porrazzi 1985, Medak 1970]. There can also be a clear perinuclear halo. The cells can appear very atypical, and the N/C ratio is high. The nucleus is enlarged and has a smooth but thick nuclear membrane. In contrast with cancer cells, the chromatin is usually pale, fine, and even [Medak 1970] but may appear coarse in the acute phase of the disease. Nucleoli are prominent and may be multiple or irregular. A bar- or bullet-shaped nucleolus is characteristic. Normal mitotic figures can be seen. The atypical cells resemble those in repair, except that the number of single cells is increased. One must be careful not to mistake these atypical cells for cancer cells.

In addition, larger cells with more abundant cytoplasm [Levin 1969] and occasionally even giant, multinucleated cells can be seen, particularly after therapy [7 I9.6] [Medak 1970]. A variable inflammatory infiltrate consisting of neutrophils, lymphocytes, or monocytes is usually present.

Other Diseases With Characteristic Changes Involving Oral Mucosa

Darier's Disease: Rough white oral papules, usually of the hard palate. Cytologic appearance includes cell-in-cell arrangements (resembling corps ronds), dyskeratosis, and orange cells with elongated nuclei (resembling grains) [Burlakow 1969, Witkop 1962]. Corps ronds and grains are characteristic histologic features of Darier's disease. These findings must be distinguished from those that characterize squamous cell carcinoma [Tiecke 1966]. Similar cell-in-cell arrangements can be seen after therapy with methotrexate, 5-fluorouracil, or radiation [Witkop 1962].

Hereditary Benign Intraepithelial Dyskeratosis: Soft white mucosa of variable thickness; may appear to fold on itself. Cytologic appearance is similar to that of Darier's disease and includes cell-in-cell arrangements and dyskeratosis [8 I9.7] [Tiecke 1966, Witkop 1962].

White Sponge Nevus: Clinical appearance similar to that of hereditary benign intraepithelial dyskeratosis but also involves other mucosae, particularly the vagina. Cytologic appearance includes parakeratosis and cells with eosinophilic or orangeophilic cytoplasmic condensations or inclusions surrounded by a halo [Morris 1988, Tiecke 1966, Witkop 1962].

Radiation

Cytology is useful in detecting recurrent carcinoma [Umiker 1965], but when there is a history of radiation, be cautious about diagnosing malignancy. The cytology of radiation change in the mouth is similar to that seen in the Pap smear (and also similar to changes caused by folate or B_{12} vitamin deficiency). Radiation produces characteristic macrocytes in which the nucleus and cytoplasm both enlarge but the N/C ratio remains relatively normal [Ogden 1989]. Radiation results in signs of regeneration (enlarged nucleus and cytoplasm, multinucleation, prominent nucleoli) and degeneration (nuclear pyknosis, karyorrhexis, karyolysis, and cytoplasmic vacuolization and amphophilia) [I9.8] [Memon 1970, Peters 1958]. Radiation changes in the mouth can persist for the patient's life [S Silverman 1967], but they revert to normal more often than radiation changes in the uterine cervix do [Ogden 1989]. Similar changes can be produced by certain chemotherapeutic agents [Koss 1993].

Deficiency Diseases

In pernicious anemia (B_{12} deficiency), megaloblastic anemias, tropical sprue, and malnutrition, the squamous cells may show significant nuclear and cytoplasmic enlargement (ie, macrocytosis) [Boen 1957, R Graham 1954, Koss 1993, Staats 1965]. (See Chapter 6 for further discussion.)

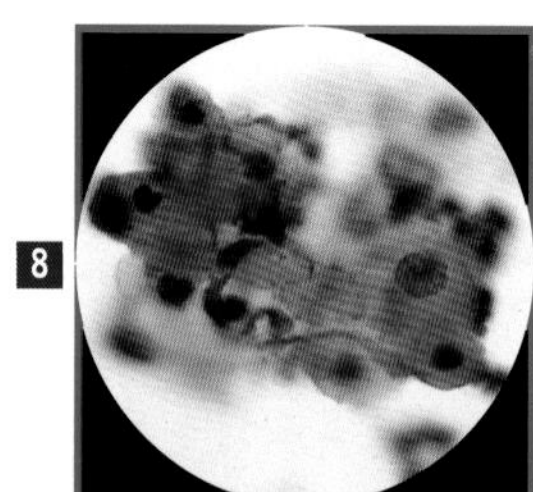
8

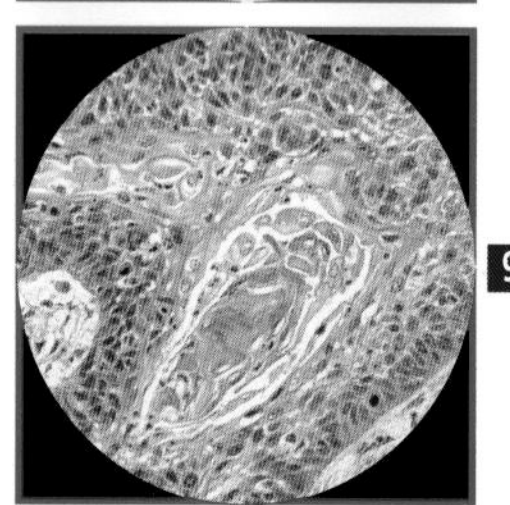
9

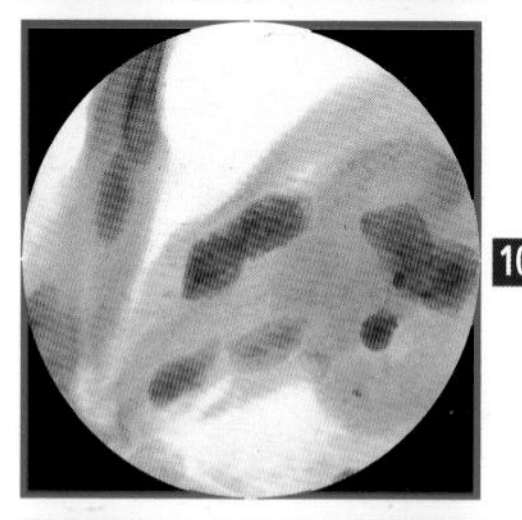
10

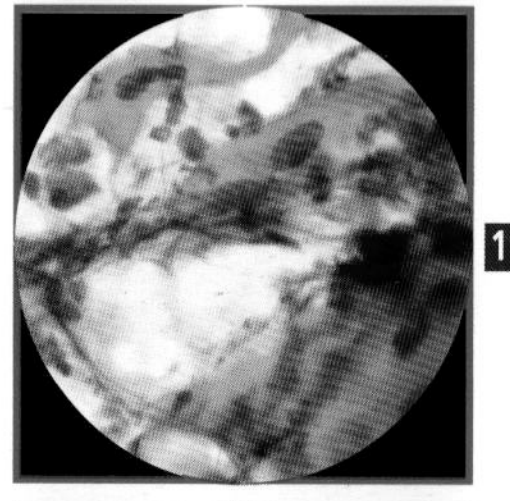
11

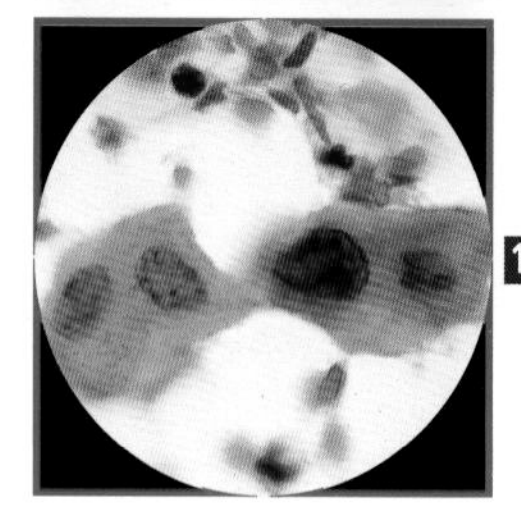
12

Cancer

Oral cancer accounts for about 2% to 3% of all visceral cancers and 1% to 2% of cancer deaths. Most oral cancers (~90%) derive from the squamous epithelium [Gardner 1965].

Squamous Cell Carcinoma

The great majority of oral malignancies are well-differentiated, keratinizing squamous cell carcinomas (SCCs) [9 I9.12]. It is important to know that the malignant features of oral SCC can be subtle [Allegra 1973], resembling what might be considered only a low-grade dysplasia, or squamous intraepithelial lesion, in the Pap smear. Slight nuclear enlargement, slight irregularity of the nuclear membrane, and slight abnormality of the chromatin characterize some well-differentiated SCCs [Koss 1993]. Poorly differentiated (nonkeratinizing) SCCs also occur.

The cells in squamous cell carcinoma are found singly and in clusters [10 I9.9, 11 I9.10, 12 I9.11]. They exhibit characteristic morphologic features [Sandler 1965]. The malignant cells are typically pleomorphic in size and shape (eg, snakes, tadpoles, bizarre shapes). Malignant keratin pearls are pathognomonic of keratinizing SCC. The cytoplasm is thick, often bright orange, and may show refractile keratin rings around the nucleus. The nuclei vary in size and shape, with irregular, coarse to pyknotic chromatin. Nucleoli may be seen, or they may be obscured by the dense chromatin. "Ghost" cells with heavily keratinized cytoplasm and karyolysis (dissolution of the nucleus) are frequent [Koss 1993]. Mitotic figures are rare in benign specimens, and abnormal mitotic figures are particularly important diagnostically. Nonkeratinizing SCC is recognized, as in the Pap smear, by more uniform malignant squamous cells with much less keratinization, no pearls, somewhat more open chromatin, and more prominent nucleoli. The background usually shows necrotic material, blood, and inflammation, ie, a tumor diathesis [Koss 1993].

Dysplasia and Carcinoma In Situ

Like SCC in the cervix, SCC in the mouth is thought to be preceded by an atypical, intraepithelial neoplastic lesion, ie, dysplasia and carcinoma in situ. Patients with dysplasia have an increased risk of developing oral cancer [S Silverman 1984]. Both light microscopic and ultrastructural abnormalities occur [Chomette 1986]. The premalignant lesions can be detected by cytologic techniques, which show a mixture of parabasal to intermediate-sized cells with significant nuclear enlargement and hyperchromasia [Koss 1993, Stahl 1967]. It may be difficult to distinguish dysplasia from well-differentiated squamous cell carcinoma on cytologic grounds alone. On the other hand, mild atypia and atypical parakeratosis are common benign changes in the mouth that may suggest a more significant lesion. Dysplastic changes must be differentiated from reactive changes [Elzay 1974]. Tissue confirmation is required.

Recurrent Oral Cancer

Oral cancer recurs often enough after treatment that close surveillance is indicated [Koss 1993]. Cytology is useful in detecting recurrent, or new primary, cancer that may be clinically inapparent [Hutter 1966].

Other Malignancies

A wide variety of other malignancies can occur in the mouth. They can arise from lymphoid tissue (eg, tonsils; see Chapter 18), minor salivary glands (see Chapter 16), or soft tissue (see Chapter 14). Melanomas can also occur in the oral cavity [Koss 1993].

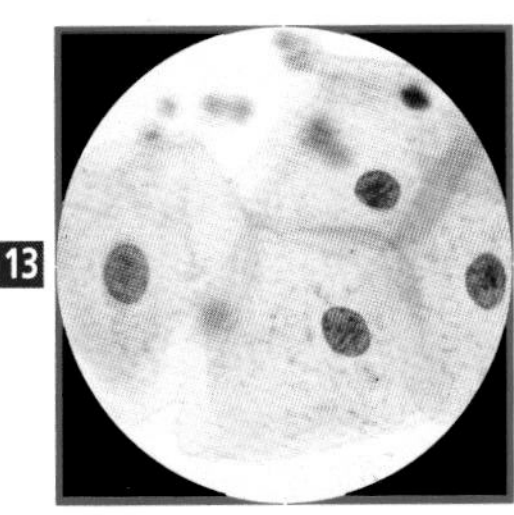
13

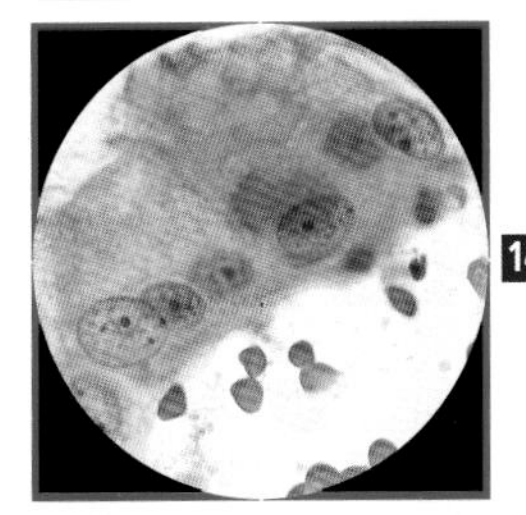
14

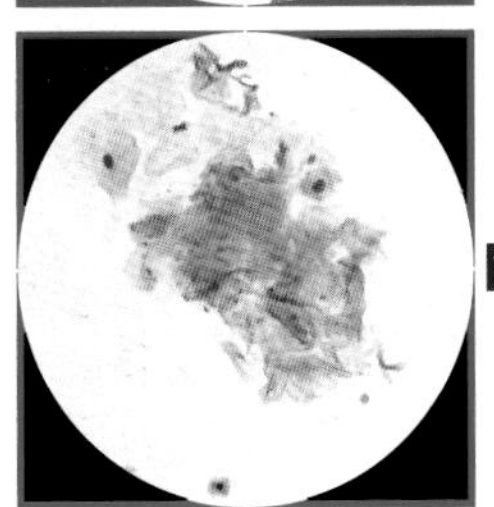
15

Esophagus

The esophagus is the gullet, ie, the muscular tube running through the neck and mediastinum connecting the mouth to the stomach. It is divided, for clinical purposes, into the upper, middle, and lower thirds. The esophagus runs near several vital structures (larynx, trachea, aorta, and heart) as well as important nerves, such as the vagus and recurrent laryngeal. The esophagus also has a rich vascular and lymphatic supply. Moreover, unlike most of the rest of the GI tract, the esophagus has no serosal lining to act as a barrier to the spread of inflammation, infection, or cancer. Consequently, lesions of the esophagus can readily disseminate to surrounding vital tissues and organs.

Most esophageal cell samples are obtained by direct endoscopic brushings. In high-risk populations, screening with an esophageal balloon has been used to detect early cancer [Berry 1981, Dawsey 1994, Greenebaum 1984, Shu 1983, Tim 1982, Tsang 1987]. The method, in essence, is to have the patient swallow a deflated balloon, inflate it, pull it through the esophagus, deflate it, and collect cells for diagnosis.

The Cells

Squamous Cells

Most of the esophagus is lined with a nonkeratinized, stratified squamous epithelium. Cytologically, the squamous cells resemble those of the uterine cervix as seen in the Pap smear. They are mostly intermediate cells (abundant delicate cytoplasm, vesicular nucleus) with a few superficial cells (abundant cytoplasm, pyknotic nucleus) [13 I9.13] [Shu 1983]. Only rarely are cells from the deeper layers seen [Johnson 1955], although parabasal cells (smaller, denser cytoplasm; vesicular nucleus) can be seen if there is inflammation, an ulcer, or an excessively hard scrape. Normal esophageal superficial cells may contain keratohyalin granules. An occasional benign squamous pearl is also normal [Koss 1993] (see "Leukoplakia," below). Although skin appendages are not seen, melanocytes do occur. However, primary esophageal malignant melanoma is rare.

Glandular Cells

The normal esophagus has submucosal mucous glands, but they are generally inaccessible to exfoliative cytology. However, near the distal end of the esophagus, interdigitating, finger-like projections of glandular epithelium are found that are continuous with the lining epithelium of the cardia of the stomach [14 I9.14]. Gastric cardiac-type glands can also occur in the lamina propria of the upper esophagus. Glandular cells in an esophageal specimen, particularly when obtained some distance from the gastroesophageal junction, may indicate Barrett's esophagus.

During embryologic development, the esophagus is lined with ciliated epithelium. Esophageal cysts rarely contain ciliated cells [Rubio 1991]. However, ciliated cells are usually contaminants from the respiratory tract, especially if the sampling tube was inserted through the nose. Swallowed respiratory cells, including alveolar macrophages with carbon pigment, can also be seen [Johnson 1955]. Other elements (bacteria, yeast, inflammatory cells) can be present, usually due to oral contamination but sometimes due to disease. Note also that tumor cells can be swallowed or can be "pickup" contaminants, more often in blind lavage than in brush specimens.

Diseases of the Esophagus

Leukoplakia

Leukoplakia is a nonspecific clinical term for a white plaque. The causes include hyperkeratosis, parakeratosis, atypical parakeratosis, condyloma, dysplasia, and cancer [15 I9.15]. The cytology depends on the etiology (see Chapter 6). A white appearance of the distal esophagus can also be due to heavy glycogen content of the cells (glycogenic acanthosis).

Vitamin Deficiency

In pernicious anemia (B_{12} deficiency) [Brandborg 1961, Massey 1955] and folate deficiency, the squamous cells may enlarge, with nucleus and cytoplasm enlarging in concert, maintaining a relatively normal N/C ratio (ie, the cells become macrocytes). Similar changes can be associated with human papilloma virus infection or condyloma.

Esophagitis

Esophagitis, with or without ulceration, can be due to a wide variety of conditions, including irritants (eg, alcohol, smoking, lye, hot drinks), reflux, trauma, hiatal hernia, Crohn's disease, sarcoid, radiation/chemotherapy, infectious agents, uremia, and other sorts of injury [16 I9.16]. For example, achalasia (also known as cardiospasm) causes dysphagia for liquids and solids. Mechanical damage can result in inflammation and may cause ulceration. Esophagitis is also a common, early manifestation of AIDS [Koss 1993]. *Candida*, viruses, or other infective agents may be identified in the cytologic specimen (see below).

Reflux esophagitis, the most common type of esophagitis in the United States, is often associated with hiatal hernia. Reflux may also be associated with alcoholism, diabetic neuropathy, or connective tissue disease, particularly scleroderma. Reflux of gastric contents injures the esophageal mucosa and may cause superficial peptic ulceration. Inflammation is usually limited to the lamina propria, but the degree of inflammation may be difficult to assess. For this reason, the epithelial changes, which are essentially due to increased cellular proliferation, receive more emphasis in the diagnosis of reflux esophagitis.

With reflux, the mucosa becomes inflamed. The basal and parabasal cells proliferate. Papillae of connective tissue extend close to the mucosal surface. Ulceration begins at the tips of these elongated papillae, and marked reactive atypia of the epithelium may occur, which can mimic malignancy. Eventually, the squamous epithelium may be replaced by glandular gastric-type epithelium, which in turn may be replaced by intestinal-like epithelium. These glandular metaplastic changes are known as Barrett's esophagus.

Endoscopically, the mucosa is granular and red and may be ulcerated. Cytologically, increased numbers of reactive parabasal cells and reparative epithelial cells with enlarged, reactive nuclei; vesicular chromatin; prominent nucleoli and occasionally binucleation may be seen [16 I9.16, 17 I9.17] [Koss 1993]. Nuclear and cytoplasmic degenerative changes, including karyorrhexis, karyopyknosis, and cytoplasmic vacuolization may be seen [Johnson 1955]. Inflammation may be intimately admixed with the reactive cells and present in the background of the smear [16 I9.16]. With chronic esophagitis, hyperkeratosis may occur. These changes are nonspecific. Eosinophils may indicate reflux esophagitis [Lee 1985a, Tummala 1987, Winter 1982], while the presence of neutrophils suggests ulceration. Glandular cells may also be observed (see "Barrett's Esophagus" for further discussion).

Atypical cells in a "dirty," inflammatory background may suggest malignancy. Cellular cohesion, orderly cellular arrangements, relatively normal N/C ratios, fine chromatin, and smooth nuclear membranes distinguish reactive cells from malignant cells.

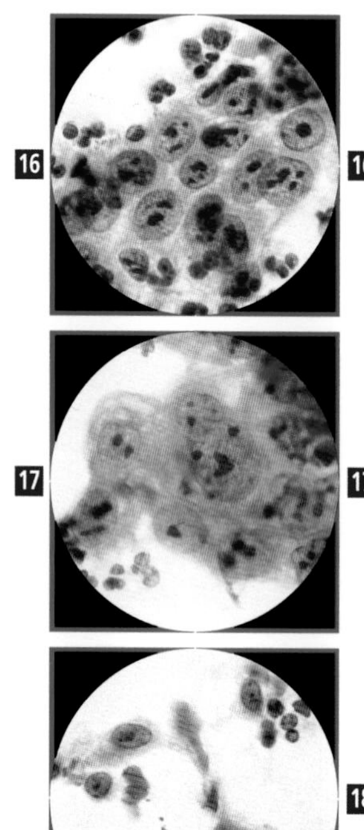

Esophageal Ulcer

Esophageal ulcers can be acute or chronic. The primary function of cytology in this setting is to distinguish benign from malignant ulcers. Sometimes a specific infectious agent can be identified.

With ulceration, basal- to parabasal-sized cells may be observed in addition to the usual superficial and intermediate cells. These cells are found singly and in cohesive clusters. They have scant to moderate amounts of cytoplasm, and the nuclei are relatively large, resulting in increased N/C ratios. The nuclei may have irregular shapes [Johnson 1955]. However, the nuclear membrane remains relatively smooth, unlike the membranes in malignant nuclei. Also, the chromatin may be clumped or marginate, which makes the nuclear membrane appear thick. Prominent nucleoli may be seen. Cells deriving from repair/regeneration, characterized by active but orderly cells with good intercellular cohesion, can be seen [16 I9.16, 17 I9.17]. Reactive mesenchymal cells may be obtained from the ulcer base [18 I9.18].

Signs of degeneration are also often present. Degenerated cytoplasm can become vacuolated or fragmented. The nuclei may become pyknotic as well as break up (karyorrhexis) or dissolve altogether (karyolysis). Inflammatory cells and necrotic debris are seen in the background. The combination of atypical cells in a necrotic background may suggest cancer. Cancer is characterized by increased single cells, coarse chromatin, and more cytologic atypia.

Granulomatous Esophagitis

Granulomatous esophagitis can be due to tuberculosis, sarcoid, syphilis, or Crohn's disease. The cytology may reveal nodular collections of epithelioid histiocytes and giant histiocytes. A specific infectious agent may be identified in some cases. Recommend special stains (eg, acid fast) and culture. Clinical history may be crucial in the final diagnosis.

Barrett's Esophagus

Barrett's esophagus, which Barrett described as the "lower esophagus lined by columnar epithelium" [Barrett 1950], is a syndrome in which the glandular epithelium extends above the lower esophageal sphincter to the distal esophagus [Spechler 1986]. The glandular extensions may be circumferential, finger-like projections, or islands. Barrett's esophagus is thought to be a protective, metaplastic reaction of the esophageal mucosa to chronic, recurrent gastric reflux. The mechanically resistant native squamous epithelium is replaced by a chemically resistant metaplastic gastrointestinal glandular epithelium that is better able to withstand the action of gastric digestive juices.

Genetic predisposition, smoking, and alcohol may also be factors in the development of Barrett's esophagus. The disease occurs predominantly among whites rather than blacks (~10:1), and more commonly in males than females (~3:1) [Skinner 1983].

Clinical symptoms may include dysphagia, heartburn, and regurgitation [Messian 1978], but Barrett's esophagus can also be asymptomatic and therefore go undiagnosed [Spechler 1986]. Esophageal stricture, ulceration, and hemorrhage are common complications. Barrett's esophagus is also considered a premalignant condition [Berenson 1978, Haggitt 1978, Hameeteman 1989, Naef 1975]. A small but significant percentage of patients (~10%) develop adenocarcinoma (Dawson's syndrome) [Hameeteman 1989, Naef 1975], a risk at least 30 to 40 (and possibly 350 or more [Robertson 1988]) times greater than that of the general population [Cameron 1985, Hameeteman 1989, Spechler 1986, Van Der Veen 1989]. In fact, almost all adenocarcinomas of the distal esophagus arise in Barrett's epithelium. Because adenocarcinoma is probably preceded by dysplasia, dysplasia of the glandular epithelium is considered an ominous finding [Skinner 1983]. Cytology is useful not only in diagnosing Barrett's esophagus but also in detecting dysplasia and cancer [Robey 1988].

The pathogenesis of Barrett's esophagus is thought to begin with esophageal ulceration followed by replacement of the normal squamous epithelium of the esophagus by a metaplastic glandular epithelium [Spechler 1986]. The normally smooth, pearly pink squamous esophageal mucosa is replaced by the velvety red appearance characteristic of gastric mucosa. This change is visible endoscopically. However, the endoscopic appearance is unreliable in the diagnosis of Barrett's esophagus, and morphologic documentation of the presence of glandular epithelium is required [Spechler 1986].

Barrett's esophagus probably represents incomplete intestinal metaplasia of gastric-type epithelium [Lee 1984]. In Barrett's esophagus, both gastric and intestinal features may be seen morphologically. Mucous cells (goblet and nongoblet types), chief cells, or parietal cells may be present [Hameeteman 1989, Paull 1976]. The intestinal, or specialized, type of epithelium, characterized by the presence of goblet cells, is the most likely to undergo malignant degeneration.

Benign cells exfoliate in large, flat, cohesive sheets. Single cells are rare when the specimen is well preserved [19 I9.19]. An important feature of benign glandular cells in Barrett's esophagus is that the sheets are distinctly outlined, with sharply defined, smooth edges [Geisinger 1992]. The cells are uniformly distributed, and although they may be somewhat crowded, there is neither loss of polarity nor significant piling-up. However, small acinar, or rosette-like, structures may be seen [Wang 1992], and villous arrangements are characteristic of intestinal-type epithelium [Robey 1988]. The nuclei are round to oval and relatively uniform, with smooth nuclear membranes; fine, even chromatin; and single nucleoli, which may be prominent in repair [Geisinger 1992, Wang 1992]. The cytoplasm is granular to nondescript or may show goblet-cell vacuolization in intestinal-type epithelium. The background is relatively clean and noninflammatory and may include squamous cells and some fresh blood.

19 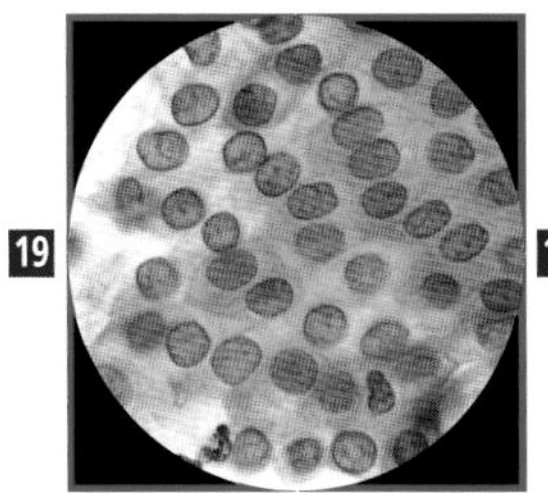 19

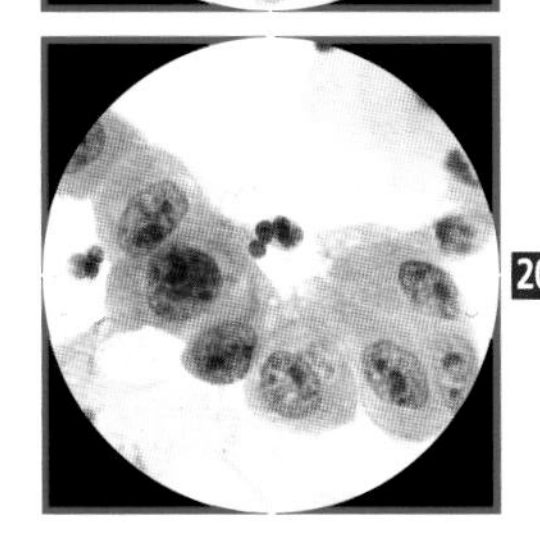 20

Reactive or reparative changes, with nuclear enlargement and pleomorphism, prominent nucleoli, and mitotic figures as well as degenerative changes, in an inflammatory background are common cytologic characteristics of Barrett's esophagus and may suggest malignancy. Maintenance of cellular cohesion and polarity, N/C ratio, round to oval nuclear shape, and fine chromatin are benign features [20 I9.20]. (See also "Glandular Dysplasia in Barrett's Esophagus, p 340.)

Nongoblet mucous cells are present in all types of Barrett's mucosa. Cytologically, gastric-type epithelium appears as cells of uniform size, shape, and staining [Robey 1988], which cannot be distinguished from normal stomach cells [Doos 1985]. The specialized-, or intestinal-type, columnar epithelium is composed of somewhat pleomorphic mucous cells in which characteristic Paneth or endocrine cells or striated borders are rarely identified [Doos 1985].

Goblet cells are present only in intestinal- (ie, specialized-) type epithelium. For this reason, they serve as markers of intestinal metaplasia [Paull 1976]. Goblet cells have single, large, clear cytoplasmic vacuoles that compress the nuclei [Wang 1992]. When seen en face, the sheets of intestinal-type cells have the appearance of Swiss cheese (the holes are due to the presence of large, pale-staining goblet cells scattered among nongoblet mucous cells) [Robey 1988]. The goblet cells in Barrett's esophagus are more variable in size and distribution than the goblet cells that characterize intestinal metaplasia in the stomach.

Both gastric- and intestinal-type mucous cells secrete neutral mucins, which stain with PAS and mucicarmine. However, goblet cells and, in many cases, the specialized mucous cells secrete acid mucins that stain intensely with alcian blue [Lee 1984] but may also stain lightly with mucicarmine [T9.1] [Robey 1988].

In essence, the cytologic diagnosis of Barrett's esophagus consists of identifying glandular cells in an esophageal specimen [19 I9.19]. In making the diagnosis of Barrett's esophagus, it is critical to verify that the specimen actually came from the esophagus rather than the gastroesophageal junction or stomach. This may not always be clear to the endoscopist. For this reason, the specimen should originate at least 2 to 3 cm above the gastroesophageal junction to be certain of a diagnosis of Barrett's esophagus. Barrett's esophagus may ulcerate,

T9.1 **Barrett's Epithelia**

Type of Epithelium	PAS	Alcian Blue
Intestinal*	(+)	(+)
Gastric	(+)	(–)

* Hallmark of Barrett's esophagus; most likely to develop adenocarcinoma [Skinner 1983].

resulting in the usual cytologic findings of peptic ulcer (reactive or reparative epithelial atypia, inflammation, and necrosis), which could suggest malignancy or dysplasia. (For further discussion, see "Adenocarcinoma," p 339, and "Glandular Dysplasia in Barrett's Esophagus," p 340.)

Radiation and Chemotherapy

Chemotherapy or radiation used in the treatment of cancer, including lung cancer and mediastinal malignancies, commonly causes clinical esophagitis with dysphagia and substernal burning. The morphologic changes can mimic cancer, and the differential diagnosis may be particularly difficult in patients who have been treated for esophageal cancer. The history of radiation or chemotherapy must be provided by the clinician for proper diagnosis.

Radiation

The changes induced by radiation (seen, eg, in patients treated for pulmonary or mediastinal disease) are similar to the changes that radiation induces in the cervix [Gephart 1959, Goldgraber 1956]. Radiation change is exemplified by the presence of macrocytes with nucleus and cytoplasm enlarged in concert, so that the N/C ratio remains within normal limits. Pale, hypochromatic or dark, hyperchromatic, degenerated nuclei with thickened or wrinkled membranes can be seen. Nucleoli are usually inconspicuous. Multinucleation can also occur in the squamous cells. The cytoplasm may be vacuolated and two-tone stained. Radiation may induce cytoplasmic keratinization or cell death. Multinucleated giant cell histiocytes may be seen.

Radiation changes may be particularly marked in young patients who have received radiation treatment for mediastinal lymphoma (eg, Hodgkin's disease, lymphoblastic lymphoma, or other diseases). Be cautious diagnosing squamous cell carcinoma in a young patient. The presence of few atypical cells and large cells with relatively normal N/C ratios, and generally insignificant hyperchromasia favors a benign process.

Chemotherapy

Chemotherapy can induce changes similar to those seen in radiation (ie, macrocytes). Chemotherapy can also produce cells that are even more markedly abnormal than in radiation. Chemotherapeutic agents may also enhance radiation reaction [Greco 1976]. The changes can include variation in nuclear size with crowding and overlapping; irregular nuclear membranes; and hyperchromatic, clumped chromatin [21 I9.22]. The N/C ratio may be increased. Multiple nucleoli of variable size and shape can also be seen. Evidence of cell death as well as keratinization may occur. These changes can mimic carcinoma [O'Morchoe 1983].

21

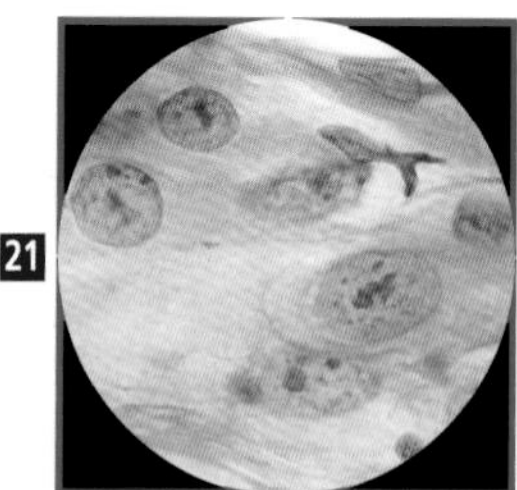

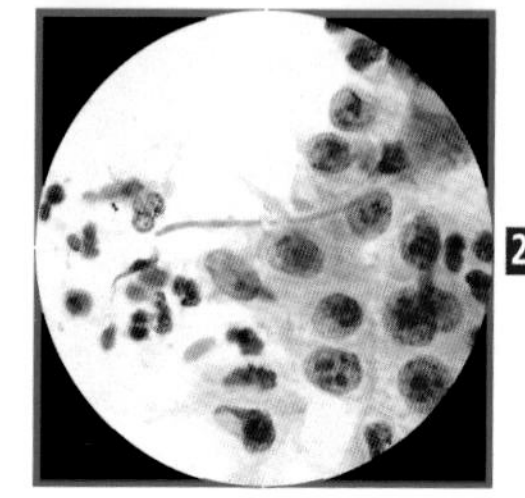

22

Infections

Bacterial Esophagitis

Primary bacterial esophagitis is uncommon but may be seen in immunocompromised patients. Secondary bacterial infections, eg, of herpetic ulcers, are more common. Bacteria, inflammation, debris, and, possibly, reparative cells are seen cytologically.

Candida

Esophageal candidiasis in immunocompromised patients (including patients with AIDS, organ transplants, diabetes, and cancer) is an increasingly important clinical problem and is the most common cause of infectious esophagitis. Esophageal candidiasis may be an early sign of AIDS and is used as a diagnostic criterion for that disease. *Candida* infection is also associated with antibiotic therapy in immunocompetent and, especially, immunosuppressed patients. Candidiasis also occurs in association with functional or mechanical obstruction of the esophagus (eg, achalasia, stricture, neoplasm) [Gefter 1981]. Occasionally, *Candida* infection occurs in otherwise apparently healthy individuals.

Esophageal candidiasis can produce mild to severe disease or can be a commensal in the upper GI tract of asymptomatic individuals. Therefore, it is important to distinguish true invasive infection from the mere presence (surface colonization) of *Candida*. The classic clinical/endoscopic appearance of candidiasis is a white plaque (or pseudomembrane) on a reddened mucosa. The lesion may ulcerate, resulting in a characteristic cobblestone appearance. The clinician must correlate the clinical and endoscopic findings with the presence of *Candida* organisms to arrive at the proper diagnosis.

Candida organisms are more readily demonstrated in cytologic brushings than in tissue biopsies [22 I9.23] [Geisinger 1995, Kodsi 1971]. Cytologically, the presence of significant numbers of *Candida* (budding yeasts, pseudohyphae) as well as necrotic debris, inflammatory cells (mostly neutrophils), reactive/reparative cells, and anucleate squames obtained from a clinically compatible lesion is consistent with invasive infection. Finding organisms that are apparently growing in squamous cells is particularly characteristic of infection [22 I9.23]. Marked necrosis or inflammation can mask the diagnostic organisms; special stains, eg, Gomori methenamine silver (GMS), may help identify them.

Aspergillus

Aspergillus is a rare cause of esophagitis. It is diagnosed cytologically by the usual features (eg, 45° branching, septate hyphae). However, it is frequently a contaminant.

Herpes

Herpes infections include both herpes simplex and varicella-zoster viruses, which produce lesions that are morphologically indistinguishable. Like candidiasis, esophageal herpes infections are becoming a more common clinical problem. Herpetic esophagitis is usually associated with immunodeficiency or debility but can be seen in otherwise apparently healthy immunocompetent patients [Ashenburg 1986, Depew 1977, Owensby 1978, Springer 1979]. Predisposing factors include an immunocompromised state (eg, AIDS or cancer, especially malignant lymphoma or leukemia [Buss 1979]), complications of anticancer or immunosuppressive therapy, achalasia, and trauma (including nasogastric intubation [Nash 1974] and burns).

Herpes causes vesicles, which frequently ulcerate and occasionally hemorrhage [Fischbein 1979]. Patients may have severe odynophagia, or they may be asymptomatic [Buss 1979]. Herpes patients are predisposed to superinfection, eg, with *Candida* [P Rosen 1971]. Because herpetic ulcers are usually superficial, they usually resolve spontaneously, without serious sequelae. Thus, superinfections, and particularly the possibility of a serious underlying disorder, may be of more clinical importance than the herpes infection itself. However, in immunocompromised hosts, dissemination of the herpes infection may occur.

Cytology facilitates a reliable diagnosis of herpes, and although cytology and tissue biopsy are complementary, cytology can be more definitive [Lightdale 1977]. Cytologic techniques reveal the usual cellular features, including the 3 Ms (multinucleation, molding, and margination) and, sometimes, acidophilic intranuclear inclusions [23 I9.24] [Lasser 1977, Shah 1977]. Ulceration may produce reactive and reparative changes in the epithelial cells, with an inflammatory or necrotic background that includes inflammatory cells and debris and may suggest a tumor diathesis. The presence of bacteria or fungi may indicate superinfection.

23

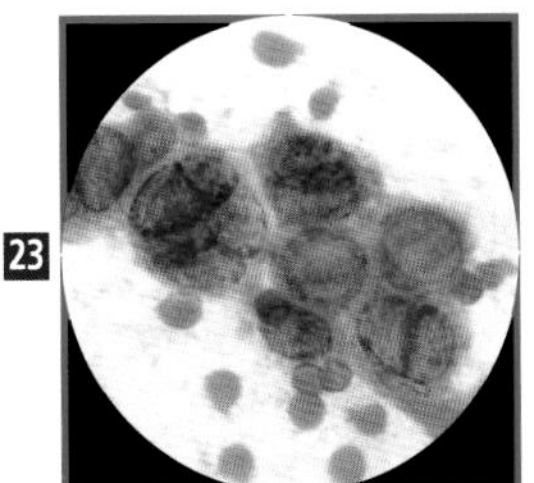

Atypical reactive/reparative changes can also occur in the squamous epithelium. Atypical pleomorphic cells with viral inclusions (resembling macronucleoli) in a necrotic background could mimic cancer. Familiarity with the morphology of herpes and the bland, ground-glass ("empty" or "viral") appearance of the chromatin should enable one to avoid this mistake. Contamination of the esophageal specimen with oral or respiratory herpes-infected cells should also be considered.

Cytomegalovirus

Cytomegalovirus (CMV) infection usually occurs in immunocompromised patients, particularly those with organ transplants or AIDS [Teot 1993]. CMV infects submucosal glands and endothelial cells and is therefore rarely seen in exfoliative (ie, surface) cytology of the esophagus unless the lesion is ulcerated. In gastrointestinal cytology, CMV is more commonly diagnosed in glandular epithelium of the stomach or intestine. Diagnostic cells are enlarged and characterized by large intranuclear inclusions with halos and may have satellite nuclear and cytoplasmic inclusions. The diagnostic cells may be sparse; tissue biopsy may be required for diagnosis.

Human Papilloma Virus

Human papilloma virus (HPV) appears to be the primary cause of squamous papillomas of the esophagus as well as flat condylomas. As in the uterine cervix, koilocytes can be detected cytologically [de Borges 1986, Rubel 1979] and are pathognomonic of HPV infection (see Chapter 6). Infection with HPV may play a role in the development of at least some squamous carcinomas of the esophagus.

Benign Neoplasms

Benign esophageal neoplasms include squamous papillomas (some may actually be inflammatory), leiomyomas, lipomas, granular cell tumors, hemangiomas, and lymphangiomas. These lesions, particularly the soft tissue tumors that occur in the submucosa, are seldom diagnosed by exfoliative cytology. Endoscopic fine needle aspiration biopsy may facilitate preoperative diagnosis of these tumors.

Malignant Neoplasms

Cancer of the esophagus accounts for only about 1% of all visceral cancers but 5% to 10% of all deaths from gastrointestinal cancer [Boring 1994]. A wide variety of malignancies can occur in or involve the esophagus, including salivary gland type tumors, lymphomas, melanomas, soft tissue sarcomas, and various carcinomas. However, the majority are squamous cell carcinomas, with adenocarcinoma a distant second; the others are rare.

Patients with a history of Plummer-Vinson syndrome; alcohol abuse; smoking; dietary problems, such as an excess of nitrites or a deficiency of vitamins A, B, or C or trace metals (eg, zinc); contamination with *Aspergillus* toxin; achalasia; webs; lye ingestion; diverticula; esophagitis; Barrett's esophagus; or head and neck malignancies have an increased risk of developing esophageal cancer. Except for squamous papilloma, the significance of human papilloma virus in the development of esophageal neoplasms remains to be elucidated [Koss 1993].

The presenting clinical sign of esophageal carcinoma is usually dysphagia. Unfortunately, by the time dysphagia develops, the cancer is often far advanced. Cytology has a higher rate of success than tissue biopsy in the diagnosis of esophageal carcinoma (~95% vs ~85%, respectively). Cytologic material is usually taken along with histologic biopsy. Together, the diagnostic yield approaches 100%.

Squamous Cell Carcinoma

Traditionally, as many as 90% to 95% of esophageal cancers are squamous cell carcinomas (SCCs). Most cases occur in black men (in a 4:1 ratio, compared with both whites and women), usually older than 50. Risk factors include alcohol and smoking as well as sclerotherapy for treatment of esophageal varices [Dina 1992]. Dysphagia and weight loss are the most common symptoms [Adelstein 1984]. Odynophagia, pain, and regurgitation are also relatively common. Squamous cell carcinoma has a propensity to occur in areas where the esophagus narrows, ie, near the thyroid cartilage, the bifurcation of the trachea, and at the level of the diaphragm. Most SCCs grow as polypoid masses, some as ulcerative cancers, and a few are diffusely infiltrative, akin to linitis plastica of the stomach. Half occur in the distal esophagus and a third occur in the middle esophagus. Because most of the esophagus has no serosa to act as a barrier, the tumor spreads easily [DeNardi 1991]. Although tumor stage and degree of differentiation are the most important prognostic indicators [Robey-Cafferty 1991], the prognosis is grim, with less than 5% of patients surviving five years, because tumors are usually detected late. Most cases can be diagnosed by cytology. Cytologic screening (eg, using an esophageal balloon) of high-risk populations could decrease the mortality by facilitating early detection of the disease.

Squamous cell carcinoma of the esophagus varies from well differentiated to poorly differentiated [Koss 1993, Shu 1983], keratinizing or nonkeratinizing[I9.28, I9.30]. The diagnostic features of keratinizing SCC usually include marked variation in cellular size and shape, including oval, spindle, irregular, and, frequently, bizarre cells [24 I9.25, 25 I9.26, I9.27] [Johnson 1955]. The nuclei are pleomorphic and hyperchromatic. A characteristic angular, crumpled-looking outline may be seen in many nuclei [Johnson 1955]. Hyperchromasia and pyknosis may obscure nuclear details such as chromatin and nucleoli, but the malignant features are usually obvious. The malignant cells show evidence of squamous differentiation—eg, cytoplasmic keratinization, orange-ophilia, and refractile ringing around the nucleus; keratin pearls; cell-in-cell arrangement; mosaic pattern; and intercellular bridges (though bridges may be difficult to appreciate in cytologic specimens).

Nonkeratinizing SCC is characterized by increased N/C ratios and enlarged nuclei with hyperchromatic, dense, coarse chromatin and irregular nuclear membranes, but the cells are generally smaller and less pleomorphic than in keratinizing cancers [26 I9.29]. Multiple, large, prominent nucleoli are more frequently observed than in keratinizing SCC [Johnson 1955]. The cytoplasm is scanty but dense, often basophilic, and has distinct cell boundaries. An occasional orange dyskeratotic cell (ie, individual cell keratinization) may be present in nonkeratinizing SCC, but malignant pearls indicate keratinizing SCC. Multinucleated malignant cells are occasionally noted [Johnson 1955]. Because squamous cell carcinomas of the esophagus are frequently ulcerated, the background often shows cytoplasmic debris, inflammation, and necrosis (ie, a tumor diathesis). When very poorly differentiated, malignant squamous cells have a basaloid appearance, with small, hyperchromatic nuclei and scant cytoplasm [27 I9.31], which must be distinguished from small-cell carcinoma. Spindle squamous cell carcinoma can be seen in the esophagus [28 I9.32].

24

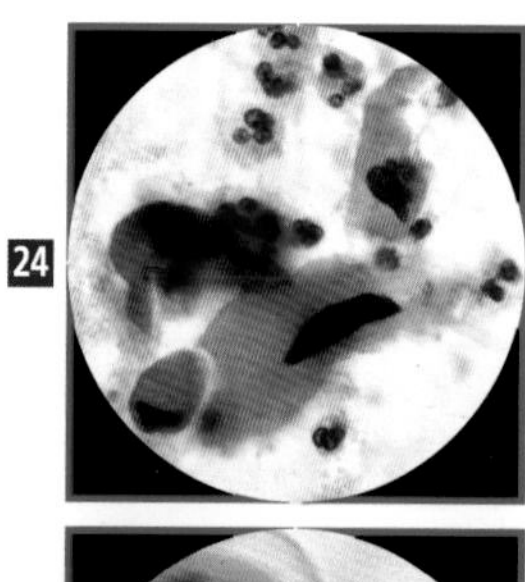

25

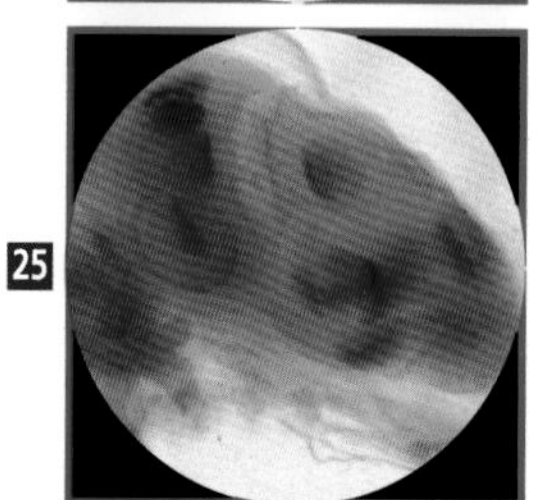

26

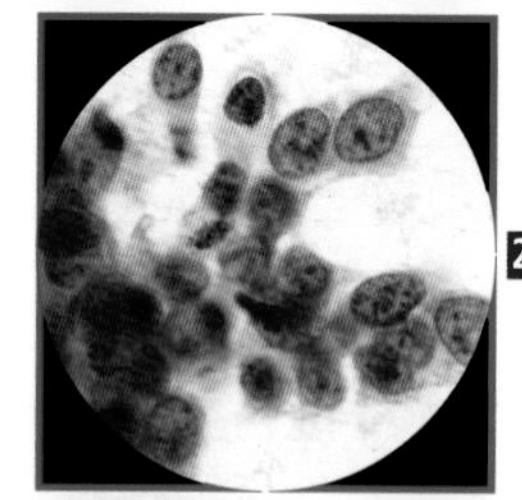

27

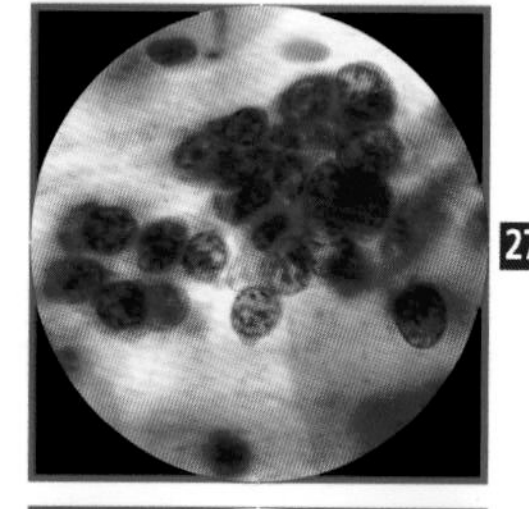

28

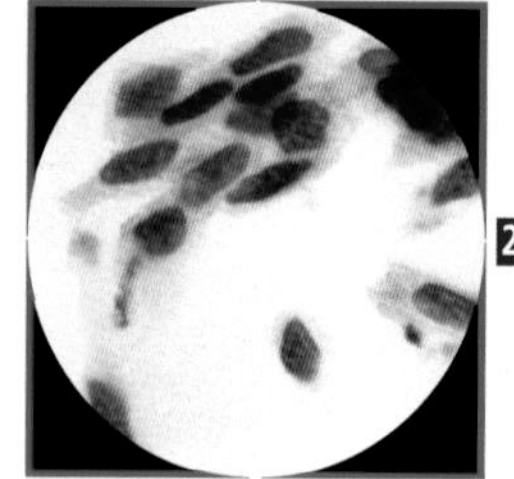

Degenerative vacuolization of the cytoplasm may occur in SCC that could be mistaken for secretory vacuoles of adenocarcinoma. Benign reactive and reparative atypia as well as radiation or chemotherapy effect can mimic SCC. Though not present in every group of cells, sharply angulated nuclei; coarse, dark chromatin; and high N/C ratios are features of cancer that distinguish it from repair [Hoover 1988]. In addition, more atypia and pleomorphism, as well as more single cells, are seen in cancer, although a few single cells can occasionally be seen in repair. Poorly differentiated squamous cell carcinoma may be difficult to distinguish from poorly differentiated adenocarcinoma.

Squamous Dysplasia and Carcinoma In Situ

As in the uterine cervix, squamous cell carcinoma of the esophagus is apparently preceded by an intraepithelial, neoplastic squamous lesion (ie, dysplasia and carcinoma in situ), which is usually asymptomatic. The mucosa may appear normal at endoscopy or there may be abnormalities, eg, white plaques (leukoplakia) or velvety red areas (erythroplasia). Although the microscopy of esophageal dysplasia has not been as thoroughly studied as that of the cervix, characteristic features have been described [Bishop 1977, Imbriglia 1949, Jacob 1990, Koss 1993, Shu 1983].

Low-grade dysplasia is characterized by enlarged, hyperchromatic nuclei in superficial- or intermediate-type cells, akin to keratinizing or mature metaplastic (large cell, nonkeratinizing) dysplasia as described in the Pap smear. The N/C ratio is only somewhat elevated, corresponding to a low-grade squamous intraepithelial lesion. Low-grade dysplasia may be difficult to distinguish from reactive atypia, since both may have somewhat enlarged, pleomorphic or hyperchromatic nuclei. In fact, these low-grade "dysplastic" changes may be more commonly associated with esophagitis than cancer [Jacob 1990].

High-grade dysplasia and carcinoma in situ are also characterized by enlarged, hyperchromatic, abnormal nuclei. However, the changes are more advanced than in low-grade dysplasia, with more hyperchromasia, coarser chromatin, more irregular nuclear membranes, and higher N/C ratios. In some cases, basal- to parabasal-sized cells with abnormal nuclei and high N/C ratios, similar to the cells characteristic of immature metaplastic dysplasia described in the Pap smear, may be seen. In other cases, moderately to markedly atypical, pleomorphic keratinized cells may be seen [Howell 1985], characteristic of high-grade keratinizing dysplasia described in the cervix. These patterns correspond to a high-grade squamous intraepithelial lesion.

In some cases, cells that appear almost malignant are seen, with markedly abnormal, irregular dark nuclei; heavy keratinization; malignant pearls; and tadpole and snake cells and other bizarre shapes. Such cases of high-grade dysplasia or carcinoma in situ may be difficult or impossible to distinguish from infiltrating SCC on cytologic grounds alone. On the other hand, infiltrating SCC of the esophagus can be very well differentiated, yielding cells that in the Pap smear might be considered only dysplastic rather than fully malignant [Barch 1986].

Adenocarcinoma

Traditionally, adenocarcinoma has accounted for approximately 10% of all esophageal cancers. Although adenocarcinoma can develop at any level of the esophagus, including the cervical portion, it is usually found in the distal esophagus, near the gastric cardia, where adenocarcinoma is actually more common than SCC. Formerly, most adenocarcinomas of the esophagus were thought to arise in the stomach and extend from there, involving the esophagus only secondarily. The current belief, however, is that adenocarcinoma arising in the distal esophagus, gastroesophageal junction, or gastric cardia is a distinctive group of tumors that share epidemiologic, clinical, and pathologic features and are usually associated with Barrett's metaplasia [Hamilton 1988, MacDonald 1972, Potet 1991, R Smith 1984, J Thompson 1983, Wang 1986]. Like Barrett's esophagus, adenocarcinoma occurs predominantly in white males, particularly those who smoke or abuse alcohol [Spechler 1986]. In striking contrast with SCC of the esophagus as well as adenocarcinoma of the stomach, adenocarcinoma of the esophagus is rare in blacks. Also, compared with ordinary gastric cancer, the patients are younger, more often men (~5:1), more frequently have hiatal hernia, but less frequently have signet ring cell tumors [Hamilton 1988, Potet 1991, R Smith 1984, Wang 1986]. Although the carcinoma usually associated with Barrett's esophagus is adenocarcinoma, sometimes other tumors, eg, squamous cell carcinoma, adenosquamous carcinoma, and adenocarcinoids, occur [R Smith 1984]. In summary, adenocarcinoma of the esophagus may account for as much as one third of all esophageal cancer and nearly two thirds of cancers occurring in the distal esophagus [Wang 1986].

Esophageal adenocarcinoma is usually an ordinary papillary or acinar cancer, relatively well differentiated, similar to the type of adenocarcinoma most common in the stomach (ie, intestinal-type adenocarcinoma, see p 346) [29 I9.36]. Three-dimensional groups, microacini, or papillae may be seen cytologically [30 I9.33, 31 I9.34, 32 I9.35]. The groups are disorderly, with loss of polarity, and loosely cohesive with irregular outlines. The malignant cells trail away from the groups [Geisinger 1992], and more single cells are usually seen than in benign lesions [Geisinger 1992, Wang 1992]. The presence of single cells is important diagnostically, although they may not be numerous in some brush preparations [Shurbaji 1991]. The cells are columnar, with polar orientation of the nucleus and cytoplasm and high N/C ratios [Wang 1992]. There is a progressive increase in the degree of nuclear abnormality from well-differentiated to poorly differentiated tumors. As the nuclei become increasingly abnormal, they lose their oval shape, becoming round or irregular. Nuclear atypia varies from subtle thickening and irregularity of the membrane, with fine chromatin, to large, irregular nuclei with hyperchromatic, coarse, irregularly distributed chromatin and obviously malignant features [Geisinger 1992]. The malignant nuclei are enlarged, usually about two to three times normal size, overlapped, and crowded, with loss of nuclear polarity. One or more prominent nucleoli are often present and may be irregular in outline [Wang 1992].

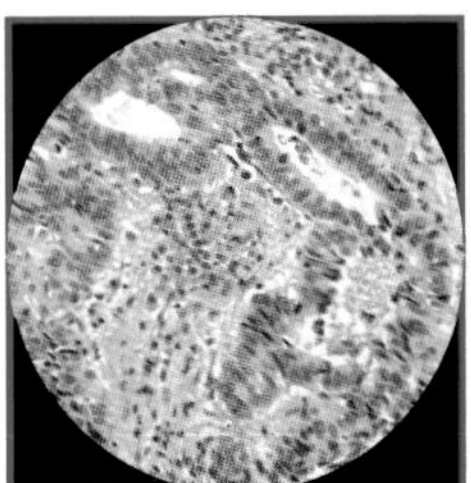
29

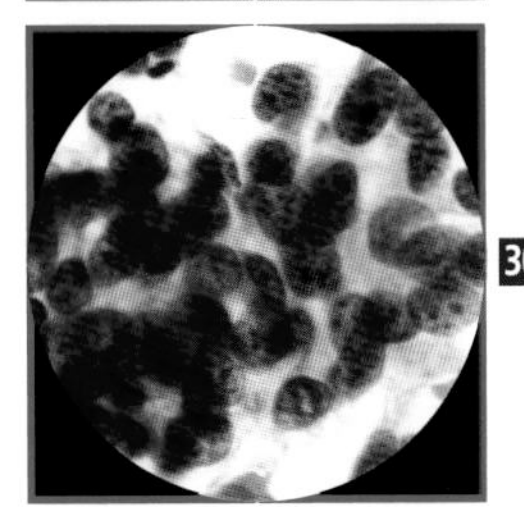
30

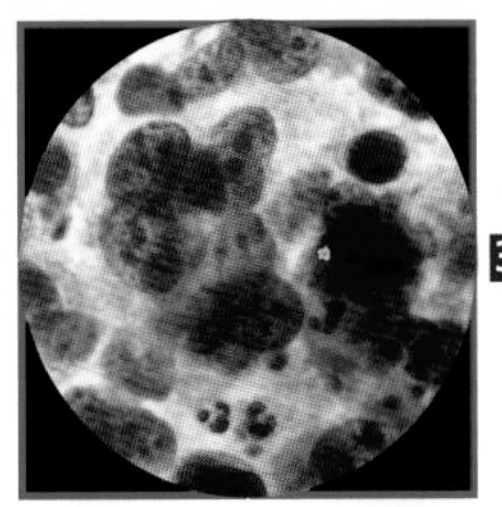
31

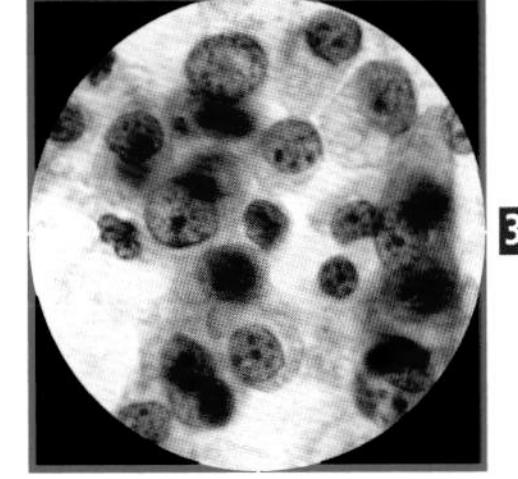
32

The cytoplasm is granular or vacuolar and mucin content is decreased. The cell borders are indistinct and molding may be seen. Occasionally, a larger or even giant tumor cell may be present. Although rudimentary cilia have been described on cells of papillary adenocarcinoma arising in Barrett's epithelium, they are so poorly developed that oil immersion or even electron microscopy is needed to see them [Rubio 1991]. Benign metaplastic and goblet cells tend to be scarce. In the background is evidence of inflammation and necrosis, ie, a tumor diathesis.

Adenocarcinoma is thought to be preceded by various degrees of dysplasia. The dysplastic cells can be fairly atypical in appearance, depending on grade, and the cytologic differential diagnosis with frank adenocarcinoma can be difficult. Moreover, reactive/regenerative atypia may also be quite marked, with large nuclei and macronucleoli, and therefore difficult to distinguish from well-differentiated adenocarcinoma or dysplasia. Orderly groups, cohesion, relatively smooth nuclear membranes, and fine chromatin favor a diagnosis of a benign reactive process. Clinical correlation and tissue biopsy may be required to differentiate among reactive, dysplastic, and neoplastic changes in some cases.

If the tumor is signet ring cell type, consider origin in the stomach with extension to the esophagus. Other types of adenocarcinoma, including adenosquamous carcinoma (presumably arising from reserve cells capable of both glandular and squamous differentiation) and salivary gland tumors (eg, adenoid-cystic carcinomas, which arise in minor salivary glands of the esophagus), may also occur but are rare.

Glandular Dysplasia in Barrett's Esophagus

Glandular dysplasia can precede or coexist with adenocarcinoma arising in Barrett's esophagus [Hamilton 1987, Reid 1988b, Schmidt 1985, Skinner 1983]. The abnormal process apparently begins in metaplasia and may advance to dysplasia and, finally, cancer. Dysplastic Barrett's mucosa, particularly when high grade, is a marker for the development of adenocarcinoma [Lee 1985b]. However, as in other sites, the natural history of Barrett's dysplasia (ie, how rapidly, how often, and in whom dysplasia will progress to invasive cancer) cannot be predicted for individual patients [Reid 1988a,b]. Thus, long-term surveillance of patients with Barrett's esophagus is currently recommended to detect the occurrence of dysplasia and potentially curable cancer [Berenson 1978, Haggitt 1978, Hamilton 1987, Reid 1988a, Robertson 1988, Schmidt 1985, Schnell 1988, Skinner 1983, R Smith 1984]. Unfortunately, Barrett's dysplasia can be visually unremarkable, and even early carcinoma may be missed endoscopically and by biopsy [Reid 1988b, Robey 1988]. For this reason, cytologic techniques, which allow for the sampling of multiple and relatively wide areas, have a potential advantage in the diagnosis and surveillance of Barrett's esophagus [Robey 1988]. Nevertheless, cytology is not a substitute for tissue biopsy but a useful adjunct in the diagnosis and management of patients with Barrett's esophagus [Robey 1988].

Dysplasia usually affects the specialized (ie, intestinal) type of epithelium [Hameeteman 1989, Hamilton 1987, Schmidt 1985]. Two basic patterns have been described histologically [Berenson 1978, Robey 1988, Schmidt 1985, Spechler 1986]. The more common pattern of dysplasia, seen also in gastrointestinal adenomas, is characterized by crowded, enlarged, elongated, hyperchromatic nuclei; increased N/C ratios; and loss of nuclear polarity [Riddell 1983, Schmidt 1985]. This pattern probably represents true glandular dysplasia. The cytology is similar to that of the usual type of endocervical adenocarcinoma in situ described in the Pap smear.

The less common pattern, similar to atypical repair/regeneration, eg, in inflammatory bowel disease, is characterized by less crowded but more pleomorphic, enlarged nuclei. These nuclei appear to be malignant, with marginated chromatin, prominent nucleoli, and an increased N/C ratio [Riddell 1983, Robey 1988, Schmidt 1985]. This pattern, in which the cells may be indistinguishable from invasive cancer, might represent frank malignancy, in which invasion is inconspicuous or absent in limited tissue biopsies. In fact, invasive cancer is more often associated with this second, less common pattern of dysplasia [Berenson 1978, Schmidt 1985]. The cytology is similar to that of the variant type of endocervical adenocarcinoma in situ described in the Pap smear. Both patterns are characterized by loss of cytoplasmic mucin. Mixed dysplasia can also occur.

Compared with benign Barrett's glandular epithelium, the dysplastic cells exfoliate in smaller, haphazardly arranged, three-dimensional groups of mildly pleomorphic cells [Wang 1992] in which nuclear crowding, piling up, and loss of polarity are conspicuous features [33 I9.21]. Occasional flat sheets and acini may also be seen. The groups are less cohesive than normal and have irregular outlines; cells seem to trail away from the groups. However, in contrast with invasive adenocarcinoma, only a few single atypical cells are present [Geisinger 1992]. The cells are enlarged and have increased N/C ratios [Wang 1992]. The nuclei are oval to elongated and are usually enlarged (often two to three times their normal size); have irregularly thickened membranes and evenly dispersed but granular, dark chromatin; and may have multiple small nucleoli [Geisinger 1992, Wang 1992]. Mitotic figures are frequent [Wang 1992]. The cytoplasmic changes include increased basophilia and decreased or absent mucin production [Reid 1988b]. Benign metaplastic and goblet cells are usually also present. There is no diathesis [Wang 1992].

33

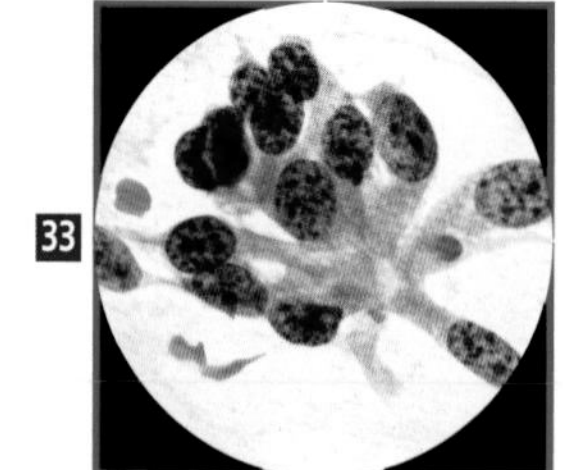

The differential diagnosis of dysplasia mainly requires distinguishing it from regeneration/repair (ie, reactive atypia) on the one hand and invasive cancer on the other. Reparative processes are common in Barrett's esophagus due to irritation and ulceration. Repair is characterized by cohesive, flat sheets of well-ordered cells with vesicular nuclei, prominent nucleoli, and N/C ratios within normal limits. Single, atypical glandular cells are rare or absent in well-preserved benign smears [Geisinger 1992, Wang 1992]. Groups of benign cells show nuclear streaming, while dysplasia shows loss of nuclear polarity, with overlapping, enlarged, pleomorphic nuclei. Macronucleoli suggest either repair or frank carcinoma rather than dysplasia. Diagnose dysplasia cautiously if there is significant inflammation.

Dysplasia and adenocarcinoma, particularly when well differentiated, may be difficult to distinguish because the morphologic features overlap [T9.2]. In general, invasive cancer shows more single cells with more obvious malignant features and a diathesis. The increased number of single atypical cells is a major diagnostic criterion of frank cancer [Geisinger 1992]. Obviously malignant-appearing cells (eg, with giant, irregular nuclei) or atypical mitotic figures suggest invasive cancer [Geisinger 1992, Wang 1992].

T9.2 **Barrett's Esophagus**

	Benign	Dysplasia/Adenocarcinoma
Cell groups	Large, cohesive, flat	Smaller, less cohesive, 3-dimensional
Outlines	Sharply defined	Irregular, cells trail away
Single cells	Rare	Few (dysplasia)/many (adenocarcinoma)
Organization	Well ordered, but may be crowded	Disorderly, loss of polarity
Nuclei	Uniform	Enlarged, pleomorphic
Shape	Oval	Elongate or round to irregular
Membrane	Smooth, uniform	Variably irregular
Chromatin	Fine, even; normal to hyperchromatic	Fine to coarse, irregular; hyperchromatic
Cytoplasm	Granular or nondescript	Decreased mucin, occasional signet rings

[Geisinger 1992, Riddell 1983, Schmidt 1985, Wang 1992]

Both benign reactive cells and malignant cells can have prominent nucleoli and mitotic figures. An increase in the number of single cells and the presence of clear-cut malignant features favor a diagnosis of adenocarcinoma rather than dysplasia. The presence of metaplastic cells and goblet cells favor a benign or dysplastic process, while the presence of a diathesis favors a diagnosis of frank malignancy.

In some cases, the cytologic features suggest dysplasia or carcinoma but are less than diagnostic. These indeterminate, or suspicious, cases should be evaluated by repeat endoscopy. In tissue biopsies, there is relatively good interobserver agreement for high-grade lesions, but results are not highly reproducible for low-grade and indeterminate lesions [Reid 1988a]. It may also be difficult to grade dysplasia using cytologic techniques [Wang 1992]. Moreover, carcinoma in situ is cytologically indistinguishable from invasive carcinoma [Belladonna 1974]. Invasion can be assessed histologically; excision of the affected segment should be considered clinically [Berenson 1978].

Small Cell Carcinoma

Primary small cell carcinoma of the esophagus is rare. Most cases actually arise in the lung and only involve the esophagus secondarily. True primary small cell carcinoma of the esophagus usually arises in the mid or distal third. As in the lung, it may be associated with hormone production and paraneoplastic syndromes. The cytology is also typical of small cell carcinoma of the lung [Hoda 1992, Horai 1978] (see Chapter 7). The cells are relatively small blue cells with scant cytoplasm, dark chromatin, and invisible or inconspicuous nucleoli. Round, oval, or spindle-shaped cells may be seen. The cells form tightly molded groups, may line up in Indian files, and may show crush artifact, particularly in specimens obtained by brushing.

The differential diagnosis of small cell carcinoma of the esophagus includes poorly differentiated squamous cell carcinoma [Y Rosen 1975], malignant carcinoid, malignant lymphoma, and, in particular, extension of small cell carcinoma from the lung [34 I9.37]. Clinical correlation may be required.

34

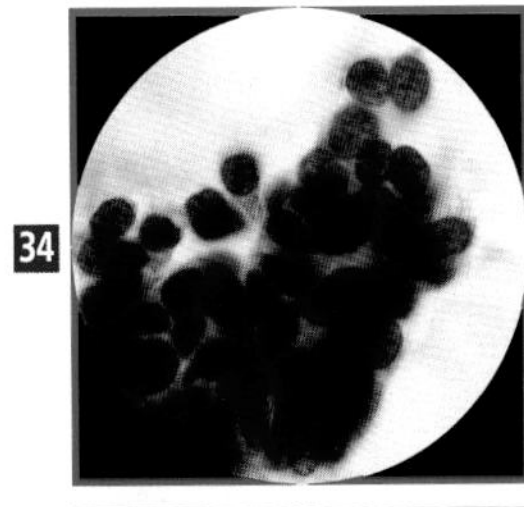

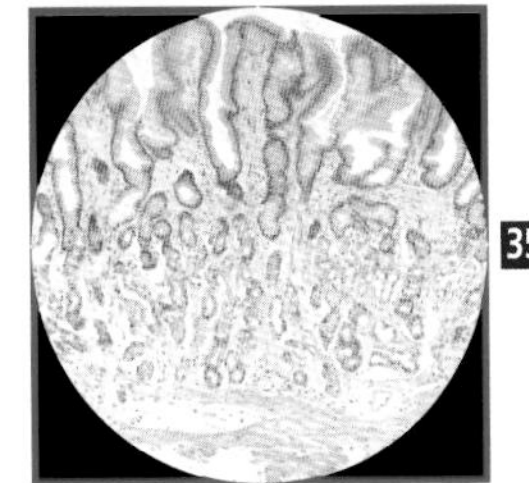

35

Miscellaneous Tumors

Salivary Gland Tumors: Arise in minor salivary glands of the esophagus, eg, adenoid cystic carcinoma.

Melanoma: Usually secondary, may be polypoid primary [Aldovini 1983, Broderick 1972].

Sarcoma: Leiomyosarcoma is most common, but virtually any type, including malignant fibrous histiocytoma [Sapi 1992] and rhabdomyosarcoma [Chetty 1991], can occur. Differential diagnosis includes pseudosarcoma (see below). Endoscopic fine needle aspiration biopsy may be helpful in obtaining diagnostic cells.

Malignant Lymphoma: Large cell non-Hodgkin's lymphoma is the most common type. Differential diagnosis includes gastric vs esophageal primary as well as benign follicular hyperplasia (eg, of tonsil).

Pseudosarcoma: Polypoid tumor, often with squamous cell carcinoma (SCC) in situ on surface [Enrile 1973].

Spindle Cell Squamous Carcinoma: Nonkeratinizing squamous cell carcinoma with spindle-shaped cells.

Choriocarcinoma: Cyto/syncytiotrophoblast, elevated βHCG [Trillo 1979].

Metastases: Lung, breast, and melanoma cancers are among the common sources [Kadakia 1992]. However, most "metastases" actually represent direct extension of lung cancer into the esophagus.

Stomach

The stomach was considered by the Ancients to be the seat of spirit and courage. For descriptive purposes, the stomach is divided into the cardia (immediately distal to the esophagus), fundus (above the gastroesophageal junction), body (largest portion), and pyloric area (which joins the duodenum at the pyloric sphincter) [35 I9.38].

Endoscopic brush specimens are preferred for cytodiagnosis. Blind lavage is obsolete because autodigestion can interfere with cell preservation. Directed washes may be helpful when both the brush cytology and histology yield negative results but malignancy is still suspected clinically (eg, in linitis plastica). Location of malignancy in the cardia or antrum, infiltrating linitis-plastica–type cancers, and recurrences are more likely to cause false-negative results [Winawer 1975a].

The Cells

The cardia and pyloric areas of the stomach are lined with mucous cells. The fundus and body contain chief and parietal cells in addition to mucous cells. However, chief and parietal cells occur in the deeper parts of the mucosa and therefore are seldom sampled by exfoliative cytology but may be seen in imprints of biopsies. In addition, heterogeneous endocrine cells, collectively referred to as Kulchitsky cells, are also present. Autolysis may result in numerous naked nuclei. In general, the cells are strongly cohesive, with few single intact cells. The groups form honeycombs, rosettes, or palisades. Tight clusters of cells are usually benign.

Mucous Cells

Mucous cells normally line the entire surface of the stomach and most of the gastric pits. Therefore, the majority of cells in a gastric specimen are usually mucous cells. The normal mucous cells of the stomach are tall columnar and have basal nuclei [36 I9.39, I9.40]. Apical cytoplasmic densities (microvilli), which look like terminal bars, may be seen, but no true cilia are present. Groups of cells are usually tightly cohesive. However, single cells may be seen, particularly with inflammation or degeneration. When seen en face, the groups form orderly honeycombs; when seen from the side, they form palisades or rosettes. The cytoplasm is relatively abundant, eosinophilic, somewhat dense, and finely granular or vacuolated. Goblet cells, with large, single mucin vacuoles, are not seen in the normal stomach but may accompany intestinal metaplasia. Normal gastric mucin is strongly PAS positive but alcian-blue negative, indicating the presence of neutral rather than acid mucin. The nuclei are very uniform, round to oval, and have fine chromatin that may become opaque due to degeneration. The nuclear membrane is smooth and distinct. Small nucleoli may be present. Naked nuclei may be a prominent feature of gastric specimens.

Chief Cells

Chief cells are zymogen-granule–containing cells similar in appearance to acinar cells of the pancreas and salivary gland [37 I9.41]. In the stomach, the zymogen granules are proenzymes of, eg, papain, renin, and lipase. Chief cells are cuboidal and characteristically have relatively coarse, basophilic cytoplasmic granules. The cytoplasm can also be vacuolated. The nuclei are round and smooth with fine chromatin.

Parietal Cells

Parietal cells secrete intrinsic factor (to absorb vitamin B_{12}) and hydrochloric acid. They vary from pyramidal or flask shaped to round and are larger than chief cells [38 I9.42]. The abundant granular or vacuolar cytoplasm characteristically is intensely eosinophilic but may be pale. The nuclei are generally single, but occasionally there may be more than one nucleus. The chromatin is relatively coarse, and a prominent nucleolus is present. Parietal cells are sometimes seen in two orderly, parallel rows.

Reactive/Reparative Cells and Degeneration

Reactive/reparative and degenerative changes are very common in the gastric epithelium and are the result of gastritis and ulcers due to a wide variety of causes. These benign diseases do not usually have specific diagnostic features.

Reactive changes can range from mild to severe, in which case they must be differentiated from cancer [I9.43, 39 I9.44]

36
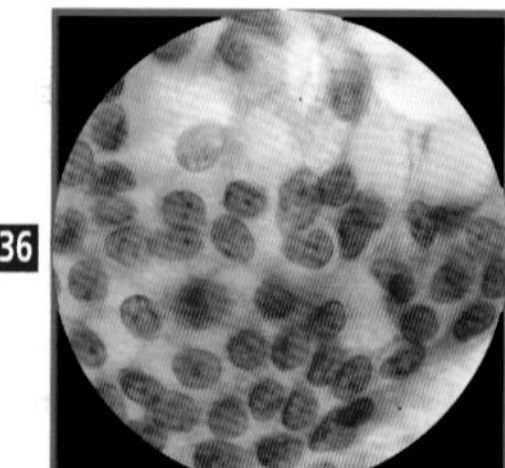

37
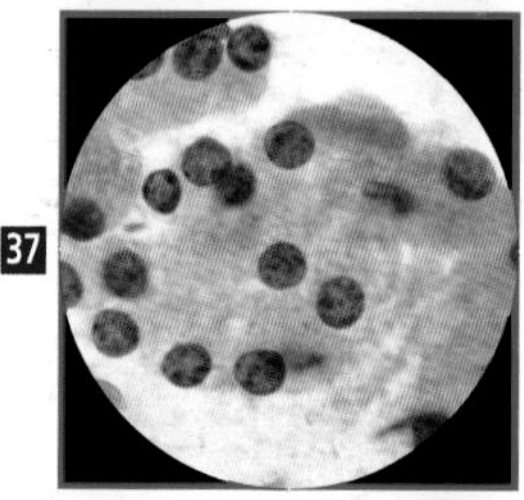

38
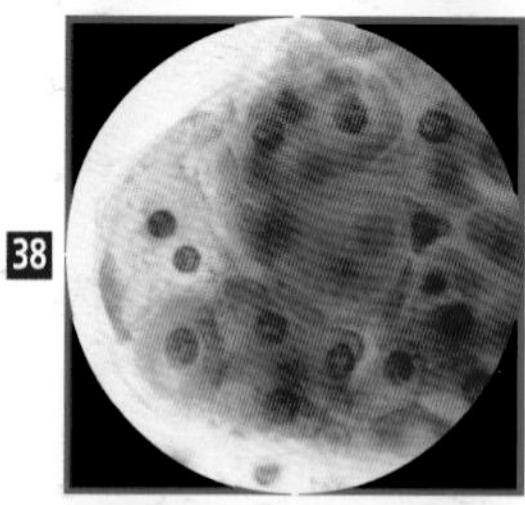

39
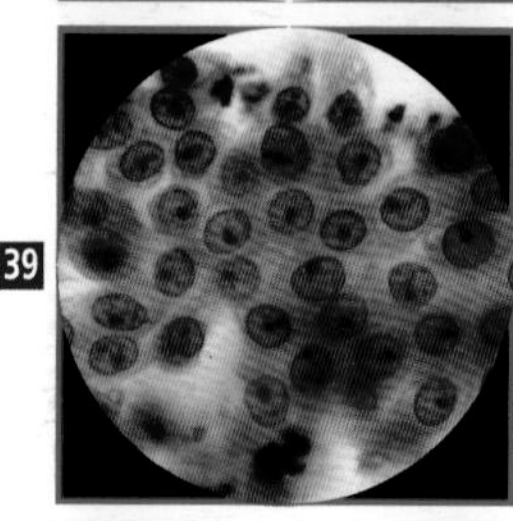

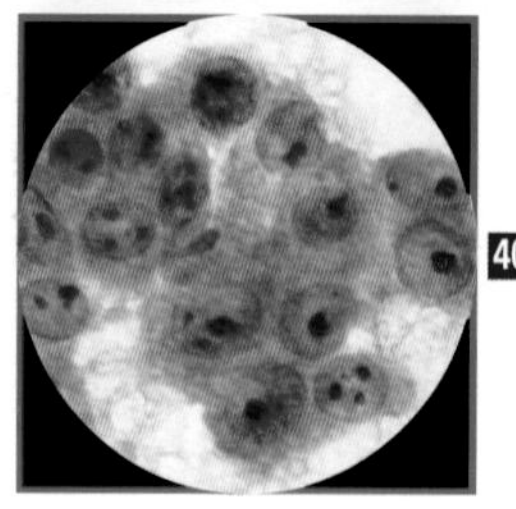
40

[R Gupta 1983, Prolla 1971a]. Reactive cells are usually present in cohesive sheets, with few single cells. The benign cells may be crowded but lack significant nuclear molding, piling up, or loss of polarity. Reactive nuclei may be atypical—ie, enlarged and hyperchromatic, with coarse chromatin, one or two prominent nucleoli, and some variation in size. Macro- or irregular nucleoli can be seen in benign cells.

Although benign and malignant cells can share some morphologic properties, gastric cancers usually have more pleomorphic nuclei and are characterized by loss of polarity, irregular nuclear membranes, and an increased number of single cells. In fact, the mere presence of atypical single cells is suspicious for cancer. In contrast, most cases of benign reactive atypia are characterized by relatively uniform, orderly nuclei with smooth nuclear membranes; intact single cells are rare. The nuclear chromatin of benign cells is more evenly distributed than in malignant cells. Atypical goblet cells may resemble cells deriving from signet ring cell carcinoma [Prolla 1971a]. Ciliated metaplasia has been observed rarely [Rubio 1988].

Repair can also occur in gastric epithelial cells [40 I9.45]. As in the repair that occurs in the uterine cervix, the reparative cells form cohesive, relatively orderly, flat sheets of cells with enlarged, sometimes pleomorphic nuclei and prominent nucleoli but relatively fine chromatin [I9.46]. Inflammation is usually present in the background of the smear as well as mixed in with the groups of cells.

Degenerative changes are common in gastric specimens. The degenerated nucleus shrinks, causing the membrane to become irregular (crenated), with variable degrees of hyperchromasia and granularity of chromatin. Degenerated cells with pyknotic or karyorrhectic nuclei may resemble plasma cells. Naked nuclei can also be seen and may either be enlarged and pale or small and dark. Degenerative vacuolization of the cytoplasm is also common.

Miscellaneous Cells

Red Blood Cells: May be fresh or old. Hemosiderin-laden macrophages indicate old bleeding.

Neutrophils: A small number are commonly present. Increased numbers are associated with acute inflammation.

Lymphocytes: May be contaminant from tonsils, adenoids. Lymphocytes are normally found in the lamina propria, but increased numbers may represent chronic inflammation. Also, lymphoid follicles are normally found in the lamina propria of the pyloric area. Malignant lymphoma should be excluded.

Eosinophils: Eosinophilic gastritis, associated with allergy or sensitivity to food or drugs (eg, penicillin). Also associated with asthma, parasites (eg, *Giardia lamblia*), ulcers, polyps, and sometimes cancer [Michán 1976].

Histiocytes: May be associated with atypical mycobacteria (need special stain to see), xanthelasma (with neutral fat and cholesterol), or malakoplakia (with Michaelis-Gutmann bodies).

Giant Cells: May be seen with granulomatous inflammation, eg, in sarcoid, tuberculosis, Crohn's disease. Histiocytes (giant or epithelioid) may be atypical (ie, characterized by nuclear pleomorphism, hyperchromasia, and irregular chromatin) and should not be mistaken for malignancy [Bennington 1968]. Syphilis can also cause granulomatous inflammation as well as reactive epithelial, histiocytic, and fibroblastic atypia, which could be mistaken for malignancy [Prolla 1970b]. Giant cells can also be seen with pneumatosis cystoides [Bhathal 1985, Koss 1952].

Contaminants: Squamous cells from the mouth or esophagus, respiratory cells (ciliated, mucous, alveolar macrophages with or without pigment [41 I9.47]) from the respiratory tract, and atypical mononuclear cells (resembling lymphoma) in patients with colds [Brandborg 1968a] may be swallowed contaminants. These swallowed cells are more commonly observed in blind lavages than in directed washing or brushing specimens. Liver and pancreas cells obtained when brushing a penetrating ulcer may show reactive atypia [Martinez-Onsurbe 1991]. Foreign material, eg, food, may also be observed. It is important to note that cancer cells can be swallowed contaminants from the mouth or lung.

Benign Diseases

Acute Gastritis and Ulcers

Acute inflammation (ie, acute gastritis) or acute ulceration can be associated with chronic analgesic use (particularly aspirin), heavy smoking or drinking, chemotherapy or radiation, staphylococcal food poisoning, severe stress (trauma, surgery, burns), shock, uremia, or infections. Although it can be fulminant, acute gastritis is usually transient and the diagnosis can be made clinically. Therefore, the lesion is seldom evaluated cytologically. Cell degeneration, debris, and acute inflammation are typical. Cytologic reactive atypia in the form of nuclear pleomorphism and prominent nucleoli can be seen.

Chronic Gastritis

Nonspecific chronic gastritis is subdivided into three phases: chronic superficial gastritis, chronic atrophic gastritis, and gastric atrophy. These form a continuum of increasingly severe inflammation and atrophy of the gastric mucosa. The changes are associated with loss of specialized cells, intestinal metaplasia, and glandular dysplasia, which predisposes to peptic ulcers and gastric cancer. Two pathogenetic forms are recognized. One involves predominantly the fundus, is thought to be autoimmune, and can result in pernicious anemia. Patients with this form of chronic gastritis may develop cancers in the body or fundus of the stomach rather than the more common pyloric antrum location [Morson 1980]. The other, much more common form of chronic gastritis involves predominantly the antrum; is thought to be due to the toxic effects of substances such as bile, alcohol, or analgesics (see also *H pylori*, p344); is usually asymptomatic; and rarely results in pernicious anemia. Mixed forms also occur.

The morphologic changes are similar in both forms of chronic gastritis. Crowded sheets of small cells with relatively high N/C ratios may be seen. The cytoplasm shows mucus depletion and increased basophilia. The nuclei become somewhat pleomorphic, enlarged, and hyperchromatic, with prominent nucleoli. These changes may reflect regeneration. Degenerative changes can also be seen. The phase of the disease cannot be determined by cytologic techniques alone. However, the primary purpose of cytology is to recognize changes as benign and exclude cancer, since most gastric cancers arise in intestinalized, atrophic epithelium.

41 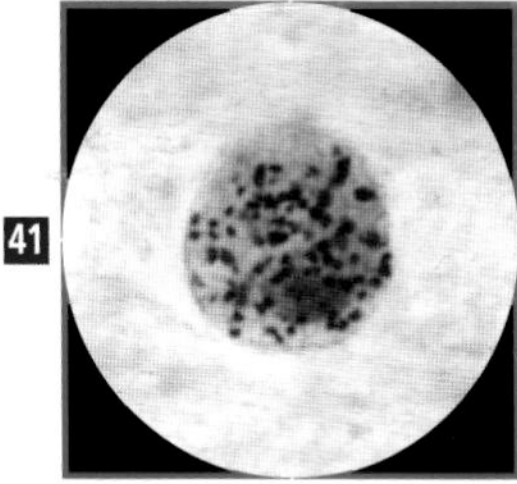

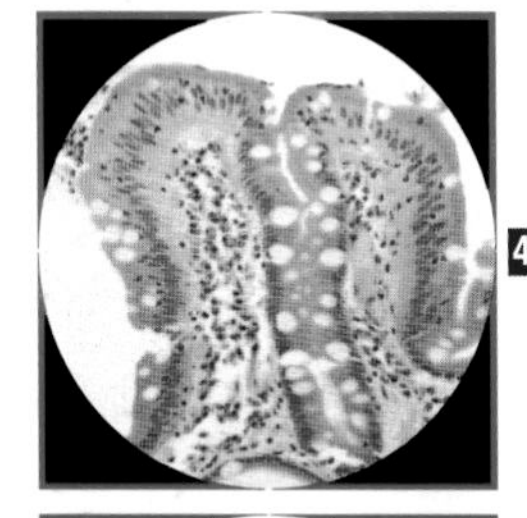 42

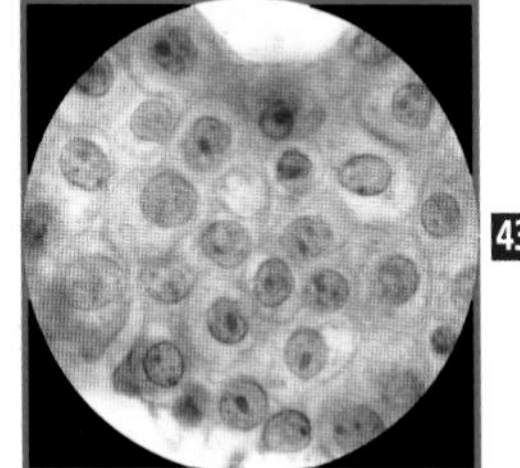 43

Intestinal Metaplasia

Intestinal metaplasia, or intestinalization, is a major diagnostic feature of chronic atrophic gastritis or gastric atrophy, as may be seen in, eg, pernicious anemia (B_{12} deficiency), folate deficiency, and radiation. Although benign, intestinal metaplasia is important because the majority of gastric cancers are thought to arise in the milieu of intestinalization. For this reason, any entity associated with intestinal metaplasia can be considered a predisposing factor to gastric cancer. The intestinal metaplastic epithelium may include mucous, goblet, and absorptive cells as well as Paneth and argyrophil cells. Goblet cells and some forms of intestinal metaplasia secrete sulfomucins. Carcinogenesis is associated with sulfomucin-producing intestinal metaplasia [42 I9.49] [Rothery 1985].

Intestinal metaplasia appears cytologically as cohesive sheets of orderly absorptive or mucous cells with irregularly scattered goblet cells [43 I9.48]. The most characteristic feature of goblet cells relates to the cytoplasm. Instead of the finely vacuolated cytoplasm of normal gastric mucous cells, the goblet cell is distended by a large secretory vacuole with slightly flattened basal nuclei, which somewhat resembles a signet ring cell. When sheets of cells are seen en face, there is a perinuclear clearing due to the pale-staining mucin vacuole. In addition, the cell borders are prominent where the cells are joined to one another. The pale goblet-cell cytoplasm contrasts with the somewhat denser surrounding cells, giving it the appearance of Swiss cheese (as described in "Barrett's Esophagus," p334). Although the goblet-cell nuclei may be enlarged, they remain uniform and bland. A small nucleolus may be present.

The absorptive cells are tall columnar, with finely granular cytoplasm, and may have a striated border (ie, a terminal bar–like border that corresponds to microvilli and glycocalyx, ultrastructurally). No cilia are present. The nucleus is more central than in mucous cells and may become larger, oval, and somewhat hyperchromatic, with more granular chromatin and prominent nucleoli. Paneth and argyrophilic cells, though present histologically, are usually not recognized in cytologic specimens.

Chronic Gastric Ulcer

Chronic gastric ulcers usually occur in intestinalized (ie, metaplastic) epithelium. They may be single or multiple, but single ulcers must be distinguished from malignant ulcers. Approximately 1% of all chronic gastric ulcers are associated with malignancy [Morson 1980]. However, if true epithelial dysplasia occurs, distinct from atypia of regeneration/repair, the patient is at high risk of developing gastric cancer (see "Gastric Dysplasia," p 347).

Chronic ulcers have an organized structure composed of four zones: a superficial layer of cell debris and necrosis overlying a zone of acute inflammation and fibrin, underneath which is granulation tissue, producing the final layer of scar.

Structure of a Chronic Ulcer

Zone I: Necrotic debris
Zone II: Fibrin, neutrophils
Zone III: Granulation tissue
Zone IV: Scar

Samples from the ulcer center may obtain only necrotic debris and inflammation (ie, the eschar). Cytologic samples should be taken from the edge of the ulcer. The cytologic findings include acute and chronic inflammation, intestinal metaplasia, and reactive/reparative and degenerative atypia. Cytologic atypia can be marked and mimic malignancy. Granulation tissue, including branching small blood vessels with reactive endothelial cells surrounded by histiocytes, may also be seen. Scattered, atypical, plump spindle/stellate myofibroblasts, with pleomorphic, active nuclei (prominent nucleoli but pale chromatin) may be associated with granulation tissue or a young scar. Similar, sometimes bizarre, stromal cells can be found in polyps and ulcers throughout the gastrointestinal tract [Shekitka 1991].

The primary use of gastric cytology is to differentiate between benign and malignant ulcers. Benign ulcers may show cells deriving from repair/regeneration, with atypia, mitoses, and necrosis. Both benign and malignant ulcers may have inflammation, degeneration, siderophages, and debris. Cohesion and few cytologic abnormalities indicate a benign process. Both usually occur in a background of intestinal metaplasia. Clinical history is also important.

Pernicious Anemia

Pernicious anemia is associated with characteristic cellular changes and autoantibodies to parietal cells and intrinsic factor. Macrocytic changes, with enlargement of the nuclei and the cytoplasm and maintenance of a relatively normal N/C ratio, may be seen in some cells [Brandborg 1961, Rubin 1955]. Similar macrocytic changes can also be caused by folate deficiency and radiation. Some of the nuclei in pernicious anemia are large and bland, with folds or creases in the nuclear membrane [Rubin 1955]. They may have nucleoli or chromocenter formation. Pernicious anemia is associated with chronic atrophic gastritis, which predisposes to gastric ulcer and cancer (see "Chronic Gastritis," p 343). Intestinal metaplasia, reactive cells associated with ulcer, or glandular dysplasia can also be seen. Reactive cells with very large nuclei, chromatin clumping, and prominent nucleoli may result in false-positive diagnoses [Foushee 1969].

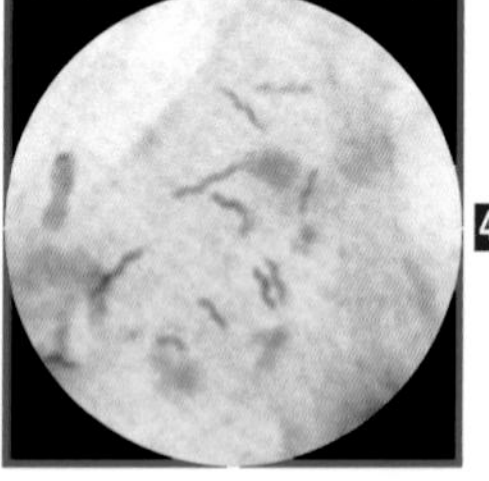

44

Aspirin Gastritis

Patients who take aspirin chronically, eg, to treat rheumatoid arthritis, may develop gastric ulcers that are sampled cytologically. Aspirin can cause markedly atypical reactive changes in gastric cells, which can mimic from adenocarcinoma. The nuclei are usually normal sized or only slightly enlarged but sometimes can be greatly enlarged.

Granulomatous Gastritis

Granulomas (epithelioid histiocytes, with or without giant cell histiocytes) may indicate any of a wide variety of diseases, including Crohn's disease, tuberculosis, sarcoid, and fungal infections. Granulomas may also be a response to peptic ulceration or cancer.

Eosinophilic Gastritis

This may be associated with hypersensitivity reactions, allergies, or vasculitis.

Malacoplakia

This is characterized by the presence of numerous histiocytes (of Von Hanseman), which may contain diagnostic Michaelis-Gutmann bodies. (See Chapter 10.)

Organisms

Candida, Actinomyces: These organisms are usually oral contaminants but may grow on ulcers.

Leptothrix: Frequently normal; commonly associated with ulcers, either benign or malignant. Fine, pink, intertwining, nonbranching filamentous bacteria, distinct from fungal hyphae and *Actinomyces* [Sanders 1991].

Helicobacter (Campylobacter) pylori is associated with chronic gastritis, Barrett's esophagus, and peptic ulcer disease [Blaser 1987, Dooley 1989, Leung 1992, Schnadig 1990]. These tiny curved or spiral-shaped bacteria, which measure between 1 and 3 µm in length, are found in the mucous coating of luminal glandular cells [Davenport 1990, De Francesco 1993, Faverly 1990]. Brushings and touch preparations of biopsies have been used to identify these microbiologic organisms [**44** I9.50] [Davenport 1990, Debongnie 1989,1994, Faverly 1990, Mendoza 1993, Pinto 1991, Schnadig 1990]. The organisms are usually visible with the Papanicolaou stain [Davenport 1990, Pinto 1991] but may stain poorly [Faverly 1990]. When stained with Giemsa or Diff-Quik, they are readily identifiable as dark-blue bacteria with highly characteristic spiral shapes [Faverly 1990]. Oil immersion may be helpful in identification [Robinson 1991]. *H pylori* produces a protease that can break down protective mucus, exposing the underlying cells to injury from digestive juices and resulting in acute inflammation and epithelial repair [Davenport 1990]. Associated with chronic gastritis, gastric and duodenal ulcers, and gastric cancer, these bacteria are rarely found on normal mucosa [Goodwin 1986, Pinto 1991, Wyatt 1991]. The differential diagnosis requires distinguishing *H pylori* from *Gastrospirillum hominis*, which is longer, more tightly coiled (like a corkscrew), and unattached to surface epithelium. *G hominis* may be associated with mild active chronic gastritis similar to that seen in some patients with *H pylori* [Wyatt 1991].

Benign Tumors

Hyperplastic Polyps

The great majority of gastric polyps, perhaps 90%, are hyperplastic or regenerative (ie, nonneoplastic) polyps [45 I9.51, 46 I9.52]. Although they are frequently present in stomachs resected for cancer, gastric polyps carry little or no risk of malignant transformation [Morson 1980]. Hyperplastic polyps are small, pedunculated, and may be multiple [T9.3]. Cytologically, relatively normal gastric mucous cells line the surface. Nonspecific reparative changes can also be seen. Consequently, a specific diagnosis cannot be made by cytology alone; clinical or endoscopic correlation is required.

Adenomatous Polyps

Adenomatous polyps are rare, neoplastic growths in the stomach. They are generally larger than hyperplastic polyps and are usually single and sessile rather than multiple or pedunculated [T9.3]. They grow as villous, tubulovillous, or, rarely, papillary structures. Cell groups in frond formation may be seen cytologically [Rubin 1955]. The polyps are usually lined by intestinal-type, columnar epithelium. Dysplastic changes may occur. Adenomatous polyps carry a significant risk of malignant transformation [Morson 1980].

Leiomyoma

The stomach is the most common site of gastrointestinal leiomyomas, which can sometimes cause gastric ulceration with symptoms related to the ulcer. However, they are usually asymptomatic. Diagnosing gastrointestinal leiomyomas by exfoliative cytology is difficult, particularly if the leiomyoma is covered by an intact mucosa. If the mucosa is ulcerated, reactive gastric cells will be obtained.

T9.3 **Gastric Polyps**

Hyperplastic	Adenomatous
More common	Rare
May be multiple	Usually single
Smaller	Larger
Pedunculated	Sessile
Gastric cells	Intestinal type cells
Repair atypia may occur	Dysplasia may occur
Almost no risk of carcinoma	Significant risk of carcinoma

45

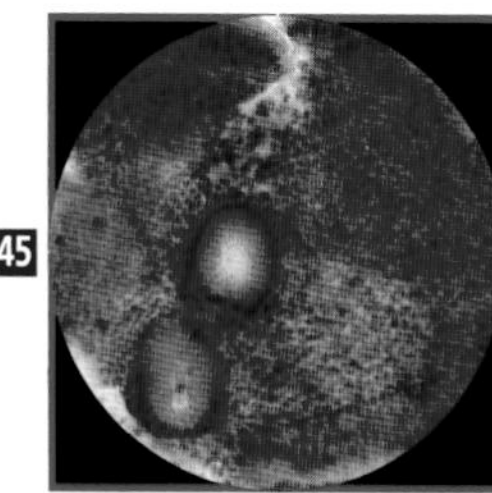

46

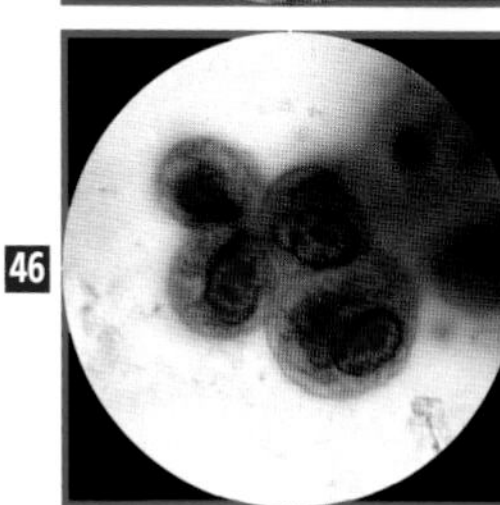

Malignant Disease

The incidence of gastric cancer in the United States has been decreasing, but it is not clear why. Environmental and dietary factors are suspected in the etiology (diet high in salt, complex carbohydrates, and nitrites but low in animal fat and protein, green leafy vegetables, and fruits). Racial and genetic factors may play a role, eg, gastric cancer is more common among blacks than whites and more common among people with type A blood.

Cytology and histology are each about 80% accurate in diagnosing gastric malignancy. However, the two techniques are complementary, and when used together, diagnostic accuracy increases to 90% or more. Because definitive therapy may be undertaken based on the cytologic diagnosis, every effort must be made to ensure that the diagnosis is accurate. A definitive diagnosis should not be rendered on only a few cells, although the specimen may be considered suspicious for malignancy. Note, however, that gastric cytology may be positive months to years before a malignant lesion is suspected clinically or demonstrated by fluoroscopy or endoscopy [Loux 1969, Schade 1959].

Gastric cancers may be flat, polypoid, or ulcerated. Malignant ulcers tend to occur on the greater curvature of the stomach [T9.4]. They are often relatively large and have

T9.4 **Differentiation of Benign From Malignant Ulcers**

Benign	Malignant
Patients tend to be younger	Patients tend to be older
M>>F	M slightly >F
Normal or increased acid	Normal or decreased acid
Usually on lesser curve	Usually on greater curve
Usually <2 cm	Often >4 cm
Responds to therapy	Incomplete or no response to therapy
Punched-out appearance	Heaped-up margins

"heaped-up" margins, compared with the "punched-out" appearance of benign ulcers. Malignant ulcers may respond, at least to some degree, to medical therapy, mimicking a healing benign ulcer.

In the United States the five-year survival of patients with gastric cancer is between 5% and 15%. However, in countries with a high incidence of gastric cancer and intensive screening programs, 40% of the cancers can be detected early, and nearly 90% of patients with early cancer survive five years or more. The majority of gastric cancers are adenocarcinomas, but other malignancies (eg, leiomyosarcomas, malignant lymphomas) also occur.

Adenocarcinoma

Adenocarcinoma of the stomach occurs in two basic cytologic forms [T9.5]: (1) intestinal type (typical papillary or acinar adenocarcinoma) [47 I9.58] and (2) gastric type (also known as diffuse, linitis plastica, or signet ring cell adenocarcinoma) [I9.60] [An-Foraker 1981, Laurén 1965, Takeda 1981]. Intestinal-type adenocarcinoma is thought to arise in intestinal metaplasia and has cytologic features that mimic those of colonic carcinoma. Gastric-type adenocarcinoma is thought to arise in ordinary gastric mucosa (akin to surface mucous cells) and may have signet ring cells or poorly differentiated pleomorphic cells [Takeda 1981]. Mixed cancers also occur, and with high-grade tumors, distinctive features may be lost. Intestinal-type adenocarcinoma is more common than gastric type, which accounts for about 10% to 20% of cases [An-Foraker 1981]. However, the incidence of the intestinal type is decreasing, while the incidence of the gastric type has remained constant. Either form can be characterized grossly by excavating tumors. Polypoid or fungating growth is twice as common with the intestinal type, and infiltrating linitis plastica is three times more common with the gastric type [Laurén 1965].

The cancers are located predominantly in the pylorus and antrum. The lesser curvature and the body of the stomach are the next most common locations, and most of the remainder are located in the cardia. The most common location of gastric cancer is the lesser curve of the pyloric antrum. Although the greater curve is uncommonly involved, ulcers on the greater curve are more suspicious (pylorus/antrum: lesser curve, body: cardia → 6 : 3 : 1 [Laurén 1965]).

Intestinal-type adenocarcinoma occurs predominantly in men, in a ratio of about 2:1. The sex distribution of the gastric type is nearly even, though men predominate slightly [Laurén 1965]. Gastric-type adenocarcinoma occurs, on average, nearly a decade earlier than the intestinal type (late 40s vs late 50s) [An-Foraker 1981, Laurén 1965]. The prognosis for intestinal-type adenocarcinoma is somewhat more favorable.

T9.5 Stomach Cancer

Growth Pattern	Intestinal Type	Gastric Type
Polyp, fungating	60%	31%
Excavating	25%	26%
Linitis plastica	15%	43%

[Laurén 1965]

47
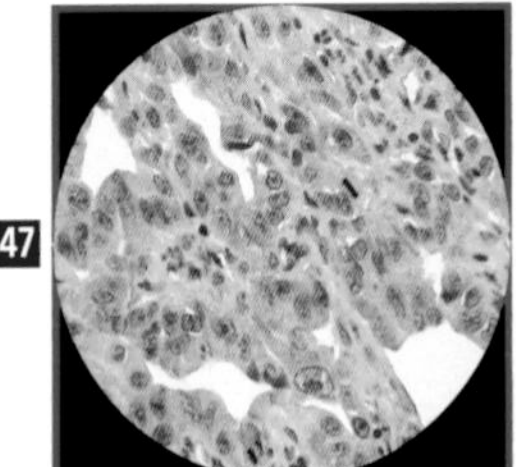

48
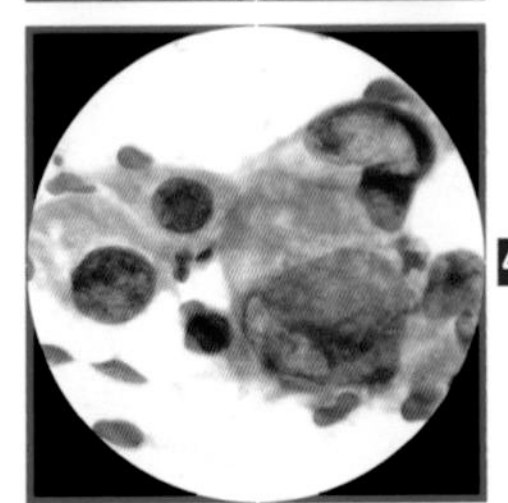

49
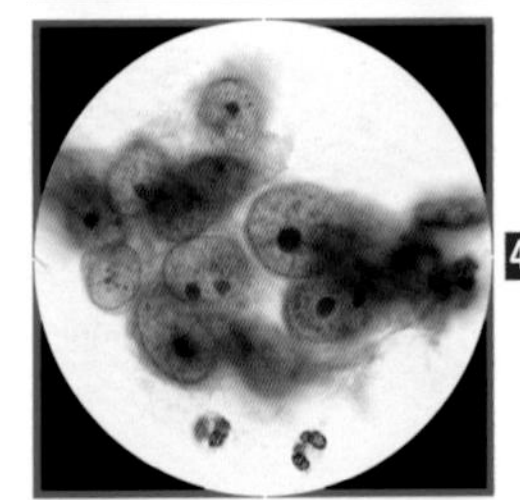

50
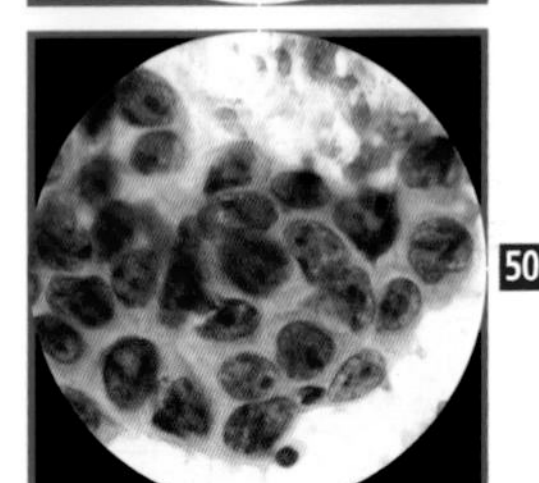

The incidence of gastric cancer in countries like the United States is too low for mass screening to be practical [MacDonald 1964]. However, screening may be successful in countries with high incidences, eg, Japan, Finland, Iceland, by facilitating the detection of early gastric cancers, which have good prognoses [E Kaneko 1977]. Screening high-risk patients may also be cost effective. For example, patients who have had a partial gastrectomy for benign disease have an increased risk of developing cancer in the gastric remnant many years after the operation [Morson 1980]. Either intestinal- or gastric-type cancer may occur in this setting, and both are detectable cytologically [Takeda 1985].

Risk Factors for Gastric Cancer

Family history of gastric cancer
Chronic atrophic gastritis
Chronic ulcers
Pernicious anemia
Partial gastrectomy
Adenomatous polyps
Ménétrier's disease

[Brandborg 1968a, Ming 1984, Morson 1980, Saraga 1987, Seifert 1979]

Intestinal-Type Adenocarcinoma: The cells of intestinal-type gastric cancer are generally fairly abundant and vary from well to poorly differentiated, ie, from relatively uniform to markedly pleomorphic [I9.58]. The cells form loosely cohesive, multilayered, disorderly, thick groups—sheets, papillae, or acini. Many of the cells are single, an important feature of malignancy [Young 1982]]. However, in intestinal-type carcinoma there are not as many single cells as are seen in gastric-type carcinoma. The cells vary from columnar (well differentiated) to cuboidal (poorly differentiated) [I9.53-I9.57] [Takeda 1981].

The nuclei are peripherally oriented [48 I9.56]. They are generally enlarged and oval to elongated or, occasionally, round and pleomorphic with a moderately increased N/C ratio. Although the nuclei are morphologically variable, they tend to fall into two groups [Pilotti 1977]. One group is characterized by fine chromatin and prominent, single nucleoli [49 I9.54]; the other is hyperchromatic with coarse chromatin and multiple smaller nucleoli [50 I9.55]. The nuclei have irregular nuclear membranes, with occasional cerebriform convolutions [Takeda 1981]. Naked nuclei are occasionally observed.

The cytoplasm is usually granular but may be vacuolated. A characteristic terminal bar–like edge on the apical aspect of the cell may be seen, particularly in well-differentiated tumors [I9.57]. This corresponds to the striated border seen in tissue. The cytoplasm contains mucins that are usually either pure acid mucin or mixed acid and neutral mucins [Laurén 1965]. Acid mucins and particularly sulfomucins (colonic type) usually predominate [Jass 1981]. This type of cancer is associated with intestinal metaplasia and dysplasia of the gastric epithelium. A tumor diathesis with necrotic debris and numerous neutrophils is common but nondiagnostic [Pilotti 1977]. The colloid variant shows cells with larger but fewer cytoplasmic vacuoles [Pilotti 1977] and pools of mucus. Multinucleated tumor giant cells are rare [Pilotti 1977].

The primary differential diagnotic problem is distinguishing intestinal-type adenocarcinoma from reactive atypia, which may be particularly difficult in some cases. Cancer is characterized by the presence of loosely cohesive clusters and syncytia of disorderly groups of atypical cells as well as single intact atypical cells. Abnormal single cells must be present to establish a diagnosis of malignancy. Reactive cells usually occur in more orderly cohesive groups. However, benign cells can also be single, which complicates the differential diagnosis. Cell-in-cell patterns, signet ring forms, high N/C ratios, and irregularly shaped cells favor a diagnosis of malignancy [Dziura 1977]. Abundant cytoplasm, smooth nuclear membranes, and lower N/C ratios favor a benign diagnosis. Macronucleoli, coarsely granular chromatin, and irregular nuclear shapes can be found in both benign and malignant cells [Dziura 1977].

Mitotic figures, unless abnormal, are not helpful in the differential diagnosis, because they can occur in both benign, regenerating epithelium and in malignancy. Similarly, a necrotic background (diathesis) can be seen with either benign or malignant ulcers, and therefore is not helpful in the differential diagnosis. Chemotherapy can induce significant cytologic atypia, including large cells with pleomorphic, intensely hyperchromatic nuclei and prominent nucleoli, which could be mistaken for malignancy [Becker 1986]. However, the N/C ratio remains relatively normal and the chromatin is smudgy rather than distinct, changes that are similar to radiation-induced atypia [Choi 1985].

Gastric-Type Adenocarcinoma: In essence, gastric- or diffuse-type stomach cancer is a signet ring cell adenocarcinoma [51 I9.60]. However, it may also contain a mixture of poorly differentiated, pleomorphic cells with scant to abundant cytoplasm [Takeda 1981]. Gastric-type cancer tends to grow diffusely in the wall of the stomach, causing a "leather bottle" deformity (linitis plastica). Gastric-type stomach cancer is not significantly associated with intestinal metaplasia or glandular dysplasia. The tumor may not be associated with mucosal ulceration. If the overlying mucosa is intact, a false-negative diagnosis may occur with exfoliative cytologic techniques.

The majority of the tumor cells are found singly or in small, loose clusters. They are generally less numerous than in intestinal-type cancer [An-Foraker 1981]. Glandular groupings or papillae are absent or rare. The cells tend to be rounded rather than columnar and relatively small and uniform. The nuclei are similar to those seen in intestinal-type cancer but tend to be smaller, rounder, and have a higher N/C ratio. There is a predominance of nuclei with large nucleoli and fine chromatin [Pilotti 1977]. The nuclei may be pushed to the side by a single large mucin vacuole or numerous small vacuoles, resulting in a characteristic signet ring cell [52 I9.59]. Pleomorphic cells may also be present [Takeda 1981]. These cells have scant to abundant granular cytoplasm, which is not characteristic of signet rings [Takeda 1981]. Most mucins (88%) are mixed neutral and acid [Laurén 1965], but neutral mucins are more abundant in gastric- than in intestinal-type cancers [Jass 1981]. Intestinal metaplastic or

51

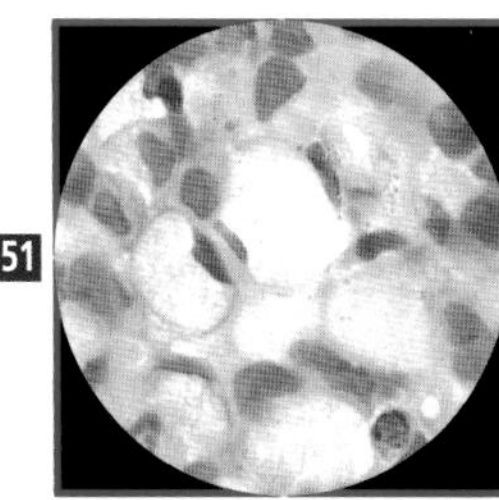

52

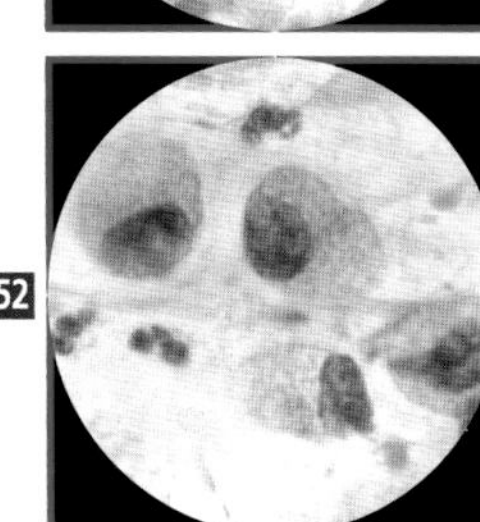

dysplastic cells are less commonly observed with the gastric-type variant [Laurén 1965, Pilotti 1977]. The background tends to be relatively clean, but lymphocytes and plasma cells are more commonly seen with this variant [Pilotti 1977]. The signet ring cells may be found in pools of mucus.

Because the diagnostic cells are typically few, small, and relatively bland, false-negative diagnoses may occur. If the lesion is ulcerated, inflammation may obscure the diagnostic cells. The differential diagnosis includes malignant lymphoma, in which the cells are exclusively single and never contain mucin, and metastatic carcinoma, particularly from the breast.

Gastric Dysplasia and Early Gastric Cancer

Gastric Dysplasia and Carcinoma In Situ: Intestinal-type carcinoma of the stomach is preceded by atrophic, metaplastic, and, particularly, dysplastic changes. Dysplasia does not seem to play a prominent role in the development of the gastric-, or diffuse-, type stomach cancer, the precancerous lesion of which remains undetected [Cuello 1979, Ming 1984]. As in other organs, it is believed that adenocarcinoma of the stomach is preceded by dysplasia/carcinoma in situ. Gastric dysplasia/ carcinoma in situ is considered a neoplastic, preinvasive lesion and is the most important precancerous change [Rugge 1991]. Dysplasia and carcinoma in situ occur most frequently in chronic atrophic gastritis (eg, in patients with pernicious anemia [Boon 1964]) and gastric ulcer and, less frequently, in patients with gastric adenomatous polyps or after a partial gastrectomy [Rugge 1991]. Patients with gastric ulcers associated with significant dysplasia have a high risk of developing cancer [Farinati 1989, Farini 1982]. Morphologically similar dysplastic changes can be seen in Barrett's esophagus [Wang 1991a], intestinal adenomas, and inflammatory bowel disease. In a small but significant number of patients undergoing endoscopy, gastric dysplasia is detected in otherwise apparently normal mucosa [Rugge 1991]. Premalignant gastric lesions are rarely diagnosed in the United States but are more commonly discovered in countries that have a high prevalence of gastric cancer and screening programs (eg, Japan).

The biologic behavior of gastric dysplasia is similar to that of dysplasia occurring in the uterine cervix. Unfortunately, as in the cervix, the behavior of a lesion in an individual patient cannot be predicted. However, the basic concept is the same—ie, the malignant potential of the dysplasia parallels the degree of cellular abnormality [Ming 1984]. The majority of cases are low grade, and low-grade lesions tend to regress but may persist or progress. The higher the grade of dysplasia, the more likely the lesion is to progress and the less likely it is to regress [Rugge 1991]. Surgery may be indicated for patients with severe gastric dysplasia, because gastric cancer develops in a high proportion of patients (as many as 75%–80%), often rapidly (ie, within a few months) [Rugge 1991, Saraga 1987]. Dysplasia can also coexist with cancer. Moreover, high-grade dysplasia and well-differentiated gastric carcinoma (intestinal type) may be difficult to distinguish by cytology. Thus, clinical correlation and tissue biopsy may be required for final diagnosis. Patients with lesions suggestive of but not diagnostic for dysplasia (ie, morphologically indefinite or suspicious lesions) should undergo repeat endoscopy.

Histology of Dysplasia and Carcinoma In Situ: Like glandular dysplasia in other areas of the gastrointestinal tract, two forms of gastric dysplasia have been described histologically [Cuello 1979, Jass 1983, Rugge 1991]. The more common, classic type of dysplasia resembles the epithelium of colonic adenomatous polyps (intestinal-type dysplasia [Rugge 1991]) and consists of markedly crowded, columnar cells with elongated (cigar-shaped), hyperchromatic, pleomorphic nuclei; inconspicuous nucleoli; and scant, amphophilic cytoplasm containing a small amount of mucin (usually sulfomucin). Goblet cells are usually absent. This type of dysplasia is associated with better-differentiated, intestinal-type adenocarcinomas.

The less common type of dysplasia (gastric-type dysplasia [Rugge 1991]) has been compared to the epithelium of hyperplastic polyps, atypia of repair/regeneration, and incomplete maturation of colonic crypts [Cuello 1979, Jass 1983, Riddell 1983]. In contrast with intestinal-type dysplasia, the cells are less crowded and have round to oval, enlarged, pleomorphic nuclei with vesicular chromatin, prominent nucleoli, and eosinophilic to pale cytoplasm. There is evidence of acid and neutral mucin secretion in various combinations. Goblet cells may be present. This form of dysplasia is associated with poorly differentiated, intestinal-type carcinomas [Jass 1983]. The two types of dysplasia may coexist, and either type can arise in areas of incomplete intestinal metaplasia [Jass 1983].

Cytology of Dysplasia and Carcinoma In Situ: Cytologically, dysplasia is characterized by mild to moderate nuclear pleomorphism and atypia [Wang 1991a]. The nuclei are somewhat but not markedly enlarged and ovoid to elongated, with focally irregular nuclear membranes, an increased N/C ratio, hyperchromasia, coarse chromatin, and loss of polarity. Nucleoli can be seen in some cells, but macronucleoli are not present. Mucous secretion is reduced or absent, with increased cytoplasmic basophilia [Ming 1984]. The groups are somewhat disorderly, crowded, and molded, and they demonstrate some degree of decreased intercellular cohesion, resulting in a few single atypical cells. The difference between dysplasia and cancer is the degree of cytologic abnormality. Cancer has more single cells, more haphazard cellular arrangements, and tends to have more obvious malignant features (eg, large, poorly differentiated, pleomorphic cells with large nuclei and prominent nucleoli) [Hustin 1994].

Qualitative, quantitative, and clinical features suggest that dysplasia should be divided into two grades—low and high—rather than three [Riddell 1983, Saraga 1987]. Mild dysplasia may be difficult to distinguish from reactive changes and frequently regresses [Saraga 1987]. Therefore, many cases of so-called mild dysplasia and even some cases of moderate dysplasia might be better categorized as reactive/regenerative (ie, nondysplastic) changes [Hustin 1994]. Both dysplasia and reactive changes can show some degree of nuclear enlargement and pleomorphism as well as mucus depletion of the cells [Riddell 1983]. One should be cautious about making a diagnosis of dysplasia, particularly low-grade dysplasia, if inflammation is present.

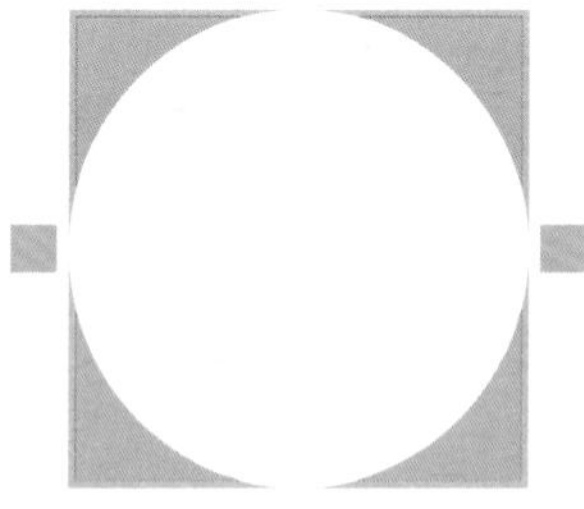

Severe dysplasia and carcinoma in situ could simply be designated high-grade dysplasia. The cases of "moderate dysplasia" remaining after reactive changes have been accounted for are divided into either low- or high-grade dysplasia, depending on morphology. It may be difficult to distinguish high-grade dysplasia from well-differentiated carcinoma. Carcinoma in situ unassociated with invasive cancer is rare in the stomach [Ming 1984]. The key to the differential diagnosis of dysplasia and carcinoma in situ lies in the nucleus (hyperchromasia, pleomorphism, loss of polarity) [Riddell 1983]. As usual, diagnosis is based on the most advanced abnormality [Morson 1980, Riddell 1983, Saraga 1987].

The advantage of the diagnostic system shown [T9.6] is that the divisions are related to the clinical management and biological behavior of the gastric lesions [Tosi 1989]. These divisions resemble the Bethesda System classifications for premalignant lesions of the uterine cervix (ie, low- and high-grade squamous intraepithelial lesions).

Early Gastric Cancer: Early gastric cancer, or superficial cancer, is restricted to the mucosa or submucosa, without penetration of the muscularis propria, although regional lymph node metastases may be present [Carter 1984]. Minute gastric cancers less than 5 mm in diameter have been discovered [Oohara 1982]. When detected early, gastric cancer can be cured. Early gastric cancer has a much better prognosis than deeply invasive, or advanced, adenocarcinoma, with a five-year survival of 80% to 90% or greater, compared with about 10% to 20% for advanced adenocarcinoma [Carter 1984, Seifert 1979]. However, even very superficial invasion can result in disseminated disease. Cases with only regional lymph node metastases have an excellent prognosis [Carter 1984]. Early gastric cancer tends to occur, on average, in patients more than two decades younger than those with advanced gastric cancer, but otherwise there may be no significant differences in endoscopic or radiologic appearance, tumor location (most are antral), presence of regional lymph node metastases, or type of resection [Carter 1984]. In particular, it may be difficult or impossible to distinguish a benign ulcer from early gastric cancer. Moreover, even malignant ulcers can

T9.6 Diagnostic System

Traditional Nomenclature	Revised Nomenclature	Cancer Risk	Guidelines for Management
Reactive changes →	Reactive changes	No risk	Treatment as indicated
Mild dysplasia (→ Reactive changes / → Low-grade dysplasia)			
Moderate dysplasia (→ Low-grade dysplasia / → High-grade dysplasia)	Low-grade dysplasia	Low risk	Careful follow-up
Severe dysplasia/CIS →	High-grade dysplasia	High risk	Surgery

appear to heal clinically [Machado 1976, Rugge 1991]. The lesions may be multifocal [Mason 1965], and multiple biopsies may be required to diagnose malignancy [Seifert 1979]. Cytologic techniques can easily sample multiple areas to detect malignancy. However, neither endoscopic biopsy nor cytology can distinguish early from more advanced gastric cancer [Vilardell 1978]. Surgery is the primary therapeutic modality; recurrences tend to be local and can be treated by local resection [Carter 1984].

Both intestinal-type and gastric-type cancers can be found at an early stage [Takeda 1981]. The cytology depends on the type of cancer [T9.7]. In intestinal-type cancer, the cells are often arranged in three-dimensional clusters or loose groups, with some loss of polarity. The cells are columnar, with finely granular cytoplasm. The nuclei are enlarged, with prominent, irregular nuclear membranes; fine chromatin; and single large or multiple small nucleoli [Howell 1985]. Gastric-type cancer has signet ring cells and a component of pleomorphic, rounded cells, which tend to occur singly or in small groups rather than in more cohesive clusters. Necrotic debris, inflammation, intestinal metaplasia, and reactive atypia can all be seen in either early gastric cancer or benign lesions [Howell 1985].

T9.7 **Adenocarcinoma of the Stomach**

	Intestinal Type	Gastric Type
Origin	Intestinal metaplasia, dysplasia	Arises de novo
Tumor grade	Better differentiated	Poorly differentiated
Incidence	Decreasing	Steady
Growth pattern	Polypoid	Diffuse
Age	>50	Slightly younger
Sex	Men, 2 to 1	Equal
Association with gastritis	Yes	No
Cells	Columnar	Signet ring

Other Carcinomas

Squamous cell carcinoma [Milstoc 1969], adenosquamous carcinoma, large-cell undifferentiated carcinoma, and small-cell carcinomas all occur but are rare. Ciliated adenocarcinoma has been described [Chan 1993].

Malignant Lymphoma

In addition to its digestive functions, the GI tract is an important lymphoid organ. Mucosa-associated lymphoid tissue (MALT) is a specific type of lymphoid tissue, which in the gastrointestinal tract may be the bursa equivalent for B-cell lymphocytes. The GI tract, particularly the stomach, is the most common extranodal site of malignant lymphoma, particularly B-cell types [53 I9.63]. Malignant lymphoma is the second most common gastric malignancy (albeit a distant second) and can be either primary or secondary [Lozowski 1984]. The incidence of GI lymphoma decreases along the GI tract (sites of GI lymphomas: stomach > small intestine > large intestine > anal). Anal lymphoma is rare but associated with AIDS. Lymphomas arising in the GI Tract generally have a better prognosis than those involving it secondarily [Hall 1991], and the prognosis is considerably better than for adenocarcinoma.

Criteria for Diagnosing Primary GI Lymphoma

No superficial lymphadenopathy
No radiologic evidence of mediastinal lymphadenopathy
Normal white blood cell count
GI lesions predominate over regional lymphadenopathy
Liver and spleen disease-free
[Hall 1991]

Gastrointestinal lymphomas can occur at any age but are most common in middle-aged and elderly patients. Predisposing factors include celiac disease, chronic inflammatory bowel disease, and immunocompromised states such as AIDS and, possibly, chronic gastritis associated with *Helicobacter pylori* [Hall 1991]. The signs and symptoms of GI lymphomas are usually indistinguishable from carcinomas occurring in the same site [Hall 1991]. The growth pattern can be diffusely infiltrating (particularly T-cell lymphomas), exophytic (particularly B-cell lymphomas), or polypoid (particularly small cleaved lymphomas in the colon). These patterns, particularly ulcerated lesions, can mimic adenocarcinoma.

53 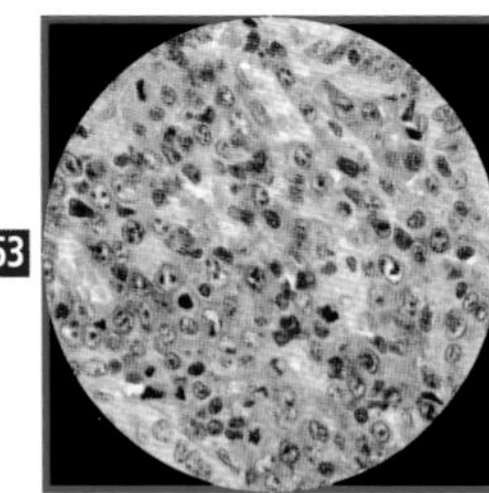

54 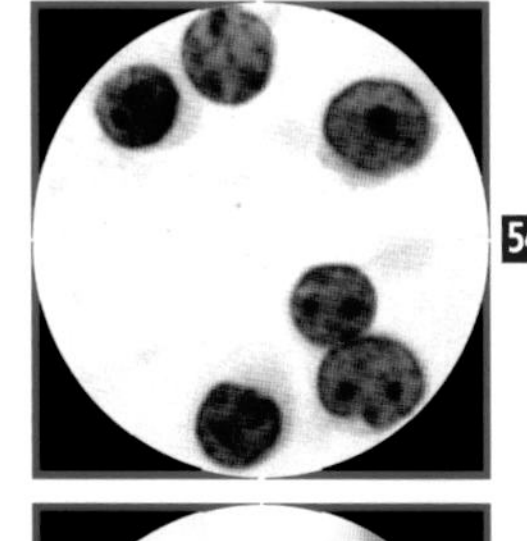

55 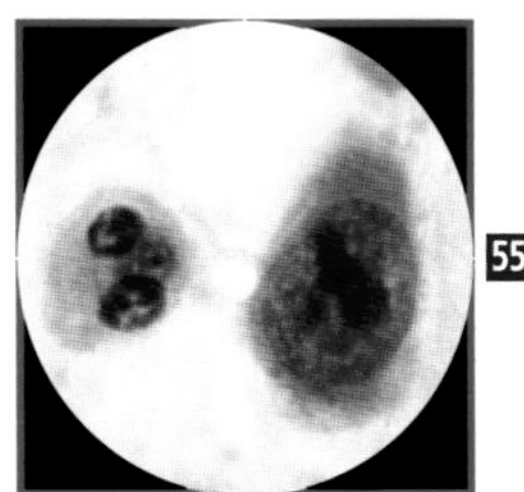

Nearly all GI lymphomas are non-Hodgkin's type [54 I9.61, 55 I9.62]. Low-grade lymphomas developing in MALT ("MALTomas") are characterized by indolent growth and a tendency to remain localized for long periods of time and then disseminate to regional lymph nodes and other mucosal (MALT) sites [Hall 1991]. However, aggressive, diffuse, large cell lymphomas, including immunoblastic lymphoma, are the most common types [Sherman 1994]. Other types of lymphomas, such as well-differentiated (small lymphocytic) and poorly differentiated (small cleaved) malignant, non-Hodgkin's lymphomas as well as Hodgkin's disease may also be seen. Small, noncleaved (Burkitt's, non-Burkitt's types), non-Hodgkin's lymphomas are more common in the ileocecal area [Van Krieken 1992].

GI Lymphomas

Most are non-Hodgkin's
Most are diffuse
Most are large cell high grade
Most are B cell

Lymphomas that ulcerate are more likely to be diagnosed by exfoliative cytology than nonulcerated tumors [Cabré-Fiol 1978, Foushee 1969, S Katz 1973]. Ulceration is more likely to occur with primary lymphomas [Lozowski 1984]. However, exfoliative cytology can be positive when tissue biopsy is negative [Posner 1975]. Deep-lying tumors may be diagnosed by endoscopic fine needle aspiration biopsy [Iishi 1986]. Because lymphoma patients are immunosuppressed, they commonly have cytologic evidence of *Candida* infection [Lozowski 1984].

The most characteristic cytologic feature of malignant lymphoma is a lack of cellular cohesion: no true tissue aggregates are formed [Kline 1973,1974, Prolla 1970a, Rubin 1954]. The cells, even from large-cell lymphomas, can be unexpectedly small due to degeneration. The nuclei are hyperchromatic and cytoplasm is scanty. Nucleoli may be prominent. Ulceration or, more precisely, the associated inflammation and debris, can mask single tumor cells.

MALTomas are characterized by a predominance of small lymphocytes with only mild to moderate atypia, presence of lymphoepithelial lesions (nondestructive invasion of glands), and an association of reactive lymphoid follicles and plasma cells [Isaacson 1986, Sherman 1994, Zukerberg 1990]. Differentiating between benign lymphoid infiltrates and MALTomas can be difficult.

Large cell lymphomas are characterized by relatively large lymphoid cells, often with irregular nuclear outlines. The chromatin appears vesicular, and multiple, often peripheral nucleoli are common [Sherman 1994]. The cytoplasm is slightly basophilic [56 I9.61].

Immunoblastic lymphoma is characterized by a more polymorphous infiltrate of large cells, with vesicular chromatin and prominent, centrally placed nucleoli. The cytoplasm is typically plasmacytoid [57 I9.62].

Small (well-differentiated) lymphocytic lymphoma is usually composed of relatively normal-appearing small lymphocytes, which may be larger than ordinary mature lymphocytes. The nuclei are monomorphic, with coarse chromatin, inconspicuous nucleoli, and smooth nuclear membranes. The cytoplasm is scant.

Lymphoplasmacytoid lymphoma is characterized by the presence of lymphoid cells intermediate in appearance between small lymphocytes and plasma cells, as well as plasma cells, lymphocytes, and occasional immunoblasts [De Gaetani 1977, Rilke 1978]. Plasmacytoid differentiation is common in GI lymphomas and should not be diagnosed as plasmacytoma unless the entire lesion is composed of plasma cells.

Small cleaved (poorly differentiated lymphocytic) lymphoma is composed of cells that are more variable in size and shape and slightly larger than normal lymphocytes. Nuclear membrane irregularities (cleavages), coarse chromatin, and small nucleoli are seen. The cytoplasm is slightly more abundant than in mature lymphocytes.

Small, noncleaved cell lymphoma is characterized by a more monomorphous population of intermediate-sized lymphoid cells, with scant, intensely basophilic cytoplasm. Numerous tingible body macrophages are present. Burkitt's lymphoma shows little nuclear variation, dispersed chromatin, and two to five nucleoli. Non-Burkitt's lymphoma shows some nuclear pleomorphism, with more vesicular chromatin and occasional prominent nucleoli [Van Krieken 1992].

Differential diagnosis includes benign chronic inflammation and pseudolymphoma. Pseudolymphoma, like follicular cervicitis seen in the Pap smear, is associated with lymphoid cells in varying stages of maturation, including mature plasma cells [Kobayashi 1970a, Prolla 1970a] and tingible body macrophages. Note that plasma cells can be seen in lymphoplasmacytic lymphoma, plasmacytoma, and Mediterranean abdominal lymphoma. Lymphocytes with plasmacytoid features indicate abnormal cellular proliferation [Rilke 1978]. Inflammation associated with ulceration may make diagnosis difficult. Recognizing small cell lymphomas (small or well-differentiated, lymphocytic, and small cleaved or poorly differentiated, lymphocytic lymphomas) may be particularly difficult. Moreover, exfoliative cytologic techniques may not yield enough information to subclassify the malignant lymphoma. Tissue biopsy and marker studies may be required for final diagnosis. (For further discussion of malignant lymphomas, see Chapter 18.)

56

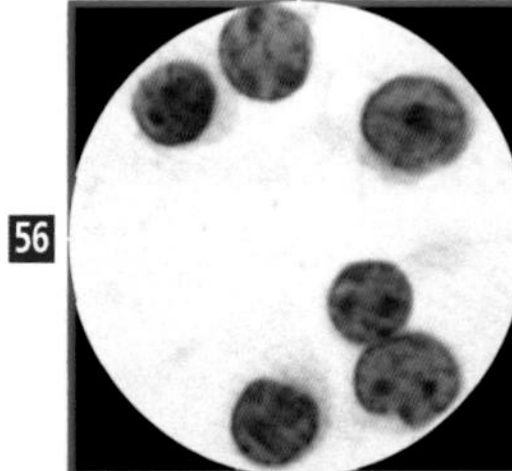

57

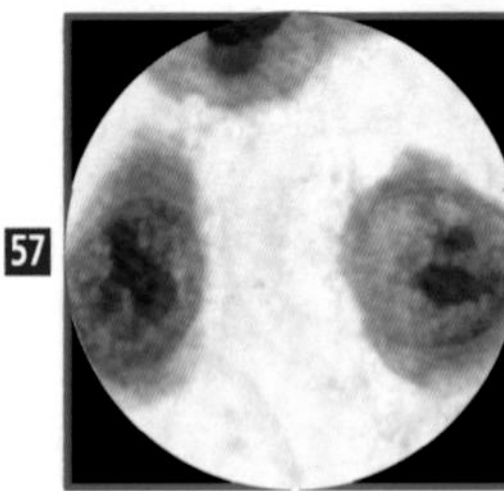

Poorly differentiated adenocarcinoma, particularly the gastric type, may show a dissociated cell pattern that can mimic malignant lymphoma. The lymphoid nature of a neoplasm may be more obvious when cytologic rather than histologic techniques are used [Wang 1991b]. The presence of true tissue aggregates or mucin production by the tumor cells excludes malignant lymphoma from diagnostic consideration [Kline 1974].

Carcinoid Tumors

Carcinoid is the second most common epithelial tumor of the stomach. Gastric carcinoids are often multiple. Combined adenocarcinomas and carcinoid (adenocarcinoids) also occur and can be diagnosed cytologically [Wheeler 1984].

Small Cell Carcinoma

Small cell carcinoma, similar to that occurring in the lung, arises rarely in the stomach. There is usually much debris, necrosis, and exudate. The malignant cells, which may be scarce and hidden in the debris, are small, about one to two times the size of a lymphocyte, and have very scant cytoplasm. The nuclei mold and nucleoli are inconspicuous. True tissue aggregates eliminate malignant lymphoma from the differential diagnosis. Before diagnosing small cell carcinoma of the stomach, one must exclude a diagnosis of metastatic small cell carcinoma from the lung.

Smooth Muscle Tumors

Leiomyomas and leiomyosarcomas grow primarily in a submucosal location. Therefore, these lesions must cause ulceration in order to be diagnosed by exfoliative cytology; a lesion that does not cause ulceration may be detected with endoscopic fine needle aspiration biopsy. The classic appearance of leiomyoma and leiomyosarcoma is a spindle cell neoplasm that, when malignant, generally has large, hyperchromatic nuclei and mitotic figures [Cabre-Fiol 1975]. Contractile filaments may be seen in some cells, which may be highlighted with special stains (eg, Masson trichrome). The main differential diagnostic problem is separating benign from malignant tumors, particularly since markedly atypical-appearing cells can occur in benign bizarre leiomyoma. Also, benign reactive myofibroblasts may be obtained from the base of a chronic ulcer and can show significant atypia.

Leiomyoblastoma, which is of uncertain histogenesis, is thought to be an epithelioid smooth muscle or possibly neural tumor [Blei 1992]. It occurs predominantly in the stomach. The cells are round and are found in loose groups and singly. The nuclei are central and round. The cytoplasm is vacuolated. The tumor cells may have a signet ring appearance.

Carney's triad is a rare, multitumoral syndrome in which patients, usually young and female, develop nonepithelial gastric tumors, pulmonary chondromas, and functioning extra-adrenal paragangliomas [Carney 1977,1983]. Most patients have gastric tumors but only one of the other two neoplasms, although they may remain at risk for developing the full syndrome [Blei 1992]. The neoplasms are commonly multicentric. When leiomyoblastoma occurs as part of Carney's triad, patients can survive for a long time, even in the face of metastatic disease. In contrast, ordinary leiomyosarcoma may have a grim prognosis, particularly after metastases have occurred.

Miscellaneous Malignancies

Sarcomas, germ cell tumors (eg, choriocarcinoma [Gorczyca 1992, Uei 1973]), etc, can arise in the stomach.

Metastases

Melanoma [Reed 1962] and breast and lung cancer are the malignancies that most commonly metastasize to the stomach.

Small Intestine

Most pathologic conditions of the small intestine that are diagnosed cytologically involve the duodenum, particularly the descending portion, which contains the ampulla of Vater with the distal common bile duct. (See also "Extrahepatic Biliary Tract," p 357.) The jejunum and ileum are not easily accessible by endoscopy. Neoplasms of the small intestine are unusual, but malignant tumors are somewhat more common than benign ones.

The Cells

Normal

The mucosal lining of the small intestine is principally composed of absorptive and goblet cells [58 I9.49]. Cytologically, sheets of honeycombed absorptive cells have interspersed, clear goblet cells [59 I9.64]. The cells are tall columnar and usually well preserved in brush specimens. The nuclei are basal and round to oval, with smooth membranes, fine chromatin, and, occasionally, small nucleoli. The cytoplasm of absorptive cells is finely granular or vacuolar and has a striated, microvillous, apical border [60 I9.65] [Orell 1972]. (Note: Although the terms "striated" and "brush" border are used interchangeably by some authors, "striated border" actually refers only to highly regular microvilli, eg, on absorptive cells of the small intestine, and "brush border" refers to less regular microvilli, eg, proximal renal tubular cells. The microvilli of the intestinal cells are about 1 μm long while those on the renal tubular cells are about 2 to 3 μm long. Neither type of adult cell is normally ciliated.) Goblet cells contain large mucin vacuoles. A few inflammatory cells may be present in the background.

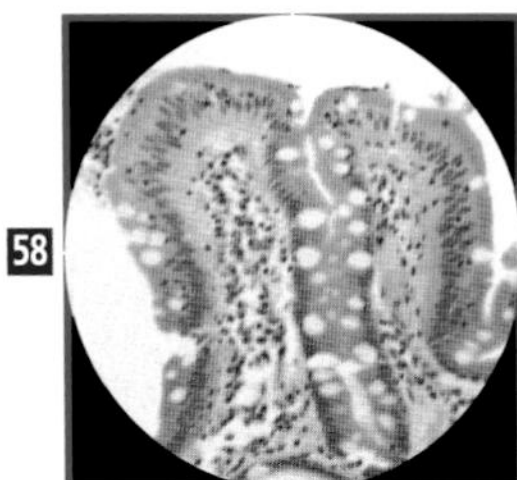
58

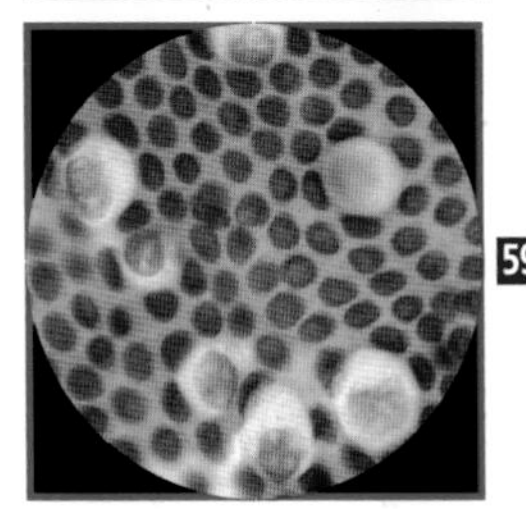
59

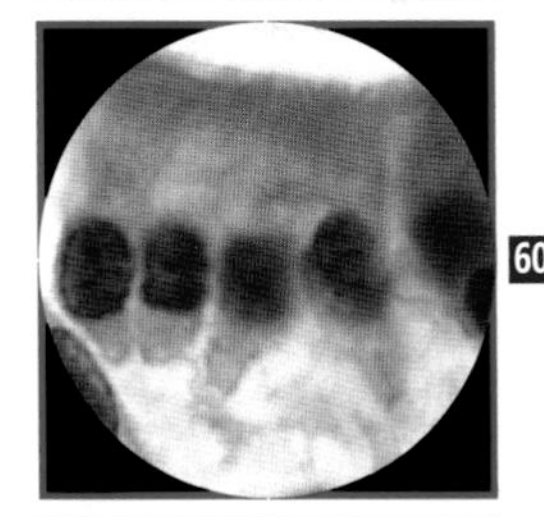
60

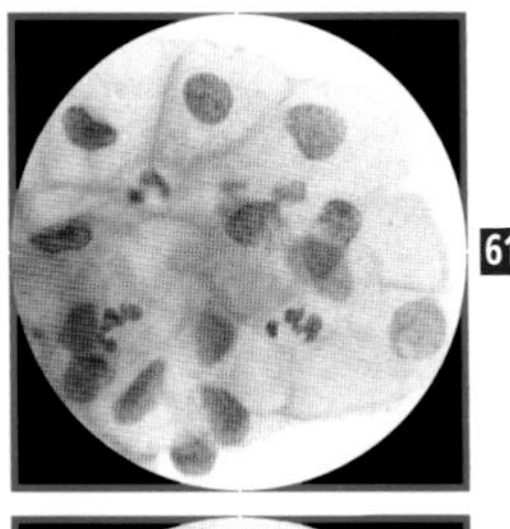
61

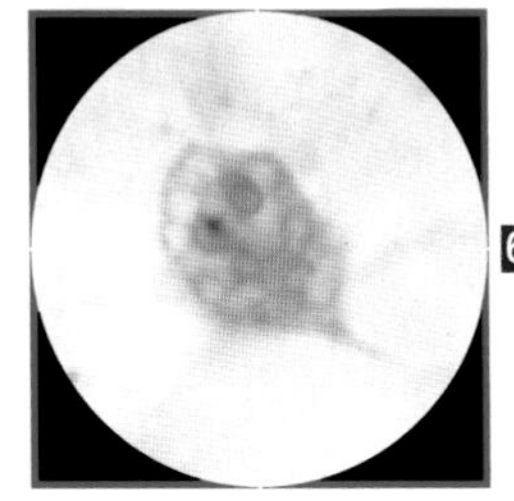
62

Reactive and Degenerative Changes

Due to ulceration or inflammation, small intestinal cells may undergo reactive/reparative or degenerative changes [61 I9.66]. The smears may be quite cellular. The cells are often poorly preserved; naked nuclei, nuclear pyknosis, and karyorrhexis are common. The cytoplasm may take on a squamoid appearance and sometimes intercellular bridges can be seen. Also, very reactive spindle myofibroblasts may be obtained from the base of an ulcer; these could suggest the presence of a spindle cell tumor, eg, leiomyosarcoma or atypical leiomyoma. Evidence of inflammation or necrosis may be seen in the background.

Infections

Giardia lamblia

Giardia lamblia is a pear-shaped organism that has a terminal flagellum and resembles *Trichomonas vaginalis* [62 I9.67]. The organism has two nuclei, each containing a prominent chromocenter [Sun 1980]. *Giardia* can be beautifully demonstrated in cytologic specimens.

Cryptosporidiosis

Cryptosporidiosis is usually seen in immunocompromised patients, particularly those with AIDS. It produces a profuse, watery diarrhea. Infection is noninvasive; the organism is free or attached to the apical border of glandular cells. *Cryptosporidium* is a round, basophilic protozoal organism, about 2 to 4 μm in diameter, which may resemble platelets (which tend to clump) or yeasts (which may bud). Although the organisms can be seen with the Papanicolaou stain, they are better appreciated with Diff-Quik [Silverman 1990].

Benign Tumors

A variety of benign tumors and tumor-like conditions can occur in the small bowel [Attanoos 1991]. Tumor-like conditions include Brunner's gland hamartoma, myoepithelial hamartoma, and hamartomatous mucosal polyps (Peutz-Jeghers, or juvenile polyposis, syndrome: autosomal dominant, multiple, generalized hamartomatous polyps of the intestinal tract associated with melanin spots on lips, in the mouth, and on fingers). These lesions would be expected to exfoliate benign-appearing glandular cells, without atypia or mitotic figures. However, dysplastic changes are occasionally seen in Peutz-Jeghers polyps, which can precede malignancy.

Duodenal adenomas are benign epithelial neoplasms that are similar to adenomas occurring in the colon. When multiple, they may be associated with familial adenomatous polyposis coli. As in the colon, adenocarcinomas may arise in the polyps.

Gangliocytic paraganglioma is a tumor that may contain neural elements, ganglion cells, and endocrine cells.

Amyloid

Amyloidosis is usually associated with a clinical history of multiple myeloma, chronic infections, or neuroendocrine tumors, or it may be a primary disease. Amyloid deposits can cause obstruction, bleeding, malabsorption, or can be asymptomatic. Amyloid is a waxy, amorphous material that is extracellular but may be adherent to benign glandular cells [Korat 1988]. To confirm the diagnosis, special stains may be used, eg, Congo red with typical apple-green birefringence [Yang 1995].

63

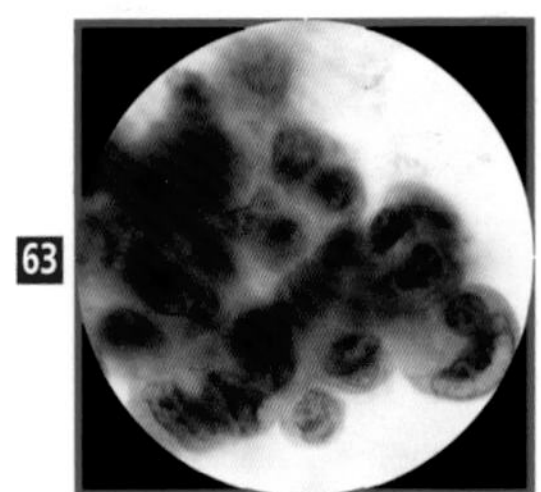

Malignant Tumors

Primary malignancies of the small bowel are unusual. At least half arise in the ileum (mostly carcinoids and malignant lymphomas). Most adenocarcinomas of the small bowel arise in the duodenum, but many actually originate in the extrahepatic biliary tract and involve the duodenum near the ampulla of Vater. Small-bowel adenocarcinomas are of the intestinal type, similar to those occurring in the colon. Adenocarcinomas arising in the ampulla of Vater, bile ducts, and pancreas are morphologically identical and cannot be differentiated on cytologic grounds alone.

Adenocarcinoma

Tumors of the ampulla of Vater or the duodenum are usually well differentiated. The cells are relatively large and are present singly or in small, crowded clusters [63 I9.68]. The nuclei are enlarged and pleomorphic, with increased N/C ratios and irregular nuclear membranes. They are usually hyperchromatic and may have enlarged, multiple, or irregular nucleoli. The cytoplasm is relatively abundant, particularly in well-differentiated tumors, and may show squamoid features, particularly in other than well-differentiated tumors. Anaplastic giant or spindle cells may be seen in some cases.

The differential diagnosis mainly requires distinguishing these tumors, which are often very well-differentiated, from reactive atypia in benign cells, particularly in cells from the biliary tract. For a firm diagnosis of malignancy, numerous cells, including single cells, should be present with the features described above. Important diagnostic features, even in well-differentiated carcinomas, are the presence of irregular nuclear membranes and increased mitotic activity. Also, abnormalities in the arrangement of the cells, ie, loss of polarity, crowding, and piling up, are associated with malignancy.

Malignant Lymphoma

Malignant lymphomas of the GI tract are described on p 349. The differential diagnosis includes metastatic carcinoma, eg, of the breast.

Carcinoid Tumors

Carcinoid tumors, or carcinoids, are potentially malignant neuroendocrine neoplasms; they may behave in a benign fashion or they may be aggressive. Carcinoids are usually single but can be multiple, particularly when part of multiple endocrine neoplasia. Carcinoids are often associated with hormone production and may produce recognizable clinical syndromes, eg, Zollinger–Ellison (ulcerogenic) syndrome due to gastrin production. A wide variety of hormones can be produced, including not only gastrin but also somatostatin, calcitonin, insulin, pancreatic polypeptide, VIP, substance P, and polypeptide YY. More than one hormone is usually produced. The typical carcinoid syndrome associated with serotonin production is rare. More commonly, local disease causes obstruction of the small bowel, with jaundice, pancreatitis, and hemorrhage. Most small-bowel carcinoids occur in the ileum and are of midgut origin. Midgut carcinoids are typically both argentaffin and argyrophil positive. The duodenum is the next most common site of small bowel carcinoid. These are of foregut origin and may be argyrophilic.

Carcinoids characteristically display monomorphic, plasmacytoid cells, singly and in loose aggregates. Spindle-shaped cells may also be seen. Few mitotic figures are present, and there is no necrosis. The nuclei are usually round and monomorphic, with salt-and-pepper chromatin and inconspicuous nucleoli. Naked nuclei are common and may resemble lymphocytes. The cytoplasm is pale, granular, and moderate in amount. Some cells may have neurosecretory granules, which can be demonstrated using special stains. Neurosecretory granules are typically metachromatic and may appear as fine, red, cytoplasmic granules when Diff-Quik stain is used.

Colon and Rectum

Cancers of the colon and rectum are the second leading cause of cancer death in the United States. Most cancers of the gastrointestinal tract are adenocarcinomas. They are thought to progress through a series of morphologically identifiable preinvasive lesions (ie, dysplasia, carcinoma in situ). In theory, using cytologic techniques to screen for colorectal cancer could significantly reduce morbidity and mortality, just as the Pap smear has done for cervical cancer. Unfortunately cytologic techniques do not easily lend themselves to mass screening, because GI endoscopy, which is relatively expensive, is necessary to collect adequate specimens from most intestinal sites. People who have a high risk of developing colorectal carcinoma can be screened in this manner. Screening for occult blood (most cancers bleed) is easy and relatively inexpensive. Unfortunately, testing for occult blood in a random stool specimen from a person on an unmodified diet is essentially worthless, because there are so many false-positive and false-negative results (eg, meat can lead to a false positive). But when used in a prescribed way in people on special diets (meat-free, high-bulk, etc), these tests (eg, Hemoccult®) can usually detect asymptomatic, early colon cancers with few false positives [Winawer 1976a,b]. Blind colonic lavage (ie, enemas) to obtain exfoliative cytologic specimens has been used for diagnosis [Raskin 1964, Rosenberg 1977]. However, the procedure is cumbersome, uncomfortable for the patient, and has lower diagnostic accuracy than colonoscopy [Vilardell 1978], although lavage could be used to complement endoscopy [Rozen 1990].

Risk Factors for Colorectal Cancer

- Ulcerative colitis
- Familial polyposis
- Gardner's syndrome
- History of adenoma
- Family or personal history of colorectal cancer
- In women, a history of breast or genital cancer
- Blood in stool (occult or otherwise)
- Changes in bowel habits

[Bardawil 1990, Fath 1983, Winawer 1978]

About 38,000 new cases of rectal cancer develop each year in the United States alone [Wingo 1995]. Cancers of the rectum can be detected cytologically; cells can be collected by simple rectal examination [Kune 1984, Linehan 1983, Soni 1991]. Most colonic adenocarcinomas arise within reach of the sigmoidoscope and therefore are accessible to tissue biopsy. Colonoscopic cytology is useful in areas beyond the reach of the sigmoidoscope, in differential diagnosis of polyps, evaluation of strictures, screening of high-risk patients (eg, patients with ulcerative colitis), and investigation of iron deficiency anemia [Brandborg 1968a, Forde 1985, Mortensen 1984, J Williams 1988]. Cytology has a potential advantage over endoscopic tissue biopsy in surveying lesions and high-risk patients, because cytologic techniques can be used to sample a relatively large area (~3 cm² vs ≤0.2 cm² for biopsy [Melville 1988]). For example, cytologic techniques could be used to detect an occult carcinoma arising in an adenoma.

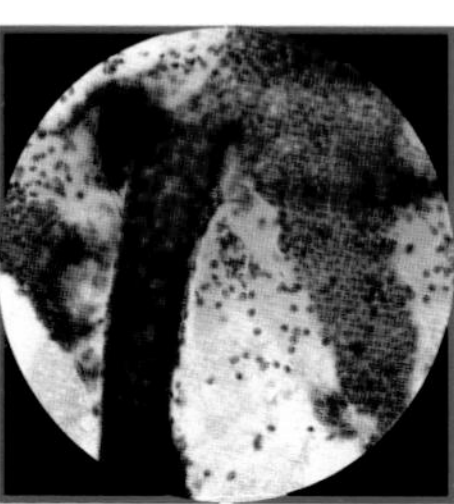

64

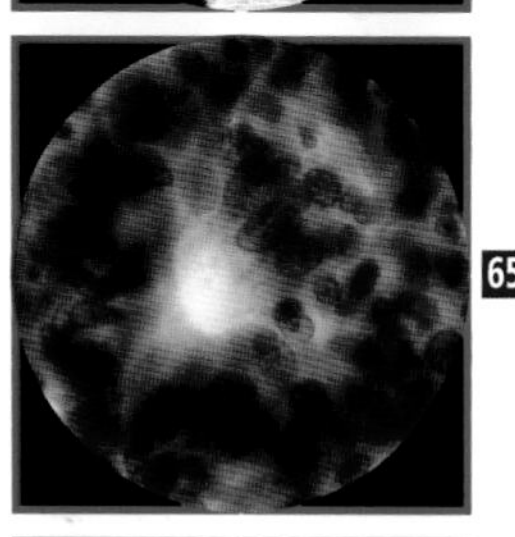

65

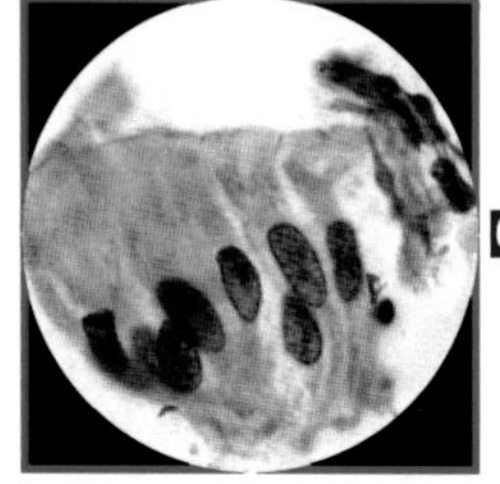

66

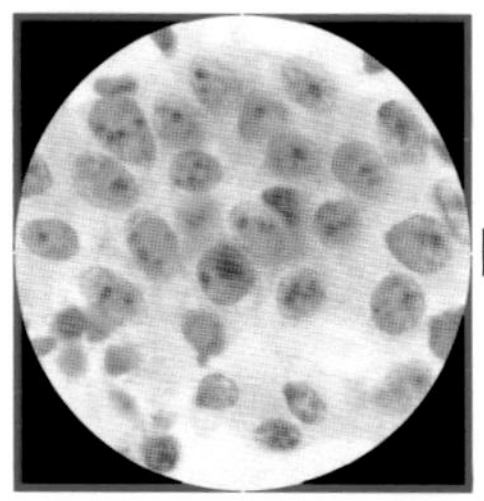

67

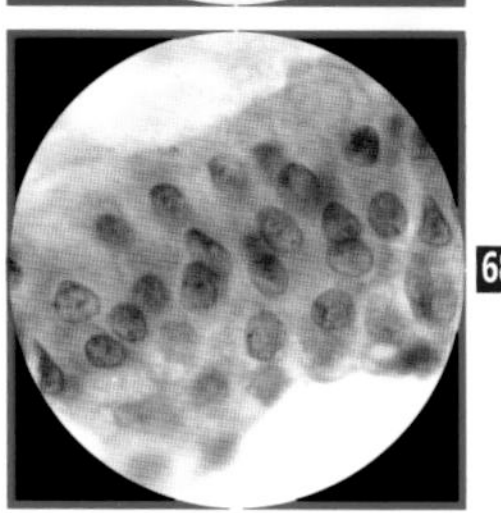

68

The Cells

Histologically, the colorectal mucosa is normally composed of an epithelium that forms straight, nonbranching, test tube–like glands. The epithelium is composed of absorptive cells and is rich in goblet cells [Bader 1952]. Occasionally, lymph follicles with germinal centers may be seen in the tissue.

Cytologically, the cells in brush specimens are exfoliated in relatively large, monolayered sheets with distinct edges. The sheets are cohesive and single cells are sparse. The cells are uniform and orderly, forming a honeycomb arrangement when seen en face and palisades when seen from the side. Well-ordered, partial or complete glandular lumens of the colonic crypts may also be seen [64 I9.69, 65 I9.70, 66 I9.71] [Ehya 1990].

The cells are tall columnar with basal nuclei and apical cytoplasm. The nuclei are round and uniform and have smooth membranes; fine, even chromatin; and inconspicuous nucleoli. Absorptive cells have a prominent striated border and granular cytoplasm [Bader 1952]. The striated border appears as terminal bar–like apical density [66 I9.71] and is a characteristic feature of colorectal cells that is maintained in well-differentiated malignancy. Goblet cells with pale cytoplasm are interspersed among the denser absorptive cells like stars in the sky. Goblet cells are distinguished by the presence of large mucin vacuoles. The background may contain a few neutrophils, lymphocytes (which are sometimes numerous), macrophages, anal squamous cells, mucus, and, possibly, undigested food and debris (caca).

Reactive Cells: Repair/Regeneration

In response to inflammation or ulceration, the colorectal cells, like other epithelial cells, may undergo reactive changes of repair/regeneration, which may mimic malignancy [I9.72, 67 I9.73, 68 I9.74]. The cells increase in size but remain cohesive and orderly [Ehya 1990]. The nuclei also enlarge and may be somewhat irregular, but the N/C ratio remains within normal limits. Although the nucleoli can be prominent, the chromatin is fine in these benign cells. Because reparative changes frequently accompany an ulcer, a dirty background (mimicking a tumor diathesis) is common and is not necessarily evidence of malignancy. Squamous metaplasia with marked reactive atypia can also occur, eg, in diverticulitis, which may be mistaken for squamous cell carcinoma.

Infectious Colitis

Infectious colitis is characterized by the presence of acute or chronic inflammation as well as reactive or degenerated epithelial cells. A specific infectious agent (ova, parasites) can sometimes be identified.

Bacillary Dysentery: Pus, blood, many bacteria [B Chapman 1959].

Amoeba: Entamoeba histolytica, characterized by ingested red blood cells.

Schistosoma: Characterized by spines (see Chapter 5).

Cytomegalovirus: Can affect all areas of the GI tract and is being diagnosed with increasing frequency. CMV is associated with immunosuppression and commonly affects AIDS patients [Meiselman 1985] and transplant patients [Foucar 1981]. CMV may cause severe ulceration and bleeding in the lower GI tract. Diagnostic cells, which are enlarged (cytomegaly), with large intranuclear viral inclusion as well as satellite nuclear and cytoplasmic inclusions, are few and single.

Other: Occasionally, other infectious agents, such as *Blastocystis hominis* [Dellers 1992], may be detected.

Chronic Idiopathic Inflammatory Bowel Disease

Chronic idiopathic inflammatory bowel disease, ie, Crohn's disease and ulcerative colitis, are characterized cytologically by reactive/reparative epithelial cells and an increased number of neutrophils. The term "idiopathic" implies not only that the cause of the disease is unknown but, more importantly, that specific diseases such as amoebic colitis have been excluded. Patients with chronic idiopathic inflammatory bowel disease, particularly those with ulcerative colitis, have an increased risk of developing colorectal adenocarcinomas. Malignant lymphomas, mostly extraintestinal, also occur in these patients [Greenstein 1992].

Ulcerative Colitis

Patients with ulcerative colitis have an increased risk of developing colorectal adenocarcinoma. Although the degree of risk is unknown and has probably been previously overestimated, it is related to the duration and extent of disease [Albert 1989, Fath 1983, Isbell 1988]. Only 1% of all cases of colorectal adenocarcinoma arise in a colitic colon [Isbell 1988]. The cancers tend to be multiple, flat, ulcerative, and infiltrative, although polypoid or nodular tumors can also occur [Isbell 1988]. Previously, it was thought that adenocarcinomas arising in patients with ulcerative colitis were more biologically aggressive. However, survival rates for age-and-stage–matched colonic cancer patients, with and without colitis, are similar. Unfortunately, however, the diagnosis of adenocarcinoma in unscreened colitic patients may be delayed because the symptoms of the two diseases are similar. It is thought that the delay in diagnosis rather than the biology of the tumor is responsible for the advanced stage at diagnosis [Isbell 1988]. Dysplasia is a precancerous change that identifies the population of patients at highest risk for developing cancer [Yardley 1974]. It is important that this high-risk population be screened for evidence of dysplasia and cancer, but cancer surveillance is difficult and expensive, and screening protocols are controversial [Albert 1989, Isbell 1988]. Cytologic techniques offer potential advantages over endoscopic biopsy: they screen a larger area and are potentially able to detect flat, early lesions or lesions obscured by inflammation [Festa 1985]. Cytology may be positive when endoscopic findings, tissue biopsy, or both are negative [S Katz 1977]. However, combining cytologic and histologic techniques yields the highest diagnostic sensitivity and specificity [Granqvist 1980].

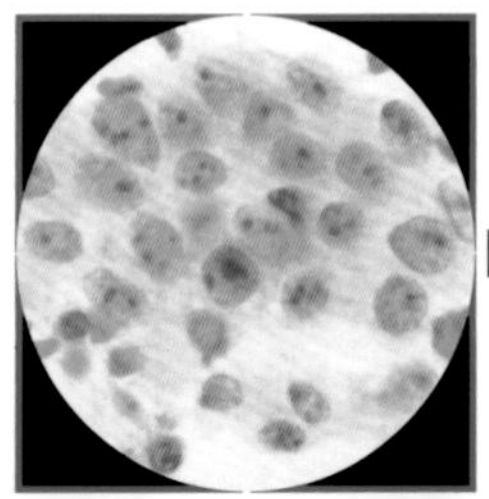
69

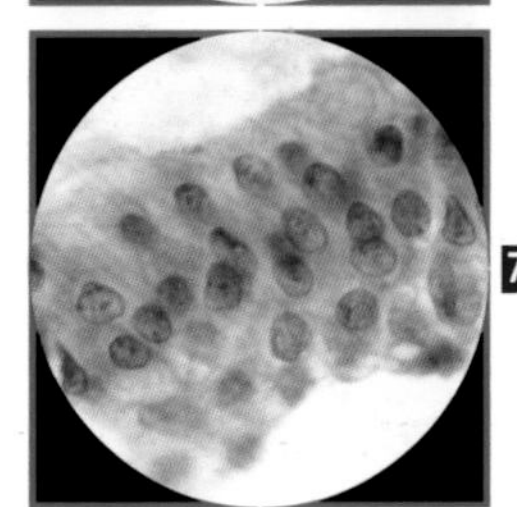
70

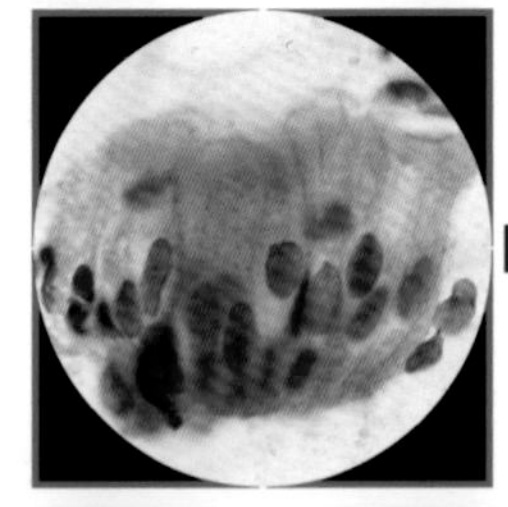
71

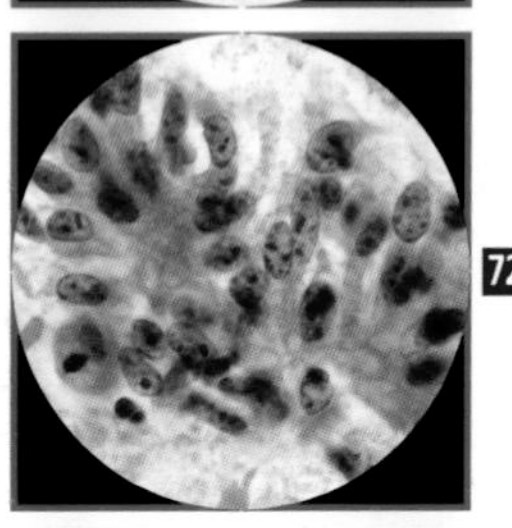
72

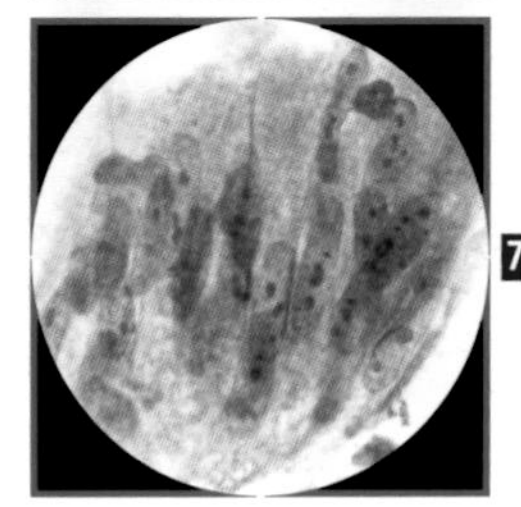
73

The cytology of inflammatory bowel disease depends on the lesions present and therefore varies from essentially normal (for quiescent disease in remission) to reactive changes in active disease, to dysplasia or cancer. However, dysplasia is seldom observed unless the patient has had the disease for several years [Festa 1985].

Large groups of cells, pus, blood, and bacteria are seen in active disease [Boddington 1956]. Evidence of epithelial repair or regeneration may also be seen [69 I9.73, 70 I9.74] [B Chapman 1959]. The cells can show pronounced enlargement of both nucleus and cytoplasm, with nuclear diameters commonly two times normal size [Galambos 1956]. The chromatin varies from fine to coarse, and nucleoli can be prominent. Occasionally, multinuclear giant epithelial cells, with nuclei up to five times normal diameter and large nucleoli can be seen [Boddington 1956, Galambos 1956]. Such changes seem to correlate with the severity of the disease rather than its chronicity, and in most instances they disappear after the ulcerative colitis heals.

Adenoma

Benign neoplastic growths, or adenomas, include adenomatous polyps [72 I9.76] and villous adenomas [73 I9.77] but not hyperplastic polyps [71 I9.75]. Adenomas are very common in the colon, but cytologic samples are rarely collected from adenomas because the lesions are usually removed when discovered. However, cytology could play an important role in the diagnosis of occult carcinoma arising in one of these lesions.

Adenomas can grow as polyps or sessile lesions. Histologically, they can be tubular, tubulovillous, or villous. Patients with adenomas have an increased risk of developing adenocarcinoma. Adenomas have malignant potential, although only a minority of adenomas actually give rise to cancer [Morson 1974]. The adenoma–carcinoma sequence is generally regarded as the primary pathway for the histogenesis of exophytic colorectal carcinomas [Morson 1974]. Infiltrative cancers, which account for approximately 40% of cases, more often appear to arise de novo in flat mucosa [Bedenne 1992]. Also, cancers in patients with inflammatory bowel disease, particularly ulcerative colitis, arise from flat, dysplastic lesions, but only affect a small number of patients.

Adenomas smaller than 1 cm in diameter rarely contain cancer. The risk increases as the size increases: about half of adenomas larger than 2 cm in diameter contain cancer [Morson 1974]. Even allowing for their generally larger size, sessile villous adenomas carry a significantly greater risk of harboring cancer (5–10 times greater) than adenomatous polyps [Morson 1974]. Dysplasia in an adenoma is probably a key risk factor for carcinoma; the more severe the dysplasia, the greater the risk [Morson 1974]. Other important risk factors include age, sex, site, environmental influences, and, possibly, genetic susceptibility [Morson 1974].

The cytology of various benign adenomas is similar, and the histologic growth pattern can rarely be predicted cytologically [Bardawil 1990, Ehya 1990]. Occasionally, a papillary structure may be seen, suggesting villous adenoma [Ehya 1990].

The cells exfoliate in cohesive, crowded sheets of relatively uniform cells. The cells are tall columnar, usually with granular cytoplasm. Goblet cells and mucin are typically decreased but not necessarily absent. The nuclear features are similar to those in mild dysplasia. The nuclei are enlarged, oval to elongated, and somewhat irregular. They are hyperchromatic and piled up, with some loss of polarity and an increased N/C ratio. Nucleoli vary from inconspicuous to prominent. Mitotic figures can be seen, but none are abnormal. No diathesis is present.

Any degree of neoplastic change, from low-grade dysplasia to invasive carcinoma, can be seen in these polyps. Dysplasia is characterized by nuclear enlargement, irregularity, loss of polarity, and prominent nucleoli. However, cell cohesiveness and uniformity are relatively maintained [Ehya 1990]. The cytologic differential diagnosis of well-differentiated invasive adenocarcinoma, which must be distinguished from benign but dysplastic adenoma, may be difficult or impossible in some cases [Galambos 1962]. However, in many cases, the distinction between benign and malignant can be made [Tidbury 1990]. The primary cytologic features to evaluate are cellularity, cohesion, and polarity. Compared with a benign adenoma, adenocarcinoma is characterized by more cells, more atypia, less cohesion (increased single cells), and loss of polarity (ie, disorderly arrangements).

Adenocarcinoma

Most adenocarcinomas of the GI tract, including the colorectum, arise in premalignant lesions or conditions, particularly in adenomas. Colorectal adenocarcinomas are usually moderately to well differentiated [74 I9.81].

Cytologically, the smears tend to be cellular. An increase in the number of single atypical cells is particularly characteristic of outspoken cancer. Small, crowded, overlapped groups of disorderly cells with loss of nuclear polarity are seen, and groups of cells may form microacinar, glandular arrangements. The cells vary from tall columnar with elongated, cigar-shaped nuclei (when well differentiated) to rounded cells with rounded nuclei (when poorly differentiated) [75 I9.78, 76 I9.79, 77 I9.80]. Nuclear atypia depends on the degree of differentiation. The nuclei are generally eccentrically located, pleomorphic, and enlarged [Bardawil 1990]. The nuclear membranes are irregular [Kline 1976]. The chromatin is generally dark and may be coarse and irregular. Prominent nucleoli are characteristic.

74
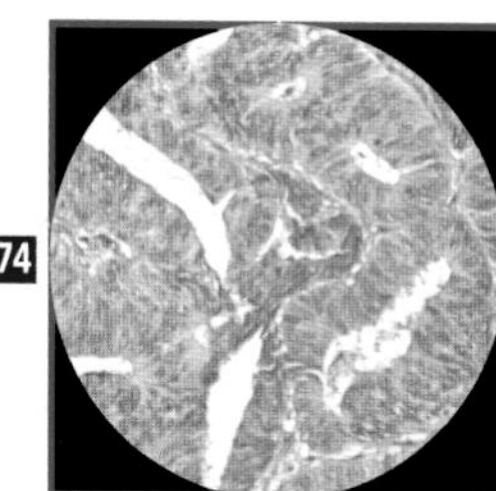

75
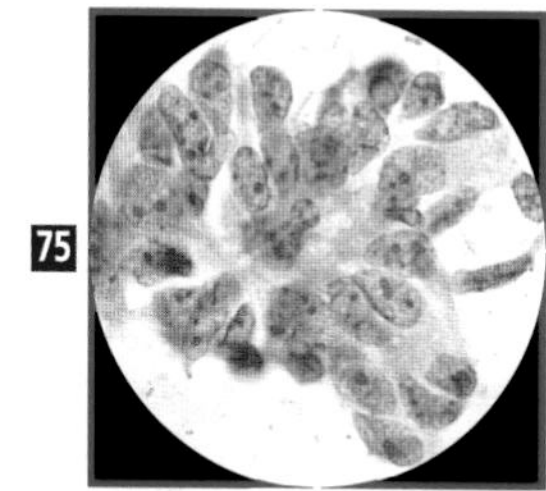

76
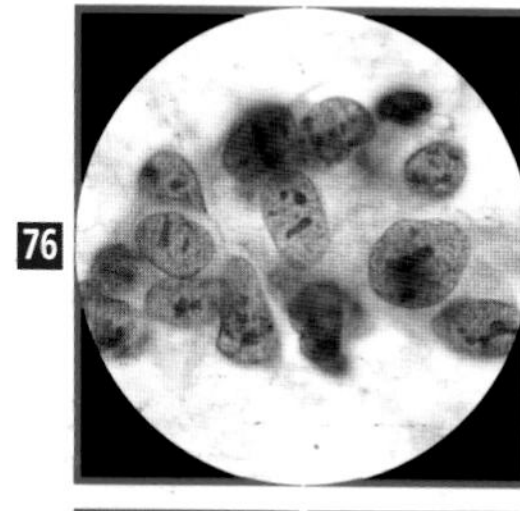

77
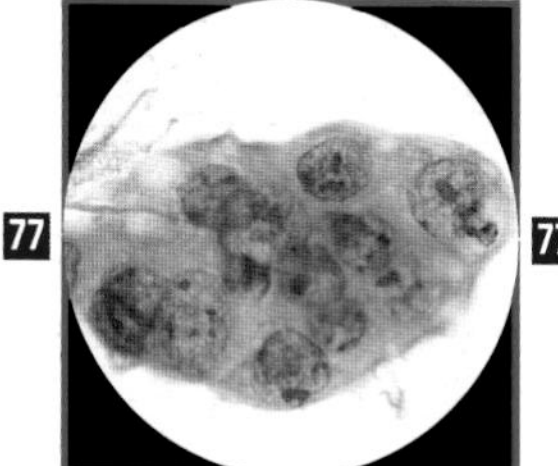
77

The cytoplasm is granular and basophilic with variable degrees of mucin vacuolization. A characteristic feature, particularly of better-differentiated tumors, is maintenance of the striated border, resulting in a terminal-bar–like density on the apical border of malignant cells [77 I9.80].

Signet ring cells may be seen in some cases [Nakahara 1992]. They may form small clusters but are predominantly single. The background shows a diathesis characteristic of invasive carcinoma. Some cases show abundant mucus in the background (colloid or mucinous carcinomas).

Ulcerated lesions may result in excessive necrotic debris, which masks the diagnostic cells. Also, differentiating between severe dysplasia and well-differentiated adenocarcinoma may be difficult or impossible. Loss of cohesion and nuclear polarity suggest a frankly malignant process (see "Ulcerative Colitis," p 354) [Bardawil 1990, Ehya 1990]. Some tumors produce abundant mucin and may cause pseudomyxoma peritonei. The differential diagnosis also includes other tumors, eg, prostatic carcinoma [Kune 1984].

Dysplasia and Carcinoma In Situ

Adenocarcinoma of the large intestine is thought to be preceded by various degrees of dysplasia. The dysplastic changes in inflammatory bowel disease are the prototype of similar changes described in the glandular epithelium of Barrett's esophagus and the stomach [Riddell 1983]. (See T9.2 and T9.6.)

In low-grade dysplasia, the cells are relatively orderly and cohesive and form flat sheets, sometimes with glandular acini. Although the nuclei are enlarged, they show little pleomorphism and the nuclear membrane remains smooth. The chromatin is granular and evenly distributed. Nucleoli may be seen in some cells [Festa 1985].

As dysplasia becomes increasingly severe, the number of single cells increases [Festa 1985]. The nuclei become more variable in size, with increased N/C ratios, loss of polarity, and irregularity of the nuclear membranes [Melville 1988]. The chromatin can vary from fine to coarse. Nucleoli can be prominent or multiple. Mitotic figures may be frequent.

Adenocarcinoma is characterized by more cells—more single cells and more groups of cells that are loosely cohesive and disorderly, with architectural anarchy [Melville 1988]. The fully malignant cells are more pleomorphic than in dysplasia, with enlarged, hyperchromatic nuclei; coarse, irregular chromatin; and prominent, multiple, or irregular nucleoli. Abnormal mitotic figures may be seen.

Low-grade dysplasia may be difficult to distinguish from reactive changes [Granqvist 1980], while high-grade dysplasia may be difficult to distinguish from cancer. Nuclear enlargement, pleomorphism, prominent nucleoli, mitotic figures, and cytoplasmic mucin depletion are common characteristics of both dysplastic and regenerative epithelium [M Cook 1975]. Cellular cohesion, regular nuclear membranes, homogeneous chromatin, and a flat, sheet-like arrangement of cells are characteristics that suggest a benign process. Single cells; pronounced pleomorphism; dense, coarse chromatin; very large nucleoli; atypical mitotic figures; and very disorderly, crowded clusters of cells suggest a malignant process [Cook 1975, Festa 1985, Melville 1988].

Carcinoid

Carcinoid tumors commonly arise in the appendix but are rarely diagnosed by exfoliative cytology. However, diagnostic cells can be obtained by endoscopic fine needle aspiration biopsy (see "Small Intestine," p 351).

Malignant Lymphoma

Malignant lymphoma may involve the large intestine either as a primary or secondary tumor. No true tissue aggregates are formed, and the diathesis associated with ordinary adenocarcinoma is usually lacking. (See "Stomach," p 341, for further discussion.)

Sarcoma

Soft tissue sarcomas, particularly leiomyosarcoma, occur rarely in the bowel wall [78 I9.82, 79 I9.83]. They are more amenable to diagnosis by endoscopic fine needle aspiration biopsy than by surface exfoliative cytology.

78
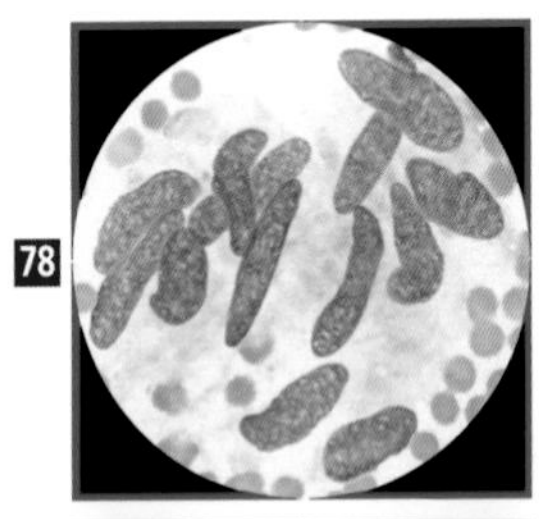

79
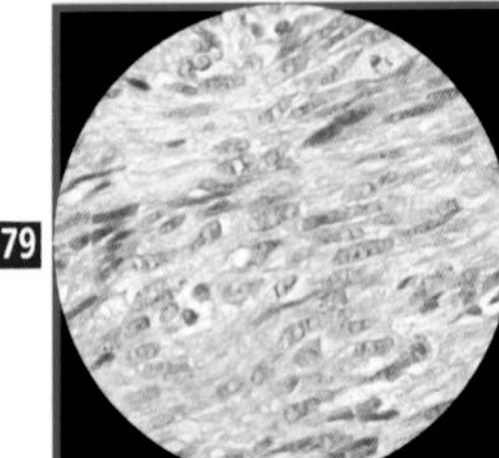

Anal Canal

The anal canal is about 3 to 4 cm in length and extends from the rectum to the perineal skin. Anal smears are easily obtainable and can be used to detect anal condylomas, dysplasia, and cancers [Fenger 1991].

The Cells

Beginning at the anorectal junction, the colonic-type glandular epithelium changes into a transitional epithelium and finally into a keratinized or nonkeratinized squamous epithelium, externally. Anal glands, which originate in cloacogenic epithelium, open into the anal canal through long tubular anal ducts. Anal ducts are lined by transitional epithelium but also contain mucus and goblet cells. Cloacogenic, or transitional, epithelium is light microscopically similar to that occurring in the urinary bladder, but ultrastructurally is more closely related to squamous epithelium. Any ultrastructural similarities to transitional epithelium are considered vestigial [J Gillespie 1978].

Anal Cancers

Anal cancer accounts for only about 2% of all colorectal malignancies. Most carcinomas of the anal canal are squamous cell carcinomas [Boman 1984], and the great majority of those are nonkeratinizing [Morson 1968]. Keratinizing squamous cell carcinoma is more likely to arise in the anal margin or the perianal skin [Fenger 1988]. Typical colonic-type adenocarcinomas commonly involve the anal canal, but most cases arise in the mucosa of the rectum and involve the anal canal by extension. In addition, a number of anal cancers, about 20% [Gillespie 1978], have been classified as cloacogenic (basaloid or transitional) carcinomas. These tumors are thought to be essentially epidermoid in nature, but they can manifest a variety of morphologies (keratinizing squamous cell carcinoma, nonkeratinizing squamous, basaloid, mucinous, and adenoid cystic carcinomas) and could simply be designated "anal carcinoma." A variety of rare tumors, including anal duct carcinoma, Paget's disease, melanoma, verrucous carcinoma, soft tissue tumors, and metastases, can also involve the anal canal. Malignant lymphomas have been described in AIDS patients.

Cancers of the anal area are relatively rare. Each type accounts for, at most, only a small percentage of all colorectal cancers. About three fourths of these cancers develop in the anal canal, and the remainder occur in the perianal area. The most common symptoms are bleeding, pain, a mass, or pruritus. However, a number of patients are asymptomatic. Cytologic techniques that can be used to detect lesions of the anal canal include direct scraping (using saline-moistened Dacron® or cotton swabs or wooden spatulas) or simply a gloved finger [Frazer 1986, Soni 1991]. A satisfactory smear should show an assessable number of reasonably well-preserved squamous, metaplastic, or glandular cells [Frazer 1986, Haye 1988].

Squamous Cell Carcinoma

Squamous cell carcinoma often arises in a preexisting lesion, eg, fistulae, long-standing hemorrhoids, chronic inflammation (including inflammatory bowel disease), radiation fibrosis, or leukoplakia. The incidence of anal cancer has increased recently, particularly among homosexual men [Daling 1987]. Receptive anal intercourse is a risk factor. The tumors are probably preceded by squamous dysplasia and carcinoma in situ.

Squamous cell carcinoma of the anal canal is also associated with a history of genital warts. Using sensitive techniques, human papilloma virus (HPV) DNA can be detected in up to 85% of anal carcinomas [Duggan 1991], which suggests that HPV plays a carcinogenic role [Melbye 1990]. HIV infection, certain other genital infections (eg, herpes, chlamydia), and cigarette smoking are also associated with the development of anal cancer or its precursors [Daling 1987, Frazer 1986, Palefsky 1990]. The cytology of squamous cell carcinoma of the anal canal is similar to that of other squamous cell carcinomas and varies from well to poorly differentiated. An extremely well-differentiated variant, verrucous carcinoma, also occurs in the anorectal region.

Condyloma, Dysplasia, and Carcinoma In Situ

Condylomas occur in the skin of the perineum and the squamous mucosa of the anal canal [Duggan 1989] and can be detected cytologically [Frazer 1986, Medley 1984, Melbye 1990]. The diagnostic features of anal condyloma are similar to those described in the Pap smear [Palefsky 1990], although the cytologic material may more closely resemble cells obtained from the vulva [Haye 1988]. Koilocytes (cytoplasmic halos, nuclear atypia) are considered pathognomonic but may be sparse [De Ruiter 1994, Haye 1988]. Dyskeratocytes as well as dysplastic squamous cells are more common but less specific. As in the uterine cervix, subclinical condylomas that are not grossly visible may be detected by cytologic techniques [De Ruiter 1994, Haye 1988].

Squamous dysplasia and carcinoma in situ (anal intraepithelial neoplasia or lesion) also occurs in this area as a precursor to squamous cell carcinomas and can be detected cytologically [De Ruiter 1994, Fenger 1991, Frazer 1986, Nash 1986]. The criteria for diagnosing anal intraepithelial neoplasia are also similar to those used to diagnose dysplasia and carcinoma in situ in the Pap smear: large, dark nuclei with elevated N/C ratios, irregular nuclear shape, hyperchromasia, and coarse chromatin [De Ruiter 1994].

Cloacogenic Carcinoma

Cloacogenic carcinoma is rare and occurs mostly in white males. The tumors are morphologically variable. Well-differentiated cloacogenic carcinoma bears a resemblance to transitional cell carcinoma of the bladder. The basaloid variant, which resembles cutaneous basal cell carcinoma, has a relatively good prognosis when well differentiated, even if lymph nodes are involved [Morson 1968]. However, poorly differentiated basaloid tumors have a very poor prognosis. True basal cell carcinoma of the hair-bearing perianal skin can occur but is rare. Squamous, mucoepidermoid, adenoid cystic, and pleomorphic morphologies can also be seen.

Small Cell Carcinoma

Although some include this tumor in the category of cloacogenic carcinoma, anal small-cell carcinomas, like their pulmonary counterparts, are highly aggressive neoplasms that may show signs of endocrine differentiation [Fenger 1988].

Anal Duct Carcinoma

Anal duct carcinoma is also rare. These tumors are well-differentiated mucus-producing, colloid carcinomas characterized by slow growth, with frequent recurrences and late metastases to inguinal lymph nodes.

Melanoma

Malignant melanoma arises from the squamous mucosa of the anus only rarely, but it is highly aggressive. These tumors may be misdiagnosed clinically as hemorrhoids or polyps.

Carcinoid

The rectum is the third most common site of GI carcinoids (the appendix and ileum are first and second). Rectal carcinoid tumors usually behave in a benign fashion. They are of hindgut origin and are variably positive with argentaffin or argyrophil silver stains.

Paget's Disease

Anal Paget's disease occurs in the perianal region but may extend up the anal canal. Clinically, signs and symptoms can range from none to florid eczema. The malignancy could arise in perianal apocrine glands or spread from a rectal adenocarcinoma. In contrast with Paget's disease of the breast, only about 50% of cases of anal Paget's disease have an underlying malignancy [Fenger 1991]. Mucin-containing malignant cells are characteristic, but histologic sampling is needed to exclude ordinary adenocarcinoma.

Extrahepatic Biliary Tract

Exfoliative cytology of the extrahepatic biliary tract, including the ampulla of Vater, common bile duct, pancreatic duct, and gallbladder, is becoming increasingly important for a variety of reasons. Benign and malignant biliary tract disease may be clinically and radiologically indistinguishable. Even if stones are detected, malignancy is not excluded [Howell 1988, Wanebo 1975]. Surgery in this area is difficult and may result in significant complications. In a significant number of patients undergoing laparotomy for clinical biliary tract obstruction (as many as one third of cases [Wanebo 1975]), the correct diagnosis of malignant disease is not made at the first surgery. Cytologic examination can not only aid in the diagnosis but can spare the patient unnecessary surgery.

In the past, duodenal drainage specimens, often with secretin stimulation to increase exfoliation of cells [Kline 1978,

Lemon 1949, McNeer 1949, Nieburgs 1962, Nundy 1974, Orell 1972, Raskin 1958, Wenger 1958], were obtained for diagnosis. However, the procedure is difficult to perform and uncomfortable for the patient. Material for cytologic examination can also be obtained from T tubes or drains [Cressman 1977, Dreiling 1960, Goldstein 1968, Lumsden 1986, Muro 1983]. Unfortunately, false-positive and false-negative diagnoses are relatively common. Poor specimens are likely and may be caused by exfoliation of too few malignant cells, reactive atypia due to inflammation and irritation, and artifacts due to digestive secretions [Soudah 1989]. Thus, drainage specimens are of limited use in the diagnosis of pancreaticobiliary carcinoma [Fitzgerald 1978, Kasugai 1978].

Techniques are now available for obtaining a more direct sampling of cells [Endo 1974, Floyd 1985, Harell 1981, Howell 1988, Kurzawinski 1993, Vilmann 1992]. These include endoscopic retrograde cholangiopancreatography (ERCP) [Cotton 1977, Ferrari 1994, Goodale 1981, Hatfield 1974,1976, Ihre 1978, Kameya 1981, Kasugai 1978, Nishimura 1973, Roberts-Thomson 1979, Rupp 1990, Sawada 1989] and percutaneous transhepatic cholangiography (PTC) [Brambs 1988, Elyaderani 1980, Klavins 1964, Mendez 1980, Nakaizumi 1992]. Intraoperative exfoliative cytology can be used to detect lesions of the gallbladder [Ishikawa 1988] and pancreaticobiliary tract [Bowden 1959, Ishikawa 1992, R Rosen 1968]. Similarly, cytologic specimens can be obtained during laparoscopy [Verma 1982] or minilaparotomy procedures [Wertlake 1976]. Endoscopically obtained exfoliative cytology is less sensitive than fine needle aspiration biopsy in the diagnosis of pancreatic cancer [Mitchell 1985]. (Percutaneous fine needle aspiration biopsy of the pancreas is discussed in Chapter 24.)

Bile, pancreatic, and duodenal juice are fragile cytologic specimens [Cobb 1985]. They should be submitted fresh and processed without delay to prevent degeneration and autolysis. Collecting and sending the specimen to the laboratory on ice and using a refrigerated centrifuge if available may help retard cellular degeneration [Kline 1978, Wertlake 1976, Yamada 1984]. In patients with external drains, specimens should be obtained directly from the catheter rather than the collection bag. Direct brushings provide richer, better-preserved cellular specimens [Osnes 1975]. On the other hand, one cannot expect to obtain diagnostic cells by brushing unless the lesion involves the mucosal surface and is directly sampled [Osnes 1979].

The Cells

The cells of the pancreatic ducts and biliary tract are cytologically similar [Kurzawinski 1993]. The specimens are often of low cellularity. Cohesive, monolayered sheets of medium-sized columnar cells are obtained [80 I9.84, 81 I9.85]. The cells form regular, honeycomb-like arrangements when seen *en face* and line up in orderly palisades when seen from the side. Single cells

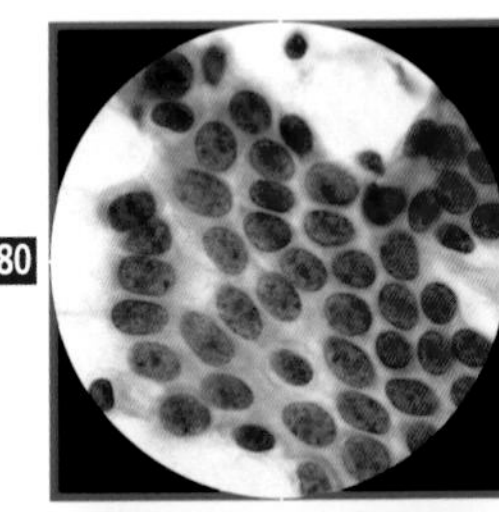
80

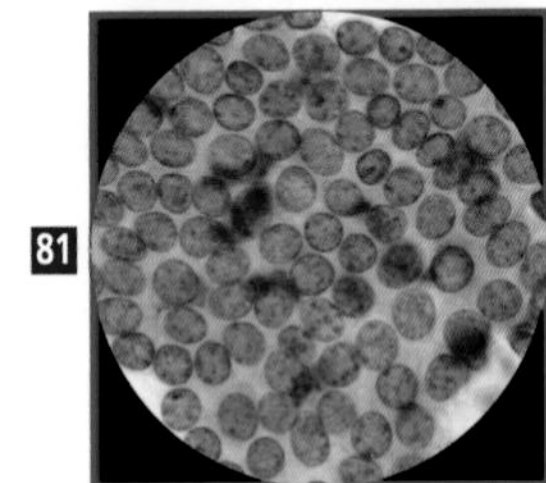
81

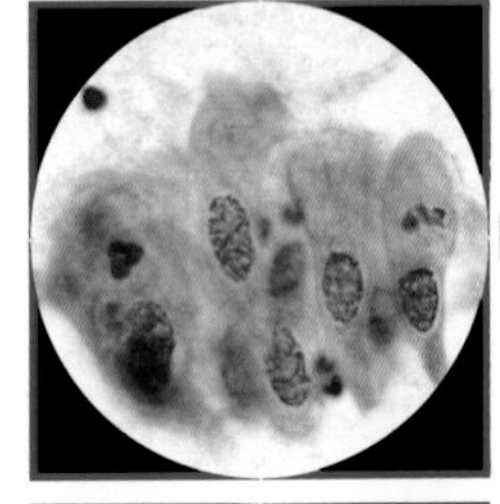
82

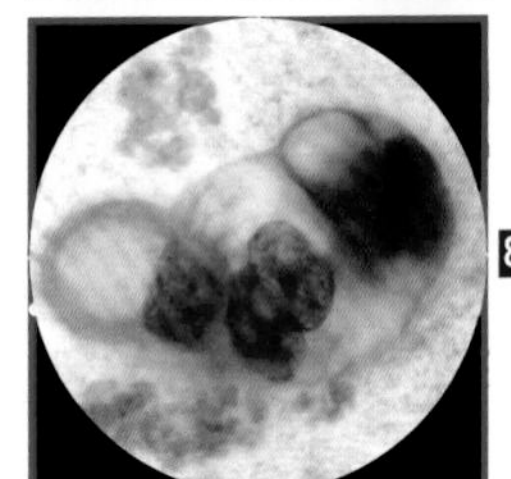
83

tend to become more rounded compared with their columnar shape in tissue. The nuclei are round to oval and "basally" located (ie, they show nucleocytoplasmic polarity). The nuclei have smooth membranes; fine, evenly distributed chromatin; and may have small nucleoli. Mitotic figures are not seen in normal cells [Rupp 1990]. The cytoplasm is pale, delicate, and moderately abundant. Goblet cells can also be seen [Kurzawinski 1993]. Golden brown, granular bile pigment is commonly present in the background.

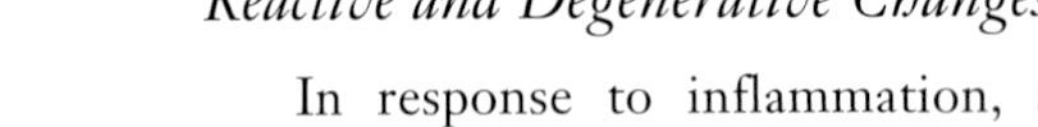

Reactive and Degenerative Changes

In response to inflammation, stones, manipulation, instrumentation, or catheters, the biliary tract epithelium may undergo significant reactive changes (hyperplasia, regeneration, degeneration), which can be suggestive of malignancy [82 I9.86, 83 I9.92] [Kurzawinski 1993, Rupp 1990]. Benign atypical cells can show marked variation in nuclear size, and enlargement of up to four or five times normal size may occur [Rupp 1990]. Hyperchromasia and degenerative changes of the chromatin may be seen. Nucleoli can become prominent and may be single or multiple. Normal mitotic figures can be seen in benign reactive cells. Cells deriving from a reparative process or squamous metaplasia as well as normal cells can all be present in reactive conditions.

Degenerative changes consisting of nuclear pyknosis, karyorrhexis, or cytoplasmic coagulation (in which the cytoplasm becomes dense and eosinophilic) are common, particularly in drainage material or pancreatitis, but can also occur in cancer [Hatfield 1976, Smithies 1977]. Degenerative changes can mimic malignancy. Degenerated cells are usually single but are occasionally found in sheets [Hatfield 1976]. Cellular degeneration occurs rapidly in duodenal juice, due to enzymatic digestion [Hatfield 1976], and in bile-stained material [Gibbs 1983]. Occasionally, "pencil" cells, which are long and thin [Evett 1964, Nishimura 1973]), or "matchstick" cells, which are elongated with bulging basal nuclei [Smithies 1977]), can also be seen. Nuclear irregularity, with angular nuclear edges, projections, and notches (ie, crenation), can result from degeneration. (However, tulip- or popcorn-like nuclear membrane irregularities or nuclear grooves are uncommon in benign disease and suggest malignancy [Mitchell 1985].) These benign nuclear abnormalities are often associated with other signs of degeneration, such as loss of nuclear detail and evidence of cytoplasmic degeneration, eg, eosinophilia [Mitchell 1985].

To help exclude malignancy, look for similar atypical changes in adjacent cells that are clearly benign [Kameya 1981]. In contrast with cancer, reactive cells occur in well-ordered, cohesive clusters or sheets, with minimal nuclear crowding or overlap [Kline 1978, Layfield 1995], and have relatively abundant cytoplasm (thus, normal N/C ratios), smooth nuclear membranes, and less abnormal chromatin.

Inflammatory Diseases

A variety of conditions, including cholangitis, pancreatitis, and cholecystitis as well as lithiasis, can be associated with inflammation and inflammatory changes. In addition to the reactive or degenerative epithelial changes described above, the smear may show evidence of inflammation, including neutrophils, macrophages, and, sometimes, specific organisms or cellular changes associated with viral infection (eg, cytomegalovirus [Rupp 1990]).

Benign Tumors

Granular cell tumor, which is a relatively rare, benign neoplasm, may cause abdominal pain or biliary obstruction and strictures mimicking malignancy [Eisen 1991]. Granular cell tumor of the bile duct is more common in blacks, young adults, and, particularly, females. Cytologic samples would be expected to show large single cells with coarsely granular cytoplasm due to lysosomes. The nuclei are usually small, central, and bland but occasionally show marked atypia. Because granular cell tumors grow in the submucosa, they are unlikely to be diagnosed by exfoliative cytology unless ulcerated. However, the tumor may also be associated with striking epithelial hyperplasia with cytologic atypia, which could result in an erroneous diagnosis of cholangiocarcinoma [Eisen 1991].

Several other benign or low-grade malignant tumors, including islet cell tumors, carcinoids [Dei Tos 1993], paragangliomas, and Brunner's gland neoplasms, can occur in and around the biliary tract. These typically grow in a submucosal location, which makes diagnosis by exfoliative cytology difficult.

Malignant Tumors

If the tumor can be directly visualized, exfoliative cytology is diagnostic in a high percentage of cases; if not, cytology is less accurate [Blackstone 1977, Cohn 1976]. In general, the further the tumor is from the site at which the specimen is taken, the less sensitive the cytologic diagnosis (ie, increased distance, decreased sensitivity) [DiMagno 1977a,b]. Also, the tumor usually must infiltrate into the ductal system or duodenum to be diagnosed by exfoliative cytology [Bourke 1972]. If the tumor is causing extrinsic compression of the ducts, exfoliative cytologic techniques may result in false negatives [Cobb 1985]. False negatives can also be due to poor sampling, enzymatic digestion of cells, fibrotic stenosis of ducts, submucosal tumor growth, improper specimen collection or processing, and very well-differentiated tumors [Cobb 1985, Ferrari 1994, Mohandas 1994]. False-positive diagnoses are related primarily to the difficulty of distinguishing malignancy from inflammatory or degenerative changes, particularly in duodenal aspirates [DiMagno 1977b]. A positive cytologic result on bile obtained directly from the biliary tract, together with characteristic findings on percutaneous transhepatic cholangiography (PTC) or endoscopic retrograde cholangiopancreatography (ERCP), is reliable in the diagnosis and localization of biliary tract carcinomas [I9.91] [Cobb 1985]. Flow cytometry may help in the diagnosis [Ryan 1994].

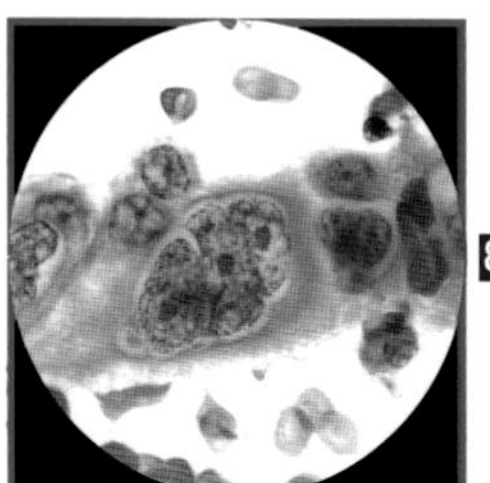
84

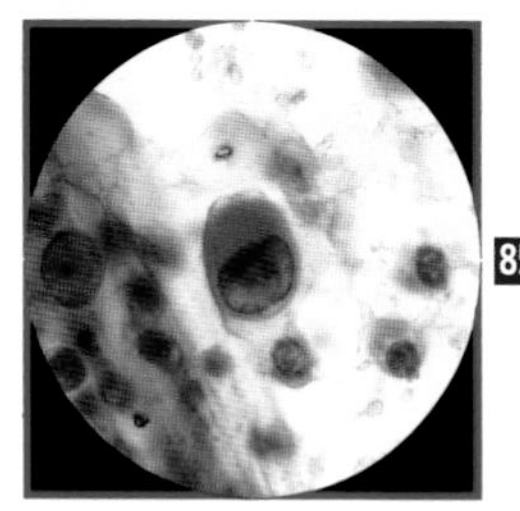
85

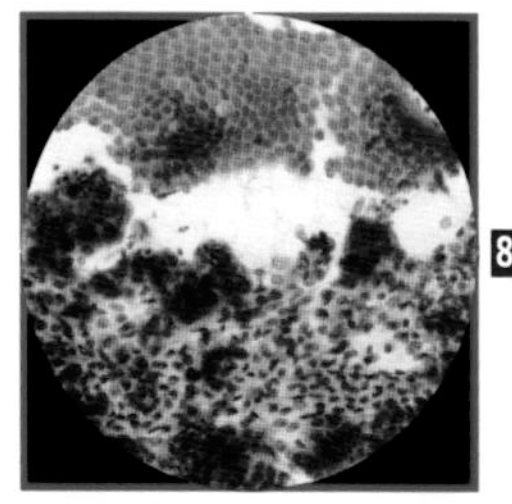
86

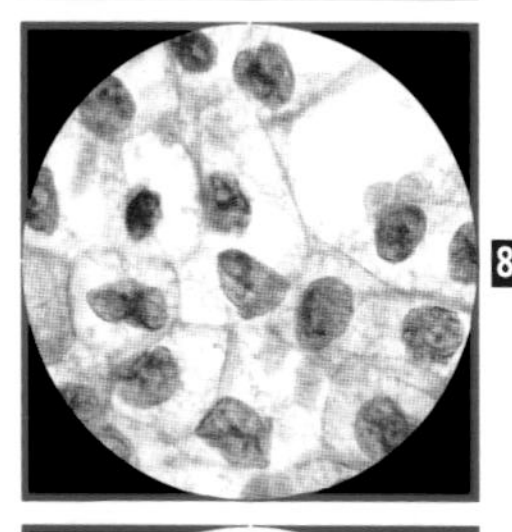
87

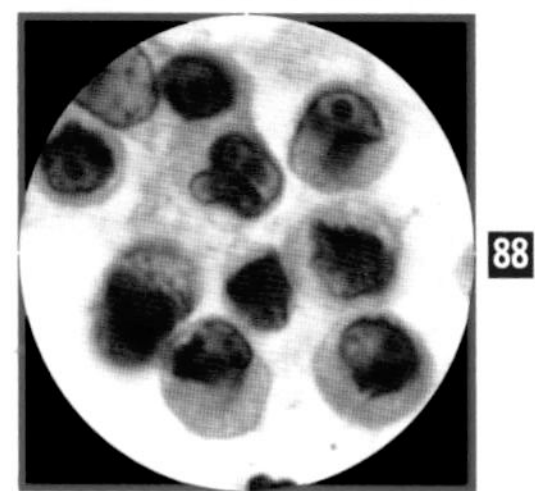
88

Unfortunately, most tumors are relatively large and far advanced by the time they are diagnosed [Wanebo 1975], but even small cancers may be lethal [Yamada 1984]. Cytologic techniques can be used to diagnose cancers of the pancreaticoduodenal and biliary tracts that are too small to be visualized by radiologic, endoscopic, or other diagnostic methods [Yamada 1984].

Carcinomas arising anywhere in the pancreaticobiliary ductal-type epithelium, including the gallbladder, are morphologically similar, and the origin of the tumor cannot be identified from cell samples alone [Cobb 1985, Floyd 1985, Kurzawinski 1993]. Most of these cancers show glandular differentiation, but squamoid features are also common, particularly in tumors that are other than well differentiated. In fact, combined adenosquamous differentiation is a characteristic feature of neoplasms arising in this type of epithelium [84 I9.89, 85 I9.90] [Raskin 1958]. Pure squamous cell carcinoma is rare.

Malignant cells are usually poorly cohesive, with an increase in the number of single atypical cells [86 I9.87, 87 I9.88, 84 I9.89, 85 I9.90, I9.93, 88 I9.94] [Layfield 1995]. Three-dimensional cell clusters are crowded, piled up, and show cellular molding and loss of polarity [86 I9.87]. Glandular-acinar structures may occur in better-differentiated tumors [Rupp 1990]. Cells in endoscopic aspirates are more likely to be in papillary groups than they are in fine needle aspiration biopsy [Mitchell 1985]. Cell-in-cell patterns may be seen in less differentiated neoplasms. In most cases, the nuclei are enlarged and pleomorphic, with high N/C ratios; irregular nuclear borders; irregular, coarse chromatin; and prominent nucleoli [84 I9.89, 88 I9.94] [Cobb 1985, Howell 1988, Kurzawinski 1993, Layfield 1995]. Adjacent nuclei may mold one another [Nakajima 1994]. Cells from endoscopic specimens may have more uniform nuclei than in fine needle aspiration biopsy [Mitchell 1985]. Abnormal mitotic figures indicating malignancy may be seen. The cytoplasm varies from delicate and vacuolated [87 I9.88, 88 I8.94] to dense and squamoid [84 I8.89, 85 I8.90]. In the background, blood, bile, inflammation, cells with degenerated nuclei, and granular necrotic debris may be seen. These findings should trigger a careful search for tumor cells [Bourke 1972, Nakajima 1994, Roberts-Thomson 1979]. However, a similar background can also be found in smears from patients with other forms of cholestatic jaundice, eg, gallstones in the common bile duct (choledocholithiasis) [Bourke 1972]. Cellular necrosis is more common in exfoliative than in aspiration biliary cytology, perhaps due to enzymatic digestion of the cells [I9.93, 88 I9.94] [Mitchell 1985].

Signet ring cells may be found in some cases [Nieburgs 1962]. Malignant giant cells and spindle cells may be present in some poorly differentiated tumors and can suggest a pleomorphic or spindle cell sarcoma. Papillary groups of neoplastic cells suggest a diagnosis of papillary carcinoma of the bile duct [Ahsan 1988]. The cells in these groups may be particularly bland, but because such architectural arrangements are abnormal, the mere presence of papillary groups suggests a papillary neoplasm. However, the frond-like appearance of a villous adenoma, which can occur in the duodenum, may be very similar cytologically [Howell 1988]. Also, papillary mucinous cystadenocarcinoma as well as solid and papillary adenocarcinoma of the pancreas must be included in the differential diagnosis of papillae.

Pancreaticobiliary tumors, particularly when detected early (eg, periampullary lesions may lead to early obstructive jaundice), can sometimes be extremely well-differentiated, or "minimal deviation," tumors [Nishimura 1973]. The cells may appear deceptively bland and uniform, but there are three important clues to a malignant process: (1) nuclear membrane irregularity; (2) increased mitotic activity; and (3) loss of normal honeycomb pattern. Normally, the cells are in highly ordered, tightly knit, honeycomb arrangements. In contrast, the malignant honeycombs can be either loosely arranged and poorly formed ("drunken" honeycombs) [89 I9.88] or irregularly crowded and piled up [90 I9.87]. The differential diagnosis is with reactive atypia, which may show the conspicuous cytologic abnormalities previously described. Other important features of malignancy include loss of polarity, enlargement and flattening of the nuclei, cell-in-cell arrangements, and bloody background [Nakajima 1994].

89

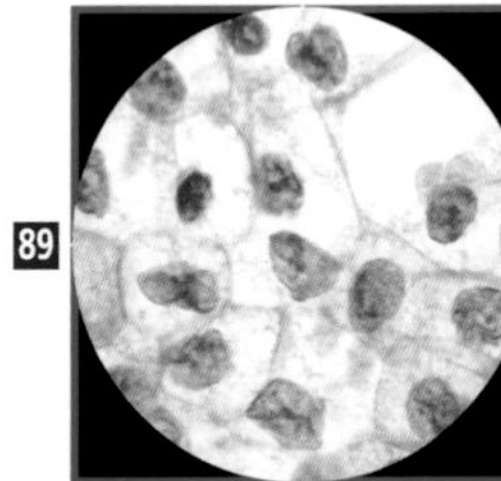

90

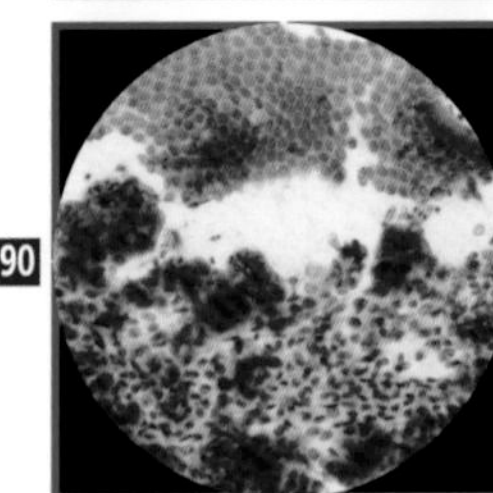

Dysplasia and Carcinoma In Situ

Dysplasia and carcinoma in situ have been described in the mucosa of the gallbladder [Albores-Saavedra 1980, Alonso de Ruiz 1982], and similar premalignant changes occur in the related pancreaticobiliary epithelium [Yamada 1984].

Dysplasia is characterized by sheets and clusters of cells that are somewhat less cohesive, more pleomorphic, and have higher N/C ratios than normal [Alonso de Ruiz 1982]. The cytologic features become progressively more abnormal as the grade of dysplasia increases but fall short of being diagnostic of malignancy. Low-grade dysplasia is characterized by mild to moderate nuclear enlargement with smooth nuclear membranes, chromatin clearing or slight coarsening, and distinct nucleoli. High-grade dysplasia shows cells with increased N/C ratios, mild nuclear membrane irregularities, coarse chromatin or clearing, and prominent nucleoli [Layfield 1995].

Carcinoma in situ is characterized by more cells with more pleomorphism and less cohesion. Syncytial aggregates can be seen. Nuclear atypia is more pronounced, with coarsely granular, irregularly distributed chromatin and large, pleomorphic, or multiple nucleoli [Alonso de Ruiz 1982]. Giant cells may be seen [Albores-Saavedra 1980]. The findings may be indistinguishable from those in invasive adenocarcinoma.

More extensive loss of cohesion and a tumor diathesis characterize frank carcinoma. The changes can be focal; cytohistologic correlation increases with the extent and severity of the lesion [Alonso de Ruiz 1982].

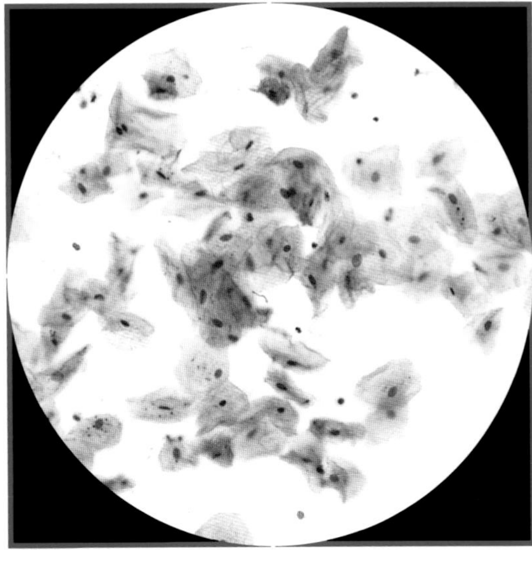

I9.1
Mature squamous cells. A smear of the nonkeratinized squamous mucosa, characteristic of most of the oral cavity, is made up predominantly of intermediate squamous cells, with few superficial cells and no parabasal cells.

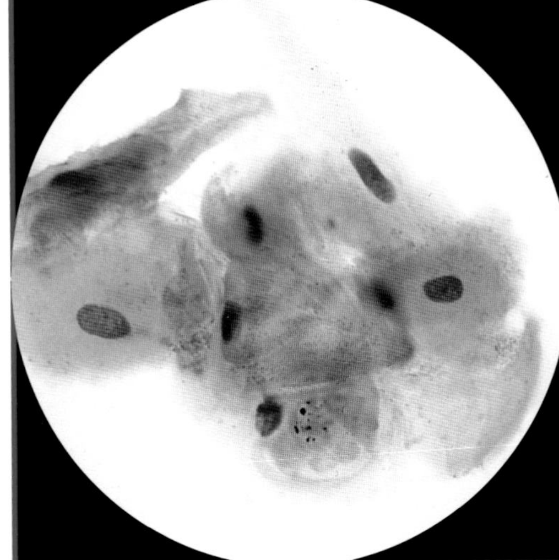

I9.2
Anucleate squames and intermediate cells. Normally, these cells can be obtained from the keratinized squamous mucosa of the oral cavity. However, hyperkeratosis is also characterized by the presence of anucleate squames. Most cases of leukoplakia are due to combinations of benign hyperkeratosis and parakeratosis, but some cases are associated with high-grade dysplasia or cancer. Unfortunately, because the keratotic lesion is a surface reaction, it may cover and mask an underlying abnormality.

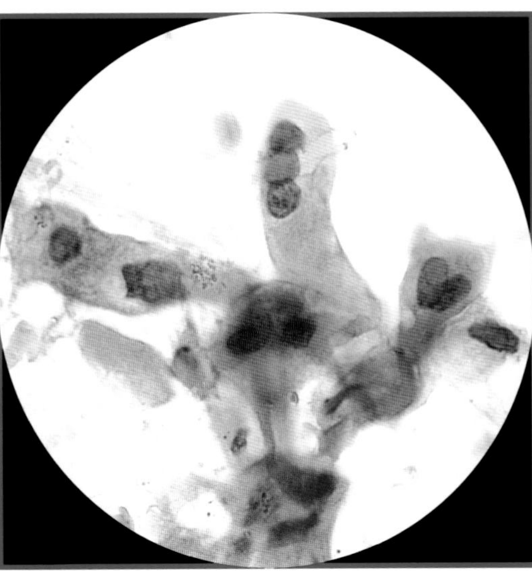

I9.3
Atypical squamous cells. The squamous epithelium may undergo various reactions related to inflammation and infection, including repair and inflammatory changes. These atypical squamous cells, mimicking dysplasia, were associated with a herpes infection (compare with well-differentiated keratinizing SCC).

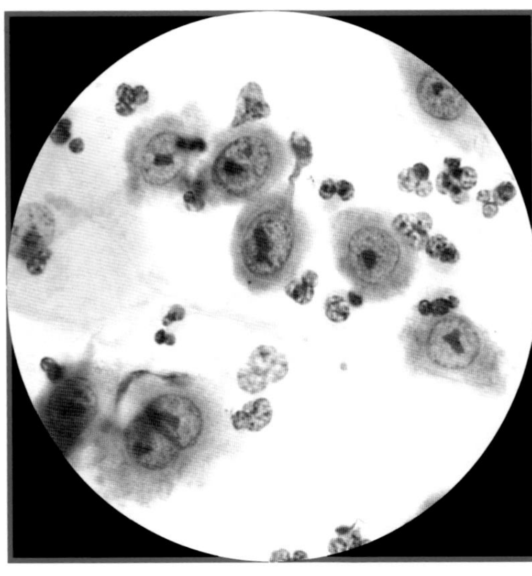

I9.4
Pemphigus vulgaris. Parabasal-sized acantholytic cells with enlarged nuclei; prominent, multiple, or irregular nucleoli; dense cytoplasm; and high N/C ratios. The appearance resembles that of repair/regeneration, except for the presence of single cells. Numerous atypical cells and poor cohesion may suggest malignancy. In contrast with cancer cells, the nuclear membranes are smooth and the chromatin fine and evenly distributed.

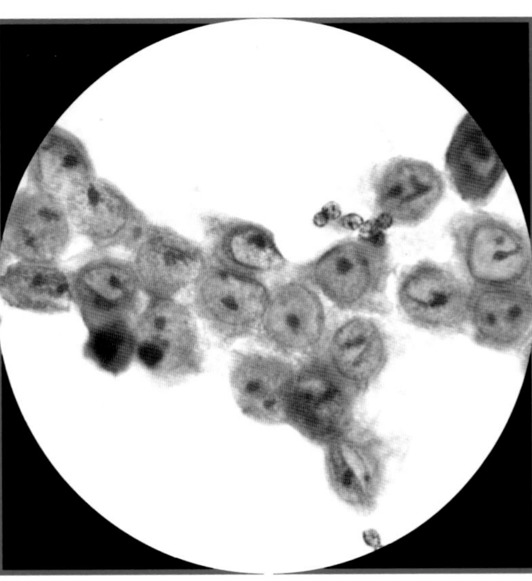

I9.5
Pemphigus vulgaris. Perinuclear acidophilic staining of the cytoplasm is a common finding.

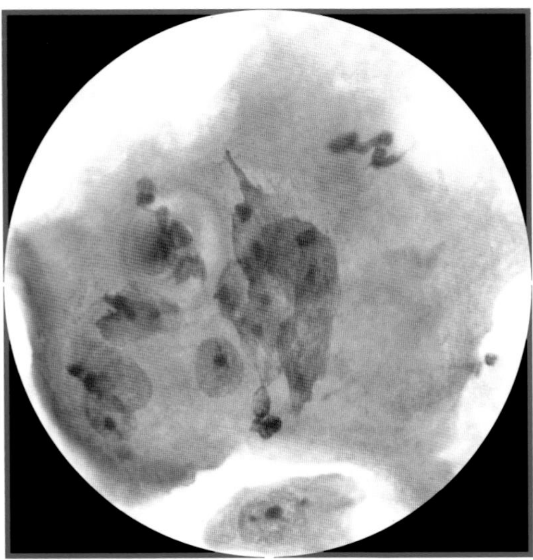

I9.6
Pemphigus vulgaris. Multinucleated giant cells can be seen, particularly after therapy.

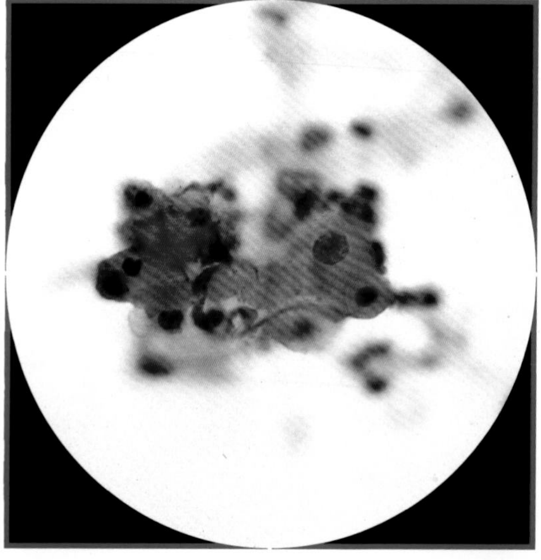

I9.7
Dyskeratocytes. Individual cell keratinization (grains, dyskeratosis) as may be seen in Darier's disease, hereditary benign intraepithelial dyskeratosis, radiation and chemotherapy, and dysplasia/cancer.

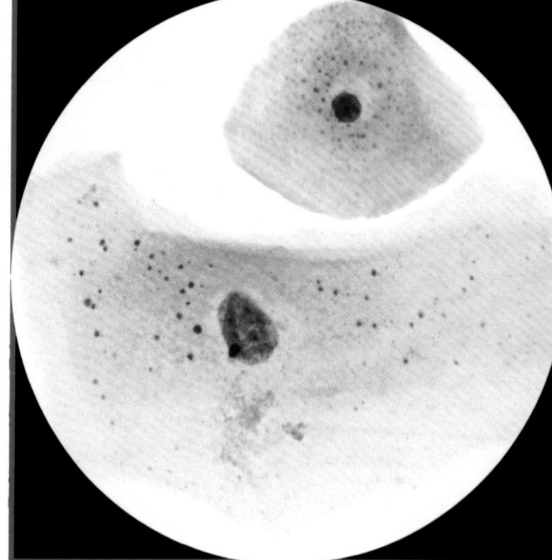

I9.8
Radiation effect. As in the Pap smear, radiation change is characterized by cytomegaly, in which the nucleus and cytoplasm enlarge in concert while maintaining a relatively normal N/C ratio (macrocytes). Signs of degeneration or regeneration can also be seen.

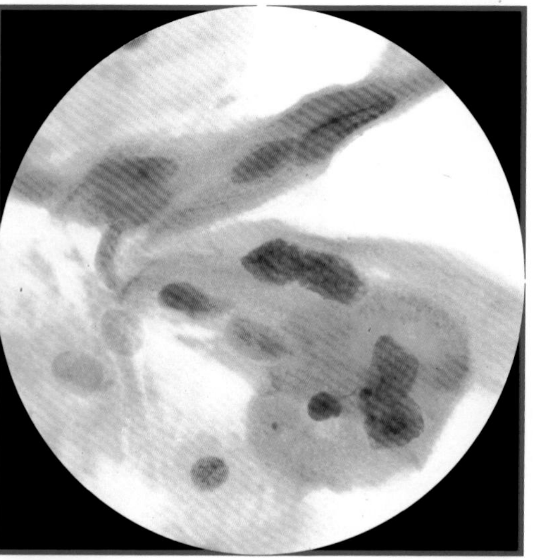

I9.9
Keratinizing squamous cell carcinoma. Most oral cancers are well-differentiated, keratinizing, squamous cell carcinomas. Malignant features in these tumors can be subtle. Cells that might represent a low-grade dysplasia in the Pap smear may represent cancer at this site. For example, compare the malignant cells illustrated here with the atypical but benign cells associated with herpes infection shown in I9.3. The nonkeratinized component in the malignancy is helpful in diagnosis.

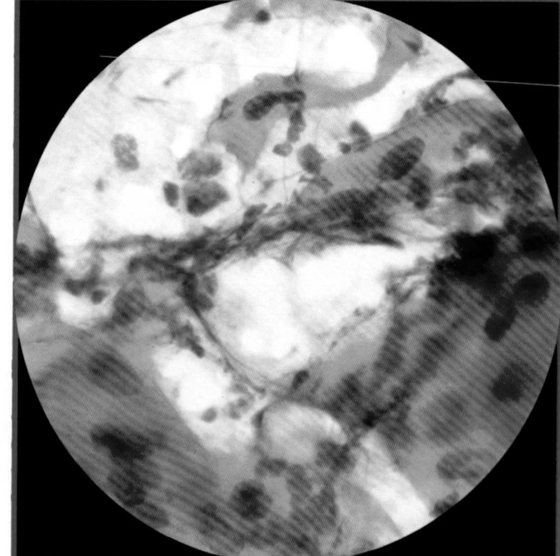

I9.10
Keratinizing squamous cell carcinoma. The tumor usually shows typical features of keratinizing SCC, including numerous single cells, bizarre cell shapes, and heavy keratinization.

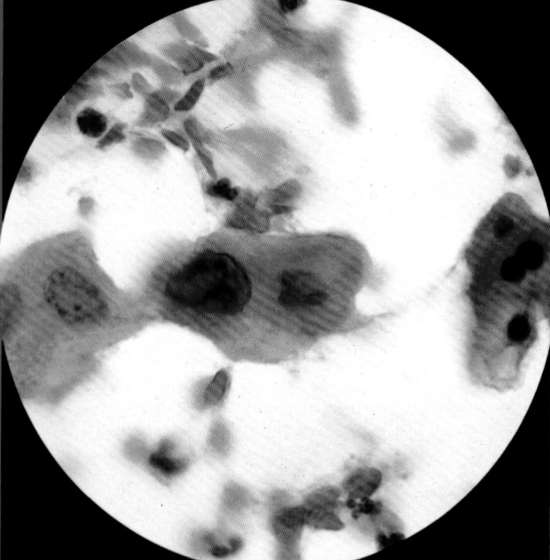

I9.11
Keratinizing squamous cell carcinoma. The nuclei are pleomorphic and hyperchromatic. Nucleoli are often obscured by the dense chromatin.

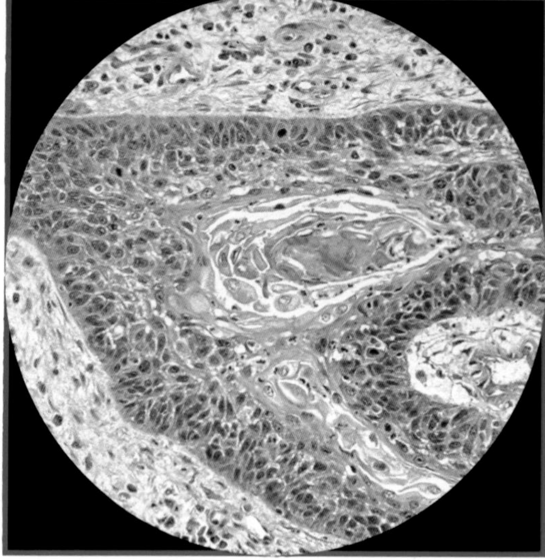

I9.12
Keratinizing squamous cell carcinoma (tissue). Note the presence of a pearl (which indicates keratinization and a high degree of differentiation) as well as the presence of nonkeratinized (ie, poorly differentiated) cells from which the keratinized component differentiated.

I9.13
Squamous cells. The esophagus is normally lined by a nonkeratinized, stratified, squamous epithelium. A scrap of the surface would reveal mostly intermediate cells, as illustrated here. A few superficial cells, sometimes with keratohyaline granules, or benign pearls, can also be seen. However, parabasal cells are not a normal finding.

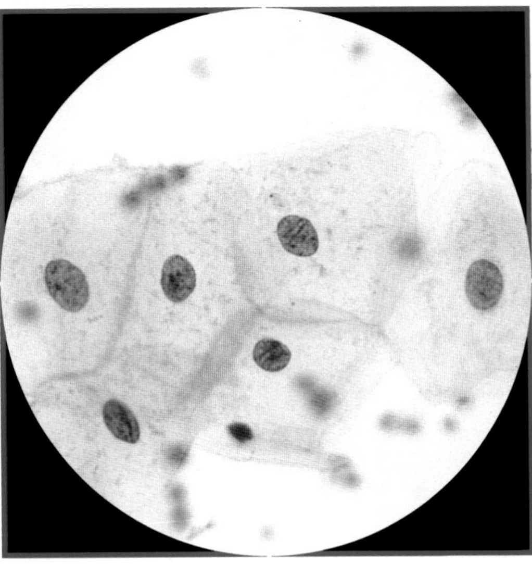

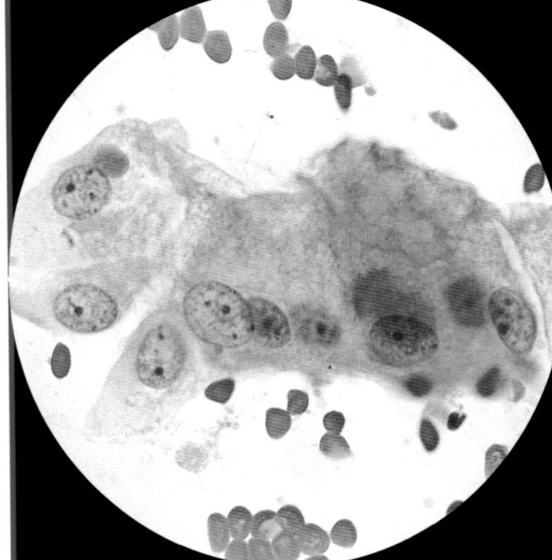

I9.14
Glandular cells. Although the esophagus has submucosal mucous glands, these are not seen in cytologic specimens. Normally, however, gastric-type cardiac glandular cells may be obtained from the distal esophagus at the gastroesophageal border. The distal esophageal cells illustrated here show mild reactive changes. Glandular cells obtained from the esophagus at other sites may indicate Barrett's esophagus.

I9.15
Leukoplakia. Nonspecific clinical term for white plaque, which can be caused by conditions ranging from benign (eg, hyperkeratosis, here illustrated) to malignant (eg, squamous cell carcinoma). Note the anucleate squames.

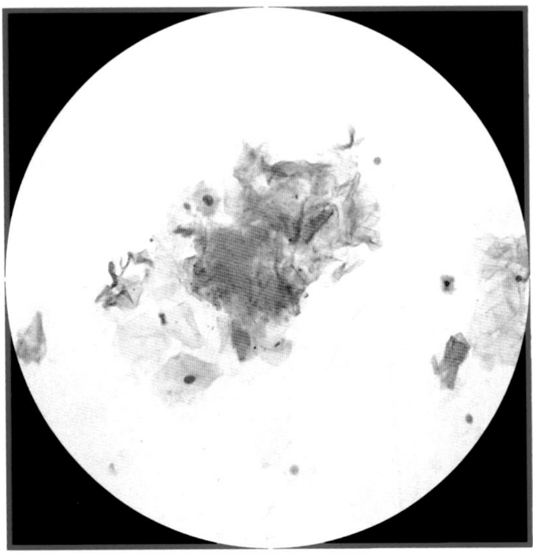

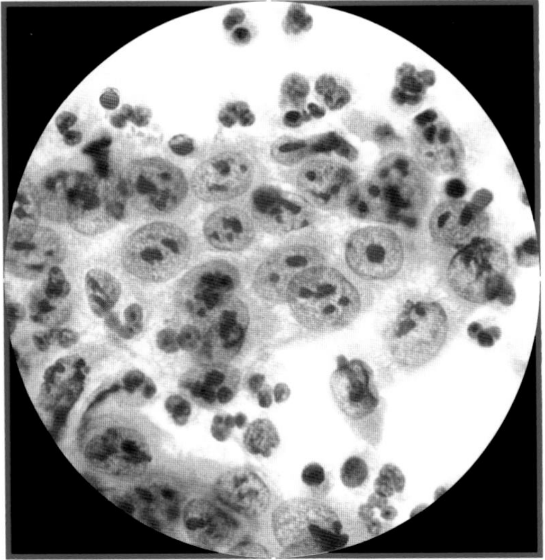

I9.16
Esophagitis. A wide variety of conditions can produce esophagitis with or without ulceration, including irritants, reflux, trauma, hernia, Crohn's disease, or infections. Reflux esophagitis, which may lead to peptic ulceration of the esophageal mucosa can result in marked reparative changes, including the nuclear enlargement and prominent nucleoli illustrated here. The reparative cells remain cohesive and orderly, the nuclear membranes are smooth, and the chromatin is fine.

I9.17
Reflux esophagitis. In some cases of severe reflux esophagitis, the marked regenerative activity results in atypical reparative cells, mimicking malignancy. However, intercellular cohesion and some degree of order is usually evident.

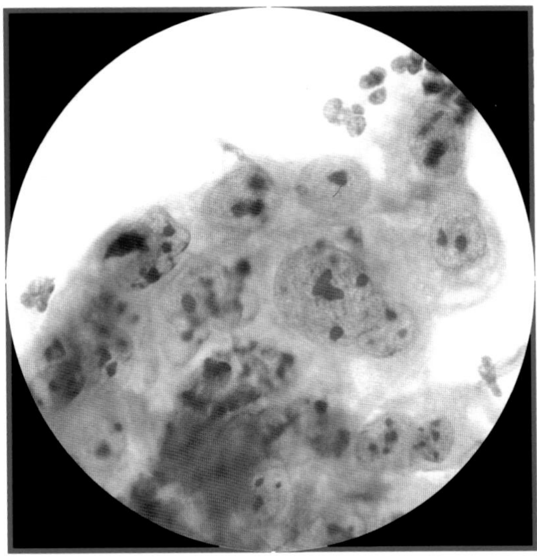

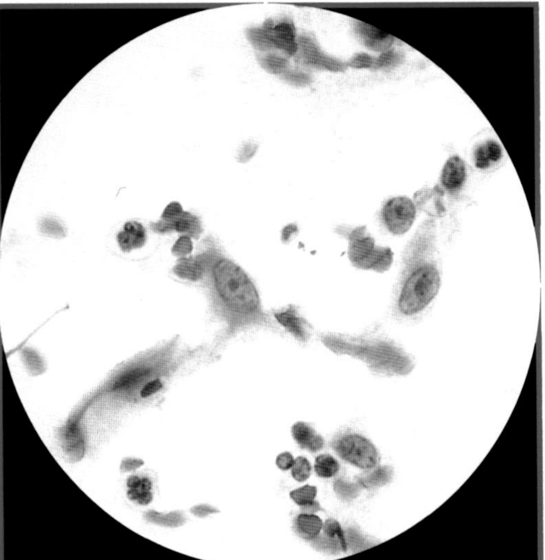

I9.18
Esophageal ulcer. In addition to the reparative epithelial changes previously illustrated, reactive mesenchymal cells may be obtained from the ulcer base. The cells are myofibroblasts, characterized by a spindle/stellate shape and oval to elongated nuclei with fine chromatin and distinct nucleoli.

I9.19
Barrett's esophagus. Defined as "lower esophagus lined by columnar epithelium," this condition is diagnosed by identifying glandular cells in an esophageal specimen. The cells may either be gastric type or intestinal type with goblet cells. Because the origin of the cells cannot be determined by cytology, it is crucial to correlate the cytology with clinical and endoscopic findings.

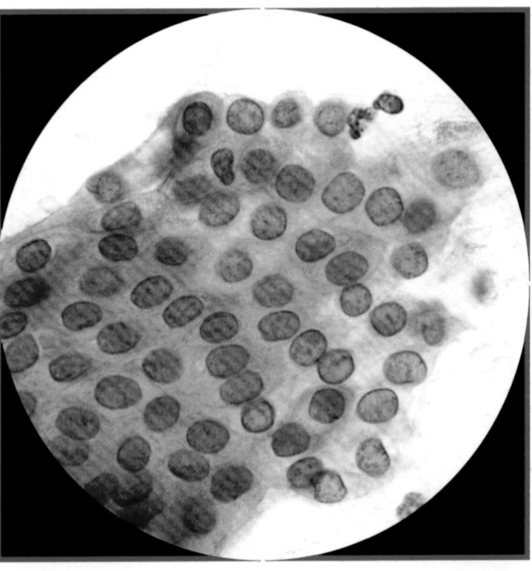

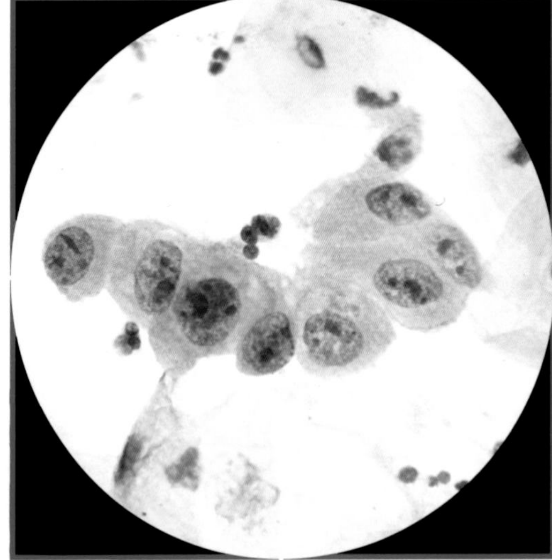

I9.20
Reactive changes in Barrett's esophagus. Various degrees of reactive/reparative change can occur in Barrett's epithelium, including nuclear enlargement, pleomorphism, and prominent nucleoli. However, the cells are still cohesive and orderly, and the chromatin is fine and pale.

I9.21
Dysplasia in Barrett's esophagus, a premalignant condition. Almost all adenocarcinomas of the distal esophagus arise in Barrett's epithelium. Adenocarcinoma is preceded by glandular dysplasia, which is characterized by crowded, enlarged, elongated, hyperchromatic nuclei; increased N/C ratios; and loss of nuclear polarity. Illustrated here is high-grade dysplasia in which a focus of invasion was found. Compare the chromatin of these cells with the reactive nuclei shown in I9.20.

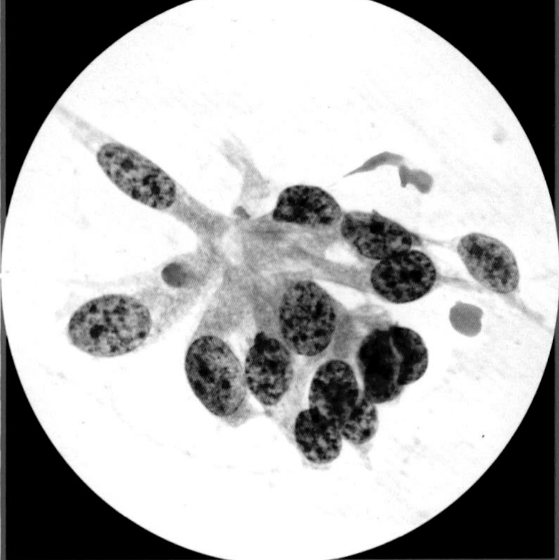

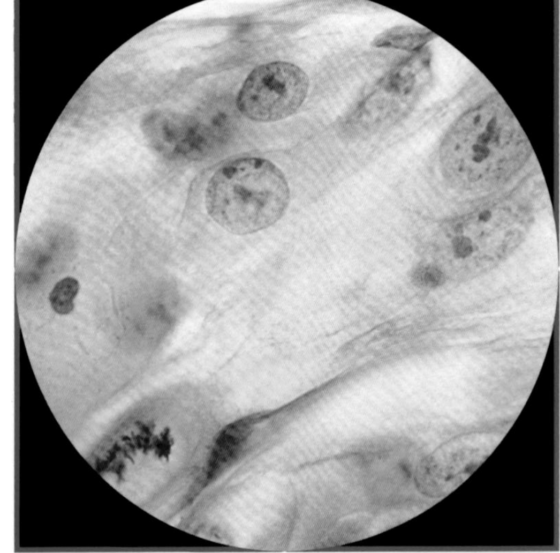

I9.22
Radiation/chemotherapy effect. Esophagitis is a common complication of radiation to the chest or systemic chemotherapy. Illustrated is an atypical reparative process due to chemotherapy for leukemia. Note that despite the nuclear pleomorphism, prominent, irregular nucleoli, and even a mildly atypical mitotic figure, the cells are cohesive, there is little nuclear overlap, each cell has adequate cytoplasm, and the chromatin is fine and pale.

I9.23
Candida esophagitis. *Candida* is the most common cause of infectious esophagitis and an increasingly common problem in immunocompromised patients. The severity of the disease can range from mild to severe, in which case there may be marked reactive changes in the epithelium. Note the presence of *Candida* (arrow). It is important to search all esophageal specimens specifically for the presence of *Candida*.

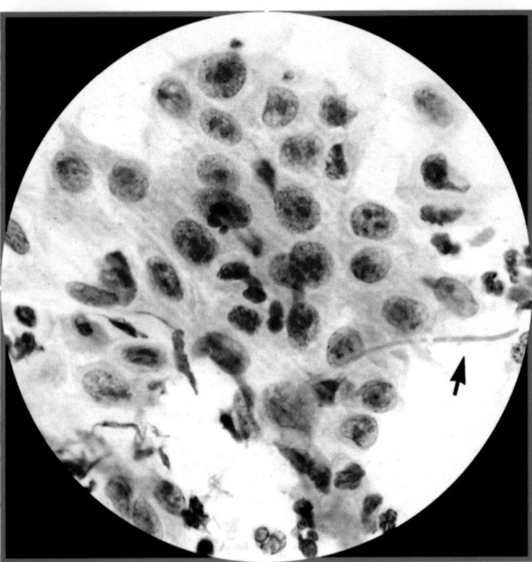

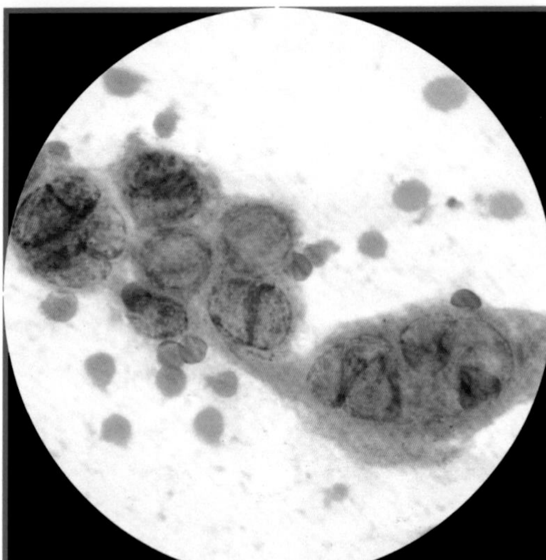

I9.24
Herpes esophagitis. Like *Candida* esophagitis, herpetic esophagitis is an increasingly important clinical problem, particularly in immunocompromised patients. However, it can also be seen in otherwise apparently healthy individuals. Characterized cytologically by multinucleation, molding, ground glass chromatin, margination of chromatin (ie, a thick nuclear membrane), and, sometimes, intranuclear inclusions.

I9.25
Keratinizing squamous cell carcinoma. Squamous cell carcinoma is the most common malignancy of the esophagus. Most cases occur in black men older than 50. Keratinizing SCC is characterized by numerous, single, heavily keratinized cells, often with bizarre spindle or tadpole shapes as illustrated here. Note the densely keratinized, orangeophilic cytoplasm; irregular cell shapes; and the densely hyperchromatic to pyknotic, angular nuclei.

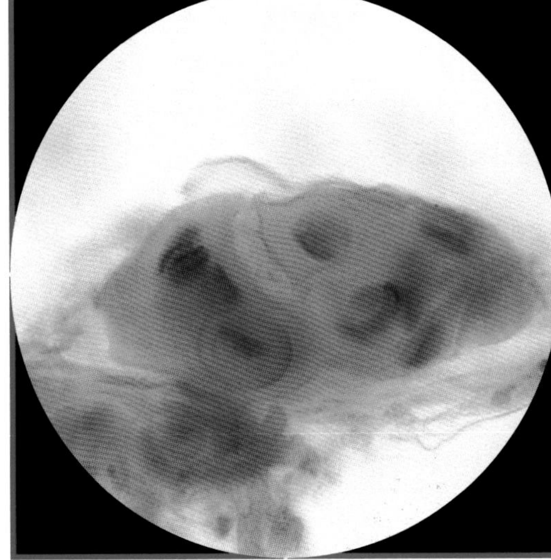

I9.26
Keratinizing squamous cell carcinoma. Cell-in-cell arrangements are characteristic. Pearl formation is pathognomonic of keratinization.

I9.27
Keratinizing squamous cell carcinoma. Keratinizing SCC is frequently associated with surface reactions of parakeratosis, hyperkeratosis, and atypical parakeratosis (illustrated).

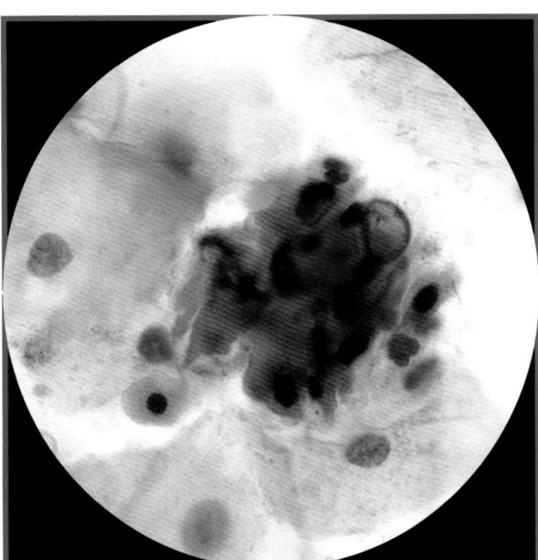

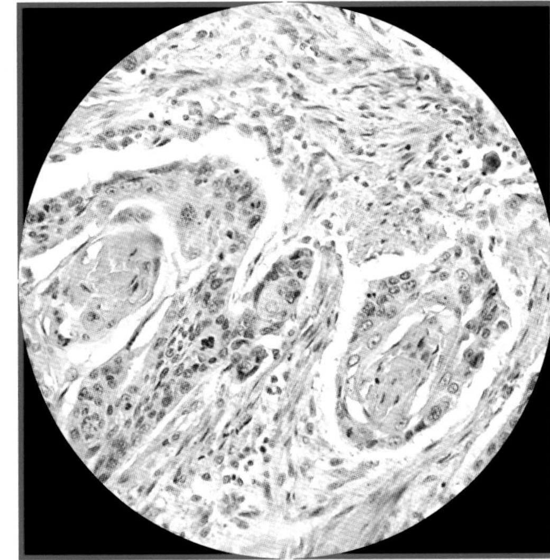

I9.28
Keratinizing squamous cell carcinoma (tissue). Invasive keratinizing SCC with classic keratin eddies, or pearls.

I9.29
Nonkeratinizing squamous cell carcinoma. Compared with keratinizing SCC, the malignant cells of nonkeratinizing SCC tend to be smaller and more uniform, with higher N/C ratios and more prominent nucleoli but scantier cytoplasm. Note the cytoplasmic basophilia and density, particularly of cells at the edge of the group. Although an occasional dyskeratotic cell indicating single cell keratinization may be seen, there are no pearls.

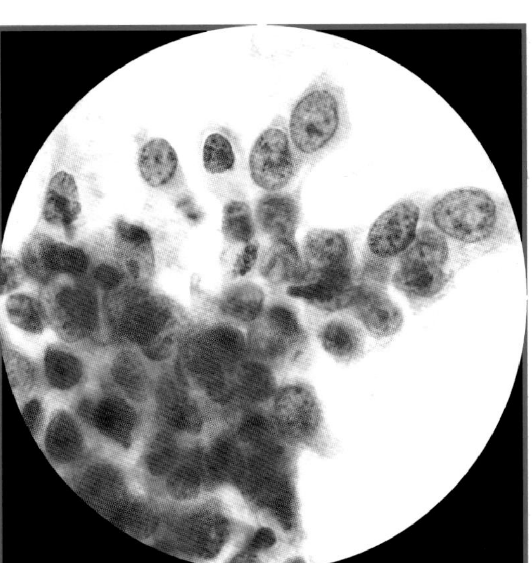

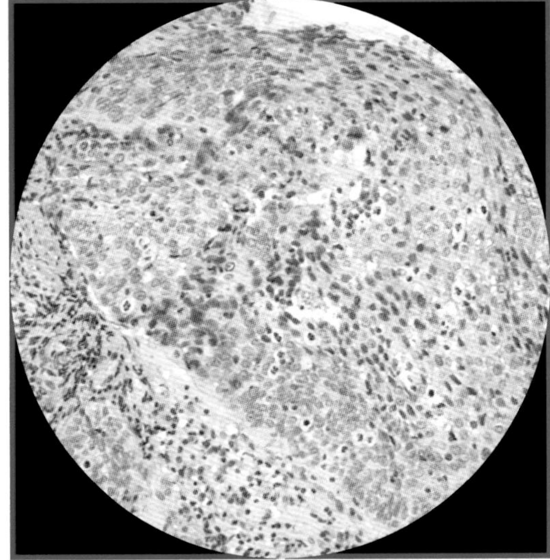

I9.30
Nonkeratinizing squamous cell carcinoma (tissue). Invasive sheets of malignant squamous cells without pearl or gland formation.

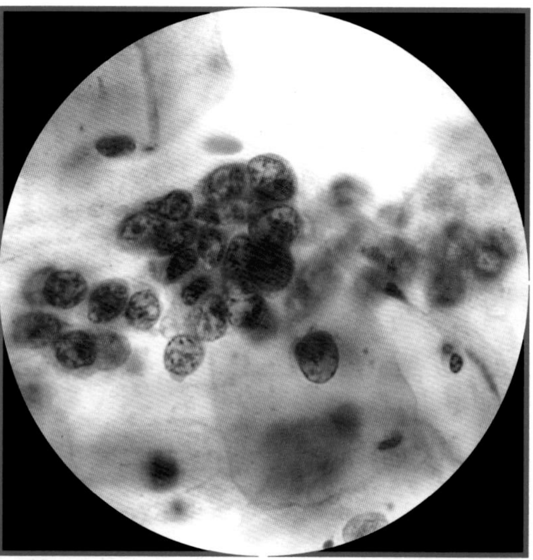

I9.31
Poorly differentiated squamous cell carcinoma. The cells are small and basaloid—about the size of the intermediate cell nuclei that are also present in the field. The nuclei are hyperchromatic and the cytoplasm is scant. The differential diagnosis is with small cell carcinoma. Prominent nucleoli; coarse, irregular chromatin; little nuclear molding; distinct, dense cytoplasm; and lack of crush artifact favor a diagnosis of poorly differentiated squamous cell carcinoma.

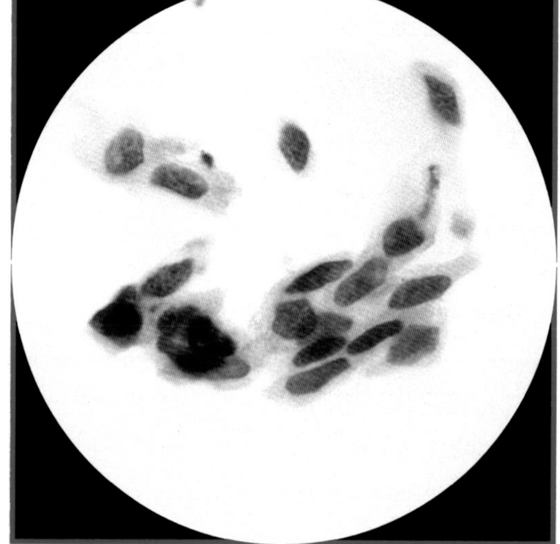

I9.32
Poorly differentiated squamous cell carcinoma. Spindling of the tumor cells can also occur, sometimes mimicking a sarcoma (spindle cell carcinoma).

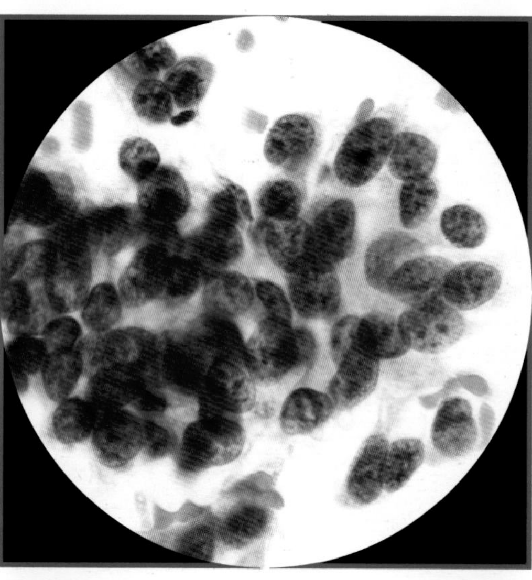

I9.33
Adenocarcinoma. Occurs most commonly in the distal esophagus, predominantly in white males. Adenocarcinoma is associated with Barrett's esophagus but can arise anywhere in the esophagus. Most cases are ordinary papillary/acinar adenocarcinomas similar in appearance to ordinary gastric cancer. Note the acinar structure, which indicates glandular differentiation. Compare the invasive adenocarcinoma shown here with dysplasia in Barrett's esophagus.

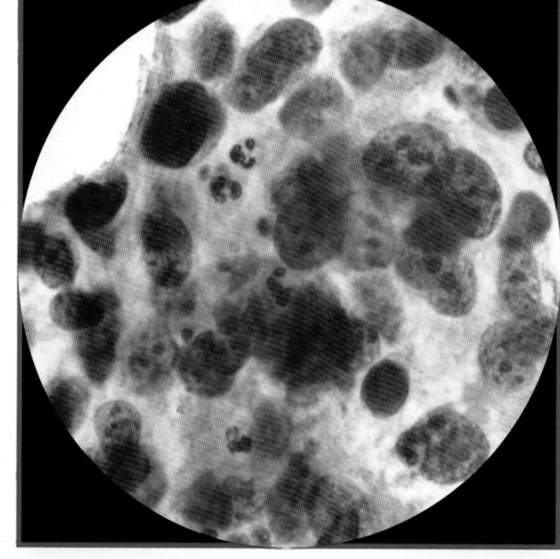

I9.34
Adenocarcinoma (esophagus). Prominent nucleoli, delicate cytoplasm, and acinar arrangements are characteristics of adenocarcinoma. Note the nuclear crowding and overlap, which are features of disorganized cellular arrangements associated with cancer.

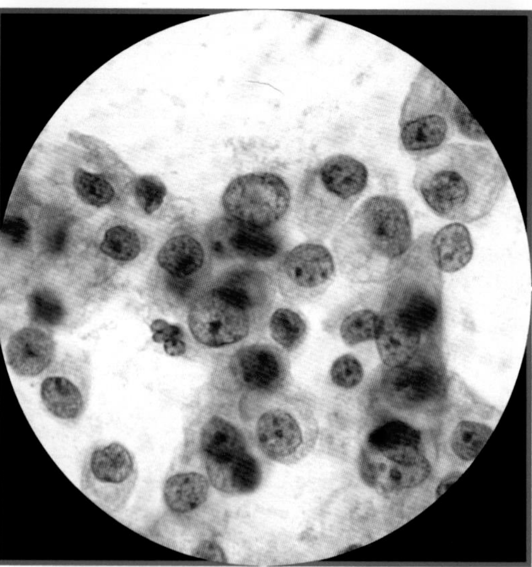

I9.35
Adenocarcinoma (esophagus). Nuclear/cytoplasmic polarity or columnar-shaped cells with delicate, foamy cytoplasm are also associated with glandular differentiation.

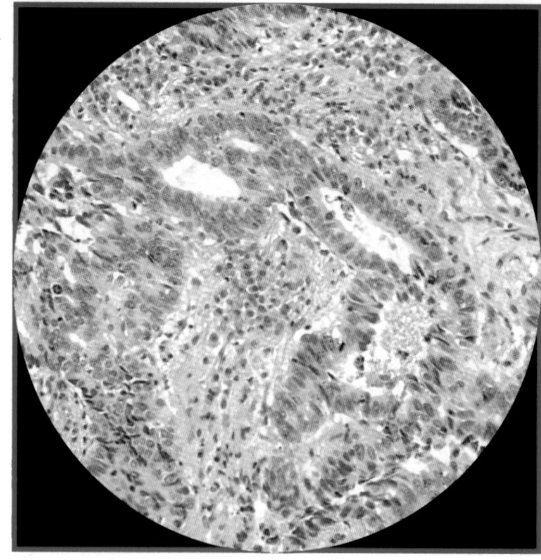

I9.36
Adenocarcinoma (esophagus tissue). Note the gland-in-gland growth pattern characteristic of adenocarcinoma.

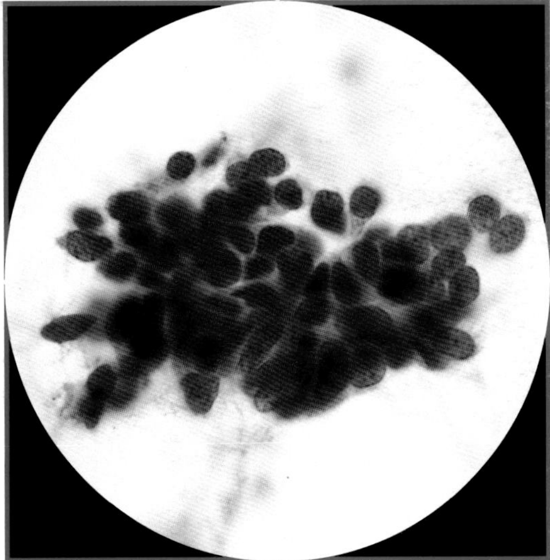

I9.37
Small cell carcinoma. Although small cell carcinoma can arise in the esophagus, far more commonly this tumor represents direct extension of a lung primary. Small blue cells, with high N/C ratios; nuclear molding; fine chromatin; inconspicuous nucleoli; and scant, delicate cytoplasm characterize small cell carcinoma. Crush artifact is also common. (Compare with poorly differentiated squamous cell carcinoma, I9.31.)

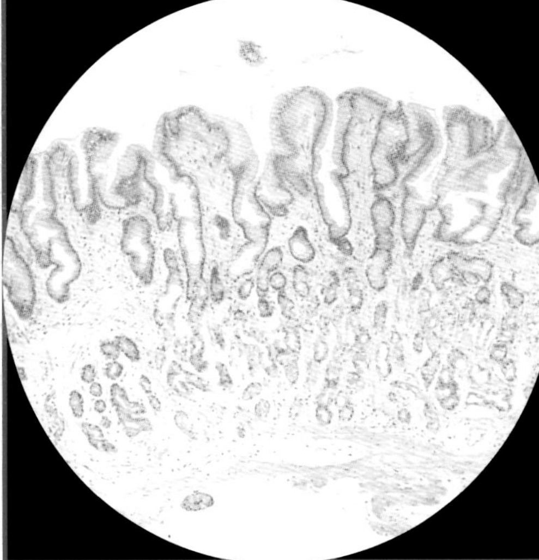

I9.38
Gastric mucosa (tissue). The surface is lined with mucous cells. There are also chief and parietal cells in the deep mucosa of the fundus and body of the stomach.

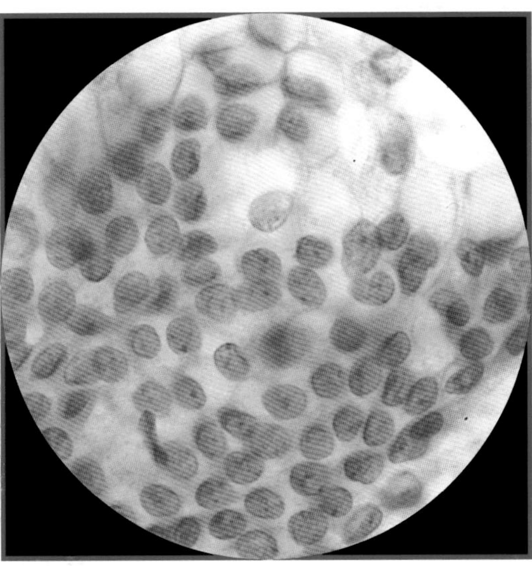

I9.39
Mucous cells. Because these cells line the gastric surface, they are usually the major cell type in gastric cytology. When viewed en face, the groups form orderly, cohesive honeycomb arrangements that resemble endocervical cell groupings.

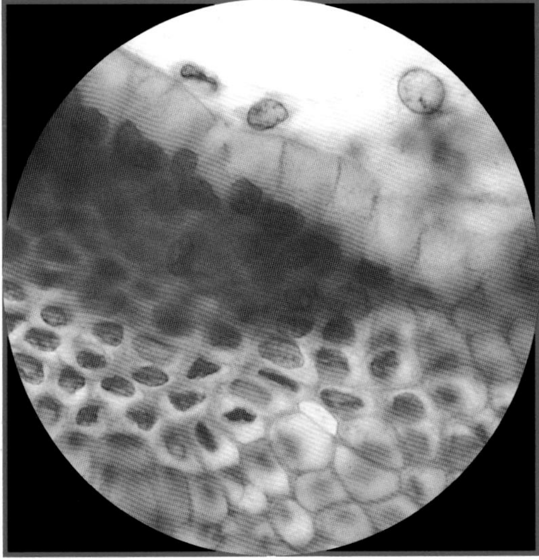

I9.40
Mucous cells. Orderly palisades are noted when the benign cells are viewed from the side. Note the uniform nuclei and mucinous cytoplasm.

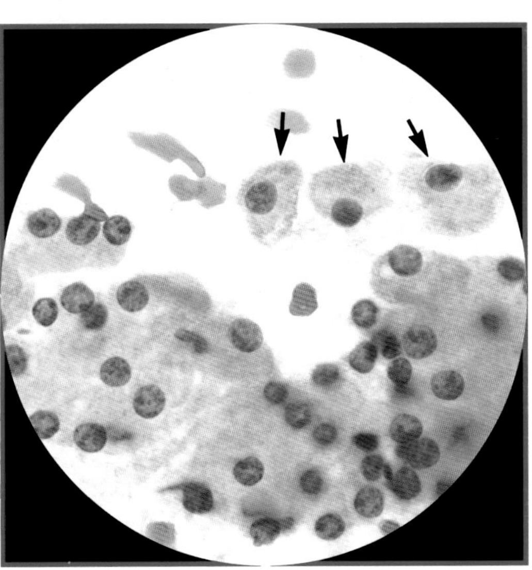

I9.41
Chief cells. The cuboidal chief cells manufacture zymogen, or proenzyme, granules, which impart a coarsely granular, basophilic quality to the cytoplasm. The cells resemble acinar cells from the pancreas. A few flask-shaped parietal cells are also seen near the top of the group, with faint eosinophilic staining (arrows).

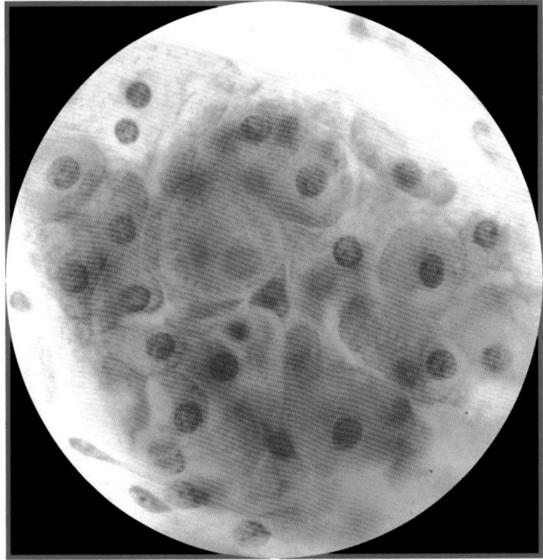

I9.42
Parietal cells. Flask-shaped cells that secrete intrinsic factor. They are larger than chief cells and tend to stain eosinophilic.

I9.43
Reactive changes. Gastric epithelium with enlarged nuclei and prominent nucleoli but fine chromatin and orderly arrangements (such as the palisade shown here).

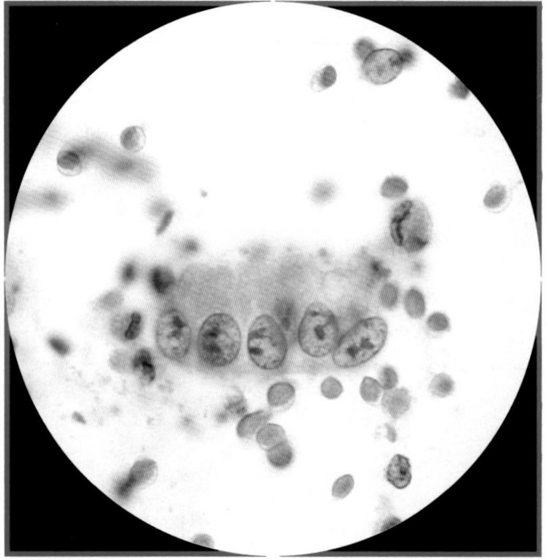

I9.44
Reactive changes (stomach). Cohesive sheets of cells that may be crowded but maintain relative orderliness. Reactive cells have enlarged nuclei with prominent nucleoli.

I9.45
Repair. As in the Pap smear, gastric repair is characterized by sheets of cells with nuclear enlargement and prominent nucleoli but fine chromatin, ample cytoplasm, and good cohesion.

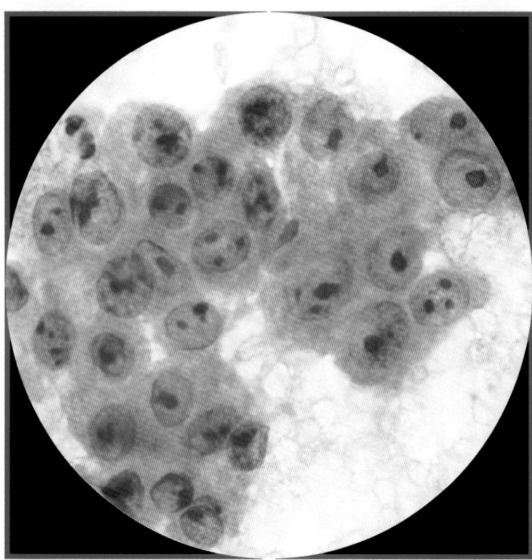

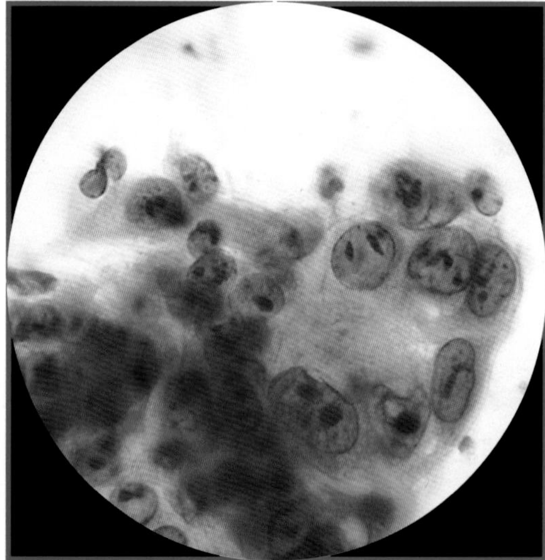

I9.46
Atypical repair. Occasionally, atypical features suggesting malignancy can be seen in a benign reparative process. Cohesion, order, and fine chromatin favor a benign process. Also, note the intimate association with more obviously benign cells.

I9.47
Contaminants (dust cells). A variety of swallowed contaminants, such as dust cells from the respiratory tract (illustrated), can be seen in gastric specimens. Note that cancer cells can also be swallowed contaminants.

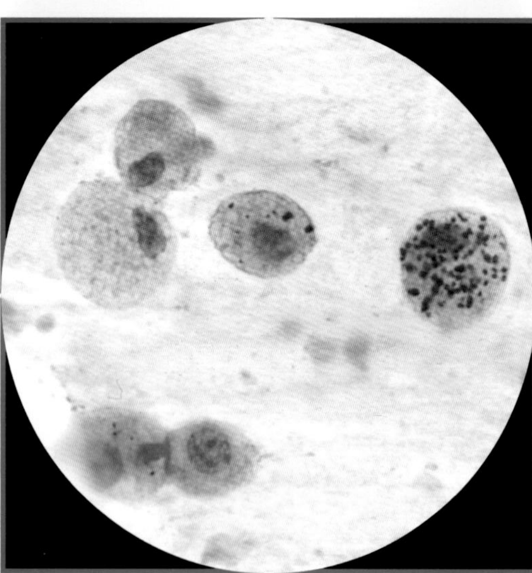

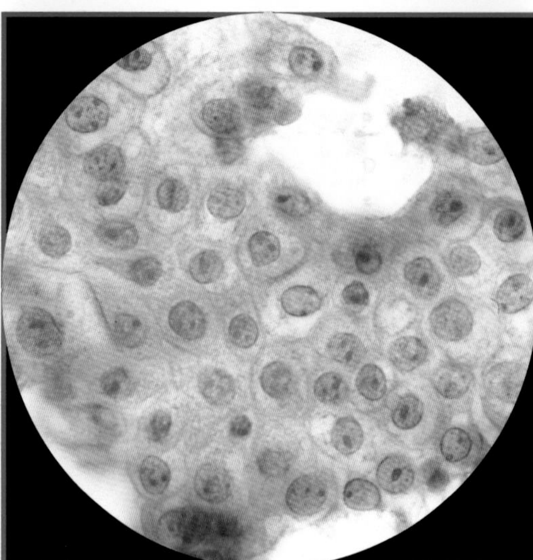

I9.48
Intestinal metaplasia. Diagnostic of chronic atrophic gastritis or gastric atrophy. Although benign, intestinal metaplasia is the milieu in which cancer may arise. Shown here are cohesive sheets of mucous cells, including goblet cells, which are characterized by perinuclear clearing and prominent cell borders.

I9.49
Intestinal metaplasia (corresponding tissue). Note the presence of absorptive cells and clear goblet cells.

I9.50
Helicobacter pylori. Associated with gastric ulcers, *H pylori* is a spiral-shaped bacteria found in luminal mucus. (Oil)

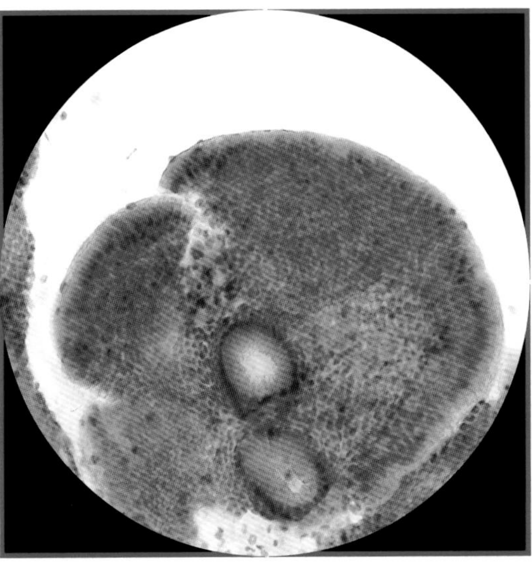

I9.51
Gastric polyp. Most gastric polyps are hyperplastic rather than neoplastic and often multiple. The specific diagnosis cannot be based on cytology, because cytologic techniques obtain relatively normal (illustrated cell block) or reactive gastric epithelium.

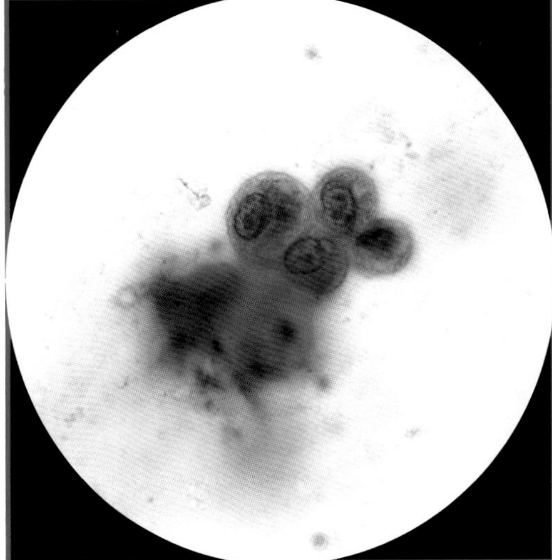

I9.52
Gastric polyp, reactive changes.

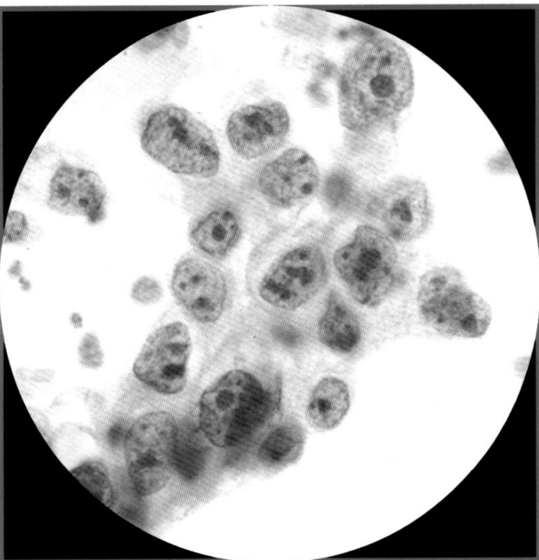

I9.53
Adenocarcinoma (stomach). The more common, intestinal type of adenocarcinoma is characterized by loosely cohesive, multilayered, disorderly groups of cells.

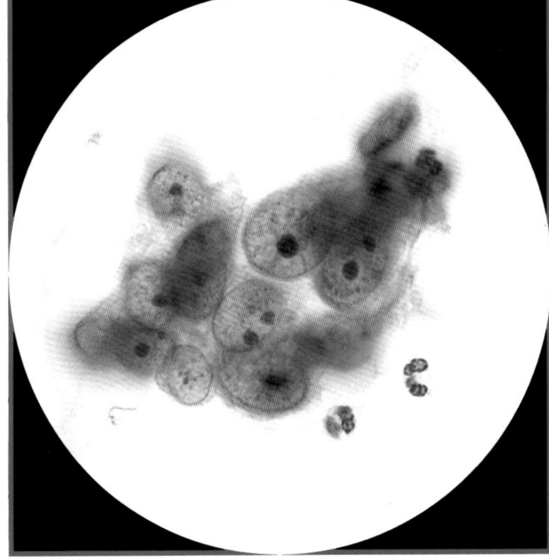

I9.54
Adenocarcinoma (stomach). Nuclear morphology in adenocarcinoma is variable but tends to fall into two groups: one with pale chromatin and prominent nucleoli and the other with dark chromatin and multiple, smaller nucleoli. Illustrated is a three-dimensional cell ball (a characteristic feature of adenocarcinoma) with pale nuclei and prominent nucleoli.

I9.55
Adenocarcinoma (stomach). The second type of nuclear appearance is characterized by hyperchromatic, coarse chromatin and multiple, smaller nucleoli.

I9.56
Adenocarcinoma (stomach). The cells range from cuboidal to columnar, with nucleocytoplasmic polarity.

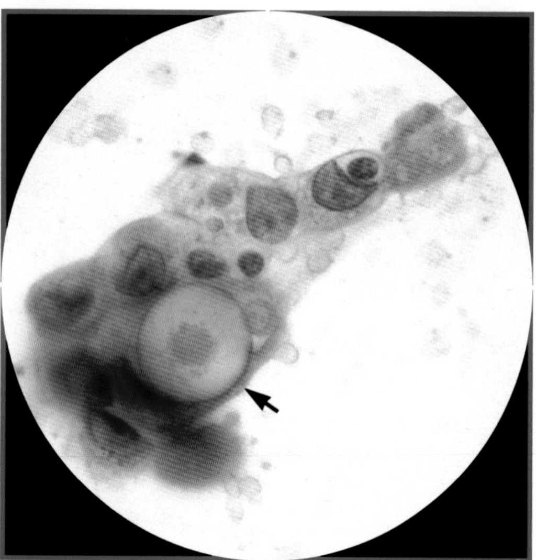

I9.57
Adenocarcinoma, intercellular gland formation. Note that the gland lumen has a terminal bar–like luminal edge (arrow), which is a characteristic feature of intestinal-type gastric adenocarcinoma.

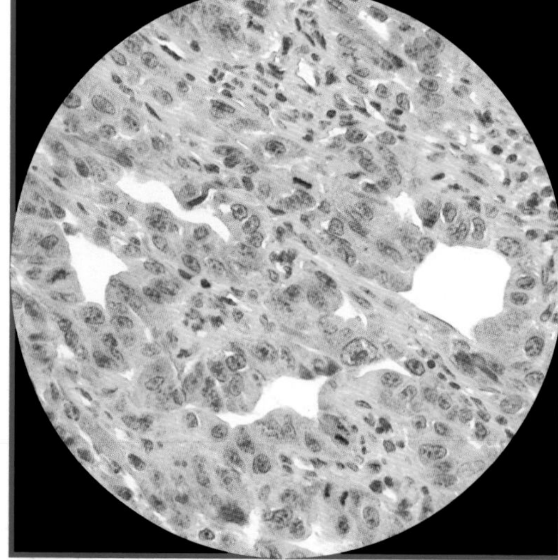

I9.58
Adenocarcinoma. Intestinal-type adenocarcinoma of the stomach (tissue).

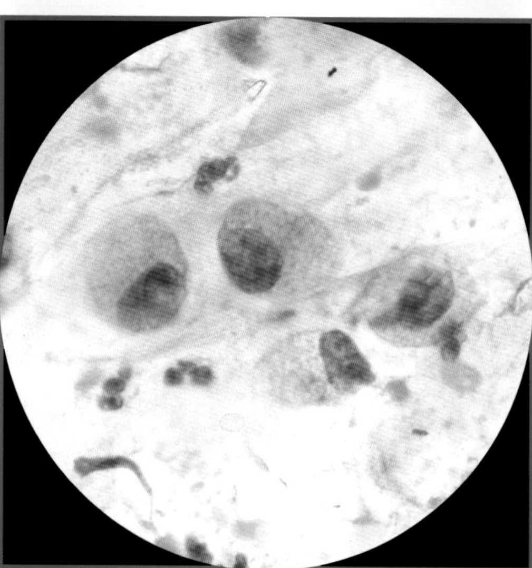

I9.59
Signet ring cell carcinoma, which is characteristic of the less common, gastric-type adenocarcinoma. The malignant cells are often found in pools of mucus, but the background is usually clean. The cells are small and nuclei appear relatively bland. The nuclei are pushed to the side by mucin vacuoles. Diagnostic cells may be sparse.

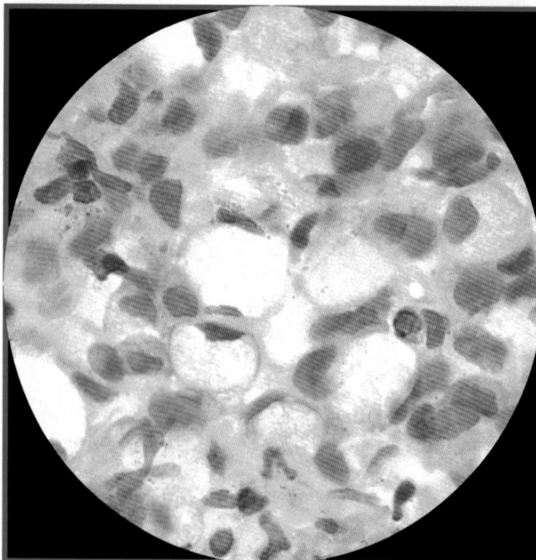

I9.60
Signet ring cell carcinoma of the stomach (corresponding tissue). The tumor commonly grows by diffuse infiltration, causing a "leather-bottle" stomach (linitis plastica). A component of pleomorphic cells can also be present. The malignant signet ring cells can also be found floating in pools of mucus.

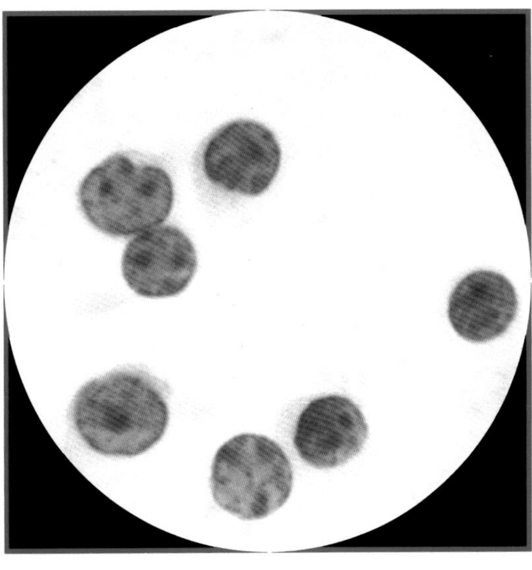

I9.61
Malignant lymphoma. The mucosa-associated lymphoid tissue (MALT) of the GI tract, particularly the stomach, is an important source of primary, extranodal lymphomas. Most are non-Hodgkin's, diffuse, large, B-cell type, as shown here. (Oil)

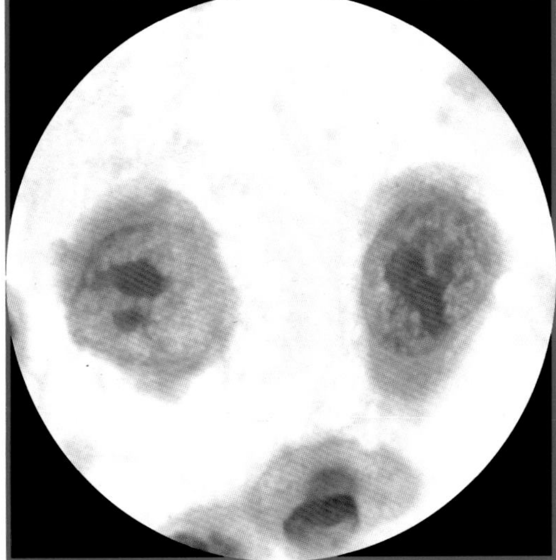

I9.62
Malignant lymphoma. Large cell immunoblastic lymphoma. Singly dispersed cells, with characteristic plasmacytoid appearance and prominent nucleoli. (Oil)

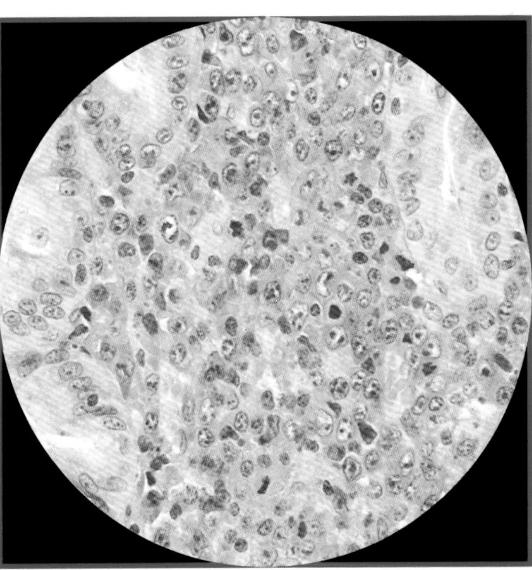

I9.63
Malignant lymphoma, corresponding tissue. The differential diagnosis includes pseudolymphoma, which in cytology shows characteristic predominance of small mature lymphocytes, a range of maturation, tingible body macrophages, and mature plasma cells. The features of pseudolymphoma are similar to those of follicular cervicitis as seen in the Pap smear.

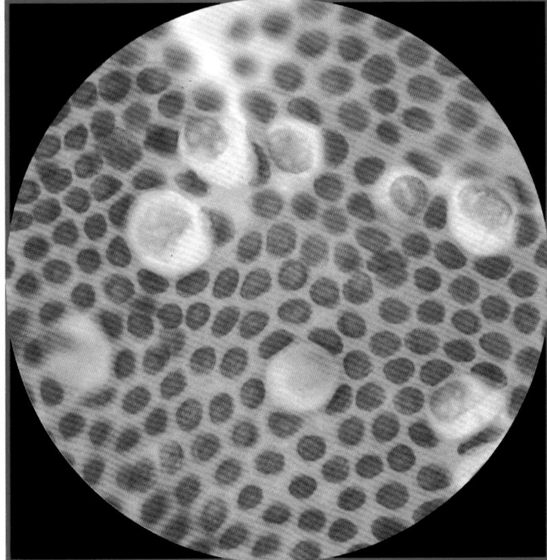

I9.64
Normal. The normal small intestinal mucosa is predominantly composed of relatively dense, granular absorptive cells with interspersed, pale-staining goblet cells. When seen en face, the goblet cells stand out as "holes" in the sheets of absorptive cells.

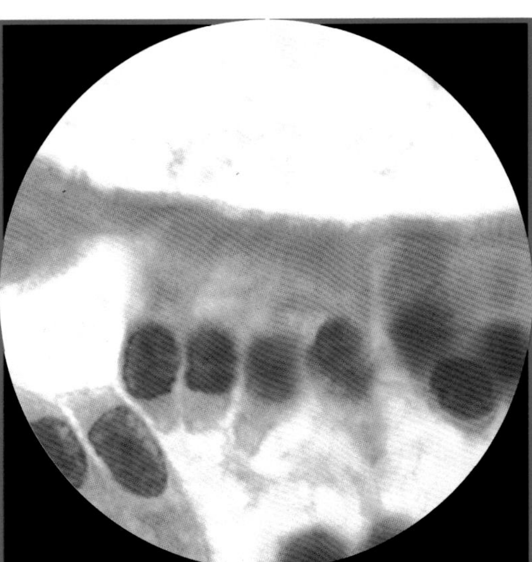

I9.65
Normal striated border (small intestinal). Absorptive cells with nucleocytoplasmic polarity. When viewed from the side under optimal conditions, a striated microvillus border can be seen. (Oil)

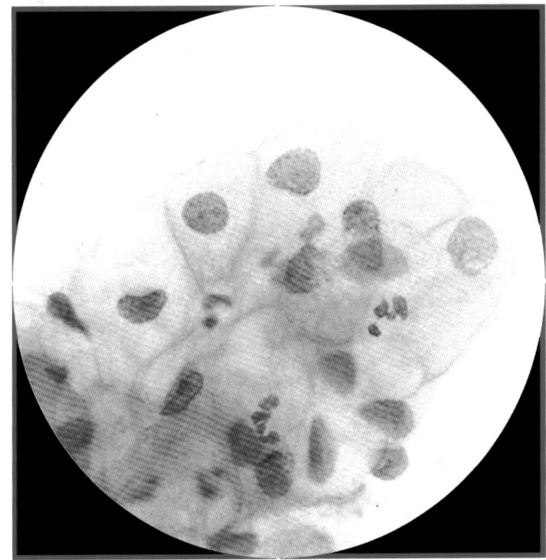

I9.66
Reactive change (small intestinal). In the epithelium, reactive changes can be seen in association with inflammation or ulceration. The cytoplasm takes on a squamoid appearance in some cases.

I9.67
Giardia lamblia. A pear-shaped, flagellated protozoan similar in appearance to *Trichomonas* but with two nuclei, each with a prominent chromocenter.

I9.68
Adenocarcinoma. Primary malignancies of the small bowel are rare; most are carcinoids and lymphomas, which have a tendency to arise in the ileum. Most adenocarcinomas arise in the duodenum, but many are actually carcinomas of the extrahepatic biliary tract that involve the duodenum secondarily. Most intestinal adenocarcinomas are relatively well differentiated; important features of malignancy are disorderly cell arrangements, single cells, and irregular nuclear membranes.

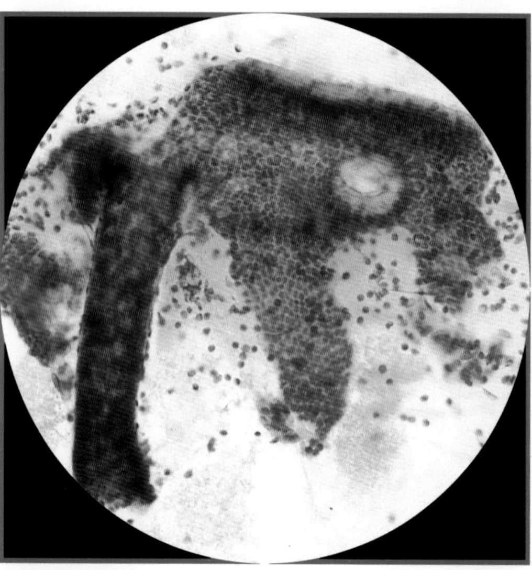

I9.69
Normal colon. Straight, nonbranching, test-tube–like glands composed of absorptive cells and many goblet cells.

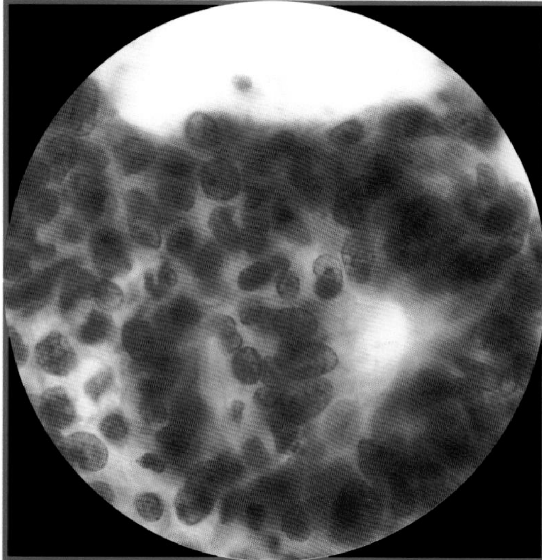

I9.70
Normal reactive colonic epithelium. Large, monolayered sheets of cells with well-ordered glandular lumens. Individual cells show reactive changes, including nuclear "atypia" and cytoplasmic loss of mucin.

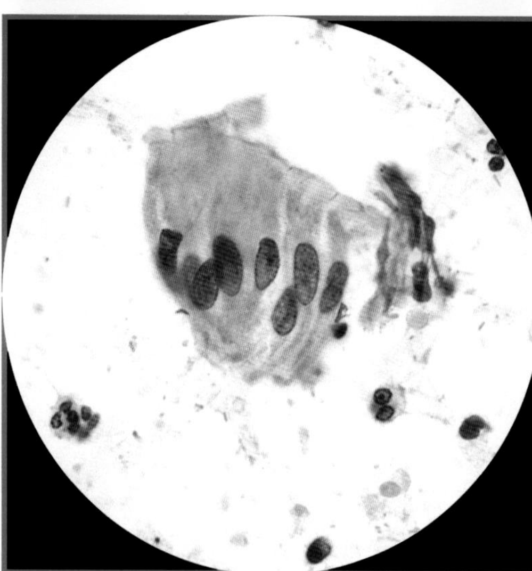

I9.71
Normal colon. Tall columnar cells with basal nuclei and apical cytoplasm. Note the terminal bar–like apical border, which is a characteristic feature of both benign and malignant colorectal cells.

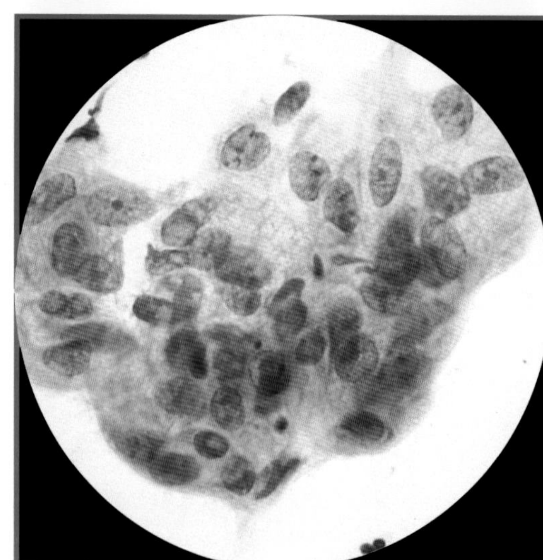

I9.72
Reactive changes. Like other epithelia, the colorectal cells can undergo reactive/reparative changes that can mimic malignancy, including nuclear enlargement with prominent nucleoli. Good cellular cohesion, maintenance of order, and fine chromatin all favor a benign process.

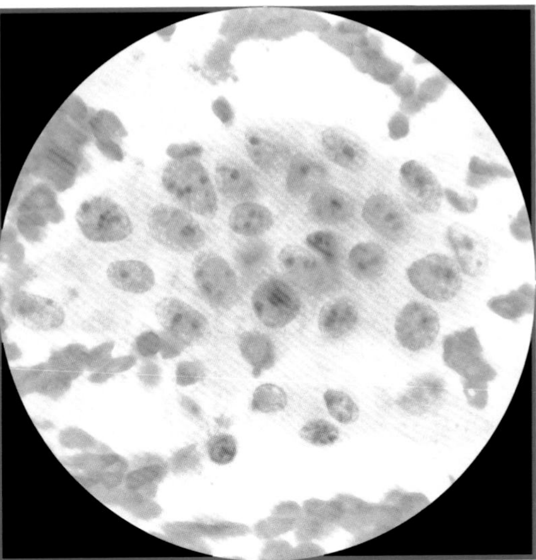

I9.73
Inflammatory bowel disease. The cytologic appearance of inflammatory bowel disease ranges from essentially normal (for quiescent disease in remission), to reactive changes (which correlate with severity of disease), to dysplasia (after several years), and, finally (in some cases) to cancer. Illustrated are severe changes with cytologic features of repair.

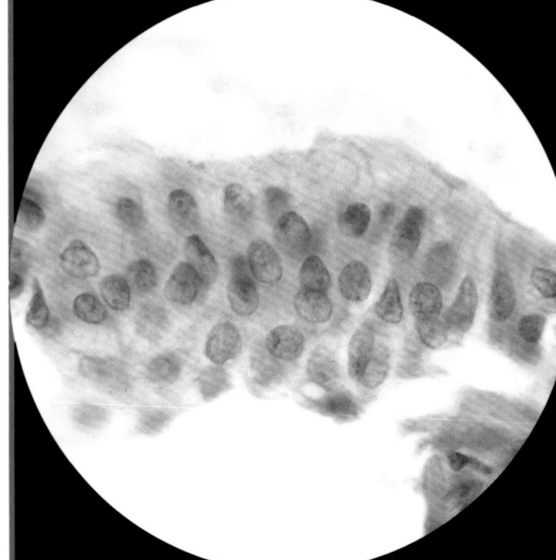

I9.74
Inflammatory bowel disease, reactive changes of less severity. Note, however, the loss of goblet cells. The changes in inflammatory bowel disease are nonspecific; essentially identical changes are seen in infectious colitis.

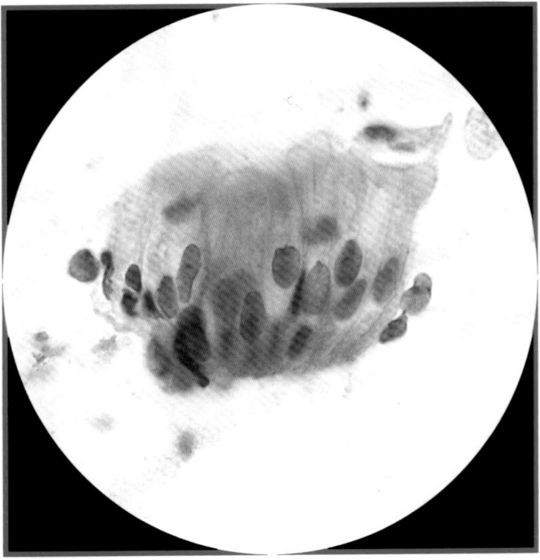

I9.75
Hyperplastic colonic polyp. Nonneoplastic polyp with reactive-appearing mucosal cells.

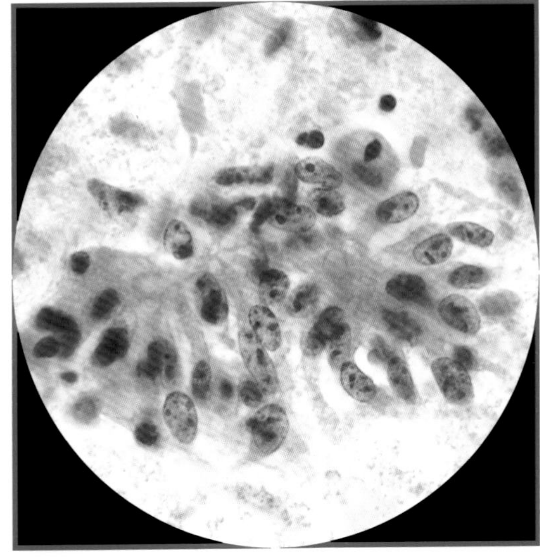

I9.76
Adenomatous polyp (colon). The cytology of benign adenomas (adenomatous polyps and villous adenomas) is similar. Cohesive but crowded groups of atypical (ie, dysplastic) tall columnar cells with loss of cytoplasmic mucin.

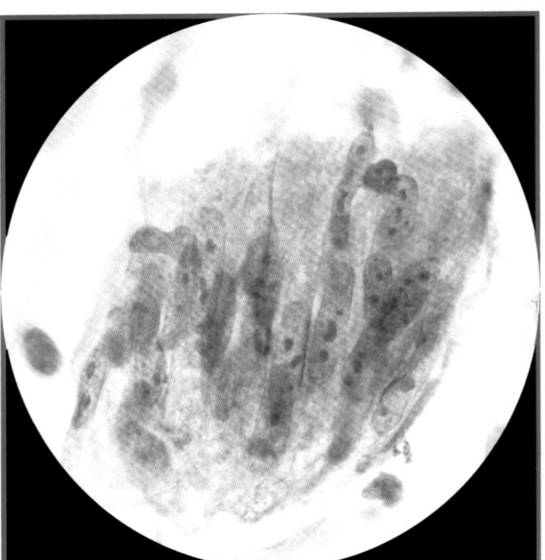

I9.77
Villous adenoma (colon). Because they pose a higher risk of malignancy than adenomatous polyps, villous adenomas may have a more atypical (ie, dysplastic) cytologic appearance, with larger nuclei, higher N/C ratios, and more pleomorphism. Cytology is useful in detecting malignant change.

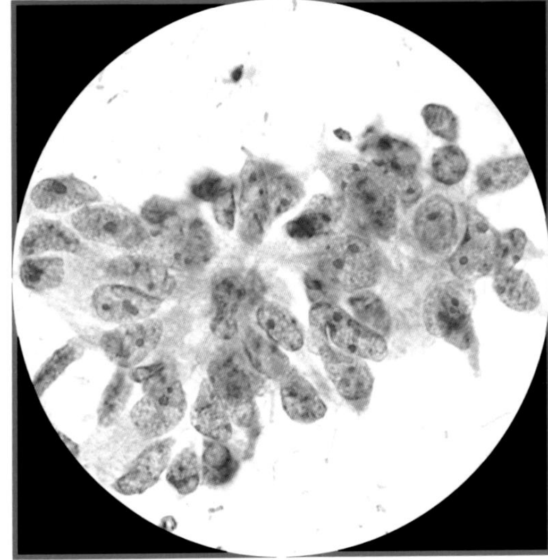

I9.78
Adenocarcinoma. Most colorectal carcinomas are moderately to well differentiated. Well-differentiated adenocarcinoma shows tall columnar cells with cigar-shaped nuclei that may be difficult to distinguish from those in dysplasia. More cells, more single cells, and loss of polarity suggest malignancy.

I9.79
Adenocarcinoma (colon). Moderately differentiated adenocarcinoma has rounded nuclei with higher N/C ratios. The cells are crowded, poorly oriented, and have prominent nucleoli.

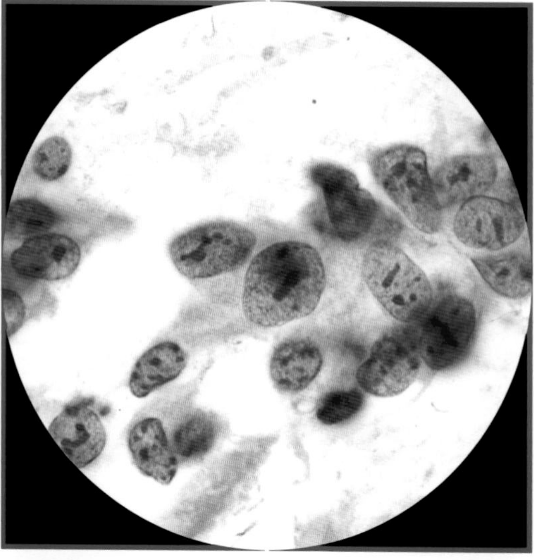

I9.80
Adenocarcinoma. Note the apical cytoplasmic densities, or "terminal bars" (arrows), which are a characteristic feature of colorectal adenocarcinoma. Ultrastructurally, terminal bars correspond with microvilli that have long, apical, cytoplasmic rootlets.

I9.81
Adenocarcinoma (colon), corresponding tissue.

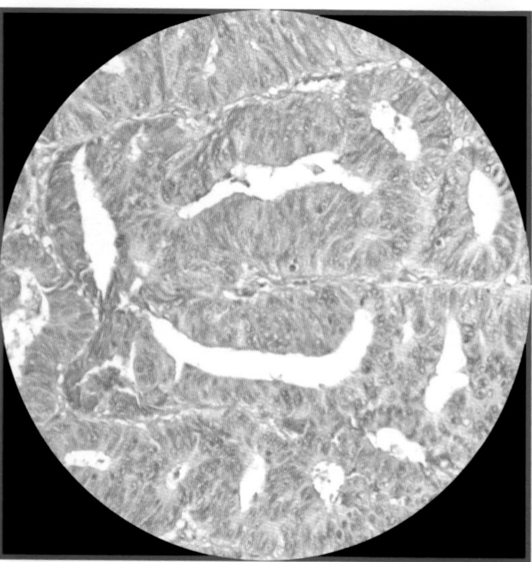

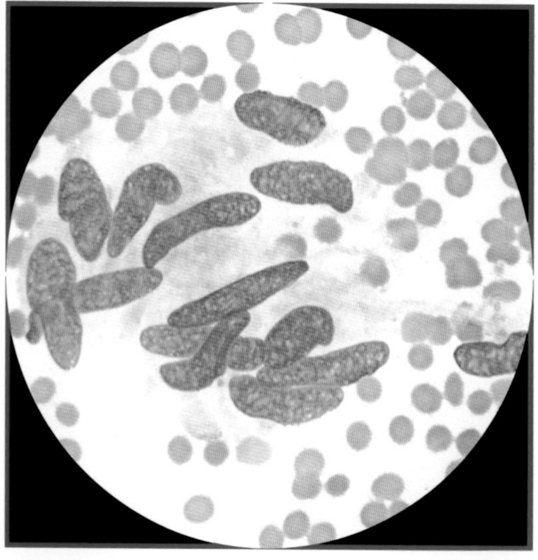

I9.82
Leiomyosarcoma. Tumors that grow submucosally are usually not amenable to diagnosis by exfoliative cytologic methods (ie, surface cytology). However, submucosal lesions can be diagnosed with endoscopic FNA biopsy, as was the spindle cell leiomyosarcoma illustrated here. (Diff-Quik®)

I9.83
Leiomyosarcoma, corresponding tissue.

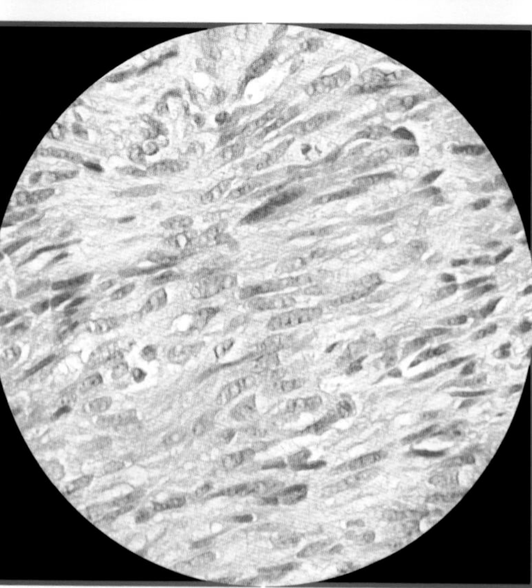

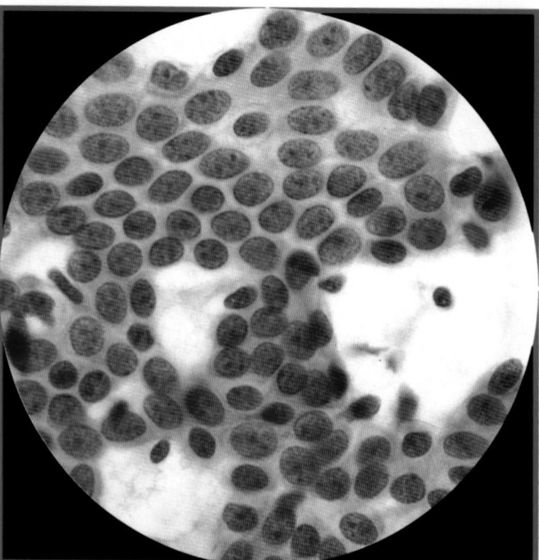

I9.84
Ductal cells. The cells of the pancreatic ducts and biliary tract are cytologically indistinguishable. They are characterized by cohesive, monolayered sheets of very orderly cells, which exhibit neither crowding nor loosening of the cellular arrangements.
(Brush specimen)

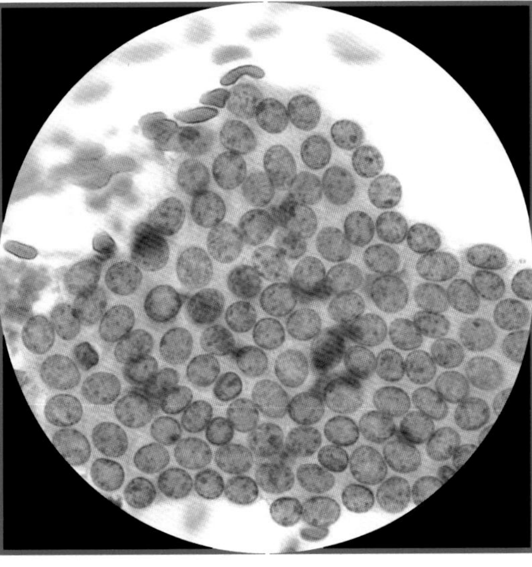

I9.85
Ductal cells. The cytoplasm is delicate and the nuclei are bland, with smooth nuclear membranes, fine chromatin, and inconspicuous or invisible nucleoli. (Brush specimen)

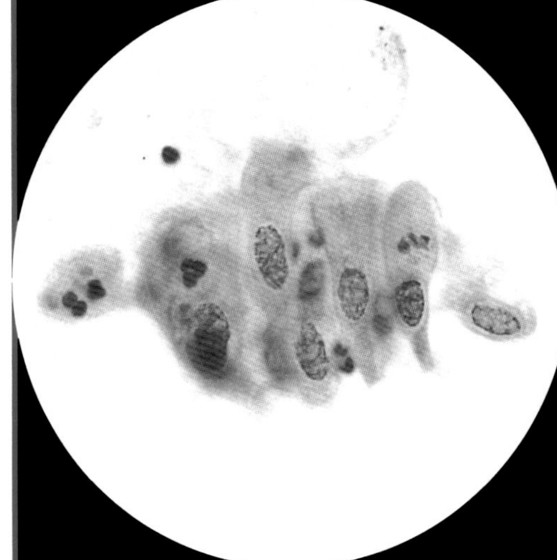

I9.86
Reactive/degenerative changes (bile duct). In response to inflammation, stones, or instrumentation, the epithelium can undergo reactive or degenerative changes. In degeneration, the chromatin may become hyperchromatic and clump (karyorrhexis), as shown here. These features sometimes suggest malignancy. (Brush specimen)

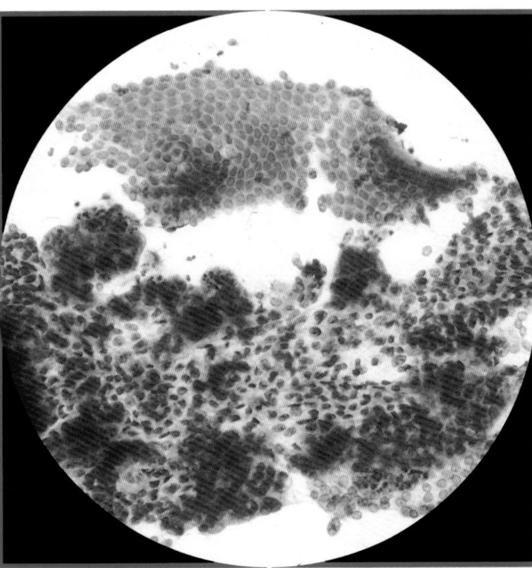

I9.87
Adenocarcinoma (bile duct). Many adenocarcinomas are very well differentiated. Important clues are loss of cohesion, irregular cellular arrangements, and irregular nuclear membranes. Compare the cohesive, orderly, smaller benign ductal cells (top) with the less cohesive, disorderly, larger malignant cells (bottom). (Brush specimen)

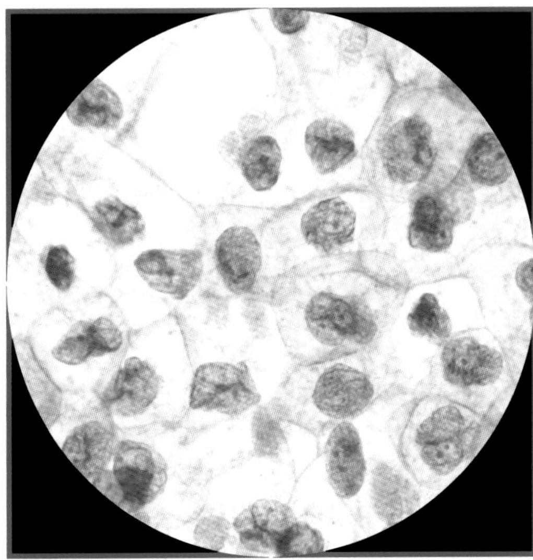

I9.88
Adenocarcinoma (bile duct). Compare the loose arrangement of this honeycomb arrangement of malignant cells with the tightly knit, extremely orderly honeycomb of benign cells. Note the irregular nuclear membranes, which are an important feature of well-differentiated cancer. (Brush specimen)

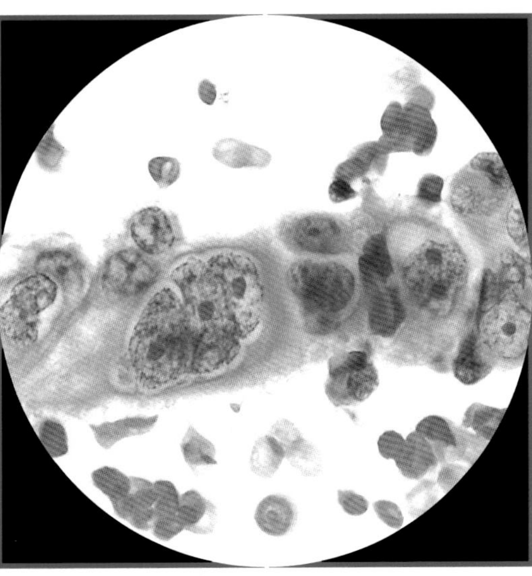

I9.89
Adenocarcinoma (bile duct). In less differentiated cancers, the cytoplasm tends to become dense and squamoid. Nuclear atypia is obvious. (Brush specimen)

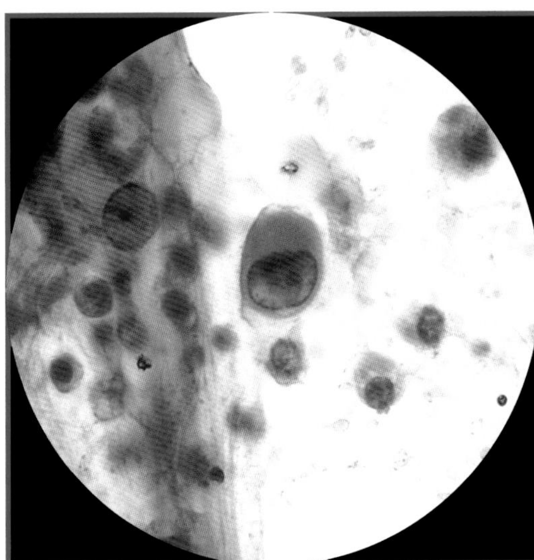

I9.90
Adenocarcinoma (bile duct). Note the nucleocytoplasmic polarity (a glandular feature) and the dense cytoplasm (a squamous feature). (Brush specimen)

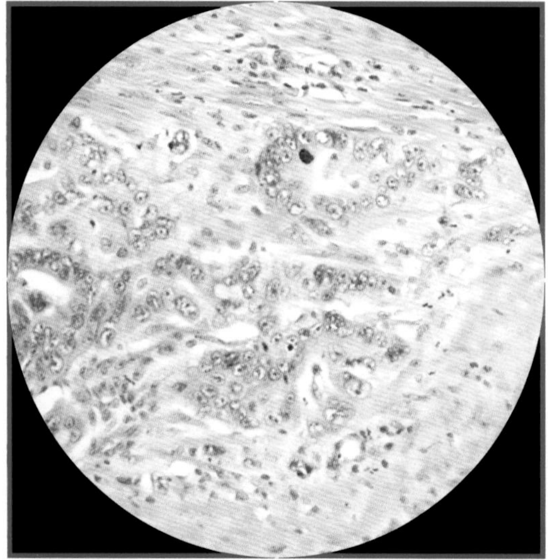

I9.91
Adenocarcinoma (bile duct), corresponding tissue.

I9.92
Ductal cells. Cells in fluids tend to become rounded and exfoliate singly or in small, cohesive groups. Reactive and degenerative changes, such as prominent nucleoli and cytoplasmic vacuolization, are common. Note the bile pigment in the background. (Bile specimen)

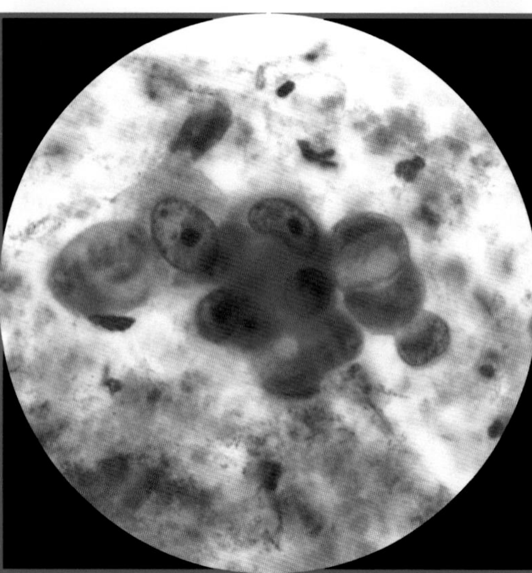

I9.93
Adenocarcinoma (bile duct). The malignant cells are poorly cohesive, form irregular crowded aggregates, and show molding. The nuclei are enlarged and pleomorphic, with prominent nucleoli. Diagnostic cells may be sparse and hidden in biliary debris. (Bile specimen)

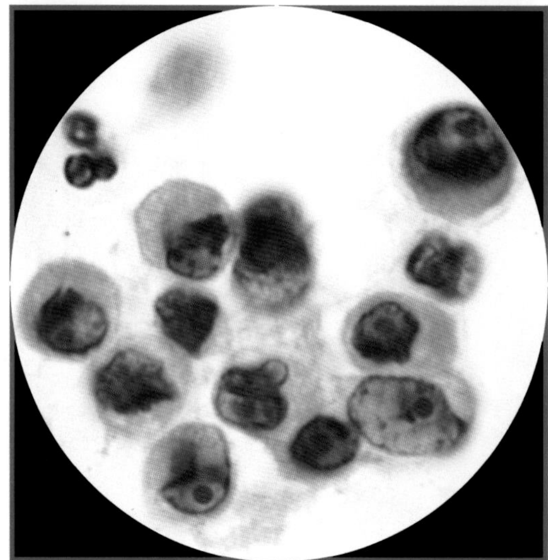

I9.94
Adenocarcinoma (bile duct). Loose aggregate of cells with malignant nuclear features, including irregular nuclear membranes, irregular chromatin, and prominent nucleoli. (Bile specimen)

References

Adelstein DJ, Forman WB, Beavers B: Esophageal Carcinoma: A Six-Year Review of the Cleveland Veterans Administration Hospital Experience. *Cancer* 54: 918–923, 1984.

Ahsan N, Berman JJ: Papillary Carcinoma of the Common Bile Duct: Diagnosis by Bile Drainage Cytology. *Acta Cytol* 32: 471–474, 1988.

Albert MB, Nochomovitz LE: Dysplasia and Cancer Surveillance in Inflammatory Bowel Disease. *Gastroenterol Clin North Am* 18: 83–97, 1989.

Albores-Saavedra J, Alcántra-Vasquez A, Cruz-Ortiz H, et al: The Precursor Lesions of Invasive Gallbladder Carcinoma: Hyperplasia, Atypical Hyperplasia and Carcinoma In Situ. *Cancer* 45: 919–927, 1980.

Aldovini D, Detassis C, Piscioli F: Primary Malignant Melanoma of the Esophagus: Brush Cytology and Histogenesis. *Acta Cytol* 27: 65–68, 1983.

Allegra SR, Broderick PA, Corvese N: Oral Cytology: Seven Year Oral Cytology Screening Program in the State of Rhode Island: Analysis of 6448 Cases. *Acta Cytol* 17: 42–48, 1973.

Alonso de Ruiz P, Albores-Saavedra J, Henson DE, et al: Cytopathology of Precursor Lesions of Invasive Carcinoma of the Gallbladder: A Study of Bile Aspirated From Surgically Excised Gallbladders. *Acta Cytol* 26: 144–152, 1982.

Anderson WR, Belding J, Pixley E: Oral Cytology: A Hormonal Evaluation. *Acta Cytol* 13: 81–83, 1969.

An-Foraker SH, Vise D: Cytodiagnosis of Gastric Carcinoma, Linitis Plastica Type (Diffuse, Infiltrating, Poorly Differentiated Adenocarcinoma). *Acta Cytol* 25: 361–366, 1981.

Ashenburg C, Rothstein FC, Dahms BB: Herpes Esophagitis in the Immunocompetent Child. *J Pediatr* 108: 584–587, 1986.

Attanoos R, Williams GT: Epithelial and Neuroendocrine Tumors of the Duodenum. *Semin Diagn Pathol* 8: 149–162, 1991.

Bader GM, Papanicolaou GN: The Application of Cytology in the Diagnosis of Cancer of the Rectum, Sigmoid, and Descending Colon. *Cancer* 5: 307–314, 1952.

Barch DH, Walloch J, Hidvegi D, et al: Histopathology of Methylbenzylnitrosamine-Induced Esophageal Carcinoma in the Rat: Comparison With Cytomorphology. *J Natl Cancer Inst* 77: 1145–1153, 1986.

Bardawil RG, D'Ambrosio FG, Hajdu SI: Colonic Cytology: A Retrospective Study With Histopathologic Correlation. *Acta Cytol* 34: 620–626, 1990.

Barrett NR: Chronic Peptic Ulcer of the Œsophagus and 'Œsophagitis'. *Br J Surg* 38: 175–182, 1950.

Batra SK, Kini SR, Schuman BM, et al: Evaluation of Brush Rinsings for the Cytologic Diagnosis of Esophageal and Gastric Cancer. *Gastrointest Endosc* 28: 23–25, 1982.

Becker SN, Sass MA, Petras RE, et al: Bizarre Atypia in Gastric Brushings Associated With Hepatic Arterial Infusion Chemotherapy. *Acta Cytol* 30: 347–350, 1986.

Bedenne L, Faivre J, Boutron MC, et al: Adenoma–Carcinoma Sequence or "De Novo" Carcinogenesis? A Study of Adenomatous Remnants in a Population-Based Series of Large Bowel Cancers. *Cancer* 69: 883–888, 1992.

Bedine MS, Cocco AE: A Comparison of Washing and Brushing Cytology and Biopsy in the Diagnosis of Malignant Disease of the Esophagus, Stomach, and Colon. *Gastrointest Endosc* 19: 75–76, 1972.

Behmard S, Sadeghi A, Bagheri SA: Diagnostic Accuracy of Endoscopy With Brushing Cytology and Biopsy in Upper Gastrointestinal Lesions. *Acta Cytol* 22: 153–154, 1978.

Belladonna JA, Hajdu SI, Bains MS, et al: Adenocarcinoma In Situ of Barrett's Esophagus Diagnosed by Endoscopic Cytology. *N Engl J Med* 291: 895–896, 1974.

Bemvenuti GA, Prolla JC, Kirsner JB, et al: Direct Vision Brushing Cytology in the Diagnosis of Colo-Rectal Malignancy. *Acta Cytol* 18: 477–481, 1974.

Bennington JL, Porus R, Ferguson B, et al: Cytology of Gastric Sarcoid: Report of a Case. *Acta Cytol* 12: 30–36, 1968.

Benya RV, Metz DC, Hijazi YM, et al: Fine Needle Aspiration Cytology of Submucosal Nodules in Patients With Zollinger-Ellison Syndrome. *Am J Gastroenterol* 88: 258–265, 1993.

Berenson MM, Riddell RH, Skinner DB, et al: Malignant Transformation of Esophageal Columnar Epithelium. *Cancer* 41: 554–561, 1978.

Berry AV, Baskind AF, Hamilton DG: Cytologic Screening for Esophageal Cancer. *Acta Cytol* 25: 135–141, 1981.

Bhasin DK, Kochhar R, Rajwanshi A, et al: Endoscopic Suction Cytology in Upper Gastrointestinal Tract Malignancy. *Acta Cytol* 32: 432–454, 1988.

Bhathal PS, Brown RW, Doyle TC, et al: Pneumatosis Cystoides Gastrica Associated With Adenocarcinoma of the Stomach. *Acta Cytol* 29: 147–150, 1985.

Bishop D, Lushpihan A, Louis C: The Cytology of Carcinoma In Situ and Early Invasive Carcinoma of the Esophagus. *Acta Cytol* 21: 298–300, 1977.

Blackstone MO, Cockerham L, Kirsner JB, et al: Intraductal Aspiration for Cytodiagnosis. *Gastrointest Endosc* 23: 145–147, 1977.

Blaser MJ: Gastric Campylobacter-like Organisms, Gastritis, and Peptic Ulcer Disease. *Gastroenterology* 93: 371–383, 1987.

Blei E, Gonzalez-Crussi F: The Intriguing Nature of Gastric Tumors in Carney's Triad: Ultrastructural and Immunohistochemical Observations. *Cancer* 69: 292–300, 1992.

Boddington MM, Truelove SC: Abnormal Epithelial Cells in Ulcerative Colitis. *Br Med J* 1: 1318–1321, 1956.

Boddington MM: Changes in Buccal Cells in the Anaemias. *J Clin Pathol* 12: 222–227, 1959a.

Boddington MM, Spriggs AI: The Epithelial Cells in Megaloblastic Anaemias. *J Clin Pathol* 12: 228–234, 1959b.

Boen ST: Changes in Nuclei of Squamous Epithelial Cells in Pernicious Anemia. *Acta Med Scand* 159: 425–431, 1957.

Boman BM, Moertel CG, O'Connell MJ, et al: Carcinoma of the Anal Canal: A Clinical and Pathologic Study of 188 Cases. *Cancer* 54: 114–125, 1984.

Boon TH, Schade ROK, Middleton GD, et al: An Attempt at Presymptomatic Diagnosis of Gastric Carcinoma in Pernicious Anaemia. *Gut* 5: 269–270, 1964.

Boring CC: Cancer Statistics. *CA Cancer J Clin* 44: 18–19, 1994.

Bourke JB, Brown CL, Swann JC, et al: Exocrine Pancreatic Function Studies, Duodenal Cytology, and Hypotonic Duodenography in the Diagnosis of Surgical Jaundice. *Lancet* (i): 605–608, 1972.

Bowden L, Papanicolaou GN: Exfoliated Pancreatic Cancer Cells in the Duct of Wirsung. *Ann Surg* 150: 296–298, 1959.

Brambs H-J, Leser HG, Salm R: Percutaneous Transhepatic Cholangioscopy: A New Diagnostic Method in Bile Duct Tumors. *Gastrointest Endosc* 34: 185, 1988.

Brandborg LL, Taniguchi L, Rubin CE: Exfoliative Cytology in Non-Malignant Conditions of the Upper Intestinal Tract. *Acta Cytol* 5: 187–190, 1961.

Brandborg LL, Wenger J: Cytological Examination in Gastrointestinal Tract Disease. *Med Clin North Am* 52: 1315–1328, 1968a.

Brandborg LL: Gastric Exfoliative Cytology: Past, Present, and Future. *Gastroenterology* 55: 632–635, 1968b.

Broderick PA, Allegra SR, Corvese N: Primary Malignant Melanoma of the Esophagus: A Case Report. *Acta Cytol* 16: 159–164, 1972.

Brown AM, Young A: The Effects of Age and Smoking on the Maturation of the Oral Mucosa. *Acta Cytol* 14: 566–569, 1970.

Burlakow P, Medak H, McGrew EA, et al: The Cytology of Vesicular Conditions Affecting the Oral Mucosa: Part 2. Keratosis Follicularis. *Acta Cytol* 13: 407–415, 1969.

Buss DH, Scharyj M: Herpesvirus Infection of the Esophagus and Other Visceral Organs in Adults: Incidence and Clinical Significance. *Am J Med* 66: 457–462, 1979.

Cabre-Fiol V, Vilardell F, Sala-Cladera E, et al: Preoperative Cytological Diagnosis of Gastric Leiomyosarcoma: A Report of Three Cases. *Gastroenterology* 68: 563–566, 1975.

Cabré-Fiol V, Vilardell F: Progress in the Cytological Diagnosis of Gastric Lymphoma: A Report of 32 Cases. *Cancer* 41: 1456–1461, 1978.

Cameron AJ, Ott BJ, Payne WP: The Incidence of Adenocarcinoma in Columnar-Lined (Barrett's) Esophagus. *N Engl J Med* 313: 857–859, 1985.

Camp R, Rutkowski MA, Atkison K, et al: A Prospective, Randomized, Blinded Trial of Cytological Yield With Disposable Cytology Brushes in Upper Gastrointestinal Tract Lesions. *Am J Gastroenterol* 87: 1439–1442, 1992.

Caos A, Olson N, Willman C, et al: Endoscopic "Salvage" Cytology in Neoplasms Metastatic to the Upper Gastrointestional (sic) Tract. *Acta Cytol* 30: 32–34, 1986.

Carney JA, Sheps SG, Go WLW, et al: The Triad of Gastric Leiomyosarcoma, Functioning Extra-Adrenal Paraganglioma and Pulmonary Chondroma. *N Engl J Med* 296: 1517–1518, 1977.

Carney JA: The Triad of Gastric Epithelioid Leiomyosarcoma, Pulmonary Chondroma, and Functioning Extra-Adrenal Paraganglioma: A Five-Year Review. *Medicine* 62: 159–169, 1983.

Carter KJ, Schaffer HA, Ritchie WP Jr: Early Gastric Cancer. *Ann Surg* 199: 604–609, 1984.

Castelli M, Gattuso P, Reyes C, et al: Fine Needle Aspiration Biopsy of Intraoral and Pharyngeal Lesions. *Acta Cytol* 37: 448–450, 1993.

Chambers LA, Clark WE II: The Endoscopic Diagnosis of Gastroesophageal Malignancy: A Cytologic Review. *Acta Cytol* 30: 110–114, 1986.

Chan WY, Hui PK, Leung KM, et al: Gastric Adenocarcinoma With Ciliated Tumor Cells. *Hum Pathol* 24: 1107–1113, 1993.

Chapman BM: Cytologic Diagnosis of Rectal and Colonic Conditions. *Gastroenterology* 36: 501–504, 1959.

Chapman DLS, Klopp CT, Platt LI: Application of Balloon Technique in Detection of Cancer. *Cancer* 6: 1174–1176, 1953.

Chen YL: The Diagnosis of Colorectal Cancer With Cytologic Brushings Under Direct Vision at Fiberoptic Colonoscopy: A Report of 59 Cases. *Dis Colon Rectum* 30: 342–344, 1987.

Chetty R, Learmonth GM, Price SK, et al: Primary Oesophageal Rhabdomyosarcoma. *Cytopathology* 2: 103–108, 1991.

Choi HY, Takeda M: Gastric Epithelial Atypia Following Hepatic Arterial Infusion Chemotherapy. *Diagn Cytopathol* 1: 241–244, 1985.

Chomette G, Auriol M, Vaillant JM: Scanning Electron Microscopy in Oral Cytology. *Diagn Cytopathol* 2: 110–117, 1986.

Cobb CJ, Floyd WN Jr: Usefulness of Bile Cytology in the Diagnostic Management of Patients With Biliary Tract Obstruction. *Acta Cytol* 29: 93–100, 1985.

Cohn I Jr: Cancer of the Pancreas: Detection and Diagnosis. *Cancer* 37: 582–588, 1976.

Connolly GN, Winn DM, Hecht SS, et al: The Reemergence of Smokeless Tobacco. *N Engl J Med* 314: 1020–1027, 1986.

Cook IJ, de Carle DJ, Haneman B, et al: The Role of Brushing Cytology in the Diagnosis of Gastric Malignancy. *Acta Cytol* 32: 461–464, 1988.

Cook MG, Goligher JC: Carcinoma and Epithelial Dysplasia Complicating Ulcerative Colitis. *Gastroenterology* 68: 1127–1136, 1975.

Cooper WA, Papanicolaou GN: Balloon Technique in the Cytological Diagnosis of Gastric Cancer. *JAMA* 10–14, 1953.

Coscia-Porrazzi L, Maiello FM, Ruocco V, et al: Cytodiagnosis of Oral Pemphigus Vulgaris. *Acta Cytol* 29: 746–749, 1985.

Cotton PB: Progress Report: ERCP. *Gut* 18: 316–341, 1977.

Cressman FK Jr, Lerman RI: Carcinoma of the Common Bile Duct Diagnosis by Cytologic Examination of T-Tube Drainage Contents (Letter). *Acta Cytol* 21: 496–497, 1977.

Cuello C, Correa P, Zarama G, et al: Histopathology of Gastric Dysplasias: Correlations With Gastric Juice Chemistry. *Am J Surg Pathol* 3: 491–500, 1979.

Cussó X, Monés-Xiol J, Vilardell F: Endoscopic Cytology of Cancer of the Esophagus and Cardia: A Long-Term Evaluation. *Gastrointest Endosc* 35: 321–323, 1989.

Cussó X, Mones J, Ocana J, et al: Is Endoscopic Gastric Cytology Worthwhile? An Evaluation of 903 Cases of Carcinoma. *J Clin Gastroenterol* 16: 336–339, 1993.

Dabelsteen E, Roed-Petersen B, Smith CJ, et al: The Limitations of Exfoliative Cytology for the Detection of Epithelial Atypia in Oral Leukoplakias. *Br J Cancer* 25: 21–24, 1971.

Daling JR, Weiss NS, Hislop TG, et al: Sexual Practices, Sexually Transmitted Diseases, and the Incidence of Anal Cancer. *N Engl J Med* 317: 973–977, 1987.

Das DK, Gulati A, Bhatt NC, et al: Fine Needle Aspiration Cytology of Oral and Pharyngeal Lesions: A Study of 45 Cases. *Acta Cytol* 37: 333–342, 1993.

Das DK, Pant CS: Fine Needle Aspiration Cytologic Diagnosis of Gastrointestinal Tract Lesions. A Study of 78 Cases. *Acta Cytol* 38: 723–729, 1994.

Davenport RD: Cytologic Diagnosis of *Campylobacter pylori*-Associated Gastritis. *Acta Cytol* 34: 211–213, 1990.

Dawsey SM, Yu Y, Taylor PR, et al: Esophageal Cytology and Subsequent Risk of Esophageal Cancer. A Prospective Follow-up Study From Linxian, China. *Acta Cytol* 38: 183–192, 1994.

Dawson MA, Schaefer JW: A Simple Method of Obtaining Cytologic Material During Esophagoscopy. *Gastrointest Endosc* 27: 76–77, 1970.

Day GL, Blot WJ: Second Primary Tumors in Patients With Oral Cancer. *Cancer* 70: 14–19, 1992.

Debongnie JC, Beyaert C, Legros G: Touch Cytology, A Useful Diagnostic Method for Diagnosis of Upper Gastrointestinal Tract Infections. *Dig Dis Sci* 34: 1025–1027, 1989.

Debongnie JC, Mairesse J, Donnay M, et al: Touch Cytology: A Quick, Simple, Sensitive Screening Test in the Diagnosis of Infections of the Gastrointestinal Mucosa. *Arch Pathol Lab Med* 118: 1115–1118, 1994.

de Borges RJ, Acevedo F, Miralles E, et al: Squamous Papilloma of the Esophagus Diagnosed by Cytology: Report of a Case With Concurrent Occult Epidermoid Carcinoma. *Acta Cytol* 30: 487–490, 1986.

De Francesco F, Nicotina PA, Picciotto M, et al: *Helicobacter pylori* in Gastroduodenal Diseases: Rapid Identification by Endoscopic Brush Cytology. *Diagn Cytopathol* 9: 430–433, 1993.

De Gaetani CF, Botticelli CS, Rigo GP: Primary Gastric Lymphoplasmacytoid Malignant Lymphoma (Gastric Plasmacytoma): An Endoscopic Cytologic Diagnosis. *Acta Cytol* 21: 465–468, 1977.

Dei Tos AP, Laurino L, De Boni, et al: Preoperative Cytodiagnosis of Primitive Carcinoid Tumor of the Wirsung Duct: A Case Report With Immunocytochemical Study. *Diagn Cytopathol* 9: 471–474, 1993.

Dellers EA, Dunn JC, DeSantis P, et al: Identification of *Blastocystis hominis* by Colonic Brush Cytology: A Case Report. *Acta Cytol* 36: 757–758, 1992.

DeNardi FG, Riddell RH: The Normal Esophagus. *Am J Surg Pathol* 15: 296–309, 1991.

Depew WT, Prentice RSA, Beck IT, et al: Herpes Simplex Ulcerative Esophagitis in a Healthy Subject. *Am J Gastroenterol* 68: 381–385, 1977.

De Ruiter A, Carter P, Katz DR, et al: A Comparison Between Cytology and Histology to Detect Anal Intraepithelial Neoplasia. *Genitourin Med* 70: 22–25, 1994.

DiMagno EP, Malagelada J-R, Taylor WF, et al: A Prospective Comparison of Current Diagnostic Tests for Pancreatic Cancer. *N Engl J Med* 297: 737–742, 1977a.

DiMagno EP, Go VLW: Cytodiagnosis of Pancreatic Cancer. *Gastrointest Endosc* 23: 173–174, 1977b.

Dina R, Cassisa A, Baroncini D, et al: Role of Esophageal Brushing Cytology in Monitoring Patients Treated With Sclerotherapy for Esophageal Varices. *Acta Cytol* 36: 477–479, 1992.

Dokumov SI, Spasov SA: A Comparison of Oral and Vaginal Smears in Women With Normal Menstrual Cycles. *Acta Cytol* 14: 31–34, 1970.

Dooley CP, Cohen H, Fitzgibbons PL, et al: Prevalence of *Helicobacter pylori* Infection and Histologic Gastritis in Asymptomatic Persons. *N Engl J Med* 321: 1562–1566, 1989.

Doos WG, Stilmant MS, Murphy JL, et al: The Cytologic Characteristics of Barrett's Epithelium (Abstract). *Gastroenterology* 88: 1368, 1985.

Douglass LE, Beaver DL: Experience With Buccal Smears in the General Cytopathology Laboratory. *Acta Cytol* 13: 595–600, 1969.

Dreiling DA, Nieburgs HE, Janowitz HD: The Combined Secretin and Cytology Test in the Diagnosis of Pancreatic and Biliary Tract Cancer. *Med Clin North Am* 44: 801–815, 1960.

Duggan MA, Boras VF, Inoue M, et al: Human Papillomavirus DNA Determination of Anal Condylomata, Dysplasias, and Squamous Carcinomas With In Situ Hybridization. *Am J Clin Pathol* 92: 16–21, 1989.

Duggan MA, Boras VF, Inoue M, et al: Human Papillomavirus DNA in Anal Carcinomas: Comparison of In Situ and Dot Blot Hybridization. *Am J Clin Pathol* 96: 318–325, 1991.

Dziura BR, Otis R, Hukill P, et al: Gastric Brushing Cytology: An Analysis of Cells From Benign and Malignant Ulcers. *Acta Cytol* 21: 187–190, 1977.

Ehya H, O'Hara BJ: Brush Cytology in the Diagnosis of Colonic Neoplasms. *Cancer* 66: 1563–1567, 1990.

Einhorn J, Wersäll J: Incidence of Oral Carcinoma in Patients With Leukoplakia of the Oral Mucosa. *Cancer* 20: 2189–2193, 1967.

Eisen RN, Kirby WM, O'Quinn JL: Granular Cell Tumor of the Biliary Tree: A Report of Two Cases and a Review of the Literature. *Am J Surg Pathol* 15: 460–465, 1991.

Elyaderani MK, Gabriele OF: Brush and Forceps Biopsy of Biliary Ducts via Percutaneous Transhepatic Catheterization. *Radiology* 134: 777–778, 1980.

Elzay RP, Frable WJ: "Accessory Oral Tonsils"—A Cytologic Dilemma. *Acta Cytol* 18: 125–129, 1974.

Endo Y, Morii T, Tamura H, et al: Cytodiagnosis of Pancreatic Malignant Tumors by Aspiration, Under Direct Vision, Using a Duodenal Fiberscope. *Gastroenterology* 67: 944–951, 1974.

Enrile FT, de Jesus PO, Bakst AA, et al: Pseudosarcoma of the Esophagus (Polypoid Carcinoma of Esophagus With Pseudosarcomatous Features). *Cancer* 31: 1197–1202, 1973.

Evett RD, Higgins JA, Brown AL Jr: The Fine Structure of Normal Mucosa in Human Gall Bladder. *Gastroenterology* 47: 49–60, 1964.

Faravelli A, Sironi M, Villa E, et al: Immunoperoxidase Study of Cytologic Smears in Oral Pemphigus. *Acta Cytol* 28: 414–418, 1984.

Farinati F, Cardin F, Di Mario F, et al: Follow-up in Gastric Dysplasia Patients. *Am J Surg Pathol* 13: 173–174, 1989.

Farini R, Farinati F, Leandro G, et al: Gastric Epithelial Dysplasia in Relapsing and Nonrelapsing Gastric Ulcer. *Am J Gastroenterol* 77: 844–853, 1982.

Fath RB Jr, Winawer SJ: Early Diagnosis of Colorectal Cancer. *Annu Rev Med* 34: 501–507, 1983.

Faverly D, Famerée, Lamy V, et al: Identification of *Campylobacter pylori* in Gastric Biopsy Smears. *Acta Cytol* 34: 205–210, 1990.

Fenger C: Anal Canal Tumors and Their Precursors. *Pathol Annu* 23(l): 45–66, 1988.

Fenger C: Anal Neoplasia and Its Precursors: Facts and Controversies. *Semin Diagn Pathol* 8: 190–201, 1991.

Ferrari AP, Lichtenstein DR, Slivka A, et al: Brush Cytology During ERCP for the Diagnosis of Biliary and Pancreatic Malignancies. *Gastrointest Endosc* 40: 140–145, 1994.

Festa VI, Hajdu SI, Winawer SJ: Colorectal Cytology in Chronic Ulcerative Colitis. *Acta Cytol* 29: 262–268, 1985.

Fischbein PG, Tuthill R, Kressel H, et al: Herpes Simplex Esophagitis: A Cause of Upper-Gastrointestinal Bleeding. *Dig Dis Sci* 24: 540–544, 1979.

Fitzgerald PJ, Fortner JG, Watson RC, et al: The Value of Diagnostic Aids in Detecting Pancreas Cancer. *Cancer* 41: 868–879, 1978.

Floyd WN Jr, Cobb C: Cholangiography and Bile Cytopathology in the Diagnosis of Biliary Tract Obstruction. *South Med J* 78: 134–137, 1985.

Folsom TC, White CP, Bromer L, et al: Oral Exfoliative Study: Review of the Literature and Report of a Three-year Study. *Oral Surg* 33: 61–74, 1972.

Forde KA, Treat MR: Colonoscopy in the Evaluation of Strictures. *Dis Colon Rectum* 28: 699–701, 1985.

Foucar E, Mukai K, Foucar K, et al: Colon Ulceration in Lethal Cytomegalovirus Infection. *Am J Clin Pathol* 76: 788–801, 1981.

Foushee JHS, Kalnins ZA, Dixon FR, et al: Gastric Cytology: Evaluation of Methods and Results in 1,670 Cases. *Acta Cytol* 13: 399–406, 1969.

Fraga-Fernández J, Vicandi-Plaza B: Diagnosis of Hairy Leukoplakia by Exfoliative Cytologic Methods. *Am J Clin Pathol* 97: 262–266, 1992.

Frazer IH, Crapper RM, Medley G, et al: Association Between Anorectal Dysplasia, Human Papillomavirus, and Human Immunodeficiency Virus Infection in Homosexual Men. *Lancet* (ii): 657–660, 1986.

Fukuda T, Shida S, Takita T, et al: Cytologic Diagnosis of Early Gastric Cancer by the Endoscope Method With Gastrofiberscope. *Acta Cytol* 11: 456–459, 1967.

Galambos JT, Massey BW, Klayman MI, et al: Exfoliative Cytology in Chronic Ulcerative Colitis. *Cancer* 9: 152–159, 1956.

Galambos JT: Cytologic Examination of Benign Colonic Lesions. *Acta Cytol* 6: 148–154, 1962.

Gardner AF: An Investigation of 890 Patients With Cancer of the Oral Cavity: Its Incidence, Etiology, Prognosis and Relationship to Oral Exfoliative Cytology. *Acta Cytol* 9: 273–281, 1965.

Gefter WB, Laufer I, Edell S, et al: Candidiasis in the Obstructed Esophagus. *Radiology* 138: 25–38, 1981.

Geisinger KR, Teot LA, Richter JE: A Comparative Cytopathologic and Histologic Study of Atypia, Dysplasia, and Adenocarcinoma in Barrett's Esophagus. *Cancer* 69: 8–16, 1992.

Geisinger KR: Endoscopic Biopsies and Cytologic Brushings of the Esophagus Are Diagnostically Complementary. *Am J Clin Pathol* 103: 295–299, 1995.

Gephart T, Graham RM: The Cellular Detection of Carcinoma of the Esophagus. *Surg Gynecol Obstet* 107: 75–82, 1959.

Gibbs DD: Degenerating Cells in Bile-Stained Gastric Aspirates. *Acta Cytol* 7: 311–314, 1963.

Gillespie GM: Renewal of Buccal Epithelium. *Oral Surg Oral Med Oral Pathol* 27: 83–89, 1969.

Gillespie JJ, MacKay B: Histogenesis of Cloacogenic Carcinoma: Fine Structure of Anal Transitional Epithelium and Cloacogenic Carcinoma. *Hum Pathol* 9: 579–587, 1978.

Goldgraber MB: The Response of Esophageal Cancer to Irradiation: A Serial Cytologic Study of Two Cases. *Gastroenterology* 30: 618–624, 1956.

Goldstein H, Ventzke LE, Wernett C: Value of Exfoliative Cytology in Pancreatic Carcinoma. *Gut* 9: 316–318, 1968.

Goodale RL, Gajl-Peczalska K, Dressel T, et al: Cytologic Studies for the Diagnosis of Pancreatic Cancer. *Cancer* 47: 1652–1655, 1981.

Goodwin CS, Armstrong JA, Marshall BJ: *Campylobacter* Pyloridis, Gastritis, and Peptic Ulceration. *J Clin Pathol* 39: 353–365, 1986.

Gorczyca W, Woyke S: Endoscopic Brushing Cytology of Primary Gastric Choriocarcinoma: A Case Report. *Acta Cytol* 36: 551–554, 1992.

Graham DY, Spjut HJ: Salvage Cytology: A New Alternative Fiberoptic Technique. *Gastrointest Endosc* 25: 137–139, 1979.

Graham DY, Tabibian N, Michaletz PA, et al: Endoscopic Needle Biopsy: A Comparative Study of Forceps Biopsy, Two Different Types of Needles, and Salvage Cytology in Gastrointestinal Cancer. *Gastrointest Endosc* 35: 207–209, 1989.

Graham RM, Rheault MH: Characteristic Cellular Changes in Epithelial Cells in Pernicious Anemia. *J Lab Clin Med* 3: 235–254, 1954.

Granqvist S, Granberg-Öhman I, Sundelin P: Colonoscopic Biopsies and Cytological Examination in Chronic Ulcerative Colitis. *Scand J Gastroenterol* 15: 282–288, 1980.

Greco FA, Brereton HD, Kent H, et al: Adriamycin and Enhanced Radiation Reaction in Normal Esophagus and Skin. *Ann Intern Med* 85: 294–298, 1976.

Green LK, Zachariah S, Graham DY: The Use of Gastric Salvage Cytology in the Diagnosis of Malignancy: A Review of 731 Cases. *Diagn Cytopathol* 6: 1–4, 1990.

Greenebaum E, Schreiber K, Shu Y-J, et al: Use of the Esophageal Balloon in the Diagnosis of Carcinomas of the Head, Neck and Upper Gastrointestinal Tract. *Acta Cytol* 28: 9–15, 1984.

Greenstein AJ, Mullin GE, Strauchen JA, et al: Lymphoma in Inflammatory Bowel Disease. *Cancer* 69: 1119–1123, 1992.

Gupta JP, Jain AK, Agrawal BK, et al: Gastroscopic Cytology and Biopsies in Diagnosis of Gastric Malignancies. *J Surg Oncol* 22: 6264, 1983.

Gupta RK, Rogers KE: Endoscopic Cytology and Biopsy in the Diagnosis of Gastroesophageal Malignancy. *Acta Cytol* 27: 17–22, 1983.

Haggitt RC, Tryzelaar J, Ellis FH, et al: Adenocarcinoma Complicating Columnar Epithelium-lined (Barrett's) Esophagus. *Am J Clin Pathol* 70: 1–5, 1978.

Hagy GW, Brodrick MM: Variation of Sex Chromatin in Human Oral Mucosa During the Menstrual Cycle. *Acta Cytol* 16: 314–321, 1972.

Hall PA, Levison DA: Malignant Lymphoma in the Gastrointestinal Tract. *Semin Diagn Pathol* 8: 163–177, 1991.

Hameeteman W, Tytgat GNJ, Houthoff HJ, et al: Barrett's Esophagus: Development of Dysplasia and Adenocarcinoma. *Gastroenterology* 96: 1249–1256, 1989.

Hamilton SR, Smith RRL: The Relationship Between Columnar Epithelial Dysplasia and Invasive Adenocarcinoma Arising in Barrett's Esophagus. *Am J Clin Pathol* 87: 301–312, 1987.

Hamilton SR, Smith RRL, Cameron JL: Prevalence and Characteristics of Barrett Esophagus in Patients With Adenocarcinoma of the Esophagus or Esophagogastric Junction. *Hum Pathol* 19: 942–948, 1988.

Hanson JT, Thoreson C, Morrissey JF: Brush Cytology in the Diagnosis of Upper Gastrointestinal Malignancy. *Gastrointest Endosc* 26: 33–35, 1980.

Harell GS, Anderson MF, Berry PF: Cytologic Bile Examination in the Diagnosis of Biliary Duct Neoplastic Strictures. *Am J Roentgenol* 137: 1123–1126, 1981.

Hatfield ARW, Whittaker R, Gibbs DD: The Collection of Pancreatic Fluid for Cytodiagnosis Using a Duodenoscope. *Gut* 15: 305–307, 1974.

Hatfield ARW, Smithies A, Wilkins R, et al: Assessment of Endoscopic Retrograde Cholangiopancreatography (ECRP) and Pure Pancreatic Juice Cytology in Patients With Pancreatic Disease. *Gut* 17: 14–21, 1976.

Haye KR, Stanbridge CM: Cytological Screening to Detect Subclinical Anal Human Papillomavirus (HPV) Infection in Homosexual Men Attending Genitourinary Medicine Clinic. *Genitourin Med* 64: 378–382, 1988.

Hayes RL, Berg GW, Ross WL: Oral Cytology: Its Value and Its Limitations. *JADA* 79: 649–657, 1969.

Hoda SA, Hajdu SI: Small Cell Carcinoma of the Esophagus: Cytology and Immunohistology in Four Cases. *Acta Cytol* 36: 113–120, 1992.

Hoover L, Berman JJ: Epithelial Repair Versus Carcinoma in Esophageal Brush Cytology. *Diagn Cytopathol* 4: 217–223, 1988.

Horai T, Kobayashi A, Tateishi R, et al: A Cytologic Study on Small Cell Carcinoma of the Esophagus. *Cancer* 41: 1890–1896, 1978.

Howell LP, Wright AL, Calafati SA, et al: Cytodiagnosis of In Situ and Early Carcinoma of the Upper Gastrointestinal Tract. *Acta Cytol* 29: 269–273, 1985.

Howell LP, Chow H-C, Russell LA: Cytodiagnosis of Extrahepatic Biliary Duct Tumors From Specimens Obtained During Cholangiography. *Diagn Cytopathol* 4: 328–334, 1988.

Hustin J, Lagneaux G, Donnay M, et al: Cytologic Patterns of Reparative Processes, True Dysplasia and Carcinoma of the Gastric Mucosa. *Acta Cytol* 38: 730–736, 1994.

Hutter RVP, Gerold FP: Cytodiagnosis of Clinically Inapparent Oral Cancer in Patients Considered to be High Risks. A Preliminary Report. *Am J Surg* 112: 541–546, 1966.

Ihre T, Pyk E, Raaschou-Nielsen, et al: Percutaneous Fine-Needle Aspiration Biopsy During Endoscopic Retrograde Cholangio-Pancreatography. *Scand J Gastroenterol* 13: 657–662, 1978.

Iishi H, Yamamoto R, Tatsuta M, et al: Evaluation of Fine-Needle Aspiration Biopsy Under Direct Vision Gastrofiberscopy in Diagnosis of Diffusely Infiltrative Carcinoma of the Stomach. *Cancer* 57: 1365–1369, 1986.

Imbriglia JE, Lopusniak MS: Cytologic Examination of Sediment From the Esophagus in a Case of Intra-Epidermal Carcinoma of the Esophagus. *Gastroenterology* 13: 457–463, 1949.

Ingoldby CJH, Mason MK, Hall RI: Endoscopic Needle Aspiration Cytology: A New Method for the Diagnosis of Upper Gastrointestinal Cancer. *Gut* 28: 1142–1144, 1987.

Isaacson PG, Spencer J, Finn T: Primary B-Cell Gastric Lymphoma. *Hum Pathol* 17:72–82, 1986.

Isbell G, Levin B: Ulcerative Colitis and Colon Cancer. *Gastroenterol Clin North Am* 17: 773–791, 1988.

Ishikawa O, Ohhigashi H, Sasaki Y, et al: The Usefulness of Saline-Irrigated Bile for the Intraoperative Cytologic Diagnosis of Tumors and Tumorlike Lesions of the Gallbladder. *Acta Cytol* 32: 475–481, 1988.

Ishikawa O, Imaoka S, Ohigashi H, et al: A New Method of Intraoperative Cytodiagnosis for More Precisely Locating the Occult Neoplasms of the Pancreas. *Surgery* 111: 294–300, 1992.

Jacob P, Kahrilas PJ, Desai T, et al: Natural History and Significance of Esophageal Squamous Cell Dysplasia. *Cancer* 65: 2731–2739, 1990.

JAMA. Joint Position Statement: Oral Cytology. *JAMA* 205: 523, 1968.

Jaskiewicz K, Venter FS, Marasas WF: Cytopathology of the Esophagus in Transkei. *J Natl Cancer Inst* 79: 961–965, 1987.

Jass JR, Filipe MI: The Mucin Profiles of Normal Gastric Mucosa, Intestinal Metaplasia and Its Variants and Gastric Carcinoma. *Histochem J* 13: 931–939, 1981.

Jass JR: A Classification of Gastric Dysplasia. *Histopathology* 7: 181–193, 1983.

Jeevanandam V, Treat MR, Forde KA: A Comparison of Direct Brush Cytology and Biopsy in the Diagnosis of Colorectal Cancer. *Gastrointest Endosc* 33: 370–371, 1987.

Johnson WD, Koss LG, Papanicolaou GN, et al: Cytology of Esophageal Washings: Evaluation of 365 Cases. *Cancer* 8: 951–957, 1955.

Kadakia SC, Parker A, Canales L: Metastatic Tumors to the Upper Gastrointestinal Tract: Endoscopic Experience. *Am J Gastroenterol* 87: 1418–1423, 1992.

Kameya S, Kuno N, Kasugai T: The Diagnosis of Pancreatic Cancer by Pancreatic Juice Cytology. *Acta Cytol* 25: 354–360, 1981.

Kaneko E, Nakamura T, Umeda N, et al: Outcome of Gastric Carcinoma Detected by Gastric Mass Survey in Japan. *Gut* 18: 626–630, 1977.

Kaneko F, Mori M, Tsukinaga I, et al: Pemphigus Vulgaris of Esophageal Mucosa. *Arch Dermatol* 121: 272–273, 1985.

Kasugai T: Evaluation of Gastric Lavage Cytology Under Direct Vision by the Fibergastroscope Employing Hanks' Solution as a Washing Solution. *Acta Cytol* 12: 345–351, 1968.

Kasugai T, Kobayashi S: Evaluation of Biopsy and Cytology in the Diagnosis of Gastric Cancer. *Am J Gastroenterol* 62: 199–203, 1974.

Kasugai T, Kobayashi S, Kuno N: Endoscopic Cytology of the Esophagus, Stomach and Pancreas. *Acta Cytol* 22: 327–330, 1978.

Katz S, Klein MS, Winawer SJ, et al: Disseminated Lymphoma Involving the Stomach: Correlation of Endoscopy With Directed Cytology and Biopsy. *Dig Dis* 18: 370–374, 1973.

Katz S, Katzka I, Platt N, et al: Cancer in Chronic Ulcerative Colitis: Diagnostic Role of Segmental Colonic Lavage. *Dig Dis* 22: 355–364, 1977.

King OH Jr, Coleman SA: Analysis of Oral Exfoliative Cytologic Accuracy by Control Biopsy Technique. *Acta Cytol* 9: 351–354, 1965.

King OH Jr: Cytology—Its Value in the Diagnosis of Oral Cancer. *Dent Clin North Am* 15: 817–826, 1971.

Klavins JV, Flemma RJ: A Method for Studying the Material of the Bile Ducts. *Acta Cytol* 8: 332–335, 1964.

Kline TS, Goldstein F: Malignant Lymphoma Involving the Stomach. *Cancer* 32: 961–968, 1973.

Kline TS, Goldstein F: The Role of Cytology in the Diagnosis of Gastric Lymphoma. *Am J Gastroenterol* 62: 193–198, 1974.

Kline TS, Yum KK: Fiberoptic Coloscopy and Cytology. *Cancer* 37: 2553–2556, 1976.

Kline TS, Joshi LP, Goldstein F: Preoperative Diagnosis of Pancreatic Malignancy by the Cytologic Examination of Duodenal Secretions. *Am J Clin Pathol* 70: 851–854, 1978.

Kobayashi S, Prolla JC, Kirsner JB: Reactive Lymphoreticular Hyperplasia of the Stomach. *Arch Intern Med* 125: 1030–1035, 1970a.

Kobayashi S, Prolla JC, Kirsner JB: Brushing Cytology of the Esophagus and Stomach Under Direct Vision by Fiberscopes. *Acta Cytol* 14: 219–223, 1970b.

Kobayashi S, Yoshii Y, Kasugai T: Selective Use of Brushing Cytology in Gastrointestinal Strictures. *Gastrointest Endosc* 19: 77–78, 1972.

Kobayashi S, Kasugai T: Brushing Cytology for the Diagnosis of Gastric Cancer Involving the Cardia or the Lower Esophagus. *Acta Cytol* 22: 155–157, 1978.

Kochhar R, Gupta SK, Malik AK, et al: Endoscopic Fine Needle Aspiration Biopsy. *Acta Cytol* 31: 481–484, 1987.

Kochhar R, Rajwanshi A, Malik AK, et al: Endoscopic Fine Needle Aspiration Biopsy of Gastroesophageal Malignancies. *Gastrointest Endosc* 34: 321–323, 1988.

Kochhar R, Bhasin DK, Rajwanshi A, et al: Crush Preparations of Gastroesophageal Biopsy Specimens in the Diagnosis of Malignancy. *Acta Cytol* 34: 214–216, 1990a.

Kochhar R, Rajwanshi A, Dev Wig J, et al: Fine Needle Aspiration Cytology of Rectal Masses. *Gut* 31: 334–336, 1990b.

Kochhar R, Rajwanshi A, Goenka MK, et al: Colonoscopic Fine Needle Aspiration Cytology in the Diagnosis of Ileocecal Tuberculosis. *Am J Gastroenterol* 86: 102–104, 1991.

Kodsi BE, Wickremesinghe PC, Kozinn PJ, et al: *Candida* Esophagitis: A Prospective Study of 27 Cases. *Gastroenterology* 71: 715–719, 1971.

Korat O, Yachnis AT, Ernst CS: Cytologic Detection of Amyloid in Duodenal and Ureteral Brushings. *Diagn Cytopathol* 4: 133–136, 1988.

Koss LG: Abdominal Gas Cysts (Pneumatosis Cystoides Intestinorum Hominis): An Analysis With a Report of a Case and a Critical Review of the Literature. *Arch Pathol* 53: 523–549, 1952.

Koss LG: Cytologic Diagnosis of Oral, Esophageal, and Peripheral Lung Cancer. *J Cell Biochem* 17F: 66–81, 1993.

Kune GA, Baird L, Lusink C: Rapid Cytological Diagnosis of Rectal Cancer. *Ann R Coll Surg Engl* 66: 85–86, 1984.

Kurzawinski T, Deery A, Davidson BR: Diagnostic Value of Cytology for Biliary Stricture. *Br J Surg* 80: 414–421, 1993.

Lan C: Critical Evaluation of the Cytodiagnosis of Fibrogastroendoscopic Samples Obtained Under Direct Vision. *Acta Cytol* 34: 217–220, 1990.

Lasser A: Herpes Simplex Virus Esophagitis. *Acta Cytol* 21: 301–302, 1977.

Laurén P: The Two Histological Main Types of Gastric Carcinoma: Diffuse and So-Called Intestinal-Type Carcinoma: An Attempt at a Histo-Clinical Classification. *Acta Pathol Microbiol Scand* 64: 31–49, 1965.

Layfield LJ, Reichman A, Weinstein WM: Endoscopically Directed Fine Needle Aspiration Biopsy of Gastric and Esophageal Lesions. *Acta Cytol* 36: 69–74, 1992.

Layfield LJ, Wax TD, Lee JG, et al: Accuracy and Morphologic Aspects of Pancreatic and Biliary Duct Brushings. *Acta Cytol* 39: 11–18, 1995.

Lee RG: Mucins in Barrett's Esophagus: A Histochemical Study. *Am J Clin Pathol* 81: 500–503, 1984.

Lee RG: Marked Eosinophilia in Esophageal Mucosal Biopsies. *Am J Surg Pathol* 9(7): 475–479, 1985a.

Lee RG: Dysplasia in Barrett's Esophagus: A Clinicopathologic Study of Six Patients. *Am J Surg Pathol* 9: 845–852, 1985b.

Lemon HM, Byrnes WW: Cancer of the Biliary Tract and Pancreas: Diagnosis From Cytology of Duodenal Aspirations. *JAMA* 141: 254–257, 1949.

Leung KM, Hui PK, Chan WY, et al: *Helicobacter pylori*–Related Gastritis and Gastric Ulcer: A Continuum of Progressive Epithelial Degeneration. *Am J Clin Pathol* 98: 569–574, 1992.

Levin ES, Lunin M: The Oral Exfoliative Cytology of Pemphigus: A Report of Two Cases. *Acta Cytol* 13: 108–110, 1969.

Libcke JH: The Cytology of Cervical Pemphigus. *Acta Cytol* 14: 42–44, 1970.

Lightdale CJ, Wolf DJ, Marcucci RA, et al: Herpetic Esophagitis in Patients With Cancer: Ante Mortem Diagnosis by Brush Cytology. *Cancer* 39: 223–226, 1977.

Lin BPC, Harmata PA: Gastric and Esophageal Brush Cytology. *Pathology* 15: 393–397, 1983.

Linehan JJ, Melcher DH, Strachan CJL: Rapid Outpatient Detection of Rectal Cancer by Gloved Digital Scrape Cytology. *Acta Cytol* 27: 146–151, 1983.

Loux HA, Zamcheck N: Cytological Evidence for the Long "Quiescent" Stage of Gastric Cancer in 2 Patients With Pernicious Anemia. *Gastroenterology* 57: 173–184, 1969.

Lozowski W, Hajdu SI: Preoperative Cytologic Diagnosis of Primary Gastrointestinal Malignant Lymphoma. *Acta Cytol* 28: 563–570, 1984.

Lumsden AB: Bile Cytology in the Diagnosing of Sclerosing Cholangitis of Sclerosing Cholangitis and Cholangiocarcinoma. *Acta Cytol* 30: 92, 1986.

MacDonald WC, Brandborg LL, Taniguchi L, et al: Exfoliative Cytological Screening for Gastric Cancer. *Cancer* 17: 163–169, 1964.

MacDonald WC: Clinical and Pathologic Features of Adenocarcinoma of the Gastric Cardia. *Cancer* 29: 724–732, 1972.

Machado G, Davies JD, Tudway AJC, et al: Superficial Carcinoma of the Stomach. *Br Med J* 2: 77–79, 1976.

Maimon HN, Dreskin RB, Cocco AE: Positive Esophageal Cytology Without Detectable Neoplasm. *Gastrointest Endosc* 20: 156–159, 1974.

Main DMG, Keat SM: Suction Sampling Technique for Obtaining Standardized Cytologic Specimens From the Oral Mucosa. *Acta Cytol* 34: 695–698, 1990.

Martinez-Onsurbe P, Ruiz-Villaespesa A, Gonzalez-Estecha A, et al: Cytodiagnosis of Gastric Ulcer Penetration of the Liver by Examination of Endoscopic Brushings. *Acta Cytol* 35: 464–466, 1991.

Mashberg A, Morrissey JB, Garfinkel L: A Study of the Appearance of Early Asymptomatic Oral Squamous Cell Carcinoma. *Cancer* 32: 1436–1445, 1973.

Mashberg A, Meyers H: Anatomical Site and Size of 222 Early Asymptomatic Oral Squamous Cell Carcinomas: II, A Continuing Prospective Study of Oral Cancer. *Cancer* 37: 2149– 2157, 1976.

Mashberg A: Erythroplasia vs. Leukoplakia in the Diagnosis of Early Asymptomatic Oral Squamous Carcinoma. *N Engl J Med* 297: 109–110, 1977.

Mashberg A: Reevaluation of Toluidine Blue Application as a Diagnostic Adjunct in the Detection of Asymptomatic Oral Squamous Carcinoma: A Continuing Prospective Study of Oral Cancer III. *Cancer* 46: 758–763, 1980.

Mashberg A, Garfinkel L, Harris S: Alcohol as a Primary Risk Factor in Oral Squamous Carcinoma. *CA Cancer J Clin* 31: 146–155, 1981.

Mashberg A, Barsa P: Screening for Oral and Oropharyngeal Squamous Carcinomas. *CA Cancer J Clin* 34: 262–268, 1984.

Mason MK: Surface Carcinoma of the Stomach. *Gut* 6: 185–193, 1965.

Massey BW, Klayman MI: Observations on Epithelial Cells Exfoliated From the Upper Gastrointestinal Tract of Patients With Pernicious Anemia, Simple Achlorhydria, and Carcinoma of the Esophagus and Stomach. *Am J Med Sci* 230: 506–514, 1955.

McNeer G, Ewing JH: Exfoliated Pancreatic Cancer Cells in Duodenal Drainage: A Case Report. *Cancer* 2: 643–645, 1949.

Medak H, Burlakow P, McGrew EA, et al: The Cytology of Vesicular Conditions Affecting the Oral Mucosa: Pemphigus Vulgaris. *Acta Cytol* 14: 11–21, 1970.

Medley G: Anal Smear Test to Diagnose Occult Anorectal Infection With Human Papillomavirus in Men. *Br J Vener Dis* 60: 205, 1984.

Meiselman MS, Cello JP, Margaretten W: Cytomegalovirus Colitis: Report of the Clinical, Endoscopic, and Pathologic Findings in Two Patients With the Acquired Immune Deficiency Syndrome. *Gastroenterology* 88: 171–175, 1985.

Melbye M, Palefsky J, Gonzales J, et al: Immune Status as a Determinant of Human Papillomavirus Detection and Its Association With Anal Epithelial Abnormalities. *Int J Cancer* 46: 203–206, 1990.

Melville DM, Richman PI, Shepherd NA, et al: Brush Cytology of the Colon and Rectum in Ulcerative Colitis: An Aid to Cancer Diagnosis. *J Clin Pathol* 41: 1180–1186, 1988.

Memon MH, Jafarey NA: Cytologic Study of Radiation Changes in Carcinoma of the Oral Cavity: Prognostic Value of Various Observations. *Acta Cytol* 14: 22–24, 1970.

Mendez G Jr, Russell E, Levi JU, et al: Percutaneous Brush Biopsy and Internal Drainage of Biliary Tree Through Endoprosthesis. *AJR* 134: 653–659, 1980.

Mendoza ML, Martín-Rabadán P, Carrión I, et al: *Helicobacter pylori* Infection: Rapid Diagnosis With Brush Cytology. *Acta Cytol* 37: 181–185, 1993.

Messian RA, Hermos JA, Robbins AH, et al: Barrett's Esophagus: Clinical Review of 26 Cases. *Am J Gastroenterol* 69: 458–466, 1978.

Micbán I: Eosinophilic Granulocytes on the Gastrocytogram. *Acta Cytol* 20: 32–34, 1976.

Miller SC, Soberman A, Stahl SS: A Study of the Cornification of the Oral Mucosa of Young Male Adults. *J Dent Res* 30: 4–11, 1951.

Milstoc M: Squamous-Cell Carcinoma of Stomach With Liver Metastasis. *NY State J Med* 69: 2913–2914, 1969.

Ming S-C, Bajtai A, Correa P, et al: Gastric Dysplasia: Significance and Pathologic Criteria. *Cancer* 54: 1794–1801, 1984.

Mitchell ML, Carney CN: Cytologic Criteria for the Diagnosis of Pancreatic Carcinoma. *Am J Clin Pathol* 83: 171–176, 1985.

Mohandas KM, Swaroop VS, Gullar SU, et al: Diagnosis of Malignant Obstructive Jaundice by Bile Cytology: Results Improved by Dilating the Bile Duct Strictures. *Gastrointest Endosc* 40: 150–154, 1994.

Montgomery PW: A Study of Exfoliative Cytology of Normal Human Oral Mucosa. *J Dent Res* 30: 12–18, 1951.

Moreno-Otero R, Martinez-Raposo A, Cantero J, et al: Exfoliative Cytodiagnosis of Gastric Adenocarcinoma: Comparison With Biopsy and Endoscopy. *Acta Cytol* 27: 485–488, 1983.

Morris R, Gansler TS, Rudisill MT, et al: White Sponge Nevus: Diagnosis by Light Microscopic and Ultrastructural Cytology. *Acta Cytol* 32: 357–361, 1988.

Morson BC, Pang LSC: Pathology of Anal Cancer. *Proc R Soc Med* 61: 623–630, 1968.

Morson BC: Evolution of Cancer of the Colon and Rectum. *Cancer* 34: 845–849, 1974.

Morson BC, Sobin LH, Grundmann E, et al: Precancerous Conditions and Epithelial Dysplasia in the Stomach. *J Clin Pathol* 33: 711–721, 1980.

Mortensen NJM, Eltringham WK, Mountford RA, et al: Direct Vision Brush Cytology With Colonoscopy: An Aid to the Accurate Diagnosis of Colonic Strictures. *Br J Surg* 71: 930–932, 1984.

Muro A, Mueller PR, Ferruci JT Jr, et al: Bile Cytology: A Routine Addition to Percutaneous Biliary Drainage. *Radiology* 149: 846–847, 1983.

Naef AP, Savary M, Ozzello L, et al: Columnar-Lined Lower Esophagus: An Acquired Lesion With Malignant Predisposition: Report on 140 Cases of Barrett's Esophagus With 12 Adenocarcinomas. *J Thorac Cardiovasc Surg* 70: 826–835, 1975.

Nakahara H, Ishikawa T, Itabashi M, et al: Diffusely Infiltrating Primary Colorectal Carcinoma of Linitis Plastica and Lymphangiosis Types. *Cancer* 69: 901–906, 1992.

Nakaizumi A, Tatsuta M, Uehara H, et al: Cytologic Examination of Pure Pancreatic Juice in the Diagnosis of Pancreatic Carcinoma: The Endoscopic Retrograde Intraductal Catheter Aspiration Cytologic Technique. *Cancer* 70: 2610–2614, 1992.

Nakajima T, Tajima Y, Sugano I, et al: Multivariate Statistical Analysis of Bile Cytology. *Acta Cytol* 38: 51–55, 1994.

Nash G, Ross JS: Herpetic Esophagitis: A Common Cause of Esophageal Ulceration. *Hum Pathol* 5: 339–345, 1974.

Nash G, Warren A, Nash S: Atypical Lesions of the Anal Mucosa in Homosexual Men. *JAMA* 256: 873–876, 1986.

Nieburgs HE, Dreiling DA, Rubio C, et al: The Morphology of Cells in Duodenal-Drainage Smears: Histologic Origin and Pathologic Significance. *Am J Dig Dis* 7: 489–505, 1962.

Nishimura A, Den N, Sato H, et al: Exfoliative Cytology of the Biliary Tract With the Use of Saline Irrigation Under Choledochoscopic Control. *Ann Surg* 178: 594–599, 1973.

Nundy S, Shirley D, Beales JSM, et al: Simultaneous Combined Pancreatic Test. *Br Med J* 1: 87–90, 1974.

O'Donoghue JM, Horgan PG, O'Donohoe MK, et al: Adjunctive Endoscopic Brush Cytology in the Detection of Upper Gastrointestinal Malignancy. *Acta Cytol* 39: 28–34, 1995.

Ogden GR, Cowpe JG, Green MW: Effect of Radiotherapy on Oral Mucosa Assessed by Quantitative Exfoliative Cytology. *J Clin Pathol* 42: 940–943, 1989.

Ogden GR, Nairn A, Franks J, et al: Do Gelatin-Coated Slides Increase Cellular Retention in Oral Exfoliative Cytology? *Acta Cytol* 35: 186–188, 1991a.

Ogden GR, Cowpe JG, Green MW: Detection of Field Change in Oral Cancer Using Oral Exfoliative Cytologic Study. *Cancer* 68: 1611–1615, 1991b.

Ogden GR, Cowpe JG, Green M: Cytobrush and Wooden Spatula for Oral Exfoliative Cytology: A Comparison. *Acta Cytol* 36: 706–710, 1992.

O'Morchoe PJ, Lee DC, Kozak CA: Esophageal Cytology in Patients Receiving Cytotoxic Drug Therapy. *Acta Cytol* 27: 630–634, 1983.

Oohara T, Tohma H, Takezoe K, et al: Minute Gastric Cancers Less Than 5 mm in Diameter. *Cancer* 50: 801–810, 1982.

Orell SR, Ohlsén P: Normal and Post-Pancreatic Cytologic Patterns of the Duodenal Juice. *Acta Cytol* 16: 165–171, 1972.

Osnes M, Serch-Hanssen A, Myren J: Endoscopic Retrograde Brush Cytology (ERBC) of the Biliary and Pancreatic Ducts. *Scand J Gastroenterol* 10: 829–831, 1975.

Osnes M, Serck-Hanssen A, Kristensen O, et al: Endoscopic Retrograde Brush Cytology in Patients With Primary and Secondary Malignancies of the Pancreas. *Gut* 20: 279–284, 1979.

Owensby LC, Stammer JL: Esophagitis Associated With Herpes Simplex Infection in an Immunocompetent Host. *Gastroenterology* 74: 1305–1306, 1978.

Palefsky JM, Gonzales J, Greenblatt RM, et al: Anal Intraepithelial Neoplasia and Anal Papillomavirus Infection Among Homosexual Males With Group IV HIV Disease. *JAMA* 263: 2911–2916, 1990.

Paull A, Trier JS, Dalton MD, et al: The Histologic Spectrum of Barrett's Esophagus. *N Engl J Med* 295: 476–480, 1976.

Peters H: Cytologic Smears From the Mouth: Cellular Changes in Disease and After Radiation. *Am J Clin Pathol* 29: 219–225, 1958.

Pilotti S, Rilke F, Clemente C, et al: The Cytologic Diagnosis of Gastric Carcinoma Related to the Histologic Type. *Acta Cytol* 21: 48–59, 1977.

Pinto MM, Meriano FV, Afridi S, et al: Cytodiagnosis of *Campylobacter Pylori* in Papanicolaou-Stained Imprints of Gastric Biopsy Specimens. *Acta Cytol* 35: 204–206, 1991.

Platt LI, Kailin EW: Buccal X-Chromatin Frequency in Numerous Diseases. *Acta Cytol* 13: 700–707, 1969.

Posner G, Lightdale CJ, Cooper M, et al: Reappraisal of Endoscopic Tissue Diagnosis in Secondary Gastric Lymphoma. *Gastrointest Endosc* 21: 123–125, 1975.

Potet F, Fléjou J-F, Gervaz H, et al: Adenocarcinoma of the Lower Esophagus and the Esophagogastric Junction. *Semin Diagn Pathol* 8: 126–136, 1991.

Prolla JC, Kobayashi S, Kirsner JB: Cytology of Malignant Lymphomas of the Stomach. *Acta Cytol* 14: 291–296, 1970a.

Prolla JC, Kobayashi S, Yoshi Y, et al: Diagnostic Cytology of the Stomach in Gastric Syphilis: Report of Two Cases. *Acta Cytol* 14: 333–337, 1970b.

Prolla JC, Xavier RG, Kirsner JB: Morphology of Exfoliated Cells in Benign Gastric Ulcer. *Acta Cytol* 15: 128–132, 1971a.

Prolla JC, Yoshi Y, Xavier RG, et al: Further Experience With Direct Vision Brushing Cytology of Malignant Tumors of Upper Gastrointestinal Tract Histopathologic With Biopsy. *Acta Cytol* 15: 375–378, 1971b.

Prolla JC, Reilly RW, Kirsner JB, et al: Direct-Vision Endoscopic Cytology and Biopsy in the Diagnosis of Esophageal and Gastric Tumors: Current Experience. *Acta Cytol* 21: 399–402, 1977.

Qizilbash AH, Castelli M, Kowalski MA, et al: Endoscopic Brush Cytology and Biopsy in the Diagnosis of Cancer of the Upper Gastrointestinal Tract. *Acta Cytol* 24: 313–318, 1980.

Raque CJ, Stein KM, Samitz MH: Pemphigus Vulgaris Involving the Esophagus. *Arch Dermatol* 102: 371–373, 1970.

Raskin HF, Wenger J, Sklar M, et al: The Diagnosis of Cancer of the Pancreas, Biliary Tract, and Duodenum by Combined Cytologic and Secretory Methods: I. Exfoliative Cytology and a Description of a Rapid Method of Duodenal Intubation. *Gastroenterology* 34: 996–1008, 1958.

Raskin HF, Pleticka S: The Cytologic Diagnosis of Cancer of the Colon. *Acta Cytol* 8: 131–140, 1964.

Reddy CRRM, Kameswari VR, Prahlad D, et al: Correlative Study of Exfoliative Cytology and Histopathology of Oral Carcinomas. *J Oral Surg* 33: 435–438, 1975.

Reed PI, Raskin HF, Graff PW: Malignant Melanoma of the Stomach. *JAMA* 182: 298–299, 1962.

Reid BJ, Haggitt RC, Rubin CE, et al: Observer Variation in the Diagnosis of Dysplasia in Barrett's Esophagus. *Hum Pathol* 19: 166–178, 1988a.

Reid BJ, Weinstein WM, Lewin KJ, et al: Endoscopic Biopsy can Detect High-Grade Dysplasia or Early Adenocarcinoma in Barrett's Esophagus Without Grossly Recognizable Neoplastic Lesions. *Gastroenterology* 94: 81–90, 1988b.

Richardson HL, Queen FB, Bishop FH: Cytohistologic Diagnosis of Material Aspirated From Stomach. *Am J Clin Pathol* 19: 328–340, 1949.

Riddell RH, Goldman H, Ransohoff DF, et al: Dysplasia in Inflammatory Bowel Disease: Standardized Classification With Provisional Clinical Applications. *Hum Pathol* 14: 931–968, 1983.

Rilke F, Pilotti S, Clemente C: Cytology of Non-Hodgkin's Malignant Lymphomas Involving the Stomach. *Acta Cytol* 22: 71–79, 1978.

Roberts-Thomson IC, Hobbs JB: Cytodiagnosis of Pancreatic and Biliary Cancer by Endoscopic Duct Aspiration. *Med J Aust* 1: 370–372, 1979.

Robertson CS, Mayberry JF, Nicholson DA, et al: Value of Endoscopic Surveillance in the Detection of Neoplastic Change in Barrett's Oesophagus. *Br J Surg* 75: 760–763, 1988.

Robey SS, Hamilton SR, Gupta PK, et al: Diagnostic Value of Cytopathology in Barrett Esophagus and Associated Carcinoma. *Am J Clin Pathol* 89: 493–498, 1988.

Robey-Cafferty SS, El-Naggar AK, Sahin AA, et al: Prognostic Factors in Esophageal Squamous Carcinoma: A Study of Histologic Features, Blood Group Expression, and DNA Ploidy. *Am J Clin Pathol* 95: 844–849, 1991.

Robinson CR: Oil Immersion for Identification of *Campylobacter pylori*. *Acta Cytol* 35: 252–253, 1991.

Rosen P, Hajdu SI: Visceral Herpesvirus Infections in Patients With Cancer. *Am J Clin Pathol* 56: 459–465, 1971.

Rosen RG, Garrett M, Aka E: Cytologic Diagnosis of Pancreatic Cancer by Ductal Aspiration. *Ann Surg* 167: 427–432, 1968.

Rosen Y, Moon S, Kim B: Small Cell Epidermoid Carcinoma of the Esophagus: An Oat-Cell-Like Carcinoma. *Cancer* 36: 1042–1049, 1975.

Rosenberg IL, Giles GR: The Value of Colonic Exfoliative Cytology in the Diagnosis of Carcinoma of the Large Intestine. *Dis Colon Rectum* 20: 1–10, 1977.

Rothery GA, Day DW: Intestinal Metaplasia in Endoscopic Biopsy Specimens of Gastric Mucosa. *J Clin Pathol* 38: 613–621, 1985.

Rovin S: An Assessment of the Negative Oral Cytologic Diagnosis. *JADA* 74: 759–762, 1967.

Rovin S: Cytology—Its Value in the Diagnosis of Oral Cancer: (Using Cytology, or How to Avoid Biopsy). *Dent Clin North Am* 15: 807–815, 1971.

Rozen P, Tobi M, Darmon E, et al: Exfoliative Colonic Cytology: A Simplified Method of Collection and Initial Results. *Acta Cytol* 34: 627–631, 1990.

Rubel LR, Reynolds RE: Cytologic Description of Squamous Cell Papilloma of the Respiratory Tract. *Acta Cytol* 23: 227–230, 1979.

Rubin CE, Massey BW: The Preoperative Diagnosis of Gastric and Duodenal Malignant Lymphoma by Exfoliative Cytology. *Cancer* 7: 271–288, 1954.

Rubin CE: The Diagnosis of Gastric Malignancy in Pernicious Anemia. *Gastroenterology* 29: 563–587, 1955.

Rubio CA, Antonioli D: Ciliated Metaplasia in the Gastric Mucosa: In an American Patient. *Am J Surg Pathol* 12: 786–789, 1988.

Rubio CA, Jessurum J, de Ruiz PA: Geographic Variations in the Histologic Characteristics of the Gastric Mucosa. *Am J Clin Pathol* 96: 330–333, 1991.

Rubio CA, Åberg B, Stemmermann G: Ciliated Cells in Papillary Adenocarcinomas of Barrett's Esophagus. *Acta Cytol* 36: 65–68, 1992.

Rugge M, Farinati F, Di Mario F, et al: Gastric Epithelial Dysplasia: A Prospective Multicenter Follow-up Study From the Interdisciplinary Group on Gastric Epithelial Dysplasia. *Hum Pathol* 22: 1002–1008, 1991.

Rupp M, Hawthorne CM, Ehya H: Brushing Cytology in Biliary Tract Obstruction. *Acta Cytol* 34: 221–226, 1990.

Ryan ME, Baldauf MC: Comparison of Flow Cytometry for DNA Content and Brush Cytology for Detection of Malignancy in Pancreaticobiliary Strictures. *Gastrointest Endosc* 40: 133–139, 1994.

Sanders DSA, Hussein KA: Filamentous Organisms in Gastric Brushings and Gastric Cancer Diagnosis. *Diagn Cytopathol* 7: 11–13, 1991.

Sandler HC: The Cytologic Diagnosis of Tumors of the Oral Cavity. *Acta Cytol* 8: 114–120, 1964.

Sandler HC: Morphological Characteristics of Malignant Cells From Mouth Lesions. *Acta Cytol* 9: 282–286, 1965.

Sandler HC: Errors of Oral Cytodiagnosis: Report of Follow-up of 1,801 Patients. *JADA* 72: 851–854, 1966.

Sápi Z, Papp I, Bodó M: Malignant Fibrous Histiocytoma of the Esophagus: Report of a Case With Cytologic, Immunohistologic and Ultrastructural Studies. *Acta Cytol* 36: 121–125, 1992.

Saraga E-P, Gardiol D, Costa J: Gastric Dysplasia: A Histological Follow-up Study. *Am J Surg Pathol* 11: 788–796, 1987.

Sawada Y, Gonda H, Hayashida Y: Combined use of Brushing Cytology and Endoscopic Retrograde Pancreatography for the Early Detection of Pancreatic Cancer. *Acta Cytol* 33: 870–874, 1989.

Schade ROK: A Critical Review of Gastric Cytology. *Acta Cytol* 3: 7–14, 1959.

Scher RL, Oostingh PE, Levine PA, et al: Role of Fine Needle Aspiration in the Diagnosis of Lesions of the Oral Cavity, Oropharynx, and Nasopharynx. *Cancer* 62: 2602–2606, 1988.

Schmidt HG, Riddell RH, Walther B, et al: Dysplasia in Barrett's Esophagus. *J Cancer Res Clin Oncol* 110: 145–152, 1985.

Schnadig VJ, Bigio EH, Gourley WK, et al: Identification of *Campylobacter pylori* by Endoscopic Brush Cytology. *Diagn Cytopathol* 6: 227–234, 1990.

Schnell T, Sontag S, Chejfec G, et al: Detection of Barrett's Esophagus (BE) and Curable Esophageal Adenocarcinoma (AdCa) by Endoscopic Screening Based on GER Symptoms: Can It Be Cost Effective? (Abstract) *Gastroenterology* 94: A411, 1988.

Seifert E, Butke H, Gail K, et al: Diagnosis of Early Gastric Cancer. *Am J Gastroenterol* 71: 563–567, 1979.

Shah SM, Schaefer RF, Araoz E: Cytologic Diagnosis of Herpetic Esophagitis: A Case Report. *Acta Cytol* 21: 109–111, 1977.

Shanghai Gastrointestinal Endoscopy Cooperative Group, People's Republic of China: Value of Biopsy and Brush Cytology in the Diagnosis of Gastric Cancer. *Gut* 23: 774–776, 1982.

Shapiro BL, Gorlin RJ: An Analysis of Oral Cytodiagnosis. *Cancer* 17: 1477–1479, 1964.

Shedd DP: Clinical Characteristics of Early Oral Cancer. *JAMA* 215: 955–956, 1971.

Shekitka KM, Helwig EB: Deceptive Bizarre Stromal Cells in Polyps and Ulcers of the Gastrointestinal Tract. *Cancer* 67: 2111–2117, 1991.

Sherman ME, Anderson C, Herman LM, et al: Utility of Gastric Brushing in the Diagnosis of Malignant Lymphoma. *Acta Cytol* 38: 169–174, 1994.

Shklar G, Meyer I, Cataldo E, et al: Correlated Study of Oral Cytology and Histopathology: Report on 2,052 Oral Lesions. *Oral Surg Oral Med Oral Pathol* 25: 61–70, 1968.

Shklar G, Cataldo E, Meyer I: Reliability of Cytologic Smear in Diagnosis of Oral Cancer: A Controlled Study. *Arch Otolaryngol* 91: 158–160, 1970.

Shroff CP, Nanivadekar SA: Endoscopic Brushing Cytology and Biopsy in the Diagnosis of Upper Gastrointestinal Tract Lesions: A Study of 350 Cases. *Acta Cytol* 32: 455–460, 1988.

Shu Y-J: Cytopathology of the Esophagus: An Overview of Esophageal Cytopathology in China. *Acta Cytol* 27: 7–16, 1983.

Shurbaji MS, Erozan YS: The Cytopathologic Diagnosis of Esophageal Adenocarcinoma. *Acta Cytol* 35: 189–194, 1991.

Silverman JF, Levine J, Finley JL, et al: Small-Intestinal Brushing Cytology in the Diagnosis of Cryptosporidiosis in AIDS. *Diagn Cytopathol* 6: 193–196, 1990.

Silverman S Jr: The Cytology of Benign Oral Lesions. *Acta Cytol* 9: 287–295, 1965.

Silverman S Jr, Sheline GE, Gillooly CJ Jr: Radiation Therapy and Oral Carcinoma: Radiation Response and Exfoliative Cytology. *Cancer* 20: 1297–1300, 1967.

Silverman S Jr, Bilimoria KF, Bhargava K, et al: Cytologic, Histologic and Clinical Correlations of Precancerous and Cancerous Oral Lesions in 57,518 Industrial Workers of Gujarat, India. *Acta Cytol* 21: 196–198, 1977.

Silverman S Jr, Gorsky M, Lozada F: Oral Leukoplakia and Malignant Transformation: A Follow-up Study of 257 Patients. *Cancer* 53: 563–568, 1984.

Silverman S Jr: Early Diagnosis of Oral Cancer. *Cancer* 62: 1796–1799, 1988.

Singh S, Macleod G, Walker T, et al: Endoscopic Fine-Needle Aspiration Cytology in the Diagnosis of Linitis Plastica. *Br J Surg* 81: 1010, 1994.

Skinner DB, Walther BC, Riddell RH, et al: Barrett's Esophagus: Comparison of Benign and Malignant Cases. *Ann Surg* 198: 554–566, 1983.

Smith MJ, Kini SR, Watson E: Fine Needle Aspiration and Endoscopic Brush Cytology: Comparison of Direct Smears and Rinsings. *Acta Cytol* 24: 456–459, 1980.

Smith RRL, Hamilton SR, Boitnott JK, et al: The Spectrum of Carcinoma Arising in Barrett's Esophagus: A Clinicopathological Study of 26 Patients. *Am J Surg Pathol* 8: 563–573, 1984.

Smithies A, Hatfield ARW, Brown BE: The Cytodiagnosis Aspects of Pure Pancreatic Juice Obtained at the Time of Endoscopic Retrograde Cholangio-Pancreatography (E.C.R.P.). *Acta Cytol* 21: 191–195, 1977.

Soni RR, Dhamne BK: Rapid Detection of Rectal Cancer by Gloved Digital-Scrape Cytology. *Acta Cytol* 35: 210–214, 1991.

Soudah B, Fritsch RS, Wittekind C, et al: Value of the Cytologic Analysis of Fine Needle Aspiration Biopsy Specimens in the Diagnosis of Pancreatic Carcinomas. *Acta Cytol* 33: 875–880, 1989.

Spechler SJ, Goyal RK: Barrett's Esophagus. *N Engl J Med* 315: 362–371, 1986.

Springer DJ, DaCosta LR, Beck IT: A Syndrome of Acute Self-Limiting Ulcerative Esophagitis in Young Adults Probably Due to Herpes Simplex Virus. *Dig Dis Sci* 24: 535–539, 1979.

Staats OJ, Goldsby JW, Butterworth CE: The Oral Exfoliative Cytology of Tropical Sprue. *Acta Cytol* 9: 228–233, 1965.

Staats OJ, Robinson LH, Butterworth CE Jr: The Effect of Systemic Therapy on Nuclear Size of Oral Epithelial Cells in Folate Related Anemias. *Acta Cytol* 13: 84–88, 1969.

Stahl SS, Koss LG, Brown RC Jr, et al: Oral Cytologic Screening in a Large Metropolitan Area. *JADA* 75: 1385–1388, 1967.

Strigle SM, Gal AA, Martin SE: Alimentary Tract Cytopathology in Human Immunodeficiency Virus Infection: A Review of Experience in Los Angeles. *Diagn Cytopathol* 6: 409–420, 1990.

Sun T: The Diagnosis of Giardiasis. *Am J Surg Pathol* 4: 265–271, 1980.

Takeda M, Gomi K, Lewis PL, et al: Two Histologic Types of Early Gastric Carcinoma and Their Cytologic Presentation. *Acta Cytol* 25: 229–236, 1981.

Takeda M, Lewis PL, Choi HY, et al: Gastric Remnant Cancer After Billroth II Procedure. *Diagn Cytopathol* 1: 194–204, 1985.

Tamura K, Masuzawa M, Akiyama T, et al: Touch Smear Cytology for Endoscopic Diagnosis of Gastric Carcinoma. *Am J Gastroenterol* 67: 463–467, 1977.

Teot LA, Ducatman BS, Geisinger KR: Cytologic Diagnosis of Cytomegaloviral Esophagitis: A Report of Three Acquired Immunodeficiency Syndrome-Related Cases. *Acta Cytol* 37: 93–96, 1993.

Thompson H, Hoare Am, Dykes PW, et al: A Prospective Randomised Trial to Compare Brush Cytology Before or After Punch Biopsy for Endoscopic Diagnosis of Gastric Cancer. *Gut* 18: 398–428, 1977.

Thompson JJ, Zinsser KR, Enterline HT: Barrett's Metaplasia and Adenocarcinoma of the Esophagus and Gastroesophageal Junction. *Hum Pathol* 14: 42–61, 1983.

Tidbury PJ, Tate JJ, Herbert A: Cytology of Colorectal Adenomas. *Cytopathology* 1: 73–78, 1990.

Tiecke RW, Blozis GG: Oral Cytology. *JADA* 72: 855–861, 1966.

Tim LO, Leiman G, Segal I, et al: A Suction-Abrasive Cytology Tube for the Diagnosis of Esophageal Carcinoma. *Cancer* 50: 782–784, 1982.

Tosi P, Baak JPA, Luzi P, et al: Morphometric Distinction of Low- and High-Grade Dysplasias in Gastric Biopsies. *Hum Pathol* 20: 839–844, 1989.

Trillo AA, Accettullo LM, Yeiter TL: Choriocarcinoma of the Esophagus: Histologic and Cytologic Findings: A Case Report. *Acta Cytol* 23: 69–74, 1979.

Tsang T-K, Hidvegi D, Horth K, et al: Reliability of Balloon-Mesh Cytology in Detecting Esophageal Carcinoma in a Population of US Veterans. *Cancer* 59: 556–559, 1987.

Tummala V, Barwick KW, Sontag SJ, et al: The Significance of Intraepithelial Eosinophils in the Histologic Diagnosis of Gastroesophageal Reflux. *Am J Clin Pathol* 87: 43–48, 1987.

Uei Y, Koketsu H, Konda C, et al: Cytodiagnosis of HCG-Secreting Choriocarcinoma of the Stomach: Report of a Case. *Acta Cytol* 17: 431–434, 1973.

Umiker W: Cytology in the Radiotherapy of Carcinoma of the Oral Cavity. *Acta Cytol* 9: 296–297, 1965.

Vallilengua C, Rodriguez Otero JC, Proske SA, et al: Imprint Cytology of the Gallbladder Mucosa: Its Use in Diagnosing Macroscopically Inapparent Carcinoma. *Acta Cytol* 39: 19–22, 1995.

Van Der Veen AH, Dees J, Blankensteijn JD, et al: Adenocarcinoma in Barrett's Oesophagus: An Overrated Risk. *Gut* 30: 14–18, 1989.

Van Krieken JHJM, Medeiros LJ, Pals ST, et al: Diffuse Aggressive B-Cell Lymphomas of the Gastrointestinal Tract: An Immunophenotypic and Gene Rearrangement Analysis of 22 Cases. *Am J Clin Pathol* 97: 170–178, 1992.

Verma K, Bhargava DK: Cytologic Examination as an Adjunct to Laparoscopy and Guided Biopsy in the Diagnosis of Hepatic and Gallbladder Neoplasia. *Acta Cytol* 26: 311–316, 1982.

Vilardell F: Cytological Diagnosis of Digestive Cancer. *Am J Gastroenterol* 70: 357–364, 1978.

Vilmann P, Jacobsen GK, Henriksen FW, et al: Endoscopic Ultrasonography With Guided Fine Needle Aspiration Biopsy in Pancreatic Disease. *Gastrointest Endosc* 38: 172–173, 1992.

von Haam E: The Historical Background of Oral Cytology. *Acta Cytol* 9: 270–272, 1965.

Waldron CA, Shafer WG: Leukoplakia Revisited: A Clinicopathologic Study 3256 Oral Leukoplakias. *Cancer* 36: 1386–1392, 1975.

Wanebo HJ, Grimes OF: Cancer of the Bile Duct: The Occult Malignancy. *Am J Surg* 130: 262–268, 1975.

Wang HH, Antonioli DA, Goldman H: Comparative Features of Esophageal and Gastric Adenocarcinoma: Recent Changes in Type and Frequency. *Hum Pathol* 17: 482–487, 1986.

Wang HH, Ducatman BS, Thibault S: Cytologic Features of Premalignant Glandular Lesions in the Upper Gastrointestinal Tract. *Acta Cytol* 35: 199–203, 1991a.

Wang HH, Jonasson JG, Ducatman BS: Brushing Cytology of the Upper Gastrointestinal Tract: Obsolete or Not? *Acta Cytol* 35: 195–198, 1991b.

Wang HH, Doria MI Jr, Purohit-Buch S, et al: Barrett's Esophagus: The Cytology of Dysplasia in Comparison to Benign and Malignant Lesions. *Acta Cytol* 36: 60–64, 1992.

Watanabe H, Numazawa M, Shoji K, et al: Diagnosis of Early Cancer of the Colon and Rectum. *Tohoku J Exp Med* 129: 183–195, 1979.

Wenger J, Raskin HF: The Diagnosis of Cancer of the Pancreas, Biliary Tract, and Duodenum by Combined Cytologic and Secretory Methods: II. The Secretin Test. *Gastroenterology* 34: 1009–1017, 1958.

Wertlake PT, Del Guercio LRM: Cytopathology of Intra-Hepatic Bile as Component of Integrated Procedure ("Minilap") for Hepatobiliary Disorders. *Acta Cytol* 20: 42–45, 1976.

Wheeler DA, Chandrasoma P, Carriere CA, et al: Cytologic Diagnosis of Gastric Composite Adenocarcinoma-Carcinoid. *Acta Cytol* 28: 706–712, 1984.

Wiersema MJ, Hawes RH, Tao L-C, et al: Endoscopic Ultrasonography as an Adjunct to Fine Needle Aspiration Cytology of the Upper and Lower Gastrointestinal Tract. *Gastrointest Endosc* 38: 35–39, 1992.

Wiersema MJ, Wiersema LM, Khusro Q, et al: Combined Endosonography and Fine-Needle Aspiration Cytology in the Evaluation of Gastrointestinal Lesions. *Gastrointest Endosc* 40: 199–206, 1994.

Williams JG, Williams LA: Colonoscopy and Brush Cytology in the Diagnosis of Colonic Strictures. *J R Coll Surg Edinb* 33: 119–123, 1988.

Winawer SJ, Posner G, Lightdale CJ, et al: Endoscopic Diagnosis of Advanced Gastric Cancer: Factors Influencing Yield. *Gastroenterology* 69: 1183–1187, 1975a.

Winawer SJ, Sherlock P, Belladonna JA, et al: Endoscopic Brush Cytology in Esophageal Cancer. *JAMA* 232: 1358, 1975b.

Winawer SJ, Melamed M, Sherlock P: Potential of Endoscopy, Biopsy and Cytology in the Diagnosis and Management of Patients With Cancer. *Clin Gastroenterol* 5: 575–595, 1976a.

Winawer SJ, Sherlock P, Hajdu SI: The Role of Upper Gastrointestinal Endoscopy in Patients With Cancer. *Cancer* 37: 440–448, 1976b.

Winawer SJ, Leidner SD, Hajdu MI, et al: Colonoscopic Biopsy and Cytology in the Diagnosis of Colon Cancer. *Cancer* 42: 2849–2853, 1978.

Wingo PA, Tong T, Bolden S: Cancer Statistics, 1995. *CA Cancer J Clin* 45: 8–30, 1995.

Winn DM, Blot WJ, Shy CM, et al: Snuff Dipping and Oral Cancer Among Women in the Southern United States. *N Engl J Med* 304: 745–749, 1981.

Winter HS, Madara JL, Stafford RJ, et al: Intraepithelial Eosinophils: A New Diagnostic Criterion for Reflux Esophagitis. *Gastroenterology* 83: 818–823, 1982.

Witkop CJ: Epithelial Intracellular Bodies Associated With Hereditary Dyskeratoses and Cancer Therapy. *Proc 1st Int Congress Exfol Cytol* 259–268, 1962.

Witzel L, Halter F, Grétillat A, et al: Evaluation of Specific Value of Endoscopic Biopsies and Brush Cytology for Malignancies of the Oesophagus and Stomach. *Gut* 17: 375–377, 1976.

Wood TA Jr, DeWitt SH, Chu EW, et al: Anitschkow Nuclear Changes Observed in Oral Smears. *Acta Cytol* 19: 434–437, 1975.

Wuerker RB, Gordon JL, Jakowatz JG: Characteristics of Cancer Cells in Gastrointestinal Lavage Specimens. *Acta Cytol* 37: 379–384, 1993.

Wyatt JI: Gastritis and Its Relation to Gastric Carcinogenesis. *Semin Diagn Pathol* 8: 137–148, 1991.

Wynder EL, Bross IJ, Feldman RM: A Study of the Etiological Factors in Cancer of the Mouth. *Cancer* 10: 1300–1323, 1957.

Yamada T, Murohisa B, Muto Y, et al: Cytologic Detection of Small Pancreaticoduodenal and Biliary Cancers in the Early Development Stage. *Acta Cytol* 28: 435–442, 1984.

Yang M: Detection of Amyloid in Gastric Brushing Material. A Case Report. *Acta Cytol* 39: 255–257, 1995.

Yardley JH, Keren DF: "Precancer" Lesions in Ulcerative Colitis: A Retrospective Study of Rectal Biopsy and Colectomy Specimens. *Cancer* 34: 835–844, 1974.

Yoshi Y, Takahashi J, Yamaoka Y, et al: Significance of Imprint Smear in Cytologic Diagnosis of Malignant Tumors of the Stomach. *Acta Cytol* 14: 249–253, 1970.

Young JA, Hughes HE: Clinical Trial: Three Year Trial of Endoscopic Cytology of the Stomach and Duodenum. *Gut* 21: 241–246, 1980.

Young JA, Hughes HE, Hole DJ: Morphological Characteristics and Distribution Patterns of Epithelial Cells in the Cytological Diagnosis of Gastric Cancer. *J Clin Pathol* 35: 585–590, 1982.

Zargar SA, Khuroo MS, Jan GM, et al: Prospective Comparison of the Value of Brushings Before and After Biopsy in the Endoscopic Diagnosis of Gastroesophageal Malignancy. *Acta Cytol* 35: 549–552, 1991a.

Zargar SA, Khuroo MS, Jan GM, et al: Endoscopic Fine Needle Aspiration Cytology in the Diagnosis of Gastro-oesophageal and Colorectal Malignancies. *Gut* 32: 745–748, 1991b.

Zukerberg LR, Ferry JA, Southern JF, et al: Lymphoid Infiltrates of the Stomach. Evaluation of Histologic Criteria for the Diagnosis of Low-Grade Gastric Lymphoma on Endoscopic Biopsy Specimens. *Am J Surg Pathol* 14: 1087–1099,1990.

10

Urine

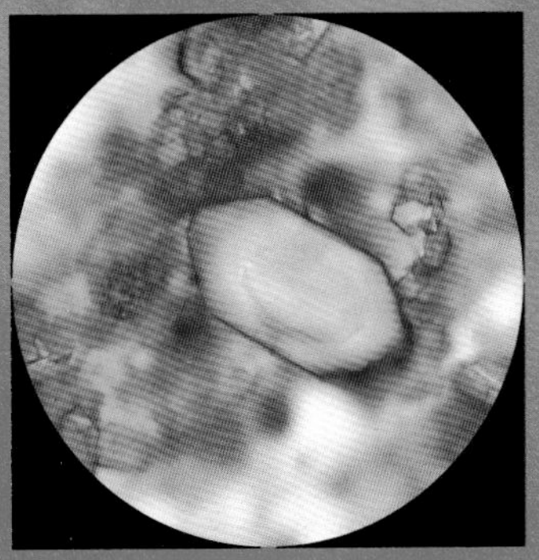

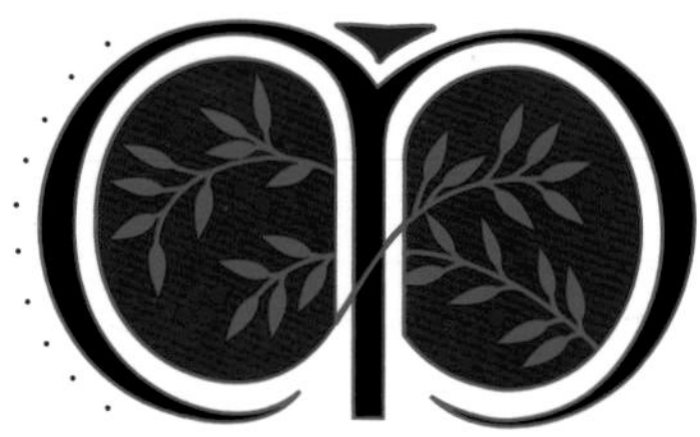

ost of the collecting and storage system of the urinary tract, including the renal pelvis, ureter, bladder, and some of the urethra (particularly in men) is lined with transitional epithelium [1 I10.1]. This epithelium was so named by Friedrich Henle, a 19th century German pathologist, because he thought that the urinary epithelium was "transitional" between squamous and glandular. It is now recognized as a specific type in its own right. Therefore, some prefer to call it "urothelium" (the terms are interchangeable). However, it is interesting that some tumors of the transitional epithelium do indeed express the ability to differentiate along squamous or glandular lines and that patches of squamous and glandular mucosa are commonly interspersed in benign transitional epithelium.

The transitional epithelium (which is the term used more often) has to be able to perform two functions. First, it maintains a barrier between the urine (which is toxic) and the blood, to prevent urine from disseminating through the blood (uremia). This is known as the blood-urine barrier, analogous to the blood-brain barrier. Second, it is able to stretch and flex, especially in the bladder, to allow for slow expansion during filling and rapid contraction during emptying. For these purposes, the transitional cell has developed a special cellular membrane, the asymmetric unit membrane. Ultrastructurally, it consists of dense plaques and flexible membranes. The outer lamina is thicker and denser than the inner (hence, asymmetric). This construction presumably plays a role in the barrier function. In addition, there are intracytoplasmic fusiform vesicles. These vesicles are continuous with the surface and apparently provide the cell with more membrane as it stretches, opening like an accordion. These two features, the asymmetric unit membrane and fusiform vesicles, are apparently unique to transitional cells. The cells are also welded together by numerous tight junctions to help make the entire epithelium water tight.

Embryologically, like the reproductive and lower gastrointestinal tracts, the bladder develops from the cloaca (Latin for sewer). Squamous epithelium lining the trigone is an essentially normal variant, particularly in women, but can also be seen in pathologic conditions. Colonic-type glandular epithelium is also frequently seen in the bladder (eg, cystitis glandularis). These features may be a reflection of the partial common origin. So it comes as no great surprise that urinary tract tumors may also show all three types of epithelium (transitional, squamous, and glandular).

Normal Number of Cell Layers

Calyces, pelvis: 2–3
Ureter: 4–5
Bladder: 6–7 (contracted) to 2–3 (maximum distention)

Bladder: Histologically, the urinary bladder (or simply the "bladder") has three zones of cells [1 I10.1]. The basal layer is one cell layer thick. Basal cells are columnar when the bladder is contracted and can change to cuboidal or flattened as the bladder fills. The intermediate cell layer, which can be up to 5 cell layers thick, depending on bladder distention, is composed of parabasal-sized cells. A single layer of superficial cells is found on the surface. Superficial transitional cells are large, usually about the size of a superficial squamous cell, but are sometimes considerably larger. Capillaries are found in the stroma immediately underneath the urothelium.

Urethra: In women the epithelium lining the urethra is mostly stratified squamous. There may be islands of pseudostratified columnar transitional epithelium. Also present are Littre's glands, which are outpouchings lined by mucus-producing columnar glandular cells.

The male urethra is divided into three zones. The proximal or prostatic zone of the urethra is about 2 cm long and lined with transitional epithelium. Many prostatic ducts and two ejaculatory ducts enter this portion of the urethra. Next is a short zone, again about 2 cm long, lined with stratified or pseudostratified columnar transitional epithelium that may also have patches of squamous mucosa. The penile portion of the urethra is the longest, about 15 cm long. It is also lined with stratified or pseudostratified columnar transitional epithelium with squamous patches especially near the meatus, where the epithelium becomes entirely stratified squamous. Littre's mucous glands, which extend from lacunae of Morgagni, are present in the penile urethra.

Ureter and Renal Pelvis: The cells of the upper urinary tract tend to be larger and have more nuclei than those found in the bladder, possibly due to decreased cellular turnover and exfoliation. Marked variation in cell shape may be seen normally: columnar, polyhedral, spindle, giant, even bizarre. (See also "Carcinoma of the Upper Urinary Tract.")

This chapter will deal for the most part with cells found in the urinary tract. For information regarding the chemical analysis and clinical microscopy of other formed elements (such as crystals, casts, etc [2 I10.2, 3 I10.3]), please see a standard text on urinalysis.

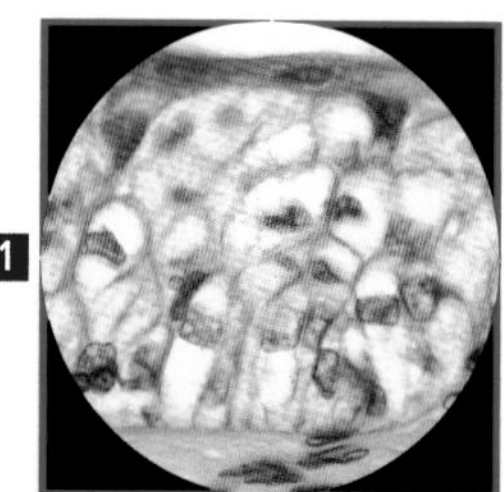
1

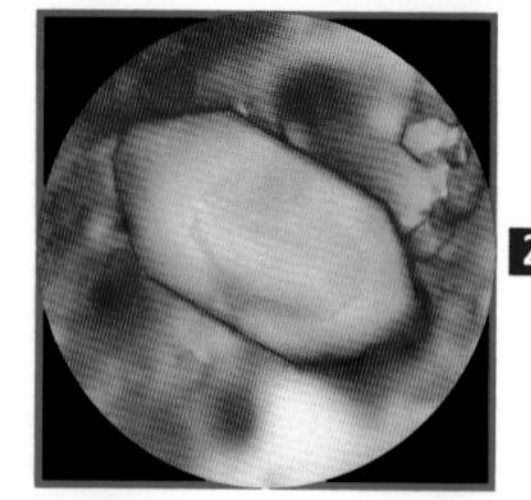
2

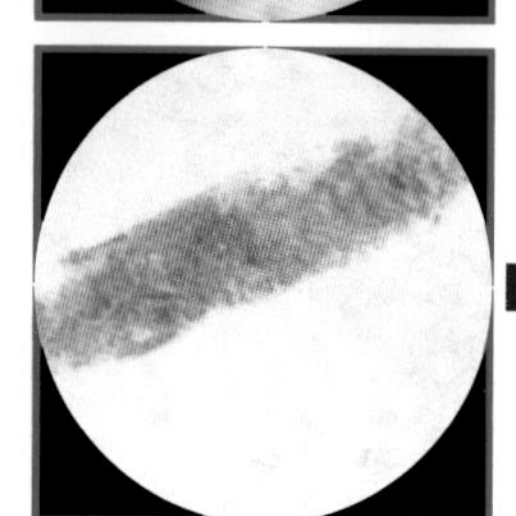
3

Urinary Tract Cytology

Cytologic examination of a urine specimen is a simple, safe, and inexpensive method that may uncover a hidden urothelial cancer [Sharma 1991]. Tumors of the urinary tract are relatively inaccessible to direct biopsy, and the tumors are often multifocal. Since the entire mucosal surface, including the farthest reaches of the urinary tract, is bathed in this easily obtained fluid, in theory, urine is the perfect specimen to examine for evidence of tumor ("survey the situation").

Urine cytology is primarily used for diagnosis of symptomatic patients, detection of cancer in high-risk patients (eg, those exposed to industrial chemicals and metals, cigarette smokers, and those with schistosomiasis), and follow-up of patients with history of urinary tract neoplasia. It complements, but does not replace, cystoscopy and biopsy. However, lesions may be detected cytologically before they can be seen cystoscopically. Urinary cytologic examination is capable of detecting small or hidden lesions (eg, in diverticuli, ureters, renal pelvis, prostatic ducts, residual urethras). Unfortunately, however, the lesions cannot be localized by cytologic study of urine.

Urinary cytology can detect most aggressive neoplasms and carcinoma in situ [Soloway 1993]. Patients with low-grade noninvasive tumors can be followed up cytologically [Thompson 1993]. Patients with negative cytologic findings have a very low risk of recurrence, while high-grade cytologic abnormalities predict an aggressive tumor course [Harving 1989]. Urine cytology is also a better indicator of the presence of concomitant urothelial atypia than preselected mucosal biopsies [Harving 1988].

Clinical history is important in proper evaluation of the specimen and should include previous diagnoses, therapy, and surgery; previous instrumentation (including catheterization); history of stones; method of specimen collection; cystoscopic findings; and any other pertinent clinical data. The most common symptoms of patients with bladder cancer are hematuria (gross or microscopic) or cystitis-like symptoms (frequency, urgency, pain). Unfortunately, the diagnosis of urinary tract specimens is less than perfect even among experts [Farrow 1990, Foot 1958, Frable 1977, Kern 1968, Koss 1985, Murphy 1990, Papanicolaou 1945]. A review of 17 published series showed that at their worst, the false-negative rates were more than 50% for primary bladder cancer and averaged nearly 75% for papillomas [El-Bolkainy 1980]. An important diagnostic principle is that the higher the grade of the tumor, the more accurate the diagnosis [DiBonito 1992, O'Donoghue 1991, Wiener 1993, Zein 1991]. Urine cytology is not reliable in detection of renal cell or prostatic carcinoma.

Indications

- Tumor detection
  - Most aggressive neoplasms
  - Carcinoma in situ
  - Small or inaccessible lesions
  - Diverticuli, ureters, pelvis
- Screen high risk asymptomatic patients
  - Industrial chemical or metal exposure
  - Others, those with schistosomiasis, smokers, etc
- Monitor tumors and therapy
  - Low-grade, noninvasive tumors
  - Carcinoma in situ
  - Ileal conduit, urethra, prostatic ducts

Note: Cytology may be positive long before cystoscopy/biopsy. Lesions cannot be localized with urine cytology alone.

As the incidence of urothelial carcinoma increases, so too does the demand for urine cytology. Accuracy of diagnosis is always important, but conservative management of bladder cancer depends on accurate cytodiagnosis. Clinical history is imperative for the reduction of misdiagnoses [DiBonito 1992, Ro 1992].

There are several reasons for diagnostic inaccuracy. Urine is an inhospitable environment for cells; consequently degenerative changes that make diagnosis difficult are common [Frable 1977]. Reactive changes caused by stones, inflammation, infection, therapy among many others, as well as "papillary clusters," are responsible for most false diagnoses (see below) [Cowen 1971, de la Rosette 1993a,b, Farrow 1990, Psihramis 1993]. In addition, transitional cells can normally show marked variation in size and shape, can be multinucleated and polyploid, and can frequently exhibit nuclear and cytoplasmic degenerative changes that can mimic malignancy. The paradox of urine cytology is that pleomorphic cells with enlarged hyperchromatic nuclei containing prominent nucleoli can be benign while cancer can be composed of nearly normal-appearing monomorphic cells with bland nuclei. The most difficult types of urinary specimens to interpret are those from the upper urinary tract (ureters and renal pelvis) [Frable 1977].

False-positive diagnoses are higher in urinary cytologic specimens than in most other cytodiagnostic specimens. However, they are of less consequence because a positive cytologic diagnosis of bladder cancer should not lead directly to radical therapy [Frable 1977]. A positive urine cytologic diagnosis should always be confirmed histologically before definitive therapy is instituted. False-positive diagnoses are commonly seen in cases involving stones, chemotherapy, radiation, viruses, reactive or degenerative changes, benign prostatic hyperplasia, prostatitis and pseudopapillary clusters.

False-negative diagnosis may be of more clinical consequence. Unfortunately, false-negative findings are also common in urine cytologic specimens. Cytologic diagnosis of papillomas and well-differentiated papillary transitional cell carcinoma (TCC) can be difficult or impossible because the cells are nearly normal-appearing [Frable 1977]. Also, cytologic examination of urine specimens is not very good for evaluation of primary tumors of the kidney or prostate, which exfoliate cells late or not at all (see also fine needle aspiration biopsy chapters).

Apparently false-positive cytologic results ("false false positives") occur when a lesion is actually present but is not confirmed histologically (which is more correctly a histologic false-negative finding). Apparent false positives can occur in urine cytology because cytologic examination can detect early lesions, sometimes long before they are cytoscopically visible for biopsy [Allegra 1966,1972, Cant 1986, Esposti 1970, Farrow 1990, Kern 1968, Lewis 1976, Lieberman 1963, Müller 1985, Murphy 1977, Orell 1969, Reichborn-Kjennerud 1972, Rife 1979, Roland 1957, Schwalb 1993, Wiener 1993]. False false positives may also occur because cytologic study can not only sample much more mucosa than histologic biopsy but can also detect tumor in hidden sites such as ureters, prostatic ducts, and diverticuli [Reichborn-Kjennerud 1972]. Furthermore, some epithelial lesions, particularly carcinomas in situ, tend to slough due to poor cellular cohesion, resulting in exfoliation of abundant tumor cells in the urine. However, sloughing of the surface epithelium can result in a nondiagnostic tissue biopsy [Boon 1986, Ro 1992]. Consequently, the biopsy findings may be negative when the cytologic findings are violently positive. Another possible explanation for false false positive cytologic findings is micrometastases in the urinary tract, which could account for the presence of tumor cells in the urine, yet be otherwise occult [Frable 1977]. Although it may take up to several years, most patients with apparently false-positive cytologic findings eventually develop histologically proven cancer [Heney

1977, Kern 1990]. Therefore, positive cytologic diagnosis requires careful follow-up [Murphy 1977, Schwalb 1993].

A variety of newer diagnostic techniques, including flow cytometry [Badalament 1987b,1988, Blomjous 1989, Collste 1980, Dean 1985, Giella 1992, Hermansen 1990, Hug 1992, Koss 1989, Melamed 1984,1990,1992, Murphy 1986, Romero 1992, Tribukait 1979, White 1986], image analysis/quantitative cytology [Alroy 1981, Amberson 1993, Blomjous 1989, Koss 1975,1977a,b, Nafe 1992], cytogenetics [Falor 1976, Lönn 1993, Olumi 1990, Pauwels 1988, Summers 1983], immunology (eg, blood group isoantigens and monoclonal antibodies to a variety of tumor-associated antigens) [Bonner 1993, Cuadrado 1986, Johnson 1980, Limas 1979, Lin 1990, Longin 1990, Sagerman 1994, Summers 1983, Yamada 1991], and molecular biology [Carter 1987] have been studied in an effort to increase diagnostic accuracy. However, at least for the moment, urinary cytopathologic examination remains one of the most clinically useful means of diagnosing urothelial cancer and predicting its biologic behavior.

Diagnoses

- False Positive
  - Instrumentation
  - Stones
  - Chemotherapy
  - Radiation
  - Virus
  - Reactive or degenerative changes
  - Benign prostatic hyperplasia
  - Pseudopapillary clusters
- False Negative
  - Low-grade papillary TCC
  - Renal carcinoma
  - Prostatic cancer
- False False Positive
  - Early detection
  - Denudation

4

5

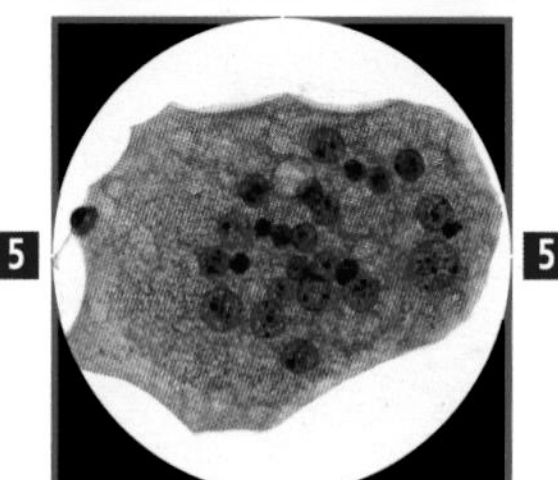

The Cells

Transitional Cells

Transitional cells are among the most pleomorphic, benign epithelial cells in the body, ranging from little basal cells somewhat larger than a lymphocyte (approximately 10 μm) to huge multinucleated superficial (umbrella) giant cells (≥100 μm), perhaps the largest benign epithelial cells in humans [4 I10.4, 5 I10.5] [Harris 1971]. Although the thickness of the urothelium varies, the cells are divided histologically into three layers (basal, intermediate, and superficial or umbrella cells). Due to expansion and contraction, the cells vary from triangular to polyhedral to rounded, or caudate to columnar. Single, mononuclear parabasal-sized cells usually predominate in voided specimens. Multinucleated umbrella cells, groups of cells, and pseudopapillary aggregates are more commonly observed in catheterized samples, including washing and brushing specimens, due to mechanical avulsion. All transitional cells may contain glycogen, and superficial cells can also contain mucin. Glycogen may be washed out during processing, resulting in a clear appearance of the cytoplasm.

Deep Transitional Cells (Basal and Intermediate)

Basal and intermediate transitional cells are cytologically similar and considered together as deep transitional cells [4 I10.4]. The cytoplasm is moderately dense with well-defined, often scalloped, cell borders. Diffuse fine vacuolization is characteristic; coarse degenerative vacuoles are also common [Harris 1971]. Transitional cells can react variably to the Pap stain, usually staining blue to gray, occasionally red to orange.

The nuclei are usually central, but occasionally are eccentrically located. They are larger than nuclei of intermediate squamous cells. The nuclear shape varies from oval to somewhat triangular or polyhedral. Binucleation is common, but multinucleation is more common in superficial (umbrella) transitional cells. The chromatin is evenly distributed and varies from finely granular to salt-and-pepper coarseness: it usually appears bland in well-preserved cells. However, polyploidy and some hyperchromasia are frequent. One or two small but conspicuous nucleoli are characteristically seen, especially in washing specimens [Harris 1971].

Reactive and degenerative changes in transitional cells may show nuclear and cytoplasmic features that can mimic cancer. Causes of reactive atypia include inflammation and stones. These two conditions are responsible for many false-positive diagnoses. Radiation, chemotherapy, and other causes are discussed later in this chapter.

Superficial Transitional Cells (Umbrella Cells)

Umbrella or superficial transitional cells take their name from their shape and the fact that they sit on the surface and cover the other cells like an umbrella, protecting them from the water [5 I10.5]. They have a rounded (convex) luminal surface and a scalloped (concave) border into which the underlying cells fit, and so umbrella cells are also shaped like the cover of an umbrella.

Umbrella cells essentially resemble other transitional cells, but are larger. They have an abundant cytoplasm and frequently two to three nuclei, but may have multiple nuclei that can vary moderately in size. Umbrella cells are usually about the size of a superficial squamous cell. However, giant forms with more than 50 nuclei can occur [Harris 1971]. Giant umbrella cells are more common in specimens from the ureter or renal pelvis, but can also be seen in the bladder. They are commonly associated with instrumentation, and in a very few cases, uremia.

Reactive umbrella cells may be seen in a variety of conditions, including cystitis and lithiasis. Their nuclei can be enlarged, but in proportion to the large amount of cytoplasm, maintaining a normal nuclear/cytoplasmic (N/C) ratio. Cytoplasmic vacuolization or clearing is common. The nuclei can be markedly atypical, including coarse chromatin and prominent nucleoli. In fact, the nuclei can be virtually identical to those seen in cells deriving from a high-grade TCC [Murphy 1990]. Umbrella cells are highly differentiated, and often polyploid.

Despite their pleomorphism and multinucleation, the N/C ratios remain low. Never render a malignant diagnosis based on the appearance of umbrella cells. Clues that a cell is an umbrella cell include abundant cytoplasm, low N/C ratio, and concave/convex cell outline. However, the mere presence of umbrella cells does not exclude malignancy, since well-differentiated neoplasms may be lined with umbrella cells [Frable 1977].

Columnar Cells

Although rare in voided urine specimens, columnar transitional cells are a normal and relatively common finding in specimens obtained by instrumentation of the bladder [6 I10.6] [Harris 1971]. They also can arise from the urethra, particularly of men, as well as in cystitis cystica. Columnar transitional cells often have a thin tail by which they are attached to the basement membrane or to each other. They can be single or form small groups. Columnar transitional cells are usually benign, but can also be seen in well-differentiated papillary neoplasms.

There are also a number of other sources of columnar cells, which are usually glandular. Columnar glandular cells may arise in the urothelium, eg, colonic-type cells associated with cystitis glandularis. Cells from Littre's glands (periurethral mucus crypts) and lacunae of Morgagni may also be seen. Extraneous glandular cells, such as those from the female genital tract (menses, also endometriosis) or the prostate (especially after prostatic massage) may be seen. Ciliated cells are observed rarely [Harris 1971, Palombini 1982]. Also, cells with stereocilia (long branching microvilli) can arise from the vas deferens or epididymis [Thompson 1993]. Renal tubular cells can also be found, but their presence indicates kidney disease.

Columnar cells in urine

- Columnar transitional cells (including neoplastic)
- Extraneous (gastrointestinal tract, female genital, prostate)
- Cystitis cystica or glandularis
- Littre's glands, lacunae of Morgagni
- Renal tubules
- Extrophy or persistence of cloacal membrane
- Intestinal metaplasia
- Cancer

6
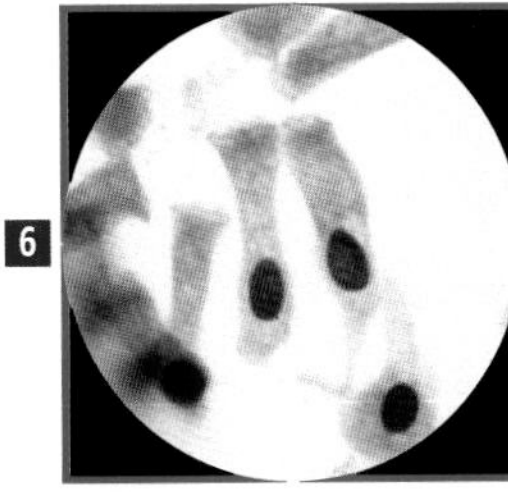

7
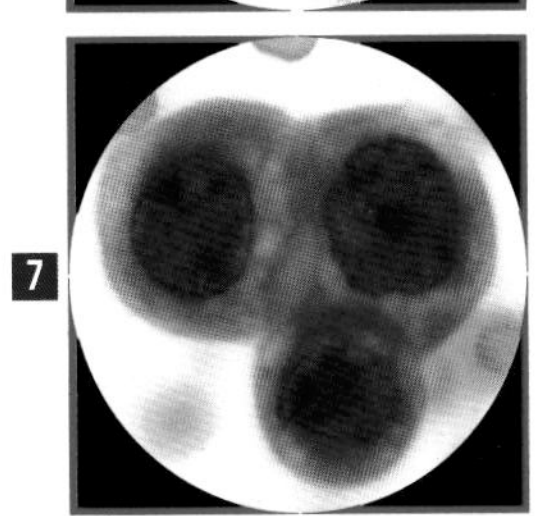

8
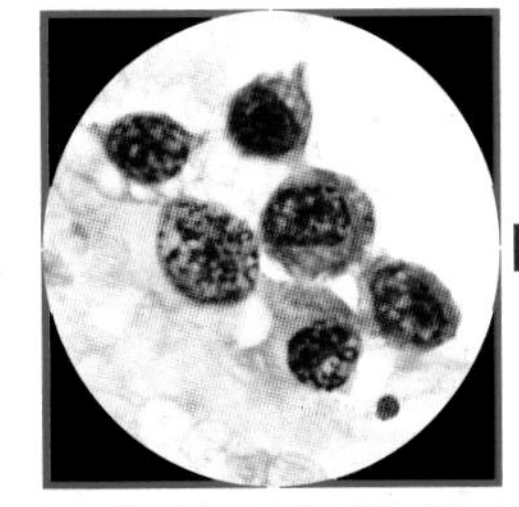

9
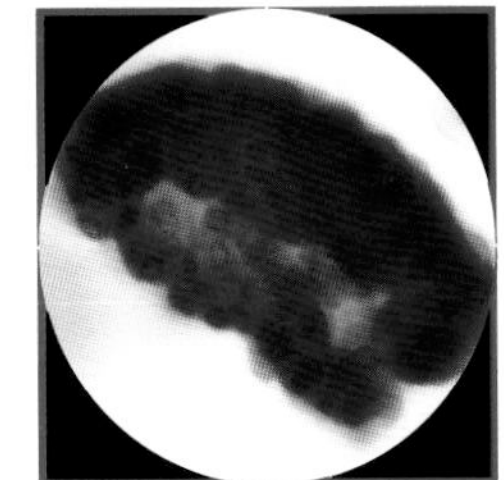

Reactive Transitional Cells

Reactive changes can be caused by a wide variety of conditions including inflammation, stones, hyperplasia, radiation/chemotherapy, viral or bacterial cystitis, drugs, or even catheterization/instrumentation. Reactive changes in transitional cells are thus very common [7 I10.15]. Superficial umbrella cells, in particular, may become frankly bizarre appearing. The nuclei increase in size and number, become more pleomorphic, and the N/C ratio may increase somewhat. Normal mitotic figures can be seen. The chromatin becomes darker and coarser, but remains evenly distributed; nucleoli become more prominent. Prominent nucleoli can be seen in either reactive transitional cells or high-grade TCC, but their presence excludes low-grade TCC [Murphy 1990]. Although the nuclear membrane usually remains smooth, it can become irregular, and frequently appears thickened due to peripheral chromatin condensation.

The cytoplasm stains deeply, and signs of cellular degeneration, particularly vacuolization, may be seen. Vacuolated cytoplasm can occur in either reactive transitional cells or high-grade TCC but is not a feature of low-grade TCC [Murphy 1990]. High-grade TCC shows obviously malignant nuclei (pleomorphism, coarse chromatin, etc) [Murphy 1985]. (See also "Stones" and "Transitional Cell Carcinoma.")

Degenerated Transitional Cells

Degeneration (caused by inflammation, stones, trauma, etc) can result in bizarre transitional cells with darkly condensed coarse or pyknotic chromatin [8 I10.14]. Although such changes can resemble cancer, the chromatin of these benign cells is usually *smudged* or degenerated. In contrast, the chromatin granules of cancerous cells are characteristically *crisp* and well preserved. Margination of the chromatin, with central clearing, is also frequent in degenerated transitional cells. Degenerated nuclei may further undergo karyolysis and karyorrhexis and become washed out or broken up. The cytoplasm may disintegrate and be merely a tag attached to the nucleus (comet cell) or absent altogether. Beware of overdiagnosing hyperchromatic nuclei with smudgy chromatin. Diagnose TCC cautiously based on findings in degenerated cells. (See also "Human Polyoma Virus" and "Decoy Cells.")

Significance of Papillary Clusters

Transitional epithelium has a marked tendency to exfoliate with the slightest trauma to the mucosa [9 I10.13]. Catheterization, bladder washing, other instrumentation, palpation of the bladder, or even vigorous exercise [Hyman 1956] can result in increased exfoliation of transitional cells and detachment of pseudopapillary tissue fragments [Farrow 1990]. Moreover, stones, postsurgical trauma, ulceration, or other inflammatory processes can lead to exfoliation of pseudopapillary aggregates with cytologic atypia (multinucleation, enlarged nuclei, coarse chromatin, prominent nucleoli). Papillary-like aggregates can also be seen in men with benign prostatic hyperplasia. The papillae from TCC tend to be disorganized and crowded, with irregular borders and mild nuclear atypia, while postinstrumentation pseudopapillae tend to be cohesive, ball-shaped, or papillary clusters with smooth (community) borders outlined by a densely staining cytoplasmic collar [Kannan 1993]. However, in practice, it can be very difficult to distinguish benign pseudopapillae from true papillae indicative of low-grade papillary transitional cell neoplasia.

As a rule, cellularity should not be used as the sole criterion for diagnosis of low-grade malignancy [Ro 1992]. Uniform central nuclei, smooth nuclear membranes, fine even chromatin, low N/C ratios, cytoplasmic vacuoles, and general lack of crowding favor a benign diagnosis [Ro 1992]. Superficial cells can line either pseudopapillary clusters or true papillae of well-differentiated neoplasms.

Pseudopapillary groups are expected with a history of trauma (catheterization, instrumentation, stones, etc). However, in patients without such a history, *the presence of papillary clusters in a spontaneously voided urine specimen warrants further investigation to rule out papillary TCC.* In the absence of trauma, the presence of papillary clusters in a spontaneously voided urine specimen is suggestive, but not diagnostic, of papillary TCC. However, the presence of papillary clusters cannot be relied on to make a diagnosis of papillary TCC, because their exfoliation is inconsistent [Wolfson 1978].

Other Cells

Renal Tubular Cells

Renal tubular cells are not a normal component of urine. Their presence is associated with kidney disease. Renal tubular cells are uniform and usually recognized in small sheets or casts [10 I10.8] [Schumann 1981a]. Cells from the convoluted tubule or collecting system can be identified [Eggensperger 1988,1989, Stella 1987]. Convoluted tubular cells are relatively large and rounded, with a low N/C ratio, and abundant granular cytoplasm (due to mitochondria). Collecting tubular cells are smaller and polygonal, with a moderate N/C ratio and finely granular cytoplasm. The nuclei of both are uniform and round, and have fine, even chromatin, which may appear slightly hyperchromatic. Nucleoli are small or absent. (See also "Renal Cell Carcinoma" and "Renal Allograft Rejection.")

Renal Tubular Cells

- Nephritis, renal damage
  - Acute tubular necrosis
  - Ischemic necrosis, infarct
  - Papillary necrosis
- Industrial chemical exposure
  - Cadmium, other heavy metals
- Renal allograft rejection
- Renal cell carcinoma

10
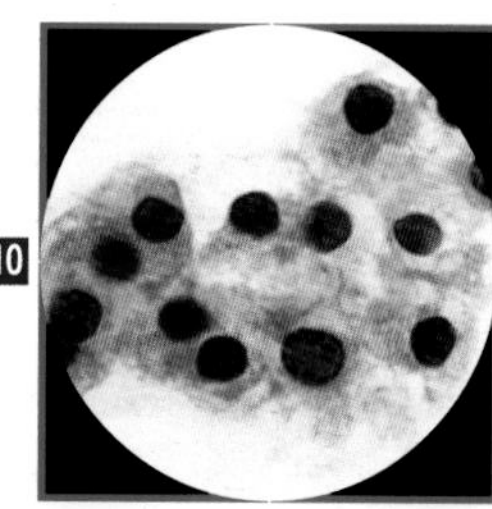

11
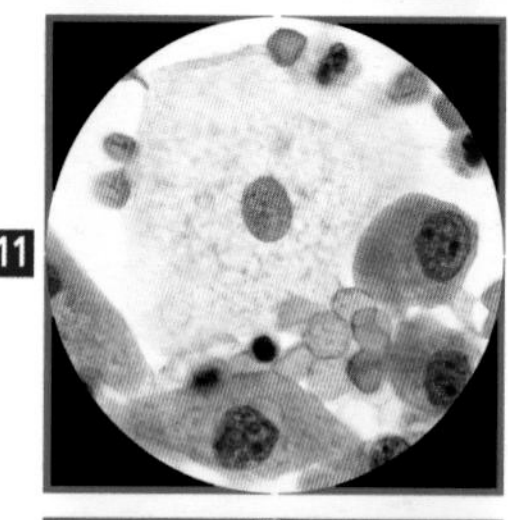

12
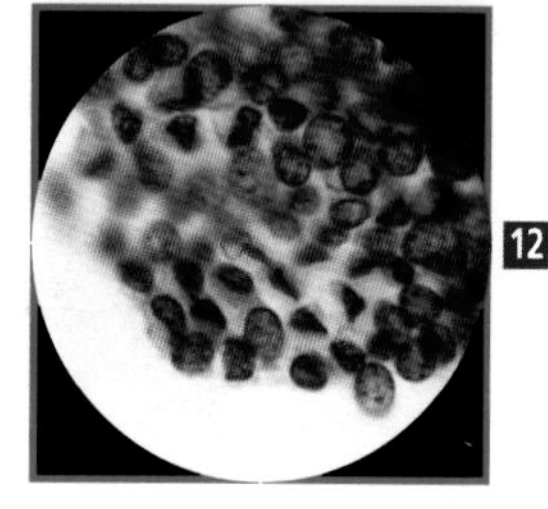

Squamous Cells and Squamous Metaplasia

Squamous cells are a common finding in urine specimens. Squamous epithelium is normally seen in the urethra of men (distal portion) and women (almost entire lining). In about 50% of women and about 5% to 10% of men, the trigone is lined by a nonkeratinizing squamous epithelium similar or identical to that of the uterine cervix [11 I10.7] [Packham 1971, Widran 1974, Wiener 1979]. A maturation index or urocytogram can be performed on these voided cells to evaluate hormonal status of patients in whom a pelvic examination might not be indicated (eg, young girls). (Also, voided urine specimens, particularly from women, often contain squamous cells from the genital tract as a contaminant.)

Squamous metaplasia of the trigone also occurs in newborn boys (due to the mother's hormones) or men being treated with estrogen (eg, for prostate cancer). In addition to hormones, chronic inflammation or irritation (eg, stones, schistosomiasis, in-dwelling catheters) can cause squamous metaplasia, which is also common in bladders of paraplegics due to chronic inflammation or stone formation.

Sources of Squamous Cells

- Contamination (voided urine)
- Urethra, meatus
- Trigone (usually women)
- Squamous metaplasia

In the context of the uterine cervix, the words "squamous metaplasia" conjure up a picture of immature, parabasal-sized cells with dense cytoplasm in a cobblestone arrangement. However, in urine cytology, the metaplastic cells are usually mature intermediate or superficial squamous cells. Squamous cells are larger than typical deep transitional cells or about the size of umbrella cells, while the squamous nuclei are smaller and may be pyknotic. Thus, the N/C ratio in a squamous cell is lower than in a transitional cell. The cytoplasm of squamous cells is thin and usually stains pink or blue, compared with the denser, gray-blue cytoplasm typical of transitional cells.

Contaminating squamous cells from the perineum, genital tract, distal urethra, etc, must be excluded to diagnose squamous metaplasia of the bladder, because the cells are identical. Thus, the diagnosis usually requires a catheterized specimen. Any degree of dysplasia or the presence of prominent nucleoli in squamous cells derived from the urinary tract is suspicious for squamous cell carcinoma, if genital tract contamination can be excluded.

Prostatic Cells

Prostatic cells rarely exfoliate spontaneously into the urine, but are more commonly found after prostatic massage. They form small sheets or clusters of cuboidal cells with uniform small, round nuclei but somewhat hyperchromatic chromatin [12 I10.9]. Small nucleoli may be seen in prostatitis, but macronucleoli suggest prostatic adenocarcinoma.

Seminal Vesicle Cells

Seminal vesicle cells, although rarely found in urine, can be strikingly atypical in appearance, particularly in older men [Voutsa 1963]. Although most seminal vesicle cells are small and degenerate, some may have a bizarre appearance, with greatly enlarged, polyploid nuclei, and dense, almost black chromatin, which could be mistaken for high-grade malignancy. In contrast to cancer, the nuclei are usually more uniform and the chromatin is degenerated and smudgy (rather than distinct). The cytoplasm of some of these benign cells contains a golden brown lipochrome pigment—an important clue to their origin in the seminal vesicles. Also, seminal vesicle cells are often found in the presence of sperm or corpora amylacea. Seminal vesicle cells, especially the highly atypical, degenerate forms, are more likely to be seen after ejaculation or prostatic massage.

Endometriosis

Women with endometriosis of the bladder may present with cyclic hematuria, dysuria, or suprapubic pain. The diagnostic cells resemble those associated with menses in the Pap smear, and may include double-contoured clusters of glandular cells and stroma as seen during exodus [Schneider 1980]. In a voided urine specimen, endometrial cells are far more commonly a contaminant (menstruation) than an indication of endometriosis. The differential diagnosis of these small dark cells includes poorly differentiated carcinoma.

Inflammatory and Blood Cells

Normally, the urine is virtually free of inflammatory cells and RBCs. Significant numbers indicate disease or trauma and, when abundant, may obscure the presence of tumor cells.

Red Blood Cells: Microhematuria can be an indication of inflammation or neoplasia. However, microhematuria is also found in a significant number (up to 100%) of random urine samples from apparently healthy people [Freni 1977, Froom 1984, Mohr 1986, Murakami 1990]. Only 1% or 2% of randomly screened people with microhematuria are found to have bladder or renal cancer. In unselected young patients, only a small percentage have serious urologic disease [Bard 1988, Mohr 1986], but the incidence increases with age [Golin 1980, Whelan 1993]. The degree of hematuria is unrelated to the seriousness of its cause [Messing 1987]. In most cases, the microhematuria originates from the renal glomeruli [Pellet 1991]. Urine cytologic examination may be helpful in differential diagnosis.

Red Blood Cells

Cancer (eg, bladder, kidney)
Primary renal disease, especially glomerulonephritis
Cystitis
Extrarenal disease
Hypertension
Trauma (including catheterization, instrumentation)
Systemic bleeding disorder
Menstrual contamination
Normal? (microhematuria only)

Note: Alkaline urine lyses RBCs, which results in background precipitate. Hypertonic urine leads to crenated/shrunken RBCs. Hypotonic urine leads to ghost or swollen RBCs.
Differential diagnosis: Do not confuse RBCs with yeast (which is more variable in size/shape and buds).

Lymphocytes: These can indicate cystitis (especially follicular) [13 I10.10], acute renal transplant rejection, or malignant lymphoma.

Plasma Cells: These can indicate chronic inflammation or multiple myeloma.

Histiocytes: These can indicate chronic inflammation (especially follicular) or radiation or BCG therapy.

Polymorphonuclear Leukocytes

Pyelonephritis
Ureteritis
Cystitis
Urethritis
Tumor

Multinucleated Giant Cells: These may be umbrella cells. They can also be multinucleated histiocytes (granulomatous inflammation), or associated with radiation or BCG therapy, virus, or renal tubular degeneration [14 I10.26].

Eosinophils: Urinary tract infection, bladder injury, including biopsy, and acute interstitial nephritis are among the most common causes of eosinophiluria [Corwin 1989, Hellstrom 1979, Nolan 1986]. Eosinophilic cystitis occurs in adults as well as children [Hellstrom 1979, Littleton 1982]. Eosinophilic aggregates can cause polypoid masses or erythema and plaques, occasionally with proliferative appearing lesions mimicking carcinoma. In some cases, eosinophils are associated with bladder cancer [Lowe 1984,1985].

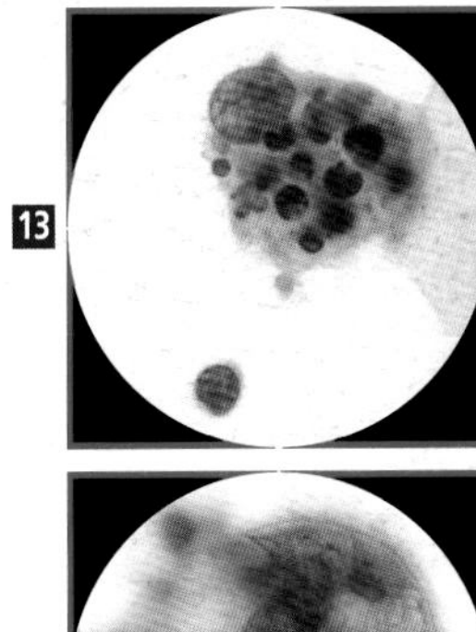

13

14

Eosinophils

Bladder injury, including biopsy, cautery
Allergies
Radiation
Acute prostatitis
Eosinophilic granuloma
Drug induced
Parasites
Nephritis
  Glomerulonephritis
  Acute interstitial nephritis
Bladder cancer

Corpora Amylacea

These are concentrically laminated (usually noncalcified) bodies of prostatic origin [15 I10.11] [Harris 1971, Long 1992]. The differential diagnosis includes psammoma bodies, which unlike corpora amylacea, are always calcified and typically surrounded by epithelial cells.

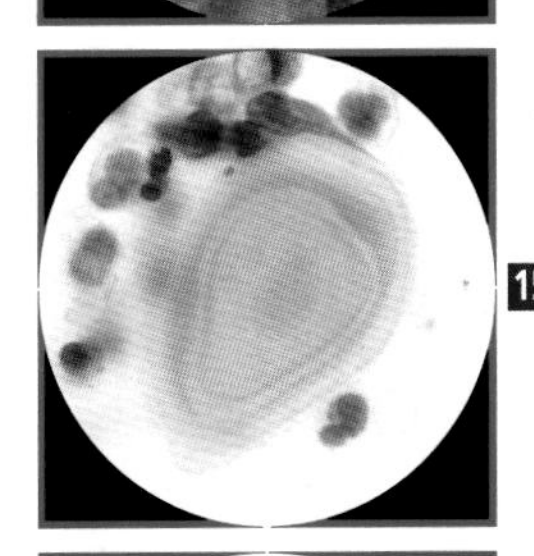

15

Globular, or Hyaline, Inclusion Bodies

Rounded cytoplasmic inclusions of variable size, single or multiple, with smooth outlines (little red or blue droplets) are commonly seen in the cytoplasm (and rarely the nuclei) of urinary tract cells [Melamed 1961, Rouse 1986]. They are often brightly eosinophilic [16 I10.12] (also known as "eosinophilic inclusion bodies"), but can also be cyanophilic, depending on the stain. They are associated with degeneration. Although the nuclei can be well preserved, they are usually degenerated or lost altogether. These inclusions are nonspecific, and specifically not viral. They may represent giant lysosomes [Nagy 1989]. They are more common in voided than catheterized specimens and are especially frequent in ileal conduit urine specimens. Similar inclusions can also occasionally be seen in specimens other than urine (such as sputum, breast cysts).

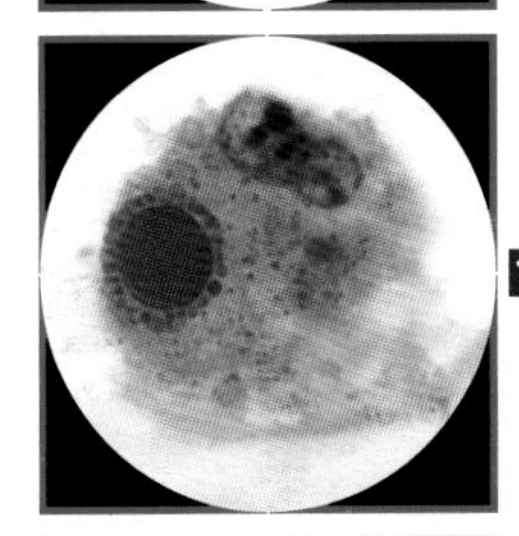

16

Other Inclusions

Nuclear or cytoplasmic inclusions can occur in a variety of conditions, including viral infections, vaccination, heavy metal toxicity [17 I10.21], immunosuppression or transplantation, cystitis, mucocutaneous lymph node syndrome (Kawasaki disease), as well as in normal individuals. Relatively large, mucin-containing inclusions can sometimes be found in transitional cells and multinucleated giant cells, particularly from the upper urinary tract (ureter, pelvis) [Dorfman 1964]. Cytoplasmic lipid inclusions (foam cells) can be seen in lipid storage disease, such as Niemann-Pick disease [Sane 1990].

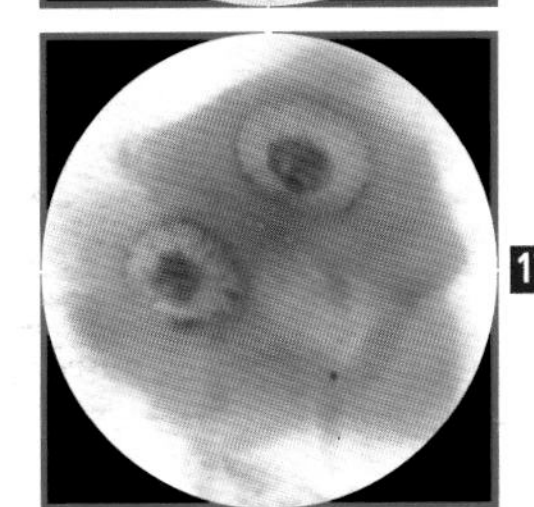

17

Intranuclear Inclusions

Globular (rarely intranuclear)
Virus (cytomegalovirus, herpes, human polyoma virus)
Heavy metals (lead, cadmium)*
Nephrotoxic drugs (gentamicin)

* Landing 1959, Rouse 1986, Schumann 1980

Miscellaneous

Sperm, crystals, casts, and various organisms as well as extraneous material including glove powder and lubricant (amorphous purplish stuff) can all be seen from time to time in urine specimens [I10.1, I10.2].

Basic Specimens

Urine cytology, being a form of exfoliative cytology, is primarily useful in diagnosing diseases that involve the mucosal surface and, therefore, the collecting system (as opposed to parenchymal diseases of the kidney or prostate). There are three basic types of exfoliated urinary tract specimens: (1) voided urine, (2) catheterized urine, and (3) brushing/ washing specimens. "Clean catch" voided urine is recommended for screening purposes [Ellwein 1990, Farrow 1990]. However, in cases in which there is a high clinical suspicion for bladder malignancy, bladder washing may is the method of choice [Ro 1992]. Directed washings or brushings may be necessary to detect lesions of the ureter or urethra. Specimens should be processed immediately or refrigerated and processed as soon as possible. If a delay is anticipated, immediate fixation with 50% ethanol may preserve the specimen for several days [Ro 1992]. However, alcohol causes cellular shrinkage, making interpretation more difficult, and the cells may adhere poorly to the slides. The Papanicolaou stain is usually preferred, since fine nuclear detail is often crucial to proper diagnosis. Romanovsky, toluidine blue, and Sternheimer-Malbin stains have also been used, often as an adjunct to routine urinalysis [Holmquist 1980,1988, Iwa 1991].

Voided Urine

No part of the void (initial, midstream, or terminal) is consistently richer in benign or malignant cells [Hastie 1990]. However, a voided urine specimen is often contaminated with cells from the perineum or the genital tract, particularly in women.

Normal voided urine usually contains only a few cells, which are mostly single. Increased cellularity may be seen, eg, with instrumentation, stones, or neoplasms. Although all cells in fluids tend to round up, transitional cells frequently have a somewhat trapezoidal (truncated pyramid or trapezium) shape. The transitional cells in a voided urine specimen are generally relatively uniform. However, the cells can vary from parabasal to relatively large. The nuclei are round to oval with smooth nuclear membranes. The chromatin is delicate or condensed, depending on the preservation. Small nucleoli may be seen. There is usually a moderate amount of variably stained cytoplasm that ranges from blue-gray to red-orange.

Degenerative changes, particularly increased nuclear and cytoplasmic density, are common in voided urine specimens. Factors causing degeneration include high acidity and variable osmolality of the urine [Crabtree 1980]. Also, the life cycle of a transitional cell is about 1 year [Murphy 1990]; thus, few cells are exfoliated and many of the degenerative changes may be related to the biological reasons the cell was exfoliated in the first place.

Although theoretically more cellular, the first morning voided urine specimen is not a good one, due to degenerative changes [Farrow 1990, Murphy 1985]. Similarly, urine specimens from a collection bag should not be submitted for cytologic examination (although malignant cells may still be recoverable from untreated urine which has been standing for 3 days in a warm room [Cowen 1971, Crabbe 1961, Umiker 1964]). To minimize diagnostic errors, some recommend that the patient be well hydrated and that the urine be acidified to an optimum pH of 5 (eg, by taking 1 g of vitamin C) to help preserve the cells [Pearson 1981, Ro 1992]. Ideally, a very fresh specimen should be sent to the cytology laboratory and processed immediately. However, specimens keep reasonably well for a short time (hours) with simple refrigeration; alcohol is probably not necessary for preservation. A well-prepared, concentrated specimen is critical to diagnosis [Dhundee 1990, Farrow 1990, Toivonen 1991, Trott 1967]. Direct (unconcentrated) smears of the urine are unsatisfactory for evaluation.

The optimum number of voided urine samples to submit is three. Of the neoplasms that can be diagnosed with voided urine cytology, about 80% will be on the first specimen, 15% on the second, and the rest on the third [Koss 1985].

Catheterization

Simple catheterization increases the cellularity over voided urine specimens, and the specimen may be somewhat better preserved. However, it makes the diagnosis of low-grade lesions more difficult because pseudopapillary clusters may be present, and lesions in the urethra may be missed. Urethral cytology is important in cancer surveillance because many patients who fail to respond to intravesical chemotherapy have residual disease in this area, particularly in the prostatic urethra in men [Droller 1986] (therefore, also submit a freshly voided specimen).

Bladder Washes

Bladder wash specimens are diagnostically superior to voided urine specimens [Badalament 1987b, Matzkin 1992, Trott 1973]. The specimens are better preserved and more cellular than voided urine. It is important that the urologist submit both the saline wash and the urine present in the bladder at cystoscopy ("cysto urine"). Although bladder washing alone has a greater diagnostic yield than cysto urine alone [Frable 1977], cysto urine does pick up a significant number of additional cases of cancer [Murphy 1981a, NCI 1977]. A freshly voided urine specimen should be submitted to detect lesions in the urethra. Although bladder washing is superior to voided urine in diagnosis, it is inconvenient, uncomfortable, relatively expensive, and has a risk of infection, especially in men. There may also be a risk of spreading the tumor [Ozono 1986, Wallace 1984, Weldon 1975]. The advantages and disadvantages of the two basic specimens are summarized [T10.1].

T10.1 **Advantages and Disadvantages of Voided Urine and Bladder Washing**

Advantages	Disadvantages
Voided urine	
Easy to obtain specimen	Degeneration
Good sensitivity for high-grade tumor	Few cells, particularly in low-grade tumor
Sample entire tract	Contamination, especially from female genital tract
Bladder washing	
Excellent preservation	Inconvenient, uncomfortable, expensive
High sensitivity, including low-grade tumors	Possible risk of infection, spread of tumor
Almost no contamination	Limited sample (ie, urethra, upper urinary tract)

Diseases and Conditions Associated With the Urinary Tract

Stones (Urinary Tract Lithiasis)

The presence of urinary tract stones can be clinically undetected; patients may have only hematuria or radiologically detected filling defects. In cases in which the stone is passed, the patient may have excruciating pain. Stones can cause an increase in cellularity even in voided urine specimens, including mechanical avulsion of pseudopapillary groups of transitional epithelium with smooth or irregular borders mimicking papillary TCC [Highman 1982]. The presence of umbrella cells may not be helpful, since well-differentiated papillary TCC can be lined with them. Stones can also be responsible for significant cellular atypia comparable to that seen in high-grade malignancy in some cases [18 I10.14, 19 I10.15] [Beyer-Boon 1978, Highman 1982]. The nuclei may be enlarged and pleomorphic, irregular in size and shape, with an increased N/C ratio. The chromatin can be coarse and variably hyperchromatic. Prominent nucleoli as well as mitotic figures can be seen. Inflammation, blood, and necrosis may be present in the background, mimicking a tumor diathesis. Columnar and multinucleated transitional cells are common. Squamous, and occasionally glandular, metaplasia occurs in long-standing cases [Beyer-Boon 1978, Salm 1969]. When squamous metaplasia is found in men, consider lithiasis.

18
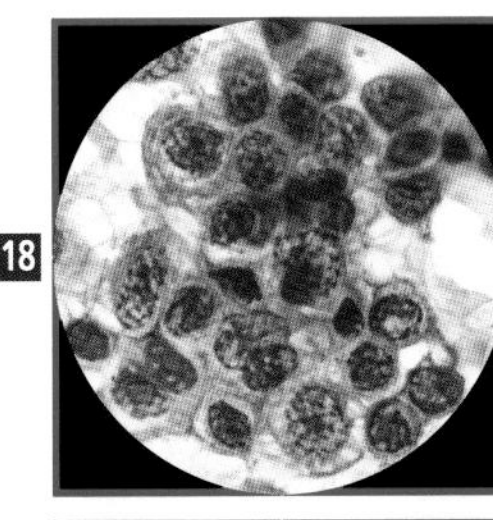

19
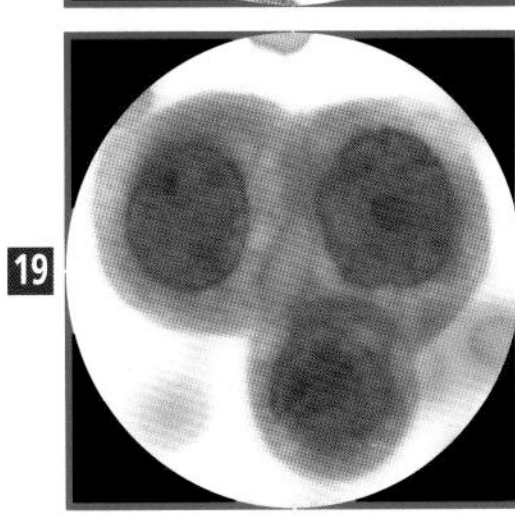

Reactive changes closely mimic malignancy. The clinical history of lithiasis is critical in proper evaluation of the specimen. Be cautious when diagnosing cancer in the presence of stones. However, cancer can coexist with stones, which may even be a predisposing factor to the development of cancer [Wynder 1977]. Beware of overdiagnosing hyperchromatic nuclei in which the chromatin is smudgy or degenerated. Multinucleated cells, both typical and atypical, are more frequent in benign reactive change than in cancer [Beyer-Boon 1978]. Factors favoring a diagnosis of carcinoma include more cells, more single cells, more clusters (ie, papillae of TCC), more disorganization, and more malignant features. If in doubt about the coexistence of stones and cancer, remove the stone; the cytologic appearance should not revert to normal if no cancer is present.

Cystitis

Cystitis is usually caused by fecal flora, particularly *Escherichia coli*, and also *Proteus*, *Klebsiella*, *Enterobacter*, *Streptococcus faecalis*, *Staphylococcus*, and *Pseudomonas*. The urine specimen contains polymorphonuclear leukocytes, histiocytes, red blood cells, and necrotic debris as the diagnostic features. There may be an increased number of cells and, of particular note, clusters of cells may be present.

The transitional cells can be quite atypical, with irregular outlines, enlarged hyperchromatic nuclei, prominent nucleoli, and coarse chromatin with clearing. Transitional cells are often poorly preserved in cystitis. The cytoplasm is often degenerated, vacuolated, or lost altogether. Neutrophils may infiltrate the cytoplasm.

Do not unequivocally diagnose cancer on poorly preserved cells. A diagnosis of cancer should ideally be based on well-preserved cells. Reactive or regenerative atypia of cystitis lacks truly malignant-appearing chromatin and macronucleoli. The nuclei may be dark, but the chromatin often has a smudgy rather than crisp and distinct appearance. Malignancy may have more necrosis, but usually less inflammation, than cystitis. However, inflammation does not rule out cancer, which may ulcerate. In doubtful cases, cytologic examination can be repeated after treating the inflammation, or the patient can be referred for cystoscopy.

Brunn's Nests, Cystitis Cystica, and Glandularis

With prolonged chronic inflammation, a progression from Brunn's nests (solid buds of transitional cells) to cystitis cystica (small cysts lined with transitional cells), then to cystitis glandularis (cysts lined with metaplastic glandular cells) may occur. (Similar processes can also occur in the ureter and renal pelvis, and are designated ureteritis or pyelitis, respectively.) Brunn's nests and cystitis cystica are so common as to be considered essentially normal variants [Wiener 1979]. The specific cytologic diagnosis of Brunn's nests or cystitis cystica is probably not possible, but a diagnosis of cystitis glandularis may be suggested by the presence of benign colonic-type columnar cells [Dabbs 1992]. The differential diagnosis includes adenocarcinoma.

Interstitial (Hunner's) Cystitis

Interstitial cystitis is of unknown etiology, primarily affects middle-aged women, and may be debilitating in some cases. Patients present with clinical symptoms of cystitis, with sterile urine, thus raising the possibility of cancer as an explanation for the symptoms [B Smith 1972]. Cystoscopically, this lesion and carcinoma in situ may resemble one another [Fall 1987]. There may be a marked but nonspecific increase in the number of reactive transitional cells, but no cancer cells are identified. An increase in the number of mast cells in the bladder wall has been reported in biopsy [Feltis 1987] and bladder washing [Fall 1987] specimens of some patients, but their diagnostic significance is disputed [Hanno 1990].

20

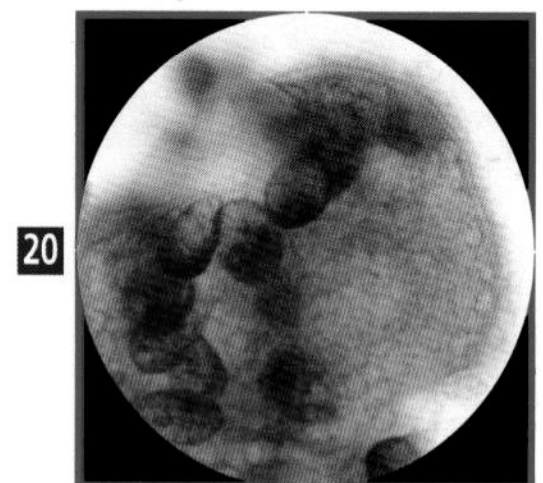

Specific Infections

Tuberculosis

Tuberculosis of the urinary tract is usually secondary to tuberculosis of the kidney. Multinucleated giant cell histiocytes, often with peripheral nuclei (Langhans' cells), may be identified [Piscioli 1985a]. They should not be mistaken for umbrella cells. Clusters of epithelioid histiocytes that often have a spindle or carrot shape may be found [Kapila 1984]. The nuclei are round to oval with fine chromatin, and the cytoplasm is finely vacuolated with indistinct borders. Phagocytosed material may be seen in the giant cells. Acid-fast bacilli or positive urine cultures confirm the diagnosis [Kapila 1984].

Mild to severe reactive epithelial atypia may also be associated with the infection, which must be differentiated from malignancy. The transitional cells can be abnormally shaped and have increased N/C ratios. The nuclei can be large and moderately hyperchromatic, but have a tendency to smudgy chromatin. Similar findings can also be seen in patients treated with bacillus Calmette Guérin (BCG)[20 I10.26] for TCC or after bladder surgery [Spagnolo 1986].

Fungus Infections

Fungal infections of the urinary tract can be an isolated finding or detected as part of systemic fungal disease. They are more commonly seen in immunosuppressed or diabetic patients, but also occur in some immunocompetent patients taking broad-spectrum antibiotics. Most common types of fungi have been reported, including *Blastomyces*, *Cryptococcus*, *Aspergillus*, and *Candida* [Orr 1972]. A polymorphonuclear leukocytic response may be seen in the urine. The most useful diagnostic information comes from urine culture.

Candida: Candida is usually a contaminant that arises from the female genital tract. Candidiasis of the urinary tract is most commonly found in diabetic or elderly patients. Candidiasis can be a serious problem in immunosuppressed patients. Urinary candidiasis can cause ureteral obstruction, possibly resulting in uremia, or generalized infection. *Candida* is usually present in urine as budding yeasts, rather than pseudohyphae. Polymorphonuclear leukocytes may be seen.

Parasites

Trichomonas: Usually a contaminant arising from the female genital tract, *Trichomonas* can occasionally be found in the urinary tract. In men, it may cause a significant number of cases of nongonococcal urethritis or prostatitis [Krieger 1981, Summers 1972]. It has the same morphologic appearance as in the Pap smear.

Ameba: Usually fecal contaminant.

Schistosomiasis: Usually caused by *Schistosoma haematobium*, occasionally *Schistosoma mansoni* (which is more commonly associated with gastrointestinal tract disease), schistosomiasis is rare in this country; it is more common in Egypt [Clements 1983]. It is associated with squamous cell carcinoma of the bladder. Schistosomal ova can sometimes be found in the urine [Dimmette 1955, Houston 1966]. The differential diagnosis includes the lemon drop form of uric acid crystal (polarized light aids in the diagnosis).

Viruses

Herpes: Herpes can infect transitional cells [Masukawa 1972]. It usually has limited significance and is usually associated with genital herpes [Person 1973]. However, herpes may be more ominous in immunosuppressed patients (such as transplant recipients) [Bossen 1975].

The diagnosis is based on multinucleation, molding, margination (of chromatin with ground glass appearance), with or without nuclear viral inclusions [Gomousa-Michael 1992, Murphy 1976].

Cytomegalovirus: In the past, urine was more commonly examined for detection of cytomegalovirus [Bancroft 1961, Bolande 1959, Chang 1970]. Because infected cells derive mostly from the renal tubules, few diagnostic cells are found in the urine. A careful search of several specimens may be needed to make the diagnosis. Cytomegalovirus is potentially fatal in infants, and immunosuppressed patients such as those with transplants [Bossen

1969,1970, Johnston 1969], cancer, especially lymphoma/ leukemia, and AIDS. However, it may not be as ominous in otherwise healthy adults, who may simply be carriers [Lang 1974].

The classic diagnostic cell is large (cytomegaly), with a large basophilic nuclear viral inclusion with halo and thick-appearing nuclear membrane, with or without small round intracytoplasmic or intranuclear satellite inclusions. Usually mononucleated, multinucleated cells occur.

Human Polyoma Virus: Human polyoma virus, not to be confused with its relative, human papilloma virus, is a member of the papovavirus (**pa**pilloma **po**lyoma **va**cuolating SV-40 virus) family. They are DNA viruses also related to progressive multifocal leukoencephalopathy, JC virus, and human papilloma viruses [Suhrland 1987]. Human polyoma virus is also known as BK virus (initials of the first patient) [Gardner 1971]. Infected cells are a relatively common cause of diagnostic error. The cells have enlarged dark nuclei mimicking cancer, particularly carcinoma in situ ("decoy cells") and sometimes short, cytoplasmic tails (known as "comet cells") [Chappell 1976, Crabbe 1971, Kupper 1993, Minassian 1994]. Some patients are immunocompromised (such as patients with transplants and cancer, patients receiving chemotherapy or corticoids, diabetics, pregnant women, patients with autoimmune disease and AIDS, as well as infants and the elderly) [Arthur 1986, Kahan 1980, Koss 1987, Minassian 1994]. However, a number of patients have no known predisposing condition (idiopathic) and these patients may be otherwise normal [Koss 1987]. The infection can be asymptomatic or associated with hematuria, and spontaneously resolves, without sequelae, within a few months [Minassian 1994].

The number of diagnostic cells in the urine specimen varies from sparse to abundant [21 I10.16, 22 I10.17, 23 I10.18]. They are enlarged, about twice the size of deep transitional cells (25 to 45 µm), and have scanty basophilic cytoplasm with high N/C ratios. They are usually mononucleated, occasionally multinucleated. The most characteristic feature is the presence of a large, round, homogeneous, opaque blue/black viral inclusion in the nucleus [Coleman 1973,1975]. The inclusion body can appear to fill the entire nucleus, so it looks like a smudgy dot, or there may be a very thin clear rim or halo between the inclusion and a thick-appearing nuclear membrane. However, the viral inclusion often partially leaches out, leaving a coarse chromatin network, or the inclusions may leach away entirely, leaving nuclei with a bland, washed out or empty ("viral") look.

The differential diagnosis includes cytomegalovirus. Compared with cytomegalovirus, human polyoma virus–infected cells are usually smaller, the peri-inclusion halo is much thinner or absent, there are no satellite (nuclear or cytoplasmic) inclusions, and the cytoplasm is less abundant. The diagnosis can be confirmed with electron microscopy or immunocytologic techniques [Akura 1988].

The cells are not related to the development of cancer, though they can mimic it. When nuclei are smudged, be cautious diagnosing cancer. Also, in contrast with cancer, the cells of human polyoma virus infection are exclusively single and not found in clusters [Boon 1989]. Compare with cancer cell [24 I10.19].

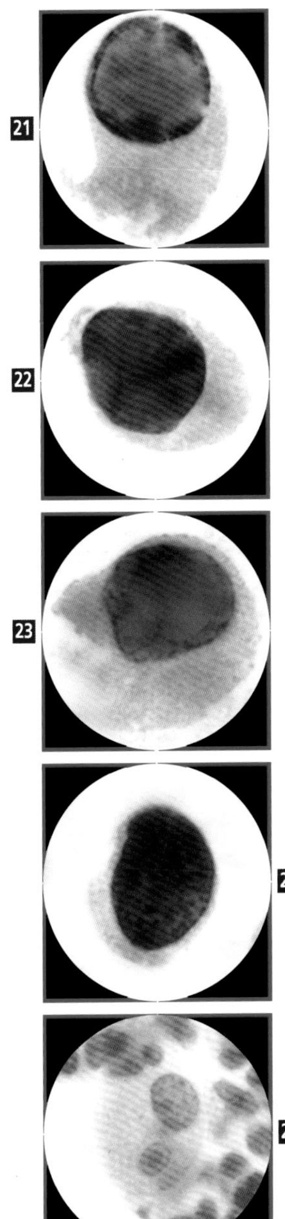

Other Viruses: Other urinary infections/organisms that can be seen include adenovirus, measles, and human papillomavirus. Adenovirus is characterized by nonspecific sterile cystitis and one or more intracytoplasmic inclusions. In measles, giant cells may be seen, with one or more intracytoplasmic inclusions; symptoms are nonspecific. Human papilloma virus causes condylomata, which can occur in the bladder (see also "Condyloma").

Malacoplakia

Malacoplakia is a rare, chronic granulomatous disease typically seen in women older than 30 years, but which can affect any age and either sex [Sinclair-Smith 1975, Stanton 1981]. On gross examination, soft yellow plaques, about 3 to 4 cm in diameter, occur in the bladder (where they can be seen cystoscopically) and occasionally elsewhere (including kidney, prostate, adrenal glands, liver, colon, lungs, bones, brain) [Chalvardjian 1985, Ho 1989, Robertson 1991]. The soft plaques can sometimes cause ureteral obstruction and, rarely, death. Immunodeficiency due to defective phagocytosis or phagolysosomes results in incomplete digestion of bacteria, which become mineralized and lead to formation of characteristic Michaelis-Gutmann bodies [25 I10.20] [Curran 1987, Ho 1989, Lewin 1974]. Dense, granulomatous collections of histiocytes in the lamina propria and muscularis occur in the bladder. Lymphocytes and plasma cells may be seen. Occasionally, multinucleated giant cells are formed.

The giant cells, known as von Hansemann histiocytes, have an abundant, granular, periodic acid–Schiff (PAS)–positive cytoplasm due to the presence of phagolysosomes containing undigested debris of bacterial origin. Some histiocytes contain characteristic Michaelis-Gutmann bodies [Ashton 1970, Melamed 1962]. These are round, laminated, usually basophilic, but occasionally eosinophilic, calcified cytoplasmic inclusions about 5 to 10 µm in diameter. They can be seen in voided urine, but usually only after biopsy [Melamed 1962]. The typical bull's eye appearance is best appreciated in larger inclusions. Michaelis-Gutmann bodies are PAS-positive and also stain for iron and calcium. Similar structures can be seen in patients with hypercalciuria, but are exclusively extracellular [Melamed 1962].

Intravenous and Retrograde Pyelogram Effect

Exposure of transitional cells to certain radiologic contrast materials ("dyes") is known to alter the morphologic appearance of the cells and possibly compromise the accuracy of cytodiagnosis [Andriole 1989, Barry 1978, Bibbo 1974, Prall 1972]. A few days after an intravenous pyelogram a number of abnormalities may be seen in exfoliated transitional cells that can mimic malignancy. Sheets of reactive or degenerated transitional cells (pseudopapillae) may be shed. In addition, single, atypical cells with nuclear enlargement, increased binucleation, coarse, hyperchromatic chromatin, and distinct nucleoli may be seen. However, in contrast with cancer, the N/C ratio remains within normal limits. Degenerative changes including nuclear pyknosis, karyorrhexis, or karyolysis, and cytoplasmic vacuolization and eosinophilic inclusions can occur [Fischer 1982]. Similar changes can be seen in transitional cells after retrograde pyelography [McClennan 1978]. Some contrast materials used in intravenous pyelography may be found in the cytoplasm of large transitional cells, resulting in large, poorly stained gray cells. Free dye can occasionally be seen as spheroid globules or rectangular plates that are colorless to slightly yellow.

Heavy Metal Poisoning (Bismuth, Lead)

In heavy metal poisoning, such as lead poisoning in children, the renal tubular cells may contain red intranuclear inclusions that resemble viral inclusions or macronucleoli [26 I10.21]. These nuclear inclusions are homogeneous but irregular in shape. They are usually single, with a well-defined halo. Unlike viral inclusions or nucleoli, these stain acid fast–positive (ie, red).

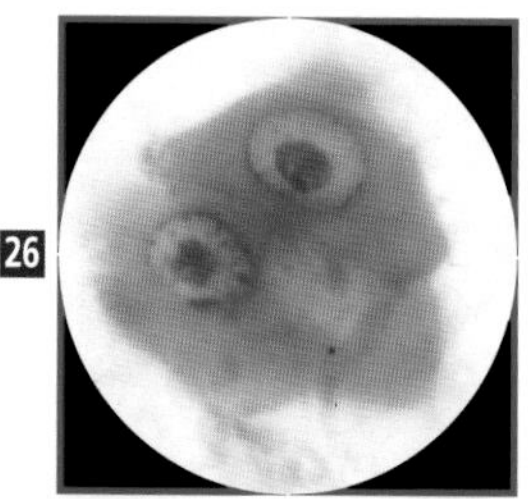
26

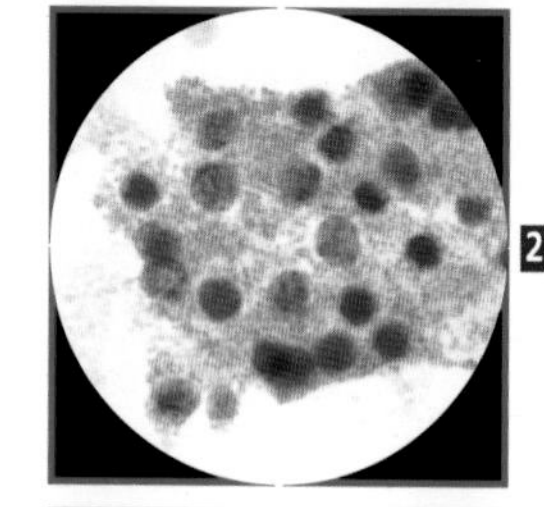
27

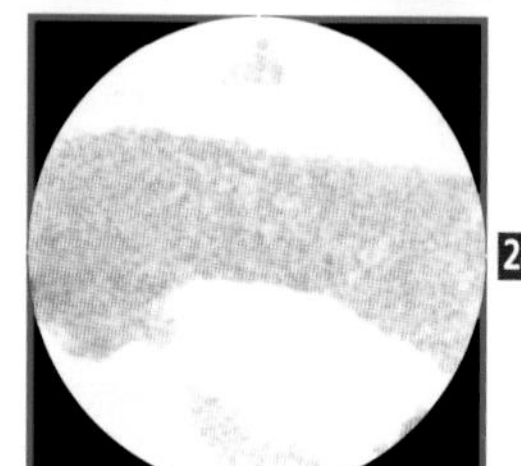
28

Renal Transplant

The urine specimen can be used to monitor patients with renal transplants and predict acute rejection, which may be reversed with prompt therapy [I10.22].

First 2 Weeks After Transplantation: In the first hours after the transplantation, the patient has gross hematuria, which gradually diminishes to microscopic hematuria over the next few days, and subsides altogether 10 days after surgery. Small to moderate numbers of large renal tubular cells, with large, active, vesicular oval nuclei, smooth nuclear membranes, and prominent nucleoli as well as delicate, vacuolated cytoplasm are present in the urine specimen [Taft 1966]. A few WBCs or granular casts may be seen at first, but the background should clear within a few days. After that, the urine sample should return to normal. If activated lymphocytes are seen or renal tubular cells are increased, it may indicate the beginning of rejection.

Recovery: If the graft is successful, spontaneously shed renal tubular cells are sparse [Taft 1966]. However, transplant recipients are immunocompromised, so it is important to look for cytomegalovirus, herpes, other viruses, or fungi [Bossen 1969, Traystman 1980]. Infections may be more life threatening than graft rejection. Transplant recipients are also at increased risk of developing malignancy, particularly squamous cell carcinoma of the skin, lip, and cervix [Kay 1970]. Also, cyclophosphamide (Cytoxan), which is carcinogenic, is sometimes used in patients who cannot tolerate other immunosuppressive drugs. Human polyoma virus infections with decoy cells may occur and should not be mistaken for malignancy in the urine specimen [Kootte 1987].

Rejection: Clinically, acute rejection is characterized by fever, local abdominal pain (due to swelling and tenderness of the kidney), and renal failure, with falling urine output, weight gain, hypertension, proteinuria, and increasing serum creatinine. Urine cytology is most helpful in predicting incipient rejection before the patient reaches this overt stage. Also, negative cytologic findings may help exclude rejection in transplant patients with fever of unknown origin.

One of the most important features for diagnosis of rejection is an increase in the number of renal tubular cells exfoliated in the urine [27 I10.22] [Eggensperger 1988, O'Morchoe 1976b, Schumann 1977, 1981b, Taft 1966]. Renal tubular cells are large columnar cells with eccentric nuclei that often show reactive changes (increased N/C ratio and enlarged nucleoli) or degenerative changes (pyknotic, smudgy nuclei and degenerated cytoplasm). They can be seen singly, in small clusters, in tubules, or in sheets of cells that may be attached to a cast. The cells become more numerous as rejection progresses. Mitotic figures may be observed in renal tubular cells as another feature of rejection.

Lymphocyturia is another important feature that is usually observed in rejection [Krishna 1982, Sandoz 1986]. Plasmacytoid, pyroninophilic, immunologically active lymphocytes, with enlarged nuclei and prominent nucleoli, are among the earliest and the most important signs of acute renal allograft rejection [Anderson 1986, Bossen 1977]. These activated lymphocytes may be accompanied by macrophages. Increasing erthyrocyturia (fresh and old RBCs) is another feature of rejection. Typically, the background is dirty, consisting of cell debris and amorphous, granular proteinaceous precipitate [O'Morchoe 1976b]. The presence of casts (hyaline, renal tubular, lymphocytic, mixed) is another feature of rejection [28 I10.22]. Mixed cell clusters consisting of pyknotic renal tubular cells, and sometimes lymphocytes or neutrophils as well as debris can also be seen. Hour glass–shaped oxalate crystals may occur.

Features of Transplant Rejection

- Increased renal tubular cells (most important diagnostic feature, especially with degenerative or reactive changes)
- Increased lymphocytes, especially reactive
- Dirty, granular background
- Casts
- RBCs
- Mixed cell clusters
- Oxalate crystals
- Mitoses

In summary, suspect rejection if the urine specimen becomes cellular. Changes are best judged against the patient's own baseline. Increased renal tubular cells and increased reactive lymphocytes are two important signs of rejection. Also, if increased renal tubular cells and two or more of the other features are present, rejection is indicated [Winkelmann 1985]. The differential diagnosis is an inflammatory process somewhere in the urinary tract. If the renal transplant recipient has undergone radiotherapy, changes associated with radiation, consisting of nuclear enlargement, multinucleation, irregular nuclear membranes, and vacuolated cytoplasm, may be superimposed on those attributable to immunologic rejection [O'Morchoe 1976a].

Cellular Reaction to Therapeutic Agents

Chemotherapy

Some drugs (eg, cyclophosphamide, busulfan [Myleran]) can cause marked atypia [29 I10.23]. Other drugs (eg, thiotepa) cause reactive atypia that usually is not mistaken for malignancy 30 I10.24]. Some drugs (eg, mitomycin C, thiotepa, cyclophosphamide) are administered intravesically and act locally. Others (eg, cyclophosphamide, busulfan) may be given systemically and become concentrated in the urine where they may remain in contact with transitional cells for prolonged periods. Systemically active drugs are used not only in cancer treatment but also to induce immunosuppression, as in severe systemic lupus erythematosus or psoriasis, or for transplantation. Cyclophosphamide, busulfan, thiotepa, and mitomycin C are alkylating agents that bind nucleic acids and prevent DNA replication. It is imperative that the clinician provide appropriate clinical history.

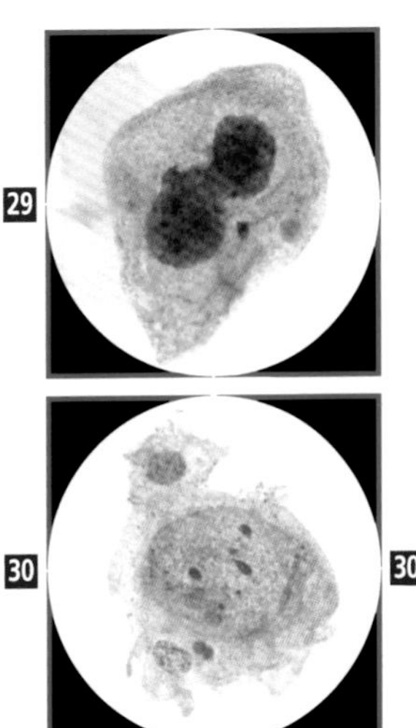

Cyclophosphamide (Cytoxan)

Cyclophosphamide is a nitrogen mustard used for cancer therapy or as an immunosuppressant. The active form of the drug is concentrated in the urine, where it can cause hemorrhagic cystitis. In some patients, severe, even life-threatening, hematuria may occur [Stillwell 1988]. Symptoms of bladder irritation are also common. Epithelial necrosis is followed by atypical repair and regeneration.

The urine can show mildly to severely atypical cells that can closely mimic cancer [29 I10.23] [Forni 1964, Stella 1990,1992]. Although both the cell and nucleus enlarge, the nucleus enlarges more, and an increase in the N/C ratio may occur (in contrast with radiation change, where the N/C ratio remains relatively constant). Cells with bizarre shapes may be seen.

The enlarged nuclei are usually eccentrically located, and may have slightly irregular nuclear membranes. Some cells may be multinucleated. The chromatin is usually markedly hyperchromatic and varies from coarse to homogeneous (ie, smudged or pyknotic). One or two large nucleoli are frequently present; occasionally, irregular macronucleoli can be seen [Forni 1964].

The cytoplasm also increases and becomes vacuolated. The vacuoles may contain debris or WBCs [Forni 1964]. In addition to the marked cellular changes, the background may contain WBCs, RBCs, and debris.

Cyclophosphamide causes cellular atypia that can closely mimic cancer. The presence of multinucleated cells with signs of nuclear degeneration (karyorrhexis, lysis, and nuclear vacuolization) suggests chemotherapy effect. The drug affects cancer cells and benign cells similarly. The cytologic abnormalities are usually transient. However, this drug, which is used to treat cancer, is itself carcinogenic and can cause bladder cancer, even in patients treated for nonmalignant disease [Dale 1974, Fuchs 1981, McDougal 1981, Seo 1985]. Therefore, the possibility of a second primary (transitional or squamous cell carcinoma) should be kept in mind. Atypical changes suggesting malignancy should be reported as suspicious [Murphy 1985]. If it looks like cancer, it probably is.

The differential diagnosis also includes viral infection, which patients with cancer are at increased risk of developing. Viral changes may include large, dark nuclei, but the nucleus usually has a homogeneous or ground glass appearance; in contrast, the chromatin is usually more granular with cyclophosphamide effect. The presence of intranuclear inclusions favors viral effect [Colandrea 1990].

Busulfan (Myleran)

Busulfan causes systemic changes that are similar to those caused by cyclophosphamide [Koss 1965, Stella 1990]. Although it predominantly affects the lung, busulfan can also affect the bladder, although less commonly than cyclophosphamide. Busulfan can cause marked atypia in renal tubular and transitional cells (cell enlargement with large, atypical nuclei) closely mimicking high-grade TCC.

Thiotepa, Mitomycin C, and others

Triethylene thiophosphoramide (thiotepa) and other drugs, such as mitomycin C, are used for intravesical therapy of superficial TCC. Their contact with the mucosa is limited since they are soon voided. In high-grade tumors, particularly carcinoma in situ, positive urine cytology following therapy is an ominous prognostic factor [30 I10.24] [Cant 1986].

Thiotepa and mitomycin C initially cause increased cell turnover and exfoliation that may persist for several weeks. Because of the marked exfoliation of cells, cystoscopic and histologic diagnoses are difficult, making urine cytology particularly important in tumor detection. Later, with subsequent installations, these drugs cause suppression of bladder tumor growth, and fewer cells appear in the urine sample. This provides an important diagnostic clue, since unsuccessful therapy, particularly of carcinoma in situ, may be associated with continued increased cellularity of the urine [Murphy 1978,1981c].

Thiotepa and mitomycin may be associated with reactive, but usually not malignant-appearing, cytologic atypia [**31** I10.24] [Murphy 1978,1981c]. The effects are reminiscent of repair (as seen in the Pap smear). These drugs affect mostly superficial umbrella cells, causing enlargement of the nucleus and cell, usually proportionately, resulting in atypical cells, but with a preserved N/C ratio [Koshikawa 1989, Rasmussen 1980]. The nuclei are round to oval and may be moderately enlarged and multiple. The nuclear membranes are usually smooth but may be wrinkled due to degeneration (crenation) [Droller 1985]. Nuclei are usually not hyperchromatic, but those that are usually have smudgy appearing chromatin [Rasmussen 1980]. Multiple small nucleoli are common. The cytoplasm is degenerated, vacuolated, and frayed.

Cells with bizarre nuclei, as can be seen with cyclophosphamide therapy, are usually not present, or are rare, and can usually be distinguished from cancer. Significant cytologic atypia or frankly malignant-appearing cells should be carefully investigated. Cancer cells generally have elevated N/C ratios, hyperchromatic nuclei, and coarse chromatin.

Cyclosporine A

Cyclosporine A, used as an immunosuppressant, can cause nephrotoxic side effects. Increased numbers of tubular cells or clusters of ill-defined renal cells may be seen in the urine specimen, suggesting ongoing renal tubular injury [Pecorella 1992]. Papillary tissue fragments may also be exfoliated. The tubular cells can show cytoplasmic inclusions (giant mitochondria) and vacuolization. Microcalcifications can also occur [Stilmant 1987].

Radiation

Pelvic irradiation, whether with external beam or implants, is commonly used in the treatment of cancer, such as bladder cancer, cervical carcinoma, and other pelvic malignancies. The effects of radiation run the gamut from no obvious change to total tissue necrosis. Radiation can cause radiation cystitis and cellular atypia, which may be mistaken for malignancy [**32** I10.25] [Wiggishoff 1972]. Clinical history is essential to diagnosis.

Radiation can also cause changes similar to those described in the Pap smear. The most reliable criterion of radiation effect is marked enlargement of the cell or cytomegaly, ie, macrocytes [Harris 1971, Loveless 1973]. Macrocytes range up to five times the size of normal transitional cells. The cells are denser and have more irregular shapes than do ordinary umbrella cells. There is nuclear enlargement and multinucleation. Macronucleoli may appear. The nuclei usually are pale with fine, even chromatin, although they may be hyperchromatic and pyknotic or karyorrhectic.

The amount of cytoplasm increases in proportion to the nuclear enlargement, so the N/C ratio remains within normal limits. Cytoplasmic vacuolization and polychromasia (two-tone staining) or eosinophilia are also characteristic findings in radiation change. Elongated, enlarged cells with big nuclei may also be seen. The background of the smear may contain debris, inflammatory cells, and proteinaceous material.

Distinguishing radiation effect from cancer can be difficult in some cases [Cowen 1971]. If numerous bizarre cells appear long after radiation, or if there has been an interim period when cytologic appearances were normal, then recurrence is strongly suggested [Cowen 1975]. Cells with high N/C ratios and the usual nuclear features of malignancy (hyperchromasia, abnormal chromatin, etc) favor cancer [Loveless 1973], while large cells with nuclei having regular chromatin patterns and abundant vacuolated cytoplasm favor radiation change. Note also that many of the changes associated with radiation (hyperchromasia, pyknosis, karyorrhexis, vacuolization, polychromasia) are commonly seen in normal or reactive transitional cells, especially in superficial umbrella cells. Radiation can cause squamous differentiation in TCC [Neumann 1986].

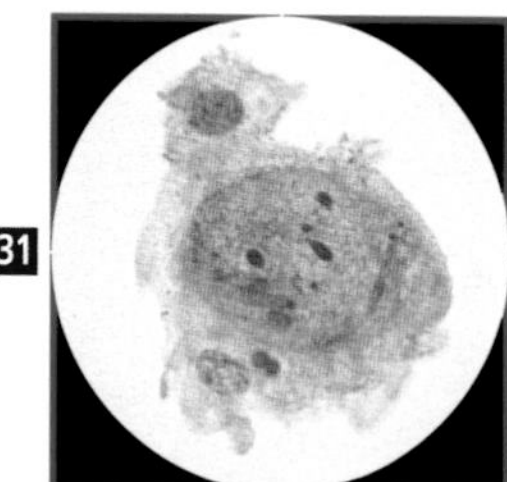

31

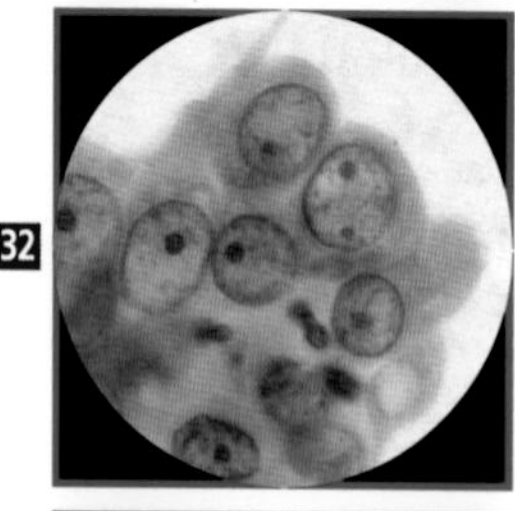

32

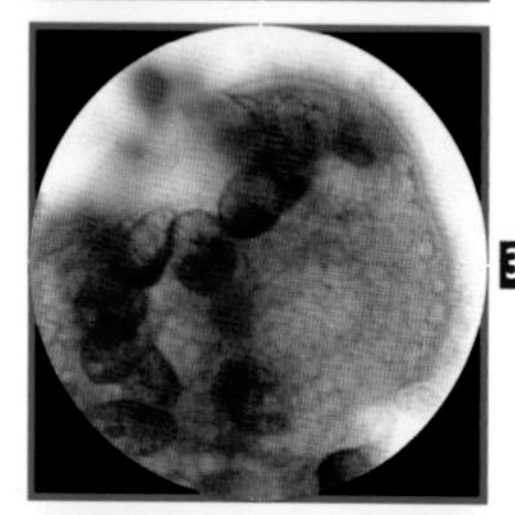

33

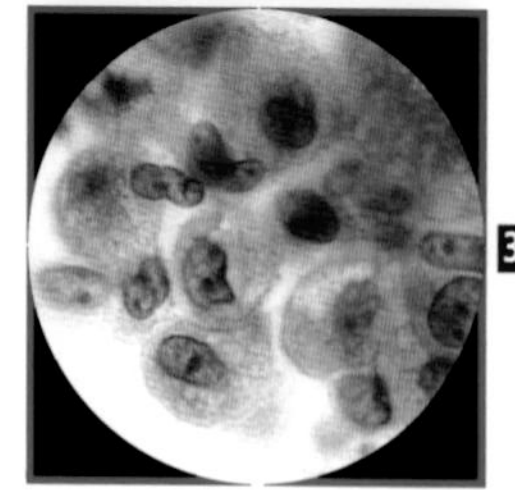

34

Bacillus Calmette-Guérin

BCG vaccine is an increasingly common therapeutic agent for bladder cancer that is particularly effective in treating carcinoma in situ. BCG vaccine derives from an attenuated strain of *Mycobacterium bovis*. Cytologic examination is useful in monitoring therapy and detecting tumor recurrence [Schwalb 1994]. During the course of therapy, the epithelium is denuded and both caseating and noncaseating granulomas may develop in the underlying stroma [Spagnolo 1986].

The cytologic findings closely parallel the histologic findings in biopsy specimens [I10.26] [Betz 1993]. Up to three quarters of patients have histiocytic aggregates [**33** I10.26] and as many as half have giant cells [**34** I10.26] in bladder washing specimens [Betz 1993, Cohen 1991]. Neutrophils predominate by the first week after induction of therapy. Later, lymphocytes and macrophages appear [Pagano 1989]. BCG therapy can also cause epithelial atypia, including slight nuclear hyperchromasia with cytoplasmic basophilia [Lage 1986]. In contrast with cancer, the N/C ratio is preserved and the nuclear membranes are smooth. Significant nuclear pleomorphism, prominent nucleoli, or cytomegaly are not seen in the transitional cells.

Laser Therapy

Laser therapy is a relatively new mode of treatment for TCC. After therapy, bladder washings often show striking spindle cell artifact, probably in response to heat [I10.60] [Fanning 1993]. The spindle cells occur singly and in groups. Single spindle cells have elongated nuclei with uniformly dense chromatin. Groups show layers of cells with indistinct borders. The differential diagnosis includes smooth muscle cells and transitional cell neoplasms with spindle cells, such as papillomas and spindle TCC. To avoid a mistake, a firm diagnosis of TCC should not be rendered on artifactually distorted cells [Staerkel 1989].

Urinary Tract Cancer

More than 50,000 new cases of bladder cancer (about 5% of all visceral cancers) are diagnosed each year and the incidence is increasing. Cancer of the bladder accounts for more than 11,000 deaths per year (~2% of all cancer-related deaths) [Boring 1994, Wingo 1995]. Cancer of the bladder is 10 to 20 times more common than cancer of the renal pelvis or ureter; it is about three times more common in men than in women, and twice as common among whites as among blacks. The average patient is 65 to 70 years old, and most patients are older than 50 years [Rife 1979]. Although bladder cancer is rare before age 40 years, it has even been reported in teenagers [Alcaraz 1991]. Since the average patient is elderly, half the patients die of unrelated disease.

Clinically, the most common presenting symptom is painless hematuria. Nonspecific cystitis-like symptoms (eg, frequency, urgency, dysuria) occur late and may indicate invasive disease.

In essence, there are two forms of transitional cell neoplasia. The first is low-grade papillary lesions, which although they may recur, usually do not become invasive, and are unlikely to kill the patient. The other is high-grade in situ or invasive malignancies. Most patients who die of bladder cancer already have carcinoma in situ or invasive carcinoma at the time of their original diagnosis. Up to 90% of all bladder tumors seen by urologists are papillary transitional cell neoplasms. These lesions are rarely occult. The vascular papillary fronds may break off, resulting in hematuria. Although the cytologic diagnosis can be difficult or impossible, the papillae can be readily visualized cystoscopically. In contrast, the much more significant lesion of carcinoma in situ is usually asymptomatic or associated with only mild, nonspecific symptoms. These high grade in situ lesions are usually flat, and therefore, not readily detectable cystoscopically. Fortunately, cytologic examination can usually detect high-grade lesions [Koss 1988, Melamed 1960,1966]. Thus, cystoscopy and cytology are complementary diagnostic techniques.

An important feature of urothelial cancer is that it is often multifocal. Unlike some tumors that are thought to be clonal (arising from a single strain of abnormal cells as in cervical cancer), patients with urothelial carcinoma have diffusely abnormal epithelium ("field change" [Gil-Salom 1990, Murphy 1979, Nagy 1982]), as demonstrated in mapping studies [Koss 1974,1979]. The abnormalities range from hyperplasia to carcinoma in situ, both near and away from obvious tumors [Cooper 1973, Murphy 1979]. These abnormalities, particularly high-grade lesions, may be the sources of new tumors. Strictly defined, urothelial tumors seldom recur. Rather, new growths may occur after therapy.

A neoplasm generally resembles the parent tissue of origin. Thus, 80% to 90% of urinary tract neoplasms are of the transitional cell (or urothelial) type. The tumors can grow as papillae or as flat, nodular lesions, and can also be in situ or invasive. Microcystic change has also been described [Young 1991b]. TCC may show squamous or glandular differentiation, which, when forming a significant component, is designated as "mixed TCC." Also, rarely, squamous carcinoma or adenocarcinoma can occur as a more or less pure tumor. Small cell carcinoma, similar to that which occurs more commonly in the lung, as well as various sarcomas, can also arise in the urinary tract.

Tumors of urothelial origin readily exfoliate cells in the urine, especially high-grade lesions. Sarcomas and prostate or renal cell carcinomas cannot be reliably diagnosed with exfoliative cytology. Most bladder sarcomas occur in children; botryoid rhabdomyosarcoma is the most common type.

Incidence of Urinary Tract Cancer

- TCC (>80%)
  - Papillary
  - Nonpapillary (flat)
- Squamous cell carcinoma (~5%)
- Adenocarcinoma (~2%)
- Mixed TCC (~5%)
- Small cell carcinoma (~1%)
- Sarcomas (<1%)

Transitional Cell Carcinoma

Risk Factors: The bladder temporarily stores concentrated toxic products of renal excretion and is vulnerable to environmental carcinogens. Bladder cancer was the first cancer documented to be related to environmental carcinogen exposure. There are several well-known risk factors for the development of TCC, the most infamous of which are aniline dyes (containing arylamines, eg, benzidine, β-naphthylamine). Urinary cytology can be helpful in the follow-up of patients exposed to carcinogenic agents by contributing to early diagnosis of urinary tract tumors [Crosby 1991, Forni 1972, Koss 1969].

Arylamines have many uses in industry. They are used as reagents to make dyes for textiles, hair coloring, and paint; antioxidants to make rubber (for tires, cables, etc); and curing agents for epoxy resins and polyurethanes. Consequently, high-risk occupations include chemical, dye, textile, rubber, and plastic workers as well as painters and hairdressers [Cole 1972, Lower 1982]. The occupational risk can run as high as 50% for those exposed, but such patients constitute a relatively small percentage of all cases of urothelial cancer. Excess tryptophan metabolites in the urine may be an endogenous counterpart of aniline dyes or arylamines that predisposes to bladder cancer.

Cigarette smoking is a risk factor for bladder cancer that is far more significant than industrial exposure to carcinogens [Cole 1971]. Cigarette smoke also contains arylamines. Smoking may be associated with as much as 40%, perhaps more, of all urothelial cancers [Lower 1982].

Certain drugs (eg, chemotherapeutic agents, phenacetin, opiates) are also associated with the development of bladder cancer [Behmard 1981, Piper 1985, Veltman 1991]. Coffee has apparently been vindicated as a risk factor for bladder cancer [Viscoli 1993].

Chronic irritation of the urothelium (eg, stones, bladder outlet obstruction, in-dwelling catheters, schistosomiasis) is associated with development of bladder cancer, including squamous cell carcinoma. A history of transitional neoplasia is a strong risk factor for developing subsequent tumors.

Risk Factors for Bladder Cancer

- Arylamines
  - Aniline dyes
  - Tryptophan metabolites
  - Smoking
- Cyclophosphamide (Cytoxan)
- Analgesic abuse (usually phenacetin)
- Chronic irritation
- Stones
- Obstruction
- Indwelling catheters
- Schistosomiasis
- Clinical history, including papilloma

Success of Urine Cytology: Urine cytology is essential for the proper evaluation and follow-up of patients with urothelial cancer. Cytologic examination can readily detect most high-grade TCCs, the biologically malignant urothelial neoplasms. Urine cytology can also detect carcinoma in situ and many well-differentiated transitional cell neoplasms as well as squamous cell carcinoma and adenocarcinoma. Cytologic study can also find small, high-grade lesions or tumors obscured by debris (eg, after therapy). Another advantage of cytology is that the entire urinary tract can be sampled (which is important because of the multifocal nature of the disease); however, the disadvantage is the inability of localizing lesions detected cytologically.

As previously discussed, cytologic findings can be positive when histologic and cystoscopic findings are negative. This is not necessarily a false-positive cytodiagnosis, but may represent early detection of tumor. A positive cytologic diagnosis of malignancy is usually a reliable indicator of the presence of disease [Highman 1988]. A negative result must be interpreted in its clinical context [Badalament 1987a,b], but negative cytologic findings after multiple examinations virtually exclude aggressive tumor [Farrow 1979]. The inconvenience, discomfort, expense, risk of infection, and lack of complete accuracy associated with cystoscopy/biopsy make cytologic examination an attractive alternative for monitoring patients even with low-grade tumors with less frequent endoscopy [Gil-Salom 1990, D Morrison 1984].

Failure of Urine Cytology: Much of the failure of urine cytology (high rate of false-negative findings) involves the inability to detect many well-differentiated papillary transitional cell neoplasms. By definition, these papillary lesions have normal or nearly normal transitional cell morphology (grade 0 or I), making the cytologic diagnosis of these neoplasms difficult or impossible [Allegra 1966,1972, DiBonito 1992, Esposti 1970,1972, Farrow 1990, Frable 1977, Jordan 1987, Kern 1968,1975, Koss 1985, Prall 1972, Sarnacki 1971, Umiker 1962,1964].

Traditionally, most urothelial neoplasms with an exophytic, papillary growth pattern have been considered malignant, not because they are particularly dangerous but because they tend to recur. Although some authorities (such as the World Health Organization) recognize a category of benign papilloma, their definition is so restrictive that a diagnosis of papilloma can rarely be made (<1% of bladder tumors) [35 I10.28]. Moreover, separation of papilloma and grade I papillary TCC into two categories is arbitrary and cannot be reliably reproduced [Kern 1975]. Other authorities consider *all* exophytic papillary tumors malignant, and include benign papillomas among TCCs (TCC grade 0) [Bergkvist 1965]. However, if the cells of these well-differentiated papillary lesions (papillomas, TCC grade 0 and I) were not located on a fibrovascular stalk, a diagnosis of cancer would not be made [Murphy 1990]. Thus another diagnostic tack is to consider papillary lesions lined with well-differentiated, normal, or nearly normal-appearing cells as benign papillomas and all transitional cell tumors, whether papillary or not, composed of malignant appearing cells as TCCs. There is biologic justification for this approach.

Transitional Cell Neoplasia—A Two Disease System: Mortality is nil for benign papillomas and negligible for grade I papillary TCC, but mortality becomes significant for grade II or higher cancers [Farrow 1979, Gilbert 1978]. Therefore, it has been proposed that urothelial neoplasia exists as two relatively distinct entities, namely low-grade, nonaggressive neoplasms and high-grade, aggressive cancers [Bergkqvist 1965, Brawn 1982, Farrow 1979, Jordan 1987, Kern 1984, Koss 1988, Lerman 1970, Murphy 1983].

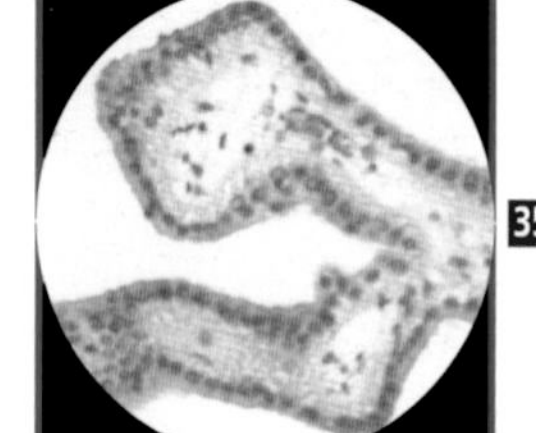
35

Low-grade transitional cell neoplasms are usually not aggressive. Very few patients who present with well-differentiated lesions initially develop aggressive cancer or die of the disease, although many of these patients have recurrences (in actuality new tumors) [Brawn 1982, Prout 1977]. Although low-grade TCCs may invade superficially, they rarely are deeply invasive [DiBonito 1992]. If the lesions are going to recur, they usually do so within 2 years. A certain number (7% to 20%) progress to more significant disease, but progression (defined as invasion or metastasis) is independent of the number of recurrences [Jordan 1987], and only about 5% of patients whose tumors were well differentiated at presentation eventually die of urothelial cancer. The most important aspect of a diagnosis of low-grade transitional cell neoplasia is that it identifies a patient who is at increased risk of developing aggressive cancer and who should be monitored closely.

High-grade carcinomas are aggressive, whether papillary or not. Almost all patients (>90%) who die of TCC present with high-grade lesions initially [Jordan 1987]. Grading correlates closely with stage [Kern 1984, Suprun 1975]. The cytologic grade of the initial tumor is highly predictive of the final outcome of the patient. Thus, the cytologic grade is a key prognostic factor, as important as depth of invasion and much more important than histologic growth pattern (ie, flat vs papillary) [Jordan 1987].

Although well-differentiated lesions are difficult or impossible to diagnose cytologically, the patient is not endangered because these lesions are rarely, if ever, lethal [Heney 1983, D Morrison 1984]. Flat carcinoma in situ and high-grade invasive cancer, not differentiated papillary carcinomas, are the dangerous lesions, and they can usually be readily detected cytologically.

There are apparently two more or less distinct pathways of development of transitional cell neoplasms. The more common form, seen in about two thirds of cases, is from dysplasia (mild to moderate atypia) to papilloma and finally low-grade (all I, some II) papillary TCC [Murphy 1984]. The cells of these low-grade lesions are morphologically similar. They are bland cytologically, usually have normal blood group isoantigens, and are predominantly diploid [Koss 1988, Murphy 1984]. The lesions frequently recur but are rarely aggressive or cause death [Murphy 1984].

The second pathway is from severe dysplasia/carcinoma in situ to aggressive high-grade TCC (all grade III, some II). The cells are clearly malignant-appearing cytologically, lack blood group antigens, may be aneuploid, and are often mitotically active [Koss 1988, Murphy 1984]. These are the lesions that are associated with invasion and mortality.

Cytologic Classification of Urothelial Malignancy: Cytologic grade is more important than histologic pattern (papillary vs flat) in determining behavior. Although low-grade lesions are more likely to be papillary and high-grade lesions more likely to be nonpapillary (flat), papillary configuration per se is not important. In essence, the lesion acts like it looks [Murphy 1990], ie, if it looks well differentiated, it behaves in a benign fashion; if it looks anaplastic, it behaves in a malignant fashion. In the present discussion, papillary lesions composed of normal or nearly normal-appearing cells are designated as papillomas rather than carcinomas. This designation includes both benign papillomas and grade I papillary TCC (as traditionally defined). Lesions composed of moderately to markedly abnormal cells are classified as carcinomas, whether papillary or not, and can be of either low- or high-grade malignancy.

Using the revised classification [T10.2], benign exophytic papillomas are not rare and comprise at least a quarter of all transitional cell neoplasms [Bergkqvist 1965, Jordan 1987].

General Principles of Cytologic Diagnosis: The higher the grade and the more extensive the tumor, the greater is the ability to make a cytologic diagnosis [Farrow 1990, Harving 1989, Kern 1975, Sarnacki 1971, Schmidlapp 1948,1950]. Disorganized tissue fragments with cellular crowding and nuclear overlapping are commonly observed in cancer. Important cytologic features of malignancy include enlarged nuclei, increased N/C ratio, coarse chromatin, and macronucleoli. The presence of elongated spindle cells may provide a clue to the diagnosis of low-grade neoplasms [Fontana 1993]. Hyperchromasia and nuclear size alone are not good diagnostic criteria: degenerated or polyploid nuclei can stain dark, and it is the N/C ratio rather than absolute nuclear size that is important in diagnosis. Mitotic figures and necrosis are factors that correlate with poor prognosis. An adenocarcinomatous component may be seen in TCC but is uncommon. A squamous component, if present, is usually well differentiated. Such mixed tumors, however, more commonly occur in high-grade TCC.

Cytologic Criteria for Diagnosis

- Disorganized groups
- Cell size and shape
- Nuclear size and shape
- Change in N/C ratio
- Chromatin (coarseness, irregularity)
- Nucleoli

T10.2 Approximate Diagnostic Equivalents in Three Systems of Classification

WHO	Bergkvist	Revised
Papilloma	TCC 0	Benign Papilloma
TCC I	TCC I	Benign Papilloma
TCC II	TCC II	Low-grade TCC
TCC III	TCC III	High-grade TCC

WHO = World Health Organization; TCC = transitional cell carcinoma.

The differential diagnosis includes atypia due to catheterization, biopsy, fulguration, therapy, cystitis, stones, radiation, and chemotherapy. Benign atypia may coexist with TCC.

Prognosis and Follow-up: The prognosis depends on the histologic tumor type and grade, the depth of invasion, presence or absence of lymphatic or blood vessel invasion, and spread to distant sites. The grade and stage of the tumor are important prognostic factors. However, TCC is a multifocal disease. Therefore the status of the residual epithelium is critically important in prognostic assessment of urothelial tumors [Koss 1988]. A voided urine specimen is cytologically sensitive to the presence of carcinoma in situ and high-grade TCC. The presence of malignant-appearing cells in the urine is strong evidence that the lesion has not responded to treatment and invasive cancer may be present [Koss 1988]. Thus, cytologic follow-up of TCC is essential.

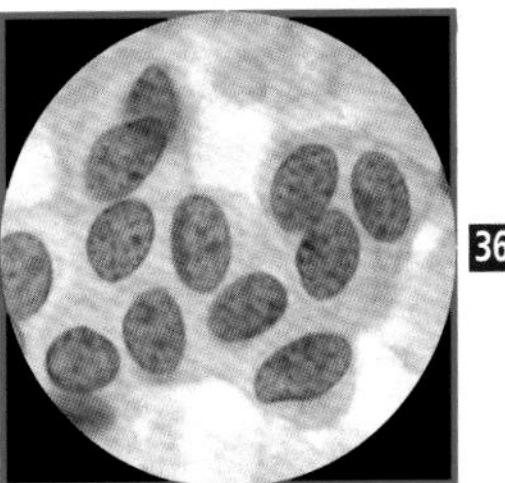
36

Papilloma (Well-Differentiated Papillary Transitional Cell Neoplasm)

Well-differentiated papillary transitional cell neoplasms are designated here as "papillomas" (lumping traditional benign papillomas and grade I papillary TCC) [I10.28] [Bergkqvist 1965, Jordan 1987]. Many papillomas are composed of cells with normal or nearly normal morphologic appearance [Murphy 1985], making cytologic diagnosis difficult or impossible. Others have morphologic features of a low-grade neoplasm. Therefore, only one third to two thirds of these lesions can be diagnosed cytologically [Kern 1988, Murphy 1990], and the higher diagnostic yield (fewer false negatives) comes at the expense of more false-positive diagnoses [Murphy 1984].

Numerous cells may be exfoliated; the number of cells correlates with the size and extent of the lesion [36 I10.27]. Loose clusters and papillary aggregates commonly occur, but must be differentiated from pseudopapillary clusters related to trauma (instrumentation, stones, etc). True papillary fronds (with fibrovascular cores) are diagnostic of papillary neoplasia [Allegra 1966,1972, Farrow 1990]. However, their presence is not essential for cytologic diagnosis.

Columnar, elongated, or spindle cells may be seen [Allegra 1972, Crabbe 1961, Harrison 1951, Highman 1986, Papanicolaou 1947, Wolinska 1985]. The cells and their nuclei are larger than normal deep transitional cells (but not superficial cells) [Murphy 1984,1990]. The cell borders are often indistinct. The cytoplasm is homogeneous rather than vacuolated. The nuclei are eccentric and have slightly irregular membranes in the form of notches or creases. The chromatin is fine and evenly distributed. Nucleoli, if present, are small [Murphy 1984,1990]. RBCs are commonly observed in the background [Wolinska 1985].

Reactive transitional cells, eg, those associated with stones, often have prominent nucleoli and vacuolated cytoplasm. These two cytologic features are usually not associated with low-grade transitional cell neoplasms [Murphy 1990]. High-grade TCC has classic malignant features. The cells of papilloma are similar to those of dysplasia, although cells from papillomas tend to be larger and more numerous, and form larger aggregates [Murphy 1981b]. The cytologic appearance of inverted papilloma is similar to that of exophytic papillomas [37 I10.29, I10.30] [Taylor 1986].

Although half or more papillomas recur (or more precisely, new tumors develop), tumors composed of cells with nearly normal morphologic appearance are rarely, if ever, aggressive [Murphy 1985]. Patients presenting with grade I tumors rarely (~2%) develop muscle invasion or metastases [Heney 1983]. However, patients with papillomas should be considered in the high-risk group and carefully monitored [Lerman 1970, Murphy 1985].

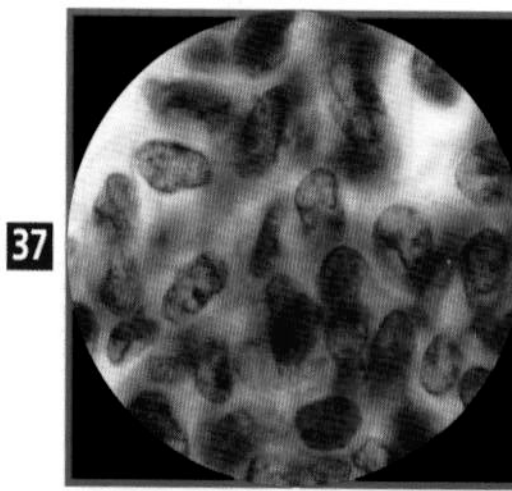

37

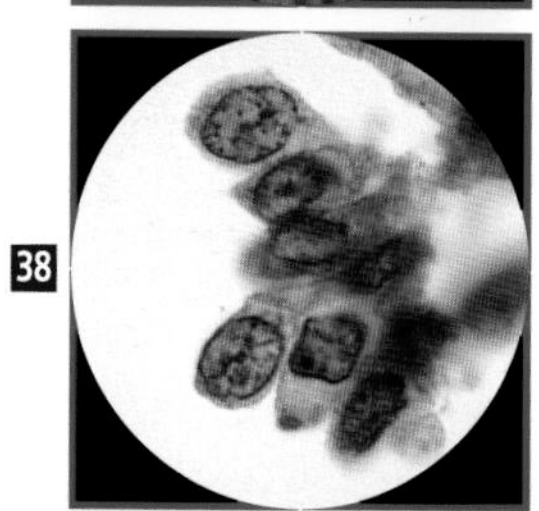

38

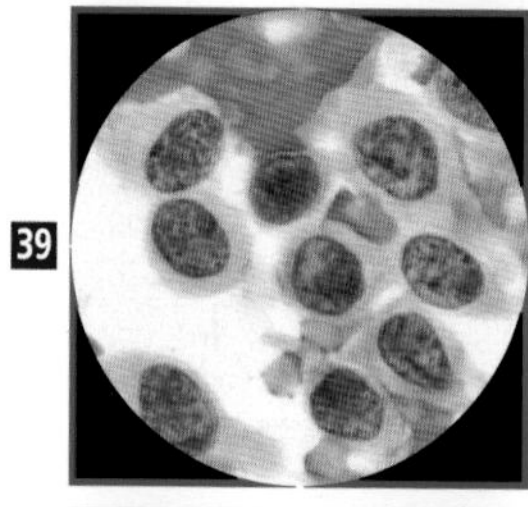

39

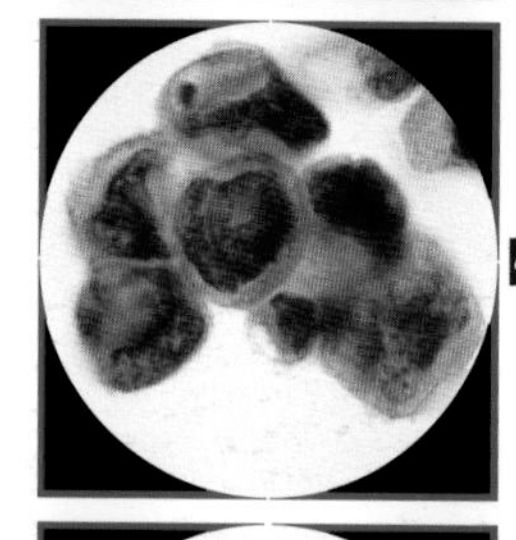

40

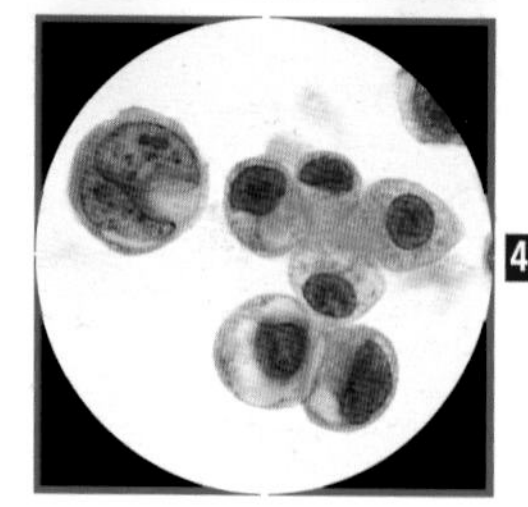

41

Low-Grade TCC

Low-grade TCC is grade II TCC as traditionally defined. [Jordan 1987, Murphy 1983]. Histologically, superficial umbrella cells are decreased or absent from the surface of these lesions [I10.34].

Many cells are shed in the urine. Increased cellularity is a suspicious finding in a voided urine specimen, which is normally sparsely cellular. The cells often form loose clusters or papillae. However, papillary fragments may fail to shed and their presence cannot be relied on to make the diagnosis. Abnormally crowded clusters are also a feature of malignancy. Columnar-shaped cells may be seen [I10.33].

Although the cells may be smaller than those of papillomas, they have higher N/C ratios [38 I10.31, 39 I10.32] [Boon 1981, Kern 1975, Murphy 1984,1990]. The nuclei are eccentrically located and show features of malignancy. Nuclear membrane irregularities are usually present and are diagnostically important [Raab 1994]. The chromatin is more granular than normal, but evenly distributed. Nucleoli are usually invisible or small, although some nuclei may have prominent nucleoli [Murphy 1985]. The cytoplasm typically appears homogeneous, rather than vacuolated [Raab 1994]

The cells appear more atypical than those of papilloma. However, significant pleomorphism, irregular chromatin distribution, or numerous large nucleoli are not seen. Mitotic figures may be observed. Focal evidence of glandular or squamous metaplasia can occur.

By statistical analysis, high N/C ratios, irregular nuclear membranes, and nonvacuolated cytoplasm were selected as three key features in the diagnosis of low-grade TCC [Raab 1994]. A background of small, pyknotic transitional cells is a warning that transitional cell carcinoma may be present [Sack 1995].

The cells lack features of aggressive neoplasms and have low malignant potential [Murphy 1985]. Although they frequently recur and may superficially invade the lamina propria, they rarely invade deeply (into muscle) or result in mortality.

High-Grade TCC

High-grade TCC is grade III (and IV) TCC as traditionally defined [Jordan 1987, Murphy 1983]. Most are nonpapillary. Metastases occur to regional lymph nodes followed by lung, liver, bone, and other sites. High-grade lesions account for almost all tumor-related deaths in TCC.

The cells are pleomorphic and often bizarre, with moderately to markedly increased N/C ratios [40 I10.39, 41 I10.40, I10.41, I10.42]. The nuclei are eccentrically located and display classic malignant features, including very irregular nuclear membranes and abnormal coarse, dark chromatin with clumping, clearing, and irregular distribution. Large nucleoli may be present. Mitotic figures are frequent and may be atypical. In contrast with well-differentiated neoplasms, the cytoplasm is often vacuolated [Murphy 1984,1990]. Glandular or squamous differentiation is more common in high-grade carcinomas [I10.45-I10.47] [DiBonito 1992, Harris 1971, Murphy 1985, Suprun 1975]. Spindle and giant cells can also be seen [I10.43, I10.44].

Reactive transitional cells can also have large nucleoli and cytoplasmic vacuolization, like high-grade TCC, but the benign nuclei lack malignant criteria. Reactive superficial cells can have malignant-appearing nuclei, but have low N/C ratios. Do not diagnose malignancy based on findings in superficial cells (ie, large cells with low N/C ratios). Compared with those of low grade TCC, the cells of high-grade TCC are obviously malignant appearing (ie, more pleomorphic, with more irregular nuclear membranes, and larger nucleoli). Poorly differentiated prostatic adenocarcinoma has relatively uniform, round nuclei with little pleomorphism. The chromatin is finer and more even. Large nucleoli are found in most cells of adenocarcinoma.

There may be some degree of discordance between histologic and cytologic classification of low- vs high-grade TCC [T10.3]. In high-grade TCC, cells at the surface may differentiate, shedding cells, leading to a false low-grade diagnosis cytologically. On the other hand, a focal high-grade area in an otherwise low-grade transitional cell neoplasm may be detected cytologically but missed histologically. Also, degenerative changes may result in misclassification, as either higher or lower grade.

Pitfalls: Umbrella cells, pseudopapillary fragments, stone atypia, ureteral/pelvic cells, ileal conduit, radiation/chemotherapy, viruses (especially polyoma), hyperplasia/papilloma, drugs.

T10.3 **Differential Diagnosis Between Reactive, Low-Grade, and High-Grade Transitional Cell Carcinoma (TCC)**

Feature	Reactive	Low-grade TCC	High-grade TCC
Groups	Pseudopapillae	Papillae; loose or crowded clusters	Loose clusters/syncytia/single
Cells	Enlarged, pleomorphic, variable in number	Enlarged, relatively uniform, often numerous, but fewer than in high-grade TCC	Enlarged, pleomorphic, usually numerous
N/C ratio*	Normal/increased	Increased† (slight to moderate)	Increased (moderate to marked)
Nucleus	Central, uniform	Eccentric, enlarged, variable	Eccentric, pleomorphic
Nuclear membrane	Smooth, "thick"	Slightly irregular,† thin	Moderately to markedly irregular, thin
Chromatin	Fine, even	Granular, even	Coarse, dark, irregular
Nucleoli	Often large	Small to none	Macronucleoli, many cells‡
Cytoplasm	Vacuolated	Homogeneous†	Often vacuolated; also squamous, glandular
Background	Inflamed or clean	Clean	Diathesis

[Kannan 1990, Murphy 1984,1985,1990, Shenoy 1985]
* Compared with deep not superficial cells.
† Key diagnostic features of low-grade TCC.
‡ Adenocarcinoma has micronucleoli in most cells.

Best Criteria: Enlarged nuclei, increased N/C ratio, irregular nuclear membranes, coarse, dark chromatin, and macronucleoli.

Dysplasia: Similar to low-grade TCC, but fewer cells.

Carcinoma In Situ: Similar to high-grade TCC; cannot reliably distinguish the two by cytology alone.

Coy Cells—The Diagnosis of Well-Differentiated Transitional Cell Neoplasms

The cytologic diagnosis of transitional cell neoplasms ranges from easy (high grade III) to difficult or even impossible (low grade, I to 0, papilloma). As previously stated, the mere presence of papillary groups in a voided urine specimen is suspicious for papillary transitional cell neoplasia (in absence of stones, instrumentation, etc). However, papillary groups are not necessarily the best place to look at the cells to make a diagnosis of low-grade TCC. Even benign cells in groups show pleomorphism (small basal to giant superficial cells). In fact, cells in benign groups can be more pleomorphic than low-grade malignancy. Add reactive changes and a few polyploid nuclei to the normal variation of transitional cell morphology, and it is apparent that pseudopapillary groups of benign cells can mimic cancer.

Instead of the groups, the diagnostic cells to look for in diagnosis of well-differentiated transitional cell neoplasms are single little cells hiding in the background ("coy cells") [42 I10.35, I10.36, 43 I10.37, 44 I10.38]. Coy cells are the opposite of decoy cells. Decoy cells look "ugly" and stand out, but on careful evaluation indicate a benign process. Coy cells are shy and innocent-looking little cells that can easily be overlooked, but on careful evaluation indicate neoplasia.

Coy cells are small and have very high N/C ratios (just a thin rim of delicate cytoplasm) and somewhat abnormal nuclei that are slightly hyperchromatic, with slightly coarse chromatin, and usually slightly irregular nuclear membranes. The nuclei look distinctly, but not markedly, different from the normal ones. (If the cells were clearly malignant looking, the diagnosis would be obvious and the lesion would not be well differentiated.) The number of these cells is variable, but increases with the grade and extent of the tumor. However, do not confuse them with benign small basaloid cells, which are expected to be present, especially in washing or brushing specimens. The primary difference is the abnormal nucleus, particularly the irregular nuclear membranes. If coy cells are present, suspect a neoplasm.

42
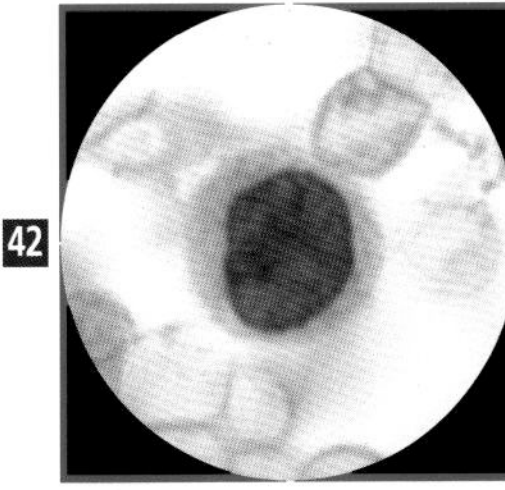

43
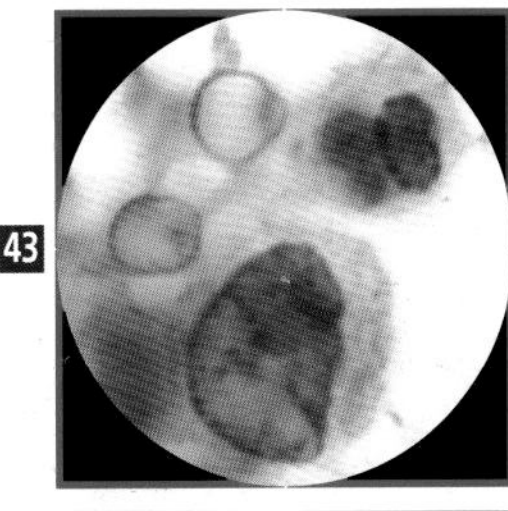

44
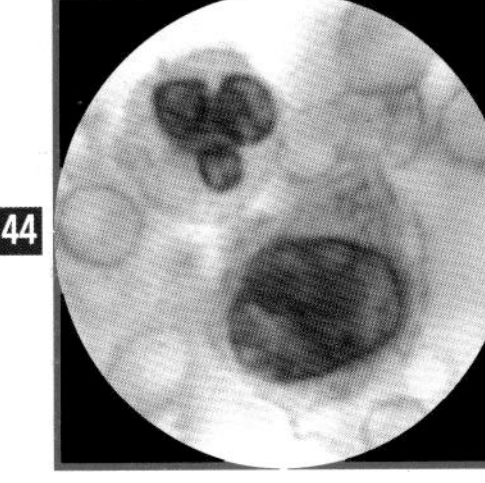

Preinvasive Lesions of the Transitional Epithelium

As with cervical carcinoma, invasive TCC is thought to be preceded by a long prodrome of hyperplasia, dysplasia, and carcinoma in situ. In theory, there should be ample opportunity to detect these preinvasive lesions. Unfortunately, in contrast with the success achieved by the Pap smear, screening of asymptomatic, low-risk patients has been largely unsuccessful [Lewis 1976]. It is not cost effective; the test may generate more false-positive than true-positive diagnoses [Gamarra 1984, A Morrison 1979]. However, screening may be useful for certain high-risk groups (eg, those with schistosomiasis or industrial exposure to aromatic amines [El-Bolkainy 1974, Gamarra 1984]).

Hyperplasia

Hyperplasia is an increase in the cell thickness of the urothelium that may show some loss of differentiation (increase in the number of basal type cells), but not atypical nuclei. This lesion cannot be detected by exfoliative cytology. Hyperplasia can precede carcinoma, but can also be associated with benign conditions such as chronic inflammation.

Dysplasia and Carcinoma In Situ

When noninvasive, this group of lesions could be referred to as low- or high-grade transitional or intraurothelial lesions [T10.4], in analogy to squamous intraepithelial lesions of the uterine cervix.

Dysplasia (Low-Grade Transitional Intraepithelial Lesion): Urothelial dysplasia is a relatively new, and somewhat controversial, area of pathology, but diagnostic criteria, both histologic and cytologic, are being defined [Murphy 1982b]. Dysplasia (or atypical hyperplasia) shows some nuclear abnormality (mild to moderate), increased mitoses, and evidence of dedifferentiation [Murphy 1981b,1982a,b]. Dysplasia is intermediate between hyperplasia and carcinoma in situ, and is often associated with carcinoma in situ. (Severe dysplasia is considered part of carcinoma in situ or high-grade transitional intraepithelial lesion.) The clinical value of grading transitional cell dysplasias has not been determined. In contrast with the uterine cervix, the worst cells determine if the lesion is dysplasia or carcinoma in situ, regardless of their histologic location in the tissue: ie, the cellular features are more important than the histologic pattern in determining biologic behavior.

The cells of dysplasia are similar to those seen in papillomas and low-grade TCC [45 I10.48] [Murphy 1982a]. Dysplastic cells may form loose clusters of up to about a dozen or so cells. The nuclei are enlarged and the N/C ratio is slightly increased. The nuclear membrane is slightly irregular, but the chromatin is fine and evenly distributed. Nucleoli are small or invisible.

These cells cannot be reliably distinguished from well-differentiated papillary transitional cell neoplasms with cytologic examination alone, although in dysplasia the cells tend to be fewer and smaller and form smaller aggregates [Murphy 1982a]. Although dysplasia may be detected cytologically, the definitive diagnosis requires correlation with cystoscopic findings (ie, absence of papillae) as well as confirmation on biopsy [Murphy 1982a]. Dysplastic cells do not have the high degree of nuclear pleomorphism, coarse chromatin, large nucleoli, or abnormal mitoses seen in carcinoma in situ. Therefore, urine cytology could be helpful in distinguishing dysplasia from carcinoma in situ.

Although dysplasia of the urinary tract has not been studied as thoroughly as dysplasia of the uterine cervix, urothelial dysplasia is a risk factor for subsequent development of transitional cell tumors [Murphy 1981b, Wolf 1983]. Patients should be carefully, but not aggressively, followed up [Murphy 1982a]. No treatment is indicated solely for (mild to moderate) dysplasia [Murphy 1982b].

Carcinoma In Situ (High-Grade Transitional Intraepithelial Lesion): Although most papillary carcinomas are noninfiltrating and in that sense in situ, carcinoma in situ is, by definition, a nonpapillary or flat lesion composed of anaplastic cells. The abnormal epithelium is highly atypical and composed of clearly malignant appearing (mainly grade III, some grade II) cells closely resembling those seen in invasive TCC [46 I10.49] [Friedell 1986]. In practice, it is difficult to draw a sharp distinction between severe dysplasia and carcinoma in situ. Therefore, severe dysplasia and carcinoma in situ can be combined into one category for purposes of clinicopathological correlations [Friedell 1986]. In sharp contrast with carcinoma in situ of the uterine cervix, carcinoma in situ of the urothelium does not require a full thickness of anaplastic cells, but rather is diagnosed by the cytologically worst appearing cells present. Invasive cancer can develop without progressing through a recognizable full thickness stage [Murphy 1981b].

T10.4 Differences Between Reactive Changes, Dysplasia, and Carcinoma In Situ (CIS)

Feature	Reactive Changes	Dysplasia*	CIS†
N/C Ratio	Normal or slightly increased	Mildly increased	Markedly increased
Nuclear membrane	Smooth	Slightly irregular	Irregular
Chromatin	Fine, even	Fine, even	Coarse, irregular
Nucleoli	Large	Small to none	Large
Cytoplasm	Vacuolated	Homogeneous	Homogeneous

* Low-grade transitional intraepithelial lesion.
† High-grade transitional intraepithelial lesion.

45
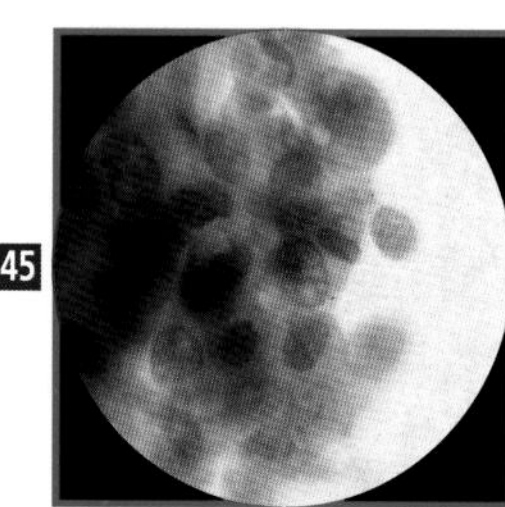

46
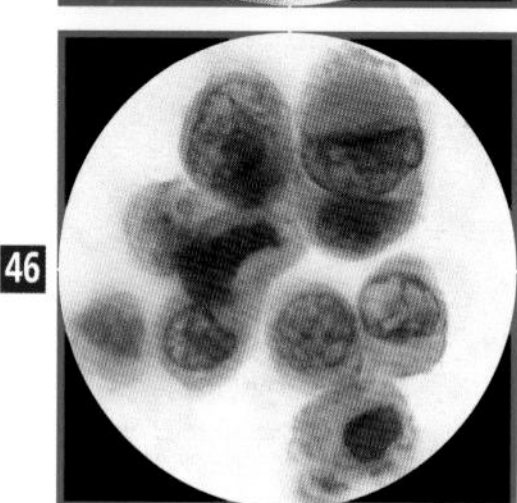

Papillary (noninvasive) TCC is not a particularly dangerous lesion. Although it tends to recur, it seldom becomes deeply invasive. Flat carcinoma in situ is the precursor lesion of deeply invasive cancers that can be lethal. Flat carcinoma in situ precedes invasive TCC by months or years. Like other urothelial neoplasms, carcinoma in situ tends to be multicentric. It is usually associated with previous or coexisting TCC and is rarely diagnosed by itself. More than 50% of cases of carcinoma in situ will eventually become invasive [Utz 1980a, Weinstein 1980]. Spontaneous regression of carcinoma in situ is very rare.

Carcinoma in situ occurs predominantly in men [Farrow 1977]. Many patients are symptomatic, but symptoms are usually mild and nonspecific [Koss 1988, Utz 1980b]. Clinically most patients present with hematuria (usually microscopic) or irritative symptoms suggestive of cystitis (frequency, urgency, dysuria). It is thought that the symptoms of carcinoma in situ relate to denudation of the epithelium, resulting in reactive inflammation (and possibly negative biopsy findings) [Boon 1986]. The severity of the symptoms is proportional to the extent of disease, but by the time symptoms occur, the disease is likely to be extensive, and may be invasive. Thus, the presence of symptoms is a poor prognostic sign.

Carcinoma in situ is generally first detected cytologically [Rife 1979]. Cystoscopically, the lesion may not be visible or may only appear red, as in cystitis. Urine cytologic examination is the single most reliable test for the diagnosis and follow up of carcinoma in situ of the bladder [Murphy 1983]. The great majority (80%–100%) of cases of carcinoma in situ can readily be recognized as malignant [Farrow 1979, Koss 1985, O'Donoghue 1991], but it cannot be reliably determined whether the disease is in situ or invasive [Shenoy 1985]. Carcinoma in situ is often multifocal and the lesions cannot be localized cytologically.

In essence, the diagnosis consists of finding many cells with marked atypia (cytologically akin to high-grade TCC) [47 I10.49]. The cells are usually easy to find, because the cells exfoliate readily due to decreased intercellular adherence, and even small lesions shed many diagnostic cells [Foot 1949, Melamed 1960]. The cells appear singly or in small clusters, but usually not in thick aggregates, in contrast with benign reactive cells [Rosa 1985, Shenoy 1985]. The cells are about the size of normal transitional cells, or slightly larger, and monomorphic [Vousta 1963]. The nuclei are somewhat enlarged and vary from rounded to angular to irregular in shape, and may be multiple [Highman 1988]. They are always hyperchromatic, with coarse chromatin. There is usually a moderate amount of delicate cytoplasm that appears normal or slightly hazy. The background is clean: few WBCs, RBCs, etc. That is, in most cases there is no diathesis [Rosa 1985].

Unfortunately, it cannot be reliably determined, by cytologic methods alone, whether a tumor is infiltrating or in situ [Murphy 1985]. Moreover, in situ and invasive lesions commonly coexist. Although the cells of carcinoma in situ are clearly malignant appearing, there is a certain uniformity about them [Rosa 1985]. Superficial umbrella cells may or may not be present on the surface of the lesion. Larger, more pleomorphic cells, more cells with prominent nucleoli, and a diathesis favor invasive carcinoma, while small, more uniform cells, with fewer nucleoli, and a clean background favor in situ carcinoma [Highman 1988, Rosa 1985, Shenoy 1985]. Finding thick sheets or large, three-dimensional clusters of abnormal cells during follow-up of carcinoma in situ suggests invasion has occurred [Highman 1988].

There can be a long latent period between carcinoma in situ and the development of invasive cancer [T10.5] [Melamed 1960]. Urine cytology is useful in detecting urothelial cancer at an early, potentially curable stage [Melamed 1966]. However, a positive cytologic diagnosis may precede by months or even years a positive histologic diagnosis, resulting in an apparent false-positive (false false-positive) cytologic diagnosis. Therefore, characterizing a cytologic result as false positive is justified only if concomitant urothelial dysplasia/carcinoma in situ can be excluded [Harving 1989]. Also, denudation of the epithelium may be responsible for a false negative biopsy result [Boon 1986].

47

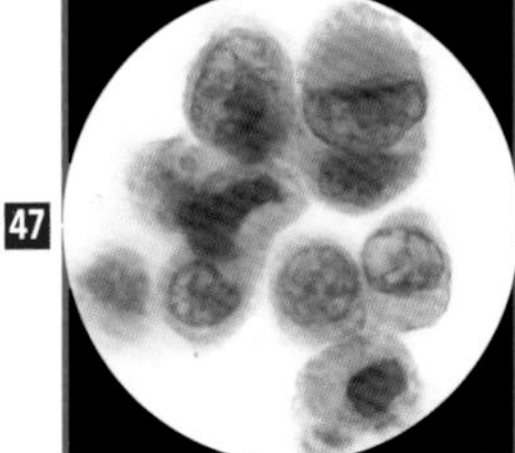

T10.5 **Diagnostic Features That Favor Carcinoma In Situ vs Invasive Transitional Cell Carcinoma (TCC)***

Feature	Carcinoma In Situ	Invasive TCC
Background	Clean	Diathesis
Cells	More uniform, smaller	More pleomorphic, larger
Nucleoli	Few	Often prominent or macronucleoli

* Cannot reliably differentiate with cytology alone.

T10.6 **Diagnostic Correlations Between Cytologic and Cystoscopic Examinations**

Cytology	Cystoscopy	Likely Diagnosis
(−)	(−)	No tumor
(−)	(+)	Well-differentiated papillary neoplasm
(+)	(−)	Carcinoma in situ* or upper tract tumor
(+)	(+)	High-grade, invasive TCC

* If cytologic findings are positive but cystoscopic findings are negative, close follow-up is indicated. Most patients will eventually develop TCC.

Other Procedures/Specimens

Cystoscopy

Cystoscopy and cytology are complementary studies [T10.6] [Farrow 1979, Ro 1992]. The low-grade papillary lesions that may be difficult to diagnose cytologically are usually easy to diagnose cystoscopically. The papillae are almost literally waving at the observer through the cystoscope; however, lesions in the dome of the bladder or upper urinary tract may not be visualized. Conversely, the high-grade flat carcinoma in situ or early invasive carcinoma, which is much more ominous, is easy to detect cytologically but may be missed cystoscopically even when extensive [Rife 1979] because it can be mistaken for hyperemia, cystitis, or even normal mucosa [Ro 1992, J Smith 1965, Wiggishoff 1972]. Thus cystoscopy may also fail for small, flat, or sessile lesions.

Failure to diagnose papilloma or low-grade papillary TCC cytologically is not a disaster because the lesions are not likely to kill the patient and can usually be found cystoscopically. The purpose of intensive endoscopic monitoring is to detect potentially lethal tumors as soon as possible; most grade II and essentially all grade III TCC can be detected cytologically.

Transabdominal ultrasonography has also been used to complement urine cytology in the detection of bladder tumors [Berlac 1992, Petersen 1989].

Ileal Conduit Urine

The ileal conduit urine specimen is usually very cellular. In the absence of cancer, most of the cells are intestinal lining cells, which exfoliate in far greater numbers than do transitional cells [Wolinska 1973]. The cells are characteristically degenerated and tend to round up, lose their columnar shape, and resemble macrophages. They may be seen singly or in sheets. The nuclei are usually degenerated and may appear hyperchromatic due to karyorrhexis and pyknosis. Many of the cells contain globular (often eosinophilic) cytoplasmic inclusions. In the background, debris, cytoplasmic fragments, granular deposits, bacteria, and crystals are found. A few RBCs and WBCs are expected, but if numerous they may indicate a problem (eg, infection).

Since urothelial cancer is usually multifocal, it is important to monitor the ileal conduit urine for recurrence of tumor in the ureter or renal pelvis [Banigo 1975]. Cancer cells in the ileal urine specimen have the same morphologic appearance as in other urine specimens, but a careful search may be necessary to find them [Wolinska 1973].

Cytologic atypia induced by chemotherapeutic agents can be a difficult diagnostic problem in this setting, particularly if radiation therapy has also been administered [Wolinska 1973]. Usually, the nuclear chromatin is poorly defined or smudgy or the cell abnormalities are so bizarre as to be unusual for cancer [Wolinska 1973]. Fresh specimens should be examined; urine from the collection bag is unsatisfactory for evaluation. Since mucus may clog filters, other preparatory techniques must be used.

Urethral Specimens

Patients who have had a cystectomy (without urethrectomy) for bladder cancer have a relatively high risk of recurrence in the residual urethra. About 20% of patients develop recurrent TCC, in situ or invasive, and still more may have atypia [Wolinska 1977]. Cytology is the most effective method available for screening the urethra for recurrent tumor [Freeman 1994]. In addition, urethral specimens from men can be used to detect various sexually transmitted diseases, such as *Chlamydia*, gonorrhea, herpes, *Trichomonas*, *Candida*, and condyloma [Fralick 1994, Giacomini 1989].

A specimen can be obtained by washing the urethra with saline or by direct swabbing with a saline-moistened cotton applicator. The normal cytologic appearance of the urethra includes not only transitional cells but also squamous cells and columnar cells (both glandular and transitional). Leukocytes are normally absent [Giacomini 1989].

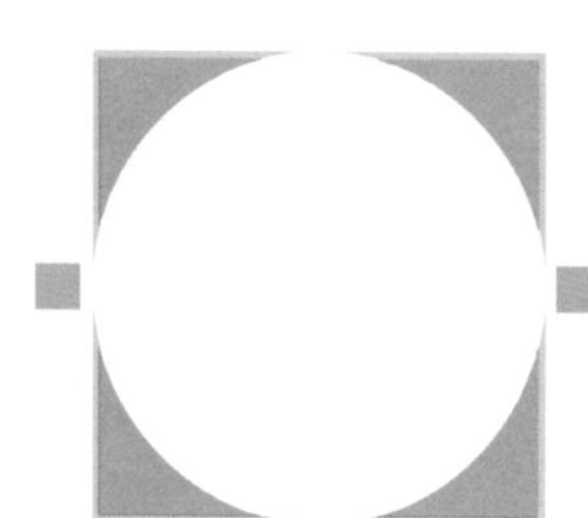

Carcinoma of the Upper Urinary Tract (Renal Pelvis and Ureter)

About 5% to 10% of urothelial tumors occur in the upper urinary tract (renal pelvis and ureter). Most of the tumors are papillary transitional cell neoplasms. Clinically, the patients are similar to those with bladder cancer in terms of age, sex, risk factors, etc [Blute 1989]. The diagnosis of cancer often entails major surgery. However, conservative therapy is not only possible in low-grade, low-stage disease, but may be required (eg, in patients with only one kidney). Thus, accurate cytodiagnosis is critical. Unfortunately, ureteral or renal pelvis specimens are among the most difficult types of urinary tract specimens to interpret [Frable 1977].

Voided Urine Specimens

In a voided urine specimen (as well as urine specimens collected by ureteral catheterization), high-grade cancer can be detected, but low-grade tumors of the upper urinary tract are difficult to detect [Erikksson 1976]. Tumors of the upper urinary tract are more likely to shed diagnostic cells only intermittently, and the cells may be markedly degenerated [Highman 1986]. False negatives may be expected in voided urine specimens from patients who have nonfunctioning kidneys or obstructed ureters [Cullen 1972]. Thus, false-negative findings in upper urinary tract tumors are common in voided urine specimens [Bibbo 1974, Cullen 1972, Grace 1967, Hawtrey 1971, Sarnacki 1971, Say 1974, Seldenrijk 1987, Zincke 1976]. The cytologic criteria for diagnosis of upper urinary tract lesions are similar to those used for bladder tumors [Cullen 1972, Naib 1961]. The location of the lesion usually cannot be determined in voided urine specimens, and many patients with upper urinary tract tumors also have disease in the bladder [Grabstald 1971, Schmidlapp 1950].

Retrograde Catheterization with Brush or Lavage

Endoscopic localization and diagnosis of upper urinary tract tumors is possible using a ureteropyeloscope [Abdel-Razzak 1994, Blute 1989]. Using retrograde catheterization with brushing or lavage (which can sample a wider area including inaccessible sites such as calyces), cytologic specimens can be directly obtained. Many tumors, particularly when high grade, can be accurately diagnosed, but low-grade tumors of the upper urinary tract are difficult to diagnose [Bibbo 1974, Gill 1973,1978, Leistenschneider 1980, Seldenrijk 1987, Zincke 1976]. The tumor grade is the most important prognostic factor. There is a significant risk of ipsilateral recurrence, depending on grade, but only about 2% recur on the contralateral side [Wallace 1981].

Specimens directly obtained from the upper urinary tract are cytologically similar to those obtained from the bladder, but with some important differences [Kannan 1990]. Transitional cells from the upper urinary tract are larger and more variable than those from the bladder [Prall 1972]. They can be polyploid and may have atypical nuclei (multiple, enlarged, hyperchromatic, sometimes with prominent nucleoli). The cells often appear in tight papillary clusters due to instrumentation. Lithiasis can also cause exfoliation of papillary clusters made up of atypical cells [Kannan 1990]. These features could be mistaken for malignancy, resulting in false-positive diagnoses [Murphy 1977,1983]. Filling defects on intravenous pyelogram may suggest malignancy, but can also be caused by benign disease such as stones.

The cytologic diagnosis of low-grade transitional cell neoplasms of the upper urinary tract is particularly difficult—or even impossible—and correlation with clinical, radiologic, endoscopic, and biopsy findings is necessary. As usual, the cytologic diagnosis of high-grade urothelial malignancy is more reliable. When evaluating specimens from the upper urinary tract, diagnostic conservation is warranted because the cells are usually more atypical in appearance than cells from the lower urinary tract. Look for clear-cut malignant changes (high N/C ratio, nuclear hyperchromasia with coarse chromatin, nuclear membrane irregularity, macronucleoli, and diathesis) to diagnose malignancy. The higher the grade, the greater are the number of cells, the number of single cells, and the degree of atypia. A specimen containing only small, bland, uniform cells is not expected in the upper urinary tract; therefore, paradoxically, this finding is suggestive of a low-grade neoplasm. The differential diagnosis, as usual, includes reactive and degenerative changes due to stones, inflammation, etc, and effects of antineoplastic therapy.

Other Lesions of the Urinary Tract

Leukoplakia

Leukoplakia is a clinical term meaning white plaque. Pathologically, leukoplakia usually corresponds to chronic inflammation, with marked squamous metaplasia and hyperkeratosis in the bladder (chronic cystitis). Leukoplakia is usually associated with one of the following: prolonged mucosal irritation (eg, stones, schistosomiasis), excess estrogens (eg, prostate cancer therapy), bladder obstruction, vitamin A deficiency, diverticuli, condyloma, or squamous cell carcinoma.

The diagnostic cells of hyperkeratosis are anucleate squames. Since these cannot be reliably differentiated from squames originating in the skin of the perineum, the diagnosis requires a catheterized specimen to be valid. The mere presence of nucleated squamous cells, particularly in a urine specimen from a woman, has little importance. Leukoplakia must be differentiated from keratinizing squamous cell carcinoma of the bladder, which may be extremely well differentiated.

Condyloma

Condylomas of the bladder are often associated with genital condylomas. Bladder condylomas may occur with increased frequency in immunocompromised patients [Del Mistro 1988, Pettersson 1976]. Human papilloma virus, particularly types 6 and 11, may be demonstrated. The virus may produce a papillary lesion (squamous papilloma). Bladder condylomas may be difficult to eradicate [Del Mistro 1988].

Scattered poorly preserved koilocytes may be seen [48 I10.50]. Highly atypical, heavily keratinized cells mimicking squamous cell carcinoma may be exfoliated in some cases [Del Mistro 1988]. In addition, some patients may actually develop squamous cell carcinoma in which HPV antigens can be demonstrated [Roussel 1991]. Rule out genital contamination.

Squamous Cell Carcinoma

Squamous differentiation is relatively frequently a component of TCC. Its presence in TCC usually implies a high-grade cancer. However, when a cancer is predominantly or completely squamous, it can then be designated squamous cell carcinoma [I10.54]. Squamous cell carcinoma accounts for no more than 5% of bladder cancers in the United States [Young 1991a]. However, squamous cell carcinoma is more common than TCC in Egypt, where squamous cell carcinoma is associated with schistosomiasis (usually *S haematobium*). In contrast with TCC, women are as commonly affected as men. Squamous cell carcinoma of the bladder has a poor prognosis even when well differentiated.

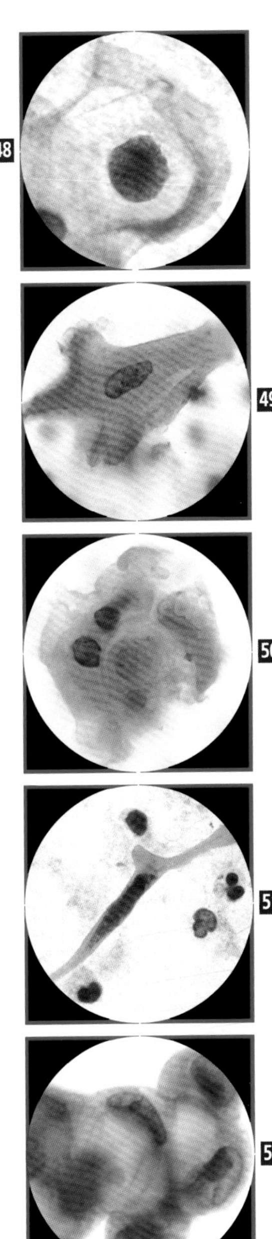

Squamous cell carcinoma usually arises in the anterior bladder wall. It is usually accompanied by squamous metaplasia (see also "leukoplakia"). Most of the tumors are fairly well differentiated, especially when associated with schistosomiasis. Very well-differentiated tumors may be difficult to diagnose cytologically.

Anucleate squames may be the only cytologic finding in some cases of squamous cell carcinoma. Finding clumps of squames, particularly if they have abnormal shapes, is suggestive of the diagnosis. Spindle or bizarre shaped cells may be seen. Single cells are more common than aggregates, particularly in well-differentiated tumors. Very well-differentiated squamous cell carcinomas may show only subtle nuclear abnormalities, suggesting low-grade squamous dysplasia rather than cancer. However, the nuclei of squamous cell carcinoma may be more pleomorphic than those usually seen in TCC. The nuclei are hyperchromatic and often degenerated [49 I10.51, 50 I10.52, 51 I10.53]. The chromatin is abnormal, and clumping and clearing is common. Prominent nucleoli may be seen in well-preserved nuclei. The cytoplasm is denser and more abundant than in TCC, and the N/C ratio is lower. The cytoplasm more commonly stains red to orange than in TCC, although it may also stain blue to green. An ectoplasmic rim may be observed. Intercellular bridges, keratin pearls, or keratohyalin granules indicate squamous differentiation. A dirty background, or tumor diathesis, is common and often correlates with deep invasion.

The differential diagnosis includes leukoplakia, secondary squamous cell carcinoma (especially from the cervix, where it could be found either as a contaminant in a voided urine specimen or as an indication of invasion of the bladder), and TCC with squamous differentiation (which is also more common than pure, primary squamous cell carcinoma of the urinary tract). Nonkeratinizing squamous cell carcinoma is cytologically similar to high-grade TCC.

Adenocarcinoma

Primary adenocarcinoma accounts for only 0.5% to 2% of bladder cancers [Young 1991a] and can also arise rarely in the upper urinary tract [Kobayashi 1985]. Mixed TCC with a component of glandular differentiation is more common. Adenocarcinoma is morphologically similar to high-grade TCC or nonkeratinizing squamous cell carcinoma. There are two basic types of primary bladder adenocarcinoma—the colonic type, the more common type, and the signet ring type, which is rare.

The cytology of adenocarcinoma is reminiscent of colorectal adenocarcinoma. Clusters of tumors cells, characterized by nuclear crowding and pleomorphism, are present [52 I10.47].

Abnormal chromatin and prominent nucleoli are characteristically seen. The cytoplasm is vacuolated and mucin may be demonstrated by special stains. However, the mere presence of mucin does not prove a malignant diagnosis, since benign mucin-positive cells can be seen in cystitis glandularis [Kobayashi 1985]. The differential diagnosis includes TCC with glandular differentiation, renal cell carcinoma, and metastatic carcinoma.

Signet Ring Cell Carcinoma: From 2% to 15% of adenocarcinomas of the bladder are signet ring cell type; about 20% to 25% of those are of urachal origin. Signet ring cell carcinoma may be pure or part of ordinary gland forming adenocarcinoma, or in some cases, TCC. However, the diagnosis of signet ring cell carcinoma should be reserved for pure, or almost pure tumors of this type [Grignon 1991, Young 1991a].

The diagnostic signet ring cells may be found in pools of mucus [53 I10.55] [DeMay 1985]. The differential diagnosis may include signet ring cell lymphoma, arising in the bladder [Siegel 1991]. Mucin positivity excludes lymphoma.

Small Cell Carcinoma

Small cell carcinoma of the urinary tract is an uncommon tumor, but is essentially similar to small cell carcinoma of the lung [54 I10.56] [Grignon 1992, Young 1991a]. The urine specimen may contain numerous small malignant cells singly or in clusters, which exhibit nuclear molding. The cells are small with high N/C ratios, hyperchromatic nuclei, and coarse chromatin [Rollins 1991]. Features of neuroendocrine differentiation may be demonstrable [Grignon 1992]. Combined small cell carcinoma with squamous cell carcinoma or adenocarcinoma also occurs, as in the pulmonary counterpart [Grignon 1992, Hom 1990]. The differential diagnosis includes high-grade TCC composed of small cells.

Lymphoma

Primary lymphoma of the urinary tract is rare [Siegelbaum 1986], but can potentially be diagnosed with urinary cytology [Cheson 1984a,b, Mincione 1982, Sano 1965, Yam 1985]. Secondary involvement is more common and can also be detected with urinary cytology [Andrion 1993, Sufrin 1977, Weimar 1981]. Leukemic cells can also occasionally be found in the urine [Kepner 1982]. The cells can be either small or large, but in either case are usually smaller than epithelial malignancies [55 I10.57]. The cells have a relatively high N/C ratio, coarse to vesicular chromatin, and may have prominent nucleoli. The most characteristic feature is the absence of true tissue aggregates. The differential diagnosis includes severe chronic inflammation, follicular cystitis, and benign lymphoid proliferations, such as Rosai Dorfman disease [Rangwala 1990]. Rarely, Hodgkin's disease involves the urinary tract usually late in the course of the disease and can potentially be diagnosed with urine cytology by the presence of Reed-Sternberg cells or variants [Bocian 1982].

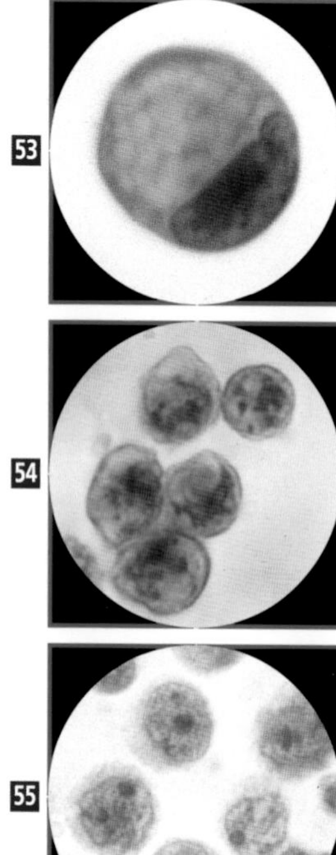

Plasmacytoma/Myeloma

Myeloma cells can be found in the urine [Neal 1985, Pringle 1974, Yang 1982], but only rarely [Geisinger 1986]. The neoplastic plasma cells may be mature or immature. They have eccentric nuclei and may show characteristic peripheral chromatin clumping ("clock face") when well differentiated. A perinuclear hof as well as an increase in binucleated cells is a further clue to plasmacytic differentiation. In contrast with plasmacytoid lymphoma, no lymphocytes are present in myeloma [Yang 1982].

More common than direct infiltration by malignant cells is renal tubular damage due to immunoglobulin deposition, or myeloma kidney, which is characterized by waxy/granular myeloma casts surrounded by reactive syncytial giant cells passed in the urine [Cheson 1985]. The differential diagnosis includes TCC with plasmacytoid cells [Sahin 1991].

Nephrogenic Adenoma

Nephrogenic adenoma of the lower urinary tract is an uncommon lesion of uncertain etiology. It appears to be a metaplastic reaction of the bladder mucosa, rather than a true neoplasm; it may, however, recur. Nephrogenic adenoma is apparently related to chronic irritation, trauma [Stilmant 1986, Troster 1986], including surgery, radiation and chemotherapy, and BCG therapy.

The typical cytologic features consist of numerous vacuolated polygonal to columnar shaped cells, singly or in loose groups [Rutgers 1988]. The nuclei are uniform, but may appear active. Cytoplasmic vacuolization, including signet ring cells, mimics that seen in adenocarcinoma [Rutgers 1988, Stilmant 1986]. Occasional glandular structures may also occur [Rutgers 1988]. Papillary fragments with peripheral palisades and community cell borders resemble papillary TCC [Troster 1986].

Secondary Tumors of the Urinary Tract

Renal Cell Carcinoma

Renal cell adenocarcinoma can be diagnosed with urine cytology [Bunge 1950a,b, Foot 1958, Harrison 1951, Papanicolaou 1947, Park 1969]. Unfortunately, the tumor cells are not shed until late in the course of the disease or the cells that are shed are nondiagnostic. Therefore, urinary cytology is of little practical value in the diagnostic evaluation of renal masses and in the detection of early stage disease [Evans 1961, Feeney 1958, Lieberman 1963, McDonald 1954, Piscioli 1983,1985b, Schmidlapp 1950, Umiker 1964]. Renal cell carcinoma can also metastasize to the bladder, and thus could be detected in the urine.

The diagnostic cells are often very degenerated, usually appear singly or in small groups, and vary from sparse to abundant. The cells typically have large, eccentric, round to oval, hyperchromatic nuclei with prominent nucleoli [Meisels 1963]. Degenerated nuclei may be pyknotic, in which case the nucleoli will be less conspicuous. When well differentiated, the cells have small, regular, bland nuclei and can be confused with normal tubular cells or other benign cells [McDonald 1954]. Clear (ie, finely vacuolated), granular, or spindle-shaped cells may be observed [Piscioli 1985b], but even clear cells appear more dense and granular than expected due to degeneration [Foot 1958].

The malignant cells may contain neutral lipid (oil red O– or Sudan IV–positive) [Daut 1947, Hajdu 1971]. Fresh, unfixed urine must be examined, since alcohol dissolves lipid [Hajdu 1971]. Lipid staining cannot be relied upon to confirm the diagnosis. Positive cells may be sparse or absent in renal cell carcinoma, while other benign and malignant cells, particularly when degenerated, including metastatic carcinomas, as well as those associated with stones, transplant rejection, and bladder outlet obstruction, can also contain lipid [Milsten 1973].

The differential diagnosis also includes benign urothelium, especially from a retrograde catheterization, and benign nephrogenic adenoma with vacuolated cytoplasm [Stilmant 1986] as well as other rare clear cell carcinomas, eg, mesonephric carcinoma of the bladder [Hausdorfer 1985] or clear cell carcinoma of the female urethra [Peven 1985]. Collecting duct carcinoma (characterized by large cells with granular cytoplasm and prominent nucleoli) has also been detected in the urine [Mauri 1994].

Prostatic Adenocarcinoma

As is true of renal carcinoma, prostate carcinoma is seldom first diagnosed in a urine specimen [Nguyen-Ho 1994, Rupp 1990], although prostate carcinoma can be diagnosed after prostatic massage in some cases [Garret 1976, Sharifi 1983]. The diagnosis of prostatic carcinoma cannot reliably be made with urine cytology. Unfortunately, by the time diagnostic cells appear in the urine, the disease is usually late and advanced.

Small round to oval glandular cells in groups or acini with large round nuclei, increased N/C ratio, and irregular nuclear membranes, as well as moderate amounts of cytoplasm may be seen [56 I10.58] [Varma 1988]. Hyperchromasia and chromatin clumping are variable. The most prominent cytologic feature is the presence of large and occasionally multiple or irregular nucleoli [Rupp 1990]. Poorly differentiated and anaplastic prostatic cancers are more likely to exfoliate and are more obviously malignant [Nguyen-Ho 1994]. However, such high-grade cells may be difficult to distinguish from poorly differentiated TCC.

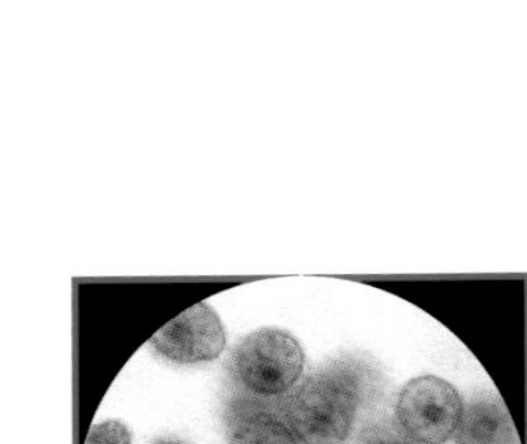

56

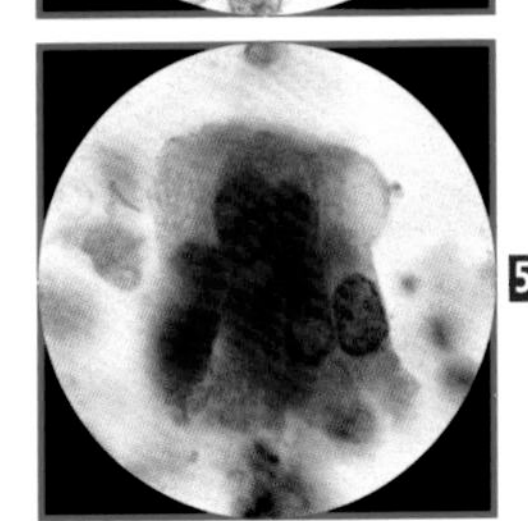

57

Melanoma

Primary melanoma of the urinary tract is rare [Gupta 1965]; secondary involvement is more common [Walsh 1966].

Melanoma cells tend to be found singly in the urine [Woodard 1978]. They have eccentric, large, vesicular nuclei with macronucleoli, and occasionally intranuclear cytoplasmic invaginations. Pigment may be observed, which must be distinguished from hemosiderin or lipofuchsin (either of which may be observed in renal tubular cells) [Piva 1964]. Melanuria, without the presence of malignant cells, may also occur in cases of melanoma as well as melanosis [Valente 1985].

Wilms' Tumor

Hematuria is one of the most common presenting complaints in patients with Wilms' tumor, which is the most common renal malignancy in children. The cells may be found singly or in clusters. The cells are oval or spindle shaped. The nuclei have slightly irregular membranes, uniform granular chromatin, and nucleoli that may be prominent. The cytoplasm is scant or absent. The differential diagnosis includes other "small blue cell tumors" of childhood.

Other Metastases

Tumors of the female genital tract, colon/rectum [57 I10.59], and prostate may involve the bladder by direct extension. Testicular tumors have also been diagnosed in the urine [Rojewska 1989, Viddeleer 1992]. The tumors are usually high grade and may be difficult to distinguish from TCC. Distant metastases, especially from lung and breast cancer, can occasionally be seen in urine specimens.

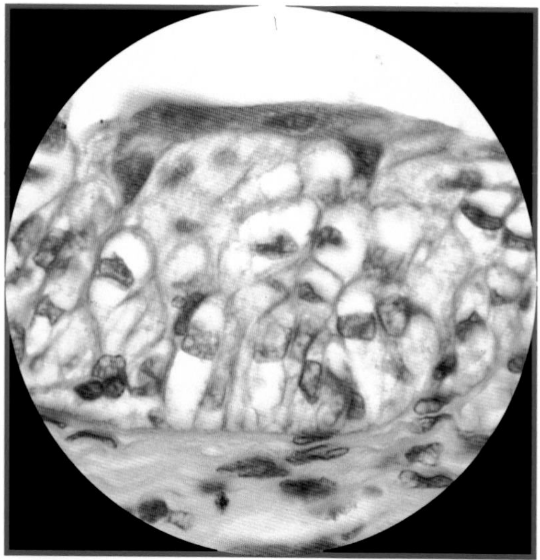

I10.1
Bladder (tissue). The mucosa is usually no more than six or seven cells thick. Note eosinophilic "umbrella" cells covering the surface.

I10.2
Crystals. A variety of crystals, including triple phosphate (illustrated), leucine, uric acid, and cystine, can be found in urine specimens.

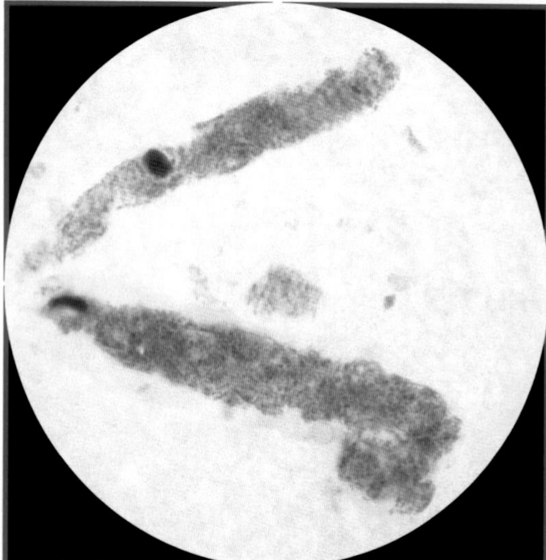

I10.3
Casts. Casts of renal tubules can be found in the urine; they may or may not indicate disease, depending on their type.

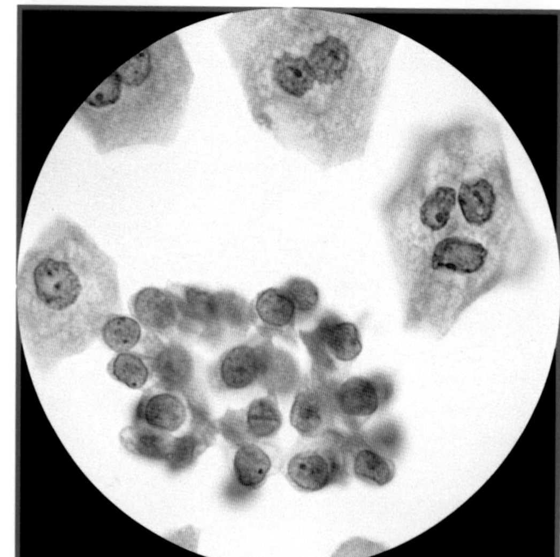

I10.4
Transitional cells. Pleomorphic, but benign, transitional cells are normal findings in bladder washing specimens (illustrated). Single, mononuclear, parabasal-sized transitional cells usually predominate in voided urine specimens. Basaloid transitional cells are seen near bottom of field.

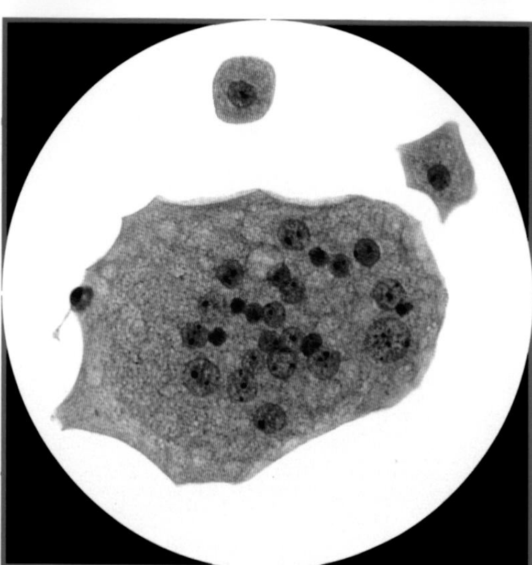

I10.5
Transitional cells. Superficial transitional cells are large and may have multiple nuclei. Note scalloping of the cytoplasm: the underlying cells fit into the concavities.

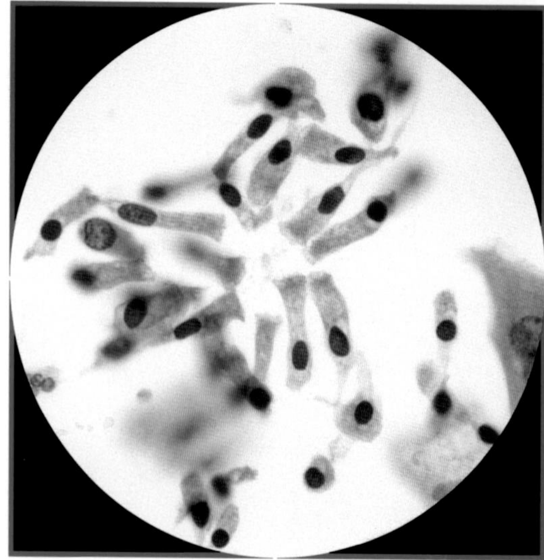

I10.6
Transitional cells. Columnar transitional cells are a normal and relatively common finding, particularly in bladder washing specimens. There are many other possible sources for columnar glandular cells in urine specimens.

I10.7
Squamous metaplasia. Recognized as fully mature squamous cells. To make the diagnosis in urine, the specimen must be obtained by catheter because the cells are indistinguishable from contaminants, eg, from the female genital tract. Compare the intermediate squamous with the transitional cells (polygonal vs scalloped outline, denser cytoplasm, larger nuclei). Squamous metaplasia can be normal, or related to hormones or chronic inflammation.

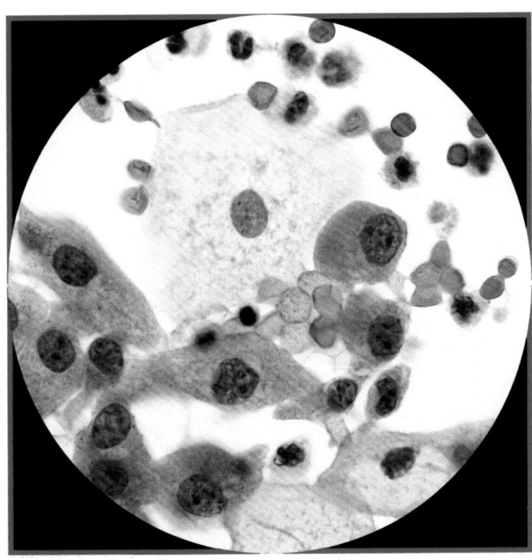

I10.8
Renal tubular cells. Uniform cells that are usually present in small sheets or casts, and vary in size and cytoplasmic granularity, depending on portion of renal tubule. Degenerative changes are common. They are not a normal component of urine; their presence implies renal parenchymal disease.

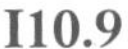

I10.9
Prostatic cells. Rarely exfoliate spontaneously, but are common after prostatic massage. They are present in small sheets of cuboidal cells; macronucleoli suggest malignancy.

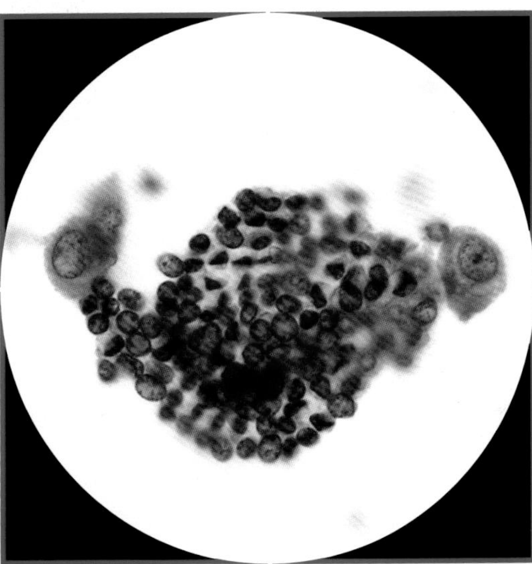

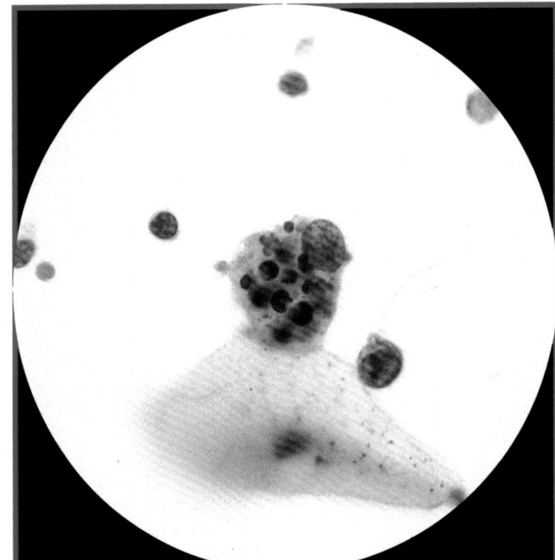

I10.10
Follicular cystitis. Normally, the urine is virtually free of inflammatory cells and RBCs. Follicular cystitis is analogous to follicular cervicitis: a range of maturation of the lymphocytes plus tingible body macrophages (illustrated) are seen.

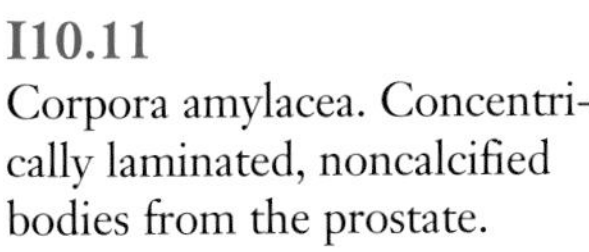

I10.11
Corpora amylacea. Concentrically laminated, noncalcified bodies from the prostate.

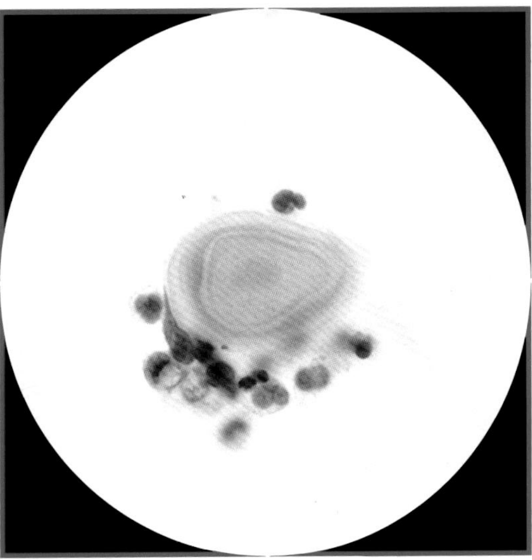

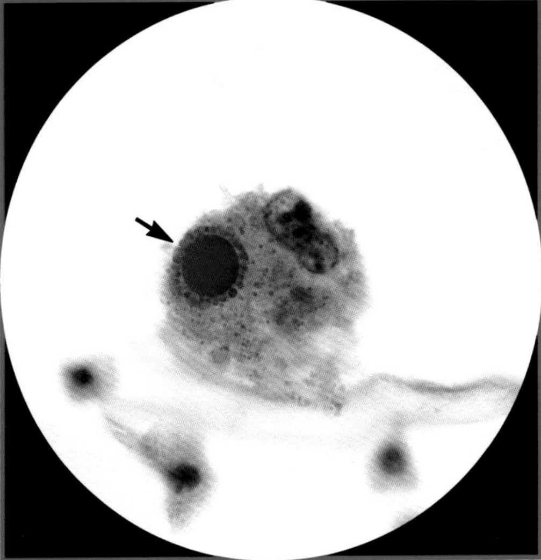

I10.12
Hyaline inclusion bodies. Also known as eosinophilic inclusion bodies, but do not necessarily stain red. They are apparently large lysosomes associated with cellular degeneration and are not virus, etc. Shown is one large inclusion surrounded by numerous smaller ones (arrow).

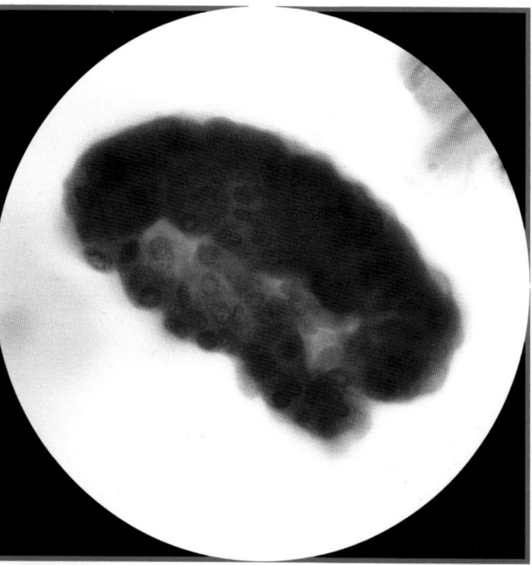

I10.13
Papillary clusters. Transitional epithelium denudes easily in response to even minor trauma. Papillary-like clusters in urine specimens obtained during or after instrumentation (or in patients with stones) have no special significance unless the cells appear abnormal. However, when papillary clusters are found in a voided urine specimen, and there is no history of trauma or instrumentation, a papillary neoplasm cannot be excluded.

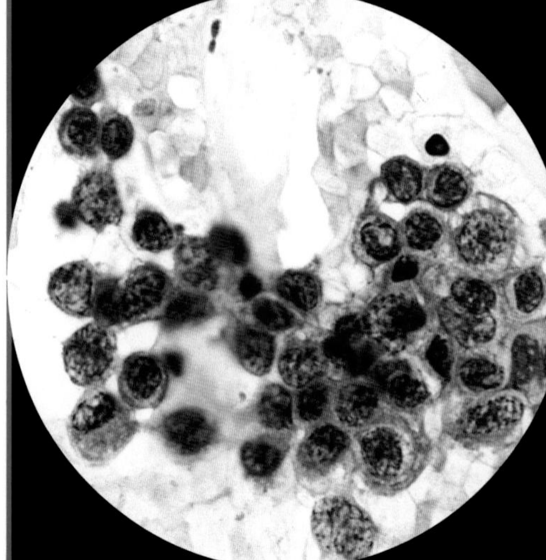

I10.14
Stone atypia. Urolithiasis can cause significant cytologic atypia sometimes comparable to high-grade malignancy, including nuclear enlargement and pleomorphism, high N/C ratios, coarse, hyperchromatic chromatin, and prominent nucleoli. Be cautious when diagnosing malignancy in patients with stones, particularly if the chromatin appears degenerated or smudgy.

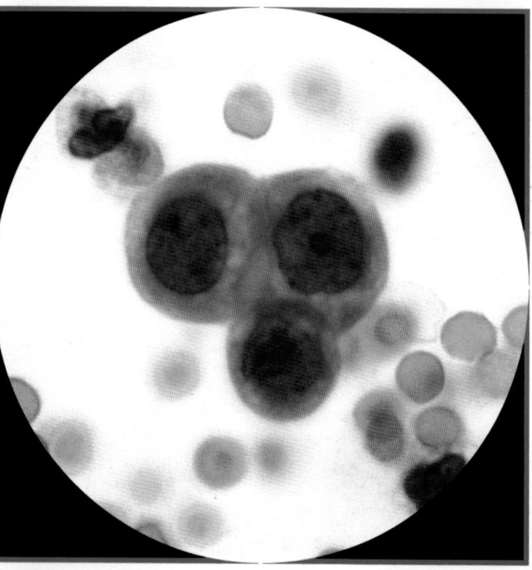

I10.15
Stone atypia. Note high N/C ratios, irregular nuclear membranes, dark chromatin, and prominent nucleoli, all features that could easily be mistaken for malignancy. Note cytoplasmic vacuolization, a feature seen in reactive cells and high-grade malignancy but usually not present in low-grade tumors.

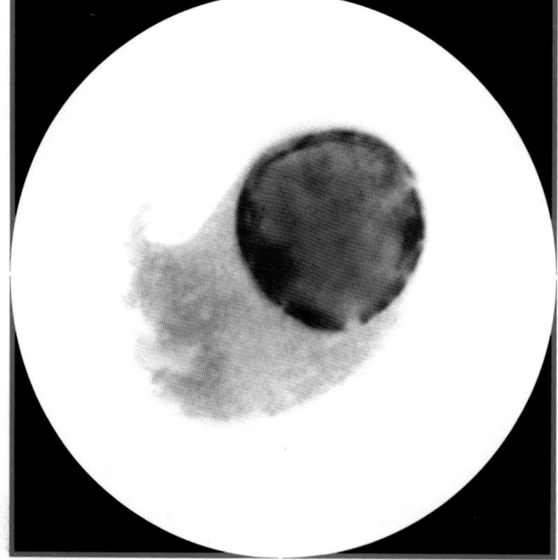

I10.16
Decoy cell. Human polyoma virus infection can result in atypical cells with enlarged, extremely hyperchromatic nuclei mimicking malignancy. (Oil)

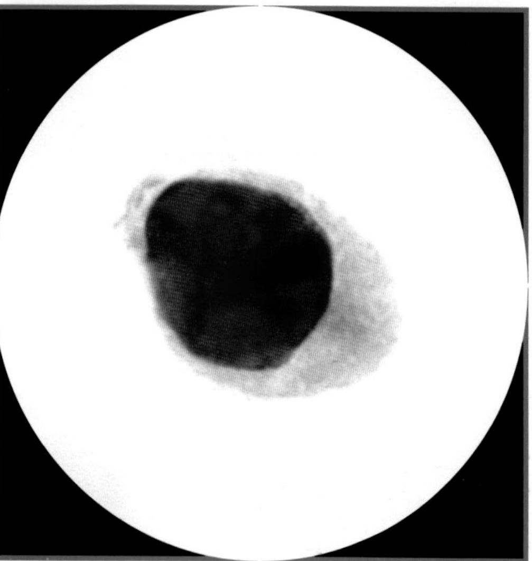

I10.17
Decoy cell. These cells, however, have smudgy chromatin or homogeneous nuclear inclusions with thick nuclear membranes.

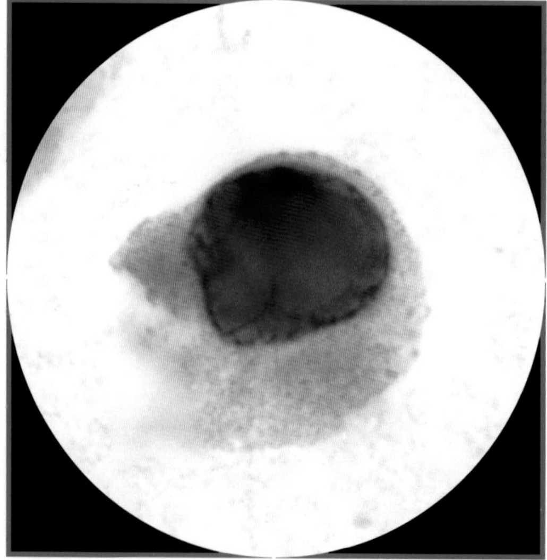

I10.18
In some cells, a washed out "viral" look may be seen. In other cells the nuclear material appears degenerated, coarse, and dark. (Oil)

I10.19
Transitional cell carcinoma. Compare the three decoy cells (I10.16-I10.18) with the real McCoy, the cancer cell with distinct, coarse chromatin. (Oil)

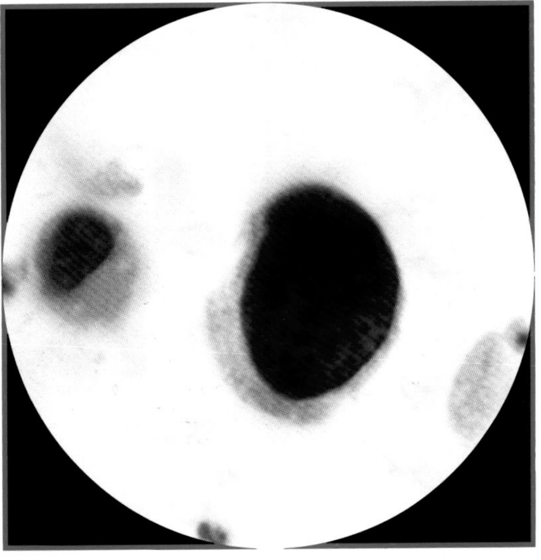

I10.20
Malacoplakia. Chronic granulomatous disease–associated incomplete intracellular digestion results in mineralization of bacteria and formation of characteristic round, laminated, basophilic intracytoplasmic inclusions about 5 to 10 μm in diameter known as Michaelis-Gutmann bodies. (arrow)

I10.21
Lead poisoning. Red, homogeneous, irregularly shaped intranuclear viral-like inclusions are seen. (Note: This patient had been shot and the bullet was not removed, a case of acute and chronic lead poisoning.)

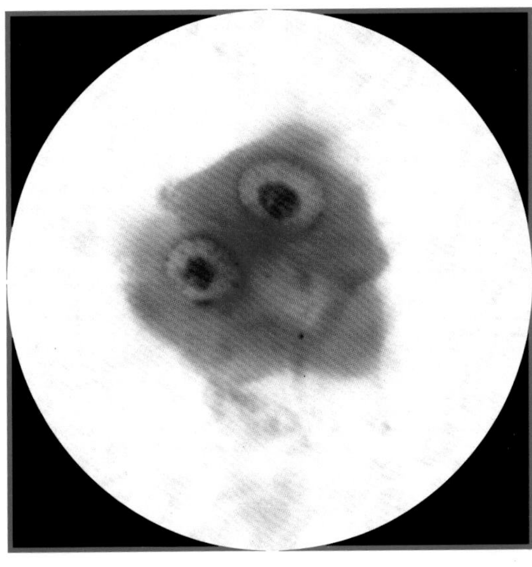

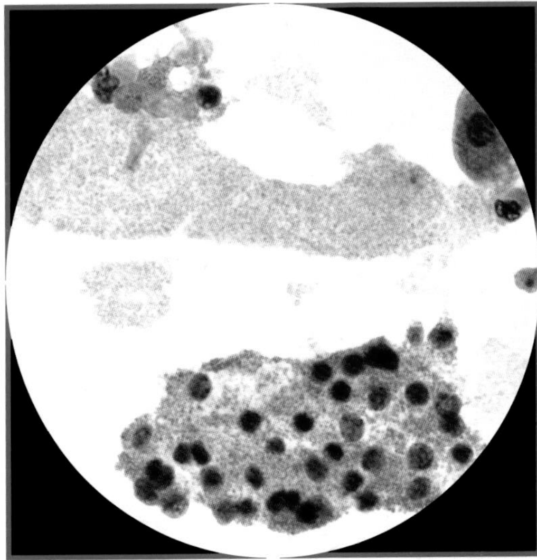

I10.22
Renal transplant rejection. Increase in number of renal tubular cells, lymphocytes (particularly reactive, plasmacytoid lymphocytes), casts, and RBCs over patient's baseline findings, accompanied by dirty background and macrophages.

I10.23
Chemotherapy. Agents such as cyclophosphamide and busulfan can cause cellular atypia mimicking malignancy.

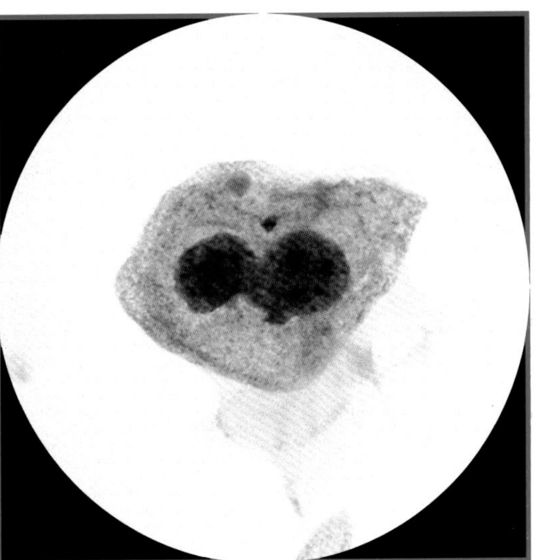

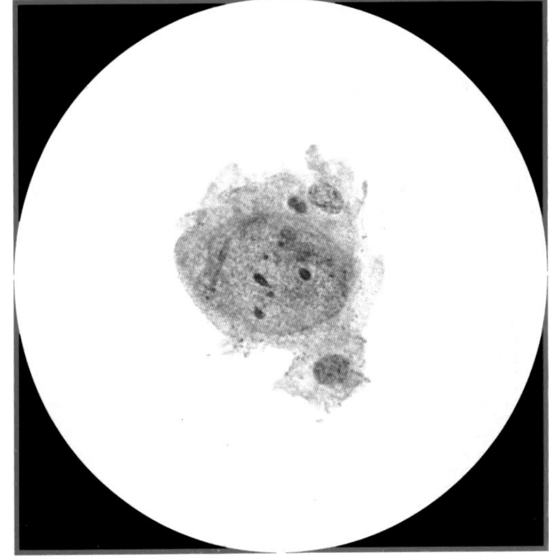

I10.24
Chemotherapy. Agents such as thiotepa and mitomycin C usually cause reactive-type cellular changes.

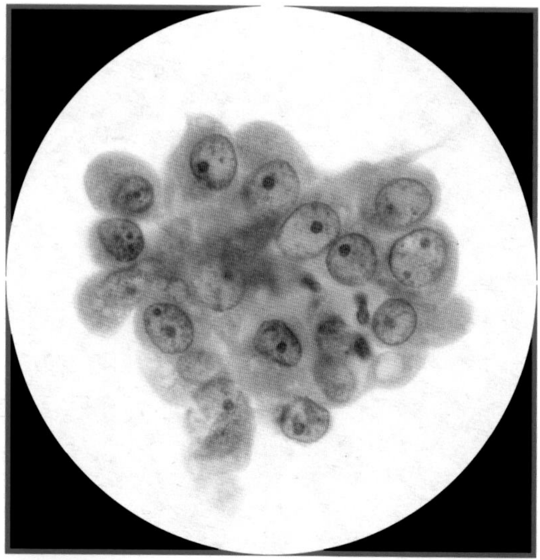

I10.25
Radiation. As in other body sites, the classic cytologic change is macrocytosis. However, radiation can also cause reactive or degenerative changes in the cells.

I10.26
BCG therapy. Histiocytic aggregates and giant cell histiocytes (arrow) associated with the granulomatous inflammation induced by this therapy are characteristic.

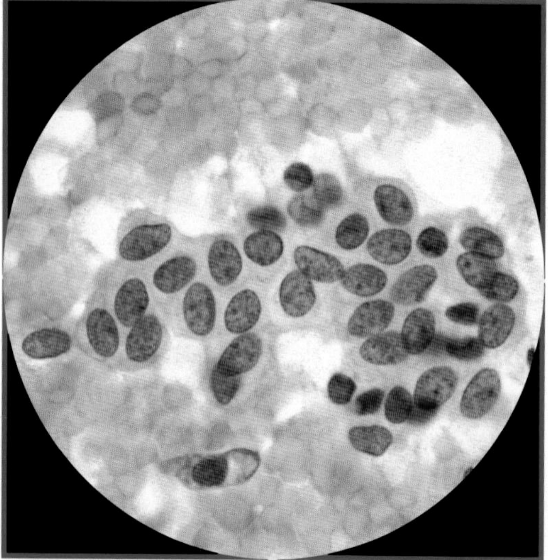

I10.27
Benign papilloma. Well-differentiated papillary neoplasm that may exfoliate cells essentially indistinguishable from normal, making cytologic diagnosis difficult or impossible.

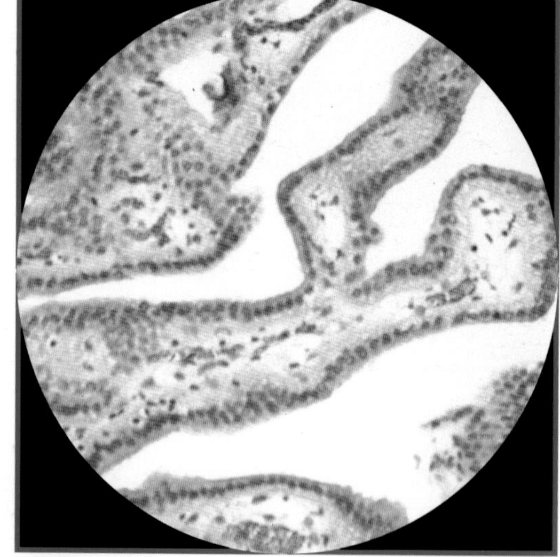

I10.28
Benign papilloma. Corresponding tissue; papillae lined by one or two layers of benign-appearing cells. Grade I transitional cell carcinomas (as defined by the WHO) with multiple layers of nearly normal-appearing cells also considered benign papillomas, in the revised classifications. Such lesions may exfoliate cells with features of a low-grade neoplasm.

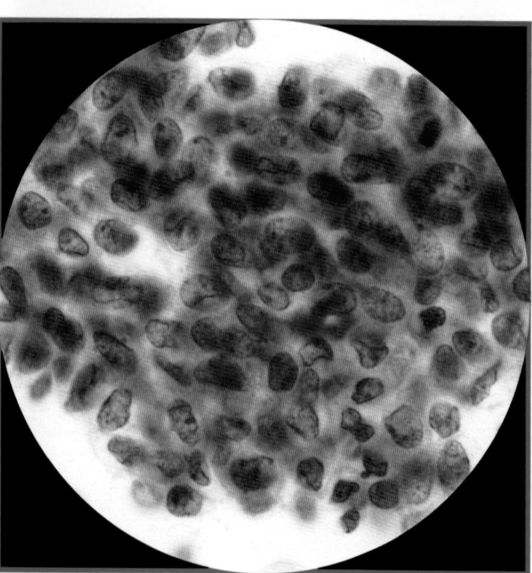

I10.29
Inverted papilloma. The cytologic findings in inverted papilloma are similar to exophytic papillomas or low-grade transitional cell carcinoma. Illustrated is cellular crowding and mild nuclear atypia. Note irregular nuclear membranes.

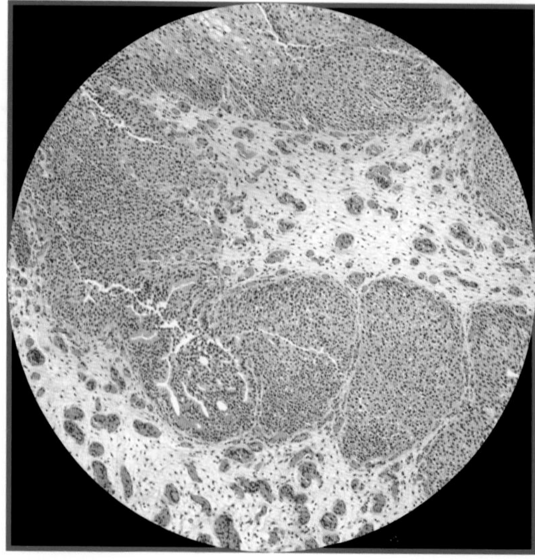

I10.30
Inverted papilloma. Surface is in left upper quadrant. Corresponding tissue.

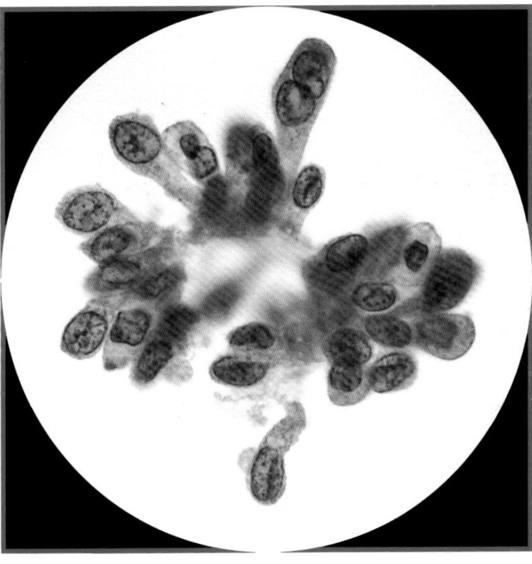

I10.31
Low-grade transitional cell carcinoma (TCC), revised classification. This is also known as papillary transitional cell carcinoma grade II (WHO). Note disorganized groups, variation in cell/nuclear size and shape, increased N/C ratio, irregular nuclear membranes, and granular chromatin.

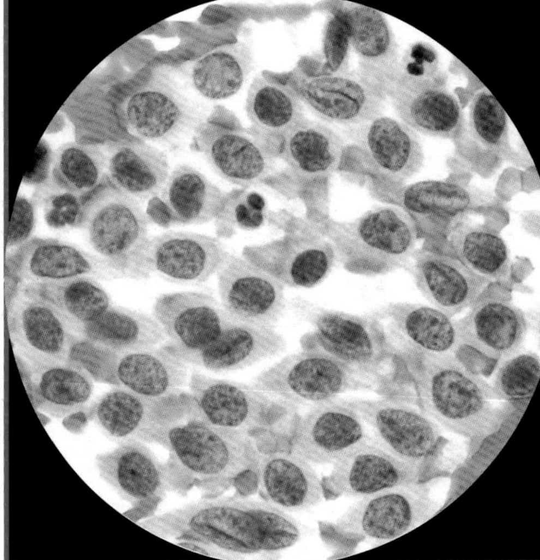

I10.32
Low-grade TCC, revised classification. Note irregular nuclear membranes, granular chromatin, and occasional micronucleolus.

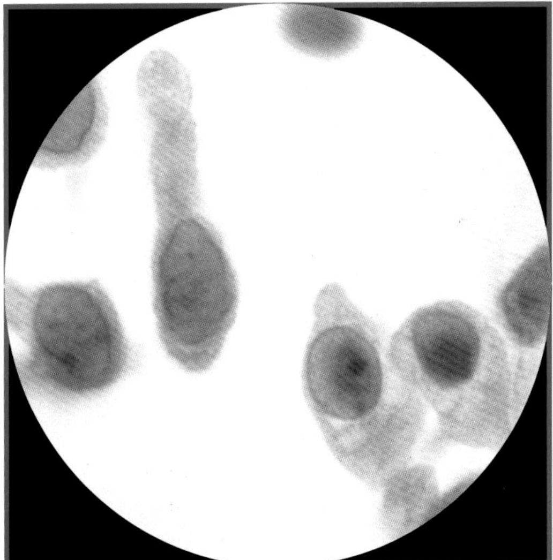

I10.33
Low-grade TCC, revised classification. Columnar, elongated, or spindle cells larger than normal deep transitional cells can be seen in well-differentiated tumors. (Oil)

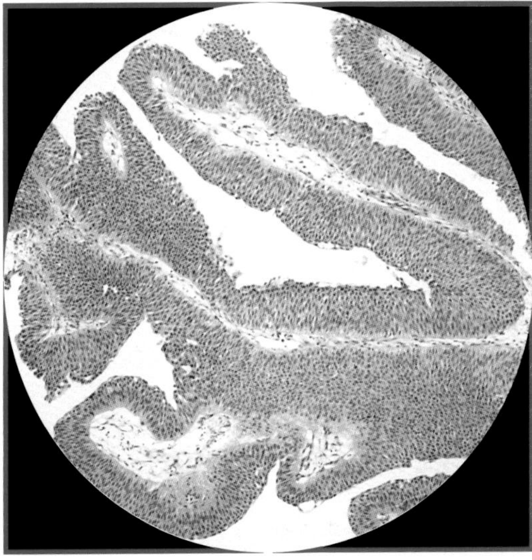

I10.34
Low-grade TCC, revised classification. Corresponding tissue.

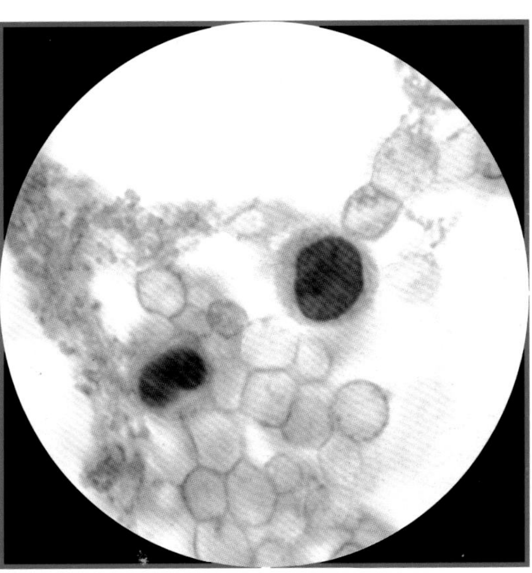

I10.35
Low-grade TCC. Individual cells are difficult to evaluate in papillary groups; even benign cells show pleomorphism. Look for single little "coy" cells in the background. (Oil)

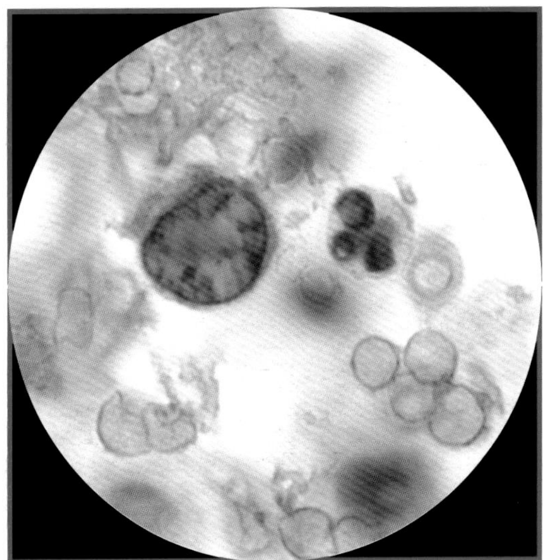

I10.36
Low-grade TCC. Single "coy" cells are easier to evaluate than cells in groups. (Oil)

I10.37
Low-grade TCC. To diagnose, look for single, small cells with high N/C ratios, and abnormal nuclei with slightly coarse chromatin and irregular nuclear membranes ("coy" cells). (Oil)

I10.38
Low-grade TCC. I10.35 to I10.38 are examples of "coy" cells exfoliated from TCC. (Oil)

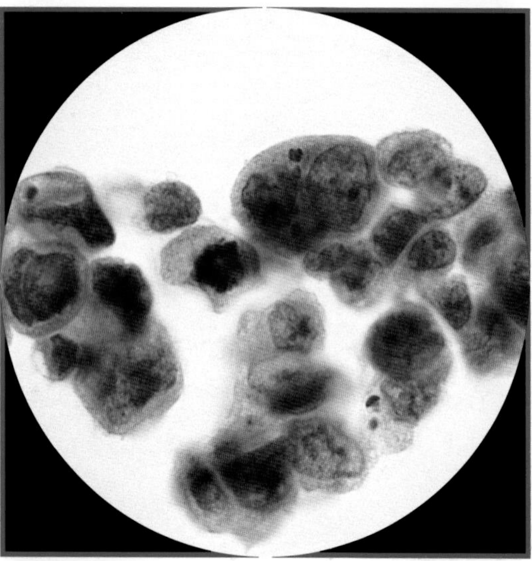

I10.39
High-grade TCC, revised classification. This is also known as TCC grade III (WHO). Numerous cells are shed in loose aggregates and singly. Malignant cytologic atypia is obvious.

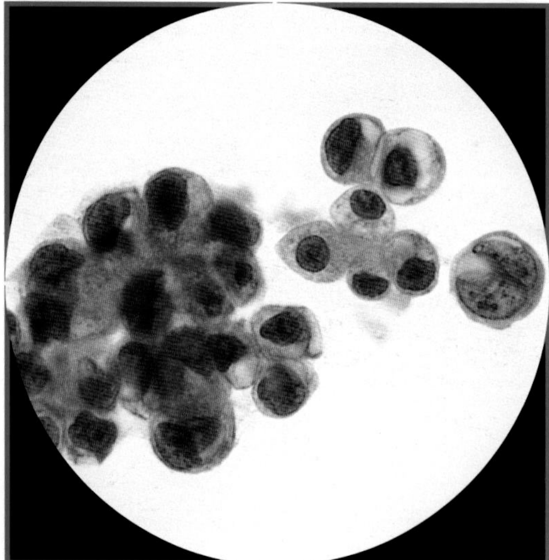

I10.40
High-grade TCC, revised classification. Eccentric nuclei with malignant atypia can be seen. Note cytoplasmic vacuolization.

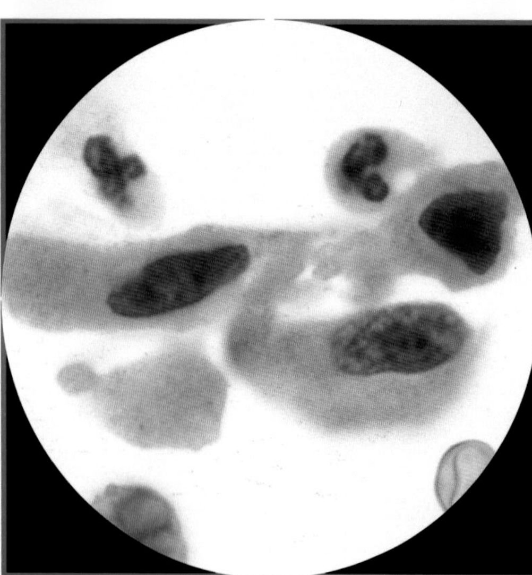

I10.41
High-grade TCC. Note dense basophilic cytoplasm characteristic of transitional cells.

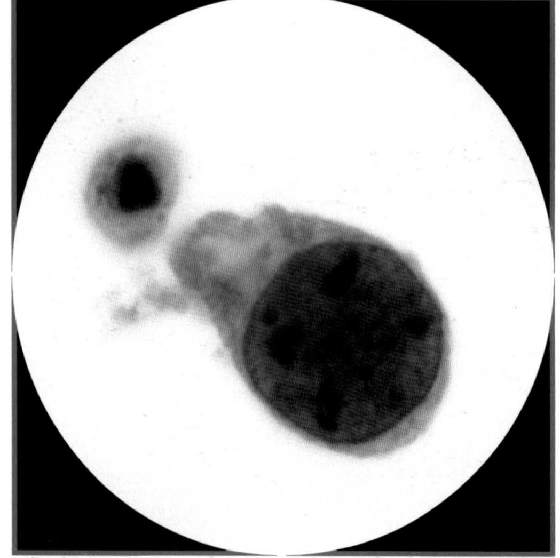

I10.42
High-grade TCC. Characterized by high N/C ratio, marked hyperchromasia, prominent, multiple nucleoli. (Oil)

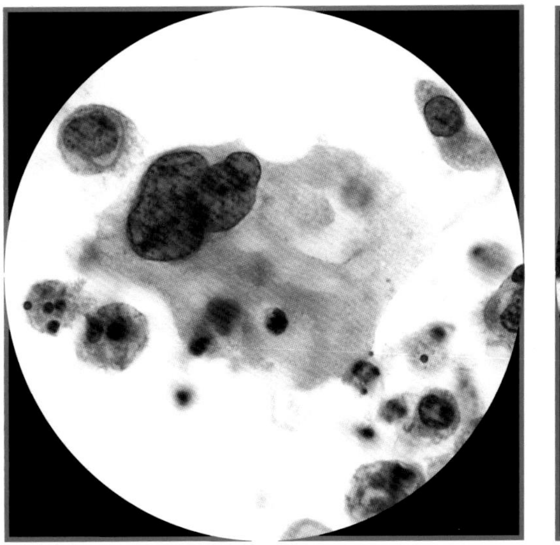

I10.43
High-grade TCC. Giant cells can be seen.

I10.44
High-grade TCC. Spindle cells can be seen.

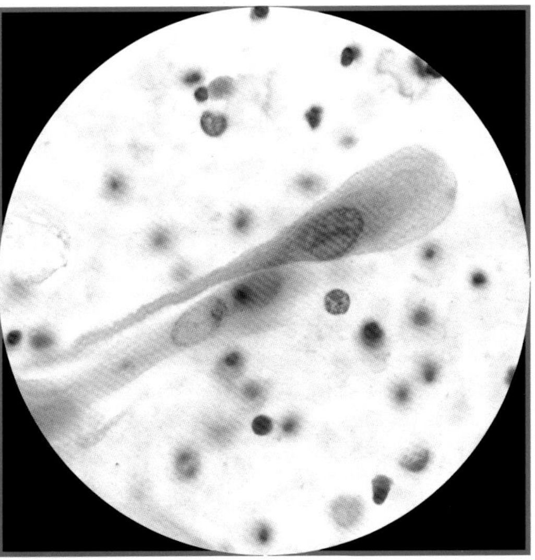

I10.45
High-grade TCC. Squamous differentiation, with bizarre keratinized cells, can be seen.

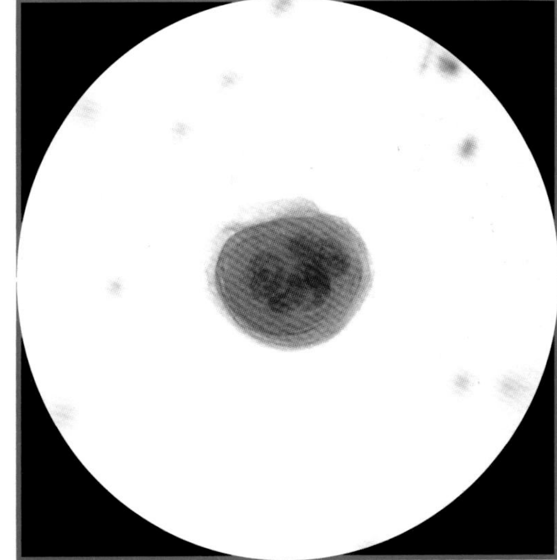

I10.46
High-grade TCC. Squamous differentiation with cell-in-cell or pearl arrangements.

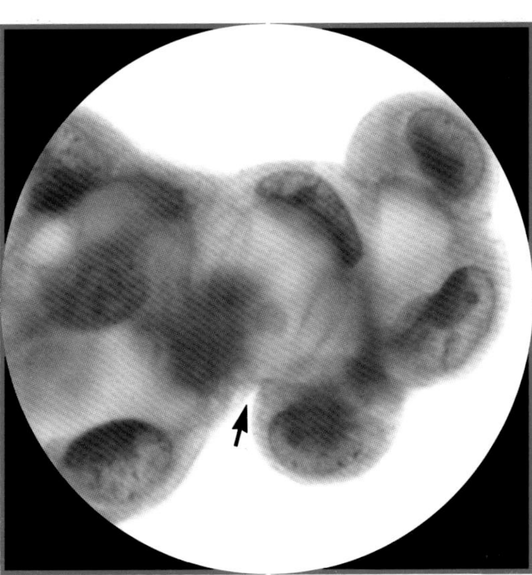

I10.47
High-grade TCC. Glandular differentiation can also occur in high-grade transitional cell carcinoma (note secretory product in cytoplasmic vacuole with mucin [arrow]). Rarely, pure adenocarcinoma arises in the bladder. Colonic type of primary adenocarcinoma is more common; pure signet ring cell carcinoma is very rare.

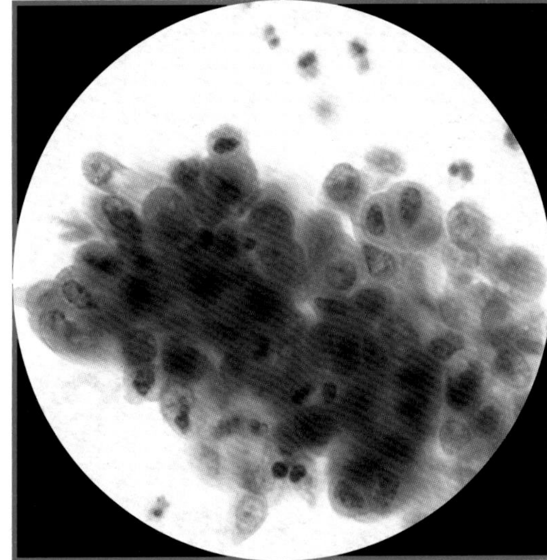

I10.48
Dysplasia. Cells are similar to low-grade transitional cell carcinoma, with mild to moderate nuclear abnormality. Diagnosis is made based on worst cells present.

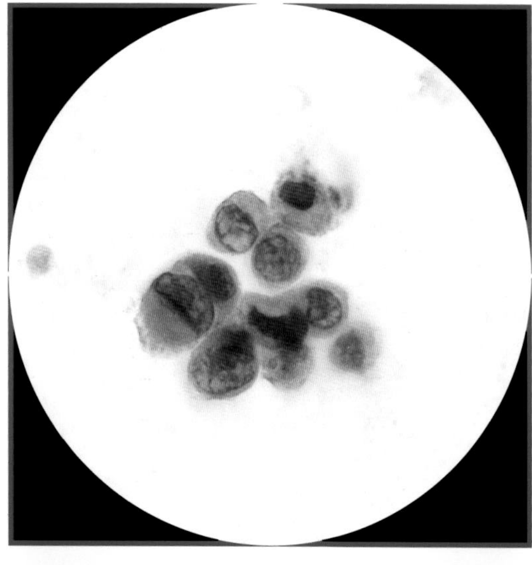

I10.49
Carcinoma in situ. Cells are similar to high-grade transitional cell carcinoma, with severe nuclear atypia. Cytologic examination alone cannot distinguish it from invasive carcinoma. The bladder may be cystoscopically unremarkable.

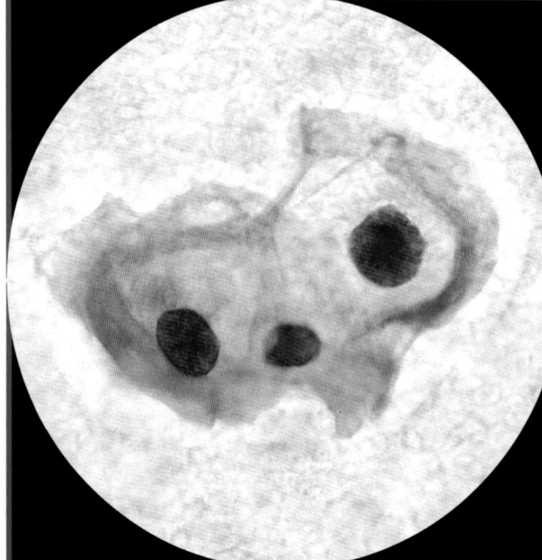

I10.50
Condyloma. Diagnostic cell is the koilocyte (distinct vacuole, nuclear atypia). It is often associated with genital condyloma; genital contamination must be excluded in diagnosis. Bladder condylomas may be difficult to eradicate.

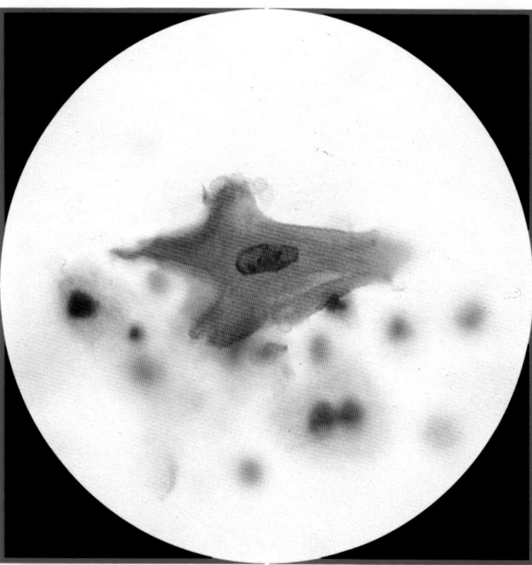

I10.51
Squamous cell carcinoma. Squamous differentiation is relatively common in transitional cell carcinoma. Squamous cell carcinoma can also involve the bladder secondarily, eg, from a cervical primary. Pure, primary squamous cell carcinoma of the bladder is rare in the US. Very well-differentiated tumors may occur, which exfoliate cells with only slight atypia (akin to mild dysplasia in the Pap smear, as illustrated).

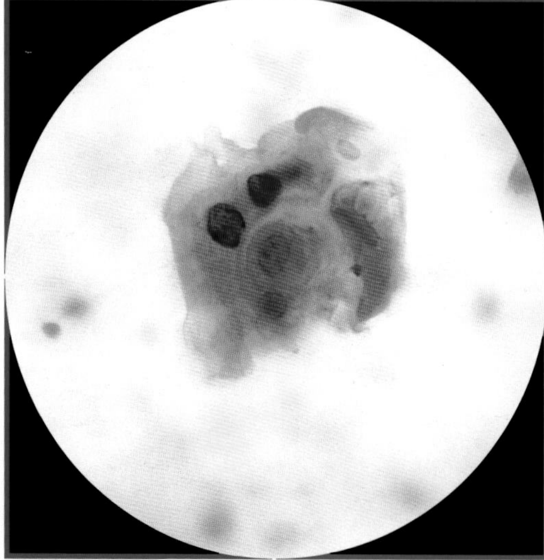

I10.52
Squamous cell carcinoma. Cell-in-cell arrangements or pearls and heavy keratinization are characteristic of well-differentiated keratinizing squamous cell carcinoma.

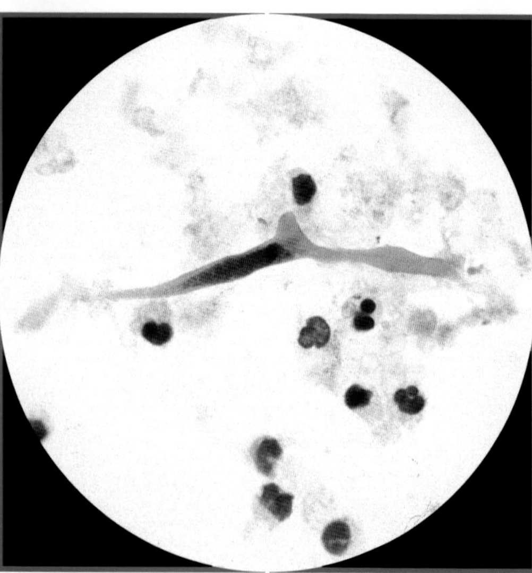

I10.53
Squamous cell carcinoma. Bizarre-shaped cells may be seen.

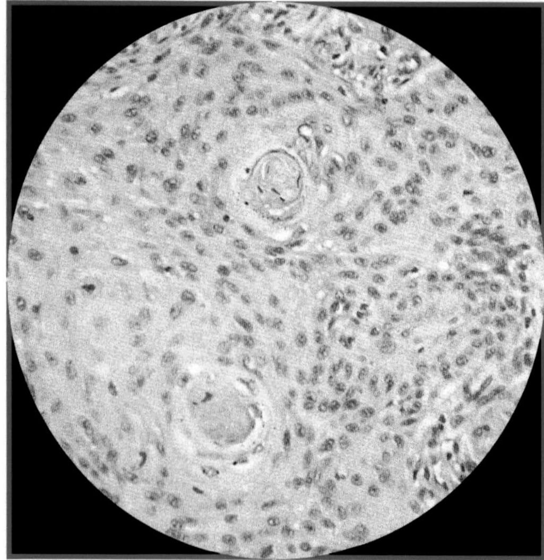

I10.54
Squamous cell carcinoma. Corresponding tissue.

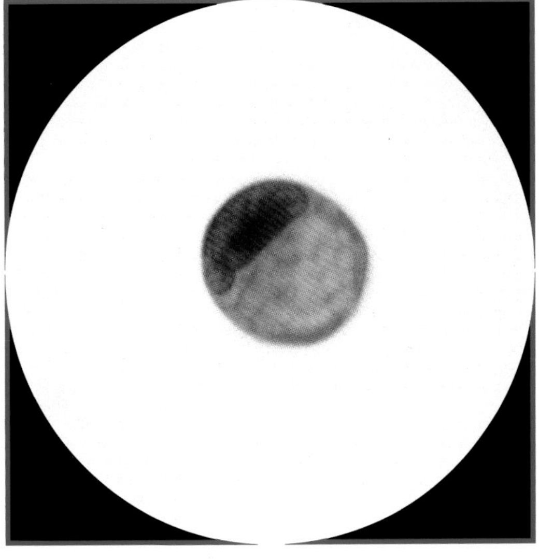

I10.55
Signet ring carcinoma. This is a rare primary tumor of the bladder that may arise from urachal remnants. The diagnosis should be reserved for pure or nearly pure signet ring cell tumors. (Oil)

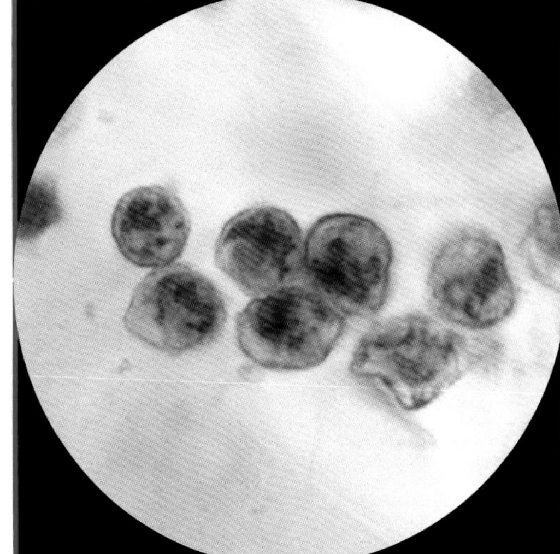

I10.56
Small cell carcinoma. This is a rare primary bladder tumor, essentially identical to the more common lung tumor of the same type, which can metastasize to the bladder. Note scant cytoplasm, high N/C ratios, molding, hyperchromasia, and inconspicuous nucleoli. (Oil)

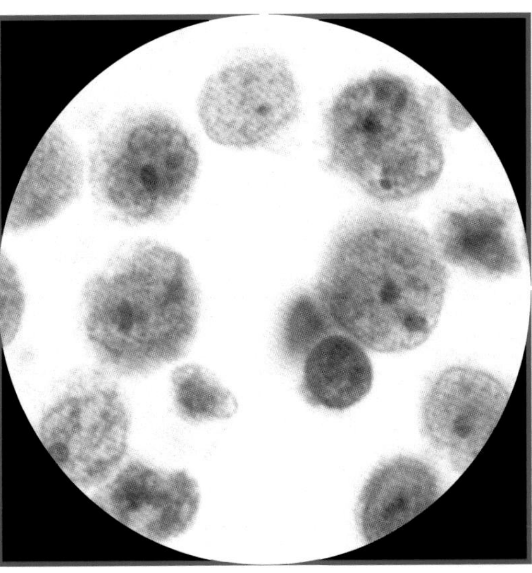

I10.57
Malignant lymphoma. Primary lymphoma of the urinary tract is rare, secondary involvement is more common. Either can potentially be diagnosed with urinary cytology. The cells are singly dispersed and even the large cell type usually has relatively small cells. (Oil)

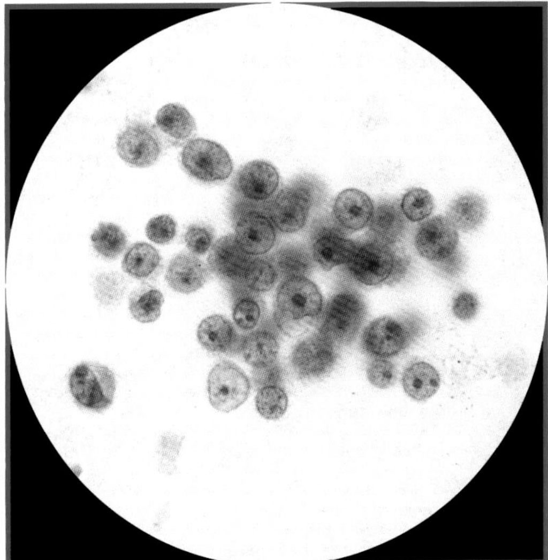

I10.58
Prostatic carcinoma. This is usually characterized by relatively uniform cells with prominent nucleoli. It is rarely first diagnosed in urine, except after prostatic massage, but can be seen late in the course of the disease.

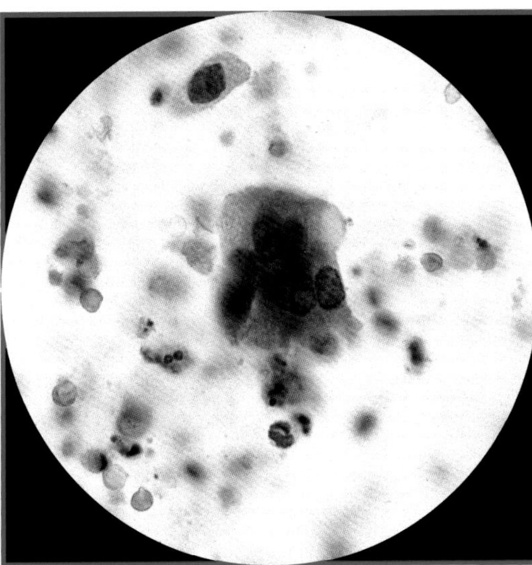

I10.59
Colonic carcinoma. The bladder may be involved by direct extension. It is characterized by tall columnar cells, with palisaded nuclei, and "terminal bar-like" apical cytoplasmic densities.

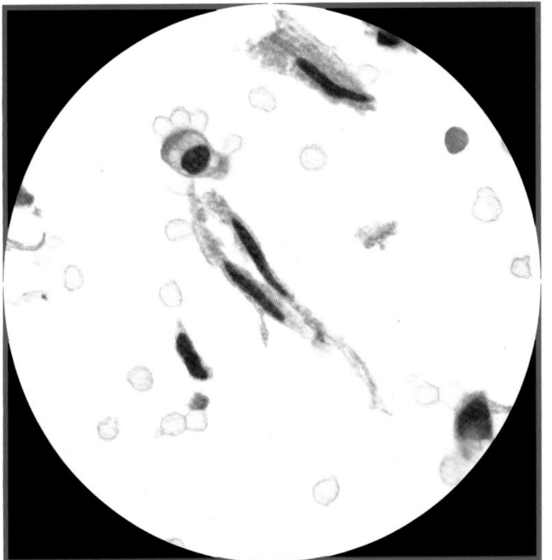

I10.60
Thermal artifact: In response to heat due to cautery or laser therapy of bladder tumors, the transitional cells may show a striking spindle cell artifact. The cells resemble smooth muscle cells, with elongated nuclei, dense, uniform chromatin, and indistinct cell borders. Spindle cells can also be seen in low grade transitional cell neoplasms, but be cautious making a malignant diagnosis on artifactually distorted cells.

References

Abdel-Razzak OM, Ehya H, Cubler-Goodman A, et al: Ureteroscopic Biopsy in the Upper Urinary Tract. *Urology* 44: 451–457, 1994.

Akura K, Hatakenaka M, Kawai K, et al: Use of Immunocytochemistry on Urinary Sediments for the Rapid Identification of Human Polyomavirus Infection: A Case Report. *Acta Cytol* 32: 247–251, 1988.

Alcaraz A, Talbot-Wright R, Samson R, et al: Vesical Tumors in Patients Under 25 Years of Age. *Eur Urol* 20: 133–135, 1991.

Allegra SR, Fanning JP, Streker JF, et al: Cytologic Diagnosis of Occult and "In-Situ" Carcinoma of the Urinary System. *Acta Cytol* 10: 340–349, 1966.

Allegra SR, Broderick PA, Corvese NL: Cytologic and Histologic Observations in Well Differentiated Transitional Cell Carcinoma of Bladder. *J Urol* 107: 777–782, 1972.

Alroy J, Pauli BU, Weinstein RS: Correlation Between Numbers of Desmosomes and the Aggressiveness of Transitional Cell Carcinoma in Human Urinary Bladder. *Cancer* 47: 104–112, 1981.

Amberson JB, Laino JP: Image Cytometric Deoxyribonucleic Acid Analysis of Urine Specimens as an Adjunct to Visual Cytology in the Detection of Urothelial Cell Carcinoma. *J Urol* 149: 42–45, 1993.

Anderson JB, Nobbs GL, Hammonds JC: Urinary Cytology and the Early Detection of Renal Allograft Rejection. *J Urol* 136: 10–12, 1986.

Andriole GL, McClennan BL, Becich MJ, et al: Effect of Low Osmolar, Ionic and Nonionic, Contrast Media on the Cytologic Features of Exfoliated Urothelial Cells. *Urol Radiol* 11: 133–135, 1989.

Andrion A, Gaglio A, Zai G: Bladder Involvement in Disseminated Malignant Lymphoma Diagnosed by Voided Urine Cytology. *Cytopathology* 4: 115–117, 1993.

Arthur RR, Shah KV, Baust SJ, et al: Association of BK Viruria With Hemorrhagic Cystitis in Recipients of Bone Marrow Transplants. *N Engl J Med* 315: 230–234, 1986.

Ashton PR, Lambird PA: Cytodiagnosis of Malakoplakia: Report of a Case. *Acta Cytol* 14: 92–94, 1970.

Badalament RA, Gay H, Cibas ES, et al: Monitoring Endoscopic Treatment of Superficial Bladder Carcinoma by Postoperative Urinary Cytology. *J Urol* 138: 760–762, 1987a.

Badalament RA, Hermansen DK, Kimmel M, et al: The Sensitivity of Bladder Wash Flow Cytometry, Bladder Wash Cytology, and Voided Cytology in the Detection of Bladder Carcinoma. *Cancer* 60: 1423–1427, 1987b.

Badalament RA, Fair WR, Whitmore WF Jr, et al: The Relative Value of Cytometry and Cytology in the Management of Bladder Cancer: The Memorial Sloan-Kettering Cancer Center Experience. *Semin Urol* 6: 22–30, 1988.

Bancroft J, Seybolt JF, Windhager HA: Cytologic Diagnosis of Cytomegalic Inclusion Disease: A Case Report. *Acta Cytol* 5: 182–186, 1961.

Banigo OG, Waisman J, Kaufman JJ: Papillary (Transitional) Carcinoma in an Ileal Conduit. *J Urol* 114: 626–627, 1975.

Bard RH: The Significance of Asymptomatic Microhematuria in Women and Its Economic Implications: A Ten-Year Study. *Arch Intern Med* 148: 2629–2632, 1988.

Barry JM, Murphy JB, Nassir E, et al: The Influence of Retrograde Contrast Medium on Urinary Cytodiagnosis: A Preliminary Report. *J Urol* 119: 633–634, 1978.

Behmard S, Sadeghi A, Mohareri M-R, et al: Positive Association of Opium Addiction and Cancer of the Bladder: Results of Urine Cytology in 3,500 Opium Addicts. *Acta Cytol* 25: 142–152, 1981.

Bergkvist A, Ljungqvist A, Moberger G: Classification of Bladder Tumours Based on the Cellular Pattern: Preliminary Report of a Clinical-Pathological Study of 300 Cases With a Minimum Follow-up of Eight Years. *Acta Chir Scand* 130: 371–378, 1965.

Berlac PA, Holm HH: Bladder Tumor Control by Abdominal Ultrasound and Urine Cytology. *J Urol* 147: 1510–1512, 1992.

Betz SA, See WA, Cohen MB: Granulomatous Inflammation in Bladder Wash Specimens After Intravesical Bacillus Calmette-Guerin Therapy for Transitional Cell Carcinoma of the Bladder. *Am J Clin Pathol* 99: 244–248, 1993.

Beyer-Boon ME, Cuypers LHRI, de Voogt JH, et al: Cytological Changes Due to Urinary Calculi: A Consideration of the Relationship Between Calculi and the Development of Urothelial Carcinoma. *Br J Urol* 50: 81–89, 1978.

Bibbo M, Gill WB, Harris MJ, et al: Retrograde Brushing as a Diagnostic Procedure of Ureteral, Renal Pelvic and Renal Calyceal Lesions: A Preliminary Report. *Acta Cytol* 18: 137–141, 1974.

Blomjous ECM, Schipper NW, Baak JPA, et al: The Value of Morphometry and DNA Flow Cytometry in Addition to Classic Prognosticators in Superficial Urinary Bladder Carcinoma. *Am J Clin Pathol* 91: 243–248, 1989.

Blute ML, Segura JW, Patterson DE, et al: Impact of Endourology on Diagnosis and Management of Upper Urinary Tract Urothelial Cancer. *J Urol* 141: 1298–1301, 1989.

Bocian JJ, Flam MS, Mendoza CA: Hodgkin's Disease Involving the Urinary Bladder Diagnosed by Urinary Cytology: A Case Report. *Cancer* 50: 2482–2485, 1982.

Bolande RP: Inclusion-Bearing Cells in the Urine in Certain Viral Infections. *Pediatrics* 24: 7–12, 1959.

Bonner RB, Hemstreet GP III, Fradet Y, et al: Bladder Cancer Risk Assessment With Quantitative Fluorescence Image Analysis of Tumor Markers in Exfoliated Bladder Cells. *Cancer* 72: 2461–2469, 1993.

Boon ME, Kurver PHJ, Baak JPA, et al: Morphometric Differences Between Urothelial Cells in Voided Urine of Patients With Grade I and Grade II Bladder Tumors. *J Clin Pathol* 34: 612–615, 1981.

Boon ME, Blomjous CEM, Zwartendijk J, et al: Carcinoma In Situ of the Urinary Bladder: Clinical Presentation, Cytologic Pattern and Stromal Changes. *Acta Cytol* 30: 360–366, 1986.

Boon ME, van Keep JPM, Kok LP: Polyomavirus Infection Versus High-Grade Bladder Carcinoma: The Importance of Cytologic and Comparative Morphometric Studies of Plastic-Embedded Voided Urine Sediments. *Acta Cytol* 33: 887–893, 1989.

Boring CC: Cancer Statistics. *CA-Cancer J Clin* 44: 18–19, 1994.

Bossen EH, Johnston WW, Amatulli J, et al: Exfoliative Cytopathologic Studies in Organ Transplantation: I. The Cytologic Diagnosis of Cytomegalic Inclusion Disease in the Urine of Renal Allograft Recipients. *Am J Clin Pathol* 52: 340–344, 1969.

Bossen EH, Johnston WW, Amatulli J, et al: Exfoliative Cytopathologic Studies in Organ Transplantation, III: The Cytologic Profile of Urine During Acute Renal Allograft Rejection. *Acta Cytol* 14: 176–181, 1970.

Bossen EH, Johnston WW: Exfoliative Cytopathologic Studies in Organ Transplantation, IV: The Cytologic Diagnosis of Herpesvirus in the Urine of Renal Allograft Recipients. *Acta Cytol* 19: 415–419, 1975.

Bossen EH, Johnston WW: Exfoliative Cytopathologic Studies in Organ Transplantation, V: The Diagnosis of Rejection in the Immediate Postoperative Period. *Acta Cytol* 21: 502–507, 1977.

Brawn PN: The Origin of Invasive Carcinoma of the Bladder. *Cancer* 50: 515–519, 1982.

Bunge RG, Kraushaar OF: Abnormal Renal Cytology. *J Urol* 63: 464–474, 1950a.

Bunge RG, Kraushaar OF: An Early Renal Malignancy, Diagnosed Preoperatively. *J Urol* 63: 475–479, 1950b.

Cant JD, Murphy WM, Soloway MS: Prognostic Significance of Urine Cytology on Initial Follow-Up After Intravesical Mitomycin C for Superficial Bladder Cancer. *Cancer* 57: 2119–2122, 1986.

Carter HB, Amberson JB, Bander NH, et al: Newer Diagnostic Techniques for Bladder Cancer. *Urol Clin North Am* 14: 763–769, 1987.

Chalvardjian A, Carydis B, Cohen S: Cytologic Diagnosis of Extravesical Malacoplakia. *Diagn Cytopathol* 1: 216–220, 1985.

Chang SC: Urinary Cytologic Diagnosis of Cytomegalic Inclusion Disease in Childhood Leukemia. *Acta Cytol* 14: 338–343, 1970.

Chappell LH, Lundin L: A Pitfall in Urine Cytology: A Case Report. *Acta Cytol* 20: 162–163, 1976.

Cheson BD, Schumann GB, Johnston JL: Urinary Cytodiagnosis of Renal Involvement in Disseminated Histiocytic Lymphoma. *Acta Cytol* 28: 148–152, 1984a.

Cheson BD, Schumann JL, Schumann GB: Urinary Cytodiagnosis Abnormalities in 50 Patients with Non-Hodgkin's Lymphomas. *Cancer* 54: 1914–1919, 1984b.

Cheson BD, De Bellis CC, Schumann GB, et al: The Urinary Myeloma Cast: Frequency of Detection and Clinical Correlations in 30 Patients With Multiple Myeloma. *Am J Clin Pathol* 83: 421–425, 1985.

Clements MHS, Oko T: Cytologic Diagnosis of Schistosomiasis in Routine Urinary Specimens: A Case Report. *Acta Cytol* 27: 277, 1983.

Cohen J-M, Szporn AH, Unger P, et al: Noncaseating Granulomata of the Bladder Following Intravesical Administration of Bacille Calmette-Guérin. *Acta Cytol* 35: 600, 1991.

Colandrea JM, Elwood L, Solomon D: Identifications of Polyoma Virus Antigens in Urine From Cyclophosphamide-Treated Patients. *Acta Cytol* 34: 710, 1990.

Cole P, Monson RR, Haning H, et al: Smoking and Cancer of the Lower Urinary Tract. *N Engl J Med* 284: 129–134, 1971.

Cole P, Hoover R, Friedell GH: Occupation and Cancer of the Lower Urinary Tract. *Cancer* 29: 1250–1260, 1972.

Coleman DV, Gardner SD, Field AM: Human Polyomavirus Infection in Renal Allograft Recipients. *Br Med J* 3: 371–375, 1973.

Coleman DV: The Cytodiagnosis of Human Polyomavirus Infection. *Acta Cytol* 19: 93–96, 1975.

Collste LG, Devonec M, Darzynkiewicz Z, et al: Bladder Cancer Diagnosis by Flow Cytometry: Correlation Between Cell Samples From Biopsy and Bladder Irrigation Fluid. *Cancer* 45: 2389–2394, 1980.

Cooper PH, Waisman J, Johnston WH, et al: Severe Atypia of Transitional Epithelium and Carcinoma of the Urinary Bladder. *Cancer* 31: 1055–1060, 1973.

Corwin HL, Bray RA, Haber MH: The Detection and Interpretation of Urinary Eosinophils. *Arch Pathol Lab Med* 113: 1256–1258, 1989.

Cowen PN: The Development of a Urological Cytodiagnosis Service and an Evaluation of Its Success. *J Clin Pathol* 24: 107–112, 1971.

Cowen PN: False Cytodiagnosis of Bladder Malignancy Due to Previous Radiotherapy. *Br J Urol* 47: 405–412, 1975.

Crabbe JGS: Cytology of Voided Urine With Special Reference to "Benign" Papilloma and Some of the Problems Encountered in the Preparation of the Smears. *Acta Cytol* 5: 233–240, 1961.

Crabbe JGS: 'Comet' or 'Decoy' Cells Found in Urinary Sediment Smears. *Acta Cytol* 15: 303–305, 1971.

Crabtree WN, Murphy WM: The Value of Ethanol as a Fixative in Urinary Cytology. *Acta Cytol* 24: 452–455, 1980.

Crosby JH, Allsbrook WC Jr, Koss LG, et al: Cytologic Detection of Urothelial Cancer and Other Abnormalities in a Cohort of Workers Exposed to Aromatic Amines. *Acta Cytol* 35: 263–268, 1991.

Cuadrado E, Rodriguez-Trinidad A, Blasco E, et al: Blood Group Isoantigens ABO (H) in Transitional Carcinoma of the Bladder: A Clinicopathological Study. *J Urol* 135: 409–415, 1986.

Cullen TH, Popham RR, Voss HJ: Urine Cytology and Primary Carcinoma of the Renal Pelvis and Ureter. *Austr N Z J Surg* 41: 230–236, 1972.

Curran FT: Malakoplakia of the Bladder. *Br J Urol* 59: 559–563, 1987.

Dabbs DJ: Cytology of Pyelitis Glandularis Cystica: A Case Report. *Acta Cytol* 36: 943–945, 1992.

Dale GA, Smith RB: Transitional Cell Carcinoma of the Bladder Associated With Cyclophosphamide. *J Urol* 112: 603–604, 1974.

Daut RV, McDonald JR: Diagnosis of Malignant Lesions of the Urinary Tract by Means of Microscopic Examination of Centrifuged Urinary Sediment. *Proc Staff Meeting, Mayo Clin* 22: 382–390, 1947.

Dean PJ, Murphy WM: Importance of Urinary Cytology and Future Role of Flow Cytometry. *Urology* 26(Suppl 4): 11–15, 1985.

de la Rosette JJMCH, Hubregtse MR, Wiersma AM, et al: Value of Urine Cytology in Screening Patients With Prostatitis Syndromes. *Acta Cytol* 37: 710–712, 1993a.

de la Rosette JJMCH, Hubregtse MR, Meuleman EJH, et al: Diagnosis and Treatment of 409 Patients With Prostatitis Syndromes. *Urology* 41: 301–307, 1993b.

Del Mistro A, Koss LG, Braunstein J, et al: Condylomata Acuminata of the Urinary Bladder: Natural History, Viral Typing, and DNA Content. *Am J Surg Pathol* 12: 205–215, 1988.

DeMay RM, Grathwohl MA: Signet-Ring-Cell (Colloid) Carcinoma of the Urinary Bladder: Cytologic, Histologic and Ultrastructural Findings in One Case. *Acta Cytol* 29: 132–136, 1985.

Dhundee J, Rigby HS: Comparison of Two Preparatory Techniques for Urine Cytology. *J Clin Pathol* 43: 1034–1035, 1990.

DiBonito L, Musse MM, Dudine S, et al: Cytology of Transitional-Cell Carcinoma of the Urinary Bladder: Diagnostic Yield and Histologic Basis. *Diagn Cytopathol* 8: 124–127, 1992.

Dimmette RM, Sproat HF, Klimt CR: Examination of Smears of Urinary Sediment for Detection of Neoplasms of Bladder: Survey of an Egyptian Village Infested With *Schistosoma hematobium*. *Am J Clin Pathol* 25: 1032–1042, 1955.

Dorfman HD, Monis B: Mucin-containing Inclusions in Multinucleated Giant Cells and Transitional Epithelial Cells of Urine: Cytochemical Observations on Exfoliated Cells. *Acta Cytol* 8: 293–301, 1964.

Droller MJ, Erozan YS: Thiotepa Effects on Urinary Cytology in the Interpretation of Transitional Cell Cancer. *J Urol* 134: 671–674, 1985.

Droller MJ: A Rose Is a Rose Is a Rose, Or Is It? *J Urol* 136: 1057–1058, 1986.

Eggensperger D, Schweitzer S, Ferriol E, et al: The Utility of Cytodiagnostic Urinalysis for Monitoring Renal Allograft Injury: A Clinicopathological Analysis of 87 Patients and Over 1,000 Urine Specimens. *Am J Nephrol* 8: 27–34, 1988.

Eggensperger DL, King C, Gaudette LE, et al: Cytodiagnostic Urinalysis: Three Years Experience With a New Laboratory Test. *Am J Clin Pathol* 91: 202–206, 1989.

El-Bolkainy MN, Ghoneim MA, El-Morsey BA, et al: Carcinoma of Bilharzial Bladder: Diagnostic Value of Urine Cytology. *Urology* 3: 319–323, 1974.

El-Bolkainy MN: Cytology of Bladder Carcinoma. *J Urol* 124: 20–22, 1980.

Ellwein LB: Bladder Cancer Screening: Lessons From a Biologically Based Model of Bladder Cancer Progression and Therapeutic Intervention. *J Occup Med* 32: 806–811, 1990.

Erikkson O, Johansson S: Urothelial Neoplasms of the Upper Urinary Tract: A Correlation Between Cytologic and Histologic Findings in 43 Patients With Urothelial Neoplasms of the Renal Pelvis or Ureter. *Acta Cytol* 20: 20–25, 1976.

Esposti PL, Moberger G, Zajicek J: The Cytologic Diagnosis of Transitional Cell Tumors of the Urinary Bladder and Its Histologic Basis: A Study of 567 Cases of Urinary-Tract Disorder Including 170 Untreated and 182 Irradiated Bladder Tumors. *Acta Cytol* 14: 145–155, 1970.

Esposti PL, Zajicke J: Grading of Transitional Cell Neoplasms of the Urinary Bladder From Smears of Bladder Washings: A Critical Review of 326 Tumors. *Acta Cytol* 16: 529–537, 1972.

Evans JA, Halpern M, Finby N: Diagnosis of Kidney Cancer: An Analysis of 100 Consecutive Cases. *JAMA* 175: 201–203, 1961.

Fall M, Johansson SL, Aldenborg F: Chronic Interstitial Cystitis: A Heterogeneous Syndrome. *J Urol* 137: 35–38, 1987.

Falor WH, Ward RM: Cytogenetic Analysis: A Potential Index for Recurrence of Early Carcinoma of the Bladder. *J Urol* 115: 49–52, 1976.

Fanning CV, Staerkel GA, Sneige N, et al: Spindling Artifact of Urothelial Cells in Post-Laser Treatment Urinary Cytology. *Diagn Cytopathol* 9: 279–281, 1993.

Farrow GM, Utz DC, Rife CC, et al: Clinical Observations of Sixty-nine Cases of In Situ Carcinoma of the Urinary Bladder. *Cancer Res* 37: 2794–2798, 1977.

Farrow GM: Pathologist's Role in Bladder Cancer. *Sem Oncol* 6: 198–206, 1979.

Farrow GM: Urine Cytology in the Detection of Bladder Cancer: A Critical Approach. *J Occup Med* 32: 817–821, 1990.

Feeney MJ, Mullenix RB, Prentiss RJ, et al: Cytological Studies of the Urine: Preliminary Report. *J Urol* 79: 589–595, 1958.

Feltis JT, Perez-Marrero R, Emerson LE: Increased Mast Cells of the Bladder in Suspected Cases of Interstitial Cystitis: A Possible Disease Marker. *J Urol* 138: 42–43, 1987.

Fischer S, Nielsen ML, Clausen S, et al: Increased Abnormal Urothelial Cells in Voided Urine Following Excretory Urography. *Acta Cytol* 26: 153–158, 1982.

Fontana P, Baiocco R: Bizarre Spindle Cells in Urine Cytology Specimens. *Diagn Cytopathol* 9: 605–606, 1993.

Foot NC, Papanicolaou GN: Early Renal Carcinoma In Situ: Detected by Means of Smears of Fixed Urinary Sediment. *JAMA* 139: 356–358, 1949.

Foot NC, Papanicolaou GN, Holmqist ND, et al: Exfoliative Cytology of Urinary Sediments: A Review of 2,829 Cases. *Cancer* 11: 127–137, 1958.

Forni AM, Koss LG, Geller W: Cytological Study of the Effect of Cyclophosphamide on the Epithelium of the Urinary Bladder in Man. *Cancer* 17: 1348–1355, 1964.

Forni A, Ghetti G, Armeli G: Urinary Cytology in Workers Exposed to Carcinogenic Aromatic Amines: A Six-Year Study. *Acta Cytol* 16: 142–145, 1972.

Frable WJ, Paxson L, Barksdale JA, et al: Current Practice of Urinary Bladder Cytology. *Cancer Res* 37: 2800–2805, 1977.

Fralick RA, Malek RS, Goellner JR, et al: Urethroscopy and Urethral Cytology in Men With External Genital Condyloma. *Urology* 43: 361–364, 1994.

Freeman JA, Esrig D, Stein JP, et al: Management of the Patient With Bladder Cancer. Urethral Recurrence. *Urol Clin North Am* 21: 645–651, 1994.

Freni SC, Freni-Titulaer LWJ: Microhematuria Found by Mass Screening of Apparently Healthy Males. *Acta Cytol* 21: 421–423, 1977.

Friedell GH, Soloway MS, Hilgar AG, et al: Summary of Workshop on Carcinoma In Situ of the Bladder. *J Urol* 136: 1047–1048, 1986.

Froom P, Ribak J, Benbassat J: Significance of Microhaematuria in Young Adults. *Br Med J* 288: 20–22, 1984.

Fuchs EF, Kay R, Poole R, et al: Uroepithelial Carcinoma in Association With Cyclophosphamide Ingestion. *J Urol* 126: 544–545, 1981.

Gamarra MC, Zein T: Cytologic Spectrum of Bladder Cancer. *Suppl Urol* 23: 23–26, 1984.

Gardner SD, Field AM, Coleman DV, et al: New Human Papovavirus (B.K.) Isolated From Urine After Renal Transplantation. *Lancet* (i): 1253–1257, 1971.

Garret M, Jassie M: Cytologic Examination of Post Prostatic Massage Specimens as an Aid in Diagnosis of Carcinoma of the Prostate. *Acta Cytol* 20: 126–131, 1976.

Geisinger KR, Buss DH, Kawamoto EH, et al: Multiple Myeloma: The Diagnostic Role and Prognostic Significance of Exfoliative Cytology. *Acta Cytol* 30: 334–340, 1986.

Giacomini G, Bianchi G, Moretti D: Detection of Sexually Transmitted Diseases, by Urethral Cytology, the Ignored Male Counterpart of Cervical Cytology. *Acta Cytol* 33: 11–15, 1989.

Giella JG, Ring K, Olsson CA, et al: The Predictive Value of Flow Cytometry and Urinary Cytology in the Follow-up of Patients With Transitional Cell Carcinoma of the Bladder. *J Urol* 148: 293–296, 1992.

Gilbert HA, Logan JL, Kagan AR, et al: The Natural History of Papillary Transitional Cell Carcinoma of the Bladder and Its Treatment in an Unselected Population on the Basis of Histologic Grading. *J Urol* 119: 488–492, 1978.

Gill WB, Lu CT, Thomsen S: Retrograde Brushing: A New Technique for Obtaining Histologic and Cytologic Material From Ureteral, Renal Pelvic and Renal Caliceal Lesions. *J Urol* 109: 573–578, 1973.

Gill WB, Lu CT, Bibbo M: Retrograde Ureteral Brushing. *Urology* 12: 279–283, 1978.

Gil-Salom M, Sánchez MC, Chuan P, et al: Multiple Mucosal Biopsies and Postoperative Urinary Cytology in Patients With Bladder Cancer. *Eur Urol* 17: 281–285, 1990.

Golin AL, Howard RS: Asymptomatic Microscopic Hematuria. *J Urol* 124: 389–391, 1980.

Gomousa-Michael M, Rammou-Kinia R: Herpesvirus Infection of the Male Urethra Identified by Cytology. *Acta Cytol* 36: 270–271, 1992.

Grabstald H, Whitmore WF, Melamed MR: Renal Pelvic Tumors. *JAMA* 218: 845–854, 1971.

Grace DA, Taylor WN, Taylor JN, et al: Carcinoma of the Renal Pelvis: A 15-Year Review. *J Urol* 98: 566–569, 1967.

Grignon DJ, Ro JY, Ayala AG, et al: Primary Signet-Ring Cell Carcinoma of the Urinary Bladder. *Am J Clin Pathol* 95: 13–20, 1991.

Grignon DJ, Ro JY, Ayala AG, et al: Small Cell Carcinoma of the Urinary Bladder: A Clinicopathologic Analysis of 22 Cases. *Cancer* 69: 527–536, 1992.

Gupta TD, Grabstald H: Melanoma of the Genitourinary Tract. *J Urol* 93: 607–614, 1965.

Hajdu SI, Savino A, Hajdu EO, et al: Cytologic Diagnosis of Renal Cell Carcinoma With the Aid of Fat Stain. *Acta Cytol* 15: 31–33, 1971.

Hanno P, Levin RM, Monson FC, et al: Diagnosis of Interstitial Cystitis. *J Urol* 143: 278–281, 1990.

Harris MJ, Schwinn CP, Morrow JW, et al: Exfoliative Cytology of the Urinary Bladder Irrigation Specimen. *Acta Cytol* 15: 385–399, 1971.

Harrison JH, Botsford TW, Tucker MR: The Use of the Smear of the Urinary Sediment in the Diagnosis and Management of Neoplasm of the Kidney and Bladder. *Surg Gynecol Obstet* 92: 129–139, 1951.

Harving N, Wolf H, Melsen F: Positive Urinary Cytology After Tumor Resection: An Indicator for Concomitant Carcinoma In Situ. *J Urol* 140: 495–497, 1988.

Harving N, Petersen SE, Melsen F, et al: Urinary Cytology in the Detection of Bladder Tumours: Influence of Concomitant Urothelial Atypia. *Scand J Urol Nephrol Suppl* 125: 127–131, 1989.

Hastie KJ, Ahmad R, Moisey CU: Fractionated Urinary Cytology in the Follow-up of Bladder Cancer. *Br J Urol* 66: 40–41, 1990.

Hausdorfer GS, Chandrasoma P, Pettross BR, et al: Cytologic Diagnosis of Mesonephric Adenocarcinoma of the Urinary Bladder. *Acta Cytol* 29: 823–826, 1985.

Hawtrey CE: Fifty-Two Cases of Primary Ureteral Carcinoma: A Clinical-Pathologic Study. *J Urol* 105: 188–193, 1971.

Hellstrom HR, Davis BK, Shonnard JW: Eosinophilic Cystitis: A Study of 16 Cases. *Am J Clin Pathol* 72: 777–784, 1979.

Heney NM, Szyfelbein WM, Daly JJ, et al: Positive Urinary Cytology in Patients Without Evident Tumor. *J Urol* 117: 223–224, 1977.

Heney NM, Ahmed S, Flanagan MJ, et al: Superficial Bladder Cancer: Progression and Recurrence. *J Urol* 130: 1083–1086, 1983.

Hermansen DK, Badalament RA, Bretton PR, et al: Voided Urine Flow Cytometry in Screening High-Risk Patients for the Presence of Bladder Cancer. *J Occup Med* 32: 894–897, 1990.

Highman W, Wilson E: Urine Cytology in Patients With Calculi. *J Clin Pathol* 35: 350–356, 1982.

Highman WJ: Transitional Carcinoma of the Upper Urinary Tract: A Histological and Cytopathological Study. *J Clin Pathol* 39: 297–305, 1986.

Highman WJ: Flat In Situ Carcinoma of the Bladder: Cytological Examination of Urine in Diagnosis, Follow Up, and Assessment of Response to Chemotherapy. *J Clin Pathol* 41: 540–546, 1988.

Ho KL: Morphogenesis of Michaelis-Gutmann Bodies in Cerebral Malacoplakia: An Ultrastructural Study. *Arch Pathol Lab Med* 113: 874–879, 1989.

Holmquist ND: Detection of Urinary Cancer With Urinalysis Sediment. *J Urol* 123: 188–189, 1980.

Holmquist ND: Detection of Urinary Tract Cancer in Urinalysis Specimens in an Outpatient Population. *Am J Clin Pathol* 89: 499–504, 1988.

Hom JD, King EB, Fraenkel R, et al: Adenocarcinoma With a Neuroendocrine Component Arising in the Urachus: A Case Report. *Acta Cytol* 34: 269–274, 1990.

Houston W, Koss LG, Melamed MR, et al: Bladder Cancer and Schistosomiasis: A Preliminary Cytological Study. *Trans Royal Soc Trop Med Hyg* 60: 89–91, 1966.

Hug EB, Donnelly SM, Shipley WU, et al: Deoxyribonucleic Acid Flow Cytometry in Invasive Bladder Carcinoma: A Possible Predictor for Successful Bladder Preservation Following Transurethral Surgery and Chemotherapy-Radiotherapy. *J Urol* 148: 47–51, 1992.

Hyman RM, Solomon C, Silberblatt J: Further Experience With Exfoliative Cytology of Urinary Tract: Increase in Exfoliation by Exercise. *Am J Clin Pathol* 26: 381–383, 1956.

Iwa N, Yutani C, Irie A, et al: Cytological Detection of Atypical Cells by Routine Urinalysis in a Cardiovascular Center. *Diagn Cytopathol* 7: 14–16, 1991.

Johnson JD, Lamm DL: Prediction of Bladder Tumor Invasion With the Mixed Cell Agglutination Test. *J Urol* 123: 25–28, 1980.

Johnston WW, Bossen EH, Amatulli J, et al: Exfoliative Cytopathologic Studies in Organ Transplantation: II. Factors in the Diagnosis of Cytomegalic Inclusion Disease in Urine of Renal Allograft Recipients. *Acta Cytol* 13: 605–610, 1969.

Jordan AM, Weingarten J, Murphy WM: Transitional Cell Neoplasms of the Urinary Bladder: Can Biologic Potential Be Predicted From Histologic Grading? *Cancer* 60: 2766–2774, 1987.

Kahan AV, Coleman DV, Koss LG: Activation of Human Polyomavirus Infection: Detection by Cytologic Technics. *Am J Clin Pathol* 74: 326–332, 1980.

Kannan V: Papillary Transitional-Cell Carcinoma of the Upper Urinary Tract: A Cytological Review. *Diagn Cytopathol* 6: 204–209, 1990.

Kannan V, Bose S: Low Grade Transitional Cell Carcinoma and Instrument Artifact: A Challenge in Urinary Cytology. *Acta Cytol* 37: 899–902, 1993.

Kapila K, Verma K: Cytologic Detection of Tuberculosis of the Urinary Bladder. *Acta Cytol* 28: 90–91, 1984.

Kay S, Frable WJ, Hume DM: Cervical Dysplasia and Cancer Developing in Women on Immunosuppression Therapy for Renal Homotransplantation. *Cancer* 26: 1048–1052, 1970.

Kepner LE, Cohen C: Monocytic Leukemia Cells in Urine: A Case Report. *Acta Cytol* 26: 335–337, 1982.

Kern WH, Bales CE, Webster WW: Cytologic Evaluation of Transitional Cell Carcinoma of the Bladder. *J Urol* 100: 616–622, 1968.

Kern WH: The Cytology of Transitional Cell Carcinoma of the Urinary Bladder. *Acta Cytol* 19: 420–428, 1975.

Kern WH: The Grade and Pathologic Stage of Bladder Cancer. *Cancer* 53: 1185–1189, 1984.

Kern WH: The Diagnostic Accuracy of Sputum and Urine Cytology. *Acta Cytol* 32: 651–654, 1988.

Kern WH: The Elusive 'False-Positive' Sputum and Urine Cytology. *Acta Cytol* 34: 587–589, 1990.

Kobayashi TK, Sugimoto T, Nishida K, et al: Intracytoplasmic Inclusions in Urinary Sediment Cells From a Patient With Mucocutaneous Lymph Node Syndrome (Kawasaki Disease): A Case Report. *Acta Cytol* 28: 687–690, 1984.

Kobayashi S, Ohmori M, Miki H, et al: Exfoliative Cytology of a Primary Adenocarcinoma of the Renal Pelvis: A Case Report. *Acta Cytol* 29: 1021–1025, 1985.

Kootte AMM, Zwartendijk J, Beekhuis-Brussee JAM, et al: Urinary Cytology in Renal Transplant Recipients With Stable Graft Functions. *Acta Cytol* 31: 620–624, 1987.

Koshikawa T, Leyh H, Schenck U: Difficulties in Evaluating Urinary Specimens After Local Mitomycin Therapy of Bladder Cancer. *Diagn Cytopathol* 5: 117–121, 1989.

Koss LG, Melamed MR, Mayer K: The Effect of Busulfan on Human Epithelia. *Am J Clin Pathol* 44: 385–397, 1965.

Koss LG, Melamed MR, Kelly RE: Further Cytologic and Histologic Studies of Bladder Lesions in Workers Exposed to Para-Aminodiphenyl: Progress Report. *J Nat Cancer Inst* 43: 233–243, 1969.

Koss LG, Tiamson EM, Robbins MA: Mapping Cancerous and Precancerous Bladder Changes: A Study of the Urothelium in Ten Surgically Removed Bladders. *JAMA* 227: 281–286,1974.

Koss LG, Bartells PH, Bibbo M, et al: Computer Discrimination Between Benign and Malignant Urothelial Cells. *Acta Cytol* 19: 378–391,1975.

Koss LG, Bartels PH, Bibbo M, et al: Computer Analysis of Atypical Urothelial Cells: I. Classification by Supervised Learning Algorithms. *Acta Cytol* 21: 247–260, 1977a.

Koss LG, Bartels PH, Sychra JJ, et al: Computer Analysis of Atypical Urothelial Cells: II. Classification by Unsupervised Learning Algorithms. *Acta Cytol* 21: 261–265, 1977b.

Koss LG: Mapping of the Urinary Bladder: Its Impact on the Concepts of Bladder Cancer. *Hum Pathol* 10: 533–548, 1979.

Koss LG, Deitch D, Ramanathan R, et al: Diagnostic Value of Cytology of Voided Urine. *Acta Cytol* 29: 810–816, 1985.

Koss LG: BK Viruria and Hemorrhagic Cystitis. *N Engl J Med* 316: 108–109, 1987.

Koss LG: Precursor Lesions of Invasive Bladder Cancer. *Eur Urol* 14 (Suppl 1): 4–6, 1988.

Koss LG, Wersto RP, Simmons DA, et al: Predictive Value of DNA Measurements in Bladder Washings: Comparison of Flow Cytometry, Image Cytophotometry, and Cytology in Patients With a Past History of Urothelial Tumors. *Cancer* 64: 916–924, 1989.

Krieger JN: Urologic Aspects of Trichomoniasis. *Invest Urol* 18: 411–417, 1981.

Krishna GG, Fellner SK: Lymphocyturia: An Important Diagnostic and Prognostic Marker in Renal Allograft Rejection. *Am J Nephrol* 2: 185–188, 1982.

Kupper T, Stoffels U, Pawlita M, et al: Morphological Changes in Urothelial Cells Replicating Human Polyomavirus BK. *Cytopathology* 4: 361–368, 1993.

Lage JM, Bauer WC, Kelley DR, et al: Histological Parameters and Pitfalls in the Interpretation of Bladder Biopsies in Bacillus Calmette-Guerin Treatment of Superficial Bladder Cancer. *J Urol* 135: 916–919, 1986.

Landing BH, Nakai H: Histochemical Properties of Renal Lead-Inclusions and Their Demonstration in Urinary Sediment. *Am J Clin Pathol* 31: 499–503, 1959.

Lang DJ, Kummer JF, Hartley DP: Cytomegalovirus in Semen: Persistence and Demonstration in Extracellular Fluids. *N Engl J Med* 291: 121–123, 1974.

Leistenschneider W, Nagel R: Lavage Cytology of the Renal Pelvis and Ureter With Special Reference to Tumors. *J Urol* 124: 597–600, 1980.

Lerman RI, Hutter RV, Whitmore WF Jr: Papilloma of the Urinary Bladder. *Cancer* 25: 333–342, 1970.

Lewin KJ, Harell GS, Lee AS, et al: Malacoplakia: An Electron-Microscopic Study: Demonstration of Bacilliform Organisms in Malacoplakic Macrophages. *Gastroenterology* 66: 28–45, 1974.

Lewis RW, Jackson AC Jr, Murphy WM, et al: Cytology in the Diagnosis and Follow-up of Transitional Cell Carcinoma of the Urothelium: A Review With a Case Series. *J Urol* 116: 43–46, 1976.

Lieberman N, Cabaud PG, Hamm FC: Value of the Urine Sediment Smear for the Diagnosis of Cancer. 89: 514–519, 1963.

Limas C, Lange P, Fraley EE, et al: A, B, H Antigens in Transitional Cell Tumors of the Urinary Bladder: Correlation With the Clinical Course. *Cancer* 44: 2099–2107, 1979.

Lin C-W, Kirley SD, Khaw AH, et al: Detection of Exfoliated Bladder Cancer Cells by Monoclonal Antibodies to Tumor-Associated Surface Antigens. *J Occup Med* 32: 910–916, 1990.

Littleton RH, Farah RN, Cerny JC: Eosinophilic Cystitis: An Uncommon form of Cystitis. *J Urol* 127: 132–133, 1982.

Long SR, Cohen MB: Classics in Cytology. V: William Sanders and Early Urinary Tract Cytology. *Diagn Cytopathol* 8: 135–136, 1992.

Longin A, Fontaniere B, Berger-Dutrieux N, et al: A Useful Monoclonal Antibody (BLs-10D1) to Identify Tumor Cells in Urine Cytology. *Cancer* 65: 1412–1417, 1990.

Lönn U, Lönn S, Nylén U, et al: Gene Amplification Detected in Carcinoma Cells From Human Urinary Bladder Washings by the Polymerase Chain Reaction Method. *Cancer* 71: 3605–3610, 1993.

Loveless KJ: The Effects of Radiation Upon the Cytology of Benign and Malignant Bladder Epithelia. *Acta Cytol* 17: 355–360, 1973.

Lowe D, Fletcher CDM, Gower RL: Tumour-Associated Eosinophilia in the Bladder. *J Clin Pathol* 37: 500–502, 1984.

Lowe D, Fletcher CDM, Carpenter G: Urine Eosinophilia in Bladder Cancer. *Acta Cytol* 29: 187, 1985.

Lower GM Jr: Concepts in Causality: Chemically Induced Human Urinary Bladder Cancer. *Cancer* 49: 1056–1066, 1982.

Masukawa T, Garancis JC, Rytel MW, et al: Herpes Genitalis Virus Isolation From Human Bladder Urine. *Acta Cytol* 16: 416–428, 1972.

Matzkin H, Moinuddin SM, Soloway MS: Value of Urine Cytology Versus Bladder Washing in Bladder Cancer. *Urology* 39: 201–203, 1992.

Mauri MF, Bonzanini M, Luciani L, et al: Renal Collecting Duct Carcinoma: Report of a Case With Urinary Cytologic Findings. *Acta Cytol* 38: 755–758, 1994.

McClennan BL, Oertel YC, Malmgren RA, et al: The Effect of Water Soluble Contrast Material on Urine Cytology. *Acta Cytol* 22: 230–233, 1978.

McDonald JR: Exfoliative Cytology in Genitourinary and Pulmonary Diseases. *Am J Clin Pathol* 24: 684–687, 1954.

McDougal WS, Cramer SF, Miller R: Invasive Carcinoma of the Renal Pelvis Following Cyclophosphamide Therapy for Nonmalignant Disease. *Cancer* 48: 691–695, 1981.

Meisels A: Cytology of Carcinoma of the Kidney. *Acta Cytol* 7: 239–244, 1963.

Melamed MR, Koss LG, Ricci A, et al: Cytohistological Observations on Developing Carcinoma of the Urinary Bladder in Man. *Cancer* 13: 67–74, 1960.

Melamed MR, Wolinska WH: On the Significance of Intracytoplasmic Inclusions in the Urinary Sediment. *Am J Pathol* 38: 711–719, 1961.

Melamed MR: The Urinary Sediment Cytology in a Case of Malakoplakia. *Acta Cytol* 6: 471–474, 1962.

Melamed MR, Whitmore WF Jr: Carcinoma In Situ of Bladder: Clinico-Pathologic Study of Case With a Suggested Approach to Detection. *J Urol* 96: 466–471, 1966.

Melamed MR, Klein FA: Flow Cytometry of Urinary Bladder Irrigation Specimens. *Hum Pathol* 15: 302–305, 1984.

Melamed MR: Flow Cytometry Detection and Evaluation of Bladder Tumors. *J Occup Med* 32: 829–833, 1990.

Melamed MR: Flow Cytometry for Detection and Evaluation of Urinary Bladder Carcinoma. *Semin Surg Oncol* 8: 300–307, 1992.

Messing EM, Young TB, Hunt VB, et al: The Significance of Asymptomatic Microhematuria in Men 50 or More Years Old: Findings of a Home Screening Study Using Urinary Dipsticks. *J Urol* 137: 919–922, 1987.

Milsten R, Frable WJ, Texter JH, et al: Evaluation of Lipid Stain in Renal Neoplasms as Adjunct to Routine Exfoliative Cytology. *J Urol* 110: 169–171, 1973.

Minassian H, Schinella R, Reilly JC: Polyomavirus in the Urine: Follow-Up Study. *Diagn Cytopathol* 10: 209–211, 1994.

Mincione GP: Primary Malignant Lymphoma of the Urinary Bladder With a Positive Cytologic Report. *Acta Cytol* 26: 69–72, 1982.

Mohr DN, Offord KP, Owen RA, et al: Asymptomatic Microhematuria and Urologic Disease: A Population-Based Study. *JAMA* 256: 224–229, 1986.

Morrison AS: Public Health Value of Using Epidemiologic Information to Identify High-Risk Groups for Bladder Cancer Screening. *Semin Oncol* 6: 184–188, 1979.

Morrison DA, Murphy WM, Ford KS, et al: Surveillance of Stage O, Grade I Bladder Cancer by Cytology Alone: Is It Acceptable? *J Urol* 132: 672–674, 1984.

Müller F, Kraft R, Zingg E: Exfoliative Cytology After Transurethral Resection of Superficial Bladder Tumors. *Br J Urol* 57: 530–534, 1985.

Murakami S, Igarashi T, Hara S, et al: Strategies for Asymptomatic Microscopic Hematuria: A Prospective Study of 1,034 Patients. *J Urol* 144: 99–101, 1990.

Murphy WM: Herpesvirus in Bladder Cancer. *Acta Cytol* 20: 207–210, 1976.

Murphy WM: Falsely Positive Urinary Cytology: Pathologist's Error or Preclinical Cancer? *J Urol* 118: 811–813, 1977.

Murphy WM, Soloway MS, Lin CJ: Morphologic Effects of Thiotepa on Mammalian Urothelium: Changes in Abnormal Cells. *Acta Cytol* 22: 550–554, 1978.

Murphy WM, Nagy GK, Rao MK, et al: 'Normal' Urothelium in Patients With Bladder Cancer: A Preliminary Report From the National Bladder Cancer Collaborative Group A. *Cancer* 44: 1050–1058, 1979.

Murphy WM, Crabtree WN, Jukkola AF, et al: The Diagnostic Value of Urine Versus Bladder Washing in Patients With Bladder Cancer. *J Urol* 126: 320–322, 1981a.

Murphy WM, Irving CC: The Cellular Features of Developing Carcinoma in Murine Urinary Bladder. *Cancer* 47: 514–522, 1981b.

Murphy WM, Soloway MS, Finebaum PJ: Pathological Changes Associated With Topical Chemotherapy for Superficial Bladder Cancer. *J Urol* 126: 461–464, 1981c.

Murphy WM, Soloway MS: Developing Carcinoma (Dysplasia) of the Urinary Bladder. *Pathol Annu* 17(1): 197–219, 1982a.

Murphy WM, Soloway MS: Urothelial Dysplasia. *J Urol* 127: 849–854, 1982b.

Murphy WM: Current Topics in the Pathology of Bladder Cancer. *Pathol Annu* 18(1): 1–25, 1983.

Murphy WM, Soloway MS, Jukkola AF, et al: Urinary Cytology and Bladder Cancer: The Cellular Features of Transitional Cell Neoplasms. *Cancer* 53: 1555–1565, 1984.

Murphy WM: Urinary Cytology in Diagnostic Pathology. *Diagn Cytopathol* 1: 173–175, 1985.

Murphy WM, Chandler RW, Trafford RM: Flow Cytometry of Deparaffinized Nuclei Compared to Histological Grading for the Pathological Evaluation of Transitional Cell Carcinomas. *J Urol* 135: 694–697, 1986.

Murphy WM: Current Status of Urinary Cytology in the Evaluation of Bladder Neoplasms. *Hum Pathol* 21: 886–896, 1990.

Nafe R, Roth S, Rathert P: Analysis of Criteria for Grading Bladder Cancer in Urine Cytological Tumor Diagnosis by Means of an Expert System. *Eur Urol* 21: 103–109, 1992.

Nagy GK, Frable WJ, Murphy WM: Classification of Premalignant Urothelial Abnormalities: A Delphi Study of the National Bladder Cancer Collaborative Group A. *Path Annu* 17(1): 219–233, 1982.

Nagy GK, Jacobs JB, Mason-Savas P, et al: Intracytoplasmic Eosinophilic Inclusion Bodies in Breast Cyst Fluids Are Giant Lysosomes. *Acta Cytol* 33: 99–103, 1989.

Naib ZM: Exfoliative Cytology of Renal Pelvic Lesions. *Cancer* 14: 1085–1087, 1961.

National Cancer Institute: Cytology and Histopathology of Bladder Cancer Cases in a Prospective Longitudinal Study: National Bladder Cancer Collaborative Group A. *Cancer Res* 37: 2911–2915, 1977.

Neal MH, Swearingen ML, Gawronski L, et al: Myeloma Cells in the Urine. *Arch Pathol Lab Med* 109: 870–872, 1985.

Neumann MP, Limas C: Transitional Cell Carcinomas of the Urinary Bladder: Effects of Preoperative Irradiation on Morphology. *Cancer* 58: 2758–2763, 1986.

Nguyen-Ho P, Nguyen G-K, Villanueva RR: Small Cell Anaplastic Carcinoma of the Prostate: Report of a Case With Positive Urine Cytology. *Diagn Cytopathol* 10: 159–161, 1994.

Nolan CR III, Anger MS, Kelleher S: Eosinophiluria: A New Method of Detection and Definition of the Clinical Spectrum. *N Engl J Med* 315: 1516–1519, 1986.

O'Donoghue JM, Horgan PG, Corcoran M, et al: Urinary Cytology in the Detection of Bladder Carcinoma. *Irish J Med Sci* 160: 352–353, 1991.

O'Morchoe PJ, Riad W, Cowles LT, et al: Urinary Cytologic Changes After Radiotherapy of Renal Transplants. *Acta Cytol* 20: 132–136, 1976a.

O'Morchoe PJ, Erozan YS, Cooke CR, et al: Exfoliative Cytology in the Diagnosis of Immunologic Rejection in the Transplanted Kidney. *Acta Cytol* 20: 454–461, 1976b.

Olumi AF, Tsai YC, Nichols PW, et al: Allelic Loss of Chromosome 17p Distinguishes High Grade From Low Grade Transitional Cell Carcinomas of the Bladder. *Cancer Res* 50: 7081–7083, 1990.

Orell SR: Transitional Cell Epithelioma of the Bladder: Correlation of Cytologic and Histologic Diagnosis. *Scand J Urol Nephrol* 3: 93–98, 1969.

Orr WA, Mulholland SG, Walzak MP Jr: Genitourinary Tract Involvement With Systemic Mycosis. *J Urol* 107: 1047–1050, 1972.

Ozono S, Lee IC, Weinstein RS, et al: Stimulation of Rat Bladder Epithelial DNA Synthesis by Intravesical Instillation of Distilled Water (42347). *Proc Soc Exper Biol Med* 182: 325–327, 1986.

Packham DA: The Epithelial Lining of the Female Trigone and Urethra. *Br J Urol* 43: 201–205, 1971.

Pagano F, Bassi P, Milani C, et al: Pathologic and Structural Changes in the Bladder After BCG Intravesical Therapy in Men. *Prog Clin Biol Res* 310: 81–91, 1989.

Palombini L: Ciliated Cells in Voided Urine. *Acta Cytol* 26: 263–264, 1982.

Papanicolaou GN, Marshall VF: Urine Sediment Smears as a Diagnostic Procedure in Cancers of the Urinary Tract. *Science* 101: 519–521, 1945.

Papanicolaou GN: Cytology of the Urine Sediment in Neoplasms of the Urinary Tract. *J Urol* 57: 375–379, 1947.

Park C-H, Britsch C, Uson AC, et al: Reliability of Positive Exfoliative Cytologic Study of the Urine in Urinary Tract Malignancy. *J Urol* 102: 91–92, 1969.

Pauwels RPE, Smeets AWGB, Schapers RFM, et al: Grading in Superficial Bladder Cancer: (2) Cytogenetic Classification. *Br J Urol* 61: 135–139, 1988.

Pearson JC, Kromhout L, King EB: Evaluation of Collection and Preservation Techniques for Urinary Cytology. *Acta Cytol* 25: 327–333, 1981.

Pecorella I, Ciardi A, Monge A, et al: Detection of Nephrotoxicity in Cyclosporine-A Amyotrophic Lateral Sclerosis Patients by Means of Urinary Cytology. *APMIS* 100: 81–86, 1992.

Pellet H, Buenerd A, Minaire E, et al: Clinical Prevalence of Glomerular Hematuria: A Nine-Year Retrospective Study. *Diagn Cytopathol* 7: 27–31, 1991.

Person DA, Kaufman RH, Gardner HL, et al: Herpesvirus Type 2 in Genitourinary Tract Infections. *Am J Obstet Gynecol* 116: 993–995, 1973.

Petersen SE, Lundbeck F, Brandsborg O, et al: Transabdominal Ultrasonography Plus Urine Cytology in Control of Benign Bladder Tumours. *Scand J Urol Nephrol Suppl* 125: 121–125, 1989.

Pettersson S, Hansson G, Blohmé I: Condyloma Acuminatum of the Bladder. *J Urol* 115: 535–536, 1976.

Peven DR, Hidvegi DF: Clear-Cell Adenocarcinoma of the Female Urethra. *Acta Cytol* 29: 142–146, 1985.

Piper JM, Tonascia J, Matanoski GM: Heavy Phenacetin Use and Bladder Cancer in Women Aged 20 to 49 Years. *N Engl J Med* 313: 292–295, 1985.

Piscioli F, Detassis C, Polla E, et al: Cytologic Presentation of Renal Adenocarcinoma in Urinary Sediment. *Acta Cytol* 27: 383–390, 1983.

Piscioli F, Pusiol T, Polla E, et al: Urinary Cytology of Tuberculosis of the Bladder. *Acta Cytol* 29: 125–131, 1985a.

Piscioli F, Pusiol T, Scappini P, et al: Urine Cytology in the Detection of Renal Adenocarcinoma. *Cancer* 56: 2251–2255, 1985b.

Piva AE, Koss LG: Cytologic Diagnosis of Metastatic Malignant Melanoma in Urinary Sediment. *Acta Cytol* 8: 398–402, 1964.

Prall RH, Wernett C, Mims MM: Diagnostic Cytology in Urinary Tract Malignancy. *Cancer* 29: 1084–1089, 1972.

Pringle JP, Graham RC, Bernier GM: Detection of Myeloma Cells in the Urine Sediment. *Blood* 43: 137–143, 1974.

Prout GR Jr: Introduction: Management (Control) of Early Bladder Lesions. *Cancer Res* 37: 2891–2894, 1977.

Psihramis KE, Hartwick W: Ureteral Fibroepithelial Polyp With Positive Urine Cytology. *Urology* 41: 387–391, 1993.

Raab SS, Lenel JC, Cohen MB: Low Grade Transitional Cell Carcinoma of the Bladder. Cytologic Diagnosis by Key Features as Identified by Logistic Regression Analysis. *Cancer* 74: 1621–1626, 1994.

Rangwala AF, Zinterhoffer LJ, Nyi KM, Ferreira PPC: Sinus Histiocytosis With Massive Lymphadenopathy and Malignant Lymphoma: An Unreported Association. *Cancer* 65: 999–1002, 1990.

Rasmussen K, Peterson BL, Jacobo E, et al: Cytologic Effects of Thiotepa and Adriamycin on Normal Canine Urothelium. *Acta Cytol* 24: 237–243, 1980.

Reichborn-Kjennerud S, Høeg K: The Value of Urine Cytology in the Diagnosis of Recurrent Bladder Tumors: A Preliminary Report. *Acta Cytol* 16: 269–272, 1972.

Rife CC, Farrow GM, Utz DC: Urine Cytology of Transitional Cell Neoplasms. *Urol Clin North Am* 6: 599–612, 1979.

Ro JY, Staerkel GA, Ayala AG: Cytologic and Histologic Features of Superficial Bladder Cancer. *Urol Clin North Am* 19: 435–453, 1992.

Robertson SJ, Higgins RB, Powell C: Malacoplakia of Liver: A Case Report. *Hum Pathol* 22: 1294–1295, 1991.

Rojewska J, Pykalo R, Czaplicki M: Urine and Semen Cytomorphology in Patients With Testicular Tumors. *Diagn Cytopathol* 5: 9–13, 1989.

Roland SI, Marshall VF: The Reliability of the Papanicolaou Technique When Cancer Cells Are Found in the Urine. *Surg Gynecol Obstet* 104: 41–44, 1957.

Rollins S, Schumann GB: Primary Urinary Cytodiagnosis of a Bladder Small-Cell Carcinoma. *Diagn Cytopathol* 7: 79–82, 1991.

Romero J, Alos L, Mallofre C, et al: Bladder Wash Cytology and Flow Cytometry for the Diagnosis of Transitional Cell Carcinoma of the Urinary Bladder. *Eur Urol* 21(Suppl 1): 13–15, 1992.

Rosa B, Cazin M, Dalian G: Urinary Cytology for Carcinoma In Situ of the Urinary Bladder. *Acta Cytol* 29: 117–124, 1985.

Rouse BA, Donaldson LD, Goellner JR: Intranuclear Inclusions in Urinary Cytology. *Acta Cytol* 30: 105–109, 1986.

Roussel F, Picquenot JM, Rousseau O: Identification of Human Papillomavirus Antigen in a Bladder Tumor. *Acta Cytol* 35: 273–276, 1991.

Rupp M, O'Hara B, McCullogh L, et al: Prostatic Carcinoma Cells in Urine Specimens: Cytologic, Histologic and Immunocytochemical Features. *Acta Cytol* 34: 744–745, 1990.

Rutgers JL, Young RH: Nephrogenic Adenoma of the Urinary Bladder: A Comparison of Its Cytologic and Histopathologic Features in Ten Cases. *Diagn Cytopathol* 4: 210–216, 1988.

Sack MJ, Artymyshyn RL, Tomaszewski JE, et al: Diagnostic Value of Bladder Wash Cytology, With Special Reference to Low Grade Urothelial Neoplasms. *Acta Cytol* 39: 187–194, 1995.

Sagerman PM, Saigo PE, Sheinfeld J, et al: Enhanced Detection of Bladder Cancer in Urine Cytology With Lewis X, M344 and 19A211 Antigens. *Acta Cytol* 38: 517–523, 1994.

Sahin AA, Myhre M, Ro JY, et al: Plasmacytoid Transitional Cell Carcinoma: Report of a Case With Initial Presentation Mimicking Multiple Myeloma. *Acta Cytol* 35: 277–280, 1991.

Salm R: Combined Intestinal and Squamous Metaplasia of the Renal Pelvis. *J Clin Pathol* 22: 187–191, 1969.

Sandoz PF, Bielmann D, Mihatsch M, et al: Value of Urinary Sediment in the Diagnosis of Interstitial Rejection in Renal Transplants. *Transplantation* 41: 343–348, 1986.

Sane SY: Urinary Sediment in Storage Diseases: Differential Diagnosis of Niemann-Pick Disease by Cytologic Means. *Diagn Cytopathol* 6: 122–123, 1990.

Sano ME, Koprowska I: Primary Cytologic Diagnosis of a Malignant Renal Lymphoma. *Acta Cytol* 9: 194–196, 1965.

Sarnacki CT, McCormack LJ, Kiser WS, et al: Urinary Cytology and the Clinical Diagnosis of Urinary Tract Malignancy: A Clinicopathologic Study of 1,400 Patients. *J Urol* 106: 761–764, 1971.

Say CC, Hori JM: Transitional Cell Carcinoma of the Renal Pelvis: Experience From 1940 to 1972 and Literature Review. *J Urol* 112: 438–442, 1974.

Schneider V, Smith MJV, Frable WJ: Urinary Cytology in Endometriosis of the Bladder. *Acta Cytol* 24: 30–33,1980.

Schmidlapp CJ II, Marshall VF: The Detection of Cancer Cells in the Urine: A Clinical Appraisal of the Papanicolaou Method. *J Urol* 59: 599–603, 1948.

Schmidlapp CJ II, Marshall VF: The Diagnostic Value of Urinary Sediment: A Review Based on the Papanicolaou Method. *N Y State J Med* 50: 56–58, 1950.

Schumann GB, Burleson RL, Henry JB, et al: Urinary Cytodiagnosis of Acute Renal Allograft Rejection Using the Cytocentrifuge. *Am J Clin Pathol* 67: 134–140, 1977.

Schumann GB, Lerner SI, Weiss MA, et al: Inclusion-Bearing Cells in Industrial Workers Exposed to Lead. *Am J Clin Pathol* 74: 192–196, 1980.

Schumann GB, Johnston JL, Weiss MA: Renal Epithelial Fragments in Urine Sediment. *Acta Cytol* 25: 147–152, 1981a.

Schumann GB, Weiss MA, Johnston JL: Cytodifferentiation of Urinary Epithelial Fragments: Papillary Transitional Cell Carcinoma in a Renal Allograft Recipient. *Acta Cytol* 25: 302–306, 1981b.

Schwalb DM, Herr HW, Fair WR: The Management of Clinically Unconfirmed Positive Urinary Cytology. *J Urol* 150: 1751–1756, 1993.

Schwalb MD, Herr HW, Sogani PC, et al: Positive Urinary Cytology Following a Complete Response to Intravesical Bacillus Calmette-Guerin Therapy: Pattern of Recurrence. *J Urol* 152: 382–387, 1994.

Seldenrijk CA, Verheggen WJHM, Veldhuizen RW, et al: Use of Cytomorphometry and Cytology in the Diagnosis of Transitional-Cell Carcinoma of the Upper Urinary Tract. *Acta Cytol* 31: 137–142, 1987.

Seo IS, Clark SA, McGovern FD, et al: Leimyosarcoma of the Urinary Bladder: 13 Years After Cyclophosphamide Therapy for Hodgkin's Disease. *Cancer* 55: 1597–1603, 1985.

Sharifi R, Shaw M, Ray V, et al: Evaluation of Cytologic Techniques for Diagnosis of Prostate Cancer. *Urology* 21: 417–420, 1983.

Sharma AK: Urinary Cytology: Simple Screening Procedure for Lymphadenopathy. *Urology* 38: 394, 1991.

Shenoy UA, Colby TV, Schumann GB: Reliability of Urinary Cytodiagnosis in Urothelial Neoplasms. *Cancer* 56: 2041–2045, 1985.

Siegel RJ, Napoli VM: Malignant Lymphoma of the Urinary Bladder: A Case With Signet-Ring Cells Simulating Urachal Adenocarcinoma. *Arch Pathol Lab Med* 115: 635–637, 1991.

Siegelbaum MH, Edmonds P, Seidmon EJ: Use of Immunohistochemistry for Identification of Primary Lymphoma of the Bladder. *J Urol* 136: 1074–1076, 1986.

Sinclair-Smith C, Kahn LB, Cywes S: Malacoplakia in Childhood: Case Report With Ultrastructural Observations and Review of the Literature. *Arch Pathol* 99: 198–203, 1975.

Smith BH, Dehner LP: Chronic Ulcerating Interstitial Cystitis (Hunner's Ulcer): A Study of 28 Cases. *Arch Pathol* 93: 76–81, 1972.

Smith JC, Badenoch AW: Carcinoma of the Bladder Simulating Chronic Cystitis. *Br J Urol* 37: 93–99, 1965.

Soloway MS: The Evaluation and Follow-Up of Patients With Ra, Tcis, and T1 Bladder Cancer. *World J Urol* 11: 153–155, 1993.

Spagnolo DV, Waring PM: Bladder Carcinoma After Bladder Surgery. *Am J Clin Pathol* 86: 430–437, 1986.

Staerkel G, Fanning C, Thomsen S, et al: Spindling Artifact of Urothelial Cells in Post-Laser Treatment Urinary Cytology. *Mod Pathol* 2: 90A, 1989.

Stanton MJ, Maxted W: Malacoplakia: A Study of the Literature and Current Concepts of Pathogenesis, Diagnosis and Treatment. *J Urol* 125: 139–146, 1981.

Stella F, Troccoli R, Stella C, et al: Urinary Cytologic Abnormalities in Bone Marrow Transplant Recipients of Cyclosporin. *Acta Cytol* 31: 615–619, 1987.

Stella F, Battistelli S, Marcheggiani F, et al: Urothelial Cell Changes Due to Busulfan and Cyclophosphamide Treatment in Bone Marrow Transplantation. *Acta Cytol* 34: 885–890, 1990.

Stella F, Battistelli S, Marcheggiani F, et al: Urothelial Toxicity Following Conditioning Therapy in Bone Marrow Transplantation and Bladder Cancer: Morphologic and Morphometric Comparison by Exfoliative Urinary Cytology. *Diagn Cytopathol* 8: 216–221, 1992.

Stillwell TJ, Benson RC Jr: Cyclophosphamide-Induced Hemorrhagic Cystitis: A Review of 100 Patients. *Cancer* 61:451–457,1988.

Stilmant MM, Murphy JL, Merriam JC: Cytology of Nephrogenic Adenoma of the Urinary Bladder: A Report of Four Cases. *Acta Cytol* 30: 35–40, 1986.

Stilmant MM, Freedlund MC, Schmitt GW: Cytologic Evaluation of Urine After Kidney Transplantation. *Acta Cytol* 31: 625–630, 1987.

Sufrin G, Keogh B, Moore RH, et al: Secondary Involvement of the Bladder in Malignant Lymphoma. *J Urol* 118: 251–253, 1977.

Suhrland MJ, Koslow M, Perchick A, et al: Cytologic Findings in Progressive Multifocal Leukoencephalopathy: Report of Two Cases. *Acta Cytol* 31: 505–511, 1987.

Summers JL, Ford ML: The Papanicolaou Smear as a Diagnostic Tool in Male Trichomoniasis. *J Urol* 107: 840–842, 1972.

Summers JL, Coon JS, Ward RM, et al: Prognosis in Carcinoma of the Urinary Bladder Based Upon Tissue Blood Group ABH and Thomsen-Friedenreich Antigen Status and Karyotype of the Initial Tumor. *Cancer Res* 43: 934–939, 1983.

Suprun H, Bitterman W: A Correlative Cytohistologic Study on the Interrelationship Between Exfoliated Urinary Bladder Carcinoma Cell Types and the Staging and Grading of These Tumors. *Acta Cytol* 19: 265–273, 1975.

Taft PD, Flax MH: Urinary Cytology in Renal Transplantation: Association of Renal Tubular Cells and Graft Rejection. *Transplantation* 4: 194–204, 1966.

Taylor FM III, Arroyo JG: Inverted Papilloma of the Renal Pelvis: Cytologic Features of Ureteral Washings. *Acta Cytol* 30: 166–168, 1986.

Thompson RA, Campbell EW Jr, Kramer HC, et al: Late Invasive Recurrence Despite Long-Term Surveillance for Superficial Bladder Cancer. *J Urol* 149: 1010–1011, 1993.

Toivonen T, Hästö AL: Large-Volume Cytocentrifuge for Processing Alcohol-Fixed Cytologic Specimens: Application in Urinary Cytology. *Acta Cytol* 35: 269–272, 1991.

Traystman MD, Gupta PK, Shah KV, et al: Identification of Viruses in the Urine of Renal Transplant Recipients by Cytomorphology. *Acta Cytol* 24: 501–510, 1980.

Tribukait B, Gustafson H, Esposti P: Ploidy and Proliferation in Human Bladder Tumors as Measured by Flow-Cytofluorometric DNA-Analysis and Its Relations to Histopathology and Cytology. *Cancer* 43: 1742–1751, 1979.

Trillo AA, Kuchler LL, Wood AC, et al: Adenocarcinoma of the Urinary Bladder: Histologic, Cytologic and Ultrastructural Features in a Case. *Acta Cytol* 25: 285–290, 1981.

Troster M, Wyatt JK, Alen-Halagah J: Nephrogenic Adenoma of the Urinary Bladder: Histologic and Cytologic Observations in a Case. *Acta Cytol* 30: 41–44, 1986.

Trott PA: Cytological Examination of Urine Using a Membrane Filter. *Br J Urol* 39: 610–614, 1967.

Trott PA, Edwards L: Comparison of Bladder Washings and Urine Cytology in the Diagnosis of Bladder Cancer. *J Urol* 110: 664–666, 1973.

Utz DC, Farrow GM: Management of Carcinoma In Situ of the Bladder: The Case for Surgical Management. *Urol Clin North Am* 7: 533–541, 1980a.

Utz DC, Farrow GM, Rife CC, et al: Carcinoma In Situ of the Bladder. *Cancer* 45: 1842–1848, 1980b.

Umiker W, Lapides J, Sourenne R: Exfoliative Cytology of Papillomas and Intra-Epithelial Carcinomas of the Urinary Bladder. *Acta Cytol* 6: 255–266, 1962.

Umiker W: Accuracy of Cytologic Diagnosis of Cancer of the Urinary Tract. *Acta Cytol* 8: 186–193, 1964.

Valente PT, Atkinson BF, Guerry D: Melanuria. *Acta Cytol* 29: 1026–1027, 1985.

Varma VA, Fekete PS, Franks MJ, et al: Cytologic Features of Prostatic Adenocarcinoma in Urine: A Clinicopathologic and Immunocytochemical Study. *Diagn Cytopathol* 4: 300–305, 1988.

Veltman GAM, Bosch FH, van der Plas-Cats MB, et al: Urine Cytology as a Screening Method for Transitional-Cell Carcinoma in Dialysis Patients With Analgesic Nephropathy. *Nephrol Dial Transplant* 6: 346–348, 1991.

Viddeleer AC, Lycklama A, Nijeholt GAB, et al: A Late Manifestation of Testicular Seminoma in the Bladder in a Renal Transplant Recipient: A Case Report. *J Urol* 148: 401–402, 1992.

Viscoli CM, Lachs MS, Horwitz RI: Bladder Cancer and Coffee Drinking: A Summary of Case-Control Research. *Lancet* 341: 1432–1437, 1993.

Vousta NG, Melamed MR: Cytology of In Situ Carcinoma of the Human Urinary Bladder. *Cancer* 16: 1307–1316, 1963.

Wallace DMA, Wallace DM, Whitfield HN, et al: The Late Results of Conservative Surgery for Upper Tract Urothelial Carcinomas. *Br J Urol* 53: 537–541, 1981.

Wallace DMA, Smith JHF, Billington S, et al: Promotion of Bladder Tumours by Endoscopic Procedures in an Animal Model. *Br J Urol* 56: 658–662, 1984.

Walsh EJ, Ockuly EA, Ockuly EF, et al: Treatment of Metastatic Melanoma of the Bladder. *J Urol* 96: 472–478, 1966.

Weimar G, Culp DA, Loening S, et al: Urogenital Involvement by Malignant Lymphomas. *J Urol* 125: 230–231, 1981.

Weinstein RS, Miller AW III, Pauli BU: Carcinoma In Situ: Comments on the Pathobiology of a Paradox. *Urol Clin North Am* 7: 523–531, 1980.

Weldon TE, Soloway MS: Susceptibility of Urothelium to Neoplastic Cellular Implantation. *Urology* 5: 824–827, 1975.

Whelan P, Britton JP, Dowell AC: Three-Year Follow-Up of Bladder Tumours Found on Screening. *Br J Urol* 72: 893–896, 1993.

White RWD, Olsson CA, Deitch AD: Flow Cytometry: Role in Monitoring Transitional Cell Carcinoma of Bladder. *Urol* 28: 15–20, 1986.

Widran J, Sanchez R, Gruhn J: Squamous Metaplasia of the Bladder: A Study of 450 Patients. *J Urol* 112: 479–482, 1974.

Wiener DP, Koss LG, Sablay B, et al: The Prevalence and Significance of Brunn's Nests, Cystitis Cystica and Squamous Metaplasia in Normal Bladders. *J Urol* 122: 317–321, 1979.

Wiener HG, Vooijs GP, van't Hof-Grootenboer B: Accuracy of Urinary Cytology in the Diagnosis of Primary and Recurrent Bladder Cancer. *Acta Cytol* 37: 163–169, 1993.

Wiggishoff CC, McDonald JH: Urinary Exfoliative Cytology in the Diagnosis of Bladder Tumors. *Acta Cytol* 16: 139–141, 1972.

Wingo PA, Tong T, Bolden S: Cancer Statistics. *CA Cancer J Clin* 45: 8–30, 1995.

Winkelmann M, Grabensee B, Pfitzer P: Differential Diagnosis of Acute Allograft Rejection and CMV-Infection in Renal Transplantation by Urinary Cytology. *Path Res Pract* 180: 161–168, 1985.

Wolf H, Højgaard K: Urothelial Dysplasia Concomitant With Bladder Tumours as a Determinant Factor for Future New Occurrences. *Lancet* (ii): 134–136, 1983.

Wolfson WL, Rosenthal DL: Cell Clusters in Urinary Cytology. *Acta Cytol* 22: 138–141, 1978.

Wolinska WH, Melamed MR: Urinary Conduit Cytology. *Cancer* 32: 1000–1006, 1973.

Wolinska WH, Melamed MR, Schellhammer PF, et al: Urethral Cytology Following Cystectomy for Bladder Carcinoma. *Am J Surg Pathol* 1: 225–234, 1977.

Wolinska WH, Melamed MR, Klein FA: Cytology of Bladder Papilloma. *Acta Cytol* 29: 817–822, 1985.

Woodard BH, Ideker RE, Johnston WW: Cytologic Detection of Malignant Melanoma in Urine: A Case Report. *Acta Cytol* 22: 350–352, 1978.

Wynder EL, Goldsmith R: The Epidemiology of Bladder Cancer: A Second Look. *Cancer* 40: 1246–1268, 1977.

Yam LT, Janckila AJ: Immunocytochemical Diagnosis of Lymphoma From Urine Sediment. *Acta Cytol* 29: 827–832, 1985.

Yamada T, Fukui I, Kobayashi T, et al: The Relationship of ABH(O) Blood Group Antigen Expression in Intraepithelial Dysplastic Lesions to Clinicopathologic Properties of Associated Transitional Cell Carcinoma of the Bladder. *Cancer* 67: 1661–1666, 1991.

Yang C, Motteram R, Sandeman TF: Extramedullary Plasmacytoma of the Bladder: A Case Report and Review of Literature. *Cancer* 50: 146–149, 1982.

Young RH, Eble JN: Unusual Forms of Carcinoma of the Urinary Bladder. *Hum Pathol* 22: 948–965, 1991a.

Young RH, Zukerberg LR: Microcystic Transitional Cell Carcinomas of the Urinary Bladder: A Report of Four Cases. *Am J Clin Pathol* 96: 635–639, 1991b.

Zein TA, Milad MF: Urine Cytology in Bladder Tumors. *Int Surg* 76: 52–54, 1991.

Zincke H, Aguilo JJ, Farrow GM, et al: Significance of Urinary Cytology in the Early Detection of Transitional Cell Cancer of the Upper Urinary Tract. *J Urol* 116: 781–783, 1976.

11

Cerebrospinal Fluid

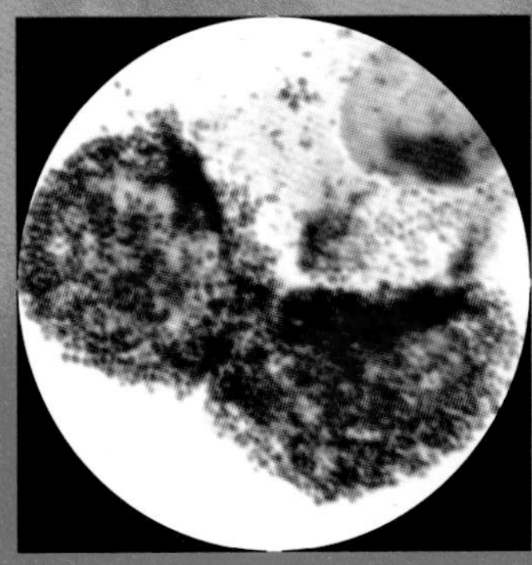

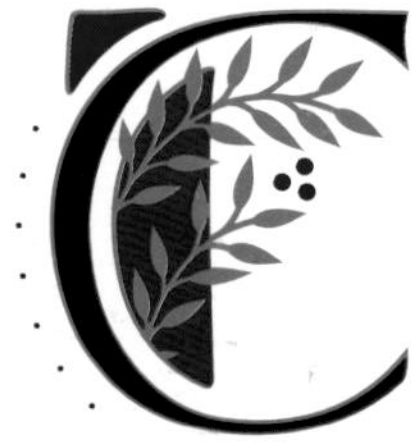erebrospinal fluid (CSF) study is not used to screen, but to investigate patients who have signs or symptoms of central nervous system (CNS) disease. CSF specimens are usually obtained by lumbar puncture, but can also be obtained from the lateral ventricles of the brain or the cisterna magna [Cumings 1954]. Cytologic examination of CSF is useful in diagnosing tumors (space-occupying lesions), infections, vascular disorders, trauma, and demyelinating diseases. It is also useful in monitoring CNS chemotherapy (eg, for lymphoma/leukemia or infections), and is part of a complete neurologic examination. Because there will seldom be tissue confirmation, accuracy in diagnosis of CSF specimens is particularly important. A complete and accurate clinical history is crucial in the diagnosis of CSF. The clinician must provide the clinical diagnosis, signs, symptoms, and pertinent laboratory and radiologic findings. For example, certain nonneoplastic diseases such as Parkinson's disease have been reported to shed atypical cells (in this case, elongated cells with markedly hyperchromatic nuclei), which could be confused with malignancy [Wertlake 1972]. It is also critical to know if other procedures have been performed recently, which could affect the CNS, causing reactive changes [T11.1].

Indications for CSF Cytology

- Tumors
  - Primary
  - Metastatic
  - Lymphoma/leukemia
- Infections
  - Meningitis
  - Encephalitis, including abscess
- Vascular disorders, trauma
  - Pathologic bleeding
  - Infarction
- Demyelinating disease
  - Multiple sclerosis
  - Guillain-Barré syndrome

Cytologic diagnosis of CSF may be difficult for several reasons [Walts 1992]. First, only a small volume of fluid is usually obtained. Moreover, the fluid often contains only a few cells, and since CSF is a rather hostile environment, the cells degenerate rapidly. For this reason, CSF specimens should be processed as soon as possible. Cells can be preserved longer (about 1 day at room temperature) in a solution of equal parts balanced salt solution and 20% human serum albumin [Veerman 1985]. Although 50% ethanol or Saccomanno fixatives allow longer preservation, they cause cell shrinkage, limit Diff-Quik® staining, and interfere with certain special stains, such as those used in diagnosis of lymphoma/leukemia (eg, Sudan black, acid phosphatase, esterase).

Specimens obtained by lumbar puncture rarely exceed 8 mL, although up to 20 mL can be withdrawn with no adverse effects [Walts 1992]. Usually, the specimen is collected in tubes and divided among various laboratories, including hematology (for cell counts and differential), chemistry, microbiology, and others (cytology, immunology, etc) as appropriate. Other special studies, such as cytochemical stains, electron microscopy, immunocytochemistry, and flow cytometry can also be performed on CSF specimens [Bach 1991,1993, Boogerd 1988, Guseo 1977, Iwa 1988, Johnston 1971, O'Hara 1985, Stark 1987, Tani 1995, Trojanowski 1986]. The cytology laboratory usually receives about 1 to 3 mL. However, when tumor is a primary diagnostic consideration, at least 3 mL, and preferably 5 mL or more, should be sent for cytologic examination. The CSF specimen should be collected in plastic tubes because cells adhere to glass. Fluid from the second or third tube is recommended for cytologic diagnosis because the first tube is more likely to be contaminated with blood and there may be insufficient material in the last tubes [Andrews 1990]. When scant specimens (in the range of 1 mL or less) are submitted, diagnostic accuracy is correspondingly diminished [Gondos 1976]. Repeated specimens may be needed to establish the diagnosis, particularly in the case of tumors [An-Foraker 1985, Mackintosh 1982, Olson 1974].

Cytopreparation: Because CSF is often sparsely cellular, even in disease, special cell-concentrating techniques, such as membrane filters or cytocentrifugation, are needed to obtain maximum cell yields. Direct smears or ordinary centrifugation are usually inadequate preparatory methods for a CSF specimen, since too few cells can be detected [Bigner 1992, Krentz 1972, McCormack 1953, Platt 1951]. Some laboratories obtain good results by sedimentation of cells directly onto the slides [Balhuizen 1974,1978, Battifora 1978, Bots 1964, Den Hartog Jager 1969, Dyken 1975,1980, Kolar 1968, Kölmel 1977, Krentz 1972]. The use of coated slides may help increase cell yield [Seyfert 1992]. Tissue culture techniques have also been applied [Kajikawa 1977], but it may be difficult to distinguish various cell types in tissue cultures [Bigner 1981a]. It is recommended that both Romanovsky (Wright, Giemsa, or Diff-Quik) and Papanicolaou-stained material be examined [Clare 1986].

Membrane filters, including gelman, millipore, and nuclepore filters, can be used for cytologic examination of CSF [Bernhardt 1961, Bigner 1981a, Del Vecchio 1959, Fleischer 1964, Gondos 1976, Hutton 1958, McAlpine 1969, McCormick 1962, Reynaud 1967, Seal 1956]. Filter preparations have the advantage of retaining a high proportion of cells (~60%–80%), while routine cytocentrifugation yields on

T11.1 **Request for Cytopathology Consultation**
Specimen Source, eg, Lumbar, Ventricular, Cisternal
Age, sex, race of patient
Clinical diagnosis, signs, symptoms
Including signs/symptoms of meningeal irritation, intracranial mass
Other CNS tests and results, particularly
Myelogram
Arteriogram
Computed tomographic (CT) scan
Magnetic resonance imaging (MRI)
Previous CSF cytology
Other
Previous therapy
Intrathecal
Radiation
Shunts, reservoirs
Previous surgery
Including biopsy (tissue, fine needle aspiration)
Cyst drainage

average about 10% to 30% [D Barrett 1976, Dyken 1980, Stark 1987]. However, although filters retain more cells, cellular detail may be compromised due to shrinkage (caused by alcohol fixation), distortion (caused by suctioning), and background staining (caused by incomplete decolorization of the filter), making the cells more difficult to diagnose [Whitmore 1982]. Also, staining is more or less limited to the Papanicolaou technique when using filter preparations [Bigner 1992]. Romanovsky-type stains do not work well with filter preparations, a significant disadvantage in classification of hematopoietic cells and diagnosis of lymphoma/leukemia. Filter preparations are also more susceptible to contamination by "floaters," possibly resulting in a false-positive diagnosis [Bigner 1984]. Another disadvantage of filters is that they require experienced, skilled personnel for successful preparations and are relatively expensive [Bigner 1992, Gondos 1986]. A theoretical advantage of filters is that the supernatant could be recovered for use in further biochemical analysis, while the supernatant in cytocentrifuged material is lost [Tutuarima 1988].

Cytocentrifugation has become the preparatory method of choice in most cytology laboratories [Bigner 1992, Choi 1979, Davey 1986, Doré 1965, Drewinko 1973, Griffin 1971, Hansen 1974, Mengel 1985, P Watson 1966, Whitmore 1982, Woodruff 1973]. Cytospin preparation is easier and faster than filters, with acceptable cell recovery when carefully performed [Kobayashi 1992, Whitmore 1982]. With cytospin preparations, cell retention on glass slides is higher with air-dried, compared with alcohol-fixed material. A broad spectrum of stains and special studies including immunocytochemistry and in situ hybridization can be applied to these preparations [Bigner 1992, O'Hara 1985]. In addition, screening the relatively large area of the filter is more tedious and time consuming than screening the smaller area produced by the cytospin. Although cytologic detail is usually excellent, cytocentrifugation may induce cellular artifacts, including cell clustering and molding, mimicking tissue aggregates, irregular nuclear outlines, and cytoplasmic vacuolization [O'Hara 1985]. In summary, cytospin preparation is simple and rapid, yields acceptable cell recovery with excellent cytologic detail, is flexible in terms of staining procedures, and is easy to screen [T11.2] [Drewinko 1973].

Physical and Chemical Properties of CSF: The brain and spinal cord are covered by a complex membrane, the meninges, which are formed by three layers separated by two spaces. The outer covering is the dura mater, the middle layer is the arachnoid, and the inner layer, which is in intimate contact with the CNS parenchyma, is the pia mater [F11.1, F11.2]. The combination of arachnoid and pia mater is known as the leptomeninges.

F11.1 Profile of Brain and Cord Showing Flow of CSF and Location of Major Structures

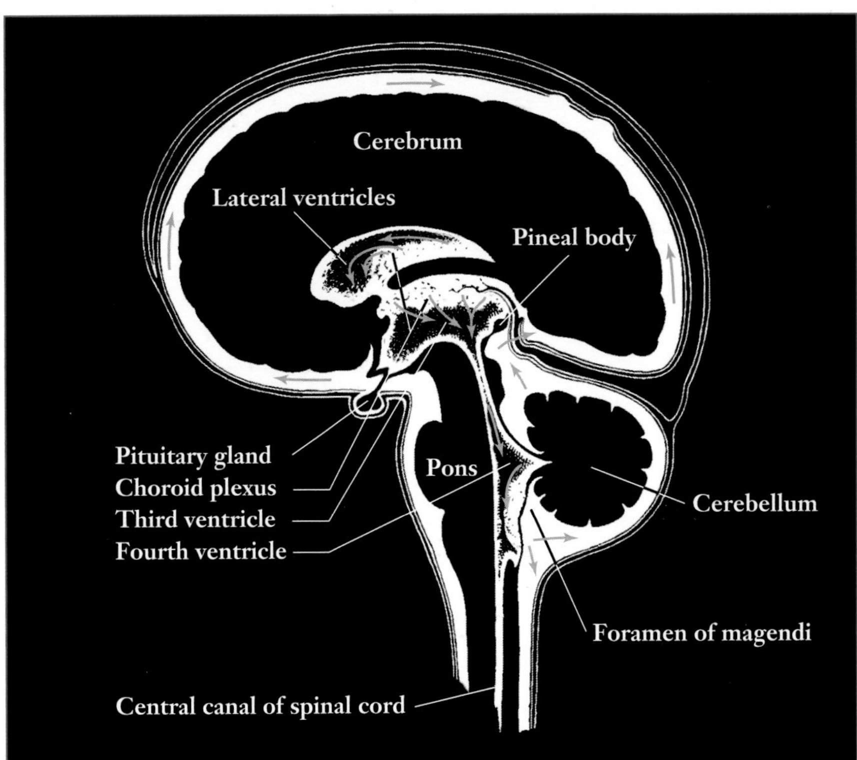

T11.2 Cytospin Preparation vs Filters in Cerebrospinal Fluid Cytology

Cytospin	Filters
Supernatant lost	Supernatant reusable
Rapid, simple processing	More complex processing
Lower cell recovery	Higher cell recovery but "floaters" more likely
Excellent cytologic detail	Cells may be distorted
Flexible staining (Pap, Diff-Quik®)	Papanicolaou only
Easier screening	Screening more difficult

CSF is found in the subarachnoid space, which is between the pia and arachnoid layers [Bering 1966]. The CSF is continually produced and absorbed, with complete turnover every 5 to 7 hours [Conly 1983]. CSF is produced by ultrafiltration of the plasma and active cation (sodium and potassium) transport. Water and anions (chloride and bicarbonate) follow passively. Most of the CSF (approximately 70% to 85%) is actively secreted by the choroid plexus (in the lateral, third, and fourth ventricles of the brain) and the ependymal lining of the ventricles and cerebral subarachnoid space. The remainder of the CSF is formed by the capillaries of the brain and metabolic water production [Conly 1983]. The CSF circulates over the cerebral hemispheres and down the spinal cord. CSF is absorbed by arachnoid villi into venous sinuses of the brain.

The choroid plexus and vascular endothelium are the anatomic basis for the blood-brain barrier, which excludes certain substances from the CNS. (Because of the blood-brain barrier, direct installation of chemotherapeutic agents, ie, intrathecal therapy, may be necessary to treat certain CNS diseases such as lymphoma/leukemia.)

F11.2 **Relationship of Meninges, Brain, and Blood Vessels**

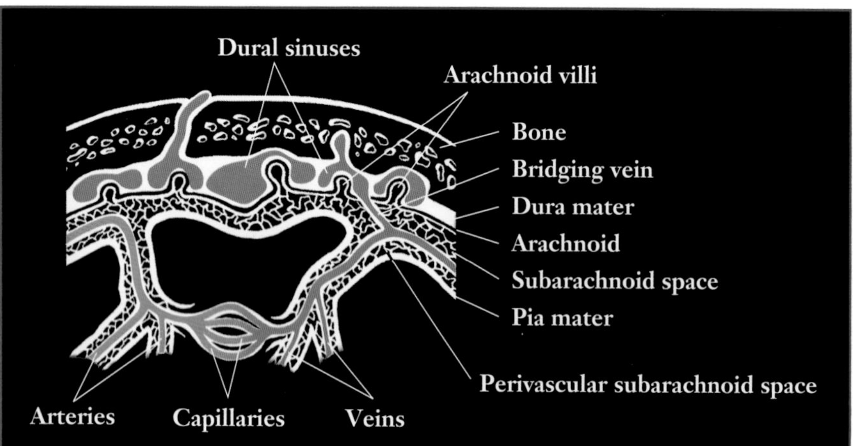

The CSF serves several important functions, including cushioning the brain by providing a bath in which the brain essentially floats. In addition, the CSF provides for circulation of nutrients and excretion of metabolites.

Functions of CSF

Cushions/lubricates
Supplies nutrients
Removes waste

The normal amount of CSF in the adult is between 90 and 150 mL; in neonates, about 10 to 60 mL. The normal CSF pressure is 100 to 200 mm H_2O in the lateral recumbent position, but varies with venous pressure and posture, up to 400 mm H_2O in a seated position. CSF pressure is elevated in meningitis, subarachnoid hemorrhage, and with space-occupying lesions (eg, brain tumor or abscess). Lead poisoning is among other possible causes of high pressure, and conditions such as hypotension or shock may cause low pressure.

Causes of Increased and Decreased CSF Pressure

Increased CSF Pressure
- Congestive heart failure
- Mass lesion (tumor, abscess)
- Inflammation
- Cerebral edema
- Superior vena cava syndrome
- Impaired resorption
- Intracranial venous thrombosis
- Increased proteins
- Acute hypo-osmolality
- Subarachnoid hemorrhage
- Lead poisoning

Decreased CSF Pressure
- Hypotension/shock
- Severe dehydration
- Spinal block
- Acute hyperosmolality

[Conly 1983]

CSF is normally clear and colorless (like water). Any other appearance is abnormal and likely to indicate disease (or a traumatic tap) [T11.3]. The specimen is normally sparsely cellular, containing only a few lymphocytes and monocytes [Marks 1960]. (See also "The Cells," p 432.)

A common problem in the diagnosis of CSF is differentiating a traumatic tap from true pathologic bleeding [T11.4] [Breuer 1982]. Traumatic taps are particularly common in infants who are difficult to restrain. The blood in a CSF specimen from a traumatic tap tends to clear in succeeding tubes, while blood from pathologic bleeding is usually evenly distributed among tubes. Other differential diagnostic features are related primarily to the length of time the blood has been present in the CSF. Generally pathologic bleeding is characterized by xanthochromia and degenerated blood, while traumatic taps show fresh, intact, well-preserved RBCs. The presence of poorly stained RBCs or RBCs ingested by macrophages suggests a pathologic bleed. Later, hemosiderin-laden macrophages may be seen [Bernad 1980]. It is important to note that a traumatic tap and a pathologic bleed are not mutually exclusive.

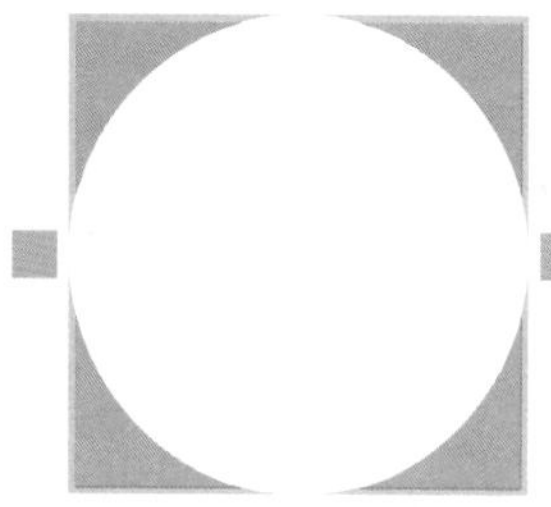

The presence of crenated RBCs microscopically is not useful in the differential diagnosis. If the CSF specimen is obtained in the first few hours after a pathologic bleed, the supernatant may be clear. Persistence of blood in repeated taps generally confirms a diagnosis of pathologic bleeding. However, blood may be present in the CSF for a few days (up to 5 days) after a very bloody traumatic tap. Therefore, repeating the procedure after a bloody traumatic tap may lead to diagnostic dilemma, since xanthochromia and preserved RBCs may coexist.

Deviations of CSF protein and glucose values from normal are reliable, but nonspecific, indicators of CNS disease. The protein concentration is normally quite low, less than 1% of the serum protein. There is a protein concentration gradient, with higher levels being found distally. (Normal: ventricles, 6–15 mg/dL; cisterna magna, 15–25 mg/dL; and lumbar, 20–50 mg/dL.) Although nonspecific, a high protein level usually indicates meningeal or CNS disease, particularly infections or tumors. Increased protein is usually, but not always, proportional to the white blood cell count. With a traumatic tap, add about 1 mg/dL per 1000 RBCs.

Protein Levels

Elevated Protein
- Tumor (Increased protein without increased WBCs)
- Inflammation/infection
- Subarachnoid hemorrhage
- Degenerative disease, especially multiple sclerosis
- Guillain-Barré syndrome
- Diabetes with peripheral neuropathy
- Drugs (particularly phenothiazines)
- Traumatic tap

Decreased Protein
- Normal in some children
- Water intoxication with increased intracranial pressure
- Some leukemias
- CSF leakage
- Hyperthyroidism
- Postpneumoencephalogram (occasional)

Immunoglobulins (γ-globulins) can be increased without an increase in total protein, particularly in multiple sclerosis, syphilis, and subacute sclerosing panencephalitis. Other causes of increased CSF γ-globulins include acute infection (bacterial meningitis), Guillain-Barré syndrome, and metastatic carcinoma. An elevation of serum γ-globulins, (eg, cirrhosis, sarcoid, myxedema, collagen vascular diseases, multiple myeloma) may also be reflected in the CSF. Other biochemical tumor markers, such as CSF β-glucuronidase (may be elevated in solid tumors) and β_2-microglobulin (elevated in hematologic malignancies) have also been reported [Van Zanten 1991].

Glucose enters the CSF by diffusion and active transport. The CSF glucose level is ordinarily about 60% to 70% of the serum (with a delay of about 1 hour), ie, normally about 50 to

T11.3 **Gross Appearance of Cerebrospinal Fluid (CSF)**

Appearance	Indication
Clear, colorless	Normal
Cloudy*	Pleocytosis, ie, WBC > 200/µL (usually >500/µL before grossly cloudy)
	Microorganisms
	Increased protein
Greenish	Purulent
Pink-red	Usually indicates blood
	Pathologic
	Subarachnoid hemorrhage
	Intracerebral hemorrhage
	Infarct
	Traumatic tap
Yellow-orange	True xanthochromia
	Bleeding (pathologic or traumatic tap)
	Jaundice
	False xanthochromia
	Increased protein (>150 mg/dL)
	Premature birth
	Hypercarotinemia
	Melanoma, other melanotic lesions
Oily	Postmyelogram
	Fat embolism (→ Fat globules)
Increased viscosity	Cryptococcal meningitis
	Ruptured nucleus pulposus
	Mucinous carcinoma
Clot	Normal CSF never clots
	Increased protein (Froin's syndrome)
	Very traumatic tap
	Suppurative meningitis

[Cumings 1954, Walts 1992]
* A "sparkling" quality = Tyndall effect.

80 mg/dL. CSF glucose may be elevated when there is hyperglycemia (including intravenous glucose therapy) as well as due to a traumatic tap. A lowered CSF glucose level is a classic finding in bacterial, tuberculous, or fungal meningitis, while the CSF glucose level is usually (but not always) normal in viral meningitis, thus providing a valuable clue to the etiology. Low CSF glucose level is also found in hypoglycemia, subarachnoid hemorrhage (due to release of glycolytic enzymes from lysed RBCs), and tumors [Little 1974, McCormack 1957, McMenemey 1959, Olson 1974]. The combination of increased protein and decreased glucose levels suggests tumor or mycobacterial or fungal infection.

Normal Values

Opening pressure: ≤190 mm H_2O
Cell count: ≤5 cells/µL (no unclassified or malignant cells)
Protein concentration: ≤45 mg/dL
Glucose level: ≥40 mg/dL

When the opening pressure, cell count (including absence of unclassified or malignant cells), and protein are all normal [Hayward 1987], additional CSF tests will rarely be useful in diagnosis (except in some cases of multiple sclerosis).

Conversely, in patients with bacterial infection, chronic infections, or malignant meningitis, results of at least one of these tests are usually abnormal (except in occasional children or patients with AIDS) [Hayward 1987].

CSF Cytology

CSF is often submitted to the cytology laboratory as part of a complete neurological evaluation of nonspecific clinical findings such as headache or seizures, in which the cytologic findings are frequently also nonspecific [Bigner 1992]. In addition, a variety of serious CNS disorders such as Alzheimer's, Jakob-Creutzfeldt, Pick's, Parkinson's, and Huntington's diseases and normal pressure hydrocephalus as well as various benign and malignant CNS tumors can be present in the face of a cytologically normal CSF specimen. Among the most common cytologic diagnoses in CSF are meningitis and secondary malignancies, including carcinomas and lymphomas/ leukemias. Certain primary brain tumors like medulloblastoma, ependymomas, and sarcomas are also seen with some frequency, depending upon the patient population [An-Foraker 1985].

A basic diagnostic principle is that if the diagnostic cells are not shed into the CSF, a cytologic diagnosis cannot be made by examining CSF ("no cells, no diagnosis"). Thus, the lesion must not only exfoliate cells, but also communicate with the leptomeninges or cerebral ventricles for diagnostic cells to be found in a CSF specimen. For example, a lesion situated deep in the parenchyma of the brain is unlikely to be diagnosable by CSF cytology unless it involves the ventricular system or meninges. On the other hand, meningiomas (benign primary neoplasms of the meninges) are ideally located, but exfoliate few, if any, diagnostic cells into the CSF.

Prerequisites for CSF Diagnosis

Exfoliation
Sheds diagnostic cells
Communication
Contact with CSF
Leptomeninges, ventricles

In the CSF specimen, even a single abnormal or foreign cell can be a significant finding. For example, neutrophils, plasma cells, macrophages, and of course, tumor cells, although sparse, may indicate a serious illness [Kolar 1968, Krentz 1972]. A corollary is that knowing the normal cytologic character of CSF is critical in avoiding diagnostic mistakes.

T11.4 **Differences in Cerebrospinal Fluid Specimens From Traumatic Tap and Pathologic Bleed**

Feature	Traumatic Tap	Pathologic Bleed
Blood distribution	Greatest in 1st tube, then decreases	Even distribution
Postcentrifuge	Clear supernatant	Xanthochromic
Clot	May clot	Does not clot
Microscopic	Well preserved RBCs	RBCs poorly stained, degenerated
	Fresh blood	Erythrophagocytosis
		Hemosiderin-laden macrophages

The Cells

Blood Cells

CSF specimens normally contain few cells; those that are present normally are almost exclusively mononuclear WBCs (ie, lymphocytes and monocytes) [1 I11.3] [Sörnäs 1972]. In adults, the normal cell count is 0 to 5/μL. Higher cell counts may be seen in normal children [Portnoy 1985] (up to 30/μL in neonates [Sarff 1976]). Thus, 1 mL of normal CSF from an adult could contain up to 5,000 WBCs [Schumann 1986]. However, cell counts in the range of 20 to 70 are common in cytospin preparations [Drewinko 1973], and many specimens are essentially acellular [Rich 1969].

Normal Cell Count

Normal
Fungal infection
Leukemic blasts
Isolated tumor cells

Lymphocytes normally outnumber monocytes by at least two to one [Sörnäs 1972]. In chamber counts, neutrophils usually comprise only a small percentage of the WBCs in adults (2% ± 5% of the total cell count). However, in cytocentrifuged specimens, neutrophils can average 10% to 15% of the cells. The upper limit of normal for neutrophils in adults may be as high as 40% [Mengel 1985, Simon 1980], and in infants, up to 60% of the cells can be neutrophils [Sarff 1976]. Nevertheless, neutrophils should not be overlooked [Bonadio 1988a,b,1990, Portnoy 1985]. Even a rare neutrophil can be an abnormal finding, particularly in adults, although a few neutrophils can be seen in CSF specimens from patients without evidence of meningeal disease. Also, even minimal blood contamination can result in the presence of a few neutrophils [Hayward 1988]. In patients with a predominance of neutrophils, bacterial meningitis should be strongly suspected [Mengel 1985]. As previously mentioned, CSF is a hostile environment for cells; WBCs may lyse if the specimen is allowed to sit before processing, particularly at room temperature. As always, clinical correlation is required for proper interpretation of results.

RBCs: RBCs are not normally present in CSF but a few are commonly seen in concentrated specimens due to capillary bleeding when the specimen was obtained. When numerous, RBCs may indicate pathologic bleeding or a traumatic tap. Since WBCs accompany RBCs, a correction must be made when assessing WBCs in the presence of fresh blood [Bonadio 1990].

Red Blood Cells

Traumatic tap
Pathologic bleeding
Rule out neoplasm

As a rule of thumb, there is normally about 1 WBC per 700 RBCs in peripheral blood [Conly 1983]. Of course, with elevated peripheral WBC counts, as seen in leukemia or leukemoid reactions, the proportion of WBCs will be higher.

Blood in the CSF irritates the meninges and may cause a pleocytosis (up to 1500 WBCs/μL), consisting mostly of neutrophils. With bleeding, monocytes are activated and erythrophagocytosis begins within a few hours. This is followed by active proliferation of leptomeningeal cells (in about 12 to 18 hours). As the phagocytosed RBCs lose their color, empty-appearing vacuoles are seen in the cytoplasm of macrophages. In a few days, hemosiderin begins to appear.

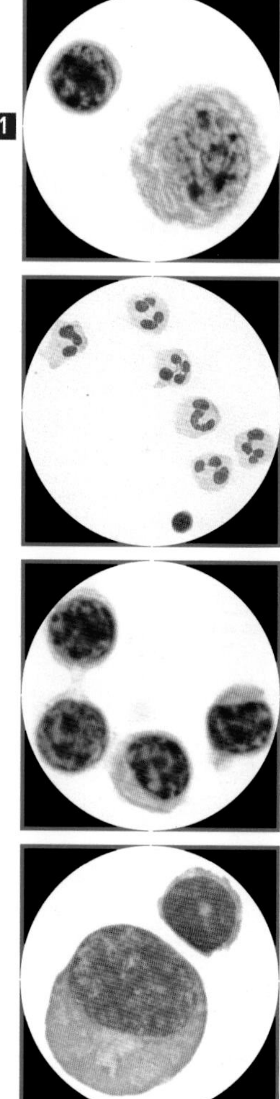

Neutrophils: Neutrophils are normally sparse in routine specimens [2 I11.1]. A primary function of neutrophils is to act against bacteria, and therefore neutrophil counts are elevated in acute bacterial infections. Acute bacterial meningitis is classically associated with marked neutrophilia accompanied by decreased CSF glucose levels (note that if the patient is receiving intravenous glucose, the sugar levels may be increased). However, neutrophilia can be seen with virtually any acute process, not necessarily infectious, including after surgery, infarcts, epileptic seizures, and previous lumbar puncture [Devinsky 1988, Puczynski 1989]. Neutrophils may also be increased early in the course of viral meningitis [Baker 1989, Walts 1992]. Neutrophils are increased when blood is present. On the other hand, neutrophils may be absent in culture-proven infectious disease, depending on factors such as etiologic organism, patient age, host immune status, and stage of disease [Hegenbarth 1990, Michael 1986, Walts 1992]. Moreover, the number of WBCs, particularly neutrophils, decreases rapidly after specimen collection due to in vitro degeneration [Steele 1986].

Neutrophils

Any acute process
Acute bacterial meningitis (classic)
Early infection with
  Mycobacteria
  Virus
  Fungus
Previous lumbar puncture
Hemorrhage
Carcinomatous meningitis
Foreign bodies, including
  Myelogram
  Intrathecal therapy
  Shunts
Epileptic seizure

Hypersegmentation of neutrophils (>6 lobes) can be seen in patients with acute pyogenic meningitis, megaloblastic anemia, and rarely, as an artifact of cytocentrifugation [Lodge-Rigal 1994].

Lymphocytes: A few lymphocytes are a normal finding in the CSF, representing roughly two thirds of the total cell count (range one third to nearly all) [3 I11.2, 1 I11.3] [Sörnäs 1972]. Most are small, mature lymphocytes, although a few may be reactive and intermediate to large. Small mature lymphocytes are characterized by small round nuclei, with smooth nuclear outlines; coarse, dense chromatin; invisible nucleoli; and relatively scant cytoplasm. Reactive lymphocytes have larger nuclei, which may be cleaved, and may have nucleoli, as well as somewhat more abundant cytoplasm [4 I11.4] [Coleman 1987].

Lymphocytes

Infections
Viral meningitis
Bacterial meningitis
  Late or treated
Tuberculosis
Syphilis
Other infections
  Leptospira (early)
  Unruptured abscess
  Fungus
  Parasites
Sarcoid
Hemorrhage, thrombosis
Lead poisoning
Uremia
Chronic nervous system disease
Brain tumor
Other

The combination of CSF lymphocytosis with decreased CSF glucose levels is classically associated with tuberculous or fungal infections, but can also be seen in some cases of viral infections as well as carcinomatous or sarcoid meningitis [Li 1992]. Lymphocytosis with normal CSF glucose is seen in viral or postinfectious meningitis as well as lead toxicity, CNS syphilis, and occasionally CNS tumors. Chronic nervous system diseases such as multiple sclerosis,

Guillain-Barré syndrome, Parkinson's disease, Duchenne's disease (tabes dorsalis), or polyneuritis may also be associated with CSF lymphocytosis. In some cases, uremia can cause a mild lymphocytosis.

Atypical Lymphocytes: In a benign, reactive condition most of the lymphocytes are small and mature [5 I11.4]. However, in some diseases there can be a spectrum of lymphocytes, including stimulated, "atypical," or "immature," lymphocytes. For example, in severe meningitis, there may be a marked elevation of the WBC count, with a shift to immature forms, sometimes even including a few blasts. These findings (elevated WBCs, blasts) do not necessarily indicate a diagnosis of lymphoma/leukemia. On the other hand, lymphoma/leukemia sometimes sheds only a few abnormal cells into the CSF; therefore, normal cell counts do not necessarily exclude lymphoma/leukemia. A mixed lymphoid population suggests a benign, reactive inflammatory infiltrate. Mixed reactions are particularly characteristic of viral infections (including herpes, cytomegalovirus) and tuberculosis. Reactive or atypical lymphocytes can be seen in viral, bacterial (including tuberculous), or fungal meningitis as well as in multiple sclerosis. In addition, atypical mononuclear cells may be seen due to radiation or chemotherapy.

Monocytes: Lymphocytes, together with monocytes, may be the only cells present in normal CSF specimens [6 I11.3]. Monocytes usually represent about 10% to 33% of the cells [Sörnäs 1972], but may be the majority in some cases. However, pure monocytosis is rare. When the monocyte count is elevated, it is usually part of a mixed pattern that includes increased lymphocytes. (The causes of monocytosis are similar to those of lymphocytosis.)

Monocytes

- Bacterial meningitis
  - Chronic or treated
- Syphilis
- Other infections
  - Mycobacterial
  - Viral
  - Fungal
  - Leptospiral
  - Amebic
- CNS hemorrhage, infarct
- Reaction to foreign material
- CNS malignancy

CSF monocytes are bone marrow–derived and identical in appearance to those seen in peripheral blood. Monocytes are the largest nonmalignant cells normally seen in CSF. Although their morphologic characteristics are somewhat variable, they generally have eccentrically located, oval to bean- to horseshoe-shaped nuclei. The chromatin is bland and typically has a "raked sand" (Diff-Quik) or "salt-and-pepper" (Papanicolaou) appearance. Nucleoli are normally invisible or tiny, although when reactive, a single, prominent nucleolus may be seen [Coleman 1987].

Macrophages: Macrophages, or histiocytes, are associated with a destructive process involving the CNS, including trauma, infarction, infections (eg, tuberculous or fungal), foreign bodies (eg, shunts, reservoirs), and invasive procedures or surgery [7 I11.6]. Macrophages are derived from transformation of monocytes [Sörnäs 1971]. Macrophages often clean up after other WBCs have appeared. Macrophages are also seen in benign cysts, histiocytoses, storage diseases, and with neoplasms.

Macrophages

- Tuberculosis
- Fungus, eg, Cryptococcus
- Resolving meningitis
- After hemorrhages such as subarachnoid hemorrhage
- After surgical or other procedures
- Shunts, reservoirs
- Also, histiocytosis (benign, malignant); cysts; neoplasms; storage diseases; idiopathic

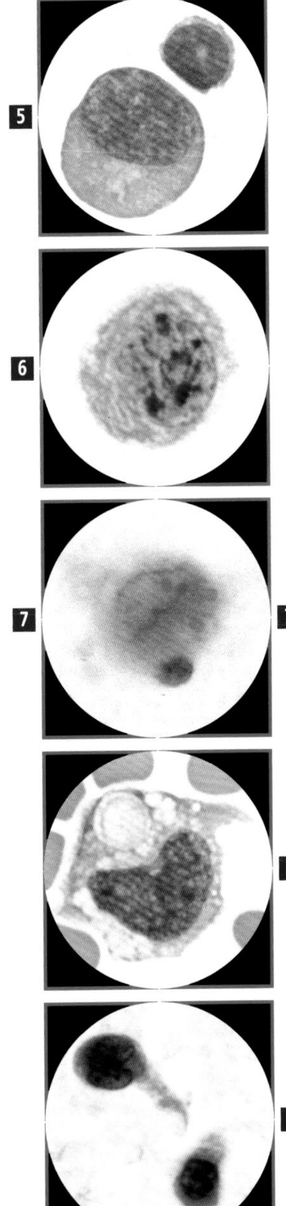

Macrophages or histiocytes are variable in size and shape, have irregular cytoplasmic borders, and may form loose clusters. The nuclei can be somewhat hyperchromatic, with clumped chromatin and occasionally, prominent nucleoli. These features (clusters of large, pleomorphic cells, with atypical nuclei) could arouse suspicion of malignancy [T Barrett 1986, Bigner 1981a, Gondos 1976, McMenemey 1959, Naylor 1961b, Takeda 1981]. However, smooth nuclear membranes, preserved N/C ratio, and characteristic chromatin pattern (as described for monocytes) as well as adequate to abundant, vacuolated cytoplasm, sometimes with inclusions, helps suggest the benign nature of the cells [Naylor 1961b,1964, Rich 1969].

Cytoplasmic inclusions may aid in differential diagnosis. For example, lipid (such as that deriving from myelin) may be seen in the macrophage cytoplasm ("lipophage") after various kinds of parenchymal destruction, including trauma and infarcts, as well as in abnormalities of myelin metabolism (eg, Tay-Sachs disease). Buhot cells, which are foamy histiocytes that contain basophilic cytoplasmic inclusions (best appreciated in Diff-Quik), can be seen in mucopolysaccharidoses (eg, Hunter, Hurler, Sanfillipo syndromes) [Bigner 1981a, Garcia-Riego 1978]. Blood [8 I11.5] or blood pigment such as hemosiderin [7 I11.6] may be seen in histiocytes after cerebral hemorrhage (siderophages) [Bernad 1980, Zaharopoulos 1987]. Siderophages can persist for months. Melanin pigment does not necessarily point to a diagnosis of melanoma, since it can also be seen in melanosis cerebri and various other tumors (see "Melanoma," p 450).

Lipophages: Also known as "gitter" (from the German for lattice) cells, lipophages are associated with parenchymal destruction (including trauma, infarct, infection, cancer), radiation, intrathecal chemotherapy, oil myelogram, and pneumoencephalogram.

Siderophages: These are seen after hemorrhage, and may persist for months [7 I11.6].

Melanophages: Melanophages are not necessarily indicative of a diagnosis of melanoma, and can also be seen with some neuroendocrine tumors, medulloblastomas, ependymomas, choroid plexus carcinomas, and melanosis cerebri.

Atypical Histiocytes: These may be seen in Langerhans' histiocytoses (histiocytosis X), particularly Hand-Schuller-Christian disease [9 I11.29]. They are also seen in malignant histiocytosis.

Plasma Cells: Plasma cells are not seen in the CSF of healthy adults [Péter 1967]. Plasma cells are particularly characteristic of multiple sclerosis or neurosyphilis [Kolar 1968, Péter 1967]. In multiple sclerosis, there may be an intense plasma cell infiltrate, including the presence of immature forms with large nuclei, more open chromatin, and promi-

Plasma Cells

- Neurosyphilis
- Tuberculosis
- Viral (some cases)
- Multiple sclerosis
- Sarcoid
- Subacute sclerosing panencephalitis
- Immune process

nent nucleoli. Plasma cells can be seen in a variety of chronic infections and tumors. Plasmacytosis may be particularly florid in infants and children with viral meningitis [Walts 1992]. In adults, plasma cell malignancies (myeloma/plasmacytoma) and plasmacytoid lymphomas sometimes involve the CSF.

Plasma cells can also be seen with late bacterial infection, Lyme disease [Razavi-Encha 1987, Sindern 1995], cysticercosis [El-Batata 1968, Wilber 1980], polyarteritis nodosa, early Guillain-Barré syndrome, Castleman's disease [Stanley 1986], myeloma, plasmacytoma, Waldenström's macroglobulinemia, and other malignancies, both primary and metastatic [Manconi 1978].

Eosinophils: Except in a traumatic tap, eosinophils are not normally found in the CSF [Bosch 1978]. Eosinophils can be differentiated from neutrophils by the distinct eosinophilic cytoplasmic granules and typical bilobed nuclei [10 I11.7]. Eosinophils are associated with introduction of foreign material (shunts [Mine 1986, Tzvetanova 1986], therapy—chemotherapy and antibiotics—and myelographic contrast material) [Holley 1979, Salberg 1980], hypersensitivity/allergy [Kolar 1968], infections (particularly parasites, eg, cysticercosis [Wilber 1980]; also, fungus, eg, *Coccidioides*; subacute meningitis, eg, tuberculosis), leukemias [Budka 1976, Catovsky 1980, Coleman 1987], lymphomas (particularly Hodgkin's disease), and occasionally primary or metastatic tumors [Conrad 1986, DeFendini 1981]; or can be idiopathic.

Eosinophils

Foreign material, including shunts
Hypersensitivity, allergy
Infections
- Parasites
- Subacute meningitis (tuberculosis)
- Fungal

Tumors
- Primary, metastatic

Lymphoma/leukemia
Idiopathic, other

Other possible associations with CSF eosinophilia include acute polyneuritis, multiple sclerosis, subacute sclerosing panencephalitis, and rarely, bacterial or viral infections and syphilis.

CNS Cells

From time to time various normal cells deriving from the CNS may be found in a CSF sample. The lining cells of the pia-arachnoid space are mesodermally derived, and include not only the pia-arachnoid cells but also fibrocytes and various free cells, ie, lymphocytes, monocytes, histiocytes, macrophages, mast cells, and plasma cells. The ventricles are lined with ependymal and choroidal cells that develop embryologically from neuroectoderm. Cells not normally in contact with the CSF include neurons and neuroglia (astrocytes and oligodendrocytes). Neurons or neuroglia may be found after a procedure that penetrates the brain substance (eg, ventricular tap) or in some diseases [Mathios 1977, Naylor 1961b]. However, normal neurons or glia are practically never found in specimens obtained by lumbar puncture [Bigner 1992].

Normal cells of the CNS are usually found singly in CSF. All cells in fluids have a tendency to round up. With degeneration, they may also imbibe water, sometimes imparting a signet ring appearance [Dalens 1982, Wagner 1960].

10

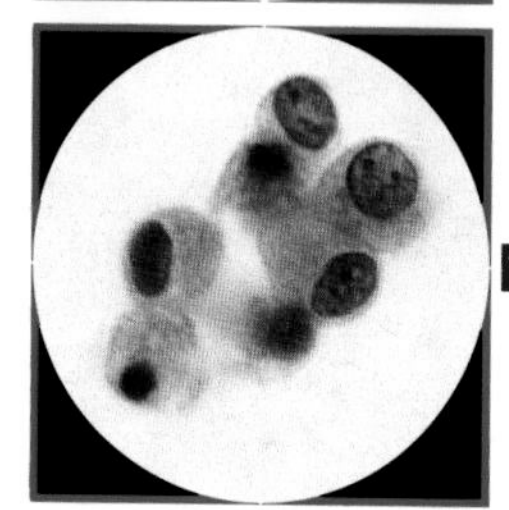

11

Mitotic figures are rarely found in CSF specimens (~1% of all cases), but when present, raise the specter of malignant disease. However, mitotic figures are not indicative of a diagnosis of malignancy unless abnormal, because they are more commonly associated with benign, reactive processes, usually being found in macrophages or monocytes [Walts 1992].

Ependymal Cells: Ependymal cells are epithelial-like cells that derive from neuroectoderm, embryologically, but are sometimes classified as glial. They line the ventricular system. Therefore, ependymal cells may be seen in ventricular fluid, but are rare in CSF obtained by lumbar puncture. Ependymal cells are more commonly seen in patients with hydrocephalus [Rich 1969, Wilkins 1974] and after trauma, surgery, or infarction [El-Batata 1968, Kolar 1968].

Ependymal cells are relatively uniform, small cuboidal to columnar cells, which usually form loose clusters, and may resemble histiocytes [Mathios 1977]. The cytoplasm is transparent, moderately abundant, and basophilic, with indistinct cell borders (Pap). Cytoplasmic vacuolization or branching cell processes may be seen. Terminal bars, cilia, or blepharoplasts (basal bodies anchoring cilia) are particularly characteristic of embryonic ependymal cells [Wertlake 1972]. Cilia are more commonly seen in infancy, and tend to become sparse with age [Mathios 1977]. The nuclei are single, central, round to oval, have delicate chromatin, and may contain a small nucleolus. Nuclear degeneration (pale to pyknotic) is common; naked nuclei may resemble lymphocytes [McGarry 1969].

Ependymal cells are difficult to distinguish from choroid plexus cells. In some cases, ependymal cells may be pleomorphic due to chronic irritation (eg, hydrocephalus), in which case they must be distinguished from tumor cells.

Choroid Plexus Cells: Choroid plexus cells are difficult to distinguish from ependymal cells [Bigner 1981a], but most such cells found in the CSF probably derive from the choroid plexus [11 I11.8] [Mathios 1977]. Both cell types (often referred to generically as choroid/ependymal cells) are much more commonly observed in ventricular or cisternal fluids than in samples obtained by lumbar puncture. They are also more common in infants and children than in adults, and frequently associated with hydrocephalus [Wilkins 1974]. They may also be associated with surgery, trauma, myelogram, ischemic infarcts, intrathecal therapy, or pneumoencephalogram. The cells usually have little diagnostic importance other than their potential to be mistaken for tumor.

Choroid plexus cells exfoliate singly and in cohesive tissue aggregates. Microacinar arrangements (best appreciated in Diff-Quik) or loose, papillary clusters may be seen, which may suggest well-differentiated adenocarcinoma [Wertlake 1972]. The cells are usually uniform, but may be distorted. The individual cells resemble macrophages and may contain hemosiderin in hemorrhagic lesions [McGarry 1969].

The nuclei are uniform, single, round to elongated, and relatively small (about the size of a small lymphocyte). The chromatin is normally delicate and even, but may be hyperchromatic due to degeneration. Nucleoli are invisible or inconspicuous.

There is a moderate amount of cytoplasm, which is usually dense but may be vacuolated or contain yellow pigment [Mathios 1977]. The cells do not have processes, and cell outlines are sharper than ependymal cells [Wilkins 1974]. Cilia, present embryologically, are not seen in adults, although ultrastructurally, peculiar club-shaped microvilli may be observed [Mathios 1977].

Pia-Arachnoid (Leptomeningeal) Cells: The arachnoid lining is the counterpart of mesothelium in other body cavities. Although the lining cells are sometimes referred to as pia-arachnoid mesothelial cells, there are no true mesothelial cells in the CSF [12 I11.9] [Mathios 1977]. Also, in contrast with mesothelial cells in effusions, pia-arachnoid (or leptomeningeal) cells are rarely exfoliated into the CSF.

The cells resemble mesothelial cells or monocytes (and are also known as monocytoid cells). They are usually sparse and single. The cytoplasm is abundant and delicate, with rounded, poorly defined cell borders. The nuclei are eccentric, round to oval to bean-shaped, with fine chromatin. Nucleoli are seldom seen. When the meninges are irritated, the cells exfoliate more readily and may assume features of macrophages, including pigment granules in their cytoplasm [McGarry 1969].

Undifferentiated Cells: Possibly of germinal matrix origin, these cells may be seen in neonates with hydrocephalus, often following intraventricular brain hemorrhage associated with prematurity [13 I11.36] [Fischer 1989]. They form molded clusters of immature blast-like cells, with round to oval, occasionally indented nuclei, containing fine, even chromatin, and single, small nucleoli. Hemosiderin-laden macrophages are often present in the background [Dalens 1982, Fischer 1989]. These primitive cells could be mistaken for malignant tumor cells such as lymphoblasts or medulloblasts. Lymphoblasts are not cohesive; medulloblasts are usually larger, but otherwise very similar [Fischer 1989].

Oligodendroglial Cells: Oligodendroglial cells may be single or may form small sheets. The cytoplasm is transparent. Elongated fine, branching processes may be seen. The nuclei are small and single, round to elongated, and hyperchromatic.

Astrocytes: Astrocytes may be seen in CSF due to bleeding (eg, cerebrovascular accident, subdural hematoma, or trauma), as well as in multiple sclerosis, encephalitis, or convulsions [Wertlake 1972]. The cells are larger and paler than oligodendroglial cells and characteristically have spindle or oval shapes with multiple branches [Wertlake 1972]. The cytoplasm of protoplasmic astrocytes (located in gray matter) is finely fibrillar, resembling a fuzzy ball [Mathios 1977]. Fibrous astrocytes, located in white matter and subpial areas, have only a few long, more discrete cytoplasmic processes [Mathios 1977]. The nuclei of both types are oval, sometimes indented, and hyperchromatic to pyknotic. They must be differentiated from tumor cells.

Neurons: Neurons may be present singly or in small clusters [14 I11.10]. They are the largest nonneoplastic cells that can be seen in CSF (usually in ventricular or cisternal fluid rather than lumbar punctures). The cells vary in size and shape, but typically have a pyramidal or multipolar body with long processes. The cytoplasm is dense and granular. The nuclei are irregular, large, and pale with finely granular, uniform chromatin. Large, central nucleoli are a characteristic feature [Mathios 1977]. The differential diagnosis is with anaplastic tumors.

12
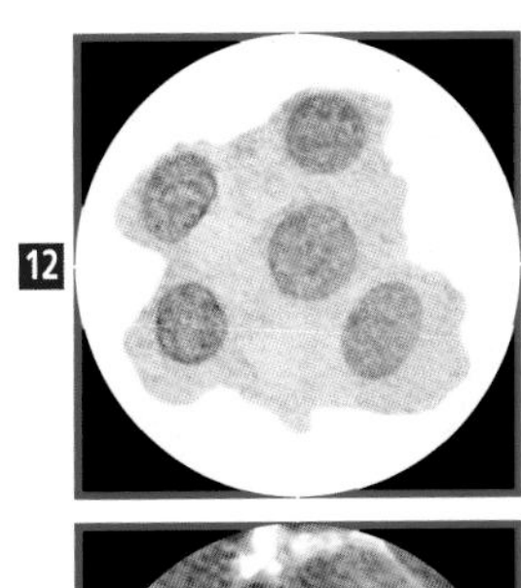

13
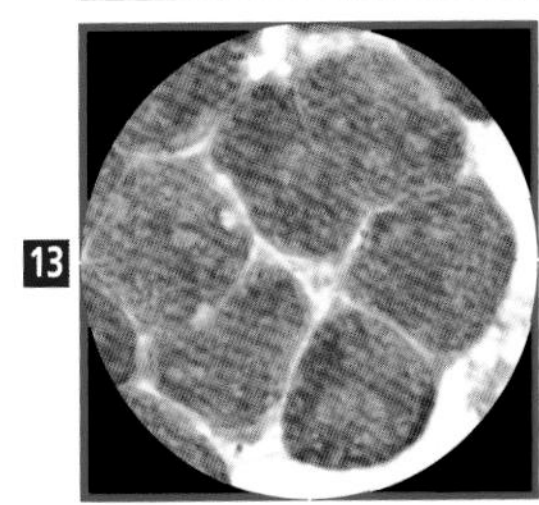

14
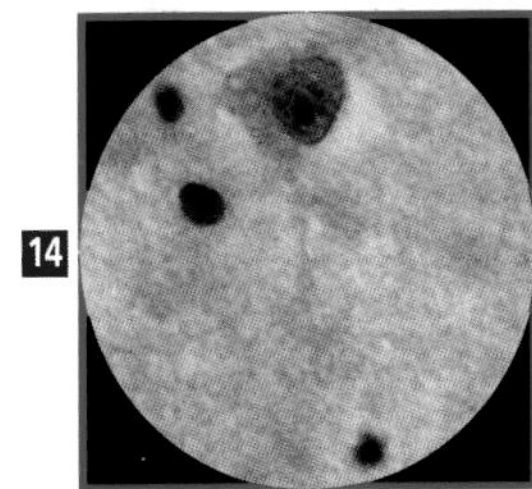

15
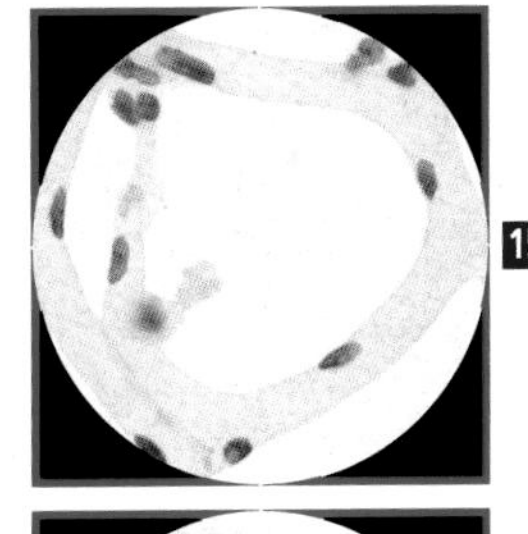

16
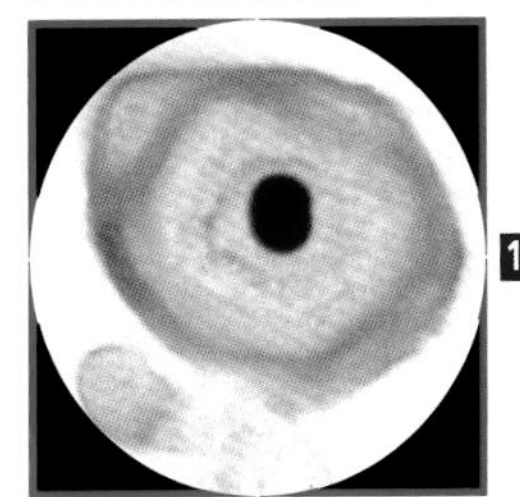

Miscellaneous Cells

From time to time, a variety of nonneoplastic cellular elements, such as squamous cells, accessory skin structures, capillaries [15 I11.14], skeletal muscle, adipose tissue, fibrous tissue, and cartilage, can be found in CSF specimens as "pick up" contaminants [Bigner 1981a, McGarry 1969, Naylor 1964].

Fibroblasts: These are single, bland spindle-shaped cells that may arise from the loose connective tissue of the leptomeninges and may resemble astrocytes.

Cartilage Cells: Cartilage cells from the vertebral column can sometimes be seen in CSF specimens [Chen 1990, Leiman 1980, Takeda 1981]. Fibrocartilage contains spindle cells and fibrillar matrix [I11.11]. Hyaline cartilage, or simply cartilage, can be either mature (adults) or immature (notochord of infants).

Mature cartilage may be seen as single cells or small clusters of two to 10 cells set in a hyalin matrix that compress each other somewhat like soap bubbles [16 I11.12]. The cells have eccentric, oval, almost pyknotic nuclei and vacuolated cytoplasm, which may give the impression of signet ring carcinoma. The cells sit in a space (lacuna) surrounded by a thick "cell wall" that is actually a thick, rigid membrane of cartilage. Cartilage is intensely metachromatic (magenta in Diff-Quik) [I11.13].

Immature cartilage usually forms tight clusters or sheets. The cytoplasm is abundant and foamy with ill-defined cell borders. The nuclei are single, oval, of variable size, and hyperchromatic. In the background is pale blue myxoid material (Pap) which is bright magenta in Diff-Quik. The differential diagnosis includes chordoma and colloid carcinoma.

Bone Marrow Elements: Immature hematopoietic cells may be seen in CSF if bone marrow is inadvertently sampled [Craver 1991, Kruskall 1983, Lane 1983, Luban 1984]. These immature cells may suggest a diagnosis of lymphoma/ leukemia, but all three hematopoietic cell lines (including myeloid and erythroid series) may be present. Diff-Quik is useful in identifying various cell lineages. The presence of megakaryocytes can be particularly helpful in suggesting the correct diagnosis.

Giant Cells: A variety of benign and malignant giant cells may be found in the CSF [I11.15] [Bigner 1985a,b].

Squamous Cells: Squamous cells in the CSF are

Giant Cells

- Benign
  - Foreign body giant cells
    - Reaction to blood, contrast or foreign material
    - Shunts [I11.15], fat, necrosis
  - Langhans' giant cells
    - Associated with tuberculosis
  - Sarcoid
  - Megakaryocytes
- Malignant
  - Glioblastoma
  - Ependymoma
  - Choroid plexus carcinoma
  - Pineal malignancies
  - Metastatic carcinoma, sarcoma, melanoma

usually contaminants. However, they may arise from squamous cell carcinoma, craniopharyngioma (usually accompanied by abundant chronic inflammation), or epidermal inclusion cysts.

Ciliated Cells: Ciliated cells are rarely found in CSF, but could be of ependymal origin, particularly in infants. Aspirates of porencephalic cysts may also contain ciliated cells [Naylor 1961a,b]. In addition, ciliated cells may be found in CSF after basilar skull fracture with torn meninges, in which the contents of the nasal sinuses may enter the subarachnoid space. In such cases, the ciliated cells may be accompanied by micro-organisms, inflammation, squamous cells, calcified debris, etc [Bigner 1981a,1985a].

Noncellular Material

Corpora Amylacea and Psammoma Bodies: Corpora amylacea are amorphous, round, polysaccharide bodies, about 8 to 25µm in diameter, which concentrate around the ventricles and pial surfaces of the elderly [Bigner 1981a]. Consequently, they may be seen in ventricular fluid specimens from older patients [Preissig 1978].

Corpora amylacea should not be mistaken for psammoma bodies or calcospherites (which are normally found in the choroid plexus). Corpora amylacea are PAS-positive, relatively homogeneous (although they may have a dense center with a paler periphery or even faint laminations), and are not calcified. In contrast, psammoma bodies are PAS-negative, distinctly laminated, and are calcified. Corpora amylacea can be extracellular or intracellular (phagocytosed by macrophages) [Bigner 1981a, Preissig 1978]. Other entities to be considered in the differential diagnosis include cryptococcal yeast forms (which may bud and have a mucoid capsule) and starch granules (which polarize, unlike corpora amylacea) [Preissig 1978].

Starch Granules: Starch granules are common contaminants of cytologic specimens, usually deriving from glove powder. Macrophages ingesting these particles may resemble cells of signet ring cancer. However, starch granules are refractile and show a characteristic Maltese cross polarization pattern [Reinhartz 1978].

Protein: This is nonspecific amorphous gray to blue to eosinophilic material, sometimes somewhat fibrillar precipitate in background of the slide [Wertlake 1972].

Reactive Conditions: Hemorrhage, Inflammation, Infection

A wide variety of procedures and conditions that affect the CNS can result in reactive changes in the CSF.

Reactive changes usually result in increased numbers of normal cell types in the CSF, particularly leptomeningeal cells and monocytes, occasionally astrocytes, but rarely neurons. If possible, it is a good idea to wait at least a week between samplings of the CSF, since even the tap itself can cause reactive changes. Although benign cells, including macrophages, can form clusters (particularly in multiple sclerosis), the finding of clusters of cells in the CSF is suspicious for malignancy.

Reactive Changes
- CNS investigation
  - Myelography
  - Previous tap
- CNS therapy
  - Radiation
  - Intrathecal chemotherapy
- Trauma, including
  - Herniated discs
  - Neonatal obstetrical trauma
  - Head injury
- Neoplasms
- Hydrocephalus
- Hemorrhage
- Infarct
- Infection
- Surgery

Hemorrhage into the subarachnoid space (eg, trauma, ruptured aneurysm, hypertension, thrombosis, arteriovenous malformation, intracerebral, or tumor) proceeds through three stages: fresh, intact RBCs → erythrophagocytosis → hemosiderin-laden macrophages. When there is associated necrosis (eg, cerebrovascular accidents, encephalomalacia), degenerated glial cells may be seen. Neutrophils may be found early in the course. Later, enlarged, reactive astrocytes with lacy cytoplasm, usually single, but occasionally forming loose clusters, may be seen. The chromatin is often granular and degenerated. Because the astrocytic cytoplasm is delicate, naked nuclei are common. Inflammatory cells, hemosiderin- or debris-laden macrophages, lipophages, and necrotic material can also be present.

Infection/Inflammation, General

Acute: Neutrophils are characteristic.

Subacute: Acute inflammation blends into chronic inflammation (ie, subacute). Likely with fungal or tuberculous infections.

Chronic: Lymphocytes.

- Exclusively small, mature lymphocytes suggest chronic, indolent inflammation.
- Range, including reactive lymphocytes, immunoblasts, and plasma cells, suggests active immune response, eg, active viral infection or multiple sclerosis.
- If neutrophils are also present (ie, together with other features of an active immune response), this implies that the inflammatory process is particularly aggressive.

Granulomatous: Rarely diagnosed in CNS. Could be seen with tuberculosis or fungus, but these usually show only chronic inflammation in CSF. Also, foreign body reaction to shunts, reservoirs.

Meningitis

Bacterial

Bacterial meningitis ordinarily proceeds through three phases—acute, exudative; proliferative; and reparative. The

Bacterial Meningitis → Pus

Newborns
- Escherichia coli
- Listeria monocytogenes

Infants, children
- Haemophilus influenzae
- Neisseria meningitidis
- Streptococcus pneumoniae ("Pneumococcus")

Adults
- Pneumococcus
- Staphylococcus
- Streptococcus
- Also, Proteus mirabilis, Pseudomonas aeruginosa, Klebsiella

acute, exudative phase occurs in the first few days. Cell counts may be 30,000 to 50,000/µL or greater, with more than 90% neutrophils and the remainder lymphocytes and monocytes. Neutrophils, attracted by bacterial toxins, emigrate through the capillary walls and ingest bacteria. In essence, the cytology shows frank pus, ie, polymorphonuclear leukocytes, fibrin, macrophages, degenerating cells and cell debris, and sometimes micro-organisms.

There is a rapid decrease in the total cell count with antibiotic therapy. In the proliferative phase, the neutrophils degenerate and activated monocytes become more numerous, many transforming into macrophages. Plasmacytoid lymphocytes and plasma cells may also be seen. Finally, in the reparative phase, the neutrophils have usually disappeared, and the cytology shows degenerated macrophages with cytoplasmic vacuolization and fewer plasma cells. The total cell count returns to normal, although there may still be an increase in the number of small lymphocytes for some time.

Brain Abscess

The CSF is usually clear and colorless in the presence of a brain abscess. However, the CSF pressure and protein levels are usually, but not always, elevated. The total cell count is less than 1,000/µL, often less than 300/µL, and may be less than 25/µL. The cytologic appearance of the CSF is similar to that of chronic meningitis. Although neutrophils are often present, lymphocytes usually predominate, and macrophages may be seen. When there is a brain mass, and CSF cytology shows inflammation, debris, and fibrin, a neoplasm must be excluded. The primary consideration in the cytologic differential diagnosis is tuberculous meningitis.

Tuberculous Meningitis

Unfortunately, there is no specific cytologic feature of tuberculous meningitis short of demonstrating diagnostic organisms. However, there is a characteristic cytologic picture. The total cell count is usually less than 1,000/µL. Neutrophils may predominate very early in the course of the disease. However, due to the insidious onset, by the time a CSF specimen is examined, transformed lymphocytes and plasma cells are the characteristic cytologic findings. Nevertheless, neutrophils continue to be present and may be numerous throughout the course of the disease [Jeren 1982, Teoh 1986].

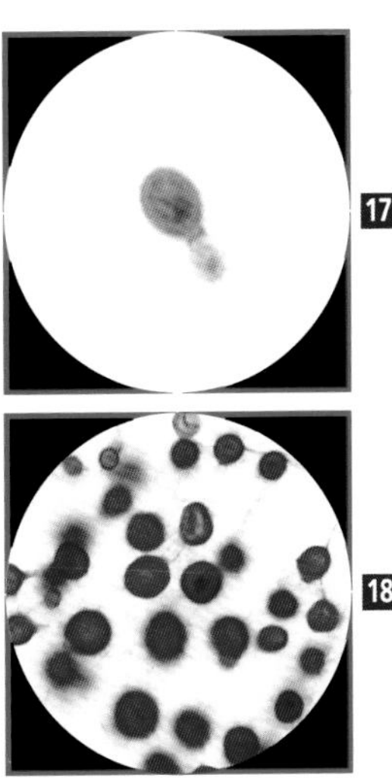
17
18

Viral Meningitis

Viral meningitis is usually a relatively benign disease, while viral encephalitis can be a serious illness. These infections are caused by such viruses as enteroviruses (coxsackie, echovirus, polio), mumps, herpes (simplex and zoster), or cytomegalovirus (as well as JC virus and SV-40 viruses associated with slow virus infections). In viral meningitis, the total cell count is generally less than 1,000/µL, although with coxsackievirus it may go up to 3,000/µL. However, the correlation between the cell count and the severity of the illness is not good, except that if the cell count is low, the patient is usually asymptomatic. With viral encephalitis the cell counts may be higher and there may also be bleeding.

The most characteristic cytologic findings are an increase in the number of small, mature lymphocytes as well as reactive (transformed) lymphocytes, plasma cells, and small macrophages [Pelc 1981]. Early in the course of the disease (first day or two), neutrophils may predominate. Later, the proportion of transformed lymphocytes diminishes, and small, mature lymphocytes and degenerated monocytes become relatively more common. Eosinophils and basophils may sometimes be seen. Although herpes may occasionally shed cells with viral inclusions [Bigner 1981a, Gupta 1972], cells with characteristic viral inclusions are generally rare in CSF specimens.

Fungal Infections

Cryptococcus: Cryptococcus is the most common fungal organism seen in CSF [17 I11.16] [Bigner 1981a,1992]. It is usually found in immunosuppressed patients, such as patients with transplants, lymphoma/leukemia, or AIDS, but is occasionally seen in patients who are otherwise apparently healthy [Saigo 1977]. The yeasts are about 5 to 15 µm in diameter, have a refractile center and mucoid capsule, and are characterized by tear drop–shaped budding. Special stains, eg, mucicarmine or Gomori-methenamine silver, as well as polarized light or fluorescence microscopy, can be useful in diagnosis [18 I11.17] [Brown 1985].

The yeasts should not be mistaken for starch crystals (budding, capsule vs Maltese cross birefringence) [Bigner 1981a, Saigo 1977]. *Cryptococcus* may incite little or no inflammatory reaction, particularly in immunosuppressed patients, and the organisms may show a poor reaction to the Papanicolaou stain. Thus, the organisms may be overlooked in screening. On the other hand, reactive lymphocytosis can occur in the CSF specimens of patients with cryptococcal meningitis. Reactive lymphocytes can suggest lymphoma/leukemia [Davies 1978]. Differentiation is critical because appropriate therapy for one may be inappropriate for the other. Marker studies may be needed in some cases to differentiate a reactive lymphocytosis from lymphoma/leukemia. In addition, these diseases are not mutually exclusive. Cryptococcal and malignant meningitis can occur during the course of lymphoma/leukemia.

Toxoplasma: Mononuclear pleocytosis with increased CSF protein in the absence of bacteria or fungus strongly suggests toxoplasmosis [DeMent 1987]. Trophozoites and cysts may be identified with Romanovsky stains (eg, Diff-Quik) [Threlkeld 1987].

Lyme Disease: Meningopolyneuritis is caused by the spirochete *Borrelia burgdorferi* which is borne by the tick *Ixodes dammini* [Benach 1983, Steere 1983a,b]; it leads to lymphocytic pleocytosis with immunoblasts and plasma cells associated with foamy macrophages [Kraft 1989, Razavi-Encha 1987, Sindern 1995]. Markedly atypical plasmacytoid mononuclear cells may suggest non-Hodgkin's lymphoma [Szyfelbein 1988].

Other Specific Infections: Blastomyces and *Histoplasma* are relatively common. Also, *Coccidioides*, *Actinomyces*, *Aspergillus*, *Phycomycetes* (*Mucor*), and *Penicillium*. Spores, rather than hyphae, are usually seen [Bigner 1981a]. *Trichomonas* has been reported [Masur 1976].

CSF Manifestations of AIDS: Human immunodeficiency virus (HIV) is apparently both lymphotropic and neurotropic; the CNS is frequently found to have pathologic abnormalities in patients with AIDS [Lobenthal 1983, Price 1986, Strigle 1991]. CSF manifestations of AIDS can be divided into three categories:

1. Primary aseptic meningoencephalitis with nonspecific, reactive, chronic inflammation, histiocytes, and occasionally multinucleated giant cells [Katz 1989].
2. Other infections, such as *Cryptococcus*, *Toxoplasma*, *Candida*, mycobacteria, or viruses such as cytomegalovirus, JC virus (a papovavirus that causes progressive multifocal leukoencephalopathy [Suhrland 1987]).
3. Malignant lymphomas, including primary CNS lymphomas, usually B-cell types (particularly large cell, including immunoblastic, and Burkitt's/non-Burkitt's types).

Although the CSF findings are usually nonspecific (eg, mild pleocytosis [Price 1986]), CSF examination can be helpful in diagnosing CNS cryptococcosis and lymphoma [Katz 1989]. Note that HIV can be recovered from CSF specimens of patients with AIDS [Hollander 1987] and therefore they are potentially infectious.

Miscellaneous Benign CNS Diseases

Systemic Lupus Erythematosus: This is associated with pleocytosis, usually mononuclear, occasionally neutrophils [Jaeckle 1982]. Lupus erythematosus (LE) cells are rare [Nosanchuk 1976].

Mollaret's Meningitis: This is a rare disease characterized by recurrent, self-limited episodes of aseptic meningitis. It may be associated with viruses such as herpes virus [Yamamoto 1991]. CSF shows marked pleocytosis, including lymphocytes and neutrophils, and large Mollaret cells, which are probably activated monocytes [H Evans 1993]. They have delicate, finely vacuolated, pale cytoplasm; eccentric, irregular, or bean-shaped nuclei; finely granular chromatin; and small nucleoli [Lowe 1982].

Tumors

Although about two thirds of all tumors occurring in the CNS are primary neoplasms, the large majority of tumors diagnosed with CSF cytology are secondary lesions—mostly lymphoma/leukemia followed by metastases. Even in the absence of diagnostic tumor cells, CNS (brain) tumors, including benign and malignant, primary and metastatic lesions, can also elicit more or less characteristic reactive changes in the CSF. The CSF is usually abnormal, although tumor cells are not necessarily identified [Olson 1974].

CSF in Tumor

Increased pressure
Increased protein
Decreased glucose
Increased cellularity
Tumor cells
CSF usually abnormal, but tumor cells not necessarily present

Most cases show elevated CSF pressure and protein levels. The glucose is usually decreased. Most cases have either normal cell counts (the majority) or only mild elevations (<25/μL). Thus, *normal cell counts do not exclude malignancy* [D Evans 1974, Kolar 1968, Nies 1965b, Olson 1974, Schumann 1986]. An important corollary is that the absence of tumor cells does not exclude malignancy, particularly in CSF specimens, which have a high false-negative rate [Glass 1979]. When high cell counts occur, neutrophils usually predominate, and in the absence of diagnostic tumor cells, the differential diagnosis would include a brain abscess. If the cancer involves the meninges (malignant meningitis), the CSF picture will look more like tuberculosis, with increased protein, low glucose, and high cell counts in which lymphocytes predominate, but tumor cells are likely to be numerous.

The rate at which CNS tumors can be diagnosed with cytologic examination of CSF depends on several factors, including the patient population and tumor type and location [Bigner 1981b, Glass 1979, Gondos 1976]. Diagnostic neoplastic cells are more likely to be found when the leptomeninges are infiltrated with tumor. Tumors (primary or secondary) exclusively involving the deep brain, extradural space, or bone, without involving the leptomeninges, rarely shed diagnostic cells into the CSF. However, when the leptomeninges are involved, there is a relatively high CSF detection rate, particularly when involvement is widespread [Glass 1979]. Cisternal taps may be positive when lumbar punctures are negative for tumor [Rogers 1992].

Although the most important factor in detection of a tumor with CSF cytology is its location, the biologic behavior and the cohesiveness of the tumor cells also play an important role in the ability to detect the lesion. In fact, most CNS tumors are benign and unlikely to shed diagnostic cells. Exfoliative cytology is generally much more useful for detecting metastases than primary tumors. Other factors have been previously discussed and are outlined [T11.5].

About 10% of positive CSF specimens come from primary tumors, about 30% from lymphoma/leukemia, and about 60% are metastatic, depending on the patient population [Ehya 1981]. Only about 15% of all primary cerebral malignancies can be detected preoperatively with CSF cytology (up to 40% postoperatively) and only about 20% of all metastatic cerebral tumors yield positive CSF cytology (preoperatively) [Balhuizen 1978]. Lymphoma/leukemia and medulloblastoma followed by metastatic carcinomas and melanomas are most likely to shed diagnostic cells [T11.6]. Primary tumors, other than medulloblastoma, and particularly benign neoplasms, are less likely to be diagnosed with CSF cytology [Gondos 1976].

The location of the tumor is also useful in differential diagnosis [T11.7]. Two of three brain tumors in children occur below the tentorium, while two of three in adults occur above the tentorium. Medulloblastoma is the most common primary CNS malignancy in children. It usually occurs in the cerebellum. Glioblastoma multiforme (a high-grade astrocytoma) is the most common primary brain tumor of the cerebral hemispheres of adults that is likely to shed diagnostic cells into the CSF (low-grade astrocytomas are unlikely to shed diagnostic cells).

The most common malignant tumor of the brain of adults is metastatic cancer. However, solitary metastases mimicking a primary tumor are relatively rare.

Cell size may be useful in differential diagnosis. In general, cancer cells in the CSF are relatively large, thus, large cells are suspicious for malignancy. Medium and large cells can be seen with epithelial, germ cell, and glial tumors, as well as with melanoma. Small and medium cells can be seen in either benign or malignant conditions, but cohesive small cells may be suspicious.

Malignant cells usually have hyperchromatic nuclei (Papanicolaou) and dark blue cytoplasm (Diff-Quik). Mitotic figures may occasionally be observed. The differential diagnosis includes monocytes and benign reactive lymphocytes, as well as blasts arriving from the peripheral blood in patients with leukemia (traumatic tap). Phagocytosis is evidence against a malignant diagnosis.

T11.5 **Cerebrospinal Fluid Positivity**

Influencing Factors	Optimum
Location of tumor	Leptomeninges infiltrated
Nature of tumor	Malignant: Lymphoma/leukemia, medulloblastoma, metastatic
Volume of fluid	At least 3 mL preferred
Type and quality of preparation	Cytospin or filters and high quality preparations
Number of examinations	More increases sensitivity

T11.6 **Likelihood of Detection of Tumors With Cerebrospinal Fluid Cytology**

Tumor Type	Likelihood of Diagnosis
Lymphoma/leukemia	High
Medulloblastoma	High
Metastasis	Medium
Gliomas	Low
Benign primary	Very low

[Choi 1979, Gondos 1976, Den Hartog Jager 1969, Kline 1962, Naylor 1964, Rich 1969]

Primary Tumors of the CNS

Benign and malignant primary tumors of the CNS account for about 9% of all neoplasms, but only 1% of all deaths. A wide variety of primary brain tumors occur, but most can be grouped into tumors of either neuronal or glial origin. Tumors of neurons include neuroblastoma or ganglion cell tumors, while glial tumors include astrocytomas (including glioblastoma multiforme), oligodendrogliomas, and ependymal and choroid plexus tumors. In addition, embryonal tumors (medulloblastoma), pituitary tumors, and nerve sheath tumors (eg, meningioma, schwannoma) also occur.

Most primary brain tumors are located deep in the CNS and do not communicate with the CSF. Moreover, primary brain tumors have less tendency to exfoliate cells than metastases. Therefore, there is a high false-negative rate for diagnosis of primary brain tumors [Bigner 1981b].

The key diagnostic feature is the presence of abnormal appearing cells. There may also be an increase in inflammatory cells. Immunocytochemistry using panels of monoclonal antibodies may be useful in distinguishing among metastatic carcinoma, lymphoma/leukemia, and various primary CNS tumors [Vick 1987, Yam 1987].

Gliomas

Gliomas are benign and malignant tumors of glia (from the Greek for glue), ie, the supporting tissues of the CNS. Gliomas are, by far, the most common primary CNS tumors in both children and adults.

Gliomas

Astrocytomas
- Including glioblastoma multiforme

Ependymoma/choroid plexus papilloma
Oligodendroglioma

In children, the majority of gliomas occur in the posterior fossa, particularly in the brain stem. Gliomas account for ~20% of primary brain tumors in the pediatric age group. In adults, most gliomas arise supratentorially. However, only about a third of all gliomas involve the leptomeninges or ventricular system. Thus, even high-grade gliomas, including glioblastoma multiforme, may be difficult to diagnose in CSF. Many gliomas

T11.7 Tumor Location

Cerebral Hemispheres
Astrocytomas, glioblastoma (most common primary)
Oligodendrogliomas, benign, malignant
Ependymal tumors
Primary lymphoma
Neuroblastoma
Metastases
Cerebellum
Most are metastases
Medulloblastoma
Astrocytoma, glioblastoma (rare)
Brain Stem
Gliomas, glioblastoma (particularly children)
Malignant ependymoma
Primary lymphoma
Metastasis
Midline
Gliomas
Pineal tumors, including germ cell tumors
Pituitary adenomas
Craniopharyngioma
Ependymoma
Cysts
Dermoid
Ependymal
Arachnoid
Metastasis
Spinal Cord
Ependymoma
Metastasis
Meninges
Meningioma
Metastasis

are low-grade tumors unlikely to exfoliate diagnostic cells. Rarely, gliomatosis cerebri, which is diffuse malignant proliferation of glial cells involving the entire cerebrum, cerebellum, brain stem, and occasionally even the spinal cord, with few or no large tumor nodules, occurs and may shed diagnostic cells into the CSF [Miller 1981].

The main consideration in the differential diagnosis is metastatic epithelial malignancy (carcinomas) [T11.8].

Astrocytomas and Glioblastoma Multiforme

Astrocytomas of all grades comprise about 80% of all primary brain tumors in adults, occurring most commonly in late middle age. Astrocytomas occur throughout the CNS, but most frequently arise in the cerebral hemispheres. Astrocytomas are also the most common primary brain tumors of children.

The behavior and morphology of astrocytoma depend upon the nature and grade of the tumor [I11.18]. Low-grade astrocytomas are slow growing and can occur at any age. High-grade astrocytomas with evidence of necrosis are designated glioblastoma multiforme; they are unusual in children. Although many of these lesions cannot be diagnosed cytologically, astrocytomas are still the most common primary CNS neoplasm detected in CSF [Bigner 1981b]. The diagnosis may be possible if the tumor is large and infiltrates the meninges or ventricular wall.

Astrocytoma: In general, astrocytoma cells tend to form clusters, but may also be single [C Watson 1977]. The cells vary in size, shape, and degree of nuclear atypia, depending on the grade of the tumor (progressive abnormality with increasing grade). Low-grade astrocytomas are unlikely to be diagnosed in the CSF because they shed only a few cells with a bland appearance. Giant tumor cells as well as anaplastic small cells may be seen with glioblastoma multiforme.

Spindle cells with fibrillar cytoplasm are typical of astrocytomas. The cytoplasm varies from scanty to abundant, and pale to deep blue depending upon how well preserved the cells are. Low-grade tumors have a delicate, lacy cytoplasm with fine vacuoles, while cells from high-grade astrocytomas have a more distinct or epithelioid cytoplasmic appearance. Short, blunt tails or cytoplasmic extensions with a fibrillary or granular quality are characteristic, but infrequent, findings [Geisinger 1984]. Gemistocytic astrocytomas have relatively abundant, finely granular, dense eosinophilic cytoplasm with slightly eccentric nuclei [An-Foraker 1985, C Watson 1977].

The nuclei also vary with the grade of the tumor, from bland (round to ovoid, pale, fine chromatin with inconspicuous nucleoli) to clearly malignant appearing (coarse, irregular chromatin with prominent, irregular nucleoli). The nuclei can be single or multiple, again depending on the degree of differentiation.

The background may show a large amount of cell debris, inflammatory cells, and protein precipitate. Fresh and old blood may also be present. Necrosis is associated with glioblastoma multiforme.

The differential diagnosis of low-grade astrocytoma includes normal or benign reactive cells in the CSF. Degenerative or reactive astrocytes may be seen in reactive gliosis, ie, around a brain abscess, and can closely resemble well-differen-

***T11.8* Differential Diagnosis Between Gliomas and Carcinoma**

Gliomas	Carcinoma
Cells	
Single	Cohesive groups
Smaller	Larger
Cytoplasm	
Scant	More abundant
Wispy	Relatively dense
Indistinct borders	Distinct borders

tiated neoplastic astrocytes. Thus, the mere presence of benign appearing astrocytes is insufficient evidence to render a diagnosis of astrocytoma. However, clusters of such cells are more suggestive than single astrocytes. Unfortunately, in practice, there may only be, at most, a few benign-appearing cells, making the diagnosis difficult or impossible. Foamy histocytes, a nonspecific reaction to any destructive lesion in the CNS, can also be a pitfall in diagnosis [Bigner 1981b].

Glioblastoma Multiforme: Glioblastoma multiforme is the most common primary malignant brain tumor of adults, who are usually older than 40 years. Glioblastoma has a dismal prognosis and is virtually always fatal. Glioblastoma multiforme, or simply glioblastoma, usually occurs in the frontal or temporal lobes. About a quarter of cases cross the corpus callosum. Only about a quarter disseminate in the spinal fluid, however, where they could be diagnosed with CSF cytology [Onda 1989]. Rarely, glioblastoma metastasizes outside the nervous system, mainly to the lung and pleura [Pasquier 1980].

Glioblastoma most commonly yields nonspecific anaplastic cells of variable size [19 I11.18] [Bigner 1992]. Large, pleomorphic, spindle- to bizarre-shaped cells with dense cytoplasm are characteristic [Watson 1977] but infrequently shed. Multinucleated giant cells, although rarely found in CSF, are suggestive of a diagnosis of glioblastoma. There may also be an anaplastic small cell component. The presence of both small and giant malignant cells in a CSF specimen is highly suggestive of glioblastoma.

Multiple, hyperchromatic, highly atypical nuclei and abnormal mitotic figures may be seen. The cytoplasm varies from granular to vacuolar to fibrillar. It is often scant and wispy, and has a tendency to trail off [Bigner 1981b]. A diagnostically important finding is the presence of necrosis, which helps separate glioblastoma from other astrocytomas, but evidence of necrosis may not be present in CSF specimens. Enlarged capillaries with marked epithelial proliferation may be seen in aspirates.

The differential diagnosis of glioblastoma includes metastatic carcinoma, sarcoma, and melanoma. Bizarre cells, giant and small cells, and wispy cytoplasm suggest glioblastoma, while more rounded cells with distinct cell borders and particularly evidence of mucin, keratin, or melanin production favor metastatic malignancy. The clinical history, as always, is very important in the differential diagnosis.

Oligodendroglioma

Oligodendroglioma is a rare tumor and it rarely sheds diagnostic cells in the CSF. However, it is the most common primary brain tumor of middle age and occurs almost exclusively in adults [Bigner 1981b]. It usually occurs in the white matter of cerebral hemispheres. There is often central cystic necrosis, and calcification is seen in up to 90% of cases. Psammoma bodies may also be seen. Oligodendroglioma is commonly mixed with astrocytoma.

19

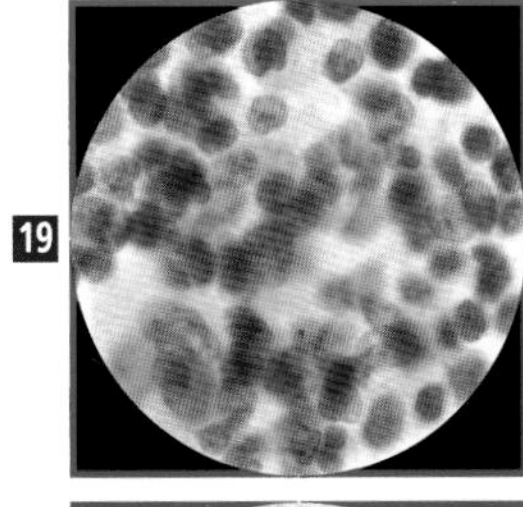

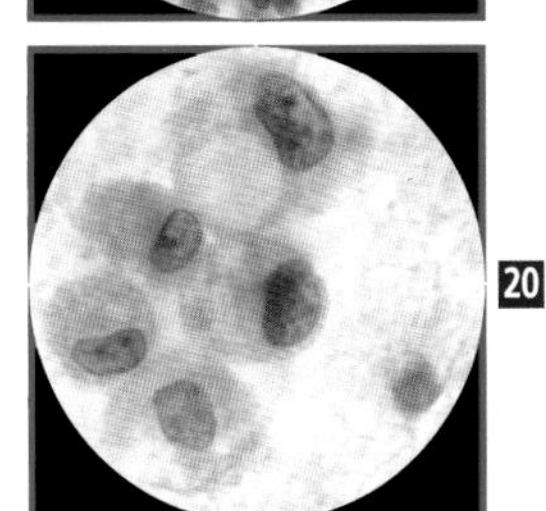

20

Although there may be slight variation in size, the cells are usually relatively uniform, round, and monotonous, and tend to cluster. Rosettes occur rarely.

The cytoplasm is delicate, wispy, indistinct, and appears syncytial. It often falls away from the nucleus. Although perinuclear halos are characteristic in the tissue pathology of oligodendroglioma, they are not always seen cytologically [Den Hartog Jager 1969].

The nuclei are eccentrically located, round, and single [C Watson 1977]. There may be slight hyperchromasia, with a salt-and-pepper appearance to the chromatin. Nucleoli are small but distinct when the cells are well preserved.

The differential diagnosis includes pituitary adenoma, ependymoma, pineal tumors, and benign ependymal or leptomeningeal cells and monocytes. Loose clusters of cells favor a diagnosis of tumor. The location of the tumor, the delicate cytoplasm, and the eccentric nuclei may help suggest oligodendroglioma.

Ependymoma

Ependymoma is an unusual tumor, but it is the most common primary tumor of the spinal cord (usually sacrolumbar). Although it can be seen at any age, it occurs predominantly in children and adolescents. It is the third most common CNS tumor in children, in whom it usually arises in the fourth ventricle of the posterior fossa. Ependymomas are usually benign tumors that arise from ependymal cells. There is a relatively good chance of making the diagnosis with exfoliative cytology because the cells shed into the CSF.

Most ependymomas are composed of cells practically indistinguishable from normal ependymal cells, except that they often form small clusters in CSF [20 I11.19] [C Watson 1977]. Rosettes occasionally occur in well-differentiated tumors. There may be many cells, particularly if the tumor arises in the fourth ventricle (ventricular fluid) or spinal cord (lumbar puncture).

The cells are cuboidal to columnar. The cells are usually bland, with little pleomorphism and no malignant features. The cytoplasm is moderate in amount, lacy, and stains blue. No glial processes are seen. Blepharoplasts, the basal bodies of cilia, stain with phosphotungstic acid hematoxylin, and are virtually pathognomonic if present.

The nuclei are eccentrically located, small, oval to slightly elongated. They are usually single, but occasionally there is binucleation or multinucleation, with only slight variation in size. The chromatin is usually bland and vesicular, but occasionally hyperchromatic to pyknotic, which is usually due to degeneration. Nucleoli are small, but conspicuous in well-preserved cells.

Myxopapillary ependymoma is a variant of ependymoma, with myxoid stroma, that occurs in the filum terminale of the spinal cord. There are also anaplastic, malignant varieties of ependymoma or ependymoblastomas. High-grade ependymoma may resemble metastatic carcinoma (particularly if the cells maintain their columnar shape) or high-grade astrocytoma or medulloblastoma.

Rosettes occur more commonly in tissue and fine needle aspiration biopsy samples than in CSF cytologic specimens. When rosettes are seen in a CSF specimen, consider a neural crest tumor, which generally has scantier cytoplasm than ependymoma. Densely packed cellular papillae, if present, aid in the diagnosis, but choroid plexus papilloma must be excluded. Oligodendroglioma usually lacks the well-defined cell borders of ependymoma, although the nuclei may be similar.

Choroid Plexus Tumors

Choroid plexus tumors—papillomas and carcinomas—are rare. They occur in the ventricular cavities where they may readily exfoliate cells into the CSF [Bigner 1981b].

Choroid Plexus Papilloma: This is a rare, benign tumor. It usually arises in the lateral ventricles of children, but may also be seen in adults, more often in the fourth ventricle. It may result in hydrocephalus due to blockage of outflow, as well as increased production, of CSF. Because of its location and the friable nature of the lesion, even these benign tumors may shed diagnostic cells into the CSF.

The diagnosis is based on finding papillae composed of relatively uniform cells, with only slight variation in size and shape. The nuclei are uniform, round, and bland and the cytoplasm is moderate in amount and granular to vacuolar. Papillomas are composed of bland, regular cells that may be indistinguishable from normal choroid plexus or ependymal cells [C Watson 1977].

Choroid plexus papilloma cannot be reliably distinguished from ependymoma by CSF cytology alone (the differential diagnosis may even require electron microscopy). Moreover, there are no reliable morphologic features or cytologic markers to distinguish papilloma from normal choroid plexus cells. This differential diagnosis may be a particular problem in ventricular fluids, which often contain numerous fragments of choroid plexus in patients without tumors. Moreover, any patient with hydrocephalus can exfoliate papillary groups of choroid plexus cells, and patients with choroid plexus papillomas often have hydrocephalus; thus the diagnostic significance of such groups may be questioned. The best guide to diagnosis is the presence or absence of an intraventricular mass [Bigner 1992].

Choroid Plexus Carcinoma: This occurs in young children of an average age of 2.5 years [K Kim 1985]. It exfoliates as tight clusters and single cells with variable nuclear anaplasia, including nuclear lobulation, irregular chromatin, and prominent nucleoli, depending on the degree of differentiation [Bigner 1992, K Kim 1985, Kline 1962, McCallum 1988, Valladares 1980]. The morphologic characteristics are essentially identical to those of metastatic (papillary) adenocarcinoma [Bigner 1981b, McCallum 1988]. However, metastatic carcinoma is an unlikely diagnosis in children [Packer 1992].

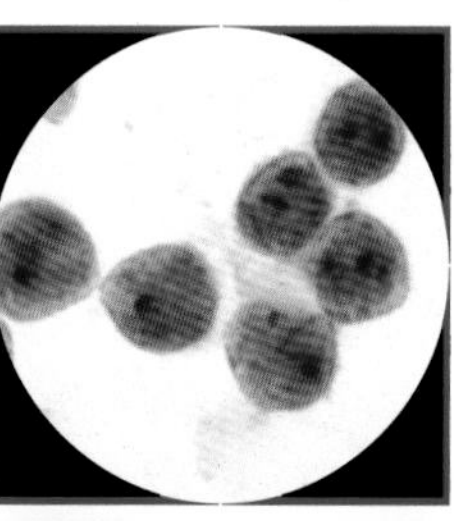
21

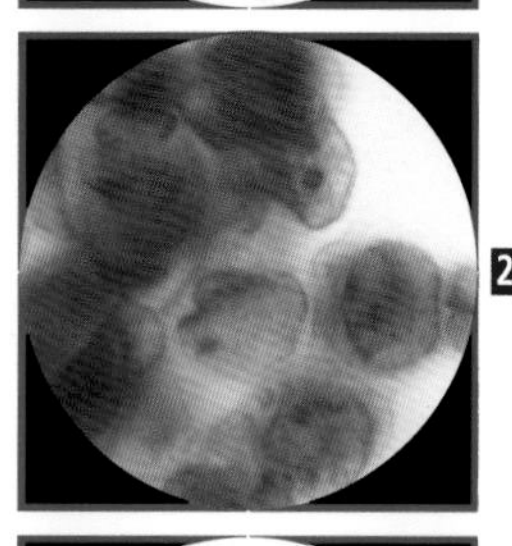
22

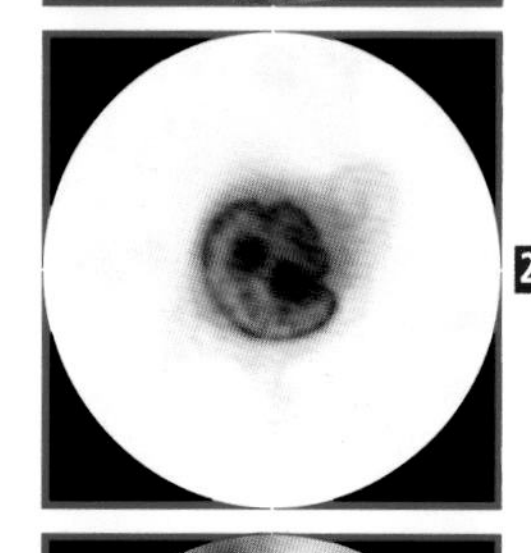
23

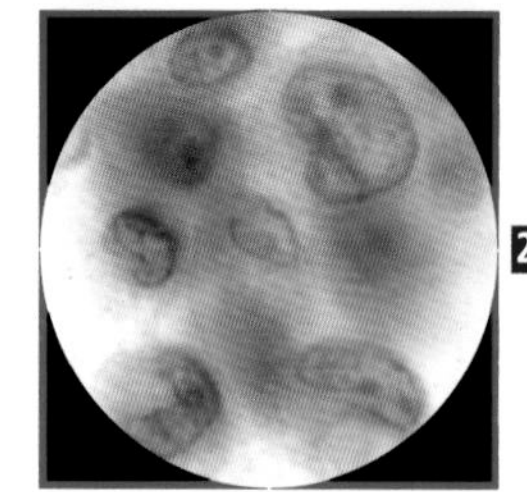
24

Neural Crest Tumors

For the most part, neural crest tumors of the CNS are neoplasms of children and young adults. Neural crest tumors are generally radiosensitive.

The cells of the various neural crest tumors are all similar in appearance (ie, small, cohesive cells with high N/C ratios, nuclear molding, hyperchromasia, and inconspicuous nucleoli), and it is probably impossible to distinguish the specific type by CSF cytology alone [21 I11.20, 22 I11.21] [Geisinger 1984]. However, knowing the clinical history, particularly the site of the tumor, may allow the specific diagnosis to be made.

Neural Crest Tumors and Sites of Origin

Medulloblastoma: Cerebellum
Retinoblastoma: Retina/eye
Pineoblastoma: Pineal gland
Neuroblastoma
  Cerebral hemisphere (rare)
  Adrenal medulla
  Peripheral ganglia
  Nasal passages (esthioneuroblastoma)
Primitive neuroectodermal tumor:
  Paravertebral

Rosettes are characteristic of neural crest tumors. However, they are rarely seen in CSF cytologic specimens and are not pathognomonic, since they can also be seen in other tumors.

Rosettes in CSF Specimens

Rosettes
  Medulloblastoma
  Retinoblastoma
  Neuroblastoma
  Ependymoma
  Pineoblastoma
No Rosettes
  Ewing's sarcoma
  Rhabdomyosarcoma
  Small cell carcinoma

The differential diagnosis includes other "small blue cell tumors." Small cell carcinoma of the lung occurs in an older age group, and although it could metastasize to any of the sites mentioned above, a lung tumor or hilar mass is usually evident. Lymphoma/leukemia does occur in this young age group and individual immature or blastic cells can closely resemble the cells of neural crest tumors. The key distinguishing feature is the presence or absence of true tissue aggregates. Cohesive clusters of cells, usually also displaying nuclear molding, must be seen to diagnose a neural crest tumor. Although blastic cells from lymphoma/leukemia may appear to aggregate, and even mold to some degree, particularly in cytospin preparations, the groups are not truly cohesive and do not show extensive molding. In addition, the cells of neural crest tumors tend to be larger and more hyperchromatic than blasts of lymphoma/leukemia. Embryonal rhabdomyosarcoma shows loosely cohesive, round to oval myoblasts, with eccentric, hyperchromatic nuclei, with one or two nuclear notches, occasional binucleation, and slightly more abundant cytoplasm [23 I11.23] [Geisinger 1984]. Ewing's sarcoma shows variable cellularity, usually single or occasionally loose clusters of cells, with very high N/C ratios, with almost no cytoplasm, and irregularly jagged nuclear outlines [24 I11.22] [Geisinger 1984]. Wilms' tumor cells are usually single, occasionally double, and rarely form organoid structures as seen in neural crest tumors. Characteristically, a biphasic population of round to polygonal cells and plump, spindle-shaped cells may be seen [Geisinger 1984]. The nuclei are hyperchromatic with occasional prominent nucleoli. Cytoplasm is scant and indistinct, but generally cyanophilic.

Other primary tumors must also be considered. Glioblastoma multiforme may have a component of small, anaplastic cells, but in contrast with medulloblastoma, almost never arises in the cerebellum. rarely, anaplastic ependymoma of the fourth ventricle occurs in children. Although the cells tend to be slightly larger than neural crest tumor cells, these lesions may be clinically and morphologically indistinguishable. Also consider benign undifferentiated germinal matrix cells in neonates (see p 435).

Medulloblastoma

Medulloblastoma occurs most commonly in children. Although it sometimes occurs in young adults, most patients are younger than 10 years. Medulloblastoma accounts for 25% of primary brain tumors in children. In children, the cerebellum is the most common site of origin. In older patients, the tumor more commonly arises in the cerebral hemispheres. Patients usually present clinically with signs and symptoms of a cerebellar mass, but may present with findings suggestive of bacterial meningitis. The tumor grows rapidly and infiltrates the leptomeninges, often disseminating numerous tumor cells into the CSF. Thus, many cases can be diagnosed with CSF cytology.

The cytologic appearance is reminiscent of other so-called "small blue cell tumors" such as small cell carcinoma of the lung or neuroblastoma [Bigner 1981b]. The tumor sheds immature neoplastic cells singly and in sheets or small, molded clusters [25 I11.20]. Although the cells are classically considered small, in fact, they often range up to about 20 µm or so in diameter and thus may actually be relatively large. The cells are similar in size and appearance to large, transformed lymphocytes or leukemic blasts, but show true tissue aggregates and nuclear molding. Homer Wright rosettes (ie, false rosettes without a well-formed central lumen) are characteristic of neural crest tumors, but are rarely seen in CSF.

The cytoplasm is very scanty, transparent (Pap), and poorly defined [C Watson 1977]. The nuclei are pleomorphic within their small size range. The chromatin is dense and dark (Pap) and varies from coarse to pyknotic depending on cellular preservation. Occasional cells may be binucleated. Nucleoli vary from inconspicuous to prominent and may be multiple. The smear also frequently shows monocytosis and an increase in other inflammatory cells as well as a background of protein precipitate.

The tumor is cytologically indistinguishable from neuroblastoma, retinoblastoma [26 I11.21], and pineoblastoma, although the site of origin is helpful in differential diagnosis, as previously mentioned. The differential diagnosis also includes metastatic Ewing's sarcoma, which characteristically sheds noncohesive cells, embryonal rhabdomyosarcoma [27 I11.23], and lymphoma/leukemia[28 I11.26]. Childhood glioblastomas may exfoliate anaplastic small cells, but virtually never arise in the cerebellum [Bigner 1981b]. However, anaplastic ependymomas of the fourth ventricle may be clinically and cytologically indistinguishable from medulloblastoma [Bigner 1981b]. Undifferentiated benign cells, thought to be of germinal matrix origin, are very similar in appearance but smaller and more uniform [29 I11.36]. In adults, metastatic small cell carcinoma is a much more likely diagnosis.

25

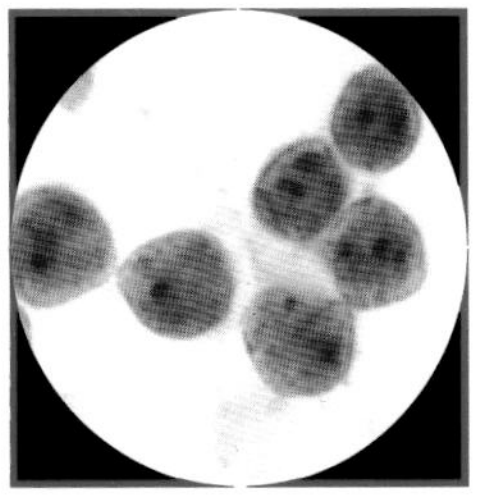

26 26

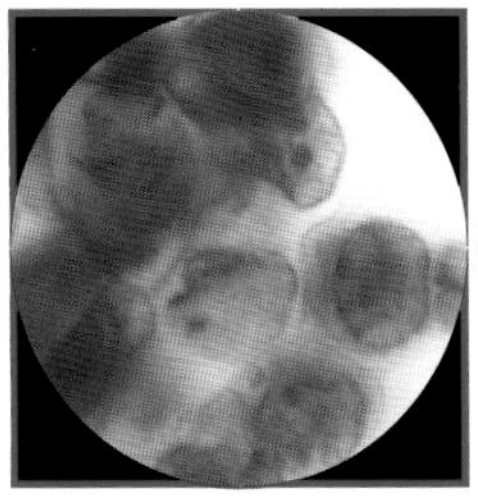

27

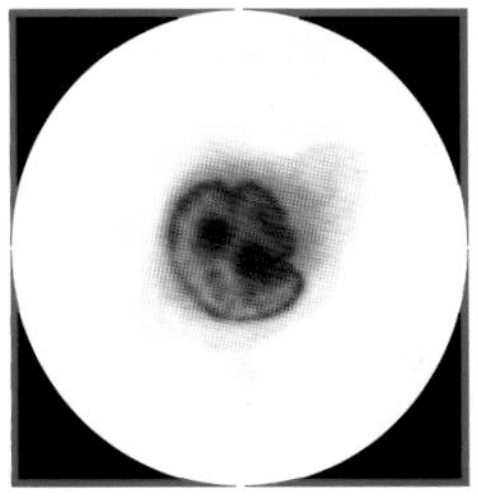

28

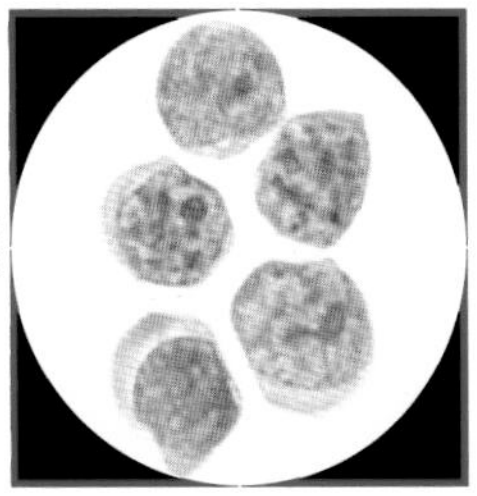

29

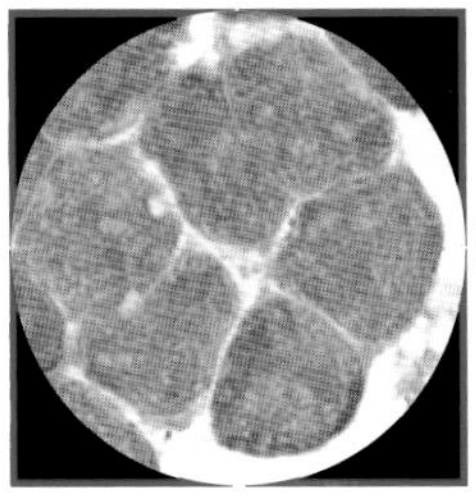

Neuroblastoma

Although neuroblastoma can arise as a primary brain tumor, it more commonly occurs in the adrenal medulla or peripheral ganglia, and then may metastasize to the brain.

Cytologic examination shows small, round to polygonal, anaplastic cells with hyperchromatic nuclei, with one or two small nucleoli, and scanty cytoplasm, in sheets or clusters, sometimes forming rosettes [Farr 1972, Gandolfi 1980, Geisinger 1984]. Neuroblastoma is indistinguishable from medulloblastoma or retinoblastoma by CSF cytology alone [Geisinger 1984, C Watson 1977].

Retinoblastoma

Retinoblastoma sheds cells virtually identical to the other neural crest tumors described herein (ie, loose clusters and sheets and single small cells with scanty cytoplasm and irregular, hyperchromatic, molded nuclei) [26 I11.21] [Greenberg 1977]. Rosettes may occur, but are seldom seen in CSF [C Watson 1977]. If the diagnosis of retinoblastoma is already known, CSF cytology may be useful in diagnosing metastasis. Cells of retinoblastoma can occasionally be found in a relatively asymptomatic patient with a no abnormal findings on brain scan.

Midline Tumors

The majority of primary midline tumors arise in boys, with the exception of pituitary adenomas, which usually occur in adults. Midline tumors may obstruct the ventricular system, causing hydrocephalus, which can compress midline structures like the brain stem or optic chiasm, resulting in corresponding symptoms. In general, these tumors are not diagnosable with exfoliative CSF cytology, except after surgery, but could be diagnosed using fine needle aspiration biopsy.

Pituitary Adenoma

Pituitary adenomas account for 10% of intracranial tumors in adults. They may be associated with an endocrine abnormality. Although benign tumors seldom exfoliate cells into the CSF [Naylor 1964], pituitary adenomas have been diagnosed in CSF [Bigner 1981b, Cairns 1931]. Also, after an incomplete resection of the tumor, cells may be found in the CSF.

The cells are present singly, in papillary clusters, or small, honeycomb sheets. The cytoplasm is relatively abundant, but variable in amount, and also varies from eosinophilic to basophilic (Pap) depending on the specific type of adenoma [Balhuizen 1974]. The nuclei are round to oval, central to eccentrically located, and usually have a bland, uniform appearance [C Watson 1977]. The chromatin varies from fine to salt-and-pepper coarseness and is regularly distributed. Nucleoli are usually small, but can be prominent [Naylor 1964]. Only a small amount of protein is seen in the background and other cells are scarce. Rarely, psammoma bodies may be seen [Wolfson 1979a]. The differential diagnosis includes oligodendroglioma and well-differentiated metastatic adenocarcinoma.

Craniopharyngioma

Craniopharyngioma is a relatively rare tumor, although it is one of the most common suprasellar tumors in children. Craniopharyngioma is a cystic neoplasm that derives from the embryonic craniopharyngeal canal (Rathke's pouch). If the tumor ruptures into the meninges, the CSF cytologic specimen may show numerous anucleate squames and benign squamous cells. These must be distinguished from contaminant squames, which are present far more commonly, but are usually less abundant. The diagnosis is facilitated if there is evidence of cellular degeneration, intense inflammatory reaction, foreign body giant cells, calcification, and cholesterol crystals [Zaharopoulos 1980]. Pearls and basaloid squamous cells may be seen [Balhuizen 1974]; their presence helps exclude contaminant squamous cells from the skin.

Pineal Gland Tumors

The pineal gland is located just posterior to the third ventricle over the brain stem. Tumors of the pineal gland may compress the cerebral aqueduct, producing hydrocephalus, which compresses the midbrain and results in aberrant eye movements. These clinical findings are relatively specific for a tumor in the pineal area.

Pineal gland tumors are very rare, comprising less than 1% of intracranial neoplasms, but can occur in either children or adults [DeGirolami 1973]. Pineal gland tumors can be either benign (pineocytoma) or malignant (pineoblastoma). Pineal germ cell tumors, which are actually the most common tumors to arise in the pineal gland, and pineal gliomas are considered separately.

Pineocytomas: These are composed of uniform cells with indistinct, vacuolated cytoplasm that varies from scanty to moderate in amount. The nuclei are relatively large and round with vesicular chromatin. The nucleoli are diagnostically important—prominent, often multiple, and vary in size and shape. The differential diagnosis includes oligodendrogliomas and germ cell tumors.

Pineoblastomas: These are even rarer than pineocytomas, but usually occur in children or young adults. The cells are pleomorphic and vary from small to giant and are present singly or in small clusters. The small cells are round to oval and have scanty, ill-defined cytoplasm. Their nuclei are round to oval, hyperchromatic, and irregular, with delicate chromatin, and tiny nucleoli. The tumor may resemble the "small blue cell" malignancies such as medulloblastoma; therefore, age and location are important in diagnosis [DeGirolami 1973, C Watson 1977].

Germ Cell Tumors

Germ cell tumors usually arise in the midline, in the pineal area, suprasellar region, pituitary fossa, or fourth ventricle. They tend to be locally destructive. Any of the gonadal type germ cell tumors can occur intracranially, but the majority resemble germinoma/seminoma. Most occur in adolescent males, particularly those arising in the pineal region [Bigner 1981b, DeGirolami 1973]. The cytologic appearance is like that of other germ cell tumors.

Germinomas: These exfoliate uniform, large round to polygonal cells with lacy or clear cytoplasm and are present singly or in loose clusters [Bigner 1981b]. The nuclei are round, with fine to coarse chromatin, and have characteristic large, prominent nucleoli [Bigner 1992, Gindhart 1979]. Although a dual population of tumor cells and lymphocytes is typical, lymphocytes are a nonspecific finding, since a reactive lymphocytosis often accompanies any type of tumor in the CSF [Bigner 1992]. The differential diagnosis includes other large cell tumors with prominent nucleoli, particularly metastatic large cell carcinoma, since cells of germinoma may look epithelial in fluid [Zaharopoulos 1980].

Immature Teratomas: These may show epithelial cell clusters, scattered squamous cells, and other elements, such as small bundles of striated muscle fibers in a background of numerous histiocytes and inflammatory cells [Kamiya 1991]. Although atypia may be slight, the presence of these cells in CSF suggests meningeal spread of the teratoma.

Lymphoma/Leukemia

Until recently primary CNS lymphoma accounted for only about 1% of all brain tumors, but has seen a dramatic increase in both high-risk groups (immunocompromised patients and those with AIDS) and in the general population [Jellinger 1992]. The majority are large B-cell, high-grade, non-Hodgkin's lymphomas; low-grade and T-cell primary CNS lymphomas, and Hodgkin's disease are rare [Jellinger 1992]. However, systemic lymphoma/leukemia is the fifth most common cause of cancer-related death in the United States, and is the single most common cause of cancer-related death in children [Wingo 1995]. Modern radiation and chemotherapy have increased survival of patients with lymphomas and leukemias, and in many cases, cure is possible. However, chemotherapeutic agents capable of producing systemic remissions may fail to pass the blood-brain barrier. Thus, with prolonged survival, CNS relapse of lymphoma/leukemia became a common problem, particularly for acute lymphoblastic leukemia, in which CNS relapse occurred in approximately 50% to 80% of cases [Aaronson 1975, Borowitz 1981, A Evans 1970, Herman 1979, Hustu 1973, Law 1977, Nies 1965a, Reske-Nielsen 1974]. However, with the institution of prophylactic CNS radiation and intrathecal chemotherapy, the incidence of CNS relapse has been markedly reduced [Aur 1971, Hutchison 1973, T Kim 1972, Lauer 1989, Simone 1972].

The meninges are often the first site of relapse, which may occur at any stage of the disease. In addition, the patients are at high risk for infections. Malignancy must be differentiated from meningitis or encephalitis as the cause of clinical CNS symptoms. Clinical symptoms suggestive of CNS involvement include vomiting, headaches, papilledema, seizures, and cranial nerve palsies [Nies 1965a]. However, it is also important to note that many patients with CNS disease are asymptomatic [Diamond 1934, Leidler 1945, Nies 1965a, Spriggs 1959]. For these reasons, cytologic examination of a CSF specimen may be particularly important in management of lymphoma/leukemia [Bigner 1981a].

Acute leukemias commonly involve the CNS [Spriggs 1959]. Conversely, CNS involvement by chronic leukemia is uncommon, except in cases of blast crisis [Bigner 1992]. CSF pleocytosis (WBC counts >10/μL) is suggestive, but not in itself diagnostic, of CNS involvement. However, pleocytosis can also be seen in benign disease (such as infections), while normal cell counts do not exclude malignancy. Thus, cytologic examination of the CSF is more sensitive and specific than mere cell counts in diagnosis.

In essence, the role of CSF cytology is to determine the presence or absence of malignant leukocytes. When the meninges are infiltrated with neoplastic leukocytes, numerous malignant cells are usually found in the CSF, particularly with malignant lymphomas. The different types of malignant hematopoietic cells may be cytologically indistinguishable, particularly with the Papanicolaou stain. The use of Romanovsky type stains is helpful in morphologic classification of the cells, eg, myeloid differentiation can be appreciated. A general rule of diagnosis is to compare the atypical cells with the patient's known malignancy to help exclude overreading reactive changes (eg, reactive histiocytes or transformed lymphocytes, neither of which has the morphologic characteristics of lymphoblasts) [Borowitz 1981]. Knowing which malignancies are likely (eg, acute lymphoblastic leukemia) and which are unlikely (eg, chronic lymphocytic leukemia) to involve the CNS is also useful.

Proportions of Lymphoma/Leukemia First Diagnosed by CSF Cytology*

Acute lymphocytic leukemia: 45%–50%
Acute nonlymphocytic leukemia: 20%–25%
Chronic leukemias: 5%–10%
Lymphoma (non-Hodgkin's): 20%–25%
Other (Hodgkin's, myeloma, etc): Rare

[Bigner 1984]
* Depends on patient population.

The cytomorphology depends on the type of lymphoma/leukemia. The malignant cells vary in size, but are usually larger than normal, small mature lymphocytes. The nuclei are enlarged and often have lobulated or irregular nuclear membranes (cleavages) or protrusions (noses, knobs) [Aaronson 1975]. Nuclear protrusions are rarely seen in normal lymphocytes. The chromatin varies from powdery fine (particularly in blasts) to coarse and hyperchromatic. Nucleoli are occasionally prominent, and may have aberrant shapes [Drewinko 1973]. Mitotic figures are sometimes seen and can be helpful in diagnosis, particularly if they are abnormal. The amount of cytoplasm varies from very scant (eg, lymphoblasts) to abundant (eg, some large cell lymphomas). Although a general feature of lymphoma/leukemia is absence of true tissue aggregates, the cells may unexpectedly cluster and may even mold to some degree as an artifact of cytocentrifugation (cytospin), particularly in air-dried specimens. Such groups must be distinguished from other "small blue cell tumors."

The diagnosis is usually fairly straightforward if there are numerous well-preserved tumor cells. However, the diagnosis can be difficult if there are only a few cells or if the cells are degenerated (eg, after therapy). An important consideration in the differential diagnosis is reactive changes in inflammatory cells such as may be seen as a result of therapy, subarachnoid hemorrhage, or intercurrent infection [Lauer 1989]. In some cases the neoplasm itself can incite a marked, but benign, inflammatory reaction in the leptomeninges.

Radiation or intrathecal chemotherapy can cause marked reactive changes as well as extensive karyorrhexis [Mayer 1980]. Patients with lymphoma/leukemia are immunosuppressed and susceptible to opportunistic infections, which may be associated with an inflammatory response. A mixed population of lymphocytes in which small, mature forms (coarse chromatin without nucleoli) predominate favors a benign reactive process. Lymphoma/leukemia is usually characterized by a predominance of immature cells (with fine chromatin and nucleoli). Plasma cells are common in reactive conditions, but rare in lymphoma/leukemia involving the CNS. Some benign conditions such as multiple sclerosis may give rise to blast-like transformed lymphocytes.

In cases of doubt, repeating the examination may be helpful. Benign processes will tend to subside in contrast with malignant disease. The use of a multiparameter approach including electron microscopy, cytochemistry, immunologic techniques, and flow cytometry may be required for an accurate and definitive diagnosis in some cases [Goodson 1979, Hovestadt 1990, Hyun 1985, Lauer 1989, Li 1986, Oehmichen 1978, O'Hara 1985, Ross 1991, Tani 1995]. Monoclonality is seen with malignancies, but because only a few malignant cells may be present together with numerous benign cells in some cases, polyclonality does not prove benignancy.

Leukemia

To unequivocally diagnose leukemia in the CSF, the clinical diagnosis should be firmly established (bone marrow biopsy, etc). Leukemic cells may be found in the CSF without clinical CNS signs or symptoms, sometimes even before a frankly leukemic blood picture develops [Nies 1965b, Spriggs 1959]. Although the peripheral blood is not necessarily involved, patients with positive CSF cytology commonly have a corresponding leukemic infiltrate in the bone marrow [Aaronson 1975].

The most common pattern of leukemic infiltration is diffuse seeding of the subarachnoid space, frequently also involving cranial and spinal nerves. Infiltration of the parenchyma of the CNS is less common, but can be seen, particularly with extreme peripheral cell counts (>100,000/μL). Acute lymphoblastic leukemia has the greatest tendency to seed the CSF, while acute myeloblastic and acute blast crisis of chronic myelocytic leukemia do so less commonly [Reske-Nielsen 1974, Wolk 1974]. It is unusual for chronic leukemias, either chronic lymphocytic or chronic myelogenous types, to involve the CSF (strongly consider reactive pleocytosis due to opportunistic infection).

The diagnosis of leukemia should be based on well-preserved cells and should not be made in the absence of blasts. Although distinguishing among the various types of blasts can be difficult or impossible, particularly using the Papanicolaou stain, it is usually not necessary for practical clinical purposes. Romanovsky type stains, such as Diff-Quik, allow for direct comparison of the CSF with leukemic cells in the peripheral blood.

When numerous blasts are present, the diagnosis is usually not difficult. However, cell counts alone are unreliable in diagnosis of lymphoma/leukemia [Aaronson 1975, A Aronson 1974, Drewinko 1973, Hyman 1965a,b, Komp 1979, Nies 1965b]. A nonmalignant pleocytosis can be caused by CNS prophylaxis (irradiation or intrathecal chemotherapy) as well as viral meningitis, leukoencephalopathy, immune recovery after therapy, posttraumatic tap, possibly as a reaction to systemic leukemia, and in some cases, with no apparent cause [Lauer 1989, McIntosh 1986]. Some cases may represent early relapse. Moreover, abnormal or atypical lymphocytes or monocytes, and even occasional blasts, can be present in severe infections (eg, bacterial, viral, fungal), or in infected immunosuppressed patients [Aaronson 1975, Kappel 1994, Nies 1965b]. However, highly immature and blast-like cells are never the predominant cell type in benign, reactive conditions. Antineoplastic therapy is not indicated for pleocytosis without evidence of leukemic cells.

On the other hand, malignant cells can be sparse, thus a normal cell count does not exclude malignancy [D Evans 1974, Nies 1965b]. A minimal leukemic infiltrate may be obscured by blood contamination or treatment with corticosteroids [McIntosh 1986]. Even a rare blast can have diagnostic significance in the appropriate clinical setting. However, whether to treat a patient based on finding only rare blasts in a specimen with low cellularity may be a difficult clinical decision [Komp 1979, Lauer 1989, McIntosh 1986]. Observing the patient clinically, with periodic examination of the CSF, will usually clarify the clinical picture [Komp 1979, McIntosh 1986].

Contamination of the CSF specimen with leukemic blood from a traumatic tap or bone marrow from vertebral bodies can result in false-positive diagnosis [Nies 1965b, Spriggs 1959]. Even a minute amount of leukemic blood, which will not discolor the fluid and therefore is visually undetectable, is sufficient to contaminate a CSF specimen [Rohlfing 1981]. The cell count can be statistically corrected by comparing the numbers of malignant cells in the blood and the fluid and relating them to the number of contaminating RBCs [Stanley 1988]. Wet fixed RBCs may lyse in 95% ethanol, but tend to be better preserved in air-dried material.

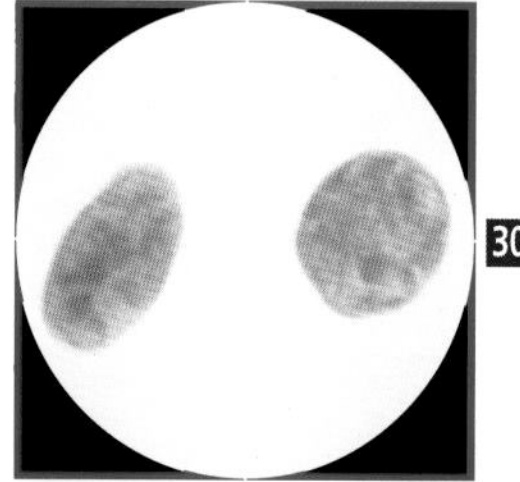
30

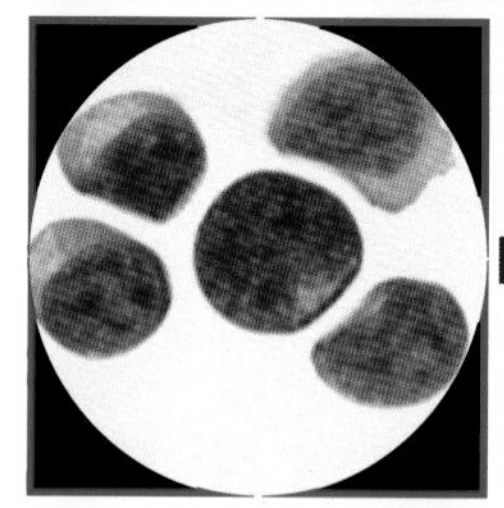
31

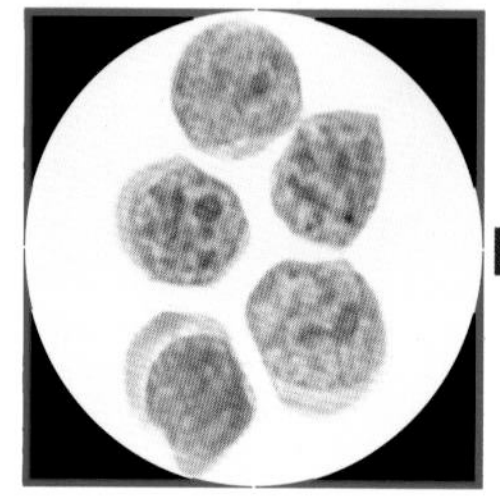
32

Acute Lymphoblastic Leukemia (ALL): This is the most common type of CNS leukemia in children and is also relatively common in adults. ALL may be impossible to distinguish from lymphoma using cytology alone.

Lymphoblasts: These are slightly larger than normal, small, mature lymphocytes, but have a higher N/C ratio because the cytoplasm is very scant. Lymphoblasts may be more pleomorphic in CSF than in the blood, bone marrow, or lymph nodes [30 I11.24, 31 I11.25, 32 I11.26]. The nuclear outline varies from case to case from smooth to convoluted. The chromatin is finer than in mature lymphocytes, but may be coarser than in myeloblasts or monoblasts. Nucleoli are usually visible, and the chromatin has a tendency to condense around them. "Hand mirror cells," with single cytoplasmic projections, are principally seen in ALL, but are occasionally also seen in chronic lymphocytic leukemia and acute myelogenous leukemia (AML), non-Hodgkin's lymphomas, and multiple myeloma, and rarely in benign conditions such as idiopathic thrombocytopenic purpura and infectious mononucleosis [Zaharopoulos 1990].

In contrast with myeloblasts, lymphoblasts never have Auer rods; although azurophilic granules may occasionally be seen (Diff-Quik) [T11.9] [Hyun 1985]. PAS stain shows coarse or block positivity, like a string of pearls around the nucleus. Common acute lymphoblastic leukemia antigen (CALLA) may aid in determining the presence of a few lymphoblasts, but occasionally CALLA tests positive in benign cells [Homans 1985]. Terminal deoxynucleotidyl transferase (TdT) is present on lymphoblasts in non-B, non-T-cell ALL and in most cases of T-cell ALL, but is rare in B-cell ALL, very rare in AML, and is never seen on benign CSF mononuclear leukocytes. Knowledge of TdT results may help in formulating a diagnosis [Casper 1983, Desai 1990].

TdT
Non-B, non-T: (+)
T-ALL: often (+)
B-ALL: rare (+)
AML: very rare (+)
Benign: always (–)

The primary differential diagnosis is with reactive lymphocytes, which may also be enlarged and have visible

T11.9 **Differential Diagnosis of Lymphoblasts, Myeloblasts, and Monoblasts**

	Cytoplasm	Auer Rods	Nuclei
Lymphoblast	Scant	No	Denser chromatin
Myeloblast	Moderate	Characteristic	More nucleoli
Monoblast	Relatively abundant	Possible	Convoluted membrane

nucleoli. Reactive lymphocytes have more cytoplasm and coarser chromatin than blasts. However, even normal lymphocytes may develop nuclear clefts or convolutions, probably an artifact of centrifugation [O'Hara 1985].

Acute Nonlymphocytic Leukemias: Acute nonlymphocytic leukemias, including AML, acute myelomonocytic, acute monocytic, and acute undifferentiated types, as well as blast crisis of chronic myelogenous leukemia, can also involve the CNS [Bigner 1985a, Kay 1976, R Meyer 1980]. AML occurs in all ages, but is more common in adults. As is true of lymphoid leukemias, the peripheral blood or bone marrow are not necessarily involved at presentation, which can result in diagnostic problems [Lagrange 1992].

Myeloblasts: Monoblasts appear similar to lymphoblasts with the Papanicolaou stain. However, using Diff-Quik, evidence of myeloid differentiation may be appreciated in maturing cells, including azurophilic granules and Auer rods [Bigner 1981a, Sindern 1994]. Myeloblasts tend to contain more nucleoli than do lymphoblasts or monoblasts [T11.9] [Hyun 1985].

Monoblasts: These may be similar in appearance to macrophages, with bean-shaped nuclei and prominent nucleoli [T11.9]. Nuclear convolutions may be particularly prominent in monoblasts. The cytoplasm is relatively abundant, greater than either lymphoblasts or myeloblasts. PAS stain may be slightly positive; if it is, the pattern is diffuse.

Using the Papanicolaou stain, the differential diagnosis of leukemic blasts includes other "small blue cell tumors," which usually form cohesive tissue aggregates and the cells are usually larger. In metastatic small cell adenocarcinomas, particularly lobular carcinoma of the breast, the cytoplasm may also show "granules" (actually intracytoplasmic mucin vacuoles).

Chronic Leukemias: Chronic leukemias, particularly chronic lymphocytic leukemia, rarely involve the CNS or shed malignant lymphocytes into the CSF [Gétaz 1979, Liepman 1981]. However, patients with chronic lymphocytic leukemia may have CNS symptoms due to infections, resulting in a benign, reactive pleocytosis which may be difficult to distinguish from malignancy [Bigner 1992, Borowitz 1981]. Small, mature lymphocytes (neoplastic vs reactive) may be indistinguishable morphologically, but in most cases, the cells will be benign.

Lymphoma

Primary CNS lymphomas are rare, but are being seen more commonly in immunosuppressed patients, including transplant recipients and patients with AIDS [Barnett 1974, Cabanillas 1987, Cho 1974, Davey 1990, Knowles 1988, Reyes 1985]. Primary CNS non-Hodgkin's lymphomas usually remain confined to the CNS [Gregory 1973, Henry 1974, Schmitt-Graff 1983]. Secondary involvement of the CNS is also rare in adults, and occurs in only 5% to 15% of all patients with non-Hodgkin's lymphoma, usually in those with widespread disease (90% of patients are stage IV, >50% have "B" symptoms) [Henry 1974, Herman 1979, Levitt 1980, Risdall 1979]. However, CNS disease may be the first sign of relapse. CNS involvement usually portends a dismal prognosis.

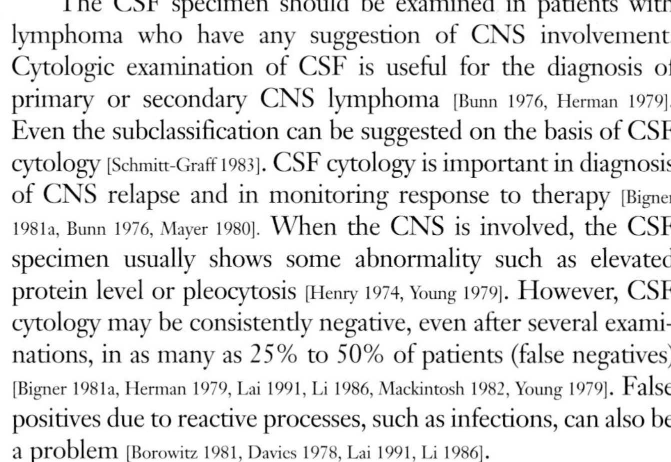

The CSF specimen should be examined in patients with lymphoma who have any suggestion of CNS involvement. Cytologic examination of CSF is useful for the diagnosis of primary or secondary CNS lymphoma [Bunn 1976, Herman 1979]. Even the subclassification can be suggested on the basis of CSF cytology [Schmitt-Graff 1983]. CSF cytology is important in diagnosis of CNS relapse and in monitoring response to therapy [Bigner 1981a, Bunn 1976, Mayer 1980]. When the CNS is involved, the CSF specimen usually shows some abnormality such as elevated protein level or pleocytosis [Henry 1974, Young 1979]. However, CSF cytology may be consistently negative, even after several examinations, in as many as 25% to 50% of patients (false negatives) [Bigner 1981a, Herman 1979, Lai 1991, Li 1986, Mackintosh 1982, Young 1979]. False positives due to reactive processes, such as infections, can also be a problem [Borowitz 1981, Davies 1978, Lai 1991, Li 1986].

In children, the most commonly diagnosed lymphomas are lymphoblastic lymphoma and small, noncleaved (Burkitt's and undifferentiated) lymphomas. In adults, diffuse large cell ("histiocytic") lymphomas including immunoblastic lymphoma, and small, cleaved cell ("poorly differentiated lymphocytic") non-Hodgkin's lymphomas are among the most common [Bunn 1976]. Burkitt's type lymphomas are also seen in patients with AIDS. Overall, the single most common CNS lymphoma diagnosed with CSF cytology is usually diffuse, large, B-cell non-Hodgkin's lymphoma.

In contrast, nodular lymphomas and small lymphocytic ("well-differentiated lymphocytic") non-Hodgkin's lymphomas, as well as Hodgkin's disease, are seldom diagnosed in the CSF [Bigner 1992, Borowitz 1981, Griffin 1971, Herman 1979]. Consider reactive pleocytosis and exclude infection in these patients.

The diagnosis of lymphoma may be difficult, particularly when malignant cells are sparse. Atypical or reactive lymphocytes associated with inflammation should not be overinterpreted as malignant lymphoma. In particular, immunocompromised patients, which include patients with lymphoma, are susceptible to opportunistic infections. Be cautious in the diagnosis of lymphoma, even when there is a history of the disease. Immunologic marker studies may be useful in some cases [Goodson 1979], but may not help in the diagnosis of a mixed inflammatory-malignant infiltrate. Most lymphomas involving the CNS are B-cell types, while most of the lymphocytes in reactive lymphocytosis are T cells.

Lymphoblastic Lymphoma: Lymphoblastic lymphoma sheds cells that are identical to those described for ALL. It is the most common type of childhood lymphoma/leukemia and has a high rate of CNS involvement.

Small Noncleaved Lymphoma: Small noncleaved (Burkitt's, non-Burkitt's) lymphoma occurs in children and is being seen with increased frequency in adults with AIDS. Many patients have CNS involvement [Janota 1966, Ziegler 1970]. The cells are actually medium-sized lymphoid cells with moderately abundant, deep blue cytoplasm which characteristically has tiny (lipid) vacuoles seen with Diff-Quik. The nuclei have fine or slightly clumped chromatin and one or more prominent nucleoli.

Large Cell Lymphoma: This is morphologically quite variable—scant to abundant cytoplasm, smooth to irregular nuclear membranes, fine to coarse chromatin, and inconspicuous to prominent nucleoli [33 I11.27, 34 I11.28]. However, it is characterized by the presence of relatively large, sometimes bizarre, noncohesive lymphoid cells. The cells must be distinguished from benign, reactive, immature lymphocytes and immunoblasts.

Small Cleaved Cell Lymphoma: This is exclusively a disease of adults. There may be many atypical small cells with coarse chromatin, visible nucleoli, and deep nuclear folds (ie, cleavages) and scant cytoplasm. Cells with bizarre twisted or irregular shapes may be encountered.

Other Lymphoreticular Diseases

Hodgkin's Disease: Hodgkin's disease rarely involves the CNS [Bigner 1981a]. When it does, the diagnosis can be suspected by the presence of large, atypical mononuclear (Hodgkin's) cells and definitively diagnosed by the presence of typical Reed-Sternberg cells [Shenoy 1987]. Reactive monocytes, lymphocytes, and eosinophils may also be seen. Primary CNS Hodgkin's disease has yet to be reported.

Myeloma: Myeloma, intradural or spinal, developing during the course of systemic multiple myeloma is encountered only rarely [Afifi 1974]. Myeloma limited to the meninges, without bone lesions or systemic disease, is rarer still [Maldonado 1970].

Plasma cells are not normally seen in the CSF; therefore, their presence, particularly when immature, is consistent with a diagnosis of plasma cell dyscrasia, including multiple myeloma, plasmacytoma, and heavy chain disease [Kumar 1988]. However, plasma cells may be found in inflammation, particularly viral infections or neurosyphilis [Bigner 1981a]. Intense plasmacytosis, including the presence of immature forms, can be seen in multiple sclerosis and certain infections such as cysticercosis, Lyme disease, and herpes [Bigner 1981a, El-Batata 1968, Kraft 1989, Péter 1967, Wilber 1980]. Circulating myeloma cells could contaminate the CSF specimen in a traumatic tap. Thus, although even rare plasma cells, particularly if they appear immature, may be suggestive of meningeal myeloma, the diagnosis must be supported by other clinical findings.

Histiocytic Proliferations: These can involve the CNS secondarily or, rarely, can be limited to the CNS [Bernard 1969, Kepes 1969, Wolfson 1979b]. The CNS is often affected in Langerhans' histiocytoses (histiocytosis X, Letterer-Siwe, and Hand-Schüller-Christian diseases), but disease confined to the CNS is rare [Bigner 1981a, Rubé 1967]. Malignant histiocytosis is a rapidly fatal disease in which CNS involvement is rare, but can occur [Bigner 1981a, Lampert 1978].

Histiocytic lesions may shed three types of cells: normal appearing histiocytes, atypical histiocytes [35 I11.29], and multinucleated histiocytes [Aozasa 1980]. The histiocytes can vary from bland to frankly malignant appearing. Evidence of phagocytosis—RBCs, WBCs, cell debris, or lipid—is a characteristic cytologic feature [Aozasa 1980, Carbone 1980, Hamilton 1982]. This unusual class of diseases should be considered in the differential diagnosis when atypical histiocytes are found in the CSF [Bigner 1981a].

33
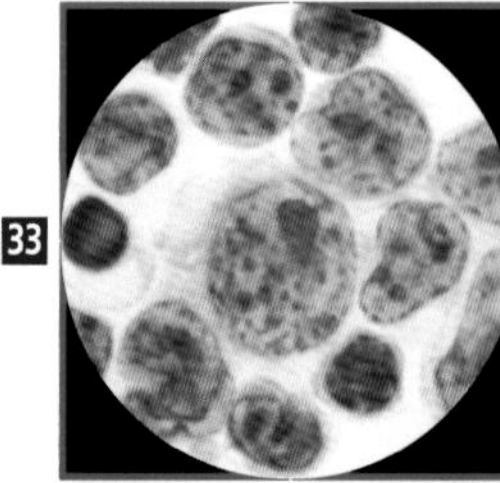

34
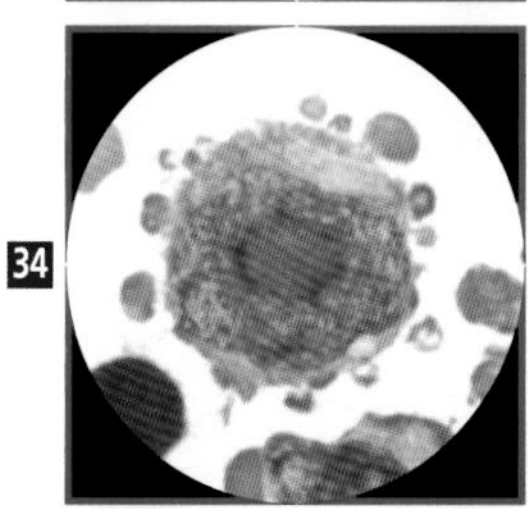

35
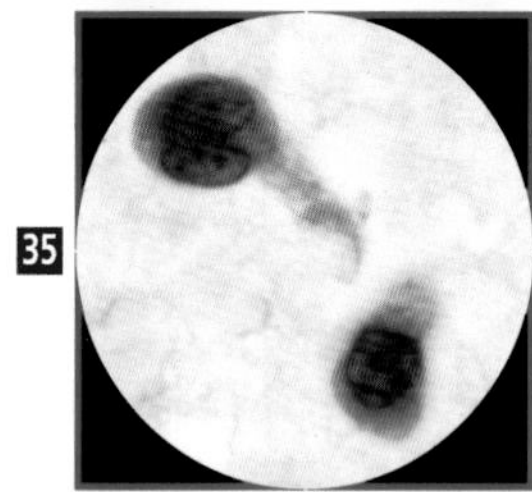

36
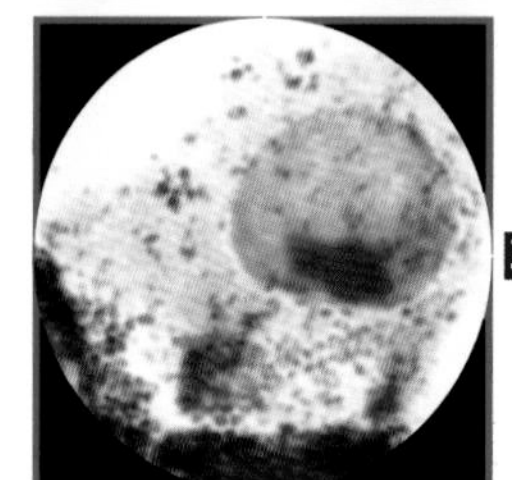

Mycosis Fungoides: This is a T-cell lymphoma that primarily affects the skin. However, it can disseminate widely, including to the CNS, resulting in positive CSF cytology. The diagnostic Sézary cells are larger than normal lymphocytes, and have hyperchromatic nuclei with deeply indented, or cerebriform, nuclear membranes [Bodensteiner 1982, Chang 1975, Gold 1976, Ludwig 1983].

Castleman's Disease: When multicentric, Castleman's disease commonly involves the CNS. The CSF may show a mixed population of lymphocytes, immunoblasts, and mature plasma cells [Stanley 1986].

Lymphomatoid Granulomatosis: This is a lymphoproliferative disorder of the lung that may also involve other organs, including the CNS [Bigner 1981a]. Lymphomatoid granulomatosis may show pleomorphic, medium-sized cells characterized by atypical nuclei, with coarse chromatin and one or more prominent nucleoli; abundant, granular cytoplasm; and cytoplasmic projections. In addition, lymphocytes, plasmacytoid lymphocytes, neutrophils, and RBCs may also be present [Saito 1978].

Miscellaneous Primary Tumors

Sarcomas, whether primary or metastatic, are uncommonly diagnosed with CSF cytology. Primary sarcomas, like meningiosarcoma or meningeal fibrosarcoma, are rare [Balhuizen 1978]. Meningeal sarcomatosis is predominantly seen in children and young adults. They shed small and large pleomorphic cells that resemble monocytes or leptomeningeal cells, but have irregular nuclear shapes, variably coarse chromatin, nucleoli, and abundant, foamy cytoplasm. Mitotic figures may be seen [Budka 1975, Garbes 1984].

Primary CNS melanoma is a rare tumor that probably arises from cells of neural crest origin in meninges, brain, or spinal cord [36 I11.35] [Bergdahl 1972, Walts 1992]. It may shed single cells with large, hyperchromatic nuclei, prominent nucleoli, and cytoplasmic pigment [Aichner 1982, An-Foraker 1985, Bigner 1984, Marks 1960, Schmidt 1988]. Despite optimal location, the CSF cytology may be (falsely) negative [Crisp 1981, Flodmark 1979].

Primary intracranial squamous cell carcinoma is a rare tumor that may represent malignant degeneration of a congenital epidermoid cyst. The most common site of these cysts is the cerebellopontine angle. The CSF may show a few isolated malignant squamous cells with large nuclei, prominent nucleoli, and abundant, hyalinized cytoplasm [Bondeson 1984].

Meningioma is a benign tumor of the meninges. Consequently, although ideally situated to shed cells into the CSF, it seldom does [Kline 1962, McMenemey 1959, Wertlake 1972, Wilkins 1966]. On rare occasions, sparse, slightly elongated cells, with moderate amounts of cytoplasm, containing ovoid nuclei with delicate chromatin and micronucleoli, and intranuclear inclusions may be seen [C Watson 1977]. When meningeal tumors exfoliate cells, they are more likely to be malignant (see "Meningeal Sarcoma").

Chordoma, a tumor of notochord, may invade the subarachnoid space and has rarely been diagnosed in the CSF [McMenemey 1959]. Physaliferous cells with bubbly cytoplasm are characteristic.

Metastatic Malignancy

Metastatic carcinoma, together with lymphoma/leukemia, are the most common tumors to be diagnosed with CSF cytology. Cancer is one of the most common causes of death in the United States and malignancies involve the CNS in up to 30% of cases [Bigner 1981a,b,1992]. The incidence of CNS involvement approaches 90% for some types of tumors such as melanoma [Bigner 1992]. CSF cytology can detect about a third of neoplasms involving the CNS [Bigner 1981b, Glass 1979, Gondos 1976]. If the leptomeninges are involved, about 50% to 60% of metastatic tumors can be diagnosed using CSF cytology [Glass 1979, Gondos 1976]. Patients usually have neurological signs or symptoms; most patients are middle aged [Olson 1974]. Positive CSF cytology is a grave prognostic sign [Ehya 1981, Little 1974].

The lung in both sexes and the breast in women are the two most common sites of origin of tumors metastatic to the brain [Bigner 1981b, Gondos 1976, Larson 1953, Little 1974, Theodore 1981, Wasserstrom 1982]. Other sites, such as the stomach, pancreas, and kidney are also common [P Meyer 1953, Naylor 1964]. In children, "small blue cell tumors" such as neuroblastoma, embryonal rhabdomyosarcoma, and Wilms' tumor are the most common sources of nonhematopoietic metastases [37 I11.22, 38 I11.23] [Vannucci 1974]. Melanoma and choriocarcinoma frequently metastasize to the brain. Either squamous carcinomas or adenocarcinomas may metastasize to the CNS, but as is also true in body cavity fluids, squamous cell carcinoma is seldom diagnosed in the CSF [Naylor 1961b,1964, Rich 1969, Weed 1975, Weithman 1987]. Although the colorectum and genitourinary tract (including ovary, endometrium, cervix, bladder [Hust 1982], and prostate) are common sources of cancers, they seldom metastasize to the CNS [S Aronson 1964]. In a small number of cases, the primary is never found.

Metastases in the CSF: The Big Three

Lung
Breast
Melanoma
[Bigner 1984, Theodore 1981]

To be detected with CSF cytology, the metastasis must involve the leptomeninges or ventricular system. Multiple samples also increase the rate of detection [Ehya 1981, Olson 1974, Wasserstrom 1982]. CSF specimens are more often positive after CNS surgery [Wilkins 1966]. Secondary malignancy in the CNS is usually associated with multiple masses (primary tumors usually produce a single mass). Meningeal carcinomatosis often sheds an abundance of malignant cells into the CSF. Positive CSF cytology in the face of no identifiable mass on CT or MRI scan suggests carcinomatous meningitis. Lung, breast, and stomach carcinomas, and occasionally sarcomas, are among the likely causes of malignant meningitis [Gonzalez-Vitale 1976, Meissner 1953].

37

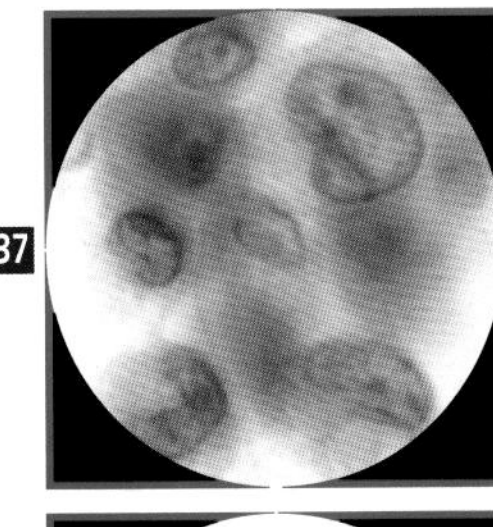

38

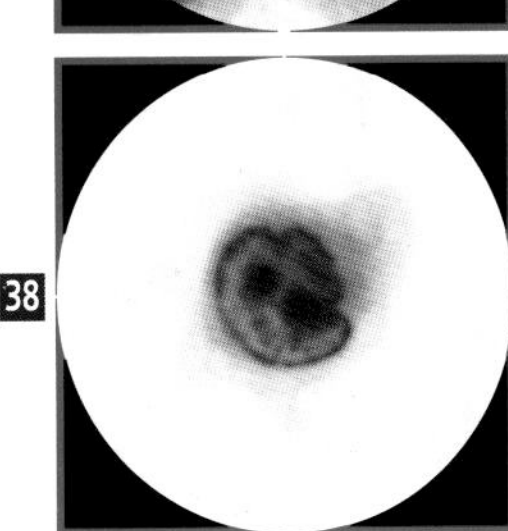

Most patients with CNS metastases have a known history of cancer, but positive CSF cytology is rarely the presenting sign. Therefore, it is usually possible, and always desirable, to compare the morphologic characteristics of the metastasis with those of the primary lesion. However, in about 10% of cases of meningeal carcinomatosis, positive CSF cytology is the initial manifestation of cancer in patients with no prior history of malignancy [Bigner 1992]. Lung, pancreas, and stomach carcinomas should be considered because they can have small, occult primaries with early metastases. Although breast carcinoma is one of the most common tumor types to involve the CNS, it rarely presents as an unknown primary in the CSF [Bigner 1984,1992, Dee 1985, Heimann 1986].

The presence of malignant cells in the CSF usually implies either multifocal or diffuse involvement of the leptomeninges by tumor [Glass 1979]. Although false negative results are common with CSF cytology, false-positive results are rare [Olson 1974]. The sparse, normal cells in the CSF are usually not confused with metastatic cancer cells [Kline 1962]. However, reactive cells such as choroid plexus cells, ependymal cells, or reticuloendothelial cells, which are particularly likely to be encountered in ventricular fluids, as well as histiocytes may lead to diagnostic confusion. On the other hand, true positive CSF cytology could result from a minute focus of metastasis, which could be missed even at autopsy (false false positive or histologic false negative) [Ehya 1981, Glass 1979, Olson 1974]. The tumor could also be eliminated with intervening therapy.

Detection of malignant cells in the CSF can be easy [Bigner 1981b, Spriggs 1954]. Even a rare foreign cell can be diagnostic of malignancy in this setting [Spriggs 1954]. The cytology is usually characterized by the presence of (only) a few atypical cells, in a clean background, although in some cases there may be protein precipitate, fresh or old blood, and cell debris. The CSF glucose is often decreased and the protein increased [Little 1974, McCormack 1953,1957]. A normal cell count does not exclude malignancy [Kolar 1968, McCormack 1957, Olson 1974, Schumann 1986].

The cytomorphologic appearance of metastatic malignancy in the CSF is similar to that seen in other fluids. True tissue aggregates with cellular disorder and nuclear crowding may be seen. However, in CSF, adenocarcinoma has a greater tendency to shed single cells rather than cells in clusters or balls [Spriggs 1954]. On the other hand, malignant cells are generally larger than any normal cell in the CSF. The malignant cells are often pleomorphic, with enlarged, irregular nuclei, prominent nucleoli, hyperchromasia, and increased N/C ratios.

It may be difficult to distinguish primary from metastatic tumors [Bigner 1981b]. Well-defined cell borders and abundant cytoplasm favor metastasis, while indistinct cell borders and scant cytoplasm suggest glioma [Naylor 1961a,b].

Nonneoplastic elements in the CSF can form loose clusters suggesting tissue aggregates, but usually lack intercellular spaces (windows) or smooth community borders. All cells in fluids tend to round up, and degenerative vacuoles, sometimes forming signet rings, may suggest cellular secretion. These features (apparent aggregates or secretion) could suggest metastatic carcinoma [Bigner 1981b, Wagner 1960]. Caution in diagnosis is advised when phagocytic activity is noted in the atypical cells, because phagocytosis suggests benign macrophages [McCormack 1957].

Lung

This is a common cancer that commonly metastasizes to the CNS and sheds diagnostic cells. The primary may be undetected clinically [Bigner 1984, Csako 1986]. Although small cell carcinoma is the most common type of lung carcinoma to metastasize to the brain, adenocarcinoma is more frequently diagnosed in CSF [Bigner 1981b,1984, Ehya 1981, Little 1974]. However, with improving survivals, small cell carcinoma may be seen more frequently in the CSF [Aisner 1979]. Squamous cell carcinoma is rare in CSF; however, dense squamoid cytoplasm is common in non–small cell lung carcinomas [Naylor 1961b].

Small Cell Carcinoma: Relatively small, cohesive cells, high N/C ratio, and nuclear molding are seen [39 I11.30] [Pedersen 1986]. Characteristic crush artifact may not be present in fluid specimens [Davenport 1990]. Differential diagnosis includes "small blue cell tumors," undifferentiated gliomas, and Merkel cell tumor [Dudley 1989]. Since small cell carcinoma of the lung is a disease of adults, pediatric tumors can be excluded.

Non–Small Cell Carcinomas: Pleomorphic cells, with large, irregular, eccentric nuclei, irregular chromatin, prominent nucleoli, and relatively dense cytoplasm can be seen. Glandular features predominate in CNS metastases. Squamous cell carcinoma has dense cytoplasm and may form pearls, but can resemble adenocarcinoma in fluid specimens [Ehya 1981]. Differential diagnosis includes high-grade gliomas, which have more delicate, wispy cytoplasm and indistinct cell borders.

Breast

This is a common tumor of women, which commonly metastasizes to the CNS and sheds diagnostic cells [Little 1974]. Cells are usually single or form loose clusters; tight balls and morulae are rare in CSF [40 I11.31] [Wallace 1982]. Indian file arrangements can be seen, but are more common in body cavity fluids [41 I11.32]. Leptomeningeal spread is particularly likely with the lobular type [Lamovec 1991].

Ductal: Medium to large cells are seen, with variation in nuclear and cytoplasmic size from case to case. However, in a given case, consistent cytologic features may give an impression of uniformity. Round to oval nuclei; fine chromatin; prominent, round nucleoli; and granular cytoplasm with well-defined cell borders are seen [Wallace 1982].

Lobular: Small, single, uniform cells with small nucleoli are seen. Intracytoplasmic lumens are characteristic (but not specific). The individual cells may resemble large cell lymphoma; look for tissue fragments or mucin vacuoles to differentiate [Ashton 1975].

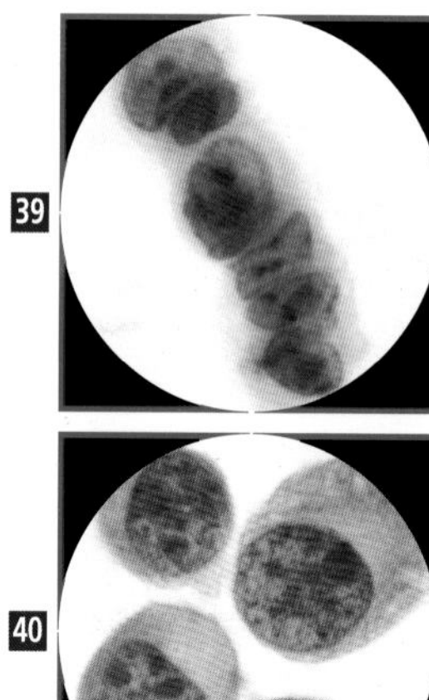

39

40

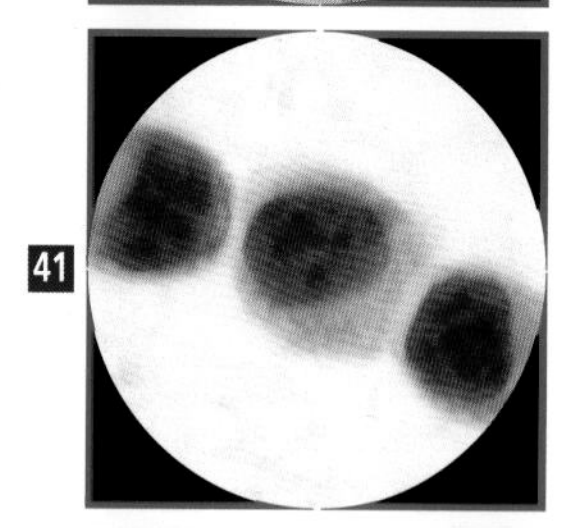

41

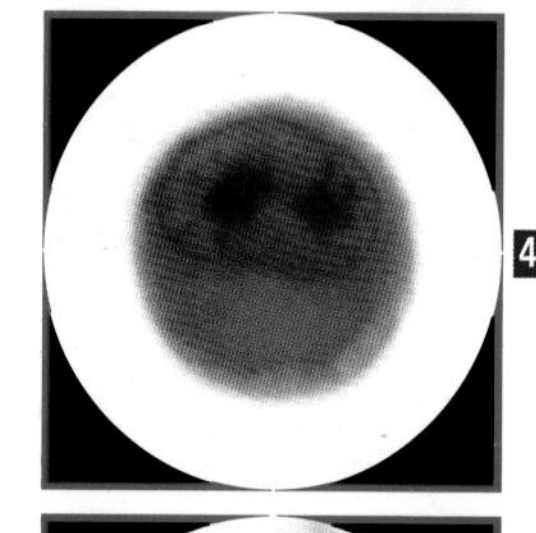

42

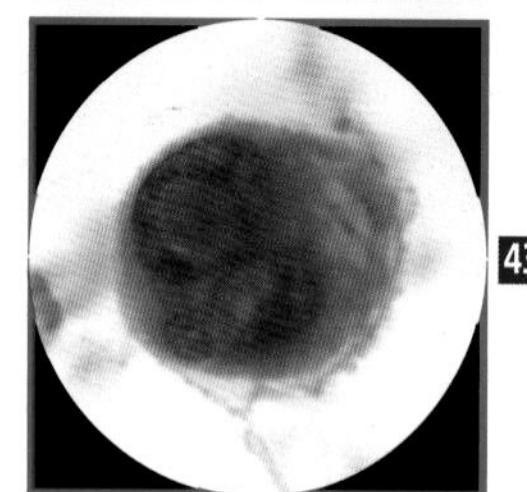

43

Stomach

This is an uncommon tumor that frequently metastasizes to the CNS, is particularly likely to spread along leptomeninges and shed abundant diagnostic cells [Meissner 1953].

The cells are small to medium sized with high N/C ratios, present singly or in small clusters, and have eccentric malignant nuclei, variable nucleoli, and a moderate amount of vacuolated cytoplasm that usually contains mucin [Iwa 1988]. Signet ring cells are classic, but not specific.

Melanoma

Melanoma is the third most common tumor (after lung and breast) to metastasize to the CNS [Amer 1978, Bigner 1984, Ehya 1981]. It frequently involves the meninges and sheds diagnostic cells. However, the primary tumor may be occult. Rarely, primary melanoma arises in the CNS, as previously discussed [I11.35].

Melanoma is characterized by large, single cells, with large, eccentric nuclei, macronucleoli, intranuclear cytoplasmic invaginations, and cytoplasmic pigment. Double mirror-image nuclei may also be seen as well as giant tumor cells [42 I11.33, 43 I11.34, I11.35].

Melanoma must be distinguished from melanosis, pigmented choroid plexus neoplasms, and ependymomas, all of which may shed pigmented cells into the CSF [Walts 1992]. In addition, nerve sheath tumors (neurofibromas, schwannomas) as well as meningiomas may contain pigmented cells, but are unlikely to shed cells into the CSF (although they may be encountered in fine needle aspiration biopsies). On the other hand, a significant number of metastatic melanomas yield poorly pigmented or nonpigmented cells.

Unknown Primary

Consider lung, stomach, and melanoma in the case of unknown primary lesions. Breast cancer is unlikely to present as an unknown primary [Bigner 1984, Dee 1985, Heimann 1986].

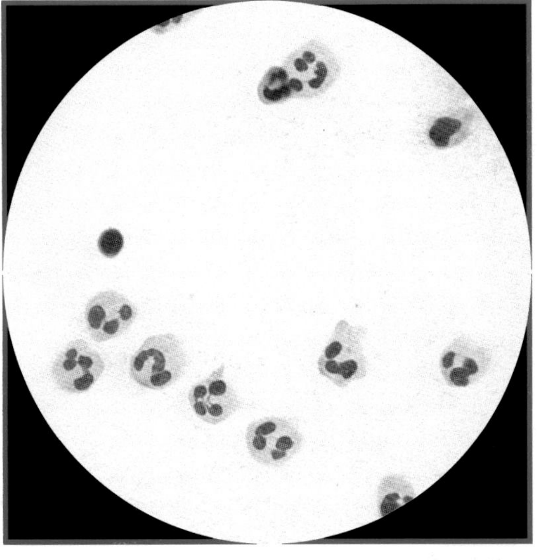

I11.1
Neutrophils. The normal CSF is sparsely cellular; most of the cells are mononuclear WBCs. Even a few neutrophils in a specimen can be an abnormal finding. When numerous, suspect bacterial meningitis.

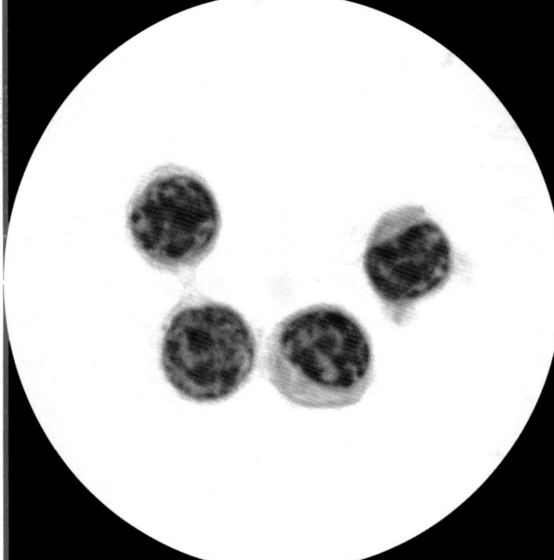

I11.2
Lymphocytes. A few lymphocytes is a normal finding in CSF; although most are small mature lymphocytes, a few reactive ones can be present normally. Lymphocytosis with decreased glucose is classically associated with tuberculosis or fungal infections. Lymphocytosis with normal glucose is associated with viral or postinfectious meningitis, as well as chronic central nervous system diseases, such as multiple sclerosis, among other entities. (Pap, oil)

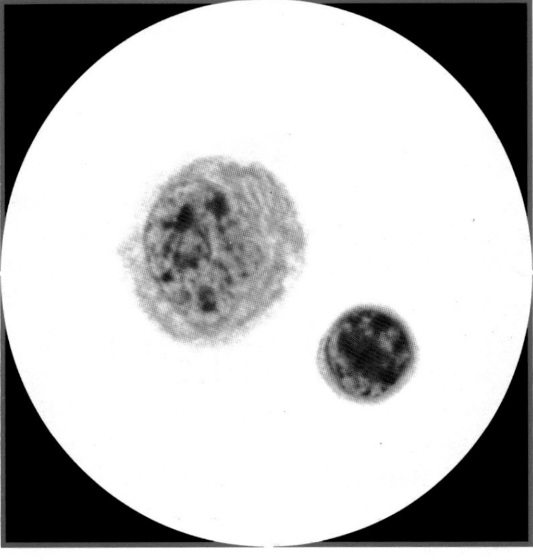

I11.3
Lymphocytes/monocytes. Lymphocytes usually outnumber monocytes by at least two to one. Monocytes have more abundant, foamy/vacuolated cytoplasm and characteristic chromatin (salt-and-pepper with Pap stain, illustrated, raked sand with Diff-Quik). (Pap, oil)

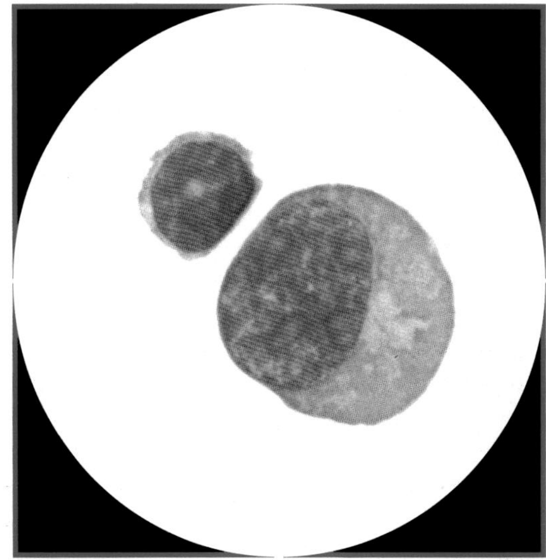

I11.4
Reactive or "atypical" lymphocytes. Immature lymphocytes can have larger nuclei, nuclear cleavages, nucleoli, and more abundant cytoplasm. They are particularly likely in viral or tuberculous infections, as well as multiple sclerosis, but can be seen in a variety of conditions. In benign, reactive conditions, small mature lymphocytes predominate. (Diff-Quik, oil)

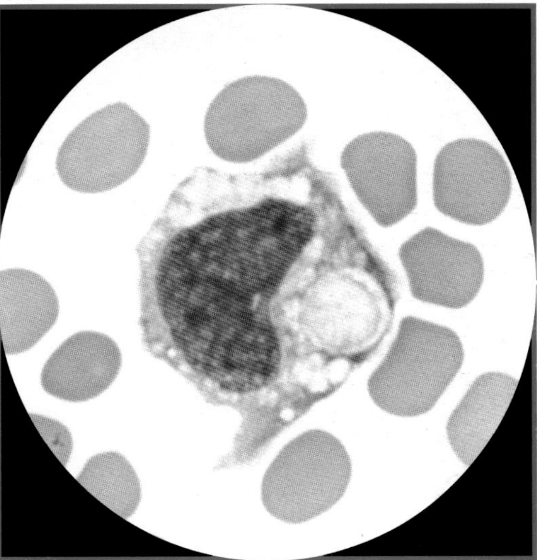

I11.5
Erythrophagocytosis. indicates recent bleeding, such as that seen in cerebral hemorrhage. (Diff-Quik, oil)

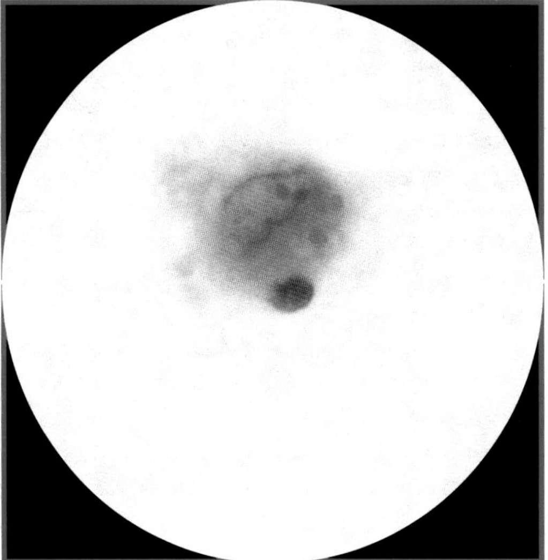

I11.6
Hemosiderin-laden macrophages. Siderophages indicate old bleeding; they may persist for months. Other substances, such as lipid, can also be found in the cytoplasm of macrophages. Lipophages are associated with parenchymal destruction. (Pap, oil)

I11.7
Eosinophils. Not normally present in CSF, eosinophils are associated with foreign bodies, allergies (including drug reactions), infections (especially parasites), and sometimes neoplasms (Hodgkin's, primary and metastatic tumors). Note bilobed nuclei and distinct reddish cytoplasmic granules (arrows) (Pap).

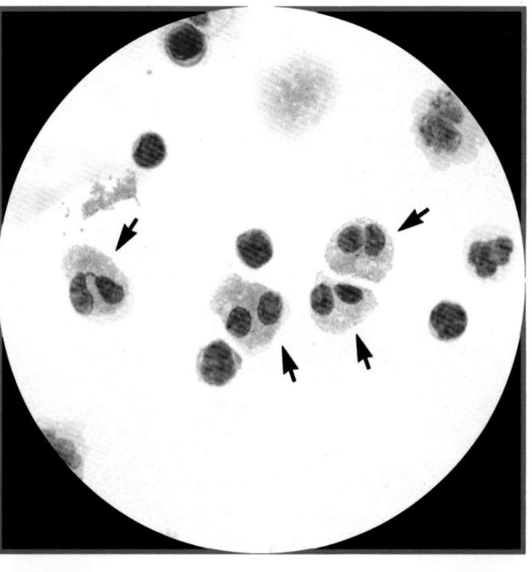

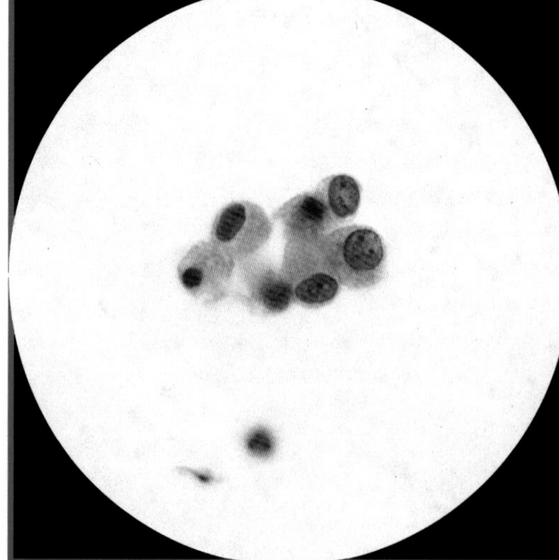

I11.8
Choroid plexus. Similar to ependymal cells (also known as choroid/ependymal cells). They are more commonly found in ventricular or cisternal fluids than lumbar punctures. Nuclei are round to elongated, small, and uniform with moderate amount of dense cytoplasm that may be vacuolated or contain yellow pigment. Acinar formation is characteristic. Primary diagnostic significance is to not mistake for malignancy. (Pap)

I11.9
Leptomeningeal cells. These cells are the counterpart of mesothelial cells in other body cavities (also known as pia-arachnoid mesothelial cells), but they are not true mesothelial cells. They have relatively abundant, delicate cytoplasm with eccentric, round to oval to bean-shaped nuclei with fine chromatin. (Pap)

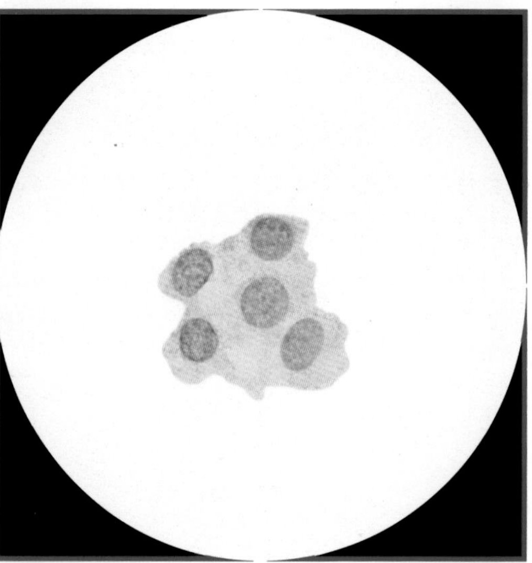

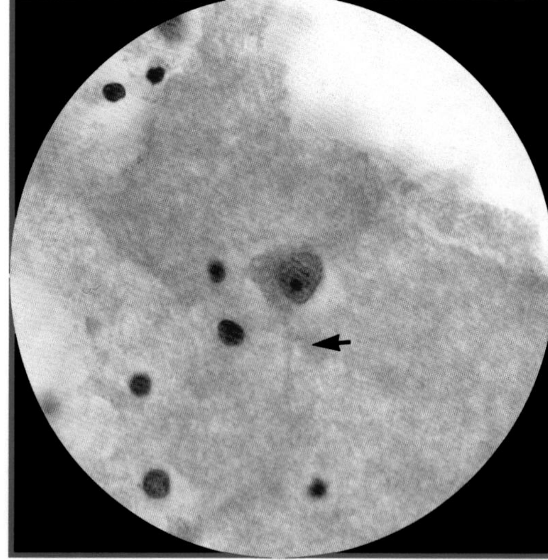

I11.10
Neurons. Neurons are the largest nonneoplastic cells seen in the CSF. They have typical pyramidal or multipolar body with long processes (arrow), dense granular cytoplasm, and nuclei with fine chromatin, but characteristic prominent nucleoli. Usually found in ventricular or cisternal fluids, rather than lumbar punctures. (Pap)

I11.11
Fibrocartilage. "Pickup" contaminant from vertebral column. (Pap)

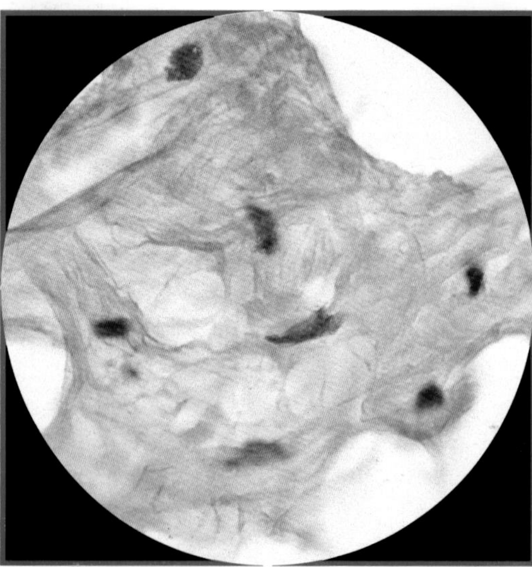

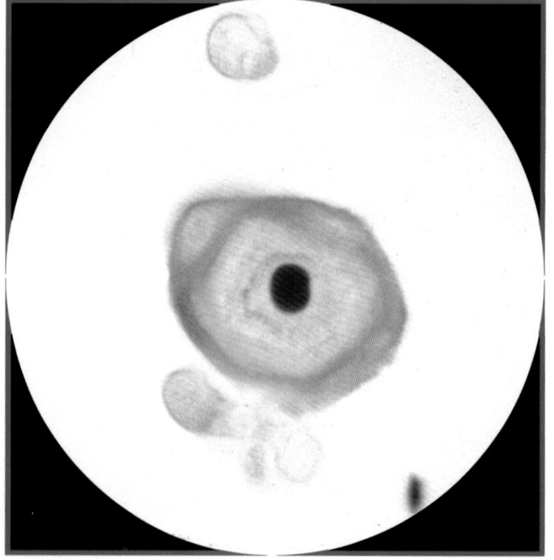

I11.12
Mature cartilage. Mature chondrocyte with pyknotic nucleus and vacuolated cytoplasm is seen in lacunar space surrounded by thick "cell wall" of cartilage. (Pap)

I11.13
Mature cartilage. Cartilage is intensely magenta (metachromatic) in Diff-Quik.

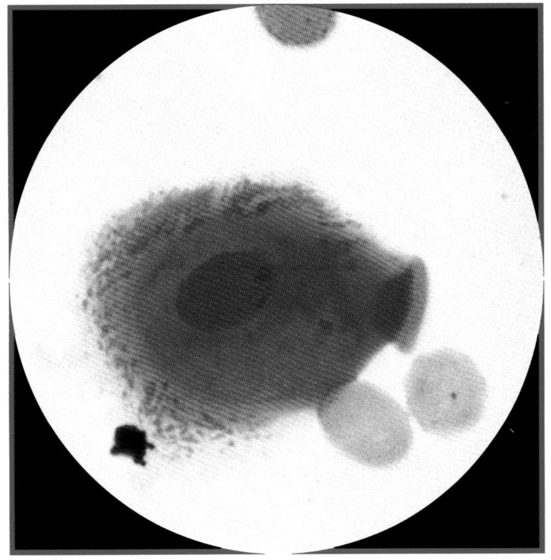

I11.14
Capillaries. Delicate tubular structures that can be seen from time to time in ventricular fluid. (Pap)

I11.15
Giant cells. Benign giant cells can be seen in granulomatous inflammation, including foreign body reaction to shunt (illustrated). Also, megakaryocytes are occasionally found as a "pick up" contaminant from bone marrow. Malignant giant cells can be seen in glioblastoma (and other primary cancers), metastases, and melanoma. Cluster of histiocytes may also be present. (Pap)

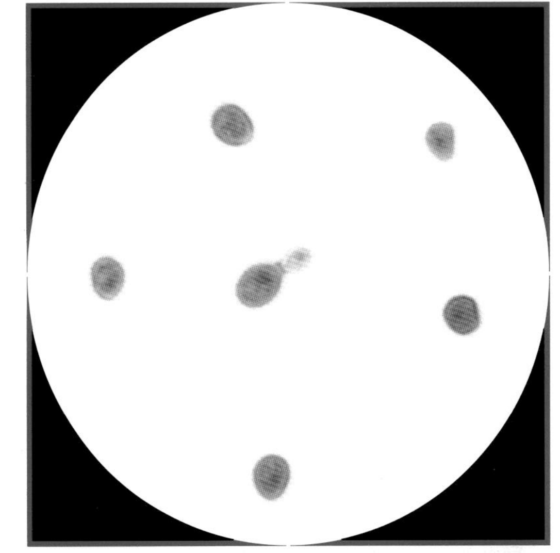

I11.16
Cryptococcus. Most common fungal organism seen in CSF. Tear drop–shaped budding is characteristic. Because they may take the Pap stain poorly, they can be missed in screening. (Pap)

I11.17
Cryptococcus. Mucoid capsule stains red with mucicarmine.

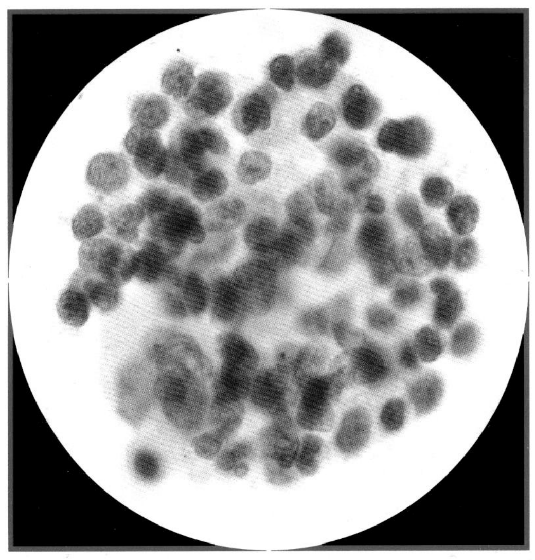

I11.18
Astrocytoma. High-grade astrocytomas and glioblastoma multiforme are the most common primary brain tumors of the cerebral hemisphere of adults that are likely to shed diagnostic cells into the CSF. Note large to giant cells with hyperchromatic nuclei and granular to fibrillar, wispy cytoplasm. Bizarre cells can be seen. Low-grade astrocytomas are unlikely to shed cells. (Pap)

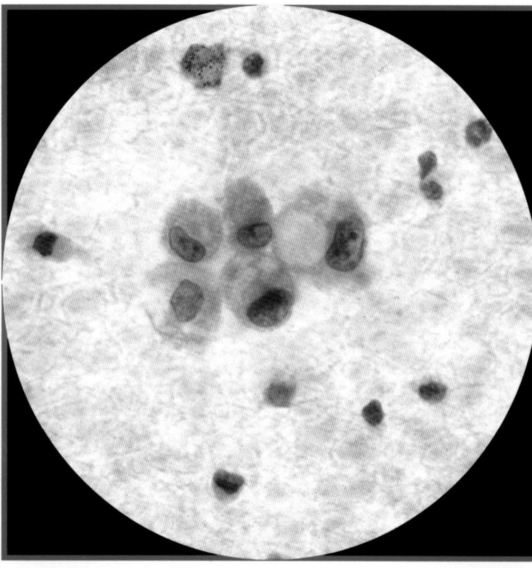

I11.19
Ependymoma. The tumor cells resemble normal ependymal cells with bland, uniform, eccentrically located nuclei and a moderate amount of lacy blue cytoplasm. Cilia and blepharoplasts (basal bodies) are virtually pathognomonic, if present. (Pap)

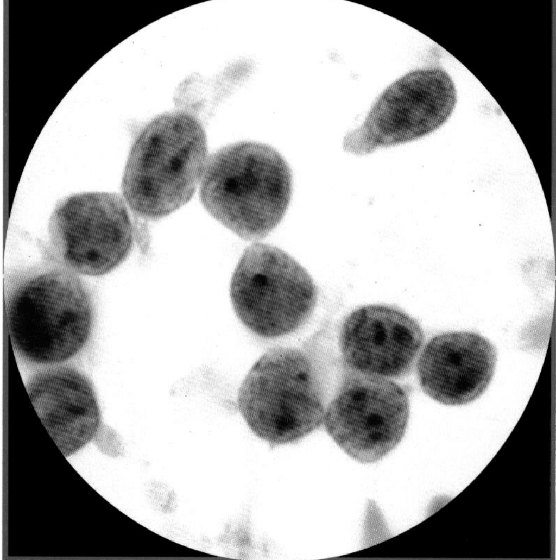

I11.20
Medulloblastoma. This tumor accounts for one quarter of primary brain tumors in children. The cytologic appearance is a classic "small blue cell tumor." The cells have scant cytoplasm, high N/C ratios, pleomorphic, dark nuclei, and form molded tissue aggregates. Nucleoli vary from inconspicuous to prominent and multiple (compare with I11.31). (Pap, oil)

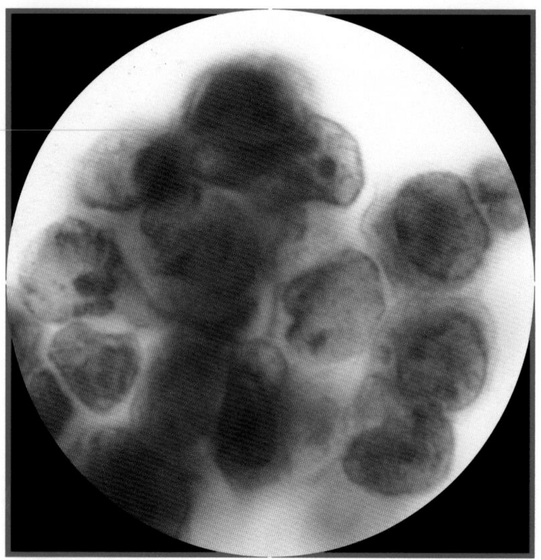

I11.21
Retinoblastoma. A family of tumors cytologically indistinguishable from medulloblastoma, including retinoblastoma (illustrated), neuroblastoma, and pineoblastoma. (Pap, oil)

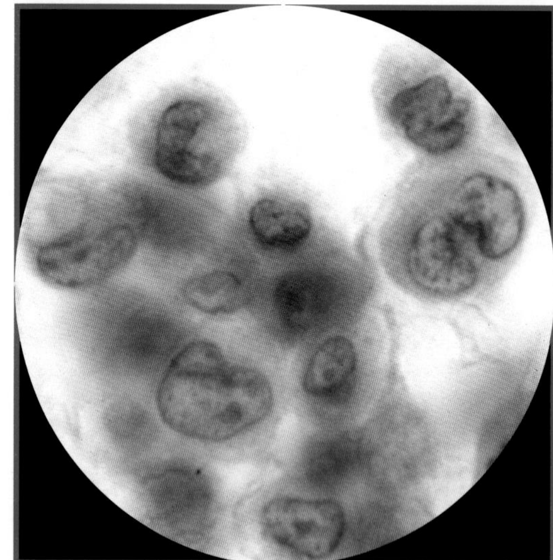

I11.22
Ewing's sarcoma. Tumors cytologically similar to medulloblastoma can metastasize to the central nervous system. Illustrated is Ewing's sarcoma, which may shed cohesive or noncohesive cells. (Oil)

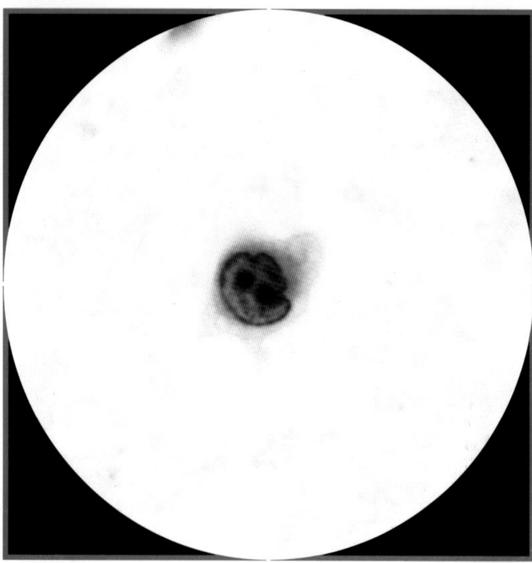

I11.23
Rhabdomyosarcoma. This is another type of "small blue cell tumor" that can be included in the differential diagnosis of primary brain tumors of children. In adults, small cell carcinoma of the lung is far and away the most likely source of malignant "small blue cells." (Pap, oil)

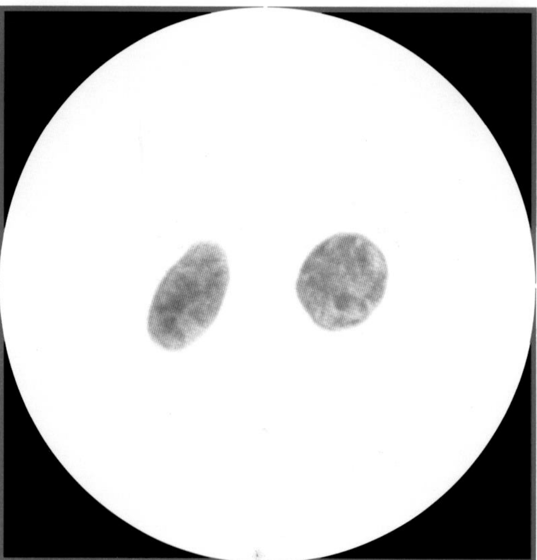

I11.24
Acute lymphoblastic leukemia. Acute leukemias commonly involve the central nervous system; acute lymphoblastic leukemia is the most common type. Lymphoblasts vary somewhat morphologically . The cytoplasm ranges from miniscule in amount (illustrated) to slightly more abundant. Nuclei can have smooth or convoluted membranes. Chromatin varies from powdery fine (illustrated) to granular in CSF. (Pap, oil)

I11.25
Acute lymphoblastic leukemia. Same case as in I11.24. Note nuclear convolutions, scant cytoplasm. (Diff-Quik, oil)

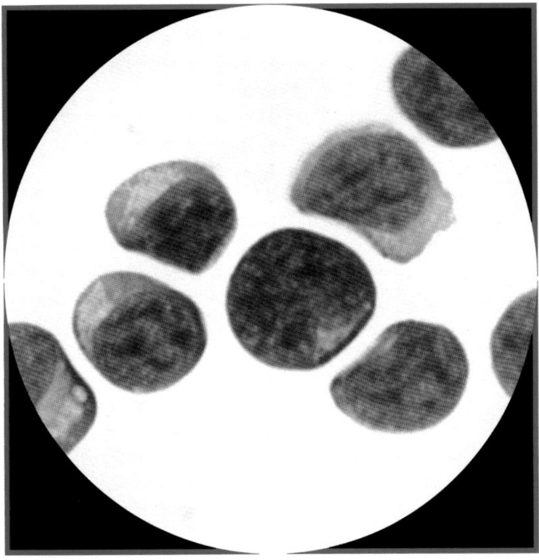

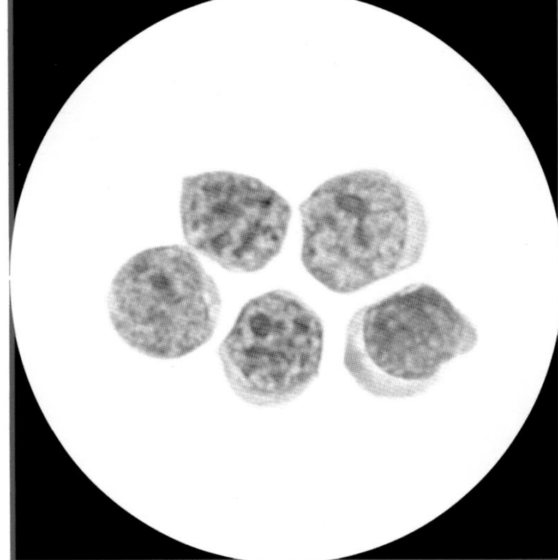

I11.26
Acute lymphoblastic leukemia. Another case, with granular chromatin and conspicuous nucleoli. No Auer rods are seen (presence would indicate myeloid differentiation). (Pap, oil)

I11.27
Large cell lymphoma. Primary central nervous system lymphomas are rare, but are being seen more commonly in patients with AIDS. They are morphologically variable, with scant to abundant cytoplasm, smooth (noncleaved) to irregular (cleaved) nuclei, and inconspicuous to prominent nucleoli. Immunoblastic lymphoma is illustrated. Note prominent central nucleoli. Note clustering of cells, an artifact of preparation. (Pap, oil)

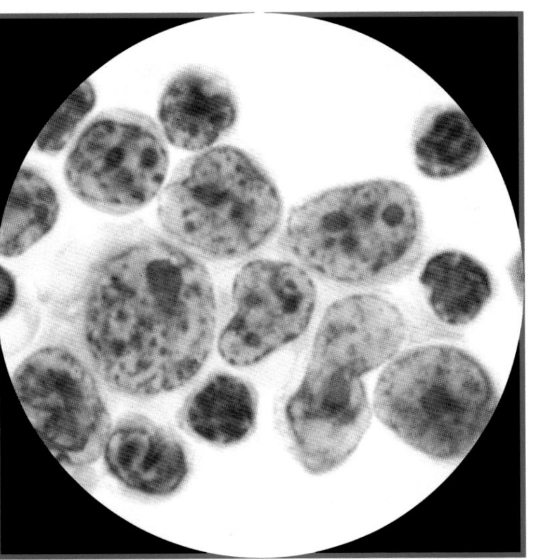

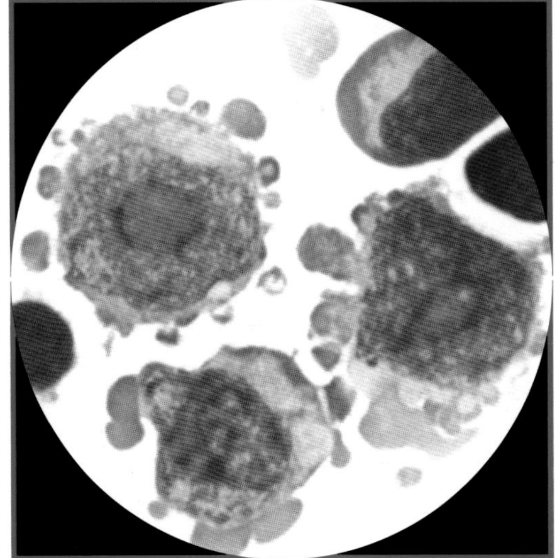

I11.28
Immunoblastic lymphoma. Same case as in I11.27. Note single, central plasmacytoid macronucleolus and plasmacytoid appearance of cytoplasm with pale staining perinuclear hof. (Diff-Quik, oil)

I11.29
Langerhans' histiocytosis (histiocytosis X). Histiocytic proliferations can shed normal appearing, atypical, or multinucleated histiocytes. Illustrated are slightly atypical appearing histiocytes. (Pap, oil)

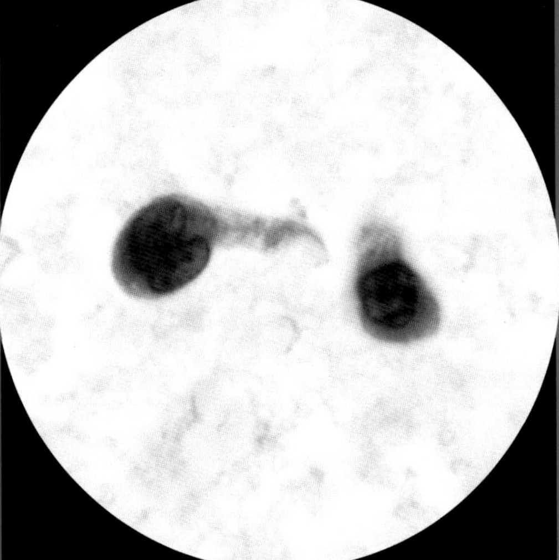

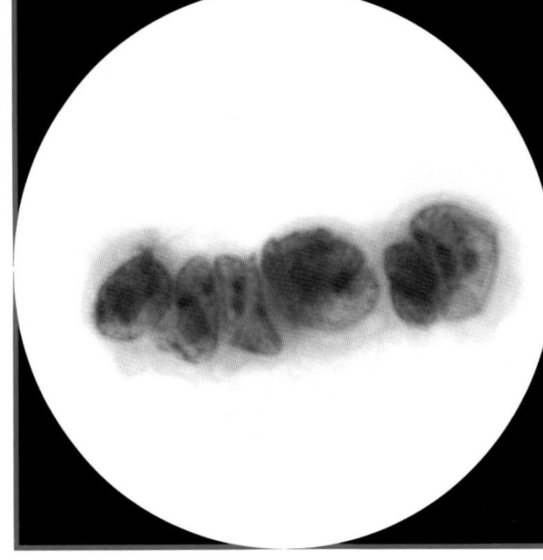

I11.30
Metastatic small cell carcinoma. Lung cancer is one of the most common sources of brain metastases. Small cell lung cancer (illustrated) is characterized by molded groups of cells with high N/C ratios. Indian file arrangements are common. Nucleoli may be somewhat more prominent in fluid specimens than expected. (Oil)

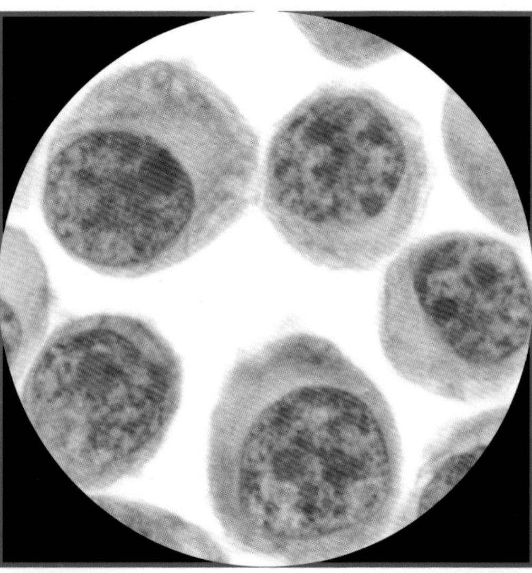

I11.31
Metastatic breast carcinoma. The key to diagnosis of metastatic carcinoma is simple: *these cells do not belong in the CSF*. They are completely unlike any normal cell that could be seen. Breast cancer is one of the most common sources of brain metastases in women. The plasmacytoid appearance (illustrated) is common. (Papanicolaou, oil)

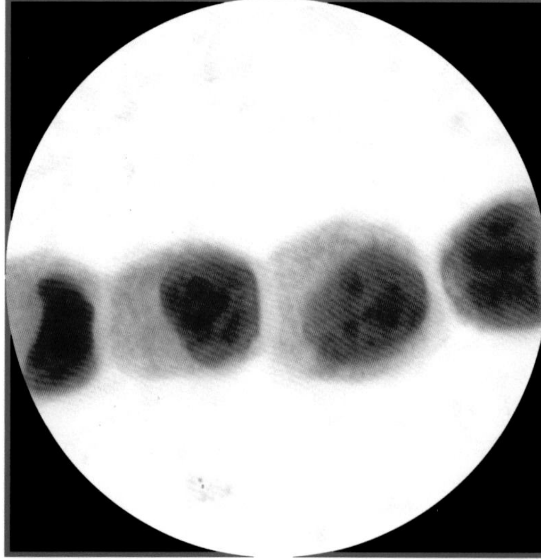

I11.32
Metastatic breast carcinoma. Indian file arrangements are common but not unique to breast carcinoma. (Pap, oil)

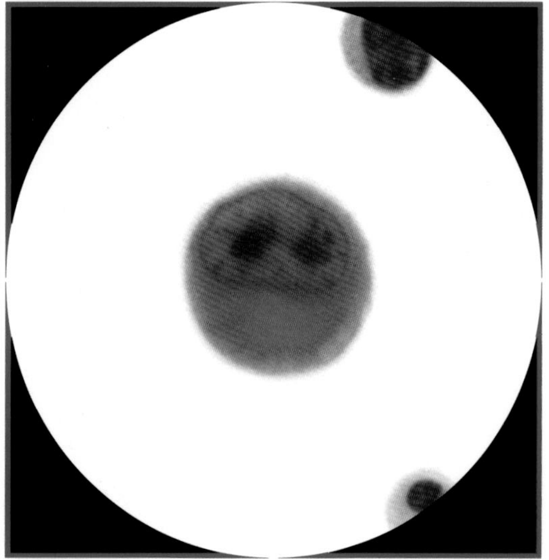

I11.33
Metastatic melanoma. Along with breast and lung cancer, metastatic melanoma rounds out the "big three" sources of brain metastases. Melanin pigment may be sparse or absent. Macronucleoli are common. (Oil)

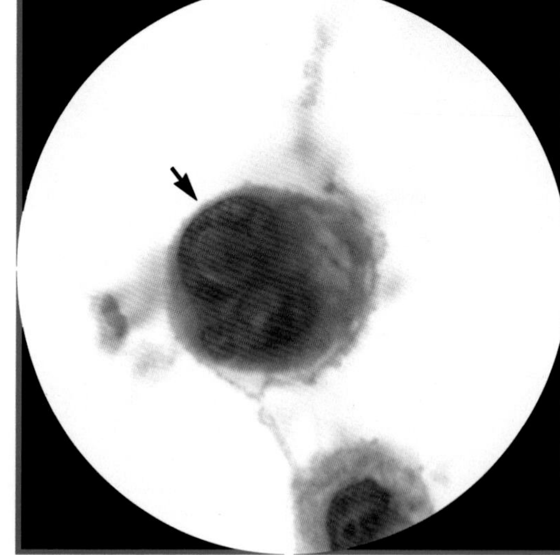

I11.34
Metastatic melanoma. Intranuclear cytoplasmic invaginations (arrow) are characteristic but not specific. (Oil)

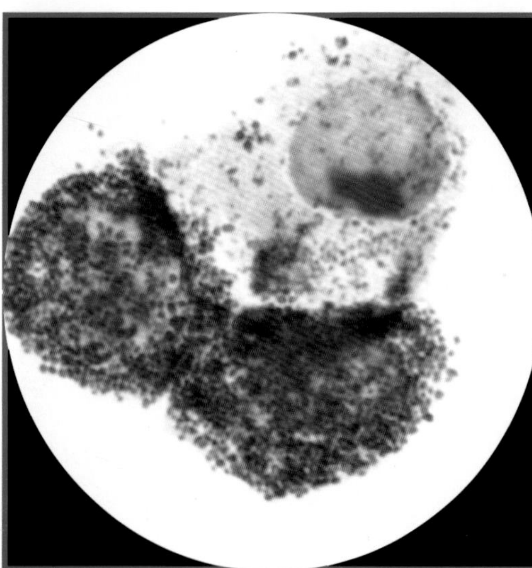

I11.35
Primary melanoma. Characteristic cytoplasmic pigmentation. (Diff-Quik, oil) (Case courtesy of Jami Walloch, MD.)

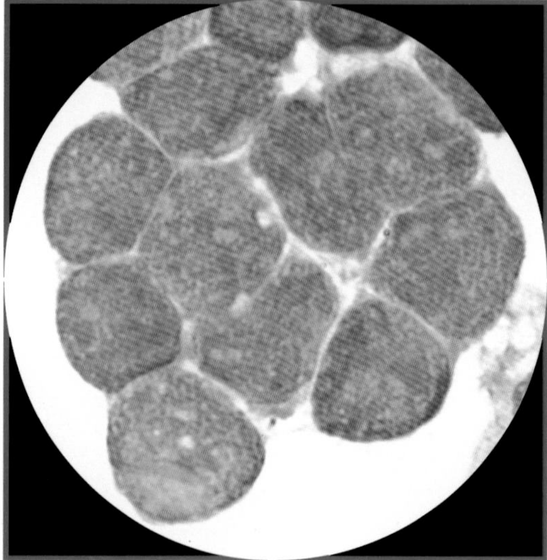

I11.36
Undifferentiated leptomeningeal cells. From neonate with intraventricular brain hemorrhage. Cells closely mimic lymphoblasts (all single cells) and, especially, medulloblasts (which may be larger and more pleomorphic but are otherwise similar).

References

Aaronson AG, Hajdu SI, Melamed MR: Spinal Fluid Cytology During Chemotherapy of Leukemia of the Central Nervous System in Children. *Am J Clin Pathol* 63: 528–537, 1975.

Afifi AM: Myeloma Cells in the Cerebrospinal Fluid in Plasma Cell Neoplasia. *J Neurol Neurosurg Psychiatry* 37: 1162–1165, 1974.

Aichner F, Schuler G: Primary Leptomeningeal Melanoma: Diagnosis by Ultrastructural Cytology of Cerebrospinal Fluid and Cranial Computed Tomography. *Cancer* 50: 1751–1756, 1982.

Aisner J, Aisner SC, Ostrow S, et al: Meningeal Carcinomatosis From Small Cell Carcinoma of the Lung: Consequence of Improved Survival. *Acta Cytol* 23: 292–296, 1979.

Amer MH, Al-Sarraf M, Baker LH, et al: Malignant Melanoma and Central Nervous System Metastases: Incidence, Diagnosis, Treatment and Survival. *Cancer* 42: 660–668, 1978.

Andrews JM, Schumann GB: Laboratory Processing of Cerebrospinal Fluid Specimens. *Diagn Cytopathol* 6: 139–143, 1990.

An-Foraker SH: Cytodiagnosis of Malignant Lesions in Cerebrospinal Fluid: Review and Cytohistologic Correlation. *Acta Cytol* 29: 286–290, 1985.

Aozasa K, Kurokawa K, Kobori Y, et al: Malignant Histiocytosis Showing Ascites and Recurrent Meningeal Infiltration. *Acta Cytol* 24: 228–231, 1980.

Aronson AS, Garwicz S, Sörnäs R: Cytology of the Cerebrospinal Fluid in Children With Acute Lymphoblastic Leukemia. *J Pediatr* 85: 222–224, 1974.

Aronson SM, Garcia JH, Aronson BE: Metastatic Neoplasms of the Brain: Their Frequency in Relation to Age. *Cancer* 17: 558–563, 1964.

Ashton PR, Hollingsworth AS Jr, Johnston WW: The Cytopathology of Metastatic Breast Cancer. *Acta Cytol* 19: 1–6, 1975.

Aur RJA, Simone JS, Hustu HO, et al: Central Nervous System Therapy and Combination Chemotherapy of Childhood Lymphocytic Leukemia. *Blood* 37: 272–281, 1971.

Bach F, Soletormos G, Dombernowsky P: Tissue Polypeptide Antigen Activity in Cerebrospinal Fluid: A Marker of Central Nervous System Metastases of Breast Cancer: *J Natl Cancer Inst* 83: 779–784, 1991.

Bach F, Bjerregaard B, Soletormos G, et al: Diagnostic Value of Cerebrospinal Fluid Cytology in Comparison With Tumor Marker Activity in Central Nervous System Metastases Secondary to Breast Cancer. *Cancer* 72: 2376–2382, 1993.

Baker RC, Lenane AM: The Predictive Value of Cerebrospinal Fluid Differential Cytology in Meningitis. *Pediatr Infect Dis J* 8: 239–330, 1989.

Balhuizen JC, Botts GTAM, Schaberg A: The Value of Cytology in the Diagnosis of Hypophyseal Tumors. *Acta Cytol* 18: 370–375, 1974.

Balhuizen JC, Bots GTAM, Schaberg A, et al: Value of Cerebrospinal Fluid Cytology for the Diagnosis of Malignancies in the Central Nervous System. *J Neurosurg* 48: 747–753, 1978.

Barnett LB, Schwartz E: Cerebral Reticulum Cell Sarcoma After Multiple Renal Transplants. *J Neurol Neurosurg Psychiatry* 37: 966–970, 1974.

Barrett DL, King EB: Comparison of Cellular Recovery Rates and Morphologic Detail Obtained Using Membrane Filter and Cytocentrifuge Techniques. *Acta Cytol* 20: 174–180, 1976.

Barrett TL, Downey EF Jr, Garvin DF: A Bizarre Mononuclear Cell Response in CSF Following Myelography. *Military Med* 151: 108–109, 1986.

Battifora H, Hidvegi D: Improved Apparatus for Spinal Fluid Cytomorphology. *Acta Cytol* 22: 170–171, 1978.

Benach JL, Bosler EM, Hanrahan JP, et al: Spirochetes Isolated From the Blood of Two Patients With Lyme Disease. *N Engl J Med* 308: 740–742, 1983.

Bergdahl L, Boquist L, Liliequist B, et al: Primary Malignant Melanoma of the Central Nervous System: A Report of 10 Cases. *Acta Neurochir* 26: 139–149, 1972.

Bering EA Jr: Cerebrospinal Fluid. *Prog Neurol Psychiatry* 21: 358– 373, 1966.

Bernad PG, Taft PD: Cytologic Diagnosis of Intraventricular Hemorrhage in a Neonate. *Acta Cytol* 24: 4–6, 1980.

Bernard JD, Aguilar MJ: Localized Hypothalamic Histiocytosis X: Report of a Case. *Arch Neurol* 20: 368–372, 1969.

Bernhardt H, Gourley RD, Young JM, et al: A Modified Membrane-Filter Technic for Detection of Cancer Cells in Body Fluids. *Am J Clin Pathol* 36: 462–464, 1961.

Bigner SH, Johnston WW: The Cytopathology of Cerebrospinal Fluid: I. Nonneoplastic Conditions, Lymphoma and Leukemia. *Acta Cytol* 25: 335–353, 1981a.

Bigner SH, Johnston WW: The Cytopathology of Cerebrospinal Fluid: II. Metastatic Cancer, Meningeal Carcinomatosis and Primary Central Nervous System Neoplasms. *Acta Cytol* 25: 461–479, 1981b.

Bigner SH, Johnston WW: The Diagnostic Challenge of Tumors Manifested Initially by the Shedding of Cells Into Cerebrospinal Fluid. *Acta Cytol* 28: 29–36, 1984.

Bigner SH, Elmore PD, Dee AL, et al: Unusual Presentations of Inflammatory Conditions in Cerebrospinal Fluid. *Acta Cytol* 29: 291–296, 1985a.

Bigner SH, Elmore PD, Dee AL, et al: The Cytopathology of Reactions to Ventricular Shunts. *Acta Cytol* 29: 391–396, 1985b.

Bigner SH: Cerebrospinal Fluid (CSF) Cytology: Current Status and Diagnostic Applications. *J Neuropathol Exp Neurol* 51: 235–245, 1992.

Bodensteiner DC, Skikne B: Central Nervous System Involvement in Mycosis Fungoides: Diagnosis, Treatment and Literature Review. *Cancer* 50: 1181–1184, 1982.

Bonadio WA: Bacterial Meningitis in Children Whose Cerebrospinal Fluid Contains Polymorphonuclear Leukocytes Without Pleocytosis. *Clin Pediatr* 27: 198–200, 1988a.

Bonadio WA, Bonadio JF: Significance of Polymorphonuclear Leukocytes in CSF of Bacteremic Children. *Pediatr Emerg Care* 4: 180–182, 1988b.

Bonadio WA, Smith DS, Goddard S, et al: Distinguishing Cerebrospinal Fluid Abnormalities in Children With Bacterial Meningitis and Traumatic Lumbar Puncture. *J Infect Dis* 162: 251–254, 1990.

Bondeson L, Fält K: Primary Intracranial Epidermoid Carcinoma. *Acta Cytol* 28: 487–489, 1984.

Boogerd W, Vroom TM, Van Heerde P, et al: CSF Cytology Versus Immunocytochemistry in Meningeal Carcinomatosis. *J Neurol Neurosurg Psychiatry* 51: 142–145, 1988.

Boring C: Cancer Statistics. *CA Cancer J Clin* 44: 18–19, 1994.

Borowitz M, Bigner SH, Johnston WW: Diagnostic Problems in the Cytologic Evaluation of Cerebrospinal Fluid for Lymphoma and Leukemia. *Acta Cytol* 25: 665–674, 1981.

Bosch I, Oehmichen M: Eosinophilic Granulocytes in Cerebrospinal Fluid: Analysis of 94 Cerebrospinal Fluid Specimens and Review of the Literature. *J Neurol* 219: 93–105, 1978.

Bots GTAM, Went LN, Schaberg A: Results of a Sedimentation Technique for Cytology of Cerebrospinal Fluid. *Acta Cytol* 8: 234–241, 1964.

Breuer AC, Tyler HR, Marzewski DJ, et al: Radicular Vessels Are the Most Probable Source of Needle-Induced Blood in Lumbar Puncture: Significance for the Thrombocytopenic Cancer Patient. *Cancer* 49: 2168–2172, 1982.

Brown RW, Clarke RJ, Gonzales MF: Cytologic Detection of *Cryptococcus neoformans* in Cerebrospinal Fluid: Rapid Screening Methods. *Acta Cytol* 29: 151–153, 1985.

Budka H, Pilz P, Guseo A: Primary Leptomeningeal Sarcomatosis: Clinicopathological Report of Six Cases. *J Neurol* 211: 77–93, 1975.

Budka H, Guseo A, Jellinger K, et al: Intermittent Meningitic Reaction With Severe Basophilia and Eosinophilia in CNS Leukemia: A Special Type of Hypersensitivity. *J Neurol Sci* 28: 459–468, 1976.

Bunn PA Jr, Schein PS, Banks PM, et al: Central Nervous System Complications in Patients With Diffuse Histiocytic and Undifferentiated Lymphoma: Leukemia Revisited. *Blood* 47: 3–10, 1976.

Cabanillas F, Pathak S, Zander A, et al: Monosomy 21, Partial Duplication of Chromosome 11, and Structural Abnormality of Chromosome 1q21 in a Case of Lymphoma Developing in a Transplant Recipient: Characteristic Abnormalities of Secondary Lymphoma? *Cancer Genet Cytogenet* 24: 7–10, 1987.

Cairns H, Russell DS: Intracranial and Spinal Metastases in Gliomas of the Brain. *J Brain* 54: 27–420, 1931.

Carbone A, Volpe R: Cerebrospinal Fluid Involvement by Malignant Histiocytosis. *Acta Cytol* 24: 172–173, 1980.

Casper JT, Lauer SJ, Kirchner PA, et al: Evaluation of Cerebrospinal Fluid Mononuclear Cells Obtained From Children With Acute Lymphocytic Leukemia: Advantages of Combining Cytomorphology and Terminal Deoxynucleotidyl Transferase. *Am J Clin Pathol* 80: 666–670, 1983.

Catovsky D, Bernasconi C, Verdonck PJ, et al: The Association of Eosinophilia With Lymphoblastic Leukemia or Lymphoma: A Study of Seven Patients. *Br J Haematol* 45: 523–534, 1980.

Chang AM, Ng ABP: The Cellular Manifestations of Mycosis Fungoides in Cerebrospinal Fluid: A Case Report. *Acta Cytol* 19: 148–151, 1975.

Chen KTK, Moseley D: Cartilage Cells in Cerebrospinal Fluid. *Arch Pathol Lab Med* 114: 212, 1990.

Cho E-S, Connolly E, Porro RS: Primary Reticulum Cell Sarcoma of the Brain in a Renal Transplantation Recipient: Case Report. *J Neurosurg* 41: 235–239, 1974.

Choi H-SH, Anderson PJ: Diagnostic Cytology of Cerebrospinal Fluid by the Cytocentrifuge Method. *Am J Clin Pathol* 72: 931–943, 1979.

Clare N, Rone R: Detection of Malignancy in Body Fluids. *Lab Med* 17: 147–150, 1986.

Coleman A, Schumann GB: Cytodiagnosis and Monitoring of Acute Lymphocytic Leukemia and Eosinophilia in Cerebrospinal Fluid. *Diagn Cytopathol* 3: 330–334, 1987.

Conly JM, Ronald AR: Cerebrospinal Fluid as a Diagnostic Body Fluid. *Am J Med* 75: 102–108, 1983.

Conrad KA, Gross JL, Trojanowski JQ: Leptomeningeal Carcinomatosis Presenting as Eosinophilic Meningitis. *Acta Cytol* 30: 29–31, 1986.

Craver RD, Carson TH: Hematopoietic Elements in Cerebrospinal Fluid in Children. *Am J Clin Pathol* 95: 532–535, 1991.

Crisp DE, Thompson JA: Primary Malignant Melanomatosis of the Meninges: Clinical Course and Computed Tomographic Findings in a Young Child. *Arch Neurol* 38: 528–529, 1981.

Csako G, Chandra P: Bronchioloalveolar Carcinoma Presenting With Meningeal Carcinomatosis: Cytologic Diagnosis in Cerebrospinal Fluid. *Acta Cytol* 30: 653–656, 1986.

Cumings JN: The Cerebrospinal Fluid in Diagnosis. *Br Med J* (i): 449–451, 1954.

Dalens B, Bezou M-J, Coulet M, et al: Cerebrospinal Fluid Cytomorphology in Neonates. *Acta Cytol* 26: 395–400, 1982.

Davenport RD: Diagnostic Value of Crush Artifact in Cytologic Specimens: Occurrence in Small Cell Carcinoma of the Lung. *Acta Cytol* 34: 502–504, 1990.

Davey DD, Foucar K, Giller R: Millipore Filter vs Cytocentrifuge for Detection of Childhood Central Nervous System Leukemia. *Arch Pathol Lab Med* 110: 705–708, 1986.

Davey DD, Gulley ML, Walker WP, et al: Cytologic Findings in Posttransplant Lymphoproliferative Disease. *Acta Cytol* 34: 304–310, 1990.

Davies SF, Gormus BJ, Yarchoan R, et al: Cryptococcal Meningitis With False-Positive Cytology in the CSF: Use of T-Cell Rosetting to Exclude Meningeal Lymphoma. *JAMA* 239: 2369–2370, 1978.

Dee AL: Carcinoma of the Breast Presenting Initially in Cerebrospinal Fluid. *Acta Cytol* 29: 909–910, 1985.

DeFendini R, Hunter SB, Schlesinger EB, et al: Eosinophilic Meningitis in a Case of Disseminated Glioblastoma. *Arch Neurol* 38: 52–53, 1981.

DeGirolami U, Schmidek H: Clinicopathological Study of 53 Tumors of the Pineal Region. *J Neurosurg* 39: 455–462, 1973.

Del Vecchio PR, DeWitt SH, Borelli JI, et al: Application of Millipore Filtration Technique to Cytologic Material. *J Natl Cancer Inst* 22: 427–431, 1959.

DeMent SH, Cox MC, Gupta PK: Diagnosis of Central Nervous System *Toxoplasma gondii* From the Cerebrospinal Fluid in a Patient With Acquired Immunodeficiency Syndrome. *Diagn Cytopathol* 3: 148–151, 1987.

Den Hartog Jager WA: Cytopathology of the Cerebrospinal Fluid Examined With the Sedimentation Technique After Sayk. *J Neurol Sci* 9: 155–177, 1969.

Desai K, Willard-Smith D, Fallon M, et al: Improving the Diagnostic Accuracy of Cerebrospinal Fluid Examinations in Acute Lymphoblastic Leukemia via High-Power Microscopy and Tdt Determinations. *Acta Cytol* 34: 749–750, 1990.

Devinsky O, Nadi NS, Theodore WH, et al: Cerebrospinal Fluid Pleocytosis Following Simple, Complex Partial, and Generalized Tonic-Clonic Seizures. *Ann Neurol* 23: 402–403, 1988.

Diamond IB: Leukemic Changes in the Brain: A Report of Fourteen Cases. *Arch Neurol Psychiatry* 32: 118–142, 1934.

Doré CF, Balfour BM: A Device for Preparing Cell Spreads. *Immunology* 9: 403–405, 1965.

Drewinko B, Sullivan MP, Martin T: Use of the Cytocentrifuge in the Diagnosis of Meningeal Leukemia. *Cancer* 31: 1331–1336, 1973.

Dudley TH Jr, Moinuddin S: Cytologic and Immunohistochemical Diagnosis of Neuroendocrine (Merkel Cell) Carcinoma in Cerebrospinal Fluid. *Am J Clin Pathol* 91: 714–717, 1989.

Dyken PR: Cerebrospinal Fluid Cytology: Practical Clinical Usefulness. *Neurology* 25: 210–217, 1975.

Dyken PR, Shirley S, Trefz J, et al: Comparison of Cytocentrifugation and Sedimentation Techniques for CSF Cytomorphology. *Acta Cytol* 24: 167–170, 1980.

Ehya H, Hajdu SI, Melamed MR: Cytopathology of Nonlymphoreticular Neoplasms Metastatic to the Central Nervous System. *Acta Cytol* 25: 599–610, 1981.

El-Batata M: Cytology of Cerebrospinal Fluid in the Diagnosis of Malignancy. *J Neurosurg* 28: 317–326, 1968.

Evans AE, Gilbert ES, Zandstra R: The Increasing Incidence of Central Nervous System Leukemia in Children (Children's Cancer Study Group A). *Cancer* 26: 404–409, 1970.

Evans DIK: CSF in Acute Childhood Leukemia: Cytocentrifuge Studies. *Arch Dis Child* 49: 496, 1974.

Evans H: Cytology of Mollaret Meningitis. *Diagn Cytopathol* 9: 373–376, 1993.

Farr GH, Hajdu SI: Exfoliative Cytology of Metastatic Neuroblastoma. *Acta Cytol* 16: 203–206, 1972.

Fischer JR, Davey DD, Gulley ML, et al: Blast-like Cells in Cerebrospinal Fluid of Neonates: Possible Germinal Matrix Origin. *Am J Clin Pathol* 91: 255–258, 1989.

Fleischer RL, Price PB, Symes EM: Novel Filter for Biological Materials. *Science* 143: 249–250, 1964.

Flodmark O, Fitz CR, Harwood-Nash DC, et al: Neuroradiological Findings in a Child With Primary Leptomeningeal Melanoma. *Neuroradiology* 18: 153–156, 1979.

Gandolfi A: The Cytology of Cerebral Neuroblastoma. *Acta Cytol* 24: 344–346, 1980.

Garbes AD: Cytologic Presentation of Primary Leptomeningeal Sarcomatosis. *Acta Cytol* 28: 709–712, 1984.

Garcia-Riego A, Prats JM, Zarranz JJ: Sanfilippo Disease: Buhot Cells in the Cerebrospinal Fluid. *Acta Cytol* 22: 282–284, 1978.

Geisinger KR, Hajdu SI, Helson L: Exfoliative Cytology of Nonlymphoreticular Neoplasms in Children. *Acta Cytol* 28: 16–28, 1984.

Gétaz EP, Miller GJ: Spinal Cord Involvement in Chronic Lymphocytic Leukemia. *Cancer* 43: 1858–1861, 1979.

Gindhart TD, Tsukahara YC: Cytologic Diagnosis of Pineal Germinoma in Cerebrospinal Fluid and Sputum. *Acta Cytol* 23: 341–346, 1979.

Glass JP, Melamed M, Chernik NL, et al: Malignant Cells in Cerebrospinal Fluid (CSF): The Meaning of a Positive CSF Cytology. *Neurology* 29: 1369–1375, 1979.

Gold JH, Shelburne JD, Bossen EH: Meningeal Mycosis Fungoides: Cytologic and Ultrastructural Aspects. *Acta Cytol* 20: 349–355, 1976.

Gondos B, King EB: Cerebrospinal Fluid Cytology: Diagnostic Accuracy and Comparison of Different Techniques. *Acta Cytol* 20: 542–547, 1976.

Gondos B: Millipore Filter vs Cytocentrifuge for Evaluation of Cerebrospinal Fluid. *Arch Pathol Lab Med* 110: 687–688, 1986.

Gonzalez-Vitale JC, Garcia-Bunuel R: Meningeal Carcinomatosis. *Cancer* 37: 2906–2911, 1976.

Goodson JD, Strauss GM: Diagnosis of Lymphomatous Leptomeningitis by Cerebrospinal Fluid Lymphocyte Cell Surface Markers. *Am J Med* 66: 1057–1059, 1979.

Greenberg ML, Goldberg L: The Value of Cerebrospinal Fluid Cytology in the Early Diagnosis of Metastatic Retinoblastoma. *Acta Cytol* 21: 735–738, 1977.

Gregory MC, Hughes JT: Intracranial Reticulum Cell Sarcoma Associated With Immunoglobulin A Deficiency. *J Neurol Neurosurg Psychiatry* 36: 769–776, 1973.

Griffin JW, Thompson RW, Mitchinson MJ, et al: Lymphomatous Leptomeningitis. *Am J Med* 51: 200–208, 1971.

Gupta PK, Gupta PC, Roy S, et al: Herpes Simplex Encephalitis, Cerebrospinal Fluid Cytology Studies: Two Case Reports. *Acta Cytol* 16: 563–565, 1972.

Guseo A, Lechner G, Bierleutgeb F: A Simple Method for Demonstrating Cells in the Cerebrospinal Fluid by Scanning Electron Microscopy. *Acta Cytol* 21: 352–355, 1977.

Hamilton SR, Gupta PK, Marshall ME, et al: Cerebrospinal Fluid Cytology in Histiocytic Proliferative Disorders. *Acta Cytol* 26: 22–28, 1982.

Hansen HH, Bender RA, Shelton BJ: The Cyto-centrifuge and Cerebrospinal Fluid Cytology. *Acta Cytol* 18: 259–262, 1974.

Hayward RA, Shapiro MF, Oye RK: Laboratory Testing on Cerebrospinal Fluid: A Reappraisal. *Lancet* (ii): 1–4, 1987.

Hayward RA, Oye RK: Are Polymorphonuclear Leukocytes an Abnormal Finding in Cerebrospinal Fluid? Results From 225 Normal Cerebrospinal Fluid Specimens. *Arch Intern Med* 148: 1623–1624, 1988.

Hegenbarth MA, Green M, Rowley AH, et al: Absent or Minimal Cerebrospinal Fluid Abnormalities in *Haemophilus influenzae* Meningitis. *Pediatr Emerg Care* 6: 191–194, 1990.

Heimann A, Merino MJ: Carcinomatous Meningitis as the Initial Manifestation of Breast Cancer. *Acta Cytol* 30: 25–28, 1986.

Henry JM, Heffner RR Jr, Dillard SH, et al: Primary Malignant Lymphomas of the Central Nervous System. *Cancer* 34: 1293–1302, 1974.

Herman TS, Hammond N, Jones SE, et al: Involvement of the Central Nervous System by Non-Hodgkin's Lymphoma: The Southwest Oncology Group Experience. *Cancer* 43: 390–397, 1979.

Hollander H, Stringari S: Human Immunodeficiency Virus-Associated Meningitis: Clinical Course and Correlations. *Am J Med* 83: 813–816, 1987.

Holley HP, Al-Ibrahim MS: CSF Eosinophilia Following Myelography. *JAMA* 242: 2432–2433, 1979.

Homans AC, Forman EN, Barker BE: Use of Monoclonal Antibodies to Identify Cerebrospinal Fluid Lymphoblasts in Children With Acute Lymphoblastic Leukemia. *Blood* 66: 1321–1325, 1985.

Hovestadt A, Henzen-Logmans SC, Vecht CJ: Immunohistochemical Analysis of the Cerebrospinal Fluid for Carcinomatous and Lymphomatous Leptomeningitis. *Br J Cancer* 62: 653–654, 1990.

Hust MH, Pfitzer P: Cerebrospinal Fluid and Metastasis of Transitional Cell Carcinoma of the Bladder. *Acta Cytol* 26: 217–223, 1982.

Hustu HO, Aur RJA, Verzosa MS, et al: Prevention of Central Nervous System Leukemia by Irradiation. *Cancer* 32: 585–597, 1973.

Hutchison JH: Treatment of Acute Lymphoblastic Leukemia: Effect of 'Prophylactic' Therapy against Central Nervous System Leukemia: Report to the Medical Research Council by the Leukemia Committee and the Working Party on Leukemia in Childhood. *Br Med J* 2: 381–384, 1973.

Hutton WE: A Survey of the Application of the 'Molecular' Membrane Filter to the Study of Cerebrospinal Fluid Cytology. *Am J Clin Pathol* 30: 407–410, 1958.

Hyman CB, Bogle JM, Brubaker CA, et al: Central Nervous System Involvement by Leukemia in Children. I. Relationship to Systemic Leukemia and Description of Clinical and Laboratory Manifestations. *Blood* 25: 1–12, 1965a.

Hyman CB, Bogle JM, Brubaker CA, et al: Central Nervous System Involvement by Leukemia in Children. II. Therapy With Intrathecal Methotrexate. *Blood* 25: 13–22, 1965b.

Hyun BH, Salazar GH: Cerebrospinal Fluid Cells in Leukemias, Lymphomas, and Myeloma. *Lab Med* 16: 667–670, 1985.

Iwa N, Yutani C, Kobayashi TK: Immunocytochemical Localization of Carcinoembryonic Antigen in Cerebrospinal Fluid With Metastatic Carcinoma of the Stomach: Report of Four Cases. *Diagn Cytopathol* 4: 312–315, 1988.

Jaeckle KA: Cerebrospinal Fluid Cytomorphology in Systemic Lupus Erythematosus With Anton's Syndrome. *Acta Cytol* 26: 532–536, 1982.

Janota I: Involvement of the Nervous System in Malignant Lymphoma in Nigeria. *Br J Cancer* 20: 47–61, 1966.

Jellinger KA, Paulus W: Primary Central Nervous System Lymphomas: An Update. J *Cancer Res Clin Oncol* 119: 7–27, 1992.

Jeren T, Beus I: Characteristics of Cerebrospinal Fluid in Tuberculous Meningitis. *Acta Cytol* 26: 678–680, 1982.

Johnston WW, Gin FL, Amatulli JM: Light and Electron Microscopic Observations on Malignant Cells in Cerebrospinal Fluid From Metastatic Alveolar Cell Carcinoma. *Acta Cytol* 15: 365–371, 1971.

Kajikawa H, Ohta T, Ohshiro H, et al: Cerebrospinal Fluid Cytology in Patients With Brain Tumors; A Simple Method Using the Cell Culture Technique. *Acta Cytol* 21: 162–167, 1977.

Kamiya M, Tateyama H, Fujiyoshi Y, et al: Cerebrospinal Fluid Cytology in Immature Teratoma of the Central Nervous System: A Case Report. *Acta Cytol* 35: 757–760, 1991.

Kappel TJ, Manivel JC, Goswitz JJ: Atypical Lymphocytes in Spinal Fluid Resembling Posttransplant Lymphoma in a Cardiac Transplant Recipient. A Case Report. *Acta Cytol* 38: 470–474, 1994.

Katz RL, Alappattu C, Glass JP, et al: Cerebrospinal Fluid Manifestations of the Neurologic Complications of Human Immunodeficiency Virus Infection. *Acta Cytol* 33: 233–244, 1989.

Kay HEM: Development of CNS Leukemia in Acute Myeloid Leukemia in Childhood. *Arch Dis Child* 51: 73–74, 1976.

Kepes JJ, Kepes M: Predominantly Cerebral Forms of Histiocytosis-X: A Reappraisal of 'Gagel's Hypothalamic Granuloma', 'Granuloma Infiltrans of the Hypothalamus' and 'Ayala's Disease' With a Report of four Cases. *Acta Neuropathol* 14: 77–98, 1969.

Kim K, Greenblatt SH, Robinson MG: Choroid Plexus Carcinoma: Report of a Case With Cytopathologic Differential Diagnosis. *Acta Cytol* 29: 846–849, 1985.

Kim T, Nesbit ME, D'Angio GD, et al: The Role of Central Nervous System Irradiation in Children With Acute Lymphoblastic Leukemia. *Radiology* 104: 635–641, 1972.

Kline TS: Cytological Examination of the Cerebrospinal Fluid. *Cancer* 15: 591–597, 1962.

Knowles DM, Chamulak GA, Subar M, et al: Lymphoid Neoplasia Associated With the Acquired Immunodeficiency Syndrome (AIDS): The New York University Medical Center Experience With 105 Patients (1981-1986). *Ann Intern Med* 108: 744–753, 1988.

Kobayashi TK, Ueda M, Yamaki T, et al: Evaluation of Cytocentrifuge Apparatus With Special Reference to the Cellular Recovery Rate. *Diagn Cytopathol* 8: 420–423, 1992.

Kolar O, Zeman W: Spinal Fluid Cytomorphology: Description of Apparatus, Technique, and Findings. *Arch Neurol* 18: 44–51, 1968.

Kölmel HW: A Method for Concentrating Cerebrospinal Fluid Cells. *Acta Cytol* 21: 154–157, 1977.

Komp DM: Diagnosis of CNS Leukemia. *Am J Pediatr Hematol Oncol* 1: 31–35, 1979.

Kraft R, Altermatt HJ, Nguyen-Tran Q: Differentialdiagnose Atypischer Plasmazellen im Liquor Cerebrospinalis. *Dtsch Med Wschr* 114: 1729–1733, 1989.

Krentz MJ, Dyken PR: Cerebrospinal Fluid Cytomorphology: Sedimentation vs Filtration. *Arch Neurol* 26: 253–257, 1972.

Kruskall MS, Carter SR, Ritz LP: Contamination of Cerebrospinal Fluid by Vertebral Bone-Marrow Cells During Lumbar Puncture. *N Engl J Med* 308: 697–700, 1983.

Kumar PV, Esfahani FN, Tabei SZ, et al: Cytopathology of Alpha Chain Disease Involving the Central Nervous System and Pleura. *Acta Cytol* 32: 902–907, 1988.

Lagrange M, Gaspard M-H, Lagrange J-L, et al: Granulocytic Sarcoma With Meningeal Leukemia but No Bone Marrow Involvement at Presentation: A Report of Two Cases With Characteristic Cerebrospinal Fluid Cytology. *Acta Cytol* 36: 319–324, 1992.

Lai AP, Wierzbicki AS, Norman PM: Immunocytological Diagnosis of Primary Cerebral Non-Hodgkin's Lymphoma. *J Clin Pathol* 44: 251–253, 1991.

Lamovec J, Zidar A: Association of Leptomeningeal Carcinomatosis in Carcinoma of the Breast With Infiltrating Lobular Carcinoma: An Autopsy Study. *Arch Pathol Lab Med* 115: 507–510, 1991.

Lampert IA, Catovsky D, Bergier N: Malignant Histiocytosis: A Clinico-pathological Study of 12 Cases. *Br J Haematol* 40: 65–77, 1978.

Lane PA, Githens JH: Contamination of Cerebrospinal Fluid With Bone-Marrow Cells During Lumbar Puncture. *N Engl J Med* 309: 434, 1983.

Larson CP, Robson JT, Reberger CC: Cytologic Diagnosis of Tumor Cells in Cerebrospinal Fluid. *J Neurosurg* 10: 337–341, 1953.

Lauer SJ, Kirchner PA, Camitta BM: Identification of Leukemic Cells in the Cerebrospinal Fluid From Children With Acute Lymphoblastic Leukemia: Advances and Dilemmas. *Am J Pediatr Hematol Oncol* 11: 64–73, 1989.

Law IP, Blom J: Adult Acute Leukemia: Frequency of Central Nervous System Involvement in Long Term Survivors. *Cancer* 40: 1304–1306, 1977.

Leidler F, Russell WO: The Brain in Leukemia: A Clinicopathologic Study of Twenty Cases With a Review of the Literature. *Arch Pathol* 40: 14–33, 1945.

Leiman G, Klein C, Berry AV: Cells of Nucleus Pulposus in Cerebrospinal Fluid: A Case Report. *Acta Cytol* 24: 347–349, 1980.

Levitt LJ, Dawson DM, Rosenthal DS, et al: CNS Involvement in the Non-Hodgkin's Lymphomas. *Cancer* 45: 545–552, 1980.

Li C-Y, Witzig TE, Phyliky RL, et al: Diagnosis of B-Cell Non-Hodgkin's Lymphoma of the Central Nervous System by Immunocytochemical Analysis of Cerebrospinal Fluid Lymphocytes. *Cancer* 57: 737–744, 1986.

Li C-Y, Yam LT: Cytologic and Immunocytochemical Studies of Cerebrospinal Fluid in Meningeal Sarcoidosis: A Case Report. *Acta Cytol* 36: 963–967, 1992.

Liepman MK, Votaw ML: Meningeal Leukemia Complicating Chronic Lymphocytic Leukemia. *Cancer* 47: 2482–2484, 1981.

Little JR, Dale AJD, Okazaki H: Meningeal Carcinomatosis: Clinical Manifestations. *Arch Neurol* 30: 138–143, 1974.

Lobenthal SW, Hajdu SI, Urmacher C: Cytologic Findings in Homosexual Males With Acquired Immunodeficiency. *Acta Cytol* 27: 597–604, 1983.

Lodge-Rigal RD, Novotny DB: Hypersegmentation of Neutrophils in the Cerebrospinal Fluid: Report of a Case With Hematologic Correlation and Review of the Literature. *Diagn Cytopathol* 11: 56–59, 1994.

Lowe E: Mollaret's Meningitis: A Case Report. *Acta Cytol* 26: 338–340, 1982.

Luban NLC, Alessi RM, Gold BG, et al: Cerebral Spinal Fluid Pleocytosis With Bone Marrow Contamination. *J Pediatr* 104: 254–256, 1984.

Ludwig RA, Balachandran I: Mycosis Fungoides: The Importance of Pulmonary Cytology in the Diagnosis of a Case With Systemic Involvement. *Acta Cytol* 27: 198–201, 1983.

Mackintosh FR, Colby TV, Podolsky WJ, et al: Central Nervous System Involvement in Non-Hodgkin's Lymphoma: An Analysis of 105 Cases. *Cancer* 49: 586–595, 1982.

Maldonado JE, Kyle RA, Ludwig J, et al: Meningeal Myeloma. *Arch Intern Med* 126: 660–663, 1970.

Manconi PE, Marrosu MG, Spissu A: Plasma Cell Reaction in Cerebrospinal Fluid: An Additional Case Report. *Neurology* 28: 856–857, 1978.

Marks V, Marrack D: Tumor Cells in the Cerebrospinal Fluid. *J Neurol Neurosurg Psychiatry* 23: 194–201, 1960.

Masur H, Hook E III, Armstrong D: A *Trichomonas* Species in a Mixed Microbial Meningitis. *JAMA* 236: 1978–1979, 1976.

Mathios AJ, Nielsen SL, Barrett D, et al: Cerebrospinal Fluid Cytomorphology Identification of Benign Cells Originating in the Central Nervous System. *Acta Cytol* 21: 403–412, 1977.

Mayer JR, Watson CW: Cytologic Monitoring of Cerebrospinal Fluid in the Treatment of Histiocytic Lymphoma Involving the Central Nervous System. *Acta Cytol* 24: 26–29, 1980.

McAlpine LL, Ellsworth B: A Modified Membrane Filter Technic for Cytodiagnosis. *Am J Clin Pathol* 52: 242–244, 1969.

McCallum S, Cooper K, Franks DN: Choroid Plexus Carcinoma: Cytologic Identification of Malignant Cells in Ascitic Fluid. *Acta Cytol* 32: 263–266, 1988.

McCormack LJ, Hazard JB, Gardner WJ, et al: Cerebrospinal Fluid Changes in Secondary Carcinoma of Meninges. *Am J Clin Pathol* 23: 470–478, 1953.

McCormack LJ, Hazard JB, Belovich D, et al: Identification of Neoplastic Cells in Cerebrospinal Fluid by a Wet-Film Method. *Cancer* 10: 1293–1299, 1957.

McCormick WF, Coleman SA: A Membrane Filter Technic for Cytology of Spinal Fluid. *Am J Clin Pathol* 38: 191–197, 1962.

McGarry P, Holmquist ND, Carmel SA: A Postmortem Study of Cerebrospinal Fluid With Histologic Correlation. *Acta Cytol* 13: 48–52, 1969.

McIntosh S, Ritchey AK: Diagnostic Problems in Cerebrospinal Fluid of Children With Lymphoid Malignancies. *Am J Pediatr Hematol Oncol* 8: 28–31, 1986.

McMenemey WH, Cumings JN: The Value of the Examination of the Cerebrospinal Fluid in the Diagnosis of Intracranial Tumors. *J Clin Pathol* 12: 400–411, 1959.

Meissner GF: Carcinoma of the Stomach With Meningeal Carcinosis: Report of Four Cases. *Cancer* 6: 313–318, 1953.

Mengel M: The Use of the Cytocentrifuge in the Diagnosis of Meningitis. *Am J Clin Pathol* 84: 212–216, 1985.

Meyer PC, Reah TG: Secondary Neoplasms of the Central Nervous System and Meninges. *Br J Cancer* 7: 438–448, 1953.

Meyer RJ, Ferreira PPC, Cuttner J, et al: Central Nervous System Involvement at Presentation in Acute Granulocytic Leukemia: A Prospective Cytocentrifuge Study. *Am J Med* 68: 691–694, 1980.

Michael M, Barrett DJ, Mehta P: Infants With Meningitis Without Cerebrospinal Fluid Pleocytosis. *Am J Dis Child* 140: 851, 1986.

Miller RR, Lin F, Mallonee MM: Cytologic Diagnosis of Gliomatosis Cerebri. *Acta Cytol* 25: 37–39, 1981.

Mine S, Sato A, Yamaura A, et al: Eosinophilia of the Cerebrospinal Fluid in a Case of Shunt Infection: Case Report. *Neurosurgery* 19: 835–836, 1986.

Naylor B: Cytologic Study of Intracranial Fluids. *Acta Cytol* 5: 198–202, 1961a.

Naylor B: An Exfoliative Cytologic Study of Intracranial Fluids. *Neurology* 11: 560–570, 1961b.

Naylor B: The Cytologic Diagnosis of Cerebrospinal Fluid. *Acta Cytol* 8: 141–149, 1964.

Nies BA, Thomas LB, Freireich EJ: Meningeal Leukemia: A Follow-up Study. *Cancer* 18: 546–553, 1965a.

Nies BA, Malmgren RA, Chu EW, et al: Cerebrospinal Fluid Cytology in Patients With Acute Leukemia. *Cancer* 18: 1385–1391, 1965b.

Nosanchuk JS, Kim CW: Lupus Erythematosus Cells in CSF. *JAMA* 236: 2883–2884, 1976.

Oehmichen M, Huber H: Supplementary Cytodiagnosis Analyses of Mononuclear Cells of the Cerebrospinal Fluid Using Cytological Markers. *J Neurol* 218: 187–196, 1978.

O'Hara MF, Cousar JB, Glick AD, et al: Multiparameter Approach to the Diagnosis of Hematopoietic-Lymphoid Neoplasms in Body Fluids. *Diagn Cytopathol* 1: 33–38, 1985.

Olson ME, Chernick NL, Posner JB: Infiltration of the Leptomeninges by Systemic Cancer: A Clinical and Pathologic Study. *Arch Neurol* 30: 122–137, 1974.

Onda K, Tanaka R, Takahashi H, et al: Cerebral Glioblastoma With Cerebrospinal Fluid Dissemination: A Clinicopathological Study of 14 Cases Examined by Complete Autopsy. *Neurosurgery* 25: 533–540, 1989.

Packer RJ, Perilongo G, Johnson D, et al: Choroid Plexus Carcinoma of Childhood. *Cancer* 69: 580–585, 1992.

Pasquier B, Pasquier D, N'golet A, et al: Extraneural Metastases of Astrocytomas and Glioblastomas: Clinicopathological Study of Two Cases and Review of Literature. *Cancer* 45: 112–125, 1980.

Pedersen AG, Olsen J, Nasiell M: Cerebrospinal Fluid Cytology Diagnosis of Meningeal Carcinomatosis in Patients With Small-Cell Carcinoma of the Lung: A Study of Interobserver and Intraobserver Variability. *Acta Cytol* 30: 648–652, 1986.

Pelc S, De Maertelaere, Denolin-Reubens R: CSF Cytology of Acute Viral Meningitis and Meningoencephalitis. *Eur Neurol* 20: 95–102, 1981.

Péter A: The Plasma Cells of the Cerebrospinal Fluid. *J Neurol Sci* 4: 227–239, 1967.

Platt WR: Exfoliative-Cell Diagnosis of Central Nervous System Lesions. *AMA Arch Neurol Psychiatry* 66: 119–144, 1951.

Portnoy JM, Olson LC: Normal Cerebrospinal Fluid Values in Children: Another Look. *Pediatrics* 75: 484–487, 1985.

Preissig SH, Buhaug J: Corpora Amylacea in Cerebrospinal Fluid: A Source of Possible Diagnostic Error. *Acta Cytol* 22: 511–514, 1978.

Price RW, Navia BA, Cho E-S: AIDS Encephalopathy. *Neurol Clin* 4: 285–301, 1986.

Puczynski MS, Fox KR, Billittier AJ, et al: CSF Pleocytosis in an Infant: A Complication of Lumbar Puncture. *Am J Emerg Med* 7: 454, 1989.

Razavi-Encha F, Fleury-Feith J, Gherardi R, et al: Cytologic Features of Cerebrospinal Fluid in Lyme Disease. *Acta Cytol* 31: 439–440, 1987.

Reinhartz T, Lijovetzky G, Levij IS: Intracellular Starch Granules in Cytologic Material. *Acta Cytol* 22: 36–37, 1978.

Reske-Nielsen E, Petersen JH, Søgaard H, et al: Leukemia of the Central Nervous System. *Lancet* (ii): 211–212, 1974.

Reyes CV: Primary Malignant Lymphoma of the Brain in Acquired Immune Deficiency Syndrome. *Acta Cytol* 29: 85–86, 1985.

Reynaud AJ, King EB: A New Filter for Diagnostic Cytology. *Acta Cytol* 11: 289–294, 1967.

Rich JR: A Survey of Cerebrospinal Fluid Cytology. *Bull Los Angeles Neurol Soc* 34: 115–131, 1969.

Risdall R, Hoppe RT, Warnke R: Non-Hodgkin's Lymphoma: A Study of the Evolution of the Disease Based Upon 92 Autopsied Cases. *Cancer* 44: 529–542, 1979.

Rogers LR, Duchesneau PM, Nunez C, et al: Comparison of Cisternal and Lumbar CSF Examination in Leptomeningeal Metastasis. *Neurology* 42: 1239–1241, 1992.

Rohlfing MB, Barton TK, Bigner SH, et al: Contamination of Cerebrospinal Fluid Specimens With Hematogenous Blasts in Patients With Leukemia. *Acta Cytol* 25: 611–615, 1981.

Ross JS, Magro C, Szyfelvein W, et al: Cerebrospinal Fluid Pleocytosis in Aseptic Meningitis: Cytomorphic and Immunocytochemical Features. *Diagn Cytopathol* 7: 532–535, 1991.

Rubé J, de la Pava S, Pickren JW: Histiocytosis X With Involvement of Brain. *Cancer* 20: 486–492, 1967.

Saigo P, Rosen PP, Kaplan MH, et al: Identification of *Cryptococcus neoformans* in Cytologic Preparations of Cerebrospinal Fluid. *Am J Clin Pathol* 67: 141–145, 1977.

Saito R: The Cytologic Manifestations of Lymphomatoid Granulomatosis in Cerebrospinal Fluid: A Case Report. *Acta Cytol* 22: 339–343, 1978.

Salberg DJ: CSF Eosinophilia Following Myelography. *JAMA* 243: 1807, 1980.

Sarff LD, Platt LH, McCracken GH Jr: Cerebrospinal Fluid Evaluation in Neonates: Comparison of High-Risk Infants With and Without Meningitis. *J Pediatr* 88: 473–477, 1976.

Schmidt P, Neuen-Jacob E, Blanke M, et al: Primary Malignant Melanoblastosis of the Meninges: Clinical, Cytologic and Neuropathologic Findings in a Case. *Acta Cytol* 32: 713–718, 1988.

Schmitt-Gräff A, Pfitzer P: Cytology of the Cerebrospinal Fluid in Primary Malignant Lymphomas of the Central Nervous System. *Acta Cytol* 27: 267–272, 1983.

Schumann GB, Crisman LG: Semiquantitative Approach to CSF Cytopathology. *Diagn Cytopathol* 2: 194–197, 1986.

Seal SH: A Method for Concentrating Cancer Cells Suspended in Large Quantities of Fluid. *Cancer* 9: 866–868, 1956.

Seyfert S, Kabbeck-Kupijai D, Marx P, et al: Cerebrospinal Fluid Cell Preparation Methods: An Evaluation. *Acta Cytol* 36: 927–931, 1992.

Shenoy UA, Kushner JP, Schumann GB: Cytologic Diagnosis and Monitoring of Hodgkin's Disease in Cerebrospinal Fluid: A Case Report. *Diagn Cytopathol* 3: 323–325, 1987.

Simon RP, Koerper MA: PMNs in Normal Spinal Fluid Examined by the Cytocentrifuge Technique. *Ann Neurol* 7: 380–381, 1980.

Simone J, Aur RJA, Hustu HO, et al: 'Total Therapy' Studies of Acute Lymphocytic Leukemia in Children: Current Results and Prospects for Cure. *Cancer* 30: 1488–1494, 1972.

Sindern E, Burghardt F, Voigtmann R, et al: Cerebrospinal Fluid Cytology in Granulocytic Sarcoma With Meningeal Extension but Without Bone Marrow Involvement. *J Neurol* 241: 320–322, 1994.

Sindern E, Malin J-P: Phenotypic Analysis of Cerebrospinal Fluid Cells Over the Course of Lyme Meningoradiculitis. *Acta Cytol* 39: 73–75, 1995.

Sörnäs R: Transformation of Mononuclear Cells in Cerebrospinal Fluid. *Acta Cytol* 15: 545–552, 1971.

Sörnäs R: The Cytology of the Normal Cerebrospinal Fluid. *Acta Neurol Scand* 48: 313–320, 1972.

Spriggs AI: Malignant Cells in Cerebrospinal Fluid. *J Clin Pathol* 7: 122–130, 1954.

Spriggs AI, Boddington MM: Leukemic Cells in Cerebrospinal Fluid. *Br J Haematol* 5: 83–91, 1959.

Stanley MW, Frizzera G, Dehner LP: Castleman's Disease, Plasma-Cell Type: Diagnosis of Central Nervous System Involvement by Cerebrospinal Fluid Cytology. *Acta Cytol* 30: 481–486, 1986.

Stanley MW, Henry MJ: The Significance of Leukemia and Lymphoma Cells in Cerebrospinal Fluid Contaminated by Blood Containing Malignant Cells: A Probabilistic Approach Based on the Poisson Frequency Distribution. *Diagn Cytopathol* 4: 193–195, 1988.

Stark E, Wurster U: Preparation Procedure for Cerebrospinal Fluid That Yields Cytologic Samples Suitable for All Types of Staining, Including Immunologic and Enzymatic Methods. *Acta Cytol* 31: 374–376, 1987.

Steele RW, Marmer DJ, O'Brien MD, et al: Leukocyte Survival in Cerebrospinal Fluid. *J Clin Microbiol* 23: 965–966, 1986.

Steere AC, Bartenhagen NH, Craft JE, et al: The Early Clinical Manifestations of Lyme Disease. *Ann Intern Med* 99: 76–82, 1983a.

Steere AC, Grodzicki RL, Kornblatt AN, et al: The Spirochetal Etiology of Lyme Disease. *N Engl J Med* 308: 733–740, 1983b.

Strigle SM, Gal AA: Review of the Central Nervous System Cytopathology in Human Immunodeficiency Virus Infection. *Diagn Cytopathol* 7: 387–401, 1991.

Suhrland MJ, Koslow M, Perchick A, et al: Cytologic Findings in Progressive Multifocal Leukoencephalopathy: Report of Two Cases. *Acta Cytol* 31: 505–511, 1987.

Szyfelbein WM, Ross JS: Lyme Disease Meningopolyneuritis Simulating Malignant Lymphoma. *Mod Pathol* 1: 464–468, 1988.

Takeda M, King DE, Choi HY, et al: Diagnostic Pitfalls in Cerebrospinal Fluid Cytology. *Acta Cytol* 25: 245–250, 1981.

Tani E, Costa I, Svedmyr E, et al: Diagnosis of Lymphoma, Leukemia, and Metastatic Tumor Involvement of the Cerebrospinal Fluid by Cytology and Immunocytochemistry. *Diagn Cytopathol* 12: 14–22, 1995.

Teoh R, O'Mahony G, Yeung VTF: Polymorphonuclear Pleocytosis in the Cerebrospinal Fluid During Chemotherapy for Tuberculous Meningitis. *J Neurol* 233: 237–241, 1986.

Theodore WH, Gendelman S: Meningeal Carcinomatosis. *Arch Neurol* 38: 696–699, 1981.

Threlkeld MG, Graves AH, Cobbs CG: Cerebrospinal Fluid Staining for the Diagnosis of Toxoplasmosis in Patients With the Acquired Immune Deficiency Syndrome. *Am J Med* 83: 599–600, 1987.

Trojanowski JQ, Atkinson B, Lee VMY: An Immunocytochemical Study of Normal and Abnormal Human Cerebrospinal Fluid With Monoclonal Antibodies to Glial Fibrillary Acidic Protein. *Acta Cytol* 30: 235–239, 1986.

Tutuarima JA, Hische EAJ, Sylva-Steenland RMR, et al: A Cytopreparatory Method for Cerebrospinal Fluid in Which the Cell Yield is High and the Fluid Is Saved for Chemical Analysis. *Acta Cytol* 32: 425–427, 1988.

Tzvetanova EM, Tzekov CT: Eosinophilia in the Cerebrospinal Fluid of Children With Shunts Implanted for the Treatment of Internal Hydrocephalus. *Acta Cytol* 30: 277–280, 1986.

Valladares JB, Perry RH, Kalbag RM: Malignant Choroid Plexus Papilloma With Extraneural Metastasis: Case Report. *J Neurosurg* 52: 251–255, 1980.

Vannucci RC, Baten M: Cerebral Metastatic Disease in Childhood. *Neurology* 24: 981–985, 1974.

Van Zanten AP, Twijnstra A, Ongerboer de Visser BW, et al: Cerebrospinal Fluid Tumor Markers in Patients Treated for Meningeal Malignancy. *J Neurol Neurosurg Psych* 54: 119–123, 1991.

Veerman AJP, Huismans L, van Zantwijk I: Storage of Cerebrospinal Fluid Samples at Room Temperature. *Acta Cytol* 29: 188–189, 1985.

Vick WW, Wikstrand CJ, Bullard DE, et al: The Use of a Panel of Monoclonal Antibodies in the Evaluation of Cytologic Specimens From the Central Nervous System. *Acta Cytol* 31: 815–824, 1987.

Wagner JA, Frost JK, Wisotzkey H Jr: Subarachnoid Neoplasia: Incidence and Problems of Diagnosis. *South Med J* 53: 1503–1508, 1960.

Wallace RM, Bigner SH, Johnston WW: Metastatic Breast Carcinoma in Cerebrospinal Fluid: A Cytomorphometric Study. *Acta Cytol* 26: 787–792, 1982.

Walts AE: Cerebrospinal Fluid Cytology: Selected Issues. *Diagn Cytopathol* 8: 394–408, 1992.

Wasserstrom WR, Glass JP, Posner JB: Diagnosis and Treatment of Leptomeningeal Metastases From Solid Tumors: Experience With 90 Patients. *Cancer* 49: 759–772, 1982.

Watson CW, Hajdu SI: Cytology of Primary Neoplasms of the Central Nervous System. *Acta Cytol* 21: 40–47, 1977.

Watson P: A Slide Centrifuge: An Apparatus for Concentrating Cells in Suspension Onto a Microscope Slide. *J Lab Clin Med* 68: 494–501, 1966.

Weed JC Jr, Creasman WT: Meningeal Carcinomatosis Secondary to Advanced Squamous Cell Carcinoma of the Cervix: A Case Report: Meningeal Metastasis of Advanced Cervical Cancer. *Gynecol Oncol* 3: 201–204, 1975.

Weithman AM, Morrison G, Ingram EA: Meningeal Metastasis of Squamous-Cell Carcinoma of the Uterine Cervix: Case Report and Review of the Literature. *Diagn Cytopathol* 3: 170–172, 1987.

Wertlake PT, Markovits BA, Stellar S: Cytologic Evaluation of Cerebrospinal Fluid With Clinical and Histologic Correlation. *Acta Cytol* 16: 224–239, 1972.

Whitmore EL, Hochberg F, Wolfson L, et al: Quantitative Cytocentrifugation in the Evaluation of Cerebrospinal Fluid. *Acta Cytol* 26: 847–850, 1982.

Wilber RR, King EB, Howes EL Jr: Cerebrospinal Fluid Cytology in Five Patients With Cerebral Cysticercosis. *Acta Cytol* 24: 421–426, 1980.

Wilkins RH, Odom GL: Cytological Changes in Cerebrospinal Fluid Associated With Resections if Intracranial Neoplasms. *J Neurosurg* 25: 24–34, 1966.

Wilkins RH, Odom GL: Ependymal-Choroidal Cells in Cerebrospinal Fluid: Increased Incidence in Hydrocephalic Infants. *J Neurosurg* 41: 555–560, 1974.

Wingo PA, Tong T, Bolden S: Cancer Statistics. *CA Cancer J Clin* 45: 8–30, 1995.

Wolfson WL, Rosenthal DL, Harney B: Psammoma Bodies in Pituitary Adenoma. *Acta Cytol* 23: 90–92, 1979a.

Wolfson WL: Cytopathologic Presentation of Cerebral Histiocytosis. *Acta Cytol* 23: 392–398, 1979b.

Wolk RW, Masse SR, Conklin R, et al: The Incidence of Central Nervous System Leukemia in Adults With Acute Leukemia. *Cancer* 33: 863–869, 1974.

Woodruff KH: Cerebrospinal Fluid Cytomorphology Using Cytocentrifugation. *Am J Clin Pathol* 60: 621–627, 1973.

Yam LT, English MC, Janckila AJ, et al: Immunocytochemistry of Cerebrospinal Fluid. *Acta Cytol* 31: 825–833, 1987.

Yamamoto LJ, Tedder DG, Ashley R, et al: Herpes Simplex Virus Type 1 DNA in Cerebrospinal Fluid of a Patient With Mollaret's Meningitis. *N Engl J Med* 325: 1082–1085, 1991.

Young RC, Howser DM, Anderson T, et al: Central Nervous System Complications of Non-Hodgkin's Lymphoma: The Potential Role for Prophylactic Therapy. *Am J Med* 66: 435–443, 1979.

Zaharopoulos P, Wong JY: Cytology of Common Primary Midline Brain Tumors. *Acta Cytol* 24: 384–390, 1980.

Zaharopoulos P, Wong JY: Hemoglobin Crystals in Fluid Specimens From Confined Body Spaces. *Acta Cytol* 31: 777–782, 1987.

Zaharopoulos P, Wong JY, Wen JW: Extramedullary Hand Mirror Cells in Pathologic Conditions of Lymphoid Tissue. *Acta Cytol* 34: 868–874, 1990.

Ziegler JL, Bluming AZ, Morrow RH, et al: Central Nervous System Involvement in Burkitt's Lymphoma. *Blood* 36: 718–728, 1970.

Index

Numbers in blue (1–462) refer to pages in Volume I, Exfoliative Cytology. Numbers in red (463–1208) refer to pages in Volume II, Aspiration Cytology. Numbers in **boldface** refer to pages on which images, tables, and figures appear.

A

Numbers in blue (1–462) refer to pages in Volume I, Exfoliative Cytology. Numbers in red (463–1208) refer to pages in Volume II, Aspiration Cytology. Numbers in **boldface** refer to pages on which images, tables, and figures appear.

Numbers in blue (1–462) refer to pages in Volume I, Exfoliative Cytology. Numbers in red (463–1208) refer to pages in Volume II, Aspiration Cytology. Numbers in **boldface** refer to pages on which images, tables, and figures appear.

B

Numbers in blue (1–462) refer to pages in Volume I, Exfoliative Cytology. Numbers in red (463–1208) refer to pages in Volume II, Aspiration Cytology. Numbers in **boldface** refer to pages on which images, tables, and figures appear.

Numbers in blue (1–462) refer to pages in Volume I, Exfoliative Cytology. Numbers in red (463–1208) refer to pages in Volume II, Aspiration Cytology. Numbers in **boldface** refer to pages on which images, tables, and figures appear.

C

Numbers in blue (1–462) refer to pages in Volume I, Exfoliative Cytology. Numbers in red (463–1208) refer to pages in Volume II, Aspiration Cytology.
Numbers in **boldface** refer to pages on which images, tables, and figures appear.

Numbers in blue (1–462) refer to pages in Volume I, Exfoliative Cytology. Numbers in red (463–1208) refer to pages in Volume II, Aspiration Cytology.
Numbers in **boldface** refer to pages on which images, tables, and figures appear.

Numbers in blue (1–462) refer to pages in Volume I, Exfoliative Cytology. Numbers in red (463–1208) refer to pages in Volume II, Aspiration Cytology.
Numbers in **boldface** refer to pages on which images, tables, and figures appear.

Numbers in blue (1–462) refer to pages in Volume I, Exfoliative Cytology. Numbers in red (463–1208) refer to pages in Volume II, Aspiration Cytology. Numbers in **boldface** refer to pages on which images, tables, and figures appear.

Numbers in blue (1–462) refer to pages in Volume I, Exfoliative Cytology. Numbers in red (463–1208) refer to pages in Volume II, Aspiration Cytology. Numbers in **boldface** refer to pages on which images, tables, and figures appear.

Numbers in blue (1–462) refer to pages in Volume I, Exfoliative Cytology. Numbers in red (463–1208) refer to pages in Volume II, Aspiration Cytology.
Numbers in **boldface** refer to pages on which images, tables, and figures appear.

Numbers in blue (1–462) refer to pages in Volume I, Exfoliative Cytology. Numbers in red (463–1208) refer to pages in Volume II, Aspiration Cytology.
Numbers in **boldface** refer to pages on which images, tables, and figures appear.

F

Numbers in blue (1–462) refer to pages in Volume I, Exfoliative Cytology. Numbers in red (463–1208) refer to pages in Volume II, Aspiration Cytology. Numbers in **boldface** refer to pages on which images, tables, and figures appear.

G

Numbers in blue (1–462) refer to pages in Volume I, Exfoliative Cytology. Numbers in red (463–1208) refer to pages in Volume II, Aspiration Cytology.
Numbers in **boldface** refer to pages on which images, tables, and figures appear.

H

Numbers in blue (1–462) refer to pages in Volume I, Exfoliative Cytology. Numbers in red (463–1208) refer to pages in Volume II, Aspiration Cytology. Numbers in **boldface** refer to pages on which images, tables, and figures appear.

Numbers in blue (1–462) refer to pages in Volume I, Exfoliative Cytology. Numbers in red (463–1208) refer to pages in Volume II, Aspiration Cytology.
Numbers in **boldface** refer to pages on which images, tables, and figures appear.

I

Numbers in blue (1–462) refer to pages in Volume I, Exfoliative Cytology. Numbers in red (463–1208) refer to pages in Volume II, Aspiration Cytology. Numbers in **boldface** refer to pages on which images, tables, and figures appear.

J

K

Numbers in blue (1–462) refer to pages in Volume I, Exfoliative Cytology. Numbers in red (463–1208) refer to pages in Volume II, Aspiration Cytology. Numbers in **boldface** refer to pages on which images, tables, and figures appear.

L

Numbers in blue (1–462) refer to pages in Volume I, Exfoliative Cytology. Numbers in red (463–1208) refer to pages in Volume II, Aspiration Cytology.
Numbers in **boldface** refer to pages on which images, tables, and figures appear.

Numbers in blue (1–462) refer to pages in Volume I, Exfoliative Cytology. Numbers in red (463–1208) refer to pages in Volume II, Aspiration Cytology.
Numbers in **boldface** refer to pages on which images, tables, and figures appear.

M

Numbers in blue (1–462) refer to pages in Volume I, Exfoliative Cytology. Numbers in red (463–1208) refer to pages in Volume II, Aspiration Cytology. Numbers in **boldface** refer to pages on which images, tables, and figures appear.

Numbers in blue (1–462) refer to pages in Volume I, Exfoliative Cytology. Numbers in red (463–1208) refer to pages in Volume II, Aspiration Cytology.
Numbers in **boldface** refer to pages on which images, tables, and figures appear.

Numbers in blue (1–462) refer to pages in Volume I, Exfoliative Cytology. Numbers in red (463–1208) refer to pages in Volume II, Aspiration Cytology. Numbers in **boldface** refer to pages on which images, tables, and figures appear.

N

Numbers in blue (1–462) refer to pages in Volume I, Exfoliative Cytology. Numbers in red (463–1208) refer to pages in Volume II, Aspiration Cytology. Numbers in **boldface** refer to pages on which images, tables, and figures appear.

O

Numbers in blue (1–462) refer to pages in Volume I, Exfoliative Cytology. Numbers in red (463–1208) refer to pages in Volume II, Aspiration Cytology. Numbers in **boldface** refer to pages on which images, tables, and figures appear.

P

Numbers in blue (1–462) refer to pages in Volume I, Exfoliative Cytology. Numbers in red (463–1208) refer to pages in Volume II, Aspiration Cytology.
Numbers in **boldface** refer to pages on which images, tables, and figures appear.

Numbers in blue (1–462) refer to pages in Volume I, Exfoliative Cytology. Numbers in red (463–1208) refer to pages in Volume II, Aspiration Cytology. Numbers in **boldface** refer to pages on which images, tables, and figures appear.

Numbers in blue (1–462) refer to pages in Volume I, Exfoliative Cytology. Numbers in red (463–1208) refer to pages in Volume II, Aspiration Cytology. Numbers in **boldface** refer to pages on which images, tables, and figures appear.

Q

R

Numbers in blue (1–462) refer to pages in Volume I, Exfoliative Cytology. Numbers in red (463–1208) refer to pages in Volume II, Aspiration Cytology. Numbers in **boldface** refer to pages on which images, tables, and figures appear.

S

Numbers in blue (1–462) refer to pages in Volume I, Exfoliative Cytology. Numbers in red (463–1208) refer to pages in Volume II, Aspiration Cytology.
Numbers in **boldface** refer to pages on which images, tables, and figures appear.

Numbers in blue (1–462) refer to pages in Volume I, Exfoliative Cytology. Numbers in red (463–1208) refer to pages in Volume II, Aspiration Cytology.
Numbers in **boldface** refer to pages on which images, tables, and figures appear.

Numbers in blue (1–462) refer to pages in Volume I, Exfoliative Cytology. Numbers in red (463–1208) refer to pages in Volume II, Aspiration Cytology. Numbers in **boldface** refer to pages on which images, tables, and figures appear.

Numbers in blue (1–462) refer to pages in Volume I, Exfoliative Cytology. Numbers in red (463–1208) refer to pages in Volume II, Aspiration Cytology. Numbers in **boldface** refer to pages on which images, tables, and figures appear.

T

Numbers in blue (1–462) refer to pages in Volume I, Exfoliative Cytology. Numbers in red (463–1208) refer to pages in Volume II, Aspiration Cytology.
Numbers in **boldface** refer to pages on which images, tables, and figures appear.

Numbers in blue (1–462) refer to pages in Volume I, Exfoliative Cytology. Numbers in red (463–1208) refer to pages in Volume II, Aspiration Cytology. Numbers in **boldface** refer to pages on which images, tables, and figures appear.

Numbers in blue (1–462) refer to pages in Volume I, Exfoliative Cytology. Numbers in red (463–1208) refer to pages in Volume II, Aspiration Cytology. Numbers in **boldface** refer to pages on which images, tables, and figures appear.

W

X

Y

Z